The NutriBase Guide to

CARBOHYDRATES, CALORIES & FAT

IN YOUR FOOD

The NutriBase Guide to

CARBOHYDRATES, CALORIES & FAT

IN YOUR FOOD

AVERY
a member of Penguin Putnam Inc.
NEW YORK

Every effort has been made to ensure that the information contained in this book is complete and accurate. However, neither the publisher nor the author is engaged in rendering professional advice or services to the individual reader. The ideas, procedures, and suggestions contained in this book are not intended as a substitute for consulting with your physician. All matters regarding health require medical supervision. Neither the author nor the publisher shall be liable or responsible for any loss, injury, or damage allegedly arising from any information or suggestion in this book.

Most Avery books are available at special quantity discounts for bulk purchase for sales promotions, premiums, fund-raising, and educational needs. Special books or book excerpts also can be created to fit specific needs. For details, write Putnam Special Markets, 375 Hudson Street, New York, NY 10014.

a member of
Penguin Putnam Inc.
375 Hudson Street
New York, NY 10014
www.penguinputnam.com

Library of Congress Cataloging-in-Publication Data

The NutriBase guide to carbohydrates, calories, and fat.—2nd ed.
p. cm.
Rev. ed. of: The NutriBase guide to carbohydrates, calories & fat in your food / Art Ulene, ©1995.
ISBN 1-58333-109-3
1. Food—Carbohydrate content—Tables. 2. Food—Caloric content—Tables. 3. Food—Fat content—Tables. I. Title: Guide to carbohydrates, calories, and fat. II. Ulene, Art. Nutribase guide to carbohydrates, calories & fat in your food. III. CyberSoft, Inc.
TX553.C28 N88   2001   2001034085
613.2'83—dc21

Printed in the United States of America
5   7   9   10   8   6

CONTENTS

INTRODUCTION

Throughout history, people have recognized the connection between the food we eat and the state of our health. But only recently have we begun to appreciate just how important this connection is. Researchers have now proven a strong relationship between excess fat consumption and obesity, high blood pressure, and stroke; between excess fat and coronary artery disease; between excess calorie consumption and premature death. The list goes on and on.

But not all of the associations are negative. Research has also shown that changing the quantity and quality of the carbohydrates and fats you consume can have a positive effect on your health. For instance, by reducing your intake of fat and cholesterol, you can lower blood cholesterol levels. By changing the carbohydrates you consume, you can reduce your risk of colon cancer and lower your blood cholesterol. And if you have diabetes, by consuming complex carbohydrates, you can more easily maintain a blood sugar level within the normal range.

Some people are surprised to learn that carbohydrates can be a useful part of a weight-loss program. Many weight-loss diet promoters advise people to shun carbohydrates in favor of protein-rich foods like steak and cheese. This is because pasta, potatoes, and breads are thought by some to be a major cause of excessive weight gain. But in fact the culprit usually isn't the pasta; it's the fat-rich sauces that go on top. In fact, carbohydrates provide dieters with a feeling of satisfaction and fullness, as well as a continuing source of energy.

This book is designed to help you make wiser choices when you buy food and when you dine out. It will help you interpret nutritional stories in the media so you can distinguish useful information from nonsense. It will give you the control you need over your personal nutrition.

Many people refer to books of this sort as "counter" books, because of the nutritional numbers that fill the pages. But this is not a book about counting. This is a book about *control* and *choices*. Use this book to learn more about the foods you should consume—or avoid—so you can meet your particular nutritional needs. Don't be intimidated by the huge number of choices listed or by all the nutritional value numbers that accompany the lists. It is not necessary to memorize these numbers. Instead, just try to familiarize yourself with the foods and food categories that are best suited to your needs.

Begin by looking up the foods that you eat most often or in the largest quantities. If these foods are not providing you with the nutrients you need, use the book to find better alternatives that are just as tasty. Once you are familiar with the nutritional content of your most common food choices, gradually look up the remainder of the foods in your diet. You'll be surprised by how easy it is to learn about these foods and to make any necessary changes.

The following section will explain some of the basics about fats, carbohydrates, and calories. After that, you will learn how to use this book to locate the information you need to improve your diet.

UNDERSTANDING CARBOHYDRATES

Carbohydrates supply the body with the energy it needs to function. Carbohydrates are metabolized, or "burned," by the body, providing 4 calories—4 units of energy—per gram. (There are 454 grams in one pound.) Carbohydrates are found almost exclusively in plant foods, such as fruits, vegetables, grains, peas, and beans. Milk is the only food derived from animals that contains a significant amount of carbohydrate.

Carbohydrates are divided into two groups: simple and complex. Simple carbohydrates, sometimes called simple sugars, include fructose (fruit sugar), sucrose (table sugar), and lactose (milk sugar), as well as several other sugars. Fruits are one of the richest natural sources of simple carbohydrates. Complex carbohydrates are also made up of sugar, but the sugar molecules are strung together to form longer, more complex chains. Complex carbohydrates include fiber and starches. Foods rich in complex carbohydrates include vegetables, whole grains, peas, and beans.

Carbohydrates are the main source of blood glucose, which is a major fuel for all of our cells, and the only source of energy for the brain and red blood cells. Except for fiber, which cannot be digested, both simple and complex carbohydrates are converted into glucose, which is either used directly to provide energy for the body, or stored in the liver for future use. When a person consumes more calories than the body is using, a portion of the carbohydrates consumed may also be stored in the body as fat.

When choosing carbohydrate-rich foods for your diet, it is a good idea to select unrefined foods, such as fruits, vegetables, peas, beans, and whole-grain products, as opposed to refined, processed foods such as soft drinks, candy, and sugar. Refined foods offer few, if any, of the vitamins and minerals that are important to your health. Also, be cautious in your use of any carbohydrate-rich foods that are combined with large quantities of fat in their preparation. These foods, which include pastries and snack foods, are usually loaded with calories far out of proportion to their overall nutritional value.

UNDERSTANDING FATS

Fats have been classified into three major categories—saturated fats, polyunsaturated fats, and monounsaturated fats. This classification is based on the number of hydrogen atoms each has in its chemical structure.

Saturated fats, which are usually solid at room temperature, are found primarily in animal products, including fatty meats like beef, veal, lamb, pork, and ham; and in dairy items such as whole milk, cream, ice cream, and cheese. For example, the white marbling you can see in a piece of beef is saturated fat. Some types of vegetable products—including coconut oil, palm kernel oil, and vegetable shortening—are also high in saturates.

The liver uses saturated fats to manufacture cholesterol. Therefore, excessive dietary intake of saturated fats can significantly raise the blood cholesterol level, especially in people who have an inherited tendency toward high blood cholesterol. Guidelines issued by the National Cholesterol Education Program (NCEP) and widely supported by most experts recommend that your intake of saturated fats should be kept below 10 percent of your total calorie intake. However, for people who have severe problems with high blood cholesterol, even that level may be too high.

Polyunsaturated fats are found in greatest abundance in corn, soybean, safflower, and sunflower oils. Certain fish oils, particularly those containing the omega-3 fatty acids, are also high in polyunsaturates. Unlike the saturated fats, polyunsaturates may actually lower your total blood cholesterol level. In doing so, however, large amounts of polyunsaturates also have a tendency to reduce your HDLs—your "good cholesterol." For this reason—and because, like all fats, polyunsaturates are high in calories for their weight and volume—the NCEP guidelines state that your intake of polyunsaturated fats should not exceed 10 percent of your total calorie intake.

Monounsaturated fats are found mostly in vegetable and nut oils such as olive, peanut, and Canola (rapeseed). These fats appear to reduce blood levels of LDL cholesterol without affecting HDLs in any way. However, this positive impact upon LDL cholesterol is relatively modest. The NCEP guidelines recommend that your intake of monounsaturated fats be kept between 10 and 15 percent of your total calorie intake.

Although most foods—including some plant-derived foods—contain a combination of all three types of fats, one of the types usually predominates. Thus, a food is considered "saturated" or "high in saturates" when it is composed primarily of saturated fatty acids. Similarly, a food composed mostly of polyunsaturated fatty acids is called "polyunsaturated," and a food composed mostly of monounsaturated fatty acids is called "monounsaturated."

One other element, *trans-fatty acids,* might also play a role in blood cholesterol levels. Trans-fatty acids occur when polyunsaturated oils are altered through hydrogenation, a process used to harden liquid vegetable oils into solid foods like margarine and shortening. One recent study found that trans-monounsaturated fatty acids raise LDL cholesterol levels, behaving much like saturated fats. Simultaneously, these trans-fatty acids reduced HDL cholesterol readings. Much more research is necessary, since some studies have not produced clear-cut conclusions about these substances. But your dietary choices could become less matter-of-fact than they now appear. For now, however, it is clear that when your goal is to lower cholesterol, polyunsaturated and monounsaturated are much more desirable than saturated fats, and are probably more desirable than any kind of hydrogenated fats.

UNDERSTANDING CALORIES

When we talk about foods, we often mention the number of calories a certain food has. Calories are not among the four basic nutrients, nor are they considered micronutrients. What, then, are calories?

A calorie is an energy unit. As already discussed, carbohydrates, protein, and fat provide the body with the energy it needs to function. This energy is measured in calories. There are, for instance, approximately four calories in every gram of protein, four calories in every gram of carbohydrate, and nine calories in every gram of fat. It is no wonder, then, that people who are trying to lose weight are often advised to cut down on fatty foods. On a gram-for-gram basis, fat is more than twice as fattening as carbohydrates or protein.

In addition to having more calories than protein or carbohydrates, dietary fat is metabolized differently. Because dietary fat is similar in chemical composition to body fat, it takes less energy to convert it to body fat. In fact, it takes only 3 percent of the calories in the fat we eat to turn that food into body fat, while it takes at least 25 percent of the calories in the carbohydrates and proteins we eat to convert them into body fat.

THE FOOD GUIDE PYRAMID

The U.S. Department of Agriculture (USDA) encourages Americans to eat a well-balanced diet, which it illustrates with a diagram known as the Food Guide Pyramid. At the base of the pyramid are breads, cereals, rice, and pasta. Six to eleven servings from this group are recommended daily—more servings than from any other group of foods in the pyramid. The next level is occupied by vegetables, with three

FOOD GUIDE PYRAMID
A Guide to Daily Food Choices

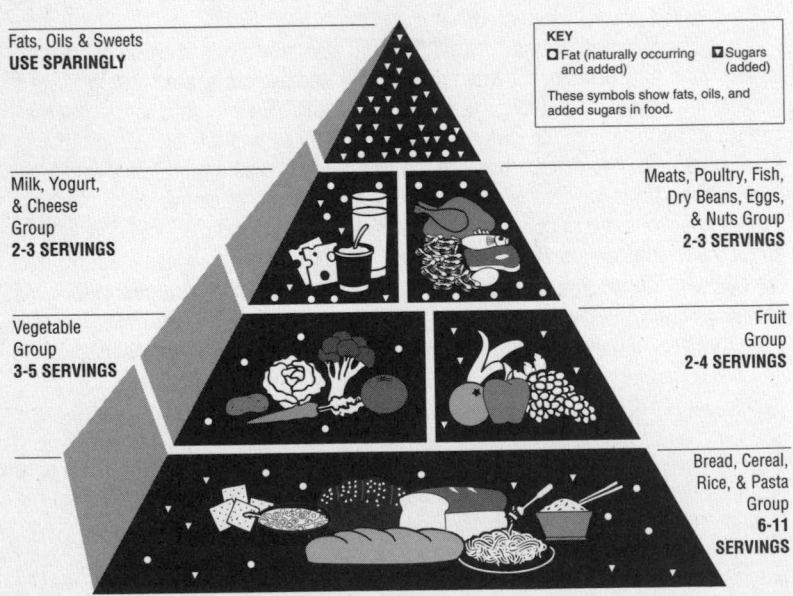

Fats, Oils & Sweets
USE SPARINGLY

KEY
☐ Fat (naturally occurring ▼ Sugars
and added)   (added)

These symbols show fats, oils, and added sugars in food.

Milk, Yogurt, & Cheese Group
2-3 SERVINGS

Meats, Poultry, Fish, Dry Beans, Eggs, & Nuts Group
2-3 SERVINGS

Vegetable Group
3-5 SERVINGS

Fruit Group
2-4 SERVINGS

Bread, Cereal, Rice, & Pasta Group
6-11 SERVINGS

Source: U.S. Department of Agriculture &
U.S. Department of Health and Human Services

to five daily servings recommended, and by fruit, with two to four servings recommended. Moving upward, the next level is shared by milk, yogurt, and cheese—two to three servings—and meat, poultry, fish, dry beans, eggs, and nuts—two to three servings. Finally, at the peak of the pyramid are fats, oils, and sweets, for which there are no recommended amounts, only a note that they should be consumed sparingly.

Government health officials recommend that no more than 30 percent of your dietary calories should come from fat. Others believe that levels of 20 to 25 percent would be even healthier. In contrast, it is recommended that about 60 percent of daily calories come from complex carbohydrates—those foods found in the two largest levels of the pyramid.

Unfortunately, most Americans—97 percent, by some estimates—are not eating a balanced diet by any definition. The standard American diet, appropriately nicknamed SAD, gets about 36 percent of its calories from fat. This is significantly higher than the government recommendation of 30 percent, and far above the 20- to 25-percent target that many physicians think is healthier.

Are Americans getting adequate amounts of carbohydrates? Studies show that Americans get only about 45 percent of their calories from carbohydrates, rather than the 60 percent now recommended. Worse, about half of those carbohydrate calories come from refined foods—soft drinks, cakes, candies, and other low-nutrient foods—rather than from unrefined foods that contain a variety of other nutrients.

GUIDELINES FOR HEALTHY EATING

The remainder of this book will help you choose foods that are low in health-compromising fat and high in nutrient-rich carbohydrates. But as the Food Guide Pyramid illustrates, to maximize your health, you must eat adequate servings from each of the pyramid's first three levels. The following guidelines should help you design and stick to a well-balanced diet:

■ When choosing breads, cereals, rice, and pasta, always choose whole-grain, high-fiber, low-fat varieties, preferably without added sugar, coloring, or unnecessary preservatives. Choose brown rice over white rice, and whole-grain pastas over pastas made from white flour.

■ Eat your vegetables and fruits fresh and, preferably, raw as often as possible. Water-soluble vitamins such as vitamin C may leach out of foods during cooking, be damaged by overprocessing, or be destroyed when foods are overcooked. Even fat-soluble vitamins, which are fairly stable during low-temperature cooking, can be affected by frying. For this reason, it is best to steam or microwave vegetables rather than boiling or frying them. And, unless produce is organically grown, be sure to peel or thoroughly wash it before eating to reduce such unwanted elements as waxes and pesticide residue.

■ Select low-fat and nonfat varieties of milk, yogurt, and cheese. These provide the most nutrients and the least amount of fat. When eating meat, poultry, or fish, choose the leanest cuts available, trim off any excess fat, and bake or broil the foods instead of frying them.

■ Select as few foods as possible from the fats, oils, and sweets category. When you do use fats and oils, choose monounsaturated and polyunsaturated fats instead of saturated ones. Limit your intake of sweets. Choose fresh fruits instead of cakes, cookies, and other high-fat desserts.

FOOD LABELING

Food labels are required to include a "Nutrition Facts" section that identifies how many servings are found in each container and how much of the following components each serving contains:

- Total calories.
- Calories from fat.
- Total fat.
- Saturated fat.
- Cholesterol.

- Sodium.
- Total carbohydrates.
- Dietary fiber.
- Sugars.
- Protein.

- Vitamin A.
- Vitamin C.
- Calcium.
- Iron.

For the last four nutrients, the amount is expressed only as a percentage of Daily Value—a recommended daily intake based on a 2,000-calorie diet. For most of the other nutrients listed, the amount is expressed both in grams or milligrams and as a percentage of its Daily Value. Reference values are provided to show how much total fat, saturated fat, cholesterol, sodium, total carbohydrates, and dietary fiber should be included in both a 2,000-calorie and a 2,500-calorie diet.

Then there are the numerous potentially confusing terms you find sprinkled across food labels. What many people do not know is that the U.S. Food and Drug Administration (FDA) has actually standardized some of the terms used on the labels of products it regulates, as well as on processed meat products that are regulated by the USDA. Following are definitions of some of the most frequently used terms:

■ **Free.** This means that the product contains no amount of, or only "physiologically inconsequential" amounts of, one or more of these components: fat, saturated fat, cholesterol, sodium, sugars, and calories. For instance, "calorie-free" means that there are fewer than 5 calories per serving. "Sugar-free" and "fat-free" indicate that there is less than 1/2 gram per serving of sugar and fat, respectively.

■ **Low.** This means the food can be eaten frequently without exceeding dietary guidelines for one or more of the following: fat, saturated fat, cholesterol, sodium, and calories. Thus, the following terms are used:

■ **Low fat.** 3 grams or less per serving.

■ **Low saturated fat.** 1 gram or less per serving.

■ **Low sodium.** Less than 140 milligrams per serving.

■ **Very low sodium.** Less than 35 milligrams per serving.

■ **Low cholesterol.** Less than 20 milligrams per serving.

■ **Low calorie.** 40 calories or less per serving.

■ **Lean and extra lean.** The following terms can be used to describe the fat content of meat, poultry, seafood, and game meats:

■ **Lean.** Less than 10 grams of fat, less than 4 grams of saturated fat, and less than 95 milligrams of cholesterol per serving and per 100 grams.

■ **Extra lean.** Less than 5 grams of fat, less than 2 grams of saturated fat, and less than 95 milligrams of cholesterol per serving and per 100 grams.

■ **High.** This means that one serving of the food contains 20 percent or more of the recommended daily intake of a particular nutrient.

■ **Good source.** This means that one serving of the food contains 10 to 19 percent of the recommended daily intake of a particular nutrient.

■ **Reduced.** This term denotes a nutritionally altered product that contains 25 percent less of a nutrient or of calories than the regular, or reference, product.

■ **Less.** This denotes a food, whether altered or not, that contains 25 percent less or a nutrient or of calories than the reference food.

■ **Light.** This designates a nutritionally altered product containing one-third fewer calories or half the fat of the reference food, or a low-calorie, low-fat food whose sodium content has been reduced by 50 percent.

■ **More.** This means that one serving of the food, altered or not, contains a nutrient in a quantity that is at least 10 percent of the recommended daily intake more than the reference food.

The following section should provide you with the details you need to better access and understand the data contained in this volume. With this information, and the information that makes up the bulk of this book, you will be equipped to learn more about your unique nutritional needs and the foods you are using to meet those needs. You should enjoy the sense of control this knowledge gives you. More important, you will make better food choices and take a major step toward better health.

HOW TO USE
THIS BOOK

This book was designed to provide comprehensive nutritional information on a wide range of foods, both generic and brand name, raw and prepared. The information provided here was gleaned from a number of government agencies, from hundreds of manufacturers, and from food trade associations. This information was compiled and later supplemented through countless hours of follow-up that involved hundreds of additional sources. Because scientific techniques are continually being improved, this book will be continually updated to reflect the most current nutritional data available.

FINDING THE LISTING YOU WANT

This easy-to-use guide is divided into two parts. The first part is an A-to-Z reference to the nutrients provided by foods. In this section, you will find the amount of calories, fat, saturated fat, and cholesterol, as well as the percentage of calories that come from fat. The second is an A-to-Z reference to the nutrient values of restaurant-chain foods. In this section, foods are listed alphabetically under the name of the appropriate restaurant, and each food item is accompanied by the amounts of the general nutrients found in that item.

The second part is an A-to-Z reference to the nutrient values of restaurant-chain foods. In this section, foods are listed alphabetically under the name of the appropriate restaurant, and each food item is accompanied by the amounts of the general nutrients found in that item.

All of the foods in this reference have been listed alphabetically. For instance, if you are looking for the nutrient values of ground beef, you would turn to the *B's* and look under *Beef.* For convenience, similar foods have sometimes been grouped together in categories such as *Baby Foods, Breads, Candies, Cereals, Cheese, Cookies, Pasta,* and *Sauces.* Therefore, if the food you are looking for is not listed individually by its own name, you should try looking it up under a logical category.

Some foods are known by two or more names. In most cases, the food is listed under just one name, and cross-references have been provided to guide you to the proper listing. For instance, chickpeas are also called garbanzo and ceci beans. In this book, you will find the nutrient information under *Chickpeas,* with cross-references under *Ceci* and *Garbanzo.*

If you are unable to find a particular food, look for the entry for a similar food. The nutritional data should be close, if not exact, for any product not listed.

After you locate the listing for the food you are interested in, you may find that abbreviations have been used to provide you with the information you need. Refer to page xvii for a key to the abbreviations used throughout this book.

When examining the nutrient values of cooked generic foods, keep in mind that unless otherwise noted, no additional ingredients have been added during cooking. For processed foods such as cake or pancake mixes, the term "prepared" signifies that the item has been prepared according to the directions on the package, with whatever additional ingredients that requires. Unless otherwise noted, the food values for fish, meats, and poultry are for meat only, and do not include skin or bones.

CODES AND ABBREVIATIONS

To provide the most comprehensive nutritional information possible, a number of codes and abbreviations have been used throughout this book. A complete translation is given below.

>	greater than		nia	niacin
<	less than		pkg	package
approx	approximately		pot	potassium
cal	calories		prep	prepared according to directions
calc	calcium		prot	protein
carbs	carbohydrates		rib	riboflavin
fl	fluid		sat fat	saturated fat
fol	folic acid		sod	sodium
gm	gram		tbsp	tablespoon
IU	international unit[1]		thi	thiamine
lb	pound		tr	trace
mag	magnesium		(tr)	may contain a trace amount
mcg	microgram(s)		tsp	teaspoon
med	medium-sized		w/	with
mg	milligram(s)		w/o	without
(mq)	may contain a measurable quantity[2]		wt	weight
na	not available		zn	zinc

[1] International units, which are used throughout this book to express vitamin A content, are a measure of fat-soluble vitamin activity. The amounts of all other nutrients are expressed in grams or milligrams, which are units of mass and weight.

[2] The food item may contain a quantity ranging from a trace amount to a substantial amount. This quantity depends upon any one of a number of variables—such as soil condition and mineral content of fertilizer used—that may have affected the food item during growing, processing, and/or preparation.

A-to-Z Listing
of Foods

A

Food Name	Serv. Size	Total Cal.	Carbs GMS	Fat GMS
ABALONE, mixed species, raw	3 oz	89	5	0.6
ABALONE MUSHROOM. See MUSHROOM, OYSTER.				
ACEROLA, RAW/Barbados cherry/Puerto Rican cherry/West Indian cherry				
raw, trimmed	1 medium	2	0	0.0
raw, untrimmed	1 cup	31	8	0.3
ACEROLA JUICE				
	1 cup	56	12	0.7
	1 fl oz	7	1	0.1
ACORN				
dried	1 oz	144	15	8.9
raw	1 oz	110	12	6.8
ACORN FLOUR. See under FLOUR.				
ACORN SQUASH. See SQUASH, ACORN.				
ADZUKI BEAN. See BEAN, ADZUKI.				
AGAR. See under SEA VEGETABLE.				
AKU. See under TUNA, SKIP JACK.				
ALARIA. See under SEA VEGETABLE.				
ALASKA KING CRAB. See under CRAB.				
ALBACORE. See under TUNA.				
ALE. See BEER, ALE, AND MALT LIQUOR.				
ALCOHOLIC BEVERAGES. See BEER, ALE, AND MALT LIQUOR; COCKTAIL; COCKTAIL MIX; SHERRY; VERMOUTH; WINE; WINE, COOKING; WINE COOLER; and individual listings.				
ALFALFA SEEDS				
(Arrowhead Mills)	1 cup	40	4	1.0
sprouted, raw	1 cup	10	1	0.2
sprouted, raw	1 tbsp	1	0	0.0
ALFALFA TABLETS (Shaklee)	10 tablets	5	0	0.0
ALGAE				
blue-green, Klamath lake algae)	1 gram	3	0	0.0
spirulina, dried	1 cup	44	4	1.2
ALLIGATOR	1 oz	41	na	0.8
ALLSPICE				
ground	1 tbsp	16	4	0.5
ground	1 tsp	5	1	0.2
ground (Durkee)	1 tsp	7	0	0.0
ground (Laurel Leaf)	1 tsp	7	0	0.0
ground (McCormick/Schilling)	1 tsp	6	1	0.0
ground (Spice Islands)	1 tsp	6	1	0.1
ground (Tone's)	1 tsp	5	1	0.2
ALMOND				
ground	1 cup	549	19	48.1
whole kernels, approx 24	1 oz	164	6	14.4
(Beer Nuts)	1 oz	180	7	14.4
(Dole)	1 oz	170	12	14.0
(Fisher)	1 oz	170	3	15.0
natural, chopped (Blue Diamond)	1 oz	172	6	14.3
natural, sliced (Blue Diamond)	1 oz	172	6	14.3
natural, unsalted (Flanigan Farms)	1 oz	170	5	14.0
natural, whole (Blue Diamond) natural	1 oz	172	6	14.3
natural, whole or sliced (Azar)	2 oz	340	12	30.0
Barbecue (Blue Diamond)	1 oz	167	5	15.0
Blanched				
pieces	1 oz	165	6	14.4

Food Name	Serv. Size	Total Cal.	Carbs GMS	Fat GMS
pieces	1 tbsp	53	2	4.6
whole kernels	1 cup	842	29	73.4
(Blue Diamond)	1 oz	175	5	14.5
(Planters)	1 oz	170	6	14.5
slivered *(Azar)*	2 oz	330	10	29.0
slivered *(Blue Diamond)*	1 oz	175	5	14.5
whole *(Blue Diamond)*	1 oz	175	5	14.5
Chili w/lemon *(Blue Diamond)*	1 oz	172	4	16.0
Dry-roasted				
whole kernels, salted	1 cup	824	27	72.9
whole kernels, salted, approx 22	1 oz	169	5	15.0
whole kernels, unsalted	1 cup	824	27	72.9
whole kernels, unsalted, approx 22	1 oz	169	5	15.0
California, whole *(Flanigan Farms)*	1/4 cup	170	6	15.0
chopped, unsalted *(Flanigan Farms)*	1/4 cup	170	6	15.0
(Planters)	1 oz	170	6	15.0
sliced, unsalted *(Flanigan Farms)*	1/4 cup	170	6	15.0
slivered, unsalted *(Flanigan Farms)*	1/4 cup	170	5	15.0
unsalted *(Blue Diamond)*	1 oz	170	5	15.1
w/tamari *(Eden Foods)*	1 oz	170	8	12.0
Honey-roasted				
unblanched	1 oz	168	8	14.1
whole kernels, unblanched	1 cup	855	40	71.9
(Blue Diamond)	1 oz	170	8	14.2
(Planters)	1 oz	170	9	13.0
Oil-roasted				
whole kernels, salted	1 cup	953	28	86.6
whole kernels, salted, approx 22	1 oz	172	5	15.6
whole kernels, unsalted	1 cup	953	28	86.6
whole kernels, unsalted, approx 22	1 oz	172	5	15.6
Raw				
sliced *(Planters)*	1 oz	170	6	15.0
slivered *(Planters)*	1 oz	170	6	15.0
whole *(Planters)*	1 oz	170	6	15.0
Roasted *(Dole)*	1 oz	170	5	14.0
Smokehouse *(Blue Diamond)*	1 oz	173	5	15.8
Unblanched				
sliced	1 cup	549	19	48.1
slivered	1 cup	624	21	54.7
whole	1 cup	821	28	71.9
Yogurt-coated, made w/real fruit juice *(Fruit Source)*	9 pieces	210	19	14.0
ALMOND BUTTER				
salted	1 cup	1583	53	147.8
salted	1 tbsp	101	3	9.5
unsalted	1 cup	1583	53	147.8
unsalted	1 tbsp	101	3	9.5
(Hain)				
blanched, toasted	2 tbsp	220	3	19.0
raw, 'Natural'	2 tbsp	190	3	18.0
(Maranatha Natural)				
organic, raw	2 tbsp	190	8	15.0
roasted	2 tbsp	190	8	15.0
(Roaster Fresh)				
gourmet	1 oz	184	6	16.0
roasted fresh, creamy, salted	1 oz	184	6	16.0
(Westbrae)				
crunchy, unsalted, 'Natural'	2 tbsp	190	7	17.0

Food Name	Serv. Size	Total Cal.	Carbs GMS	Fat GMS
smooth, unsalted, 'Natural'	2 tbsp	190	7	17.0
ALMOND DRINK original flavor *(Almond Mylk)*	8 fl oz	80	8	4.0
ALMOND MEAL				
partially defatted	4 oz	463	32.8	20.8
partially defatted, salted	4 oz	463	32.8	20.8
ALMOND OIL				
	1 cup	1927	0	218.0
	1 tbsp	120	0	13.6
(Hain)	1 tbsp	120	0	14.0
pure-pressed organic *(Spectrum)*	1 tbsp	120	0	14.0
sweet *(International Collection)*	1 tbsp	120	0	14.0
ALMOND PASTE				
	1 oz	130	14	7.9
firmly packed	1 cup	1040	109	63.0
ALOE VERA JUICE				
sodium-free, certified 100% juice *(Sunburst)*	2 fl oz	5	1	0.0
AMARANTH				
	1 cup	729	129	12.7
(Arrowhead Mills) whole-grain, organic	1/4 cup	170	29	2.0
AMARANTH DISH/ENTRÉE				
(Health Valley) w/vegetables, fat-free, 'Fast Menu'	1 cup	160	31	0.0
AMARANTH FLOUR. See under FLOUR.				
AMARANTH LEAVES				
boiled, drained	1 cup	28	5	0.2
raw	1 cup	6	1	0.1
raw	1 leaf	3	1	0.0
AMARANTH SEED *(Arrowhead Mills)*	2 oz	200	35	3.0
ANASAZI BEAN. See BEAN, ANASAZI.				
ANCHO PEPPER. See PEPPER, ANCHO.				
ANCHOVY				
Canned				
European, in oil, boneless, drained	1 oz	60	0	2.8
European, in oil, drained	2 oz	95	0	4.4
European, in oil, drained	5 medium	42	0	1.9
European, in oil, drained	1 medium	8	0	0.4
flat fillets, in olive oil *(Crown Prince)*	9 fillets	35	0	2.5
flat fillets, in olive oil, salt added *(Reese)*	6 fillets	25	0	1.5
Fresh, European, raw	3 oz	111	0	4.1
ANCHOVY PASTE				
(Reese)	1 tbsp	30	0	2.5
(Roland)	1 tbsp	30	0	2.5
ANGEL HAIR. See under PASTA; PASTA DISH/ENTRÉE.				
ANGLER FISH. See MONKFISH.				
ANISE, dried *(McCormick/Schilling)*	1 serving	18	2	0.8
ANISE SEED				
	1 tbsp	23	3	1.1
	1 tsp	7	1	0.3
(Tone's)	1 tsp	7	1	0.3
ANTELOPE				
raw	1 oz	32	0	0.6
roasted	3 oz	128	0	2.3
roasted, boneless, yield from 1 lb raw	11.9 oz	510	0	9.1
APPLE				
Canned, sweetened slices, drained	1 cup	137	34	0.9
Dehydrated, sulfured				
low moisture, stewed	1 cup	143	38	0.2
low moisture, uncooked	1 cup	208	56	0.3

Food Name	Serv. Size	Total Cal.	Carbs GMS	Fat GMS
rings, uncooked	1 ring	16	4	0.0
stewed	1 cup	145	39	0.2
uncooked	1 cup	209	57	0.3
Fresh				
boiled, peeled, sliced	1 cup	91	23	0.6
microwaved, peeled, sliced	1 cup	95	24	0.7
raw, peeled, quartered or chopped	1 cup	74	19	0.5
raw, peeled, sliced	1 cup	63	16	0.3
raw, peeled, whole, medium, approx 3 per lb	1 apple	73	19	0.4
raw, unpeeled, whole, large, approx 2 per lb	1 apple	125	32	0.8
raw, unpeeled, whole, medium, approx 3 per lb	1 apple	81	21	0.5
raw, unpeeled, whole, small, approx 4 per lb	1 apple	63	16	0.4
Frozen				
unsweetened slices, heated	1 cup	97	25	0.7
unsweetened slices, unheated	1 cup	83	21	0.6
APPLE BUTTER				
(Bama)	2 tsp	25	6	0.0
(Eden Foods)	1 tbsp	25	3	0.0
(Knudsen & Sons) organic	2 tbsp	25	6	0.0
(Lucky Leaf)	4 oz	200	49	1.0
(Musselman's)	4 oz	200	49	1.0
(Smucker's)				
'Autumn Harvest'	1 tsp	12	3	0.0
cider	1 tsp	12	3	0.0
natural	1 tsp	12	3	0.0
'Simply Fruit'	1 tsp	16	4	0.0
spiced	1 tsp	12	3	0.0
(Tap'n Apple)	1 oz	45	13	0.1
(White House)	1 oz	50	12	0.0
APPLE DISH				
escalloped, frozen (Stouffer's)	2/3 cup	182	37	3.0
escalloped, frozen (Stouffer's)	1 oz	31	7	0.5
fried (Luck's)	1/2 cup	130	33	0.0
APPLE JUICE. See also CIDER; CIDER MIX; FRUIT DRINK; FRUIT DRINK MIX; FRUIT JUICE BLEND; FRUIT JUICE DRINK.				
Canned, bottled, or boxed				
w/added vitamin C	1 cup	117	29	0.3
w/added vitamin C	1 fl oz	15	4	0.0
w/o added vitamin C	1 cup	117	29	0.3
w/o added vitamin C	1 fl oz	15	4	0.0
w/o added vitamin C	8.45 fl oz	123	31	0.3
(Flav-R-Pac)	1 cup	120	29	0.0
(Indian Summer)	6 fl oz	90	21	1.0
(J. Hungerford)				
	9.03 fl oz	128	32	0.0
50% juice	9.03 fl oz	119	30	0.0
100% juice	9.03 fl oz	112	28	0.0
(Juicy Juice)	6 fl oz	90	21	0.0
(Knudsen)				
clear	8 fl oz	110	28	0.0
Gravenstein	8 fl oz	110	28	0.0
natural	8 fl oz	120	30	0.0
(Kraft) 'Pure 100%'	6 fl oz	80	20	0.0
(Lucky Leaf)				
'Individual Portion Control'	3.8 fl oz	60	14	0.0
100% vitamin-C enriched	6 fl oz	90	21	0.0
(McCain) 100% juice 'Junior'	4.2 fl oz	50	13	0.0

Food Name	Serv. Size	Total Cal.	Carbs GMS	Fat GMS
(Mott's)	6 fl oz	88	22	0.0
(Musselman's)				
'Individual Portion Control'	3.8 fl oz	60	14	0.0
100% vitamin-C enriched	6 fl oz	90	21	0.0
(Ocean Spray)	6 fl oz	90	23	0.0
(Red Cheek)				
'Natural'	6 fl oz	97	24	0.0
'100% Pure'	6 fl oz	97	24	0.0
(S&W)				
	8 fl oz	120	30	0.0
'100% Pure Unsweetened'	6 fl oz	85	20	0.0
(S. Martinelli) 'Sparkling'	6 fl oz	100	25	0.0
(Sippin' Pak) 100% pure.	8.45 fl oz	110	28	0.0
(Tree Top) 100%	8 fl oz	120	29	0.0
(TreeSweet)	6 fl oz	90	22	0.0
(Tropicana)				
100% pure	8 fl oz	116	29	0.0
100% pure	6 fl oz	80	20	1.0
'Pure Premium' 'Orchardstand'	8 fl oz	110	27	0.0
'Season's Best'	8 fl oz	120	29	0.0
(Ultra Slim Fast) golden	8 fl oz	153	29	1.0
(Veryfine) '100%'	8 fl oz	107	27	0.0
(Welch's)				
'Orchard Cocktail'	10 fl oz	170	42	0.0
sparkling	6 fl oz	100	24	0.0
(White House)	6 fl oz	87	22	0.0
Chilled or frozen				
concentrate, w/o added vitamin C, prepared	1 cup	112	28	0.2
concentrate, w/o added vitamin C, prepared	1 fl oz	14	3	0.0
concentrate, w/added vitamin C, prepared	1 cup	112	28	0.2
concentrate, w/added vitamin C, prepared	1 fl oz	14	3	0.0
concentrate, w/added vitamin C, undiluted	6-oz can	350	87	0.8
concentrate, w/o added vitamin C, undiluted	6-oz can	350	87	0.8
(A&P) diluted as directed	6 fl oz	90	22	1.0
(Sunkist) diluted as directed	8 fl oz	79	19	0.2
APPLE KIT				
(Concord)				
candy, microwaveable, prepared	1 apple	50	14	0.0
caramel, microwaveable, prepared	1 apple	150	27	3.0
APPLE PIE SPICE. See under SEASONING MIX.				
APPLE SPREAD, no sugar added (Fifty 50)	1 tsp	2	1	0.0
APPLE SYRUP (Knudsen)	1 oz	75	15	1.0
APPLE TOPPING (Flav-R-Pac)	2 tbsp	40	10	0.0
APPLESAUCE				
canned, sweetened, w/salt	1 cup	194	51	0.5
canned, sweetened, w/o salt	1 cup	194	51	0.5
canned, sweetened, w/o salt	1 cup	194	51	0.5
canned, unsweetened, w/added vitamin C	1 cup	105	28	0.1
canned, unsweetened w/o added vitamin C	1 cup	105	28	0.1
cinnamon (Tree Top)	1/2 cup	83	21	0.0
cranberry, 'CranFruit' (Ocean Spray)	2 oz	100	23	0.0
original (Tree Top)	1/2 cup	83	21	0.0
unsweetened (Tree Top)	1/2 cup	58	15	0.0
APRICOT				
Canned				
halves, peeled, in extra light syrup, w/liquid	1 cup	121	31	0.2
halves, peeled, in heavy syrup, w/liquid	1 cup	214	55	0.2

Food Name	Serv. Size	Total Cal.	Carbs GMS	Fat GMS
halves, unpeeled, in juice, w/liquid	1 cup	117	30	0.1
halves, unpeeled, in light syrup, w/liquid	1 cup	159	42	0.1
halves, unpeeled, in water, w/liquid	1 cup	66	16	0.4
whole, peeled, in heavy syrup, w/o pits, w/liquid	1 cup	236	61	0.1
whole, peeled, in water, w/o pits, w/liquid	1 cup	50	12	0.1
whole, unpeeled, in heavy syrup, w/liquid	1 cup	199	52	0.2
whole, unpeeled, in heavy syrup, w/liquid	1/2 apricot	33	9	0.0
whole, unpeeled, in juice, w/liquid	1/2 apricot	17	4	0.0
whole, unpeeled, in light syrup, w/liquid	1/2 apricot	25	7	0.0
whole, unpeeled, in water, w/liquid	1/2 apricot	10	2	0.1
Dehydrated/sulfured				
halves, stewed	1 cup	213	55	0.4
halves, uncooked	1 cup	309	80	0.6
low-moisture, stewed	1 cup	314	81	0.6
low-moisture, uncooked	1 cup	381	99	0.7
uncooked	1/2 apricot	8	2	0.0
Fresh				
raw, halved	1 cup	74	17	0.6
raw, sliced	1 cup	79	18	0.6
raw, whole	1 med	17	4	0.1
Frozen				
sweetened	1 cup	237	61	0.2
sliced *(Flav-R-Pac)*	2/3 cup	70	18	0.0
APRICOT KERNEL OIL				
	1 cup	1927	0	218.0
	1 tbsp	120	0	13.6
(Hain)	1 tbsp	120	0	14.0
ARBORIO RICE. See under RICE.				
ARROWHEAD				
boiled, drained	1 medium	9	2	0.0
powdered *(Tone's)*	1 tsp	10	2	0.0
raw	1 large	25	5	0.1
raw	1 medium	12	2	0.0
ARROWROOT				
raw, whole	1 med root	21	4	0.1
raw, sliced	1 cup	78	16	0.2
ARROWROOT FLOUR. See under FLOUR.				
ARTICHOKE. See also ARTICHOKE, JERUSALEM.				
Canned				
globe, bottoms *(Reese)*	2 pieces	35	7	0.0
globe, hearts *(C&W)*	1/2 cup	25	4	0.0
globe, hearts, 5-7 per can *(Reese)*	2 pieces	30	6	0.0
globe, hearts, quartered *(Maria)*	1/2 cup	35	6	0.0
globe, hearts, 10-12 per can *(Reese)*	4 pieces	30	6	0.0
hearts, marinated *(Progresso)*	1/3 cup	160	6	14.0
Fresh				
globe, fresh *(Dole)*	1 large	23	5	0.1
globe or French, boiled, drained	1 medium	60	13	0.2
globe or French, hearts, boiled, drained	1/2 cup	42	9	0.1
globe or French, raw	1 large	76	17	0.2
globe or French, raw	1 medium	60	13	0.2
Frozen				
globe or French, unprepared	9-oz pkg	97	20	1.1
globe or French, w/salt, drained	9-oz pkg	108	22	1.2
globe or French, w/salt, drained	1 cup	76	15	0.8
globe or French, w/salt, drained, 1/3 of 10-oz pkg	1 serving	36	7	0.4
globe or French, w/o salt, drained	1 cup	76	15	0.8

Food Name	Serv. Size	Total Cal.	Carbs GMS	Fat GMS
globe or French, w/o salt, drained .... 9-oz pkg		108	22	1.2
globe or French, w/o salt, drained, 1/3 of 10-oz pkg .... 1 serving		36	7	0.4
hearts *(Seabrook)* .... 3 oz		25	4	0.0
hearts, 'Deluxe' *(Birds Eye)* .... 3 oz		30	7	0.0
ARTICHOKE, JERUSALEM/sunchoke				
raw, sliced .... 1 cup		114	26	0.0
ARUGULA/rucola/rugula				
raw .... 1 leaf		1	0	0.0
raw .... 1/2 cup		3	0	0.1
(Frieda of California) .... 1 oz		7	1	0.1
ASIAN PEAR/Chinese pear/sand pear				
Fresh				
raw, whole, approx 2.25x2.5-inch diam .... 1 fruit		51	13	0.3
raw, whole, approx 3-3/8x3-inch diam .... 1 fruit		116	29	0.6
ASPARAGUS				
Canned				
cuts, green, drained .... 1 cup		46	6	1.6
cuts, green, w/liquid .... 1/2 cup		18	3	0.2
cuts, green, 50% less salt, w/liquid *(Green Giant)* .... 1/2 cup		20	3	0.0
cuts, green *(Stokely)* .... 1/2 cup		20	3	0.0
cuts, green, w/liquid *(Green Giant)* .... 1/2 cup		20	3	0.0
cuts, green 'No Salt or Sugar Added' *(Stokely)* .... 1/2 cup		20	3	0.0
cuts, white, w/liquid *(Green Giant)* .... 1/2 cup		16	3	0.0
cuts and tips *(Finast)* .... 1 cup		35	6	0.0
points, green *(S&W)* .... 1/2 cup		17	3	0.0
spears, drained .... 1 med spear		3	0	0.1
green, cut *(Green Giant)* .... 1/2 cup		18	3	0.0
green, cut, 50% less salt *(Green Giant)* .... 1/2 cup		18	3	0.0
green, cut 'No Salt Added' *(Pathmark)* .... 1/2 cup		20	2	0.0
green, cut *(Pathmark)* .... 1/2 cup		20	2	0.0
green, extra large 'LeSueur' *(Green Giant)* .... 4.5 oz		20	3	0.0
green, extra long *(Green Giant)* .... 4.5 oz		20	3	0.0
green 'Fancy' *(S&W)* .... 1/2 cup		18	3	0.0
spears, colossal *(S&W)* .... 3 pieces		10	3	0.0
white *(Green Giant)* .... 1/2 cup		16	3	0.0
Fresh				
cuts, boiled, drained .... 1/2 cup		22	4	0.3
cuts, raw .... 1 cup		31	6	0.3
spears, boiled, drained, whole .... 4 med spears		14	3	0.2
spears, fresh *(Dole)* .... 5 spears		18	2	0.0
spears, raw, extra large, 8.75 to 10-inch long .... 1 spear		6	1	0.0
spears, raw, large, 7.25 to 8.5-inch long .... 1 spear		5	1	0.0
spears, raw, medium, 5.25 to 7-inch long .... 1 spear		4	1	0.0
spears, raw, small, up to 5-inch long .... 1 spear		3	1	0.0
tips, raw, 2 inches long or less .... 1 spear tip		1	0	0.0
Frozen				
cuts *(Birds Eye)* .... 3.3 oz		25	4	0.0
cuts *(Flav-R-Pac)* .... 3/4 cup		20	3	0.0
cuts *(Seabrook)* .... 3.3 oz		25	4	0.0
cuts, unprepared .... 10-oz pkg		68	12	0.7
cuts, w/salt, boiled, drained .... 10-oz pkg		82	14	1.2
cuts, w/salt, boiled, drained .... 1 cup		50	9	0.8
cuts, w/o salt, boiled, drained .... 10-oz pkg		82	14	1.2
cuts, w/o salt, boiled, drained .... 1 cup		50	9	0.8
cuts and spears *(Frosty Acres)* .... 3.3 oz		25	4	0.0
spears *(Birds Eye)* .... 3.3 oz		25	4	0.0
spears *(Finast)* .... 3.3 oz		25	4	0.0

Food Name	Serv. Size	Total Cal.	Carbs GMS	Fat GMS
spears *(Frosty Acres)*	3.3 oz	25	4	0.0
spears *(Seabrook)*	3.3 oz	25	4	0.0
spears *(Southern)*	3.5 oz	27	4	0.2
spears, boiled, drained	4 spears	17	3	0.3
spears, unprepared	4 spears	14	2	0.1

ATLANTIC COD. See under COD.
ATLANTIC MACKEREL. See under MACKEREL.
ATLANTIC OCEAN PERCH. See OCEAN PERCH.
ATLANTIC POLLACK. See POLLACK.
ATLANTIC SALMON. See under SALMON.
AUBERGINE. See EGGPLANT.
AVOCADO
ALL COMMERCIAL VARIETIES
  Fresh

Food Name	Serv. Size	Total Cal.	Carbs GMS	Fat GMS
raw, cubed	1 cup	242	11	23.0
raw, puréed	1 cup	370	17	35.2
raw, sliced	1 cup	235	11	22.4
raw, whole	1 medium	324	15	30.8

CALIFORNIA
  Fresh

Food Name	Serv. Size	Total Cal.	Carbs GMS	Fat GMS
raw, puréed	1 cup	407	16	39.9
raw, whole, peeled and pitted	1 medium	306	12	30.0

FLORIDA
  Fresh

Food Name	Serv. Size	Total Cal.	Carbs GMS	Fat GMS
raw, puréed	1 cup	258	20	20.4
raw, whole, peeled and pitted	1 medium	340	27	27.0

AVOCADO OIL

Food Name	Serv. Size	Total Cal.	Carbs GMS	Fat GMS
	1 cup	1927	0	218.0
	1 tbsp	124	0	14.0
(Hain)	1 tbsp	120	0	14.0
pure-pressed, organic *(Spectrum)*	1 tbsp	120	0	14.0

AWA/milkfish

Food Name	Serv. Size	Total Cal.	Carbs GMS	Fat GMS
baked, broiled, grilled, or microwaved	3 oz	162	0	7.3
raw	3 oz	126	0	5.7

B

Food Name	Serv. Size	Total Cal.	Carbs GMS	Fat GMS

BABASSU OIL. See PALM KERNEL OIL.
BABY FOOD
CEREAL
  Barley

Food Name	Serv. Size	Total Cal.	Carbs GMS	Fat GMS
dry	1/2 oz	55	11	0.5
dry	1 tbsp	9	2	0.1
instant *(Heinz)*	3.5 oz	370	79	3.7
instant, prepared w/0.5 oz cereal and 2.4 oz whole milk *(Gerber)*	2.9 oz	100	14	4.0
instant, prepared w/2.4 oz formula '1st Foods' *(Gerber)*	1/2 oz	110	16	4.0
prepared w/whole milk	1 oz	31	5	0.9
Cereal w/applesauce and bananas, '3rd Foods' *(Gerber)*	7 tbsp	82	18	0.6
Cereal w/egg yolks				
junior	1 jar	88	12	3.1
strained	1 oz	14	2	0.5
w/eggs	1 oz	16	2	0.4
Cereal w/egg yolks and bacon, junior	1 oz	22	2	1.4
Corn				
instant, dry 'Tropical Foods' *(Gerber)*	3.5 oz	390	81	4.6

Food Name	Serv. Size	Total Cal.	Carbs GMS	Fat GMS
instant, prepared w/milk Tropical Foods' *(Gerber)*	2.4 oz	110	15	4.0
High-protein				
instant, dry	1/2 oz	54	7	0.9
instant, dry	1 tbsp	9	1	0.1
instant, prepared w/whole milk	1 oz	31	3	1.1
w/apple and orange, instant, dry	1/2 oz	53	8	0.9
w/apple and orange, instant, dry	1 tbsp	9	1	0.2
w/apple and orange, instant, prepared w/whole milk	1 oz	32	4	1.1
Mixed				
dry	1/2 oz	57	11	0.7
dry	1 tbsp	9	2	0.1
prepared w/whole milk	1 oz	32	5	1.0
instant, dry *(Earth's Best)*	0.5 oz	60	11	0.0
instant, dry, '2nd Foods' *(Gerber)*	0.5 oz	60	11	1.0
instant *(Heinz)*	3.5 oz	373	72	4.9
instant, prepared w/apple juice, '2nd Foods' *(Gerber)*	2.4 oz	90	20	1.0
instant, prepared w/0.5 oz cereal, 2.4 oz formula, 'Stages 2' *(Beech-Nut)*	0.5 oz	120	17	4.0
instant, prepared w/0.5 oz cereal, 2.5 oz formula *(Earth's Best)*	3 oz	110	16	3.0
instant, prepared w/0.5 oz cereal, 2.4 oz whole milk, 'Stages 2' *(Beech-Nut)*	2.9 oz	100	14	3.0
w/apple and bananas, 'Stages 2' *(Beech-Nut)*	4.5 oz	90	19	1.0
w/apple and bananas, strained *(Heinz)*	3.5 oz	70	16	0.3
w/apple 'Stages 2' *(Beech-Nut)*	4 oz	70	16	0.0
w/applesauce and bananas, junior	1 oz	24	5	0.1
w/applesauce and bananas, strained	1 oz	23	5	0.1
w/applesauce and bananas, '3rd Foods' *(Gerber)*	7 tbsp	82	19	0.6
w/banana, dry	1/2 oz	59	12	0.7
w/banana, dry	1 tbsp	10	2	0.1
w/bananas, dry, '2nd Foods' *(Gerber)*	0.5 oz	60	11	1.0
w/fruit and nuts, no sugar added, 1-4 yr, dry *(Familia)*	1.5 oz	170	31	3.0
w/fruit and nuts, 100% natural, 1-4 yr, dry *(Familia)*	1.5 oz	170	32	3.0
w/fruit and nuts, 1-4 yr, prepared w/whole milk *(Familia)*	1.5 oz	270	38	8.0
w/fruit and nuts, 1-4 yr, prepared w/2/3 cup milk *(Familia)*	1.5 oz	270	39	8.0
Oatmeal				
dry	1/2 oz	60	10	1.2
dry	1 tbsp	10	2	0.2
prepared w/whole milk	1 oz	33	4	1.2
w/apple, 'Stages 2' *(Beech-Nut)*	4 oz	70	16	0.0
w/apple and bananas 'Stages 2' *(Beech-Nut)*	4.5 oz	90	17	1.0
w/apple and bananas, strained *(Heinz)*	3.5 oz	76	16	0.6
w/apple and cinnamon, instant, '3rd Foods' *(Gerber)*	1 pkt	90	16	2.0
w/applesauce and bananas, junior	1 oz	21	4	0.2
w/applesauce and bananas, strained	1 oz	21	4	0.2
w/applesauce and bananas, '3rd Foods' *(Gerber)*	7 tbsp	80	17	0.8
w/bananas, dry	1/2 oz	59	11	0.9
w/bananas, dry	1 tbsp	10	2	0.1
w/bananas, prepared w/whole milk	1 oz	33	5	1.1
w/bananas, instant '3rd Foods' *(Gerber)*	1 pkt	90	16	2.0
w/bananas, 100% natural, organic, dry *(Healthy Times)*	0.5 oz	60	12	0.0
w/bananas, organic, prepared w/2.4 oz formula *(Healthy Times)*	0.5 oz	100	17	3.0
w/fruit, toddler, instant, dry	0.75 oz	84	16	1.5
w/fruit, toddler, instant, dry	1 tbsp	21	4	0.4
w/honey, dry	1/2 oz	56	10	1.0
w/honey, dry	1 tbsp	9	2	0.2
w/honey, prepared w/whole milk	1 oz	33	4	1.1
Rice				
dry	1/2 oz	59	12	0.7

Food Name	Serv. Size	Total Cal.	Carbs GMS	Fat GMS
dry	1 tbsp	10	2	0.1
prepared w/whole milk	1 oz	33	5	1.0
prepared w/formula '1st Foods' (Gerber)	2.4 oz	110	16	4.0
(Heinz)	3.5 oz	376	78	4.1
brown, dry (Earth's Best)	0.5 oz	60	12	0.0
brown, prepared w/0.5 oz cereal, 2.5 oz formula (Earth's Best)	3 oz	110	17	3.0
instant, prepared w/0.5 oz cereal, 2.4 oz whole milk, 'Stages 1' (Beech-Nut) 'Stages 1'	2.9 oz	110	17	3.0
instant, prepared w/0.5 oz cereal, 2.4 oz formula, 'Stages 1' (Beech-Nut)	0.5 oz	120	18	4.0
sprouted (Health Valley)	1 tbsp	60	10	1.0
w/apple, instant, prepared w/0.5 oz cereal, 2.4 oz formula (Beech-Nut)	2.9 oz	120	19	4.0
w/apple, instant, prepared w/0.5 oz cereal, 2.4 oz whole milk (Beech-Nut)	2.9 oz	110	17	3.0
w/apple, 'Stages 2' (Beech-Nut)	4 oz	70	16	0.0
w/apple and bananas, 'Stages 2' (Beech-Nut)	4.5 oz	100	24	0.0
w/apple and bananas, strained (Heinz)	3.5 oz	70	16	0.2
w/applesauce and bananas, '2nd Foods' (Gerber)	7 tbsp	79	18	0.2
w/applesauce and bananas, strained	1 oz	22	5	0.1
w/applesauce and bananas, strained	1 tbsp	13	3	0.1
w/applesauce and bananas, strained, '2nd Foods' (Gerber)	4 oz jar	89	19	0.5
w/applesauce and bananas, strained, 'Strained 2' (Heinz)	4.25 oz jar	95	21	0.5
w/bananas, dry	1 tbsp	10	2	0.1
w/bananas, dry	1/2 oz	61	12	0.6
w/bananas, prepared w/whole milk	1 oz	33	5	1.0
w/bananas, dry, '2nd Foods' (Gerber)	0.5 oz	60	11	1.0
w/bananas, prepared w/0.5 oz cereal, 2.4 oz formula (Beech-Nut)	0.5 oz	120	19	4.0
w/bananas, prepared w/0.5 oz cereal, 2.4 oz whole milk (Beech-Nut)	2.9 oz	100	17	3.0
w/honey, prepared w/whole milk	1 oz	33	5	0.9
w/mango, dry, 'Tropical Foods' (Gerber)	3.5 oz	386	84	2.6
w/mango, prepared w/milk, 'Tropical Foods' (Gerber)	2.4 oz	100	15	3.0
w/mixed fruit, junior	1 oz	22	5	0.1
w/mixed fruit, junior	1 tbsp	12	3	0.0
w/mixed fruit, junior (Gerber)	6 oz	140	31	1.0
w/mixed fruit, '3rd Foods' (Gerber)	6-oz jar	134	31	0.3
DESSERTS AND SNACKS				
Apple-strawberry dessert, 'Stages 2' (Beech-Nut)	4 oz	100	23	0.0
Apple-peach-strawberry dessert, 'Stages 2' (Beech-Nut)	4 oz	100	22	0.0
Banana-pineapple dessert, 'Stages 2' (Beech-Nut)	4 oz	100	23	0.0
Banana-vanilla dessert, (Gerber) 'Tropical Foods'	7 tbsp	85	19	0.9
Cereal snack				
apple-banana, finger snacks, 'Graduates' (Gerber)	3.2 oz	405	83	4.8
apple-cinnamon, finger snacks 'Graduates' (Gerber)	3.2 oz	407	83	5.0
Cookies and crackers				
animal-shaped, baked, chunky (Gerber)	3.5 oz	443	75	13.1
apple, organic, 'Hugga Bears' (Healthy Times)	1 oz	120	17	3.0
arrowroot	1 oz	125	20	4.1
arrowroot	1 cookie	22	4	0.7
arrowroot, baked finger snacks, 'Graduates' (Gerber)	3.5 oz	452	70	15.3
arrowroot, maple, wheat-free (Healthy Times)	1 cookie	120	17	3.0
cinnamon animal cracker, baked 'Graduates' (Gerber)	3.5 oz	449	79	12.3
pretzel	1 oz	113	23	0.6
pretzel, baked, finger snacks, 'Graduates' (Gerber)	3.5 oz	403	83	3.3
strawberry, organic, 'Hugga Bears' (Healthy Times)	1 oz	120	17	3.0

Food Name	Serv. Size	Total Cal.	Carbs GMS	Fat GMS
teething biscuit	1 oz	111	22	1.2
teething biscuit	1 biscuit	43	8	0.5
teething, biscuit, baked, chunky, 'Biter Biscuit' (Gerber)	1 biscuit	50	9	1.0
teething toast (Zings!)	1 serving	35	5	1.0
zwieback	1 oz	121	21	2.8
zwieback	1 piece	30	5	0.7
zwieback toast (Gerber)	1 cracker	30	5	0.7
zwieback toast, baked, chunky (Gerber)	3.5 oz	432	69	11.5
Cottage cheese				
w/pineapple, 'Stages 2' (Beech-Nut)	4.5 oz	130	26	1.0
w/pineapple 'Stages 3' (Beech-Nut)	6 oz	170	36	2.0
w/pears, 'Stages 2' (Beech-Nut)	4 oz	120	24	1.0
w/pears, 'Stages 3' (Beech-Nut)	6 oz	180	37	2.0
Custard/pudding				
banana pudding, 'Stages 2' (Beech-Nut)	4 oz	110	26	0.0
banana pudding, strained (Heinz)	3.5 oz	74	17	0.5
cherry vanilla pudding, strained	1 oz	19	5	0.1
cherry-vanilla pudding, strained (Gerber)	4.5 oz	90	21	1.0
cherry-vanilla pudding, junior	1 oz	20	5	0.1
custard pudding, junior (Heinz)	3.5 oz	75	14	1.2
custard pudding, strained (Heinz)	3.5 oz	75	14	1.2
orange pudding, strained	1 oz	23	5	0.3
pineapple pudding, junior	1 oz	25	6	0.1
pineapple pudding, junior	1 tbsp	13	3	0.1
pineapple pudding, junior, '3rd Foods' (Gerber)	6-oz jar	148	37	0.7
pineapple pudding, strained	1 oz	23	6	0.1
pineapple pudding, strained	1 tbsp	12	3	0.0
pineapple pudding, strained, '2nd Foods'	4 oz jar	92	23	0.3
tutti frutti pudding, junior (Heinz)	3.5 oz	67	16	0.4
vanilla custard, 'Stages 2' (Beech-Nut)	4 oz	120	23	3.0
vanilla custard, 'Stages 3' (Beech-Nut)	6 oz	180	30	5.0
vanilla custard, '3rd Foods' (Gerber)	6 oz	190	32	6.0
vanilla custard, junior (Gerber)	6 oz	150	31	2.0
vanilla custard, strained (Gerber)	4.5 oz	100	22	1.0
vanilla pudding, junior	1 cup	197	40	2.2
vanilla pudding, junior	1 oz	24	5	0.3
vanilla pudding, junior	1 tbsp	12	2	0.1
vanilla pudding, junior, 'Junior 3' (Heinz)	6 oz jar	146	30	1.7
vanilla pudding, junior, 'Stages 3' (Beech-Nut)	6 oz jar	146	30	1.7
vanilla pudding, junior, '3rd Foods' (Gerber)	6 oz jar	146	30	1.7
vanilla pudding, strained	1 cup	195	37	4.6
vanilla pudding, strained	1 oz	24	5	0.6
vanilla pudding, strained	1 tbsp	12	2	0.3
vanilla pudding, strained, '2nd Foods' (Gerber)	4 oz jar	96	18	2.3
vanilla pudding, strained, 'Stages 2' (Beech-Nut)	4 oz jar	96	18	2.3
vanilla pudding, strained, 'Strained 2' (Heinz)	4 oz jar	96	18	2.3
Dutch apple dessert				
junior	1 oz	22	5	0.0
junior (Heinz)	3.5 oz	69	16	0.4
'Stages 2' (Beech-Nut)	4 oz	100	22	0.0
strained	1 oz	19	5	0.3
strained (Heinz)	3.5 oz	69	16	0.4
'3rd Foods' (Gerber)	7 tbsp	77	17	0.9
Fruit dessert				
junior (Gerber)	6 oz	130	30	1.0
junior (Heinz)	3.5 oz	65	16	0.2
junior, w/o added vitamin C	1 oz	18	5	0.0

Food Name	Serv. Size	Total Cal.	Carbs GMS	Fat GMS
junior, w/o added vitamin C	1 tbsp	9	3	0.0
junior, w/o added vitamin C, '3rd Foods' (Gerber)	6-oz jar	107	29	0.0
junior, w/o added vitamin C 'Junior 3' (Heinz)................	6-oz jar	107	29	0.0
nonfat, 'Stages 3' (Beech-Nut).............................	6 oz	120	28	0.0
strained (Gerber)	4.5 oz	100	24	1.0
strained (Heinz)	3.5 oz	66	16	0.2
strained, w/o added vitamin C	1 oz	17	5	0.0
strained, w/o added vitamin C	1 tbsp	9	2	0.0
strained, w/o added vitamin C, '2nd Foods' (Gerber)	4-oz jar	67	18	0.0
strained, w/o added vitamin C, 'Strained 2' (Heinz)	4.25-oz jar	71	19	0.0
'3rd Foods' (Gerber)	7 tbsp	73	18	0.2
Guava dessert				
tropical fruit, 'Stages 2' (Beech-Nut)	4 oz	90	22	0.0
w/tapioca 'Tropical Foods' (Gerber)	7 tbsp	69	17	0.1
Hawaiian dessert				
Hawaiian delight, '3rd Foods' (Gerber)	7 tbsp	87	20	0.1
Hawaiian delight, junior (Gerber)...........................	6 oz	150	33	1.0
strained (Gerber)	4.5 oz	120	25	1.0
Mango dessert				
tropical fruit dessert, 'Stages 2' (Beech-Nut)	4.5 oz	100	25	0.0
w/tapioca, 'Tropical Foods' (Gerber)	7 tbsp	75	18	0.2
Mango-banana dessert, w/passionfruit, 'Tropical Foods' (Gerber) ..	7 tbsp	73	18	0.1
Papaya dessert, w/tapioca, 'Tropical Foods' (Gerber)	7 tbsp	62	15	0.2
Papaya-pineapple dessert, 'Tropical Foods' (Gerber)	7 tbsp	76	19	0.0
Peach cobbler				
junior	1 oz	19	5	0.0
junior	1 tbsp	10	3	0.0
junior (Gerber)	6 oz	130	30	1.0
'2nd Foods' (Gerber)	4-oz jar	73	20	0.0
strained	1 oz	18	5	0.0
strained	1 tbsp	10	3	0.0
strained (Gerber)	4.5 oz	100	23	1.0
strained (Heinz)	3.5 oz	72	17	0.3
'Strained 2' (Heinz)	4-oz jar	73	20	0.0
'3rd Foods' (Gerber)	6-oz jar	114	31	0.0
'3rd Foods' (Gerber)	7 tbsp	77	18	0.1
Peach-mango dessert, 'Tropical Foods' (Gerber)	7 tbsp	60	17	0.2
Pineapple-banana dessert, 'Tropical Foods' (Gerber)	7 tbsp	79	19	0.1
Tropical dessert				
island fruit dessert, 'Stages 2' (Beech-Nut)	4 oz	100	23	0.0
mango dessert, Stages 2' (Beech-Nut)	4 oz	110	26	0.0
medley, 'Tropical Foods' (Gerber)	7 tbsp	64	15	0.1
papaya dessert, 'Stages 2' (Beech-Nut)	4 oz	100	22	0.0
w/tapioca, strained (Gerber)	4.5 oz	80	20	0.0
Yogurt				
apple,'Stages 2' (Beech-Nut).............................	4 oz	100	22	1.0
apple, 'Breakfast' (Earth's Best)	4.5 oz	100	17	2.0
banana, 'Stages 2' (Beech-Nut)............................	4 oz	120	24	2.0
banana, strained (Heinz)	3.5 oz	83	19	0.5
blueberry, 'Breakfast' (Earth's Best)	4.5 oz	100	16	2.0
mixed fruit, 'Stages 2' (Beech-Nut)	4 oz	100	21	0.0
mixed fruit, 'Stages 3' (Beech-Nut)	6 oz	170	30	0.0
peach, '2nd Foods' (Gerber)	7 tbsp	76	17	0.4
peach, 'Stages 2' (Beech-Nut)	4.5 oz	120	25	2.0
pear, 'Stages 2' (Beech-Nut)	4.5 oz	130	29	2.0
pear, strained (Heinz)	3.5 oz	80	18	0.4
tropical, 'Breakfast' (Earth's Best)	4.5 oz	110	19	2.0

Food Name	Serv. Size	Total Cal.	Carbs GMS	Fat GMS
DINNERS AND MAIN DISHES				
Apple and chicken dinner				
'Simple Recipe' '2nd Foods' *(Gerber)*	4 oz	70	12	1.5
'Simple Dinner' 'Stage 2' *(Beech-Nut)*	4 oz	73	12	1.6
strained	1 oz	18	3	0.4
Apple and ham dinner				
'Simple Recipe' '2nd Foods' *(Gerber)*	4 oz	80	12	2.0
strained	1 tbsp	9	2	0.1
Apple and turkey dinner				
'Simple Recipe' '2nd Foods' *(Gerber)*	4 oz	80	13	2.0
strained	1 tbsp	10	2	0.2
Beans and rice dinner, 'Tropical Foods' *(Gerber)*	7 tbsp	52	7	1.5
Beef and rice dinner, toddler	1 oz	23	2	0.8
Beef and vegetable dinner				
lean meat, junior *(Gerber)*	4.5 oz	100	10	3.0
lean meat, strained *(Gerber)*	4.5 oz	90	9	3.0
'Stage 2' *(Beech-Nut)*	4.5 oz	90	10	4.0
'Stage 3' *(Beech-Nut)*	6 oz	160	16	7.0
Beef dinner				
junior *(Gerber)*	2.5 oz	80	1	4.0
'Stage 1' *(Beech-Nut)*	2.8 oz	90	0	5.0
'Stage 3' *(Beech-Nut)*	6 oz	150	14	8.0
'3rd Foods' *(Gerber)*	7 tbsp	103	0	4.6
Beef lasagna dinner, toddler	1 oz	22	3	0.6
Beef noodle dinner				
chunky, 'Homestyle' *(Gerber)*	7 tbsp	88	10	3.5
junior	1 oz	16	2	0.5
junior	1 tbsp	9	1	0.3
'Step 3' *(Heinz)*	6 oz	97	13	3.2
strained	1 oz	18	2	0.6
strained	1 tbsp	10	1	0.4
w/egg noodles, '2nd Foods' *(Gerber)*	7 tbsp	62	8	2.0
w/egg noodles, 'Stage 2' *(Beech-Nut)*	4 oz	100	8	6.0
w/egg noodles, 'Stage 3' *(Beech-Nut)*	6 oz	130	13	6.0
w/egg noodles, 'Step 2' *(Heinz)*	3.5 oz	49	6	1.8
w/egg noodles, '3rd Foods' *(Gerber)*	6 oz	130	18	1.9
Beef stew				
'Table Time' *(Beech-Nut)*	6 oz	150	16	6.0
toddler	1 oz	14	2	0.3
Broccoli and chicken dinner				
'Simple Recipe' '2nd Foods' *(Gerber)*	4 oz	45	3	2.0
'Step 2' *(Heinz)*	4 oz	47	4	1.7
strained	1 oz	12	1	0.4
Carrot and beef dinner				
'Simple Recipe' '2nd Foods' *(Gerber)*	4 oz	70	6	3.5
strained	1 tbsp	9	1	0.4
Chicken and rice dinner				
'Stage 2' *(Beech-Nut)*	4 oz	80	9	3.0
'Tropical Foods' *(Gerber)*	7 tbsp	48	7	1.3
Chicken and vegetable dinner				
'Stage 2' *(Beech-Nut)*	4.5 oz	90	14	3.0
'Stage 3' *(Beech-Nut)*	6 oz	90	13	2.0
w/broccoli, simple recipe, '2nd Foods' *(Gerber)*	7 tbsp	42	3	1.5
Chicken dinner				
junior *(Gerber)*	2.5 oz	110	1	7.0
'3rd Foods' *(Gerber)*	7 tbsp	132	0	7.9
w/vegetables, lean meat, junior *(Gerber)*	4.5 oz	90	10	3.0

Food Name	Serv. Size	Total Cal.	Carbs GMS	Fat GMS
w/vegetables, lean meat, strained *(Gerber)*	4.5 oz	90	8	3.0
Chicken noodle dinner				
junior	1 oz	16	2	0.3
junior	1 tbsp	9	1	0.2
'2nd Foods' *(Gerber)*	4 oz	80	11	2.5
'Step 2' *(Heinz)*	4 oz	75	10	2.3
'Step 3' *(Heinz)*	6 oz	94	15	2.0
'Stage 2' *(Beech-Nut)*	4 oz	70	7	4.0
'Stage 3' *(Beech-Nut)*	6 oz	110	14	4.0
strained	1 oz	19	3	0.6
strained	1 tbsp	11	1	0.3
'3rd Foods' *(Gerber)*	6 oz	110	16	3.5
w/carrots and peas, chunky *(Gerber)*	7 tbsp	65	9	1.5
Chicken stew				
toddler	1 oz	22	2	1.0
toddler	1 tbsp	12	1	0.6
w/noodles 'Graduates' *(Gerber)*	3.2 oz	69	9	2.0
Green bean and rice dinner *(Earth's Best)*	4.5 oz	70	14	0.0
Green bean and turkey dinner				
'Simple Recipe' '2nd Foods' *(Gerber)*	7 tbsp	55	7	1.5
'Step 2' *(Heinz)*	4 oz	60	6	2.1
strained	1 oz	15	2	0.5
Ham and vegetable dinner				
lean meat, junior *(Gerber)*	4.5 oz	110	11	4.0
lean meat, strained *(Gerber)*	4.5 oz	100	10	4.0
'Stage 2' *(Beech-Nut)*	4.5 oz	80	12	3.0
Lamb and vegetable dinner, 'Stage 2' *(Beech-Nut)*	4.5 oz	90	13	4.0
Macaroni and beef dinner				
in sauce, 'Graduates' *(Gerber)*	3.2 oz	78	11	1.7
'Stage 2' *(Beech-Nut)*	4.5 oz	90	13	4.0
'Stage 3' *(Beech-Nut)*	6 oz	130	14	6.0
Macaroni and cheese				
(Earth's Best)	4.5 oz	100	12	4.0
junior	1 oz	17	2	0.6
strained	1 oz	19	3	0.6
'Table Time' *(Beech-Nut)*	6 oz	200	21	12.0
Macaroni, tomato, and beef dinner				
junior	1 oz	17	3	0.3
junior	1 tbsp	9	2	0.2
'2nd Foods' *(Gerber)*	4 oz	70	11	1.0
strained	1 oz	17	3	0.4
strained	1 tbsp	10	2	0.2
'Step 2' *(Heinz)*	4 oz	69	11	1.7
'3rd Foods' *(Gerber)*	7 tbsp	60	10	0.9
Pasta dinner				
alphabet pasta w/beef and tomato sauce, chunky *(Gerber)*	7 tbsp	80	11	2.0
(Earth's Best)	4.5 oz	90	13	3.0
pasta w/vegetables *(Gerber)*	4 oz	68	9	2.4
seashells in tomato sauce, 'Table Time' *(Beech-Nut)*	6 oz	150	25	4.0
Potato and green bean dinner *(Earth's Best)*	4.5 oz	100	13	3.0
Ravioli				
w/beef and sauce, 'Graduates' *(Gerber)*	3.2 oz	97	16	2.0
w/beef and sauce, micro cup, 'Graduates' *(Gerber)*	6 oz	170	28	4.0
w/cheese and sauce, 'Graduates' *(Gerber)*	3.2 oz	99	16	2.2
w/cheese and sauce, micro cup, 'Graduates' *(Gerber)*	6 oz	170	28	4.0
Rice and beef dinner, w/tomato sauce, chunky *(Gerber)*	7 tbsp	79	12	1.9
Rice and chicken dinner, saucy, chunky *(Gerber)*	7 tbsp	67	10	1.5

Food Name	Serv. Size	Total Cal.	Carbs GMS	Fat GMS
Rice and lentil dinner *(Earth's Best)*	4.5 oz	80	13	2.0
Spaghetti				
in tomato sauce w/beef, '3rd Foods' *(Gerber)*	6 oz	140	20	4.5
rings w/meat sauce, 'Table Time' *(Beech-Nut)*	6 oz	160	20	6.0
w/beef, chunky *(Gerber)*	7 tbsp	85	13	1.9
w/beef, junior *(Gerber)*	6 oz	120	19	3.0
w/beef, 'Stage 3' *(Beech-Nut)*	6 oz	130	16	6.0
w/beef, '3rd Foods' *(Gerber)*	7 tbsp	64	11	1.2
w/meat, junior *(Heinz)*	3.5 oz	58	10	1.3
w/mini meatballs, 'Graduates' *(Gerber)*	6 oz	160	21	5.0
w/tomato and meat, junior	1 oz	19	3	0.4
w/tomato and meat, junior	1 tbsp	11	2	0.2
w/tomato and meat, 'Step 3' *(Heinz)*	6 oz	116	19	2.3
w/tomato and meat, toddler	1 oz	21	3	0.3
Sweet potato and chicken dinner				
(Earth's Best)	4.5 oz	90	13	2.0
'Stage 2' *(Beech-Nut)*	4 oz	84	12	2.5
strained	1 tbsp	12	2	0.3
Turkey and barley dinner *(Gerber)*	4-oz jar	60	9	1.2
Turkey and rice dinner				
junior	1 oz	16	3	0.3
junior	1 tbsp	9	2	0.1
'2nd Foods' *(Gerber)*	4 oz	60	9	1.5
'Stage 2' *(Beech-Nut)*	4 oz	70	8	3.0
'Stage 3' *(Beech-Nut)*	6 oz	100	13	3.0
strained	1 oz	15	2	0.4
strained	1 tbsp	8	1	0.2
w/vegetables, 'Step 2' *(Heinz)*	4 oz	59	9	1.4
w/vegetables, 'Step 3' *(Heinz)*	6 oz	95	16	1.6
'3rd Foods' *(Gerber)*	6 oz	100	14	3.5
Turkey and vegetable dinner				
lean meat, junior *(Gerber)*	4.5 oz	100	10	4.0
lean meat, strained *(Gerber)*	4.5 oz	100	9	4.0
Turkey dinner				
junior *(Gerber)*	2.5 oz	100	1	6.0
supreme, 'Stage 2' *(Beech-Nut)*	4 oz	90	9	4.0
Turkey stew				
w/rice, 'Graduates' *(Gerber)*	3.2 oz	59	8	1.0
w/rice, 'Table Time' *(Beech-Nut)*	6 oz	150	14	7.0
Vegetable and bacon dinner				
junior	1 oz	20	2	1.1
junior	1 tbsp	11	1	0.6
'Step 2' *(Heinz)*	4 oz	80	10	3.3
'Step 3' *(Heinz)*	6 oz	121	13	6.6
'2nd Foods' *(Gerber)*	4 oz	80	10	3.5
strained	1 oz	20	2	0.8
strained	1 tbsp	11	1	0.5
Vegetable and beef dinner				
chunky *(Gerber)*	7 tbsp	70	9	2.0
(Earth's Best)	4.5 oz	90	11	3.0
junior	1 oz	18	3	0.5
junior	1 tbsp	10	1	0.3
'2nd Foods' *(Gerber)*	4 oz	70	10	2.5
'Stage 2' *(Beech-Nut)*	4 oz	80	8	4.0
'Stage 3' *(Beech-Nut)*	6 oz	130	14	6.0
'Step 2' *(Heinz)*	4 oz	71	9	2.7
'Step 3' *(Heinz)*	6 oz	105	15	3.1

Food Name	Serv. Size	Total Cal.	Carbs GMS	Fat GMS
strained	1 oz	18	2	0.7
strained	1 tbsp	10	1	0.4
'3rd Foods' *(Gerber)*	6 oz	110	15	3.5
Vegetable and chicken dinner				
junior	1 oz	15	2	0.3
junior	1 tbsp	8	1	0.2
'2nd Foods' *(Gerber)*	4 oz	70	10	2.0
'Stage 2' *(Beech-Nut)*	4 oz	80	8	4.0
'Stage 3' *(Beech-Nut)*	6 oz	110	14	4.0
'Step 2' *(Heinz)*	4-oz jar	67	10	2.0
strained	1 oz	17	2	0.5
strained	1 tbsp	9	1	0.3
'3rd Foods' *(Gerber)*	6 oz	100	15	3.0
Vegetable and dumpling dinner				
w/beef, 'Step 2' *(Heinz)*	3.5 oz	49	9	1.3
w/beef, 'Step 3' *(Heinz)*	3.5 oz	47	7	1.2
Vegetable and ham dinner				
chunky *(Gerber)*	7 tbsp	70	9	2.3
junior	1 oz	17	2	0.5
junior	1 tbsp	10	1	0.3
'2nd Foods' *(Gerber)*	4 oz	70	10	2.5
'Stage 2' *(Beech-Nut)*	4 oz	80	9	3.0
'Step 2' *(Heinz)*	4 oz	67	9	2.4
'Step 3' *(Heinz)*	6 oz	102	15	3.2
strained	1 oz	17	2	0.6
strained	1 tbsp	9	1	0.3
'3rd Foods' *(Gerber)*	6 oz	120	16	4.0
Vegetable and lamb dinner				
junior	1 oz	14	2	0.5
strained	1 oz	15	2	0.6
strained	1 tbsp	8	1	0.3
'Step 2' *(Heinz)*	4 oz	59	8	2.3
Vegetable and noodle dinner				
w/chicken, 'Step 2' *(Heinz)*	3.5 oz	54	8	1.7
w/chicken, 'Step 3' *(Heinz)*	3.5 oz	57	9	1.8
w/turkey, 'Step 2' *(Heinz)*	3.5 oz	47	7	1.6
w/turkey, 'Step 3' *(Heinz)*	3.5 oz	48	6	2.0
Vegetable and turkey dinner				
(Earth's Best)	4.5 oz	60	11	1.0
junior	1 oz	15	2	0.5
junior	1 tbsp	8	1	0.3
strained	1 oz	14	2	0.3
strained	1 tbsp	8	1	0.1
'2nd Foods' *(Gerber)*	4 oz	60	10	1.0
'3rd Foods' *(Gerber)*	6 oz	110	16	3.5
toddler	1 oz	23	2	1.0
Vegetable dinner, 'Summer' *(Earth's Best)*	4.5 oz	90	12	3.0
Vegetable stew				
w/beef, 'Graduates' *(Gerber)*	6 oz	120	15	2.5
w/beef, 'Table Time' *(Beech-Nut)*	6 oz	110	16	3.0
w/chicken, 'Table Time' *(Beech-Nut)*	6 oz	190	23	8.0
Vegetable and beef dinner				
w/macaroni 'Stage 2' *(Beech-Nut)*	4 oz	110	9	6.0
w/dumpling, junior	1 oz	14	2	0.2
w/dumpling, strained	1 oz	14	2	0.3
Vegetable, noodle, and chicken dinner				
junior	1 oz	18	3	0.6

Food Name	Serv. Size	Total Cal.	Carbs GMS	Fat GMS
strained	1 oz	18	2	0.7
Vegetable, noodle, and turkey dinner				
junior	1 oz	15	2	0.4
strained	1 oz	12	2	0.3
EGG YOLKS				
(Gerber) '2nd Foods'	7 tbsp	193	1	16.8
FORMULA				
Infant formula, mix				
liquid, w/iron 'Enfamil' *(Mead Johnson)*	1 fl oz	41	4	2.2
liquid concentrate, low-iron, 'Enfamil' *(Mead Johnson)*	1 fl oz	41	4	2.2
liquid concentrate, low-iron *(Gerber)*	1 fl oz	40	4	2.1
liquid concentrate, low-iron, 'Similac' *(Ross)*	1 fl oz	40	4	2.2
liquid concentrate, low-iron, 'SMA' *(Wyeth-Ayerst)*	1 fl oz	41	4	2.2
liquid concentrate, w/iron, 'Alsoy' *(Carnation)*	1 fl oz	41	4	2.3
liquid concentrate, w/iron, 'Enfamil Nutramigen'				
(Mead Johnson)	1 fl oz	41	5	2.1
liquid concentrate, w/iron, 'Enfamil ProSobee' *(Mead Johnson)*	1 fl oz	40	4	2.1
liquid concentrate, w/iron, 'Follow-Up' *(Carnation)*	1 fl oz	41	5	1.7
liquid concentrate, w/iron, 'Follow-Up Soy' *(Carnation)*	1 fl oz	42	4	2.3
liquid concentrate, w/iron *(Gerber)*	1 fl oz	40	4	2.1
liquid concentrate, w/iron, 'Good Start' *(Carnation)*	1 fl oz	40	4	2.0
liquid concentrate, w/iron, 'Isomil' *(Ross)*	1 fl oz	40	4	2.2
liquid concentrate, w/iron, 'Isomil DF' *(Ross)*	1 fl oz	40	4	2.2
liquid concentrate, w/iron, 'Nursoy' *(Wyeth-Ayerst)*	1 fl oz	41	4	2.2
liquid concentrate, w/iron, 'Similac with Iron' *(Ross)*	1 fl oz	40	4	2.2
liquid concentrate, w/iron, 'SMA' *(Wyeth-Ayerst)*	1 fl oz	41	4	2.2
powder, low-iron, 'Enfamil' *(Mead Johnson)*	1 scoop	44	5	2.3
powder, low-iron *(Gerber)*	1 scoop	44	5	2.4
powder, low-iron 'Similac' *(Ross)*	1 scoop	46	5	2.5
powder, low-iron 'SMA' *(Wyeth-Ayerst)*	1 scoop	45	5	2.4
powder, soy, w/iron, milk-free, prepared *(Gerber)*	5 fl oz	100	10	5.3
powder, soy, w/iron, milk-free, prepared 'ProSobee'				
(Mead Johnson)	5 fl oz	100	10	5.3
powder, soy, w/iron, milk-free (Isomil), prepared	5 fl oz	100	10	5.5
powder, w/iron, 'Alsoy' *(Carnation)*	1 scoop	22	2	1.2
powder, w/iron, 'Enfamil' *(Mead Johnson)*	1 scoop	44	5	2.3
powder, w/iron, 'Enfamil Nutramigen' *(Mead Johnson)*	1 scoop	48	5	2.4
powder, w/iron, 'Follow-Up' *(Carnation)*	1 scoop	44	6	1.8
powder, w/iron, *(Gerber)*	1 scoop	44	5	2.4
powder, w/iron, 'Good Start' *(Carnation)*.	1 scoop	45	5	2.3
powder, w/iron, 'Isomil' *(Ross)*	1 scoop	45	5	2.5
powder, w/iron, 'Lofenalac' *(Mead Johnson)*	1 scoop	44	6	1.7
powder, w/iron, 'Nursoy' *(Wyeth-Ayerst)*	1 scoop	44	5	2.4
powder, w/iron, 'Portagen' *(Mead Johnson)*	1 scoop	44	5	2.2
powder, w/iron, 'Pregestimil' *(Mead Johnson)*	1 scoop	44	4	2.5
powder, w/iron, prepared, 'Lofenalac' *(Mead Johnson)*	1 fl oz	20	3	0.8
powder, w/iron, prepared 'Portagen' *(Mead Johnson)*	1 fl oz	20	2	1.0
powder, w/iron, prepared 'Enfamil Pregestimil' *(Mead Johnson)*	1 fl oz	20	2	1.1
powder, w/iron, 'ProSobee' *(Mead Johnson)*	1 scoop	44	4	2.3
powder, w/iron, 'SAM' *(Wyeth-Ayerst)*	1 scoop	45	5	2.4
powder, w/iron, 'Similac' *(Ross)*	1 scoop	46	5	2.5
powder, w/iron, 'Soylac' *(Carnation)*	1 scoop	22	2	1.2
Infant formula, ready to use				
low-iron 'Alimentum' *(Ross)*	1 fl oz	20	2	1.1
low-iron, 'Enfamil' *(Mead Johnson)*	1 fl oz	20	2	1.1
low-iron *(Gerber)*	1 fl oz	20	2	1.1
low-iron 'Similac' *(Ross)*	1 fl oz	20	2	1.1

Food Name	Serv. Size	Total Cal.	Carbs GMS	Fat GMS
low-iron, 'SMA' *(Wyeth-Ayerst)*	1 fl oz	20	2	1.1
low-iron 'Similac Natural Care' *(Ross)*	1 fl oz	24	3	1.3
w/iron, 'Similac with Iron' *(Ross)*	1 fl oz	24	3	1.3
soy, w/iron, 'Alsoy' *(Carnation)*	1 fl oz	20	2	1.1
soy, w/iron, 'Follow-Up Soy' *(Carnation)*	1 fl oz	20	2	1.1
soy, w/iron, milk-free, 'Enfamil ProSobee' *(Mead Johnson)*	5 fl oz	100	10	5.3
soy, w/iron, milk-free *(Gerber)*	5 fl oz	100	10	5.3
soy, w/iron, milk-free, 'Isomil' *(Ross)*	5 fl oz	100	10	5.4
soy, w/iron, milk-free, 'Nursoy' *(Wyeth-Ayerst)*	5 fl oz	100	10	5.3
soy, w/iron, 'Nursoy' *(Wyeth-Ayerst)*	1 fl oz	20	2	1.1
w/iron, 'Enfamil Nutramigen' *(Mead Johnson)*	1 fl oz	20	2	1.0
w/iron, 'Enfamil with Iron' *(Mead Johnson)*	1 fl oz	20	2	1.1
w/iron, 'Follow-Up' *(Carnation)*	1 fl oz	20	3	0.8
w/iron *(Gerber)*	1 fl oz	20	2	1.1
w/iron, 'Good Start' *(Carnation)*	1 fl oz	20	2	1.0
w/iron, 'Isomil' *(Ross)*	1 fl oz	20	2	1.1
w/iron, 'Isomil DM' *(Ross)*	1 fl oz	20	2	1.1
w/iron, 'Similac' *(Ross)*	1 fl oz	20	2	1.1
w/iron, 'SMA' *(Wyeth-Ayerst)*	1 fl oz	20	2	1.1
Toddler formula, mix				
liquid, prepared, 'Next Step' *(Mead Johnson)*	1 fl oz	20	2	1.1
powder, soy, prepared, 'Next Step Soy' *(Mead Johnson)*	1 fl oz	20	2	0.9
Toddler formula, ready to use				
w/iron *(Pediasure)*	1 fl oz	29	3	1.5
FRUIT				
Apple *(Earth's Best)*	4.5 oz	60	14	1.0
Apple and apricot				
'Stage 2' *(Beech-Nut)*	4 oz	70	17	0.0
(Earth's Best)	4.5 oz	70	15	1.0
strained *(Heinz)*	3.5 oz	55	13	0.3
Apple and banana				
(Earth's Best)	4.5 oz	80	18	1.0
'2nd Foods' *(Gerber)*	4 oz	60	15	0.0
'Stage 2' *(Beech-Nut)*	4 oz	60	14	0.0
'Stage 3' *(Beech-Nut)*	6 oz	90	21	0.0
Apple and blueberry				
(Earth's Best)	4.5 oz	60	14	1.0
junior	1 oz	18	5	0.1
'2nd Foods' *(Gerber)*	4 oz	60	14	2.0
'Stage 2' *(Beech-Nut)*	4 oz	70	17	0.0
strained	1 oz	17	5	0.1
'3rd Foods' *(Gerber)*	6 oz	80	19	1.0
Apple and cherry, 'Stage 3' *(Beech-Nut)*	6 oz	110	26	0.0
Apple and cranberry, w/tapioca, strained *(Heinz)*	3.5 oz	66	16	0.3
Apple and pear				
'Stage 2' *(Beech-Nut)*	4 oz	80	19	0.0
'Step 3' *(Heinz)*	3.5 oz	57	13	0.2
Apple and plum, *(Earth's Best)*	4.5 oz	70	16	1.0
Apple and raspberry				
w/sugar, junior	1 oz	16	4	0.1
w/sugar, strained	1 oz	16	4	0.1
Apple and sweet potato, 'Tender Harvest' *(Gerber)*	4 oz	71	17	0.2
Applesauce				
(Earth's Best)	4.5 oz	52	14	0.3
'1st Foods' *(Gerber)*	2.5 oz	35	9	0.0
golden delicious, 'Stage 1' *(Beech-Nut)*	2.5 oz	50	11	0.0
junior *(Heinz)*	3.5 oz	53	12	0.2

Food Name	Serv. Size	Total Cal.	Carbs GMS	Fat GMS
junior	1 oz	10	3	0.0
junior	1 tbsp	6	2	0.0
'2nd Foods' *(Gerber)*	4 oz	60	14	1.0
'Stage 3' *(Beech-Nut)*	6 oz	100	23	0.0
'Step 1' *(Heinz)*	3.5 oz	73	18	0.1
'Step 2' *(Heinz)*	4 oz	46	12	0.2
'Step 3' *(Heinz)*	6 oz	63	18	0.0
strained	1 oz	12	3	0.1
strained	1 tbsp	7	2	0.0
'3rd Foods' *(Gerber)*	6 oz	90	20	1.0
w/apricot	1 oz	13	4	0.1
w/apricot	1 tbsp	8	2	0.0
w/apricot, '2nd Foods' *(Gerber)*	7 tbsp	53	13	0.2
w/apricot, 'Stage 2' *(Beech-Nut)*	4.5 oz	80	19	0.0
w/apricot, 'Step 2' *(Heinz)*	4 oz	51	13	0.2
w/apricot, 'Step 3' *(Heinz)*	6 oz	80	21	0.3
w/apricot, strained *(Earth's Best)*	4.5 oz	58	15	0.3
w/apricot, strained	1 oz	13	3	0.1
w/apricot, strained	1 tbsp	7	2	0.0
w/banana, 'Stage 2' *(Beech-Nut)*	4.5 oz	80	18	0.0
w/banana, 'Stage 3' *(Beech-Nut)*	6 oz	100	25	0.0
w/banana, strained	1 tbsp	11	3	0.0
w/cherry, 'Stage 2' *(Beech-Nut)*	4.5 oz	70	18	0.0
w/cherry, 'Stage 3' *(Beech-Nut)*	6 oz	100	24	0.0
w/cherry, junior	1 oz	16	4	0.0
w/cherry, strained	1 oz	14	4	0.0
w/pineapple, junior	1 oz	11	3	0.0
w/pineapple, strained	1 oz	10	3	0.0
Apricot				
w/pear, 'Stage 3' *(Beech-Nut)*	6 oz	120	27	0.0
w/pear and apple, 'Stage 3' *(Beech-Nut)*	6 oz	130	32	0.0
w/pear and applesauce, 'Stage 2' *(Beech-Nut)*	4.5 oz	90	21	0.0
w/tapioca, junior	3.5 oz	66	16	0.2
w/tapioca, junior	1 tbsp	9	3	0.0
w/tapioca, '2nd Foods' *(Gerber)*	4 oz	90	20	1.0
w/tapioca, 'Step 2' *(Heinz)*	4.25 oz	72	20	0.0
w/tapioca, 'Step 3' *(Heinz)*	6 oz	107	29	0.0
w/tapioca, strained	3.5 oz	64	15	0.2
w/tapioca, strained	1 tbsp	9	2	0.0
w/tapioca, '3rd Foods' *(Gerber)*	6 oz	130	29	1.0
Banana				
(Earth's Best)	4.5 oz	100	22	0.0
'1st Foods' *(Gerber)*	2.5 oz	70	17	0.0
Chiquita, 'Baby's First' *(Beech-Nut)*	2.5 oz	70	16	0.0
Chiquita, 'Stage 3' *(Beech-Nut)*	6 oz	160	33	0.0
'Step 1' *(Heinz)*	3.5 oz	107	25	0.2
w/pineapple and tapioca, '2nd Foods' *(Gerber)*	7 tbsp	52	12	0.1
w/pineapple and tapioca, '3rd Foods' *(Gerber)*	7 tbsp	52	12	0.1
w/tapioca, junior	1 oz	19	5	0.1
w/tapioca, junior	1 tbsp	10	3	0.0
w/tapioca, '2nd Foods' *(Gerber)*	4 oz	110	24	1.0
w/tapioca, 'Step 2' *(Heinz)*	3.5 oz	73	18	0.2
w/tapioca, 'Step 3' *(Heinz)*	3.5 oz	73	18	0.2
w/tapioca, strained	1 oz	16	4	0.0
w/tapioca, strained	1 tbsp	9	2	0.0
w/tapioca, '3rd Foods' *(Gerber)*	6 oz	140	31	1.0
Banana and apple, strained *(Gerber)*	4.5 oz	90	20	1.0

Food Name	Serv. Size	Total Cal.	Carbs GMS	Fat GMS
Banana and pear, w/applesauce, 'Stage 2' *(Beech-Nut)*	4.5 oz	100	24	0.0
Banana and pineapple				
'Stage 2' *(Beech-Nut)*	4.5 oz	110	27	0.0
w/tapioca, junior	1 oz	19	5	0.0
w/tapioca, junior	1 tbsp	10	3	0.0
w/tapioca, '2nd Foods' *(Gerber)*	4.5 oz	60	15	0.0
w/tapioca, 'Step 2' *(Heinz)*	3.5 oz	64	15	0.2
w/tapioca, 'Step 3' *(Heinz)*	6 oz	116	31	0.2
w/tapioca, strained	1 oz	18	5	0.0
w/tapioca, '3rd Foods' *(Gerber)*	6 oz	90	20	1.0
Guava				
w/tapioca, '2nd Foods' *(Gerber)*	4 oz	90	20	1.0
w/tapioca, 'Stage 2' *(Beech-Nut)*	4.5 oz	100	24	0.0
w/tapioca, strained	1 oz	19	5	0.0
Guava and papaya, w/tapioca, strained	1 oz	18	5	0.0
Mango				
w/tapioca, '2nd Foods' *(Gerber)*	4 oz	90	21	1.0
w/tapioca, strained	1 oz	23	6	0.1
w/tapioca, strained	1 tbsp	12	3	0.0
Mango and banana				
w/passionfruit and tapioca, '2nd Foods' *(Gerber)*	4.5 oz	100	25	0.0
Mixed fruit				
apple, peach, and strawberries 'Stages 2' *(Beech-Nut)*	4.5 oz	100	24	0.0
apple, pear, and banana 'Stages 2' *(Beech-Nut)*	4.5 oz	100	24	0.0
Papaya				
'Stage 2' *(Beech-Nut)*	4.5 oz	100	24	0.0
w/tapioca, '2nd Foods' *(Gerber)*	4 oz	80	19	1.0
Papaya and applesauce, w/tapioca, strained	1 oz	20	5	0.0
Peach				
'1st Foods' *(Gerber)*	2.5 oz	30	7	0.0
'2nd Foods' *(Gerber)*	4 oz	90	19	1.0
'Stage 3' *(Beech-Nut)*	6 oz	100	21	0.0
'Step 1' *(Heinz)*	3.5 oz	80	18	0.2
'Step 2' *(Heinz)*	3.5 oz	68	15	0.3
'Step 3' *(Heinz)*	3.5 oz	68	15	0.3
'3rd Foods' *(Gerber)*	6 oz	110	25	1.0
w/banana, 'Stage 2' *(Beech-Nut)*	4 oz	70	15	0.0
w/mango and tapioca, '2nd Foods' *(Gerber)*	4 oz	100	24	1.0
w/oatmeal and banana *(Earth's Best)*	4.5 oz	70	15	1.0
w/sugar, '1st Foods' *(Gerber)*	2.5 oz	30	7	0.0
w/sugar, junior	1 oz	20	5	0.1
w/sugar, junior	1 tbsp	11	3	0.0
w/sugar, '2nd Foods' *(Gerber)*	4 oz	70	17	0.0
w/sugar, 'Stage 1' *(Beech-Nut)*	2.5 oz	50	13	0.1
w/sugar, 'Stage 3' *(Beech-Nut)*	6 oz	121	32	0.3
w/sugar, 'Step 1' *(Heinz)*	2.5 oz	50	13	0.1
w/sugar, 'Step 2' *(Heinz)*	4 oz	80	21	0.2
w/sugar, 'Step 3' *(Heinz)*	6 oz	121	32	0.3
w/sugar, strained	1 oz	20	5	0.1
w/sugar, strained	1 tbsp	11	3	0.0
w/sugar, '3rd Foods' *(Gerber)*	6 oz	110	26	0.0
w/yogurt 'Stage 2' *(Beech-Nut)*	4.5 oz	120	25	2.0
yellow cling, 'Stage 1' *(Beech-Nut)*	2.5 oz	45	10	0.0
Pear				
Bartlett, 'Stage 1' *(Beech-Nut)*	2.5 oz	50	12	0.0
Bartlett, 'Stage 3' *(Beech-Nut)*	6 oz	110	27	0.0
Bartlett, w/applesauce, 'Stage 2' *(Beech-Nut)*	4 oz	80	20	0.0

Food Name	Serv. Size	Total Cal.	Carbs GMS	Fat GMS
(Earth's Best)	4.5 oz	60	14	0.0
'1st Foods' (Gerber)	2.5 oz	40	11	0.0
junior	1 oz	12	3	0.0
junior	1 tbsp	7	2	0.0
'2nd Foods' (Gerber)	4 oz	80	16	1.0
'Step 1' (Heinz)	3.5 oz	76	18	0.2
'Step 2' (Heinz)	3.5 oz	60	14	0.2
'Step 3' (Heinz)	3.5 oz	60	14	0.2
strained	1 oz	12	3	0.1
strained	1 tbsp	7	2	0.0
'3rd Foods' (Gerber)	6 oz	100	21	1.0
Pear and pineapple				
junior	1 oz	12	3	0.1
junior	1 tbsp	7	2	0.0
'2nd Foods' (Gerber)	7 tbsp	55	13	0.2
'Stage 2' (Beech-Nut)	4 oz	46	12	0.1
'Step 2' (Heinz)	4 oz	46	12	0.1
strained	1 oz	12	3	0.0
strained	1 tbsp	7	2	0.0
'3rd Foods' (Gerber)	6 oz	100	21	1.0
Pear and raspberry, (Earth's Best)	4.5 oz	60	15	0.0
Plum				
w/tapioca, junior	1 oz	21	6	0.0
w/tapioca, junior	1 tbsp	11	3	0.0
(Gerber) '3rd Foods'	6 oz	120	28	0.0
w/tapioca, '2nd Foods' (Gerber)	4 oz	80	19	0.0
w/tapioca, strained	1 oz	20	6	0.0
w/tapioca, strained	1 tbsp	11	3	0.0
w/tapioca, 'Step 2' (Heinz)	4 oz	80	22	0.0
Prune				
'1st Foods' (Gerber)	2.5 oz	70	17	0.0
w/oatmeal (Earth's Best)	4.5 oz	100	24	0.0
w/pear, 'Stage 2' (Beech-Nut)	4 oz	110	24	0.0
w/tapioca, junior	1 oz	20	5	0.0
w/tapioca, '2nd Foods' (Gerber)	4 oz	100	22	1.0
w/tapioca, 'Step 2' (Heinz)	3.5 oz	90	22	0.2
w/tapioca, strained	1 oz	20	5	0.0
w/tapioca, strained	1 tbsp	11	3	0.0
Tropical fruit, junior	1 oz	17	5	0.0
JUICE				
Apple				
	1 fl oz	15	4	0.0
beginner, 'Step 1' (Heinz)	4 fl oz	59	15	0.1
(Earth's Best)	4.2 fl oz	62	15	0.1
(Gerber)	4 fl oz	60	14	0.1
100% juice, 'Junior' (McCain)	4.2 fl oz	50	13	0.0
'Stage 1' (Beech-Nut)	4 fl oz	60	15	0.1
strained, 'Saver Size' (Heinz)	4.2 fl oz	70	17	0.0
Apple-apricot, strained, 'Step 2' (Heinz)	3.5 fl oz	47	11	0.2
Apple-banana				
	1 fl oz	16	4	0.0
(Earth's Best)	4.2 fl oz	60	14	0.0
(Gerber)	4 fl oz	60	15	0.1
strained, 'Step 2' (Heinz)	3.5 fl oz	52	13	0.2
w/calcium, 'Graduates' (Gerber)	6 fl oz	100	24	0.0
w/vitamin C, 'Stage 2' (Beech-Nut)	4 fl oz	70	16	0.0

Food Name	Serv. Size	Total Cal.	Carbs GMS	Fat GMS
Apple-cherry				
.... 1 fl oz	1 fl oz	13	3	0.1
'Graduates' (Gerber)	6 fl oz	80	21	0.0
100% juice, 'Junior' (McCain)	4.2 fl oz	50	13	0.0
strained, 'Step 2' (Heinz)	3.5 fl oz	45	11	0.2
w/vitamin C., 'Stage 2' (Beech-Nut)	4 fl oz	70	17	0.0
Apple-cranberry, strained, 'Step 2' (Heinz)	3.5 fl oz	48	12	0.2
Apple-grape				
....	1 fl oz	14	4	0.1
(Earth's Best)	4.2 fl oz	60	15	0.3
(Gerber)	4 fl oz	60	15	0.0
strained, 'Step 2' (Heinz)	4 fl oz	58	14	0.3
w/calcium, 'Graduates' (Gerber)	6 fl oz	98	24	0.2
Apple-peach				
.... 1 fl oz	1 fl oz	13	3	0.0
(Gerber)	3.2 fl oz	47	11	0.1
strained, 'Step 2' (Heinz)	3.5 fl oz	44	10	0.2
Apple-pineapple, strained, 'Step 2' (Heinz)	3.5 fl oz	47	11	0.2
Apple-plum				
.... 1 fl oz	1 fl oz	15	4	0.0
(Gerber)	3.2 fl oz	48	12	0.1
Apple-prune				
....	4 fl oz	91	23	0.1
....	1 fl oz	23	6	0.0
strained, 'Step 2' (Heinz)	3.5 fl oz	50	12	0.2
Apple-white grape, 'Stage 2' (Beech-Nut)	4 fl oz	58	14	0.3
Fruit punch, w/calcium, 'Graduates' (Gerber)	6 fl oz	98	24	0.2
Grape				
'Juice Plus' 'Stage 2' (Beech-Nut)	4 fl oz	100	23	0.0
white (Gerber)	4 fl oz	80	20	0.0
white, 'Stage 1' (Beech-Nut)	4 fl oz	100	23	0.0
white, strained, 'Step 2' (Heinz)	3.5 fl oz	58	14	0.2
Guava, w/mixed fruit, 'Tropical Foods' (Gerber)	3.2 fl oz	58	14	0.1
Mango				
w/mixed fruit, 'Tropical Foods' (Gerber)	3.2 fl oz	59	14	0.1
nectar, w/grape and pear juice, 'Stage 2' (Beech-Nut)	4 fl oz	80	19	0.0
Mixed fruit				
.... 1 fl oz	1 fl oz	15	4	0.0
....	4 fl oz	59	15	0.1
100% juice, 'Junior' (McCain)	4.2 fl oz	60	15	0.0
strained, 'Step 2' (Heinz)	3.5 fl oz	50	12	0.2
Orange				
.... 1 fl oz	1 fl oz	14	3	0.1
'2nd Foods' (Gerber)	4 fl oz	60	13	0.4
strained, 'Step 2' (Heinz)	4 fl oz	55	13	0.4
Orange-apple				
.... 1 fl oz	1 fl oz	13	3	0.1
strained, 'Step 2' (Heinz)	3.5 fl oz	50	11	0.3
Orange-apple-banana				
.... 1 fl oz	1 fl oz	15	4	0.0
strained, 'Step 2' (Heinz)	4 fl oz	59	14	0.1
Orange-apricot	1 fl oz	14	3	0.0
Orange-banana	1 fl oz	16	4	0.0
Orange-carrot, '3rd Foods' (Gerber)	3.2 fl oz	43	10	0.1
Orange-pineapple	1 fl oz	15	4	0.0
Papaya				
nectar, w/pear and grape juice 'Stage 2' (Beech-Nut)	4 fl oz	70	17	0.0

Food Name	Serv. Size	Total Cal.	Carbs GMS	Fat GMS
Pear				
(Earth's Best)	4.2 fl oz	60	15	0.0
'1st Foods' (Gerber)	3.2 fl oz	46	11	0.1
'Stage 1' (Beech-Nut)	4 fl oz	60	15	0.0
strained, 'Saver Size' (Heinz)	4.2 fl oz	70	15	1.0
strained, 'Step 2' (Heinz)	3.5 fl oz	49	12	0.2
Pineapple-carrot, '3rd Foods' (Gerber)	3.2 fl oz	47	11	0.1
Prune-orange	1 fl oz	22	5	0.1
Tropical blend				
nectar, 'Stage 2' (Beech-Nut)	4 fl oz	90	21	0.0
'Stage 2' (Beech-Nut)	4 fl oz	90	19	0.0
MEAT				
Beef				
and beef gravy, '2nd Foods' (Gerber)	2.5 oz	70	3	3.5
junior	1 oz	30	0	1.4
junior	1 tbsp	16	0	0.7
junior, 'Step 3' (Heinz)	2.5 oz	75	0	3.5
strained	1 oz	30	0	1.5
strained	1 tbsp	16	0	0.8
strained, 'Step 2' (Heinz)	2.5 oz	76	0	3.8
'3rd Foods' (Gerber)	7 tbsp	103	0	4.6
w/broth, 'Stage 1' (Beech-Nut)	2.5 oz	76	0	3.8
w/broth, strained, 'Step 2' (Heinz)	3.5 oz	123	0	7.2
w/egg yolks (Gerber)	2.5 oz	80	0	4.0
Chicken				
and chicken gravy, '2nd Foods' (Gerber)	2.5 oz	80	2	4.5
junior	1 oz	42	0	2.7
junior	1 tbsp	22	0	1.4
'Stage 1' (Beech-Nut)	2.8 oz	80	0	4.0
strained	1 oz	37	0	2.2
strained	1 tbsp	20	0	1.2
strained, 'Step 2' (Heinz)	2.5 oz	92	0	5.6
'3rd Foods' (Gerber)	7 tbsp	132	0	7.9
w/broth, junior, 'Step 3' (Heinz)	3.5 oz	143	1	9.7
Chicken stick, 'Graduates' (Gerber)	2.5 oz	100	1	5.0
Ham				
and ham gravy, '2nd Foods' (Gerber)	2.5 oz	79	0	4.1
junior	1 oz	35	0	1.9
strained	1 oz	31	0	1.6
strained	1 tbsp	17	0	0.9
'3rd Foods' (Gerber)	7 tbsp	123	0	7.2
w/egg yolks, strained (Gerber)	2.5 oz	90	1	5.0
Lamb				
and lamb gravy, '2nd Foods' (Gerber)	2.5 oz	70	2	3.0
junior	1 oz	32	0	1.5
'Stage 1' (Beech-Nut)	2.8 oz	70	0	3.0
strained	1 oz	29	0	1.3
strained	1 tbsp	15	0	0.7
strained, 'Step 2' (Heinz)	2.5 oz jar	73	0	3.3
w/broth, strained, 'Step 2' (Heinz)	3.5 oz	129	0	7.6
w/egg yolks, strained (Gerber)	2.5 oz	70	1	3.0
Liver, w/broth, strained, 'Step 2' (Heinz)	3.5 oz	100	4	3.2
Meat stick				
'Graduates' (Gerber)	2.5 oz	100	1	7.0
junior	1 stick	18	0	1.5
Pork, strained	1 oz	35	0	2.0

Food Name	Serv. Size	Total Cal.	Carbs GMS	Fat GMS
Turkey				
and turkey gravy, '2nd Foods' (Gerber)	2.5 oz	70	2	4.0
'Stage 1' (Beech-Nut)	2.8 oz	100	0	6.0
strained, 'Step 2' (Heinz)	2.5 oz	81	0	4.1
junior	1 oz	37	0	2.0
junior	1 tbsp	19	0	1.1
strained	1 oz	32	0	1.6
strained	1 tbsp	17	0	0.9
'3rd Foods' (Gerber)	7 tbsp	115	0	6.1
w/egg yolks, strained (Gerber)	2.5 oz	100	1	6.0
Turkey stick				
'Graduates' (Gerber)	2.5 oz	100	1	7.0
junior	1 stick	18	0	1.4
Veal				
and veal gravy, '2nd Foods' (Gerber)	2.5 oz	90	2	6.0
junior	1 oz	31	0	1.4
'Stage 1' (Beech-Nut)	2.8 oz	60	0	2.0
strained, 'Step 2' (Heinz)	2.5 oz	72	0	3.4
strained	1 oz	29	0	1.4
strained	1 tbsp	15	0	0.7
'3rd Foods' (Gerber)	7 tbsp	108	0	5.0
w/broth, strained, 'Step 2' (Heinz)	3.5 oz	130	0	7.9
w/egg yolks, strained (Gerber)	2.5 oz	80	1	4.0
Veal and beef				
junior (Gerber)	6 oz	110	16	3.0
strained (Gerber)	4.5 oz	90	11	4.0
Veal and ham				
junior (Gerber)	6 oz	120	17	4.0
strained (Gerber) strained	4.5 oz	80	11	3.0
Veal and turkey				
junior (Gerber)	6 oz	100	15	3.0
strained (Gerber)	4.5 oz	70	10	2.0
SOUP				
Chicken				
'Stage 2' (Beech-Nut)	4 oz jar	57	8	1.9
strained	1 oz	14	2	0.5
strained, 'Step 2' (Heinz)	3.5 oz	49	7	1.7
w/stars, 'Table Time' (Beech-Nut)	6 oz	150	17	6.0
Cream of broccoli, '3rd Foods' (Gerber)	3.2 oz	26	3	1.1
Cream of potato, '3rd Foods' (Gerber)	3.2 oz	33	5	0.8
Cream of tomato, '3rd Foods' (Gerber)	3.2 oz	41	7	0.7
Cream of vegetable, '3rd Foods' (Gerber)	3.2 oz	29	4	0.8
VEGETABLES				
Beets				
'2nd Foods' (Gerber)	7 tbsp	39	8	0.2
strained	1 oz	10	2	0.0
strained	1 tbsp	5	1	0.0
strained (Gerber)	4.5 oz	60	11	1.0
strained, 'Step 2' (Heinz)	3.5 oz	40	8	0.2
Carrots				
beginner, 'Step 1' (Heinz)	2.5 oz	19	4	0.1
(Earth's Best)	1 tbsp	4	1	0.0
(Earth's Best)	4.5 oz	40	7	0.0
'1st Foods' (Gerber)	2.5 oz	25	5	0.0
junior	1 oz	9	2	0.1
junior	1 tbsp	4	1	0.0
junior, 'Step 3' (Heinz)	6 oz	54	12	0.3

Food Name	Serv. Size	Total Cal.	Carbs GMS	Fat GMS
'2nd Foods' *(Gerber)*	4 oz	35	7	0.0
'Stage 1' *(Beech-Nut)*	2.5 oz	25	6	0.0
'Stage 3' *(Beech-Nut)*	6 oz	70	15	0.0
strained	1 oz	8	2	0.0
strained, 'Step 2' *(Heinz)*	4 oz	31	7	0.1
'3rd Foods' *(Gerber)*	6 oz	50	11	0.0
'Vegetable Dices' 'Graduates' *(Gerber)*	2.5 oz	22	4	0.0
Carrots and parsnips *(Earth's Best)*	4.5 oz	60	14	0.0
Carrots and peas *(Beech-Nut)*	4 oz	50	10	0.0
Corn and butternut squash *(Earth's Best)*	4.5 oz	90	15	2.0
Corn, creamed				
junior	1 oz	18	5	0.1
junior	1 tbsp	10	2	0.1
junior, 'Step 3' *(Heinz)*	6 oz	111	28	0.7
'Stage 2' *(Beech-Nut)*	4 oz	90	18	0.0
'2nd Foods' *(Gerber)*	4 oz	70	14	0.5
strained	1 oz	16	4	0.1
strained	1 tbsp	9	2	0.1
strained, 'Step 2' *(Heinz)*	4 oz	64	16	0.5
Beans, green				
beginner, 'Step 1' *(Heinz)*	2.5 oz	18	4	0.1
creamed, junior	1 oz	9	2	0.1
creamed, junior	1 tbsp	5	1	0.1
creamed, junior *(Gerber)*	6 oz	80	16	1.0
creamed, junior, 'Step 3' *(Heinz)*	6 oz	54	12	0.7
creamed, '3rd Foods' *(Gerber)*	7 tbsp	45	9	0.2
'1st Foods' *(Gerber)*	2.5 oz	25	4	0.0
junior	1 oz	7	2	0.0
junior	1 tbsp	4	1	0.0
'2nd Foods' *(Gerber)*	4 oz	40	6	0.0
'Stage 1' *(Beech-Nut)*	4 oz	35	6	0.0
'Stage 3' *(Beech-Nut)*	6 oz	50	10	0.0
strained	1 oz	7	2	0.0
strained	1 tbsp	4	1	0.0
strained, 'Step 2' *(Heinz)*	3.5 oz	25	5	0.2
'Vegetable Dices' 'Graduates' *(Gerber)*	2.5 oz	21	4	0.1
w/potatoes *(Gerber)*	4 oz	71	11	2.1
w/rice, '3rd Foods' *(Gerber)*	6 oz	70	15	0.0
Garden vegetables				
(Earth's Best)	4.5 oz	70	15	0.0
strained.	1 oz	10	2	0.1
'2nd Foods' *(Gerber)*	4 oz	45	7	0.5
'Stage 2' *(Beech-Nut)*	4.5 oz	60	11	0.0
Mixed vegetables				
junior	1 oz	12	2	0.1
junior	1 tbsp	6	1	0.1
'2nd Foods' *(Gerber)*	4 oz	45	9	0.0
'Stage 2' *(Beech-Nut)*	4.5 oz	50	12	0.0
strained	1 oz	12	2	0.1
strained, 'Step 2' *(Heinz)*	3.5 oz	44	9	0.4
'3rd Foods' *(Gerber)*	6 oz	70	14	1.0
'Vegetable Dices' 'Graduates' *(Gerber)*	2.5 oz	35	6	0.0
Peas				
beginner, 'Step 1' *(Heinz)*	2.5 oz	28	6	0.2
creamed, strained	1 oz	15	3	0.5
creamed, strained	1 tbsp	8	1	0.3
creamed, strained, 'Step 2' *(Heinz)*	4 oz	60	10	2.1

Food Name	Serv. Size	Total Cal.	Carbs GMS	Fat GMS
'1st Foods' *(Gerber)*	2.5 oz	30	6	0.0
'2nd Foods' *(Gerber)*	4 oz	60	10	1.0
strained	1 oz	11	2	0.1
strained	1 tbsp	6	1	0.0
strained, 'Step 2' *(Heinz)*	4 oz	45	9	0.3
tender, sweet, 'Stage 1' *(Beech-Nut)*	2.5 oz	28	6	0.2
tender, sweet, 'Stage 1' *(Beech-Nut)*	4 oz	45	9	0.3
w/brown rice *(Earth's Best)*	4.5 oz	80	16	0.0
w/rice, '3rd Foods' *(Gerber)*	6 oz	90	16	1.0
Potato				
'Graduates' *(Gerber)*	3.2 oz	38	9	0.1
toddler	1 tbsp	5	1	0.0
Spinach				
creamed, '2nd Foods' *(Gerber)*	4 oz	50	8	1.0
creamed, strained	1 oz	10	2	0.4
creamed, strained	1 tbsp	6	1	0.2
w/potato *(Earth's Best)*	4.5 oz	60	8	2.0
Squash				
beginner, 'Step 1' *(Heinz)*	2.5 oz	17	4	0.1
butternut, 'Stage 1' *(Beech-Nut)*	2.5 oz	30	7	0.0
'1st Foods' *(Gerber)*	2.5 oz	25	5	0.0
junior	1 oz	7	2	0.1
junior	1 tbsp	3	1	0.0
'2nd Foods' *(Gerber)*	4 oz	35	7	0.0
'Stage 1' *(Beech-Nut)*	4 oz jar	27	6	0.2
strained	1 oz	7	2	0.1
strained *(Earth's Best)*	4.5 oz	31	7	0.3
strained, 'Step 2' *(Heinz)*	4 oz	27	6	0.2
'3rd Foods' *(Gerber)* junior	6 oz	60	11	1.0
w/corn *(Gerber)*	4 oz	57	11	0.7
winter *(Earth's Best)*	4.5 oz	50	12	0.0
Sweet potato				
beginner, 'Step 1' *(Heinz)*	2.5 oz	40	9	0.1
(Earth's Best)	4.5 oz	60	12	1.0
'1st Foods' *(Gerber)*	2.5 oz	45	10	0.0
junior	1 oz	17	4	0.0
junior	1 tbsp	8	2	0.0
junior, 'Step 3' *(Heinz)*	6 oz	102	24	0.2
'2nd Foods' *(Gerber)*	4.5 oz	70	16	0.0
'Stage 1' *(Beech-Nut)*	2.5 oz	50	11	0.0
'Stage 3' *(Beech-Nut)*	6 oz	110	25	0.0
strained	1 oz	16	4	0.0
strained *(Earth's Best)*	1 tbsp	8	2	0.0
strained, 'Step 2' *(Heinz)*	4 oz	64	15	0.1
'3rd Foods' *(Gerber)* junior	6 oz	110	24	1.0
WATER, w/fluoride, sodium-free *(Beech-Nut)*	4 oz	0	0	0.0
BACON				
cured, approx 12 slices per lb, raw	1 slice	211	0	21.9
cured, approx 20 slices per lb, raw	3 slices	378	0	39.1
cured, broiled, pan-fried, or roasted	3 med slices	109	0	9.4
(Hormel)				
'Black Label'	1 oz	142	2	14.0
'Black Label' low-salt	1.76 oz	250	2	25.0
'Black Label' sliced, cooked	2 slices	60	0	5.0
'Range' thick-sliced	1 oz	152	2	16.0
(Hickory Ridge) cured, hickory flavor	2 slices	80	0	6.0

Food Name	Serv. Size	Total Cal.	Carbs GMS	Fat GMS
(JM)				
cooked	2 slices	100	1	9.0
'Lower Sodium' cooked	2 slices	100	1	9.0
'Lower Sodium' raw	2 slices	290	1	30.0
raw	2 slices	280	1	29.0
(Jones Dairy Farm) raw	1 slice	165	0	17.0
(Louis Rich) turkey, cooked	1 slice	34	0	2.7
(Oscar Mayer)				
	1 slice	70	0	6.0
approx 0.2-oz slices, cooked	1 slice	33	0	2.8
'Center Cut' approx 0.2-oz slices, cooked	1 slice	25	0	1.8
'Center Cut' cooked, yield from 1 lb raw	6 oz	852	4	62.5
cooked, yield from 16-oz pkg, raw	5 oz	784	3	64.9
lower salt	1 slice	70	1	5.0
thick-cut, cooked	1 slice	60	0	5.0
(Range Brand) 'Sliced' cooked	2 slices	110	0	9.0
(Red Label) cooked	3 slices	110	0	10.0
(West Virginia)				
cured, smoked flavor, cooked	2 slices	80	0	7.0
thick-sliced, cooked	1 slice	80	0	7.0
BACON, CANADIAN STYLE				
cured, grilled, yield from 6-oz pkg	5.9 oz	257	2	11.7
cured, raw	6 oz	267	3	11.8
cured, 6 slices per 6 oz, grilled	2 slices	86	1	3.9
cured, 6 slices per 6 oz, raw	2 slices	89	1	4.0
(Hormel) sliced	1 oz	45	0	2.0
(Jones Dairy Farm) unheated	1 slice	25	0	1.0
(Light & Lean)	2 slices	35	0	1.0
(Oscar Mayer)	1 slice	50	0	1.5
BACON BITS				
*(Bac*Os)*				
imitation	2 tsp	25	2	1.0
imitation, bits, cholesterol-free	1 tbsp	30	2	1.0
(Bac' N Pieces) imitation, chips cholesterol-free	1 1/2 tbsp	30	2	1.0
(Hormel)				
	1 oz	117	1	7.0
	1 tbsp	30	0	2.0
50% less fat	1 tsp	30	0	1.5
(Oscar Mayer) real	1 tbsp	25	0	1.5
(Schilling) imitation, 'Bac'N Pieces'	1 tsp	26	2	0.4
(Tone's) imitation	1 tsp	7	0	0.3
BACON DISH/ENTRÉE *(Stouffer's)* strata, frozen	1 oz	52	3	3.5
BACON PIECES (Hormel)	1 oz	94	2	5.0
BACON SUBSTITUTE				
(Healthy Favorites) turkey, w/pork 'Breakfast Strips'	11 grams	18	0	1.0
(Heartline)				
Canadian style, vegetarian, nonfat, lite	0.5 oz	22	1	0.0
Canadian style, vegetarian, yield from 4 oz cooked	2 oz	176	9	7.0
(JM)				
beef, heated	2 slices	100	1	7.0
beef, raw	2 slices	200	1	18.0
(Louis Rich) turkey	1 slice	30	0	2.5
(Morningstar Farms) vegetarian, 'Breakfast Strips'	2 strips	56	2	4.4
(Mr. Turkey) turkey, 70% less fat	1 slice	25	0	2.0
(Sizzlean)				
beef, heated	2 strips	70	0	5.0
pork, brown sugar cured, heated	2 strips	110	2	9.0

Food Name	Serv. Size	Total Cal.	Carbs GMS	Fat GMS
pork, heated	2 strips	90	0	8.0
(White Wave SoyFood) vegetarian, 'Healthy'	1 oz	27	4	1.0
(Worthington) vegetarian, 'Stripples'	2 strips	56	2	4.4
BAGEL				
BLUEBERRY				
(Earth Grains) 3 oz	1 bagel	245	48	0.0
(Lender's)				
4-inch diam, frozen, 'Bagel Shop'	1 bagel	264	53	1.5
3.13 oz, frozen, 'Big'n Crusty'	1 serving	214	46	0.8
3-inch diam, 'Premium'	1 bagel	209	43	1.3
2.5 oz, frozen	1 bagel	190	38	1.0
(Western Bagel)	1 bagel	240	43	4.0
CINNAMON-RAISIN				
(Earth Grains) 3 oz	1 bagel	245	48	0.0
(Finast) w/cinnamon & honey, 2.5 oz	1 bagel	200	40	1.0
(Lender's) 'Big'n Crusty' 3 1/8 oz	1 bagel	250	49	2.0
(Sara Lee)				
2.5 oz	1 bagel	200	39	2.0
3.1 oz	1 bagel	240	48	2.0
(Thomas')				
	1 bagel	160	36	1.0
'Deli Style'	1 bagel	170	33	2.0
(Western Bagel)	1 bagel	230	40	4.0
EGG				
4.5-inch diam	1 bagel	306	58	2.3
3-inch diam	1 bagel	158	30	1.2
(Lender's)				
'Bakery Style'	1 bagel	210	41	2.0
3.13 oz, frozen, 'Big'n Crusty'	1 bagel	250	47	2.0
2 oz, frozen	1 bagel	160	32	1.0
(Sara Lee)				
3.1 oz, frozen	1 bagel	250	48	2.0
2.5 oz, frozen	1 bagel	200	38	2.0
(Thomas')	1 bagel	170	35	1.5
HONEY RAISIN *(Lender's)* 2.5 oz	1 bagel	200	40	1.0
HONEY WHEAT *(Earth Grains)* 3 oz	1 bagel	240	45	0.0
MULTIGRAIN *(Thomas')*	1 bagel	170	35	1.5
OAT BRAN				
(Lender's) 2.5 oz, frozen	1 bagel	170	36	2.0
(Sara Lee)				
3 oz, frozen	1 bagel	220	47	1.0
2.5 oz, frozen	1 bagel	180	38	1.0
ONION				
4.5-inch diam	1 bagel	303	59	1.8
3-inch diam	1 bagel	157	30	0.9
(Earth Grains) 3 oz bagel	1 bagel	240	45	0.0
(Lender's)				
3.13 oz, frozen, 'Big'n Crusty'	1 bagel	230	46	1.0
2 oz, frozen	1 bagel	160	31	1.0
0.9 oz, frozen, 'Bagelettes'	1 bagel	70	14	1.0
(Sara Lee) 3.1 oz, frozen	1 bagel	230	45	1.0
2.5 oz, frozen	1 bagel	190	37	1.0
(Sprouted Wheat Bagels) w/poppy seeds, organic	1 bagel	250	50	1.0
(Thomas')	1 bagel	170	35	1.5
(Western Bagel)	1 bagel	220	39	4.0
ORGANIC *(Bible Bagels)*	1 bagel	180	29	2.0

Food Name	Serv. Size	Total Cal.	Carbs GMS	Fat GMS
PLAIN				
4.5-inch diam	1 bagel	303	59	1.8
4-inch diam	1 bagel	245	48	1.4
3-inch diam	1 bagel	157	30	0.9
2.5-inch diam	1 bagel	72	14	0.4
(Earth Grains) 3 oz bagel	1 bagel	240	45	0.0
(Lender's)				
'Bakery Style'	1 bagel	210	42	2.0
soft, 2.5 oz, frozen	1 bagel	210	36	3.0
3.13 oz, frozen, 'Big'n Crusty'	1 bagel	240	47	1.0
2 oz, frozen	1 bagel	150	30	1.0
0.9 oz, frozen, 'Bagelettes'	1 bagel	70	13	1.0
(Sara Lee)				
3.1 oz, frozen	1 bagel	230	46	1.0
2.5 oz, frozen	1 bagel	190	38	1.0
(Thomas')	1 serving	160	35	1.0
POPPY SEED				
4.5-inch diam	1 bagel	303	59	1.8
4-inch diam	1 bagel	245	48	1.4
3-inch diam	1 bagel	157	30	0.9
(Lender's) 2 oz, frozen	1 bagel	160	29	1.0
(Sara Lee)				
3.1 oz, frozen	1 bagel	230	46	1.0
2.5 oz, frozen	1 bagel	190	37	1.0
PUMPERNICKEL *(Lender's)* 2 oz, frozen	1 bagel	160	31	1.0
RAISIN				
(Lender's)				
'Bakery Style'	1 bagel	220	44	2.0
0.9 oz, frozen, 'Bagelettes'	1 bagel	70	14	1.0
RYE *(Lender's)* 2 oz, frozen	1 bagel	150	30	1.0
SESAME SEED				
4.5-inch diam	1 bagel	303	59	1.8
4-inch diam	1 bagel	245	48	1.4
3-inch diam	1 bagel	157	30	0.9
(Sprouted Wheat Bagels)	1 bagel	250	50	1.0
SPELT *(Rudi's)* organic	1 bagel	280	54	2.0
WATER *(Western Bagel)*	1 bagel	230	41	4.0
WHEAT *(Lender's)* w/raisin, 2.5 oz	1 bagel	190	39	1.0
WHOLE GRAIN (Natural Ovens)	1 bagel	190	36	2.0
BAGEL CHIPS				
cinnamon raisin *(Original Bagel Crisps)*	1 oz	130	20	4.0
garlic *(Original Bagel Crisps)*	1 oz	130	20	4.0
BAGEL MIX gluten-free *(Gluten Free Pantry)*	1 serving	150	36	0.0
BAKED BEANS, CANNED				
(B&M)				
red kidney	8 oz	250	42	7.0
yellow eye	8 oz	326	50	7.0
(Beanee Weenee) w/sliced hot dogs	1 cup	30	35	14.0
(Bearitos)				
black beans, nonfat.	1/2 cup	110	22	0.0
vegetarian, organic, fat-free, original	1/2 cup	130	26	0.0
(Green Giant)				
barbecue, dry beans in brine	1/2 cup	140	28	0.5
honey bacon, dry beans in brine	1/2 cup	160	34	0.5
(Friends)				
red kidney	8 oz	340	57	4.0
red kidney, w/pork	8 oz	270	55	4.0

Food Name	Serv. Size	Total Cal.	Carbs GMS	Fat GMS
(Green Giant)				
dry beans in brine	1/2 cup	160	31	1.5
w/onion, dry beans in brine	1/2 cup	150	28	1.5
(Health Valley) honey baked, nonfat	1/2 cup	110	24	0.0
(Heinz) vegetarian, in tomato sauce	8 oz	230	41	1.0
(Homestyle) pork and beans, food service product.	1/2 cup	157	27	4.8
(Joan of Arc)				
barbecue, dry beans in brine	1/2 cup	140	28	0.5
dry beans in brine	1/2 cup	160	31	1.5
honey bacon, dry beans in brine	1/2 cup	160	34	0.5
w/onion, dry beans in brine	1/2 cup	150	28	1.5
(Luck's)				
October, seasoned w/pork	1/2 cup	140	20	3.0
pork and beans in tomato sauce.	1/2 cup	150	28	1.0
(Ranch Style) pork & beans	1/2 cup	140	28	0.5
(S&W) 'Brick Oven'.	1/2 cup	160	32	0.5
(Van Camp's)				
nonfat, seasoned w/brown sugar	1/2 cup	130	28	0.0
w/brown sugar and bacon	1/2 cup	140	29	1.0
w/pork, in tomato sauce	1/2 cup	110	24	1.5
w/beef	1 cup	322	45	9.2
w/franks.	1 cup	368	40	17.0
w/pork	1 cup	268	51	3.9
w/pork and sweet sauce	1 cup	281	53	3.7
w/pork and tomato sauce	1 cup	248	49	2.6
w/pork and tomato sauce	1 tbsp	15	3	0.2
BAKER'S YEAST. See under YEAST.				
BAKING CHOCOLATE. See CHOCOLATE, BAKING.				
BAKING MIX				
general purpose, whole wheat, dry *(Insta-Bake)*	1/3 cup	150	25	5.0
BAKING POWDER				
Double-acting				
(Clabber Girl)	1/4 tsp	3	1	0.0
(Rumford)	1/4 tsp	3	1	0.0
sodium aluminum sulfate	1 tsp	2	1	0.0
sodium aluminum sulfate	1/2 tsp	1	1	0.0
straight phosphate	1 tsp	2	1	0.0
straight phosphate	1/2 tsp	1	1	0.0
Low-sodium				
	1 tsp	5	2	0.0
	1/2 tsp	2	1	0.0
(Featherweight)	1 tsp	8	2	0.0
Regular				
(Calumet)	1/4 tsp	0	0	0.0
(Davis)	1 tsp	6	2	0.0
(Tone's)	1 tsp	5	1	0.0
BAKING SODA				
	1 tsp	0	0	0.0
	1/2 tsp	0	0	0.0
(Arm & Hammer)	1/2 tsp	0	0	0.0
(Tone's)	1 tsp	0	0	0.0
BALSAM PEAR/bitter gourd				
Leafy tips				
boiled, drained	1 cup	20	4	0.1
raw	1/2 cup	7	1	0.2
raw	1 med leaf	1	0	0.0
Pods				
boiled, drained, 1/2-inch pieces	1 cup	24	5	0.2

Food Name	Serv. Size	Total Cal.	Carbs GMS	Fat GMS
boiled, drained 1/2-inch pieces	1/2 cup	12	3	0.1
raw	21	6	0	8%
raw, 1/2-inch pieces	1 cup	16	3	0.2
BAMBOO SHOOTS				
Canned				
(La Choy)	2 tbsp	3	1	0.1
drained, 1/8-inch slices	1 cup	25	4	0.5
sliced (China Boy)	1/2 cup	15	3	0.0
Fresh				
boiled, drained	1 med shoot	17	3	0.3
boiled, drained, 1/2-inch slices	1 cup	14	2	0.3
raw, 1/2-inch pieces	1/2 cup	21	4	0.2
raw, 1/2-inch slices	1 cup	41	8	0.5
BANANA				
Dehydrated or powdered				
	1 cup	346	88	1.8
	1 tbsp	21	5	0.1
Fresh, raw				
mashed	1 cup	207	53	1.1
sliced	1 cup	138	35	0.7
whole, extra large, 9 inches long and up	1 banana	140	36	0.7
whole, extra small, up to 6 inches long	1 banana	75	19	0.4
whole, large, 8 to 8 7/8 inches long	1 banana	125	32	0.7
whole, medium, 7 to 7 7/8 inches long	1 banana	109	28	0.6
whole, small, 6 to 6 7/8 inches long	1 banana	93	24	0.5
BANANA CHIPS				
	3 oz	441	50	28.6
	1.5 oz	218	25	14.1
	1 oz	147	17	9.5
BANANA PEPPER. See PEPPER, BANANA.				
BANANA SQUASH. See SQUASH, BANANA.				
BARBADOS CHERRY. See ACEROLA.				
BARBECUE SPICE. See under SEASONING MIX.				
BARLEY				
	1 cup	651	135	4.2
pearled, cooked	1 cup	193	44	0.7
pearled, cooked (Tone's)	1 tsp	8	2	0.1
pearled, quick, raw, 'Scotch Brand' (Quaker)	1/3 cup	172	36	0.5
pearled, raw	1 cup	704	155	2.3
pearled, raw (Arrowhead Mills)	2 oz	200	45	1.0
BARLEY FLAKES rolled (Arrowhead Mills)	1/3 cup	110	28	1.0
BARLEY FLOUR. See under FLOUR.				
BARLEY MALT, natural, organic (Eden Foods)	1/2 tsp	10	2	0.0
BARLEY MALT FLOUR. See under FLOUR.				
BARLEY MIX, organic (Ener-G Foods)	1 cup	396	85	1.6
BASELLA. See SPINACH, VINE.				
BASIL				
Dried				
(Golden Dipt)	2 grams	8	1	0.0
(McCormick/Schilling)	1 tsp	3	0	0.0
crumbled (Spice Islands)	1 tsp	3	1	0.1
crumbled (Tone's)	1 tsp	4	1	0.1
ground	1 tbsp	11	3	0.2
ground	1 tsp	4	1	0.1
Fresh				
chopped	2 tbsp	1	0	0.0
ground (Durkee)	1 tsp	5	0	0.0

Food Name	Serv. Size	Total Cal.	Carbs GMS	Fat GMS
ground *(Laurel Leaf)*	1 tsp	5	0	0.0
whole leaves	5 med leaves	1	0	0.0
BASMATI RICE. See under RICE.				
BASS, CALICO. See SUNFISH.				
BASS, FRESHWATER				
mixed species, baked, broiled, grilled, or microwaved	3 oz	124	0	4.0
mixed species, raw	3 oz	97	0	3.1
BASS, SEA				
mixed species, baked, broiled, grilled, or microwaved	3 oz	105	0	2.2
mixed species, raw	3 oz	82	0	1.7
BASS, STRIPED				
mixed species, baked, broiled, grilled, or microwaved	3 oz	105	0	2.5
mixed species, raw	3 oz	82	0	2.0
BATTER MIX, ALL PURPOSE				
all-purpose, no MSG, dry mix *(Don's Chuck Wagon)*	1/4 cup	100	20	0.0
beer, dry mix *(Golden Dipt)*	1 oz	100	22	0.0
corn dog, dry mix *(Golden Dipt)*	1 oz	100	22	0.0
fish and chips, no MSG, dry mix *(Don's Chuck Wagon)*	1/4 cup	100	21	0.0
fish and chips, dry mix *(Golden Dipt)*	1.25 oz	120	27	0.0
golden mushroom, no MSG, dry mix *(Don's Chuck Wagon)*	1/4 cup	95	21	0.0
onion ring, no MSG, dry mix *(Don's Chuck Wagon)*	1/4 cup	100	21	0.0
onion ring, dry mix (Golden Dipt)	1 oz	100	22	0.0
tempura, dry mix (Golden Dipt)	1 oz	100	22	0.0
BAY LEAF				
dried *(McCormick/Schilling)*	1 tsp	2	0	0.0
dried, crumbled	1 tbsp	6	1	0.2
dried, crumbled	1 tsp	2	0	0.1
dried, crumbled *(Durkee)*	1 tsp	2	0	0.0
dried, crumbled *(Laurel Leaf)*	1 tsp	2	0	0.0
dried, crumbled *(Spice Islands)*	1 tsp	5	0	0.1
dried, crumbled *(Tone's)*	1 tsp	2	1	0.1
BEAN, ADZUKI				
Canned				
mature seeds, sweetened	1 cup	702	163	0.1
organic, no salt added, very low sodium *(Eden Foods)*	1/2 cup	80	18	1.0
organic, w/liquid *(Eden Foods)*	1/2 cup	100	17	1.0
Fresh				
mature seeds, boiled	1 cup	294	57	0.2
mature seeds, raw	1 cup	648	124	1.0
raw *(Arrowhead Mills)*	2 oz	190	35	1.0
Jarred, organic *(Eden Foods)*	1/2 cup	90	16	0.0
BEAN, ANASAZI, dry *(Arrowhead Mills)*	1/4 cup	150	27	0.5
BEAN, BLACK/black turtle bean				
Canned				
(Green Giant)	1/2 cup	90	21	0.0
(Joan of Arc)	1/2 cup	90	21	0.0
(Old El Paso)	1/2 cup	100	17	1.0
(Progresso)	1/2 cup	100	17	1.0
(Ranch Style)	1/2 cup	100	19	0.0
(S&W)	1/2 cup	70	17	0.0
'Fiesta' style *(Stokely)*	1/2 cup	100	17	0.5
50% less salt *(S&W)*	1/2 cup	70	17	0.0
'Sun Vista' *(S&W)*	1/2 cup	70	20	1.0
organic, no salt added, very low sodium *(Eden Foods)*	1/2 cup	70	17	1.0
Dry				
mature seeds, boiled	1 cup	227	41	0.9
mature seeds, raw	1 cup	662	121	2.8

Food Name	Serv. Size	Total Cal.	Carbs GMS	Fat GMS
mature seeds, raw	1 tbsp	41	8	0.2
raw *(Arrowhead Mills)*	2 oz	190	35	1.0
BEAN, BLACK TURTLE. See BEAN, BLACK.				
BEAN, BROAD. See BEAN, FAVA.				
BEAN, CANNELLINI, CANNED				
(Progresso)	1/2 cup	100	18	0.5
white *(Pathmark)*	1/2 cup	100	18	0.0
BEAN, CRANBERRY/borlotti/Roman bean/rose coco bean				
Canned *(Progresso)*.	1/2 cup	110	18	1.0
Dried				
mature seeds, boiled	1 cup	241	43	0.8
mature seeds, canned	1 cup	216	39	0.7
mature seeds, raw	1 cup	653	117	2.4
BEAN, FAVA/broad bean/horse bean/jack bean				
Canned				
(Progresso)	1/2 cup	110	20	0.5
mature seeds	1 cup	182	32	0.6
Fresh				
immature seeds, raw	1 med bean	6	1	0.0
immature seeds, raw	1 cup	78	13	0.7
mature seeds, boiled	1 cup	187	33	0.7
mature seeds, raw	1 cup	512	87	2.3
mature seeds, raw	1 tbsp	32	5	0.1
raw, in pod	1 cup	111	22	0.9
raw, in pod	1 med pod	5	1	0.0
BEAN, FRENCH/haricots. See also BEAN, GREEN.				
Fresh				
boiled	1 cup	228	43	1.3
raw	1 cup	631	118	3.7
BEAN, GARBANZO. See CHICKPEA.				
BEAN, GOA. See BEAN, WINGED.				
BEAN, GREAT NORTHERN				
Canned				
(A&P)	1 cup	210	38	1.0
(Allens)	1/2 cup	105	17	1.0
(Bush's Best)	1/2 cup	70	16	0.0
(Green Giant)	1/2 cup	80	18	1.0
(Joan of Arc)	1/2 cup	80	18	1.0
mature seeds	1 cup	299	55	1.0
mature seeds, no salt added	1 cup	209	37	0.8
organic, w/liquid *(Eden Foods)*	1/2 cup	110	20	1.0
seasoned, w/pork *(Luck's)*	1/2 cup	140	20	3.0
'Sun-Vista' *(S&W)*	1/2 cup	70	17	0.0
w/pork *(Allens)*	1/2 cup	100	19	1.0
w/pork *(Luck's)*	7.25 oz	220	32	5.0
Dried				
mature seeds, boiled	1 cup	209	37	0.8
mature seeds, raw	1 cup	620	114	2.1
BEAN, GREEN/string bean/snap bean				
Canned				
(Pathmark)	1/2 cup	20	5	0.0
(Stokely)	1/2 cup	20	4	0.0
almandine *(Green Giant)*	1/2 cup	45	5	3.0
Blue Lake, cut *(Bush's Best)*	1/2 cup	20	5	0.0
Blue Lake, cut *(Pathmark)*	1/2 cup	20	4	0.0
Blue Lake, cut, 'Premium' *(S&W)*	1/2 cup	20	4	0.0
Blue Lake, French style, *(Pathmark)*	1/2 cup	20	4	0.0

Food Name	Serv. Size	Total Cal.	Carbs GMS	Fat GMS
Blue Lake, French style, 'Premium' *(S&W)*	1/2 cup	20	4	0.0
cut *(A&P)*	1/2 cup	20	4	1.0
cut *(Allens)*	1/2 cup	20	4	1.0
cut *(Bush's Best)*	1/2 cup	20	5	0.0
cut *(Featherweight)*	1/2 cup	25	5	0.0
cut *(Finast)*	1/2 cup	20	4	0.0
cut *(Freshlike)*	1/2 cup	20	4	0.0
cut *(Green Giant)*	1/2 cup	16	4	0.0
cut *(IGA)*	1/2 cup	20	5	0.0
cut *(Pathmark)*	1/2 cup	20	4	0.0
cut *(S&W)*	1/2 cup	20	4	0.0
cut *(Stokely)*	1/2 cup	20	4	0.0
cut *(Veg-All)*	1/2 cup	20	4	0.0
cut, 'No Frills' *(Pathmark)*	1 cup	35	8	0.0
cut, 'Pantry Express' *(Green Giant)*	1/2 cup	12	3	0.0
cut, 'Veri-Green' *(Finast)*	1/2 cup	20	4	0.0
cut, 50% less salt *(Green Giant)*	1/2 cup	16	4	0.0
cut, no salt added *(Finast)*	1/2 cup	20	4	0.0
cut, no salt added *(Freshlike)*	1/2 cup	20	4	0.0
cut, stringless, w/liquid *(S&W)*	1/2 cup	20	4	0.0
cut, water packed, w/o salt *(Freshlike)*	1/2 cup	20	4	0.0
cut, water packed, w/o sugar or salt *(Freshlike)*	1/2 cup	20	4	0.0
cut, w/liquid *(Del Monte)*	1/2 cup	20	4	0.0
cut, w/liquid, no salt added *(Del Monte)*	1/2 cup	20	4	0.0
dilled *(S&W)*	1 oz	20	5	0.0
European, slender, whole *(Stokely)*	1/2 cup	20	4	0.0
50% less salt *(Green Giant)*	1/2 cup	18	4	0.0
French style *(A&P)*	1/2 cup	20	4	1.0
French style *(Allens)*	1/2 cup	20	4	1.0
French style *(Bush's Best)*	1/2 cup	20	5	0.0
French style *(Finast)*	1/2 cup	20	4	0.0
French style *(Freshlike)*	1/2 cup	20	4	0.0
French style *(Green Giant)*	1/2 cup	16	4	0.0
French style *(Stokely)*	1/2 cup	20	4	0.0
French style *(Veg-All)*	1/2 cup	20	4	0.0
French style, 'No Frills' *(Pathmark)*	1 cup	35	8	0.0
French style, cut *(TenderSweet)*	1/2 cup	20	4	0.0
French style, cut, no salt added *(TenderSweet)*	1/2 cup	20	4	0.0
French style, no salt added *(A&P)*	1/2 cup	20	4	1.0
French style, no salt added *(Freshlike)*	1/2 cup	20	4	0.0
French style, no salt added *(Pathmark)*	1/2 cup	20	5	0.0
French style, seasoned, w/liquid *(Del Monte)*	1/2 cup	20	4	0.0
French style, stringless, w/liquid *(S&W)*	1/2 cup	20	4	0.0
French style, water packed, no salt added *(Freshlike)*	1/2 cup	20	4	0.0
Italian, flat, cut *(Stokely)*	1/2 cup	20	4	0.0
Italian style *(Allens)*	1/2 cup	18	3	1.0
Italian style, cut *(Del Monte)*	1/2 cup	25	6	0.0
kitchen-sliced *(Green Giant)*	1/2 cup	16	4	0.0
kitchen-sliced, 50% less salt *(Green Giant)*	1/2 cup	20	4	0.0
no salt added *(A&P)*	1/2 cup	20	4	1.0
no salt added *(Pathmark)*	1/2 cup	20	5	0.0
no salt added, cut, drained	1 cup	27	6	0.1
no salt added, whole, drained	10 med beans	12	3	0.1
no salt or sugar *(Stokely)*	1/2 cup	20	4	0.0
regular pack, cut, drained	1 cup	27	6	0.1
regular pack, cut, w/liquid	1/2 cup	18	4	0.1
w/shelly beans, cut *(Bush's Best)*	1/2 cup	35	8	0.0

Food Name	Serv. Size	Total Cal.	Carbs GMS	Fat GMS
whole *(A&P)*	1/2 cup	20	4	1.0
whole *(Bush's Best)*	1/2 cup	20	5	0.0
whole *(Finast)*	1/2 cup	25	4	0.0
whole *(Freshlike)*	1/2 cup	20	4	0.0
whole *(IGA)*	1 cup	45	8	0.0
whole *(Pathmark)*	1/2 cup	20	4	0.0
whole, stringless, w/liquid *(S&W)*	1/2 cup	20	4	0.0
whole, w/liquid *(Del Monte)*	1/2 cup	20	4	0.0
Freeze-Dried *(Mountain House)* prepared as directed	1/2 cup	35	6	0.0
Fresh				
boiled, drained	1 cup	44	10	0.3
raw, cut	1 cup	34	8	0.1
raw, whole, approx 4-inch long	10 beans	17	4	0.1
Frozen				
(Flav-R-Pac)	2/3 cup	25	4	0.0
cut *(A&P)*	3 oz	25	6	1.0
cut *(Birds Eye)*	3 oz	25	6	0.0
cut *(Finast)*	3 oz	25	6	0.0
cut *(Freshlike)*	3 oz	25	6	0.0
cut *(Frosty Acres)*	3 oz	25	6	0.0
cut *(Green Giant)*	3/4 cup	25	5	0.0
cut *(Pictsweet)*	2/3 cup	25	4	0.0
cut *(Seabrook)*	3 oz	25	6	0.0
cut *(Veg-All)*	3 oz	25	6	0.0
cut, 'Portion Pack' *(Birds Eye)*	3 oz	25	6	0.0
cut, 'Singles' *(Stokely)*	3 oz	30	6	1.0
French cut *(C&W)*	2/3 cup	30	5	0.0
French cut *(Flav-R-Pac)*	1 cup	25	4	0.0
French style *(A&P)*	3 oz	25	6	1.0
French style *(Birds Eye)*	3 oz	25	6	0.0
French style *(Finast)*	3 oz	25	6	0.0
French style *(Freshlike)*	3 oz	25	6	0.0
French style *(Frosty Acres)*	3 oz	25	6	0.0
French style *(Pictsweet)*	1 cup	25	4	0.0
French style *(Seabrook)*	3 oz	25	6	0.0
French style *(Southern)*	3.5 oz	34	7	0.1
French style *(Veg-All)*	3 oz	25	6	0.0
French style, w/almonds, 'Combination Vegetable' *(Birds Eye)*	3 oz	50	8	2.0
Italian cut *(C&W)*	3/4 cup	25	4	0.0
Italian cut *(Finast)*	3 oz	30	7	0.0
Italian style *(Birds Eye)*	3 oz	30	7	0.0
Italian style *(Freshlike)*	3 oz	30	7	0.0
Italian style *(Frosty Acres)*	3 oz	30	7	0.0
Italian style *(Seabrook)*	3 oz	30	7	0.0
Italian style *(Veg-All)*	3 oz	30	7	0.0
no salt added, drained	1 cup	38	9	0.2
petite, 'Deluxe' *(Birds Eye)*	2.6 oz	20	5	0.0
petite, whole *(C&W)*	3/4 cup	25	4	0.0
petite, whole *(Flav-R-Pac)*	3/4 cup	25	4	0.0
'Plain Polybag' *(Green Giant)*	1/2 cup	14	4	0.0
whole *(Flav-R-Pac)*	3/4 cup	25	4	0.0
whole *(Freshlike)*	3 oz	25	5	0.0
whole *(Seabrook)*	3 oz	25	5	0.0
whole *(Southern)*	3.5 oz	33	7	0.1
whole *(Veg-All)*	3 oz	25	5	0.0
whole, 'Deluxe' *(Birds Eye)*	3 oz	25	5	0.0
whole 'Farm Fresh' *(Birds Eye)*	4 oz	30	7	0.0

Food Name	Serv. Size	Total Cal.	Carbs GMS	Fat GMS
w/almonds 'Harvest Fresh' *(Green Giant)*	2/3 cup	60	5	3.0
w/creamy mushroom 'Garden Gourmet' *(Green Giant)*	1 pkg	220	29	11.0
w/salt, drained	1 cup	38	9	0.2
BEAN, HORSE. See BEAN, FAVA.				
BEAN, HYACINTH				
immature seeds, boiled, drained	1 cup	44	8	0.2
immature seeds, raw	1 cup	37	7	0.2
mature seeds, boiled, drained	1 cup	227	40	1.1
mature seeds, raw	1 cup	722	128	3.5
BEAN, ITALIAN				
dry beans in brine *(Green Giant)*	1/2 cup	130	24	1.0
dry beans in brine *(Joan of Arc)*	1/2 cup	130	24	1.0
BEAN, JACK. See BEAN, FAVA.				
BEAN, KIDNEY				
CALIFORNIA RED				
Dried				
mature seeds, boiled	1 cup	219	40	0.2
mature seeds	1 cup	607	110	0.5
DARK RED				
Canned				
(Allens)	1/2 cup	105	20	1.0
(Bush's Best)	1/2 cup	70	17	0.0
(Finast)	1/2 cup	110	20	2.0
(Green Giant)	1/2 cup	90	20	1.0
(Joan of Arc)	1/2 cup	90	20	1.0
(Pathmark)	1/2 cup	110	18	0.0
(Progresso)	1/2 cup	110	20	0.5
(Stokely)	1/2 cup	120	21	0.5
(Stokely)	1/2 cup	110	20	1.0
(Van Camp's)	1 cup	182	35	0.5
50% less salt *(Green Giant)*	1/2 cup	90	20	1.0
50% less salt *(Joan of Arc)*	1/2 cup	90	20	1.0
50% less salt, 'Lite' *(S&W)*	1/2 cup	120	22	1.0
'Premium' *(S&W)*	1/2 cup	120	22	1.0
LIGHT RED				
Canned				
(Allens)	1/2 cup	105	2	1.0
(Bush's Best)	1/2 cup	70	17	0.0
(Finast) light	1/2 cup	110	20	2.0
(Green Giant)	1/2 cup	90	20	1.0
(Joan of Arc)	1/2 cup	90	20	1.0
(Stokely)	1/2 cup	110	20	1.0
(Stokely)	1/2 cup	120	21	0.5
(Van Camp's)	1 cup	184	36	0.5
50% less salt *(Green Giant)*	1/2 cup	90	20	1.0
50% less salt *(Joan of Arc)*	1/2 cup	90	20	1.0
RED				
Canned				
(A&P)	1/2 cup	110	20	1.0
(Green Giant)	1/2 cup	90	20	0.0
(Hunt's)	1/2 cup	95	20	0.5
(Joan of Arc)	1/2 cup	90	20	0.0
(Pathmark)	1/2 cup	110	20	0.0
(Pathmark)	1/2 cup	110	18	0.0
(Progresso)	1/2 cup	100	21	1.0
(Stokely)	1/2 cup	110	20	1.0
(Van Camp's)	1 cup	184	36	0.5

Food Name	Serv. Size	Total Cal.	Carbs GMS	Fat GMS
50% less salt, 'Lite' (S&W)	1/2 cup	120	22	1.0
mature seeds	1 cup	218	40	0.9
mature seeds	1 tbsp	14	2	0.1
New Orleans style (Van Camp's)	1 cup	178	34	0.6
'Nutradiet' (S&W)	1/2 cup	90	16	1.0
organic, very low-sodium, no salt added (Eden Foods)	1/2 cup	60	18	1.0
'Premium' (S&W)	1/2 cup	120	22	1.0
Dried				
boiled (A&P)	1 cup	230	41	1.0
mature seeds, boiled	1 cup	225	40	0.9
mature seeds, boiled	1 tbsp	14	3	0.1
mature seeds, raw	1 cup	613	110	1.5
mature seeds, raw	1 cup	620	113	1.9
mature seeds, raw	1 tbsp	41	7	0.1
raw (Arrowhead Mills)	2 oz	190	35	1.0
Sprouted, mature seeds	1 cup	53	8	0.9
ROYAL RED				
Dried				
mature seeds, boiled	1 cup	218	39	0.3
mature seeds, raw	1 cup	605	107	0.8
BEAN, LIMA/butterbean				
Canned				
(A&P)	1/2 cup	110	20	1.0
(Featherweight)	1/2 cup	80	16	0.0
(Freshlike)	1/2 cup	80	16	0.0
(Green Giant)	1/2 cup	80	16	0.0
(Joan of Arc)	1/2 cup	80	16	0.0
(S&W)	1/2 cup	100	19	1.0
(Stokely)	1/2 cup	80	16	0.0
(Van Camp's)	1 cup	162	30	0.5
(Veg-All)	1/2 cup	80	16	0.0
baby (Bush's Best)	1/2 cup	70	16	0.0
all green (Bush's Best)	1/2 cup	90	17	0.0
baby (C&W)	1/2 cup	90	15	0.5
Fordhook (Stokely)	1/2 cup	80	14	0.0
gem, green and white (Bush's Best)	1/2 cup	80	17	0.0
green (A&P)	1/2 cup	80	15	1.0
giant, seasoned w/pork (Luck's)	1/2 cup	150	23	3.0
green, small, 'Fancy' (S&W)	1/2 cup	80	16	0.0
green, small, w/pork (Luck's)	7.5 oz	220	33	7.0
green, tiny (Allens)	1/2 cup	90	15	1.0
green, w/liquid (Del Monte)	1/2 cup	70	14	0.0
green and white (Allens)	1/2 cup	90	15	1.0
'Harvest Fresh' (Green Giant)	1/2 cup	80	15	0.0
immature seeds, no salt added, w/liquid	1/2 cup	88	17	0.4
immature seeds, regular pack, w/liquid	1/2 cup	88	17	0.4
large (Allens)	1/2 cup	110	18	1.0
large (Bush's Best)	1/2 cup	70	16	0.0
large, mature seeds	1 cup	190	36	0.4
'No Salt or Sugar Added' (Stokely)	1/2 cup	80	16	0.0
seasoned w/pork (Luck's)	1/2 cup	140	23	2.0
speckled (Bush's Best)	1/2 cup	70	17	0.0
speckled, seasoned w/pork (Luck's)	1/2 cup	140	22	3.0
water packed, w/o salt (Freshlike)	1/2 cup	80	16	0.0
w/ham (Dennison's)	7.5 oz	250	33	7.0
w/pork (Luck's)	7.5 oz	230	34	7.0
Dried				
baby, boiled	1 cup	229	42	0.7

Food Name	Serv. Size	Total Cal.	Carbs GMS	Fat GMS
baby, boiled (A&P)	1 cup	230	40	1.0
baby, raw	1 cup	677	127	1.9
immature seeds, boiled, drained	1 cup	209	40	0.5
immature seeds, raw	1 cup	176	31	1.3
large, mature seeds, boiled	1 cup	216	39	0.7
large, mature seeds, boiled	1 tbsp	13	2	0.0
mature seeds, raw	1 cup	602	113	1.2
mature seeds, raw	1 tbsp	38	7	0.1
Frozen				
(Flav-R-Pac)	1/2 cup	100	20	0.0
(Green Giant)	1/2 cup	100	19	0.0
(Health Valley)	1/2 cup	94	18	0.0
baby (Birds Eye)	3.3 oz	130	24	0.0
baby (Freshlike)	3.3 oz	130	24	1.0
baby (Frosty Acres)	3.3 oz	130	24	0.0
baby (Seabrook)	3.3 oz	130	24	0.0
baby (Southern)	3.5 oz	135	25	0.5
baby (Veg-All)	3.3 oz	130	24	1.0
baby, butter (Seabrook)	3.3 oz	140	26	1.0
baby, green (A&P)	3.3 oz	130	24	1.0
Fordhook (A&P)	3.3 oz	100	19	1.0
Fordhook (Birds Eye)	3.3 oz	100	19	0.0
Fordhook (Flav-R-Pac).	1/2 cup	90	17	0.0
Fordhook (Frosty Acres)	3.3 oz	100	19	0.0
Fordhook (Seabrook)	3.3 oz	100	19	0.0
Fordhook, immature seeds, no salt added, boiled, drained	1/2 cup	85	16	0.3
Fordhook, immature seeds, no salt added, boiled, drained	10-oz pkg	311	58	1.1
Fordhook, immature seeds, unprepared	1/2 cup	85	16	0.3
Fordhook, immature seeds, unprepared	10-oz pkg	301	56	1.0
'Harvest Fresh' (Green Giant)	1/2 cup	80	18	0.0
immature seeds, drained	1/2 cup	95	18	0.3
immature seeds, drained, 10-oz pkg	1 pkg	327	60	0.9
immature seeds, no salt added, drained	1/2 cup	95	18	0.3
immature seeds, no salt added, drained	10-oz pkg	327	60	0.9
speckled (Seabrook)	3.3 oz	120	23	0.0
speckled (Southern)	3.5 oz	135	25	0.4
tiny (Seabrook)	3.3 oz	110	21	1.0
BEAN, MARROW				
regular, boiled	4 oz	158	28.5	0.4
regular, boiled	1/2 cup	125	22.5	0.3
regular, raw	1/2 cup	337	60.9	0.9
regular, raw	1 oz	94	17.1	0.2
small, boiled	4 oz	161	29.3	0.7
small, boiled	1/2 cup	127	23.2	0.6
small, raw	1/2 cup	363	67.2	1.3
small, raw	1 oz	95	17.6	0.3
BEAN, MOTH				
mature seeds, boiled	1 cup	207	37	1.0
mature seeds, raw	1 cup	672	121	3.2
BEAN, MUNG				
Canned				
mature seeds, sprouted, drained	1 cup	15	3	0.1
sprouted (La Choy)	2 oz	8	1	0.1
Dried				
mature seeds, boiled	1 cup	212	39	0.8
mature seeds, raw	1 cup	718	130	2.4
mature seeds, raw	1 tbsp	45	8	0.1

Food Name	Serv. Size	Total Cal.	Carbs GMS	Fat GMS
Sprouted				
mature seeds, raw	1 cup	31	6	0.2
mature seeds, raw	12-oz pkg	102	20	0.6
mature seeds, stir-fried	1 cup	62	13	0.3
BEAN, MUNGO				
mature seeds, boiled	1 cup	189	33	1.0
mature seeds, raw	1 cup	706	122	3.4
BEAN, NAVY				
Dry				
mature seeds, boiled	1 cup	258	48	1.0
mature seeds, raw	1 cup	697	126	2.7
'Michigan #1' cooked *(A&P)*	1 cup	220	40	1.0
Canned				
(Allens)	1/2 cup	160	24	1.0
(Bush's Best)	1/2 cup	60	17	0.0
flavored w/bacon *(Trappey's)*	1/2 cup	130	28	0.0
mature seeds	1 cup	296	54	1.1
organic, no salt added, very low sodium *(Eden Foods)*	1/2 cup	70	18	1.0
seasoned w/pork *(Luck's)*	1/2 cup	140	19	4.0
w/ham, 'Homestyle' *(Hunt's)*	9.03 oz	239	38	2.7
Sprouted, mature seeds, raw	1 cup	70	14	0.7
BEAN, PINK				
mature seeds, boiled	1 cup	252	47	0.8
mature seeds, raw	1 cup	720	135	2.4
BEAN, PINTO				
Dried				
boiled *(A&P)*	1 cup	230	42	1.0
mature seeds, boiled	1 cup	234	44	0.9
mature seeds, boiled	1 tbsp	15	3	0.1
mature seeds, raw	1 cup	656	122	2.2
mature seeds, raw	1 tbsp	41	8	0.1
raw *(Arrowhead Mills)*	2 oz	200	36	1.0
raw *(Evans)*	1 cup	660	121	2.0
Canned				
(Allens)	1/2 cup	105	18	1.0
(Bush's Best)	1/2 cup	60	15	0.0
(Gebhardt)	1/2 cup	92	18	1.2
(Green Giant)	1/2 cup	90	20	1.0
(Joan of Arc)	1/2 cup	90	20	1.0
(Old El Paso)	1/2 cup	100	19	0.0
(Progresso)	1/2 cup	110	7	1.0
(Ranch Style)	1/2 cup	100	19	0.0
baked style, w/pork, 15-oz can *(Luck's)*	7.5 oz	220	30	6.0
baked style, w/pork, 29 oz can *(Luck's)*	7.25 oz	220	30	6.0
mature seeds	1 cup	206	37	1.9
organic, no salt added, very low sodium *(Eden Foods)*	1/2 cup	70	17	1.0
organic, w/liquid (Eden Foods)	1/2 cup	110	20	1.0
picante style *(Green Giant)*	1/2 cup	100	21	1.0
picante style *(Joan of Arc)*	1/2 cup	100	21	1.0
seasoned w/pork *(Luck's)*	1/2 cup	140	19	4.0
'Sun-Vista' *(S&W)*	1/2 cup	80	12	0.5
w/jalapeño peppers *(Ranch Style)*	1/2 cup	110	21	0.0
w/onions, seasoned w/pork *(Luck's)*	1/2 cup	150	24	3.0
Frozen				
(Seabrook)	3.2 oz	160	29	0.0
immature seeds, frozen, no salt added, drained 10-oz pkg	1 pkg	460	88	1.4
immature seeds, unprepared, 10-oz pkg	1 pkg	483	92	1.4

Food Name	Serv. Size	Total Cal.	Carbs GMS	Fat GMS
immature seeds, w/salt, drained, 10-oz pkg .... 1 pkg		460	88	1.4
Jarred, organic, low-sodium *(Eden Foods)* .... 1/2 cup		120	22	0.0
BEAN, RED				
Canned				
(A&P) .... 1/2 cup		120	23	1.0
(Allens) .... 1/2 cup		115	20	1.0
(Bush's Best) .... 1/2 cup		70	17	0.0
(Green Giant) .... 1/2 cup		90	19	1.0
(Joan of Arc) .... 1/2 cup		90	19	1.0
(Van Camp's) .... 1 cup		194	38	0.6
small *(Hunt's)* .... 4 oz		91	18	0.0
small, baked-style *(B&M)* .... 8 oz		223	36	5.0
BEAN, ROMAN. See BEAN, CRANBERRY.				
BEAN, ROSE COCO. See BEAN, CRANBERRY.				
BEAN, SHELLY				
Canned				
(Allens) .... 1/2 cup		35	6	1.0
(Stokely) .... 1/2 cup		35	7	0.0
w/liquid .... 1 cup		74	15	0.5
BEAN, SNAP. See BEAN, GREEN; BEAN, WAX.				
BEAN, SOYA. See SOYBEAN.				
BEAN, STRING. See BEAN, GREEN; BEAN, WAX.				
BEAN, WAX/yellow snap bean				
Canned				
(Allens) .... 1/2 cup		15	3	1.0
(Stokely) .... 1/2 cup		20	4	0.0
cut *(S&W)* .... 1/2 cup		20	4	0.0
cut, 'Premium Golden' *(S&W)* .... 1/2 cup		20	5	0.0
cut, water packed, w/o salt *(Freshlike)* .... 1/2 cup		18	4	0.0
cut, water packed, w/o sugar or salt *(Freshlike)* .... 1/2 cup		18	4	0.0
golden, cut *(Del Monte)* .... 1/2 cup		20	4	0.0
golden, French style *(Del Monte)* .... 1/2 cup		20	4	0.0
no salt added, cut, drained .... 1/2 cup		14	3	0.1
no salt added, w/liquid .... 1/2 cup		18	4	0.1
no salt or sugar *(Stokely)* .... 1/2 cup		20	4	0.0
regular pack, cut, drained .... 1 cup		27	6	0.1
regular pack, whole, drained .... 10 med beans		12	3	0.1
regular pack, cut, w/liquid .... 1/2 cup		18	4	0.1
Fresh				
boiled, drained .... 1 cup		44	10	0.3
raw .... 1 cup		34	8	0.1
Frozen				
(Flav-R-Pac) .... 2/3 cup		25	4	0.0
(Frosty Acres) .... 3 oz		25	5	0.0
cut *(Seabrook)* .... 3 oz		25	5	0.0
no salt added, drained .... 1 cup		38	9	0.2
w/salt, drained .... 1 cup		38	9	0.2
BEAN, WHITE. See also BEAN, CANNELLINI, CANNED.				
Dried				
mature seeds, boiled .... 1 cup		249	45	0.6
mature seeds, boiled .... 1 tbsp		16	3	0.0
mature seeds, raw .... 1 cup		673	122	1.7
mature seeds, raw .... 1 tbsp		42	8	0.1
small white, mature seeds, boiled .... 1 cup		254	46	1.1
small white, mature seeds, raw .... 1 cup		722	134	2.5
Canned, mature seeds .... 1 cup		307	57	0.8

Food Name	Serv. Size	Total Cal.	Carbs GMS	Fat GMS
BEAN, WINGED/goa bean				
immature seeds, boiled, drained	1 cup	24	2	0.4
immature seeds, raw	1 med pod	8	1	0.1
immature seeds, raw, sliced	1 cup	22	2	0.4
mature seeds, boiled	1 cup	255	45	1.9
mature seeds, boiled	1 cup	253	26	10.0
mature seeds, raw	1 cup	744	76	29.7
BEAN, YARDLONG				
boiled, drained	1 med pod	7	1	0.0
boiled, drained, sliced	1 cup	49	10	0.1
boiled, mature seeds	1 cup	202	36	0.8
mature seeds, raw	1 cup	579	103	2.2
raw	1 med pod	6	1	0.0
raw, sliced	1 cup	43	8	0.4
BEAN, YELLOW, dried, mature seeds, raw	1 cup	676	119	5.1

BEAN DISH/ENTRÉE. See also BAKED BEANS, CANNED; BEAN SALAD, CANNED; BEANS, CHILI; BURRITO; CHILI; ENCHILADA.

Food Name	Serv. Size	Total Cal.	Carbs GMS	Fat GMS
(Amy's Kitchen)				
meatless 'Salisbury steak,' 'Country Dinner'	1 entrée	420	63	16.0
(Banquet) beans and frankfurters, frozen	10 oz	520	57	25.0
(Bearitos)				
refried beans, low-fat, no salt	1 serving	80	14	2.0
refried beans, nonfat	1 serving	70	14	0.0
refried beans, organic, canned	1 oz	30	5	0.5
refried beans, organic, no salt, canned	1 oz	29	5	0.5
refried beans, spicy, organic, canned	1 oz	31	5	0.6
refried beans, vegetarian, spicy, low-fat, canned	3.2 oz	80	14	2.0
refried beans, w/black beans, low-fat	1 serving	80	14	1.0
refried beans, w/green chilies, nonfat	1/2 cup	40	8	0.0
(Bush's Best) mixed, canned	1/2 cup	70	17	0.0
(Chi-Chi's) refried beans	7.5 oz	250	29	11.0
(Del Monte)				
refried beans, canned	1/2 cup	130	20	2.0
refried beans, spicy, canned	1/2 cup	130	20	2.0
(Flav-R-Pac)				
beans Parisian, frozen	1 cup	25	4	0.0
beans Parisian w/buttery sauce, frozen	1/2 cup	50	8	2.5
beans supreme, frozen	2/3 cup	50	9	0.0
four bean salad, frozen	1/3 cup	70	17	0.5
green beans w/onions and ham, 'Grande Classics'	1/2 cup	40	6	2.0
Oregon bean medley, frozen	2/3 cup	45	8	0.0
(Gebhardt)				
refried beans	1/2 cup	109	20	2.8
refried beans, food service product	1/2 cup	109	20	2.8
refried beans, jalapeño	1/2 cup	105	19	3.0
refried beans, nonfat	1/2 cup	92	20	0.5
refried beans, vegetarian	1/2 cup	118	21	2.3
(Green Giant)				
Mexican beans, canned, dry beans in brine	1/2 cup	120	21	1.5
three bean salad, canned	1/2 cup	70	16	0.0
(Health Valley)				
black beans w/garden vegetables, western, 'Fast Menu'	7.5 oz	120	14	1.0
(Homestyle)				
beans 'n fixins, food service product	1/2 cup	125	30	2.8
country kettle beans, food service product	1/2 cup	131	26	2.0
(Hunt's) beans and fixin's, 'Big John's'	1/2 cup	127	23	3.5
(Joan of Arc) Mexican beans, canned, dry beans in brine	1/2 cup	120	21	1.5

Food Name	Serv. Size	Total Cal.	Carbs GMS	Fat GMS
(Kid's Kitchen) beans and wieners, microwave cup	7.5 oz	310	36	13.0
(Lean Cuisine) three bean chili w/rice	1 entrée	210	32	6.0
(Libby's)				
beans and frankfurters in sauce, micro cup, 'Diner'	7.75 oz	330	38	15.0
(Lipton)				
beans and chicken w/sauce, mix, dry	1/4 pkg	120	26	1.0
beans and chicken w/sauce, mix, prepared	1/2 cup	150	26	4.0
(Little Pancho)				
refried beans, w/green chilies, nonfat, canned	1/2 cup	80	15	0.0
(Luck's) pinto and great northern, seasoned w/pork	1/2 cup	130	22	2.0
(Morningstar Farms) 'Spicy Black Bean Burger'	1 patty	110	16	1.0
(Morton) beans and frankfurters, frozen	10 oz	350	46	13.0
(Natural Touch)				
'Spicy Black Bean Burger'	1 patty	110	15	1.0
'Nine Bean Loaf'	1 slice	160	14	8.0
(Old El Paso)				
refried beans, canned	1/4 cup	55	8	1.0
refried beans, nonfat	1/2 cup	110	20	0.0
refried beans, spicy, canned	1/4 cup	35	5	1.0
refried beans, vegetarian, spicy, canned	1/4 cup	70	15	1.0
refried beans, w/cheese, canned	1/4 cup	36	4	1.0
refried beans, w/green chilies, canned	1/4 cup	49	8	1.0
refried beans, w/sausage, canned	1/2 cup	200	14	13.0
(Rice A Roni) red beans and rice	2.5 oz	158	29	4.0
(Rosarita)				
refried beans	1/2 cup	125	22	2.7
refried beans, nacho cheese	1/2 cup	137	24	3.2
refried beans, no fat	1/2 cup	123	28	0.5
refried beans, original, food service product	1/2 cup	109	20	2.8
refried beans, quick cooking, food service product	1/2 cup	185	31	6.7
refried beans, spicy	1/2 cup	118	22	2.7
refried beans, spicy, food service product	1/2 cup	109	20	2.6
refried beans, vegetarian	1/2 cup	121	23	2.1
refried beans, vegetarian, food service product	1/2 cup	118	21	2.3
refried beans, vegetarian, spicy, canned	4 oz	120	19	2.0
refried beans, vegetarian, w/canola oil	4 oz	100	18	2.0
refried beans, vegetarian, w/soybean oil	4 oz	100	18	2.0
refried beans, w/bacon	1/2 cup	116	19	3.1
refried beans, w/black beans, low-fat	1/2 cup	107	23	0.6
refried beans, w/green chilies	1/2 cup	110	20	2.9
refried beans, w/green chilies, no fat	1/2 cup	101	22	0.1
refried beans, w/onions	1/2 cup	114	21	2.8
salsa refried beans, no fat	1/2 cup	99	22	0.5
(S&W)				
bean salad, deli style, canned	1/2 cup	80	20	0.0
kidney, garbanzo and green beans in vinaigrette, canned	1/2 cup	90	17	1.0
(Santiago)				
refried beans, smooth	1/2 cup	174	24	5.8
refried beans, whole bean style	1/2 cup	174	24	5.8
(Stouffer's) green bean-mushroom casserole	1/2 cup	140	13	8.0
(Swanson) beans and frankfurters frozen	10.5 oz	440	53	19.0
(Weight Watchers) white beans and vegetables Parisian	1 entrée	220	23	9.0
BEAN DISH/ENTRÉE MIX				
(Fantastic Foods)				
black beans, instant, prepared	1/3 cup	160	29	1.5
refried beans, instant, prepared	1/3 cup	160	29	1.0
refried beans, instant, prepared w/o added ingredients	1/2 cup	157	28	2.0

Food Name	Serv. Size	Total Cal.	Carbs GMS	Fat GMS
BEAN SALAD. See under BEAN DISH/ENTRÉE.				
BEAN SPROUTS				
Canned				
(Chun King)	85 grams	5	0	0.0
(La Choy)	1 cup	14	1	0.1
(La Choy) food service product	1 cup	12	2	0.1
BEANS, CHILI				
Canned				
(Gebhardt)	1/2 cup	134	31	1.0
(Hunt's)	1/2 cup	87	17	1.0
(S&W)	1/2 cup	110	23	1.0
(Sun Vista)	1/2 cup	110	24	1.0
extra spicy (Green Giant)	1/2 cup	100	21	1.0
extra spicy (Joan of Arc)	1/2 cup	100	21	1.0
50% less salt (Green Giant)	1/2 cup	100	21	1.0
50% less salt (Joan of Arc)	1/2 cup	100	21	1.0
hot (Bush's Best)	1/2 cup	70	20	0.0
spiced (Gebhardt)	1/2 cup	100	19	1.6
BEANS, REFRIED. See under BEAN DISH/ENTRÉE.				
BEAR				
raw	1 oz	46	0	2.4
simmered	3 oz	220	0	11.4
simmered, yield from 1 lb raw, boneless	8 oz	717	0	37.1
BEAVER, RAW				
raw	1 oz	41	0	1.4
roasted	3 oz	180	0	5.9
roasted, yield from 1 lb raw, boneless	11 oz	664	0	21.8
BEECHNUT, dried	1 oz	163	9	14.2
BEEF. See also under LUNCHEON MEAT.				
(NOTE: TRIMMED = Lean; separable fat removed after cooking. UNTRIMMED = Separable fat not removed.)				
BRAIN				
pan-fried	3 oz	167	0	13.5
raw	4 oz	142	0	10.5
simmered	3 oz	136	0	10.7
BRISKET				
choice, shredded (Cripple Creek)	3 oz	180	6	12.0
choice, sliced (Cripple Creek)	3 oz	120	6	6.0
chopped (Cripple Creek)	3 oz	180	6	12.0
BRISKET, FLAT HALF				
Trimmed				
all grades, 0-inch fat, braised	3 oz	162	0	5.3
all grades, 1/4-inch fat, braised	3 oz	189	0	8.2
all grades, 1/4-inch fat, raw	1 oz	42	0	1.8
Untrimmed				
all grades, 0-inch fat, braised	3 oz	183	0	8.0
all grades, 1/8-inch fat, braised	3 oz	263	0	18.0
all grades, 1/8-inch fat, raw	4 oz	266	0	19.1
all grades, 1/4-inch fat, braised	3 oz	309	0	24.2
all grades, 1/4-inch fat, raw	4 oz	328	0	26.7
BRISKET, POINT HALF				
Trimmed				
all grades, 0-inch fat, braised	3 oz	207	0	11.7
all grades, 1/4-inch fat, braised	3 oz	222	0	13.3
all grades, 1/4-inch fat, raw	1 oz	46	0	2.4
Untrimmed				
all grades, 0-inch fat, braised	3 oz	304	0	24.2

Food Name	Serv. Size	Total Cal.	Carbs GMS	Fat GMS
all grades, 1/8-inch fat, braised	3 oz	297	0	23.1
all grades, 1/8-inch fat, raw	1 oz	75	0	5.9
all grades, 1/4-inch fat, braised	3 oz	343	0	29.1
all grades, 1/4-inch fat, raw	1 oz	94	0	8.2
BRISKET, WHOLE				
Trimmed				
all grades, 0-inch fat, braised,	3 oz	185	0	8.6
all grades, 1/4-inch fat, braised	3 oz	206	0	10.8
all grades, raw	1 oz	44	0	2.1
Untrimmed				
all grades, 0-inch fat, braised	3 oz	247	0	16.6
all grades, 1/8-inch fat, braised	3 oz	281	0	20.8
all grades, 1/8-inch fat, raw	1 oz	71	0	5.4
all grades, 1/4-inch fat, braised	3 oz	327	0	26.8
all grades, 1/4-inch fat, raw	1 oz	88	0	7.5
CHOPPED, canned *(Armour)*	3 oz	280	3	24.0
CHUCK, ARM POT ROAST				
Trimmed				
all grades, 0-inch fat, braised	3 oz	179	0	6.5
all grades, 1/4-inch fat, braised	3 oz	184	0	7.1
all grades, 1/4-inch fat, raw	1 oz	37	0	1.2
choice, 0-inch fat, braised	3 oz	186	0	7.4
choice, 1/4-inch fat, braised	3 oz	191	0	7.9
choice, 1/4-inch fat, raw	1 oz	39	0	1.4
prime, 1/2-inch fat, braised	3 oz	222	0	11.4
prime, 1/2-inch fat, raw	1 oz	44	0	2.0
select, 0-inch fat, braised	3 oz	168	0	5.4
select, 1/4-inch fat, braised	3 oz	175	0	6.1
select, 1/4-inch fat, raw	1 oz	35	0	1.0
Untrimmed				
all grades, 0-inch fat, braised	3 oz	238	0	14.5
all grades, 1/8-inch fat, braised	3 oz	263	0	17.6
all grades, 1/8-inch fat, raw	1 oz	69	0	5.2
all grades, 1/4-inch fat, braised	3 oz	282	0	20.2
all grades, 1/4-inch fat, raw	1 oz	69	0	5.2
choice, 1/4-inch fat, braised	3 oz	296	0	21.9
choice, 1/4-inch fat, raw	1 oz	72	0	5.5
prime, 1/2-inch fat, braised	3 oz	332	0	26.3
prime, 1/2-inch fat, raw	1 oz	83	0	6.8
select, 1/8-inch fat, raw	1 oz	62	0	4.4
select, 1/4-inch fat, braised	3 oz	268	0	18.5
select, 1/4-inch fat, raw	1 oz	66	0	4.8
CHUCK, BLADE ROAST				
Trimmed				
all grades, 0-inch fat, braised	3 oz	215	0	11.3
all grades, 1/4-inch fat, braised	3 oz	213	0	11.1
all grades, 1/4-inch fat, raw	1 oz	42	0	2.1
choice, 0-inch fat, braised	3 oz	225	0	12.5
choice, 1/4-inch fat, braised	3 oz	224	0	12.2
choice, 1/4-inch fat, raw	1 oz	45	0	2.4
prime, 1/2-inch fat, braised	3 oz	270	0	17.5
prime, 1/2-inch fat, raw	1 oz	58	0	3.8
select, 0-inch fat, braised	3 oz	202	0	9.9
select, 1/4-inch fat, braised	3 oz	201	0	9.9
select, 1/4-inch fat, raw	1 oz	39	0	1.8
Untrimmed				
all grades, 0-inch fat, braised	3 oz	284	0	20.5

Food Name	Serv. Size	Total Cal.	Carbs GMS	Fat GMS
all grades, 1/8-inch fat, braised	3 oz	290	0	21.4
all grades, 1/8-inch fat, raw	1 oz	70	0	5.5
all grades, 1/4-inch fat, braised	3 oz	293	0	21.8
all grades, 1/4-inch fat, raw	1 oz	72	0	5.7
choice, 1/8-inch fat, braised	3 oz	305	0	23.2
choice, 1/8-inch fat, raw	1 oz	75	0	6.0
choice, 1/4-inch fat, braised	3 oz	309	0	23.6
choice, 1/4-inch fat, raw	1 oz	77	0	6.3
prime, 1/2-inch fat, braised	3 oz	354	0	29.0
prime, 1/2-inch fat, raw	1 oz	93	0	8.1
select, 1/8-inch fat, braised	3 oz	270	0	19.0
select, 1/8-inch fat, raw	1 oz	65	0	4.9
select, 1/4-inch fat, braised	3 oz	277	0	19.8
select, 1/4-inch fat, raw	1 oz	67	0	5.1
CUBE STEAK, lean cuts, raw *(Lean and Free)*	4 oz	109	0	1.0
FLANK				
Trimmed				
choice, 0-inch fat, broiled	3 oz	176	0	8.6
choice, 0-inch fat, raw	1 oz	44	0	2.1
Untrimmed				
choice, 0-inch fat, braised	3 oz	201	0	11.1
choice, 0-inch fat, broiled	3 oz	192	0	10.7
choice, 0-inch fat, raw	4 oz	203	0	12.0
GROUND				
Extra lean, 17% fat				
baked, medium	3 oz	213	0	13.7
baked, well done	3 oz	233	0	13.6
broiled, medium	3 oz	218	0	13.9
broiled, well done	3 oz	225	0	13.4
pan-fried, medium	3 oz	217	0	14.0
pan-fried, well done	3 oz	224	0	13.6
raw	4 oz	264	0	19.3
raw	1 oz	66	0	4.8
Lean, 21% fat				
baked, medium	3 oz	228	0	15.6
baked, well done	3 oz	248	0	15.6
broiled, medium	3 oz	231	0	15.7
broiled, well done	3 oz	238	0	15.0
lean cuts, raw *(Lean and Free)*	4 oz	161	0	7.5
pan-fried, medium	3 oz	234	0	16.2
pan-fried, well done	3 oz	235	0	15.0
raw	4 oz	298	0	23.4
raw	1 oz	75	0	5.9
Regular, 27% fat				
baked, medium	3 oz	244	0	17.8
baked, well done	3 oz	269	0	18.2
broiled, medium	3 oz	246	0	17.6
broiled, well done	3 oz	248	0	16.5
1/4-pound patties *(Bar-S)*	1 patty	330	0	28.0
1/4-pound patties *(Chuck Wagon)*	1 patty	400	5	35.0
1/4-pound patties *(Manor House)*	1 patty	330	0	28.0
pan-fried, medium	3 oz	260	0	19.2
pan-fried, well done	3 oz	243	0	16.1
raw	4 oz	350	0	30.0
raw	1 oz	88	0	7.5
HEART				
raw	4 oz	132	3	4.3

Food Name	Serv. Size	Total Cal.	Carbs GMS	Fat GMS
simmered	3 oz	149	0	4.8
KIDNEY				
raw	1 oz	30	1	0.9
simmered	3 oz	122	1	2.9
LIVER				
braised	3 oz	137	3	4.2
pan-fried	3 oz	184	7	6.8
raw	4 oz	162	7	4.4
LOIN, TOP				
Trimmed				
all grades, 0-inch fat, broiled	3 oz	168	0	7.1
all grades, 1/4-inch fat, broiled	3 oz	176	0	8.0
all grades, 1/4-inch fat, raw	1 oz	40	0	1.6
choice, 0-inch fat, broiled	3 oz	178	0	8.2
choice, 1/4-inch fat, broiled	3 oz	182	0	8.6
choice, 1/4-inch fat, raw	1 oz	43	0	1.8
prime, 1/4-inch fat, broiled	3 oz	208	0	11.6
prime, 1/4-inch fat, raw	1 oz	54	0	3.0
prime, 1/2-inch fat, raw	3 oz	208	0	11.6
select, 0-inch fat, broiled	3 oz	156	0	5.9
select, 1/4-inch fat, broiled	3 oz	164	0	6.6
select, 1/4-inch fat, raw	1 oz	38	0	1.3
Untrimmed				
all grades, 0-inch fat, broiled	3 oz	180	0	8.7
all grades, 1/8-inch fat, broiled	3 oz	228	0	14.7
all grades, 1/4-inch fat, broiled	3 oz	244	0	16.8
choice, 0-inch fat, broiled	3 oz	194	0	10.2
choice, 1/8-inch fat, broiled	3 oz	241	0	16.3
choice, 1/4-inch fat, broiled	3 oz	253	0	17.8
prime, 1/8-inch fat, broiled	3 oz	264	0	18.8
prime, 1/4-inch fat, broiled	3 oz	275	0	20.2
prime, 1/2-inch fat, broiled	3 oz	288	0	22.0
select, 0-inch fat, broiled	3 oz	169	0	7.5
select, 1/8-inch fat, broiled	3 oz	215	0	13.2
select, 1/4-inch fat, broiled	3 oz	226	0	14.6
LUNGS				
braised	3 oz	102	0	3.1
raw	4 oz	104	0	2.8
PANCREAS				
braised	3 oz	230	0	14.6
raw	4 oz	266	0	21.0
PORTERHOUSE				
Trimmed				
all grades, 0-inch fat, broiled	3 oz	183	0	9.9
all grades, 1/4-inch fat, broiled	3 oz	180	0	9.3
all grades, 1/4-inch fat, raw	1 oz	45	0	2.1
choice, 0-inch fat, broiled	3 oz	190	0	10.9
choice, 1/4-inch fat, broiled	3 oz	183	0	9.8
choice, 1/4-inch fat, raw	1 oz	45	0	2.3
select, 0-inch fat, broiled	3 oz	165	0	7.5
select, 1/4-inch fat, broiled	3 oz	173	0	8.2
select, 1/4-inch fat, raw	1 oz	42	0	1.6
Untrimmed				
all grades, 0-inch fat, broiled	3 oz	237	0	16.7
all grades, 1/8-inch fat, broiled	3 oz	252	0	18.6
all grades, 1/8-inch fat, raw	1 oz	70	0	5.2
all grades, 1/4-inch fat, broiled	3 oz	273	0	21.1

Food Name	Serv. Size	Total Cal.	Carbs GMS	Fat GMS
all grades, 1/4-inch fat, raw	1 oz	73	0	5.6
choice, 1/8-inch fat, broiled	3 oz	254	0	18.8
choice, 1/8-inch fat, raw	1 oz	73	0	5.7
choice, 1/4-inch fat, broiled	3 oz	278	0	21.8
choice, 1/4-inch fat, raw	1 oz	73	0	5.7
select, 0-inch fat, broiled	3 oz	227	0	15.3
select, 1/8-inch fat, broiled	3 oz	250	0	18.0
select, 1/8-inch fat, raw	1 oz	63	0	4.2
select, 1/4-inch fat, broiled	3 oz	262	0	19.6
select, 1/4-inch fat, raw	1 oz	63	0	4.2
RIB, LARGE END				
Trimmed				
all grades, ribs 6-9, 0-inch fat, roasted	3 oz	202	0	11.4
all grades, ribs 6-9, 1/4-inch fat, broiled	3 oz	190	0	11.0
all grades, ribs 6-9, 1/4-inch fat, raw	1 oz	47	0	2.6
all grades, ribs 6-9, 1/4-inch fat, roasted	3 oz	201	0	11.2
choice, ribs 6-9, 0-inch fat, roasted	3 oz	215	0	12.8
choice, ribs 6-9, 1/4-inch fat, broiled	3 oz	204	0	12.5
choice, ribs 6-9, 1/4-inch fat, raw	1 oz	50	0	2.9
choice, ribs 6-9, 1/4-inch fat, roasted	3 oz	213	0	12.5
prime, ribs 6-9, 1/4-inch fat, broiled	3 oz	250	0	17.7
prime, ribs 6-9, 1/4-inch fat, raw	1 oz	60	0	4.0
prime, ribs 6-9, 1/4-inch fat, roasted	3 oz	241	0	15.6
prime, ribs 6-9, 1/2-inch fat, broiled	3 oz	250	0	17.7
prime, ribs 6-9, 1/2-inch fat, roasted	3 oz	241	0	15.6
select, ribs 6-9, 0-inch fat, roasted	3 oz	187	0	9.7
select, ribs 6-9, 1/4-inch fat, broiled	3 oz	175	0	9.3
select, ribs 6-9, 1/4-inch fat, raw	1 oz	43	0	2.2
select, ribs 6-9, 1/4-inch fat, roasted	3 oz	187	0	9.7
Untrimmed				
all grades, ribs 6-9, 0-inch fat, roasted	3 oz	300	0	24.0
all grades, ribs 6-9, 1/8-inch fat, broiled	3 oz	287	0	23.1
all grades, ribs 6-9, 1/8-inch fat, raw	1 oz	90	0	7.7
all grades, ribs 6-9, 1/8-inch fat, roasted	3 oz	302	0	24.2
all grades, ribs 6-9, 1/4-inch fat, broiled	3 oz	295	0	24.2
all grades, ribs 6-9, 1/4-inch fat, raw	1 oz	92	0	8.0
all grades, ribs 6-9, 1/4-inch fat, roasted	3 oz	310	0	25.3
choice, ribs 6-9, 0-inch fat, roasted	3 oz	316	0	25.9
choice, ribs 6-9, 1/8-inch fat, broiled	3 oz	315	0	26.5
choice, ribs 6-9, 1/8-inch fat, raw	1 oz	94	0	8.3
choice, ribs 6-9, 1/8-inch fat, roasted	3 oz	334	0	27.8
choice, ribs 6-9, 1/4-inch fat, broiled	3 oz	312	0	26.2
choice, ribs 6-9, 1/4-inch fat, raw	1 oz	98	0	8.7
choice, ribs 6-9, 1/4-inch fat, roasted	3 oz	326	0	27.2
prime, ribs 6-9, 1/8-inch fat, broiled	3 oz	343	0	29.7
prime, ribs 6-9, 1/8-inch fat, raw	1 oz	104	0	9.4
prime, ribs 6-9, 1/4-inch fat, broiled	3 oz	351	0	30.8
prime, ribs 6-9, 1/4-inch fat, raw	1 oz	107	0	9.8
prime, ribs 6-9, 1/4-inch fat, roasted	3 oz	342	0	28.8
prime, ribs 6-9, 1/2-inch fat, broiled	3 oz	361	0	32.1
prime, ribs 6-9, 1/2-inch fat, raw	1 oz	109	0	10.0
prime, ribs 6-9, 1/2-inch fat, roasted	3 oz	346	0	29.4
select, ribs 6-9, 1/8-inch fat, broiled	3 oz	275	0	21.9
select, ribs 6-9, 1/8-inch fat, raw	1 oz	84	0	7.0
select, ribs 6-9, 1/8-inch fat, roasted	3 oz	283	0	22.0
select, ribs 6-9, 1/4-inch fat, broiled	3 oz	275	0	21.9
select, ribs 6-9, 1/4-inch fat, raw	1 oz	86	0	7.4
select, ribs 6-9, 1/4-inch fat, roasted	3 oz	289	0	22.7

Food Name	Serv. Size	Total Cal.	Carbs GMS	Fat GMS
RIB, SHORTRIB				
Trimmed				
choice, braised	3 oz	251	0	15.4
choice, raw	1 oz	49	0	2.9
Untrimmed				
choice, braised	3 oz	400	0	35.7
choice, raw	1 oz	110	0	10.3
RIB, SMALL END				
Trimmed				
all grades, ribs 10-12, 0-inch fat, broiled	3 oz	181	0	8.8
all grades, ribs 10-12, 1/4-inch fat, broiled	3 oz	188	0	9.5
all grades, ribs 10-12, 1/4-inch fat, raw	1 oz	43	0	2.1
all grades, ribs 10-12, 1/4-inch fat, roasted	3 oz	185	0	9.8
choice, ribs 10-12, 0-inch fat, broiled	3 oz	191	0	9.9
choice, ribs 10-12, 1/4-inch fat, broiled	3 oz	198	0	10.7
choice, ribs 10-12, 1/4-inch fat, raw	1 oz	46	0	2.4
choice, ribs 10-12, 1/4-inch fat, roasted	3 oz	197	0	11.1
prime, ribs 10-12, 1/4-inch fat, broiled	3 oz	221	0	13.2
prime, ribs 10-12, 1/4-inch fat, raw	1 oz	57	0	3.6
prime, ribs 10-12, 1/4-inch fat, roasted	3 oz	258	0	17.9
prime, ribs 10-12, 1/2-inch fat, broiled	3 oz	221	0	13.2
prime, ribs 10-12, 1/2-inch fat, roasted	3 oz	258	0	17.9
select, ribs 10-12, 0-inch fat, broiled	3 oz	168	0	7.4
select, ribs 10-12, 1/4-inch fat, broiled	3 oz	176	0	8.2
select, ribs 10-12, 1/4-inch fat, raw	1 oz	40	0	1.8
select, ribs 10-12, 1/4-inch fat, roasted	3 oz	173	0	8.3
Untrimmed				
all grades, ribs 10-12, 0-inch fat, broiled	3 oz	252	0	17.9
all grades, ribs 10-12, 1/8-inch fat, broiled	3 oz	281	0	21.4
all grades, ribs 10-12, 1/8-inch fat, raw	1 oz	82	0	6.9
all grades, ribs 10-12, 1/8-inch fat, roasted	3 oz	290	0	23.1
all grades, ribs 10-12, 1/4-inch fat, broiled	3 oz	286	0	22.1
all grades, ribs 10-12, 1/4-inch fat, raw	1 oz	84	0	7.1
all grades, ribs 10-12, 1/4-inch fat, roasted	3 oz	295	0	23.8
choice, ribs 10-12, 1/8-inch fat, broiled	3 oz	292	0	22.8
choice, ribs 10-12, 1/8-inch fat, raw	1 oz	86	0	7.3
choice, ribs 10-12, 1/8-inch fat, roasted	3 oz	305	0	24.8
choice, ribs 10-12, 1/4-inch fat, broiled	3 oz	297	0	23.5
choice, ribs 10-12, 1/4-inch fat, raw	1 oz	89	0	7.7
choice, ribs 10-12, 1/4-inch fat, roasted	3 oz	312	0	25.7
prime, ribs 10-12, 1/8-inch fat, broiled	3 oz	301	0	23.7
prime, ribs 10-12, 1/8-inch fat, raw	1 oz	95	0	8.3
prime, ribs 10-12, 1/8-inch fat, roasted	3 oz	349	0	29.9
prime, ribs 10-12, 1/4-inch fat, broiled	3 oz	307	0	24.4
prime, ribs 10-12, 1/4-inch fat, raw	1 oz	97	0	8.5
prime, ribs 10-12, 1/4-inch fat, roasted	3 oz	354	0	30.5
prime, ribs 10-12, 1/2-inch fat, broiled	3 oz	309	0	24.8
prime, ribs 10-12, 1/2-inch fat, raw	1 oz	99	0	8.8
prime, ribs 10-12, 1/2-inch fat, roasted	3 oz	357	0	30.8
select, ribs 10-12, 1/8-inch fat, broiled	3 oz	268	0	20.0
select, ribs 10-12, 1/8-inch fat, raw	1 oz	78	0	6.4
select, ribs 10-12, 1/8-inch fat, roasted	3 oz	275	0	21.3
select, ribs 10-12, 1/4-inch fat, broiled	3 oz	273	0	20.6
select, ribs 10-12, 1/4-inch fat, raw	1 oz	81	0	6.7
select, ribs 10-12, 1/4-inch fat, roasted	3 oz	281	0	22.2
RIB, WHOLE				
Trimmed				
all grades, ribs 6-12, 1/4-inch fat, broiled	3 oz	190	0	10.4

Food Name	Serv. Size	Total Cal.	Carbs GMS	Fat GMS
all grades, ribs 6-12, 1/4-inch fat, raw	1 oz	45	0	2.4
all grades, ribs 6-12, 1/4-inch fat, roasted	3 oz	195	0	10.6
choice, ribs 6-12, 1/4-inch fat, broiled	3 oz	201	0	11.7
choice, ribs 6-12, 1/4-inch fat, raw	1 oz	48	0	2.7
choice, ribs 6-12, 1/4-inch fat, roasted	3 oz	207	0	11.9
prime, ribs 6-12, 1/4-inch fat, broiled	3 oz	238	0	15.9
prime, ribs 6-12, 1/4-inch fat, raw	1 oz	58	0	3.8
prime, ribs 6-12, 1/4-inch fat, roasted	3 oz	248	0	16.5
prime, ribs 6-12, 1/2-inch fat, broiled	3 oz	238	0	15.9
prime, ribs 6-12, 1/2-inch fat, roasted	3 oz	248	0	16.5
select, ribs 6-12, 1/4-inch fat, broiled	3 oz	175	0	8.9
select, ribs 6-12, 1/4-inch fat, raw	1 oz	42	0	2.0
select, ribs 6-12, 1/4-inch fat, roasted	3 oz	181	0	9.1
Untrimmed				
all grades, ribs 6-12, 1/8-inch fat, broiled	3 oz	286	0	22.7
all grades, ribs 6-12, 1/8-inch fat, raw	1 oz	87	0	7.4
all grades, ribs 6-12, 1/8-inch fat, roasted	3 oz	298	0	23.9
all grades, ribs 6-12, 1/4-inch fat, broiled	3 oz	291	0	23.3
all grades, ribs 6-12, 1/4-inch fat, raw	1 oz	89	0	7.6
all grades, ribs 6-12, 1/4-inch fat, roasted	3 oz	304	0	24.7
choice, ribs 6-12, 1/8-inch fat, broiled	3 oz	299	0	24.2
choice, ribs 6-12, 1/8-inch fat, raw	1 oz	91	0	7.9
choice, ribs 6-12, 1/8-inch fat, roasted	3 oz	310	0	25.3
choice, ribs 6-12, 1/4-inch fat, broiled	3 oz	306	0	25.1
choice, ribs 6-12, 1/4-inch fat, raw	1 oz	94	0	8.3
choice, ribs 6-12, 1/4-inch fat, roasted	3 oz	320	0	26.5
prime, ribs 6-12, 1/8-inch fat, broiled	3 oz	328	0	27.5
prime, ribs 6-12, 1/8-inch fat, raw	1 oz	101	0	9.0
prime, ribs 6-12, 1/8-inch fat, roasted	3 oz	340	0	28.6
prime, ribs 6-12, 1/4-inch fat, broiled	3 oz	333	0	28.2
prime, ribs 6-12, 1/4-inch fat, raw	1 oz	103	0	9.3
prime, ribs 6-12, 1/4-inch fat, roasted	3 oz	348	0	29.6
prime, ribs 6-12, 1/2-inch fat, broiled	3 oz	347	0	29.9
prime, ribs 6-12, 1/2-inch fat, raw	1 oz	105	0	9.5
prime, ribs 6-12, 1/2-inch fat, roasted	3 oz	361	0	31.4
select, ribs 6-12, 1/8-inch fat, broiled	3 oz	268	0	20.6
select, ribs 6-12, 1/8-inch fat, raw	1 oz	82	0	6.8
select, ribs 6-12, 1/8-inch fat, roasted	3 oz	281	0	21.8
select, ribs 6-12, 1/4-inch fat, broiled	3 oz	275	0	21.4
select, ribs 6-12, 1/4-inch fat, raw	1 oz	84	0	7.1
select, ribs 6-12, 1/4-inch fat, roasted	3 oz	286	0	22.5
RIB EYE, SMALL END				
Trimmed				
choice, ribs 10-12, 0-inch fat, broiled	3 oz	191	0	9.9
choice, ribs 10-12, 0-inch fat, raw	1 oz	46	0	2.4
lean cuts, raw *(Lean and Free)*	4 oz	121	0	2.6
Untrimmed				
choice, ribs 10-12, 0-inch fat, broiled	3 oz	261	0	18.9
choice, ribs 10-12, 0-inch fat, raw	1 oz	78	0	6.3
choice, ribs 10-12, 1/8-inch fat, broiled	3 oz	255	0	18.1
choice, ribs 10-12, 1/8-inch fat, raw	1 oz	74	0	5.8
ROLLED, lean cuts, raw *(Lean and Free)*	4 oz	125	0	2.8
ROUND, BOTTOM				
Trimmed				
all grades, 0-inch fat, braised	3 oz	173	0	6.5
all grades, 0-inch fat, roasted	3 oz	156	0	5.7
all grades, 1/4-inch fat, braised	3 oz	178	0	7.0

Food Name	Serv. Size	Total Cal.	Carbs GMS	Fat GMS
all grades, 1/4-inch fat, raw	1 oz	41	0	1.6
all grades, 1/4-inch fat, roasted	3 oz	161	0	6.3
choice, 0-inch fat, braised	3 oz	181	0	7.4
choice, 0-inch fat, roasted	3 oz	164	0	6.6
choice, 1/4-inch fat, braised	3 oz	187	0	8.0
choice, 1/4-inch fat, raw	1 oz	43	0	1.8
choice, 1/4-inch fat, roasted	3 oz	168	0	7.0
prime, 1/2-inch fat, broiled	3 oz	212	0	10.8
prime, 1/2-inch fat, raw	1 oz	45	0	2.1
select, 0-inch fat, braised	3 oz	163	0	5.4
select, 0-inch fat, roasted	3 oz	145	0	4.6
select, 1/4-inch fat, braised	3 oz	167	0	5.8
select, 1/4-inch fat, raw	1 oz	39	0	1.3
select, 1/4-inch fat, roasted	3 oz	152	0	5.3
Untrimmed				
all grades, 0-inch fat, braised	3 oz	181	0	7.5
all grades, 0-inch fat, roasted	3 oz	160	0	6.2
all grades, 1/8-inch fat, braised	3 oz	218	0	12.2
all grades, 1/8-inch fat, raw	1 oz	54	0	3.2
all grades, 1/8-inch fat, roasted	3 oz	195	0	10.6
all grades, 1/4-inch fat, braised	3 oz	234	0	14.4
all grades, 1/4-inch fat, raw	1 oz	59	0	3.8
all grades, 1/4-inch fat, roasted	3 oz	211	0	12.7
choice, 0-inch fat, braised	3 oz	193	0	9.0
choice, 0-inch fat, roasted	3 oz	173	0	7.7
choice, 1/8-inch fat, braised	3 oz	228	0	13.5
choice, 1/8-inch fat, raw	1 oz	57	0	3.5
choice, 1/8-inch fat, roasted	3 oz	205	0	11.8
choice, 1/4-inch fat, braised	3 oz	241	0	15.2
choice, 1/4-inch fat, raw	1 oz	62	0	4.2
choice, 1/4-inch fat, roasted	3 oz	221	0	13.9
prime, 1/2-inch fat, braised	3 oz	252	0	16.2
prime, 1/2-inch fat, raw	1 oz	64	0	4.4
select, 0-inch fat, braised	3 oz	171	0	6.4
select, 0-inch fat, roasted	3 oz	150	0	5.1
select, 1/8-inch fat, braised	3 oz	208	0	11.2
select, 1/8-inch fat, raw	1 oz	51	0	2.9
select, 1/8-inch fat, roasted	3 oz	186	0	9.6
select, 1/4-inch fat, braised	3 oz	220	0	12.8
select, 1/4-inch fat, raw	1 oz	55	0	3.4
select, 1/4-inch fat, roasted	3 oz	199	0	11.3
ROUND, EYE OF				
Trimmed				
all grades, 0-inch fat, roasted	3 oz	141	0	4.0
all grades, 1/4-inch fat, raw	1 oz	37	0	1.2
all grades, 1/4-inch fat, roasted	3 oz	143	0	4.2
choice, 0-inch fat, roasted	3 oz	149	0	4.8
choice, 1/4-inch fat, raw	1 oz	39	0	1.4
choice, 1/4-inch fat, roasted	3 oz	149	0	4.8
prime, 1/2-inch fat, raw	1 oz	42	0	1.8
prime, 1/2-inch fat, roasted	3 oz	168	0	7.0
select, 0-inch fat, roasted	3 oz	132	0	3.0
select, 1/4-inch fat, raw	1 oz	35	0	1.0
select, 1/4-inch fat, roasted	3 oz	136	0	3.4
Untrimmed				
all grades, 0-inch fat, roasted	3 oz	145	0	4.6
all grades, 1/8-inch fat, raw	1 oz	47	0	2.4

Food Name	Serv. Size	Total Cal.	Carbs GMS	Fat GMS
all grades, 1/8-inch fat, roasted	3 oz	165	0	6.9
all grades, 1/4-inch fat, raw	1 oz	60	0	4.1
all grades, 1/4-inch fat, roasted	3 oz	195	0	10.8
choice, 0-inch fat, roasted	3 oz	153	0	5.4
choice, 1/8-inch fat, raw	1 oz	49	0	2.6
choice, 1/8-inch fat, roasted	3 oz	170	0	7.6
choice, 1/4-inch fat, raw	1 oz	62	0	4.2
choice, 1/4-inch fat, roasted	3 oz	205	0	12.0
select, 1/8-inch fat, raw	1 oz	45	0	2.2
select, 1/8-inch fat, roasted	3 oz	158	0	6.2
select, 1/4-inch fat, raw	1 oz	57	0	3.7
select, 1/4-inch fat, roasted	3 oz	184	0	9.6
prime, 1/2-inch fat, raw	1 oz	63	0	4.3
prime, 1/2-inch fat, roasted	3 oz	213	0	12.7
ROUND, FULL CUT				
Trimmed				
choice, 1/4-inch fat, broiled	3 oz	162	0	6.2
choice, 1/4-inch fat, raw	1 oz	39	0	1.4
select, 1/4-inch fat, broiled	3 oz	146	0	4.4
select, 1/4-inch fat, raw	1 oz	36	0	1.0
Untrimmed				
choice, 1/8-Inch fat, broiled	3 oz	200	0	11.0
choice, 1/8-inch fat, raw	1 oz	55	0	3.4
choice, 1/4-inch fat, broiled	3 oz	204	0	11.6
choice, 1/4-inch fat, raw	1 oz	58	0	3.6
select, 1/8-inch fat, broiled	3 oz	185	0	9.4
select, 1/8-inch fat, raw	1 oz	52	0	3.0
select, 1/4-inch fat, broiled	3 oz	190	0	10.0
select, 1/4-inch fat, raw	1 oz	54	0	3.3
ROUND, TOP				
Trimmed				
all grades, 0-inch fat, braised	3 oz	169	0	4.3
all grades, 1/4-inch fat, braised	3 oz	174	0	4.8
all grades, 1/4-inch fat, broiled	3 oz	153	0	4.2
all grades, 1/4-inch fat, raw	1 oz	36	0	0.9
choice, 0-inch fat, braised	3 oz	176	0	4.9
choice, 1/4-inch fat, braised	3 oz	181	0	5.5
choice, 1/4-inch fat, broiled	3 oz	161	0	5.0
choice, 1/4-inch fat, pan-fried	3 oz	193	0	7.3
choice, 1/4-inch fat, raw	1 oz	37	0	1.1
prime, 1/2-inch fat, broiled	3 oz	183	0	7.5
prime, 1/4-inch fat, broiled	3 oz	183	0	7.5
prime, 1/4-inch fat, raw	1 oz	43	0	1.8
lean cuts, raw *(Lean Limousin)*	4 oz	134	0	4.5
select, 0-inch fat, braised	3 oz	162	0	3.4
select, 1/4-inch fat, braised	3 oz	167	0	3.9
select, 1/4-inch fat, broiled	3 oz	144	0	3.1
select, 1/4-inch fat, raw	1 oz	34	0	0.7
Untrimmed				
all grades, 0-inch fat, braised	3 oz	178	0	5.4
all grades, 1/8-inch fat, braised	3 oz	202	0	8.6
all grades, 1/8-inch fat, broiled	3 oz	176	0	7.2
all grades, 1/8-inch fat, raw	1 oz	46	0	2.2
all grades, 1/4-inch fat, braised	3 oz	211	0	9.7
all grades, 1/4-inch fat, broiled	3 oz	184	0	8.2
all grades, 1/4-inch fat, raw	1 oz	50	0	2.7
choice, 0-inch fat, braised	3 oz	184	0	6.0

Food Name	Serv. Size	Total Cal.	Carbs GMS	Fat GMS
choice, 1/8-inch fat, braised	3 oz	213	0	9.9
choice, 1/8-inch fat, broiled	3 oz	184	0	8.0
choice, 1/8-inch fat, pan-fried	3 oz	226	0	11.8
choice, 1/8-inch fat, raw	1 oz	48	0	2.4
choice, 1/4-inch fat, braised	3 oz	221	0	10.9
choice, 1/4-inch fat, broiled	3 oz	190	0	9.0
choice, 1/4-inch fat, pan-fried	3 oz	235	0	13.1
choice, 1/4-inch fat, raw	1 oz	51	0	2.8
prime, 1/2-inch fat, broiled	3 oz	201	0	9.9
prime, 1/2-inch fat, raw	1 oz	53	0	3.0
prime, 1/8-inch fat, broiled	3 oz	191	0	8.6
prime, 1/8-inch fat, raw	1 oz	49	0	2.5
prime, 1/4-inch fat, broiled	3 oz	195	0	9.1
prime, 1/4-inch fat, raw	1 oz	51	0	2.7
select, 0-inch fat, braised	3 oz	170	0	4.5
select, 1/8-inch fat, braised	3 oz	191	0	7.3
select, 1/8-inch fat, broiled	3 oz	167	0	6.2
select, 1/8-inch fat, raw	1 oz	44	0	2.0
select, 1/4-inch fat, braised	3 oz	199	0	8.4
select, 1/4-inch fat, broiled	3 oz	175	0	7.2
select, 1/4-inch fat, raw	1 oz	46	0	2.3
ROUND TIP				
Trimmed				
all grades, 0-inch fat, roasted	3 oz	150	0	5.0
all grades, 1/4-inch fat, raw	1 oz	35	0	1.1
all grades, 1/4-inch fat, roasted	3 oz	157	0	5.9
choice, 0-inch fat, roasted	3 oz	153	0	5.4
choice, 1/4-inch fat, raw	1 oz	37	0	1.2
choice, 1/4-inch fat, roasted	3 oz	160	0	6.2
prime, 1/4-inch fat, raw	1 oz	41	0	1.7
prime, 1/2-inch fat, roasted	3 oz	181	0	8.6
prime, 1/4-inch fat, roasted	3 oz	181	0	8.6
select, 0-inch fat, roasted	3 oz	145	0	4.5
select, 1/4-inch fat, raw	1 oz	34	0	0.9
select, 1/4-inch fat, roasted	3 oz	153	0	5.4
Untrimmed				
all grades, 0-inch fat, roasted	3 oz	162	0	6.7
all grades, 1/8-inch fat, raw	1 oz	54	0	3.3
all grades, 1/8-inch fat, roasted	3 oz	186	0	9.6
all grades, 1/4-inch fat, raw	1 oz	57	0	3.7
all grades, 1/4-inch fat, roasted	3 oz	199	0	11.3
choice, 0-inch fat, roasted	3 oz	170	0	7.6
choice, 1/8-inch fat, raw	1 oz	56	0	3.6
choice, 1/8-inch fat, roasted	3 oz	194	0	10.5
choice, 1/4-inch fat, raw	1 oz	60	0	4.1
choice, 1/4-inch fat, roasted	3 oz	210	0	12.6
prime, 1/4-inch fat, raw	1 oz	61	0	4.1
prime, 1/4-inch fat, roasted	3 oz	233	0	15.2
prime, 1/2-inch fat, raw	1 oz	63	0	4.6
prime, 1/2-inch fat, roasted	3 oz	241	0	16.3
select, 1/8-inch fat, raw	1 oz	50	0	2.9
select, 1/8-inch fat, roasted	3 oz	179	0	8.7
select, 1/4-inch fat, raw	1 oz	53	0	3.2
select, 1/4-inch fat, roasted	3 oz	191	0	10.3
ROUND STEAK, lean cuts, raw *(Lean and Free)*	4 oz	111	0	1.1
SHANK CROSSCUTS				
Trimmed				
choice, 1/4-inch fat, raw	1 oz	36	0	1.1

Food Name	Serv. Size	Total Cal.	Carbs GMS	Fat GMS
choice, 1/4-inch fat, simmered	3 oz	171	0	5.4
Untrimmed				
choice, 1/4-inch fat, raw	3 oz	150	0	8.4
choice, 1/4-inch fat, simmered	3 oz	224	0	12.5
SIRLOIN, TOP				
Trimmed				
all grades, 0-inch fat, broiled	3 oz	162	0	5.8
all grades, 1/4-inch fat, broiled	3 oz	166	0	6.1
all grades, 1/4-inch fat, raw	1 oz	37	0	1.2
choice, 0-inch fat, broiled	3 oz	170	0	6.6
choice, 1/4-inch fat, broiled	3 oz	172	0	6.8
choice, 1/4-inch fat, pan-fried	3 oz	202	0	9.3
choice, 1/4-inch fat, raw	1 oz	39	0	1.4
select, 0-inch fat, broiled	3 oz	153	0	4.8
select, 1/4-inch fat, broiled	3 oz	158	0	5.3
select, 1/4-inch fat, raw	1 oz	35	0	1.0
Untrimmed				
all grades, 0-inch fat, broiled	3 oz	183	0	8.5
all grades, 1/8-inch fat, broiled	3 oz	211	0	12.0
all grades, 1/8-inch fat, raw	1 oz	58	0	3.8
all grades, 1/4-inch fat, broiled	3 oz	219	0	13.1
all grades, 1/4-inch fat, raw	1 oz	62	0	4.3
choice, 0-inch fat, broiled	3 oz	195	0	9.8
choice, 1/8-inch fat, broiled	3 oz	220	0	13.2
choice, 1/8-inch fat, pan-fried	3 oz	266	0	17.9
choice, 1/8-inch fat, raw	1 oz	60	0	4.1
choice, 1/4-inch fat, broiled	3 oz	229	0	14.2
choice, 1/4-inch fat, pan-fried	3 oz	277	0	19.4
choice, 1/4-inch fat, raw	1 oz	64	0	4.6
select, 0-inch fat, broiled	3 oz	166	0	6.4
select, 1/8-inch fat, broiled	3 oz	204	0	11.3
select, 1/8-inch fat, raw	1 oz	55	0	3.5
select, 1/4-inch fat, broiled	3 oz	208	0	11.8
select, 1/4-inch fat, raw	1 oz	59	0	3.9
SIRLOIN STEAK, lean cuts, raw *(Lean and Free)*	4 oz	111	0	1.8
SIRLOIN TIP, lean cuts, raw *(Lean and Free)*	4 oz	110	0	1.2
SPLEEN				
braised	3 oz	123	0	3.6
raw	4 oz	119	0	3.4
STRIP LOIN STEAK, lean cuts, raw *(Lean and Free)*	4 oz	113	0	1.8
T-BONE				
Trimmed				
all grades, 0-inch fat, broiled	3 oz	163	0	7.6
all grades, 1/4-inch fat, broiled	3 oz	173	0	8.3
all grades, 1/4-inch fat, raw	1 oz	42	0	1.8
choice, 0-inch fat, broiled	3 oz	168	0	8.2
choice, 1/4-inch fat, broiled	3 oz	174	0	8.5
choice, 1/4-inch fat, raw	1 oz	44	0	2.1
lean cuts, raw *(Lean and Free)*	4 oz	125	0	2.7
select, 0-inch fat, broiled	3 oz	150	0	6.3
select, 1/4-inch fat, broiled	3 oz	168	0	7.6
select, 1/4-inch fat, raw	1 oz	37	0	1.3
Untrimmed				
all grades, 0-inch fat, broiled	3 oz	210	0	13.5
all grades, 1/8-inch fat, broiled	3 oz	238	0	16.5
all grades, 1/8-inch fat, raw	1 oz	62	0	4.3
all grades, 1/4-inch fat, broiled	3 oz	256	0	18.8

Food Name	Serv. Size	Total Cal.	Carbs GMS	Fat GMS
all grades, 1/4-inch fat, raw	1 oz	64	0	4.5
choice, 0-inch fat, broiled	3 oz	217	0	14.4
choice, 1/8-inch fat, broiled	3 oz	243	0	17.3
choice, 1/8-inch fat, raw	1 oz	66	0	4.8
choice, 1/4-inch fat, broiled	3 oz	263	0	19.8
choice, 1/4-inch fat, raw	1 oz	67	0	4.9
select, 0-inch fat, broiled	3 oz	194	0	11.6
select, 1/8-inch fat, broiled	3 oz	225	0	14.9
select, 1/8-inch fat, raw	1 oz	54	0	3.4
select, 1/4-inch fat, broiled	3 oz	238	0	16.5
select, 1/4-inch fat, raw	1 oz	56	0	3.5
TENDERLOIN				
Trimmed				
all grades, 0-inch fat, broiled	3 oz	175	0	8.1
all grades, 1/4-inch fat, broiled	3 oz	179	0	8.5
all grades, 1/4-inch fat, raw	1 oz	45	0	2.2
all grades, 1/4-inch fat, roasted	3 oz	189	0	9.8
choice, 0-inch fat, broiled	3 oz	180	0	8.6
choice, 1/4-inch fat, broiled	3 oz	189	0	9.5
choice, 1/4-inch fat, raw	1 oz	47	0	2.4
choice, 1/4-inch fat, roasted	3 oz	196	0	10.6
fillet steak, lean cuts, raw *(Lean and Free)*	4 oz	116	0	2.4
prime, 1/4-inch fat, broiled	3 oz	197	0	10.5
prime, 1/4-inch fat, raw	1 oz	48	0	2.5
prime, 1/4-inch fat, roasted	3 oz	217	0	13.0
prime, short loin, 1/2-inch fat, broiled	3 oz	197	0	10.5
prime, short loin, 1/2-inch fat, roasted	3 oz	217	0	13.0
select, 0-inch fat, broiled	3 oz	170	0	7.5
select, 1/4-inch fat, broiled	3 oz	169	0	7.4
select, 1/4-inch fat, raw	1 oz	43	0	2.0
select, 1/4-inch fat, roasted	3 oz	179	0	8.8
Untrimmed				
all grades, 0-inch fat, broiled	3 oz	200	0	11.2
all grades, 1/8-inch fat, broiled	3 oz	239	0	16.2
all grades, 1/8-inch fat, raw	1 oz	77	0	6.2
all grades, 1/8-inch fat, roasted	3 oz	275	0	20.9
all grades, 1/4-inch fat, broiled	3 oz	247	0	17.2
all grades, 1/4-inch fat, raw	1 oz	80	0	6.5
all grades, 1/4-inch fat, roasted	3 oz	282	0	21.8
choice, 0-inch fat, broiled	3 oz	207	0	12.2
choice, 1/8-inch fat	3 oz	251	0	17.6
choice, 1/8-inch fat, raw	1 oz	79	0	6.3
choice, 1/8-inch fat, roasted	3 oz	281	0	21.6
choice, 1/4-inch fat, broiled	3 oz	258	0	18.6
choice, 1/4-inch fat, raw	1 oz	82	0	6.7
choice, 1/4-inch fat, roasted	3 oz	288	0	22.4
prime, 1/8-inch fat, broiled	3 oz	262	0	18.9
prime, 1/8-inch fat, raw	1 oz	78	0	6.2
prime, 1/8-inch fat, roasted	3 oz	292	0	22.7
prime, 1/4-inch fat, broiled	3 oz	269	0	19.9
prime, 1/4-inch fat, raw	1 oz	81	0	6.5
prime, 1/4-inch fat, roasted	3 oz	300	0	23.7
prime, short loin, 1/2-inch fat, broiled	3 oz	270	0	19.9
prime, short loin, 1/2-inch fat, roasted	3 oz	304	0	24.4
select, 0-inch fat, broiled	3 oz	195	0	10.6
select, 1/8-inch fat, broiled	3 oz	226	0	14.7
select, 1/8-inch fat, raw	1 oz	76	0	6.0

Food Name	Serv. Size	Total Cal.	Carbs GMS	Fat GMS
select, 1/8-inch fat, roasted	3 oz	269	0	20.1
select, 1/4-inch fat, broiled	3 oz	230	0	15.2
select, 1/4-inch fat, raw	1 oz	79	0	6.4
select, 1/4-inch fat, roasted	3 oz	275	0	21.0
THYMUS				
braised	3 oz	271	0	21.2
raw	4 oz	267	0	23.0
TONGUE				
raw	4 oz	253	4	18.2
raw	1 oz	64	1	4.6
simmered	3 oz	241	0	17.6
TRIPE				
canned *(Armour)*	6 oz	180	1	4.0
raw	4 oz	111	0	4.5
raw	1 oz	28	0	1.1
BEEF, CORNED. See also under HASH.				
Canned				
cured	1 oz	71	0	4.2
cured, sliced, 0.75-oz slices	1 slice	53	0	3.1
(Dinty Moore)	2 oz	130	0	8.0
Fresh				
brisket, cured, cooked	3 oz	213	0	16.1
brisket, cured, raw	1 oz	56	0	4.2
(Eckrich) 'Slender Sliced'	1 oz	40	1	1.0
(Healthy Deli)	1 oz	35	1	1.0
(Healthy Deli) 'St. Paddy's'	1 oz	24	1	0.4
(Hillshire Farm)	1 oz	31	1	0.4
(Oscar Mayer)	0.6 oz	17	0	0.3
BEEF, CORNED, SPREAD, canned *(Hormel)*	0.5 oz	35	0	3.0
BEEF, DRIED, SLICED				
(Armour)	1.1 oz	60	2	2.0
ground and formed, extra lean *(Hormel)*	10 slices	50	1	1.5
BEEF DINNER/ENTRÉE. See also BEEF, CORNED; BURRITO; CHILI; CHIMICHANGA; HAMBURGER ENTRÉE MIX; MEAT LOAF DINNER/ENTRÉE; RAVIOLI DISH/ENTRÉE; SANDWICH.				
(Armour)				
pepper steak, frozen, 'Classics Lite'	11.25 oz	220	29	4.0
pot roast, Yankee, frozen, 'Classics'	10 oz	310	26	12.0
Salisbury steak, frozen, 'Classics'	11.25 oz	350	26	17.0
Salisbury steak, frozen, 'Classics Lite'	11.5 oz	300	29	2.0
Salisbury steak, Parmigiana frozen, 'Classics'	11.5 oz	410	32	21.0
sirloin, roast, frozen, 'Classics'	10.45 oz	190	21	4.0
sirloin tips, frozen, 'Classics'	10.25 oz	230	20	7.0
stew, canned	8 oz	210	16	11.0
stew, microwave	7.5 oz	150	15	5.0
Stroganoff, 'Classics Lite'	11.25 oz	250	33	6.0
(Banquet)				
barbecue beef, homestyle 'Healthy Balance'	10.25 oz	270	43	5.0
barbecue beef, sliced, w/sauce, 'Cookin' Bags'	4 oz	100	11	2.0
beef enchilada and tamale entrée	1 entrée	400	56	15.0
beef entrée, frozen, 'Extra Helping'	16 oz	870	50	61.0
beef entrée, frozen, 'Platters'	10 oz	460	20	34.0
beef pie, frozen	7 oz	510	39	33.0
beef pie, frozen, 'Supreme Microwave'	7 oz	440	30	29.0
beef w/gravy, potatoes, peas in sauce	1 pkg	270	19	10.0
chicken-fried steak	1 entrée	420	39	23.0
chopped beef entrée, frozen	11 oz	420	14	32.0
creamed, chipped beef, frozen, 'Cookin' Bags'	4 oz	100	9	4.0

Food Name	Serv. Size	Total Cal.	Carbs GMS	Fat GMS
meat loaf entrée (Banquet)	1 entrée	280	23	16.0
patty, charbroiled, w/mushroom and onion gravy, frozen	8 oz	300	14	21.0
patty, charbroiled, w/mushroom gravy, frozen	8 oz	290	13	21.0
patty, w/country-style vegetables	1 entrée	310	22	20.0
patty, Western style	1 entrée	380	28	23.0
pot roast 'Yankee'	1 entrée	231	20	10.0
Salisbury steak, frozen	1 entrée	380	28	24.0
Salisbury steak, frozen	11 oz	500	26	34.0
Salisbury steak, frozen, 'Extra Helping'	18 oz	910	49	60.0
Salisbury steak, w/gravy, frozen, 'Cookin' Bags'	5 oz	190	8	14.0
Salisbury steak, w/gravy, frozen, 'Family Entrées'	8 oz	300	12	22.0
Salisbury steak, w/gravy, potatoes, corn in sauce	1 pkg	398	28	25.0
Salisbury steak, w/gravy, potatoes, corn in sauce, 'Extra Helping'	1 pkg	782	47	54.1
Salisbury steak, w/mushroom gravy, frozen, 'Extra Helping'	18 oz	890	48	58.0
Salisbury steak, charbroiled, frozen, 'Healthy Balance'	10.5 oz	270	34	8.0
sliced beef entrée	1 entrée	270	19	10.0
sliced beef, w/gravy, frozen, 'Cookin' Bags'	4 oz	100	5	5.0
stew, frozen, 'Family Entrées'	7 oz	140	18	5.0
Stroganoff, homestyle, 'Healthy Balance'	11.3 oz	360	49	12.0
Stroganoff sauce, w/noodles, 'Family Entrées'	7 oz	190	18	6.0
(Budget Gourmet)				
beef Stroganoff	1 entrée	250	30	7.0
beef Stroganoff, 'Light'	1 entrée	290	32	7.0
beef Stroganoff, frozen, 'Special Selections'	1 entrée	260	28	8.0
meatballs w/gravy, 'Light & Healthy'	1 dinner	310	37	8.0
Mexicana, frozen	12.8 oz	560	56	23.0
Oriental, 'Light'	1 entrée	270	35	8.0
pepper steak, w/rice	1 entrée	290	38	8.0
pot roast, Yankee	1 entrée	230	30	5.0
pot roast, Yankee, frozen	11 oz	380	22	21.0
roast beef w/mashed potato and gravy, frozen	1 entrée	340	33	17.0
sirloin, roast, frozen	9.5 oz	330	36	14.0
sirloin, roast, frozen, 'Supreme'	1 entrée	300	32	13.0
Salisbury steak	1 entrée	240	27	8.0
Salisbury steak, beef sirloin, 'Light'	1 entrée	240	28	5.0
Salisbury steak, w/seasoned potatoes	1 entrée	240	30	6.0
sirloin, in herb sauce, 'Light'	1 entrée	260	30	7.0
sirloin entrée, frozen, 'Light & Healthy'	1 dinner	330	40	8.0
sirloin of beef, special recipe	1 entrée	270	36	5.0
sirloin tips, in burgundy sauce, frozen	11 oz	310	28	11.0
sirloin tips, w/country style vegetables, frozen	10 oz	310	21	18.0
sirloin-cheddar melt w/potato wedges, frozen	1 entrée	370	29	21.0
stir-fry w/red potato and vegetables, 'Light & Healthy'	1 dinner	261	34	5.9
(Bryan Foods) puréed beef	1/3 cup	120	0	7.0
(Castleberry Premium)				
stew	1 pkg	918	56	58.5
stew	1 serving	331	20	21.1
(Chun King)				
teriyaki beef, frozen	13 oz	380	68	2.0
pepper beef Oriental, frozen	13 oz	310	53	3.0
Szechwan beef, frozen	13 oz	340	57	3.0
(Cripple Creek)				
beef brisket, choice, chopped, w/sauce	3 oz	150	6	9.0
(Dining Lite)				
pepper steak, frozen	9 oz	260	33	6.0
Salisbury steak, frozen	9 oz	200	14	8.0

Food Name	Serv. Size	Total Cal.	Carbs GMS	Fat GMS
teriyaki beef, frozen	9 oz	270	36	5.0
(Dinty Moore)				
beef entrée, packaged, 'Micro Meal'	1 bowl	260	21	13.0
meat loaf, w/gravy and mashed potatoes, canned	1 bowl	300	27	13.0
meat loaf w/mashed potatoes and gravy, 'American Classics'	10 oz	262	26	9.0
roasted beef, w/gravy and mashed potatoes, canned	1 bowl	240	25	5.0
roasted beef, w/gravy and potatoes, microwave, 'Classics'	10 oz	260	26	6.0
stew, canned	1 cup	222	16	13.1
stew, microwave bowl	10 oz	260	19	14.0
stew, microwave cup	7.5 oz	180	15	9.0
(Estee) stew, canned	7.5 oz	210	15	11.0
(Featherweight) stew, canned	7.5 oz	160	17	3.0
(Freezer Queen)				
beef patty, charbroiled, frozen	10 oz	300	20	17.0
beef patty, charbroiled, w/mushroom and onion gravy, frozen	7 oz	200	10	12.0
beef patty, charbroiled, w/mushroom gravy, frozen	7 oz	180	9	11.0
beef w/peppers in sauce, w/rice, 'Single Serve'	9 oz	260	38	3.0
creamed, chipped beef, frozen, 'Cook-In-Pouch'	5 oz	80	11	2.0
meat loaf, w/tomato sauce, frozen, 'Family Suppers'	7 oz	230	15	13.0
Salisbury steak, frozen	10 oz	380	28	22.0
Salisbury steak, w/gravy, frozen, 'Cook-In-Pouch'	5 oz	160	7	11.0
Salisbury steak, w/gravy, frozen 'Family Suppers'	7 oz	200	9	13.0
Salisbury steak, charbroiled, w/vegetable medley, frozen	9 oz	330	14	22.0
sliced beef w/gravy, frozen	10 oz	210	18	7.0
sliced beef w/gravy, frozen, 'Cook-In-Pouch'	4 oz	60	4	1.0
sliced beef w/gravy, 'Deluxe Family Suppers'	7 oz	130	10	3.0
sliced beef w/mashed potatoes and carrots	1 pkg	207	26	4.8
stew, frozen, 'Family Suppers'	7 oz	150	15	6.0
(Gebhardt)				
beef tamale	1 serving	134	9	10.3
beef tamale, food service product	1 serving	321	26	24.2
(Green Giant)				
burgers, Italian style, frozen	1 burger	140	8	4.5
burgers, original, frozen	1 burger	140	8	4.0
burgers, Southwest style, frozen	1 burger	140	9	4.0
(Healthy Choice)				
barbecue beef, sirloin w/sauce	11 oz	280	44	4.0
beef Bejing, w/broccoli	1 entrée	300	45	4.5
beef Cantonese, w/peppers	1 entrée	280	32	7.0
beef casserole w/macaroni	1 entrée	220	34	4.0
beef dinner w/mesquite, w/barbecue sauce, mashed potato, corn	1 pkg	320	38	9.0
beef macaroni, frozen	1 serving	211	33	2.2
beef patty, charbroiled	1 entrée	280	41	6.0
beef ribs, boneless, w/barbecue sauce, frozen, 11 oz	1 serving	330	40	6.0
beef Stroganoff	1 entrée	310	44	7.0
beef tips, 'Traditional'	1 entrée	260	32	6.0
beef tips Francais	1 entrée	300	40	7.0
meat loaf, 'Traditional'	1 entrée	330	52	7.0
mesquite barbecue beef	1 entrée	320	38	9.0
pepper steak, frozen	9.5 oz	250	36	4.0
pepper steak, Oriental (Healthy Choice)	1 entrée	260	34	5.0
peppercorn steak patty, grilled	1 entrée	220	26	6.0
pot roast 'Yankee'	1 entrée	290	38	7.0
roasted beef, chopped and formed, 'Fresh Trak'	1 slice	30	1	1.0
Salisbury steak, w/mushroom gravy, mashed potato, corn, frozen	1 entrée	326	48	6.9

Food Name	Serv. Size	Total Cal.	Carbs GMS	Fat GMS
sirloin tips, traditional, frozen	1 meal	260	32	5.0
(Hereford)				
roasted beef w/gravy, canned, ready-to-serve	2/3 cup	165	12	3.0
(Hormel)				
beef steak, breaded, frozen	4 oz	370	13	30.0
beef w/mushrooms, micro cup, 'Health Selections'	7 oz	210	25	3.0
dried beef, sliced, ground and formed, extra lean	10 slices	50	1	1.5
stew, microwave cup	7.5 oz	230	11	15.0
(La Choy)				
beef chow mein, bi-pack	1 cup	105	15	1.7
beef chow mein, canned *(LaChoy)*	3/4 cup	40	5	2.0
beef pepper Oriental, bi-pack	1 cup	104	11	2.7
beef pepper Oriental, frozen, food service product	1 cup	150	30	0.7
beef w/broccoli and rice, frozen, 'Fresh & Lite'	11 oz	260	42	5.0
pepper beef, canned	3/4 cup	100	12	4.0
pepper steak.	1 serving	175	37	0.8
pepper steak, frozen	3.81 oz	36	7	0.2
pepper steak, frozen, w/rice and vegetables, 'Fresh & Lite'	10 oz	280	33	8.0
teriyaki beef, w/rice and vegetables, frozen, 'Fresh & Lite'	10 oz	240	40	5.0
(Le Menu)				
pepper steak, frozen	11.5 oz	370	36	13.0
Salisbury steak, frozen	10.5 oz	370	28	20.0
Salisbury steak, frozen, 'Lightstyle'	10 oz	280	31	9.0
sirloin, chopped, frozen	12.25 oz	430	28	24.0
sirloin tips, frozen	11.5 oz	400	29	18.0
Stroganoff	10 oz	430	28	24.0
(Lean Cuisine)				
beef chop suey, frozen	1 oz	16	2	0.5
beef Oriental	1 entrée	250	30	8.0
beef patty and whipped potatoes, 'Hearty Portions'	1 entrée	370	43	9.0
beef tips barbecue	1 entrée	290	47	6.0
beef w/peppercorns	1 entrée	220	23	7.0
homestyle beef and noodles, 'Hearty Portions'	1 entrée	330	46	7.0
meat loaf	1 entrée	250	30	6.0
meat loaf, w/macaroni and cheese, frozen	9 3/8 oz	280	26	8.0
meat loaf, w/whipped potatoes	1 entrée	250	25	7.0
Oriental beef, w/vegetables and rice, frozen	1 entrée	242	36	4.8
oven roasted beef	1 entrée	260	28	8.0
pot roast	1 entrée	210	25	6.0
pot roast w/whipped potatoes	1 entrée	210	21	7.0
Salisbury steak, w/gravy, frozen, food service product	1 oz	34	2	1.4
Salisbury steak, w/gravy and scalloped potatoes, frozen	9.5 oz	240	22	7.0
Salisbury steak, w/macaroni and cheese, frozen	1 entrée	270	27	8.0
sirloin, peppercorn, frozen, 'Cafe Classics'	1 pkg	210	24	7.0
(Lean Magic)				
mesquite beef patty, flame-broiled	1 piece	138	3	6.4
Salisbury steak, flame broiled	1 piece	148	4	7.2
Salisbury steak, flame broiled, '30'	1 piece	110	4	3.7
(Libby's)				
beef and macaroni, microwave cup, 'Diner'	7.75 oz	230	34	6.0
roasted beef w/gravy	2/3 cup	140	2	3.0
stew, canned, 15 oz package	7.5 oz	160	18	5.0
stew, microwave cup, 'Diner'	7.75 oz	240	22	12.0
stew, hearty, 'Microeasy' prepared	1/4 pkg	370	14	20.0
(Lunch Bucket) stew, hearty, microwave cup	7.5 oz	180	13	11.0
(Lunch Express) beef Oriental	1 entrée	290	43	8.0
(Lloyd's) barbecue beef, w/hickory smoked sauce	1/2 cup	200	21	7.0

Food Name	Serv. Size	Total Cal.	Carbs GMS	Fat GMS
(Marie Callender's)				
meat loaf, w/mashed potatoes and gravy	14 oz	540	42	30.0
pot roast, old fashioned, w/gravy	1 cup	260	31	7.0
Salisbury steak, sirloin, w/gravy	14 oz	550	51	25.0
Yankee pot pie	10-oz pie	690	57	44.0
(Michelina's) Cantonese chow mein, 'Lean n Tasty'	1 entrée	250	42	4.5
(Morton)				
Salisbury steak, frozen	10 oz	300	23	17.0
sliced beef, frozen	10 oz	220	20	5.0
(Mountain House)				
beef w/rice and onions, freeze-dried, prepared.	1 cup	330	42	12.0
stew, freeze-dried, prepared	1 cup	260	26	9.0
Stroganoff, freeze-dried, prepared	1 cup	270	26	13.0
(Myers)				
beef pie, frozen	3.5 oz	123	10	6.0
creamed, chipped beef, frozen	3.5 oz	136	7	8.0
Stroganoff	3.5 oz	112	7	6.0
(Nalley's)				
stew, canned, 'Big Chunk'	7.5 oz	200	24	7.0
stew, canned, 'Homestyle'	8 oz	180	22	5.0
(Nestlé)				
stew, 'Chef-Mate'	1 pkg	2305	228	74.0
stew, 'Chef-Mate'	1 cup	192	19	6.1
(Pathmark) stew, canned, 'No Frills'	8 oz	190	25	4.0
(Pierre)				
beef and onion patty, breaded, flame-broiled, frozen, 'Two-Fers'	1 piece	96	1	7.8
beef and onion patty, flame-broiled, frozen, product 3879	1 piece	161	2	9.8
beef and onion patty, flame-broiled, frozen, product 9675	1 piece	177	2	11.7
beef and onion patty, flame-broiled, frozen, product 9680	1 piece	473	4	38.4
beef finger, country-fried, frozen, product 3714	1 piece	79	3	5.5
beef finger, country-fried, frozen, product 3813	1 piece	82	4	5.5
beef finger, country-fried, frozen, product 3814	1 piece	100	4	7.0
beef nugget, country-fried, frozen, product 1910	1 piece	54	2	4.0
beef nugget, country-fried, frozen, product 1935	1 piece	49	2	3.4
beef nugget, country-fried, frozen, product 3711	1 piece	47	2	3.1
beef nugget, country-fried, frozen, product 3811	1 piece	51	2	3.1
beef patty, country-fried, frozen, product 1840	1 piece	356	16	24.8
beef patty, country-fried, frozen, product 1845	1 piece	292	14	20.3
beef patty, country-fried, frozen, product 3712	1 piece	306	16	20.1
beef patty, country-fried, frozen, product 3713	1 piece	360	17	24.6
beef patty, country-fried, frozen, product 3812	1 piece	304	15	19.9
beef patty, deluxe, flame-broiled, frozen, product 9100	1 piece	216	2	15.9
beef patty, deluxe, flame-broiled, frozen, product 9110	1 piece	160	1	11.8
beef patty, flame-broiled, frozen, product 3771	1 piece	153	2	8.9
beef patty, flame-broiled, frozen, product 3774	1 piece	211	2	12.3
beef patty, flame-broiled, frozen, product 3781	1 piece	154	2	9.0
beef patty, flame-broiled, frozen, product 3871	1 piece	158	2	9.5
beef patty, flame-broiled, frozen, product 3874	1 piece	218	2	13.1
beef patty, flame-broiled, frozen, product 3881	1 piece	158	2	9.6
beef patty, flame-broiled, frozen, product 9220	1 piece	186	2	15.1
beef patty, flame-broiled, frozen, product 9230	1 piece	229	2	18.6
beef patty, jalapeño, flame-broiled, product 3778	1 piece	154	2	9.0
beef patty, jalapeño, flame-broiled, frozen, product 3878	1 piece	159	2	9.6
beef patty, less fat, flame-broiled, product 3772	1 piece	143	2	7.9
beef patty, mesquite, deluxe, flame-broiled, frozen, product 9103	1 piece	216	2	16.3

Food Name	Serv. Size	Total Cal.	Carbs GMS	Fat GMS
beef patty, mesquite, flame-broiled, frozen, product 3870	1 piece	158	2	9.5
beef patty, mesquite, flame-broiled, frozen, product 3880	1 piece	159	2	9.6
beef patty, mesquite, flame-broiled, product 3770	1 piece	153	2	8.9
beef patty, mesquite, flame-broiled, product 3780	1 piece	154	2	9.0
beef patty w/onions, flame-broiled, product 3779	1 piece	153	2	8.8
beef steak, country-fried, frozen, product 3710	1 piece	315	14	21.0
beef steak, country-fried, frozen, product 1610	1 piece	356	14	25.6
beef steak, country-fried, frozen, product 3810	1 piece	343	16	21.1
beef steak, flame-broiled, frozen, product 9010	1 piece	249	0	18.9
beef steak, flame-broiled, frozen, product 9017	1 piece	237	1	17.4
beef steak, flame-broiled, frozen, product 9503	1 piece	177	1	12.0
beef steak, flame-broiled, product 3760	1 piece	164	1	10.2
beef steak, flame-broiled, product 3765	1 piece	164	1	10.2
beef steak, flame-broiled, product 3860	1 piece	189	1	12.8
beef steak, mesquite, flame-broiled, frozen, product 3863	1 piece	194	1	13.1
beef steak, mesquite, flame-broiled, product 3763	1 piece	169	1	10.5
flame-broiled, frozen, 'Two-Fers' product 9684	1 piece	98	1	7.8
meat loaf, flame-broiled, product 3724	1 piece	162	4	9.1
meat loaf, flame-broiled, product 3725	1 piece	152	4	8.2
meat loaf, flame-broiled, frozen, product 3824	1 piece	170	4	10.1
mesquite beef patty, flame-broiled, less fat, product 3773	1 piece	145	3	7.9
New York strip, flame-broiled, frozen, product 3877	1 piece	164	2	10.2
New York strip, flame-broiled, product 3777	1 piece	159	2	9.5
Salisbury steak, flame-broiled, frozen, product 3820	1 piece	161	3	9.8
Salisbury steak, flame-broiled, frozen, product 9600	1 piece	186	2	12.4
Salisbury steak, flame-broiled, less fat	1 piece	147	3	8.2
Salisbury steak, flame-broiled, product 3720	1 piece	157	2	9.3
(Pillsbury) casserole, frozen, 'Microwave Classic'	1 pkg	430	34	25.0
(Rib-B-Q)				
beef and onion patty, flame-broiled, frozen, 'Lean Magic'	1 piece	138	2	6.7
beef and turkey barbecue, flame-broiled, frozen, product				
9126, 'Lean Magic 30'	1 piece	116	8	3.1
beef and turkey patty, flame-broiled, w/tangy glaze,				
'Lean Magic 30'	1 piece	120	7	3.1
beef and turkey patty, flame-broiled, w/teriyaki sauce,				
'Lean Magic 30'	1 piece	28	2	0.7
beef barbecue, flame-broiled, frozen, product 3732,				
'Lean Magic 30'	1 piece	139	4	7.3
beef patty, flame-broiled, 'Lean Magic'	1 piece	136	2	6.5
beef rib barbecue, flame-broiled, frozen, product 3733	1 piece	154	3	8.6
beef rib barbecue, flame-broiled, frozen, product 3833	1 piece	175	3	10.7
beef rib barbecue, flame-broiled, frozen, product 4150	1 piece	204	3	15.9
beef rib barbecue, flame-broiled, frozen, product 3832,				
'Lean Magic'	1 piece	156	3	9.0
(Rice A Roni)				
beef and mushroom rice dish, prepared	2.5 oz	164	29	3.4
(Right Course)				
Dijon beef, w/pasta and vegetables, frozen	9.5 oz	290	31	9.0
fiesta, w/corn pasta	8 7/8 oz	270	33	7.0
pot roast, homestyle, frozen	9.25 oz	220	22	7.0
ragout, w/rice pilaf, frozen	10 oz	300	38	8.0
(Steak-Umm) sandwich steak	2 oz	180	0	16.0
(Stouffer's)				
beef pie.	1 entrée	450	36	26.0
beef pot pie.	1 pie	415	41	23.0
beef stew, frozen, food service product	1 oz	23	2	1.0
beef Stroganoff, frozen, food service product	1 oz	41	1	2.7

Food Name	Serv. Size	Total Cal.	Carbs GMS	Fat GMS
beef Stroganoff w/noodles	1 entrée	390	30	20.0
creamed chipped beef entrée	1 entrée	160	6	11.0
creamed chipped beef, frozen	1 pkg	435	18	29.5
creamed chipped beef, frozen	1 serving	175	7	11.9
creamed chipped beef, frozen, food service product	1 oz	40	1	2.8
homestyle beef w/noodles, gravy, vegetable	8 3/8 oz	230	26	7.0
meat loaf, w/whipped potatoes, 'Homestyle'	1 entrée	390	24	24.0
pepper steak, beef w/rice, frozen.	10.5 oz	310	35	10.0
Salisbury steak, w/gravy, macaroni and cheese, frozen	9 5/8 oz	350	23	17.0
Salisbury steak w/gravy, macaroni and cheese, 'Homestyle'	1 pkg	386	26	21.2
steak w/green pepper	1 entrée	330	45	9.0
(Swanson)				
barbecue beef w/sauce	11 oz	460	51	17.0
beef enchilada entrée	1 entrée	500	68	16.0
beef entrée, frozen	11.25 oz	310	38	6.0
beef pot pie, 'Hungry Man'	1 pie	660	70	31.0
beef w/gravy.	1 entrée	370	40	15.0
chopped beef steak, frozen, 'Hungry Man'	16.75 oz	640	41	37.0
chopped sirloin w/gravy	1 entrée	380	37	14.0
meat loaf	1 entrée	380	37	14.0
Salisbury steak	1 entrée	340	35	15.0
Salisbury steak, frozen, 'Homestyle Recipe'	10 oz	320	22	16.0
Salisbury steak, in gravy, w/mashed potatoes, frozen	1 entrée	330	24	18.0
Salisbury steak, frozen, 'Hungry Man'.	1 entrée	610	46	33.0
sirloin, chopped, frozen	10.75 oz	340	28	16.0
sirloin tips, in burgundy sauce, frozen, 'Homestyle Recipe'	7 oz	160	16	5.0
sirloin tips, w/noodles and beef gravy, frozen	1 entrée	290	34	11.0
sliced beef, frozen, 'Hungry Man'	15.25 oz	450	49	12.0
(Top Shelf)				
beef and potatoes, microwave bowl	1 serving	254	22	6.0
beef entrée, packaged	10 oz	320	22	15.0
beef ribs, boneless, packaged, microwave bowl	1 serving	440	29	24.0
beef sukiyaki, packaged, microwave bowl	1 serving	330	36	10.0
Oriental beef entrée, packaged, microwave bowl	1 serving	290	25	10.0
roasted beef, tender, frozen	10 oz	240	19	6.0
roasted beef, tender, packaged, microwave bowl	1 serving	240	18	7.0
Stroganoff, microwave bowl	1 serving	320	24	12.0
(Tyson)				
champignon, frozen, 'Gourmet Selection'	10.5 oz	370	31	15.0
pepper steak, beef, frozen, 'Gourmet Selection'	11.25 oz	330	38	11.0
pot roast w/potatoes, 'Homestyle'	1 entrée	270	25	10.0
Salisbury steak, supreme, frozen, 'Gourmet Selection'	10 oz	430	34	26.0
short ribs in gravy, frozen	9 oz	350	12	20.0
short ribs, frozen, 'Gourmet Selection'	11 oz	470	38	24.0
stir-fry, w/rice, Oriental vegetables, frozen	1 pkg	867	142	10.0
stir-fry, w/rice, Oriental vegetables, frozen	1 serving	433	71	5.0
(Ultra Slim-Fast)				
beef w/mushroom gravy, frozen	10.5 oz	290	44	5.0
meat loaf, beef, w/tomato sauce, frozen	10.5 oz	340	52	9.0
pepper steak, beef, w/parsley rice, frozen	12 oz	270	36	4.0
(Weight Watchers)				
beef Cantonese, w/rice, frozen, 'Stir Fry'	9 oz	200	27	4.0
beef Romanoff, supreme, w/pasta and vegetables, frozen	9 oz	230	29	7.0
beef stir-fry, frozen, 'Jade Garden'	9 oz	150	17	3.0
London broil, frozen, 'Ultimate 200'	7.5 oz	110	4	3.0
London broil, in mushroom sauce, frozen	7.37 oz	140	9	3.0
pepper steak	1 entrée	240	33	4.5

Food Name	Serv. Size	Total Cal.	Carbs GMS	Fat GMS
Salisbury steak, grilled, w/gravy	1 entrée	260	24	10.0
sirloin tips, frozen, 'Ultimate 200'	7.5 oz	200	20	6.0
stew, chunky, microwave cup	7.5 oz	120	14	2.0
(Wolf Brand) stew, canned	1 cup	179	18	7.5
(Yu Sing)				
beef and pepper Oriental, w/rice	1 container	230	38	5.0
BEEF DINNER/ENTRÉE MIX. See also HAMBURGER ENTRÉE MIX.				
(Hamburger Helper) meat loaf mix, prepared	1 slice	270	11	14.0
(Lipton)				
meat loaf mix, homestyle, mix only, 'Microeasy'	1/4 pkg	90	15	1.0
meat loaf mix, homestyle, prepared w/ground beef,				
'Microeasy'	1/4 pkg	390	15	22.0
BEEF JERKY				
chopped and formed	1 oz	116	3	7.3
cured, dried	1 oz	47	0	1.1
(Eagle)				
kippered beefsteak	0.8 oz	50	1	0.5
kippered beefsteak, hot	0.8 oz	50	2	0.5
kippered turkey steak	0.8 oz	60	2	1.5
(Frito-Lay's)				
	0.21-oz piece	25	1	1.0
'Tender'	0.7 oz	120	2	10.0
(Hickory Farms)	1 oz	100	4	3.0
(Hormel) 'Lumberjack'	1 oz	101	0	9.0
(Pemmican)				
'Arrowhead'	0.7-oz piece	70	2	3.0
'Steakers'	0.14-oz piece	40	2	1.0
jalapeno	0.25 oz	25	1	1.0
natural	0.25 oz	25	1	1.0
peppered	0.25 oz	25	1	1.0
Tabasco	0.25 oz	25	1	1.0
'Tender Brave'	1 oz	80	2	2.0
'Tender Chief'	1 oz	80	2	2.0
'Tender Tomahawk'	0.25 oz	20	1	1.0
'Tender Trail'	1 oz	80	2	2.0
'Tender Tribe'	1 oz	80	2	2.0
teriyaki	0.25 oz	20	1	1.0
(Rustlers Roundup)	5 servings	20	1	1.5
(Slim Jim)				
'Big Jerk'	0.25-oz piece	25	1	1.0
'Giant Jerk'	0.63-oz piece	60	2	2.0
	0.14-oz piece	20	1	1.0
regular, 'Super Jerk'	0.31-oz piece	30	1	1.0
Tabasco 'Super Jerk'	0.31-oz piece	30	1	1.0
(Tumen)				
hot pepperoni style	1/2 oz	50	2	2.0
smoked ham style	1/2 oz	50	2	2.0
spicy Italian style	1/2 oz	50	2	2.0
BEEF SEASONING. See under HAMBURGER ENTRÉE MIX; MARINADE; MARINADE MIX; SEASONING MIX.				
BEEF STEW. See under BEEF DINNER/ENTRÉE.				
BEEF SPREAD				
(Hormel) roast beef, canned	0.5 oz	31	0	2.0
(Underwood)				
roast beef, canned	2 1/8 oz	140	1	11.0
roast beef, canned, 'Light'	2 1/8 oz	90	2	6.0
roast beef, canned, mesquite smoked	2 1/8 oz	126	1	11.0

Food Name	Serv. Size	Total Cal.	Carbs GMS	Fat GMS
BEEF STICK				
(Eagle)	1 oz	110	1	9.0
(Eagle) pepperoni sausage	1.25 oz	150	3	11.0
BEEF SUBSTITUTE				
(Heartline)				
lite, vegetarian, 'Beef Fillet Style'	0.5 oz	22	1	0.0
lite, vegetarian, 'Ground Beef Style'	0.5 oz	22	1	0.0
vegetarian, 'Beef Fillet Style'	2 oz	176	9	7.0
vegetarian, 'Ground Beef Style'	2 oz	176	9	7.0
vegetarian, 'Teriyaki Beef Style'	2 oz	176	9	7.0
(Morningstar Farms)				
ground beef substitute, vegetarian, 'Burger Style Recipe Crumbles'	2/3 cup	80	4	2.5
ground beef substitute, vegetarian, 'Ground Meatless'	1/2 cup	60	4	0.0
(Worthington)				
beef style, vegetarian, meatless	1 slice	113	4	6.8
corned beef style, vegetarian, roll, frozen	2.5 oz	150	9	7.0
corned beef style, vegetarian, frozen, approx 2-oz slices	4 slices	120	8	6.0
ground beef style, vegetarian, 'Burger Crumbles'	1 pkg	3809	109	213.1
ground beef style, vegetarian, 'Burger Crumbles'	1 cup	231	7	12.9
ground beef style, vegetarian, 'Burger Crumbles'	1 serving	116	3	6.5
roll, vegetarian, frozen, approx 2.5-oz slices	4 slices	130	7	6.0
smoked, roll, frozen, approx. 2-oz slices	3 slices	120	7	6.0
steak style, 'Stakelets'	1 serving	144	6	8.0
(White Wave)				
roast beef style, vegetarian, sandwich sliced	1 slice	90	8	0.0
BEEF SUBSTITUTE DINNER/ENTRÉE				
(Amy's Kitchen)				
burger, vegetarian, 'California'	1 serving	100	17	3.0
burger, vegetarian, organic, frozen	2.5-oz burger	173	22	4.0
Salisbury steak, meatless, 'Country Dinner'	1 entrée	420	63	16.0
(Boca Burger)				
burger, vegetarian, frozen, 'Chef Max's Favorite'	1 burger	110	9	0.0
burger, vegetarian, original, frozen	1 burger	84	9	0.0
(Fantastic Foods)				
burger, tofu, vegetarian, prepared w/o cooking fat	3.4-oz burger	133	14	5.0
(Gardenburger)				
burger, vegetarian, original	2.5 oz	130	18	2.9
burger, vegetarian, soy-free	2.5 oz	140	21	2.5
burger, Greek, classic, vegetarian, 'Gourmet'	2.5 oz	121	17	2.9
hamburger style, vegetarian, low-fat	2.5 oz	115	7	2.6
veggie medley patty, vegetarian	2.5 oz	100	17	0.7
zesty bean patty, vegetarian	2.5 oz	120	19	2.5
(Green Giant)				
burger, vegetable protein, vegetarian, original, 'Harvest Burger'	1 pkg	552	28	16.7
burger, vegetable protein, vegetarian, original, 'Harvest Burger'	1 patty	137	7	4.1
burger, vegetarian, all-vegetable, Southwestern style, 'Harvest Burger'	1 patty	140	9	4.0
(Heartline) burger, vegetarian, meatless	4 oz	176	9	7.0
(Ken & Robert's)				
burger, vegetarian	1 serving	130	26	1.0
burger, vegetarian, frozen, 2.5 oz, 'Truly Amazing'	1 patty	110	19	2.0
(Legume)				
stew, beef style	1 cup	150	29	0.0
tamale, beef style, vegetarian, low-fat	3 tamales	220	40	2.5
(Loma Linda)				
burger, vegetarian, dry mix, 'Patty Mix'	1/3 cup	90	7	1.0

Food Name	Serv. Size	Total Cal.	Carbs GMS	Fat GMS
dinner loaf, dry mix, 'Savory Dinner Loaf' .... 1/3 cup		90	7	1.5
(Love Natural Foods)				
burger, vegetarian, prepared, 'Loveburger' .... 4-oz burger		245	20	11.0
(Morningstar Farms)				
burger, vegetarian, 'Better'N Burgers' .... 1 patty		80	8	0.0
burger, vegetarian, 'Grillers' .... 1 patty		140	5	6.0
burger, vegetarian, 'Hard Rock Café All-Natural Veggie Burgers' .... 1 patty		170	18	8.0
burger, vegetarian, 'Harvest Burgers' Italian style .... 1 patty		140	8	4.5
burger, vegetarian, 'Harvest Burgers' original flavor .... 1 patty		140	8	4.0
burger, vegetarian, 'Harvest Burgers' Southwestern style .... 1 patty		140	9	4.0
burger, vegetarian, 'Harvest Burgers' recipe crumbles .... 1/2 cup		70	5	0.0
burger, vegetarian, frozen, 'Oven Roasted Veggie Burgers' ..... 1 patty		120	40	8.0
burger, vegetarian, 'Quarter Prime' .... 1 patty		140	6	2.0
burger, vegetarian, and cheese, 'Stuffed Sandwiches' ...... 1 sandwich		290	10	8.0
(Natural Touch)				
burger, vegetarian, 'Hard Rock Cafe All Natural Veggie Burgers' .... 1 patty		170	18	8.0
burger, vegetarian, 'Vegan Burger' .... 1 patty		70	6	0.0
'Loaf Mix' dry mix .... 4 tbsp		100	10	0.5
'Stroganoff Mix' dry mix .... 4 tbsp		90	10	3.5
(Naturally Tofu) burger, vegetarian, meatless .... 4 oz		165	25	2.0
(Nature's Burger)				
burger, vegetarian, prepared w/o cooking fat, 'Original' ..... 3-oz burger		152	21	4.0
burger, barbecue, vegetarian, prepared w/o cooking fat .... 3-oz burger		117	24	0.8
burger, pizza, vegetarian, prepared w/o cooking fat .... 3-oz burger		121	24	1.0
(Tempeh) burger, soy and rice, vegetarian, frozen .... 2 2/3 oz		140	13	5.0
(White Wave)				
burger, vegetarian, 'Veggielife' .... 1 serving		130	20	3.5
tempeh burger, vegetarian .... 1 serving		110	10	2.5
(Worthington)				
burger, vegetarian, 'FriPats' .... 1 patty		132	4	6.3
burger, vegetarian, 'Vegetarian Burger' .... 1/4 cup		60	2	2.0
'Meatless Corned Beef' 72-oz roll .... 3/8-inch slice		130	4	9.0
'Meatless Corned Beef' 8-oz carton .... 4 slices		140	5	9.0
'Meatless Smoked Beef' .... 6 slices		120	6	6.0
pie, vegetarian, frozen .... 8 oz		360	44	16.0
stew, vegetarian, 'Country Stew' .... 1 cup		210	20	9.0
roast, vegetarian, 'Dinner Roast' .... 3/4-inch slice		180	5	12.0
sliced, vegetarian, 'Savory Slices' .... 3 slices		150	6	9.0
steak, vegetarian, 'Prime Stakes' .... 1 piece		136	4	9.3
steak, vegetarian, 'Stakelets' .... 1 piece		140	6	8.0
steak, vegetarian, 'Vegetable Steaks' .... 2 slices		80	3	1.5
BEEF SUBSTITUTE DINNER/ENTRÉE MIX				
(Fantastic Foods)				
Stroganoff, creamy, 'Tofu Classics' mix only .... 1/2 cup		190	35	5.0
(Loma Linda) vegetarian 'Vita-Burger Chunks' .... 1/4 cup		75	6	1.1
(Tofu Classics)				
Stroganoff, creamy, vegetarian, prepared w/tofu .... 1/2 cup		94	11	3.0
Stroganoff, creamy, vegetarian, prepared w/tofu, 2 tbsp salted butter .... 1/2 cup		127	11	7.0
BEEF SUBSTITUTE JERKY				
original flavor, meatless *(Pemmican)* .... 1 pkg		420	59	13.0
vegetarian, 'Spicy Italian Style' *(Cajun Jerky)* .... 0.5 oz		50	2	2.0
vegetable protein, 'Jerquee' *(Stonewall's)* .... 0.5 oz		50	2	2.0
BEEF TALLOW				
.... 1 cup		1849	0	205.0
.... 1 tbsp		115	0	12.8

Food Name	Serv. Size	Total Cal.	Carbs GMS	Fat GMS
BEEFALO				
composite of cuts, raw	1 oz	41	0	1.4
composite of cuts, roasted	3 oz	160	0	5.4
BEER, ALE				
ALE				
(McSorley's)	12 fl oz	166	15	0.0
(Tiger Head)	12 fl oz	166	15	0.0
BEER				
....	12 fl oz	146	13	0.0
light	12 fl oz	99	5	0.0
(Anheuser Marzen)	12 fl oz	168	15	0.0
(Beck's)	12 fl oz	148	10	0.0
(Budweiser)				
....	12 fl oz	144	11	0.0
light, 'Bud Light'	12 fl oz	110	7	0.0
(Busch)	12 fl oz	144	12	0.0
(Carlsberg)				
....	12 fl oz	149	12	0.0
light	12 fl oz	110	7	0.0
(Coors)				
....	12 fl oz	137	12	0.0
'Coors Dry'	12 fl oz	119	6	0.0
'Extra Gold'	12 fl oz	151	13	0.0
light, 'Coors Light'	12 fl oz	103	5	0.0
3.2%	12 fl oz	119	10	0.0
3.2%, 'Coors Dry'	12 fl oz	101	5	0.0
3.2%, 'Extra Gold'	12 fl oz	121	10	0.0
3.2, light, 'Coors Light'	12 fl oz	98	5	0.0
(Cutter) nonalcoholic	12 fl oz	76	20	0.0
(Dribeck's)	12 fl oz	94	7	0.0
(Kaliber) nonalcoholic	12 fl oz	71	11	0.0
(Keystone)				
....	12 fl oz	121	7	0.0
'Keystone Dry'	12 fl oz	121	6	0.0
light, 'Keystone Light'	12 fl oz	100	4	0.0
3.2%	12 fl oz	104	6	0.0
3.2%, light, 'Keystone Light'	12 fl oz	99	5	0.0
(Killian's)				
....	12 fl oz	161	15	0.0
3.2%	12 fl oz	128	11	0.0
(Knickerbocker)	12 fl oz	140	12	0.0
(LA) light alcohol	12 fl oz	114	16	0.0
(Lite)				
....	12 fl oz	96	3	0.0
'Genuine Draft'	12 fl oz	98	4	0.0
(Lowenbrau)				
'Dark Special'	12 fl oz	158	14	0.0
'Special'	12 fl oz	158	14	0.0
(Meister Brau)				
....	12 fl oz	141	13	0.0
light	12 fl oz	98	4	0.0
(Michelob)				
....	12 fl oz	156	14	0.0
'Classic Dark'	12 fl oz	158	14	0.0
'Dry'	12 fl oz	133	8	0.0
light	12 fl oz	134	12	0.0
(Miller)				
'Genuine Draft'	12 fl oz	147	13	0.0

Food Name	Serv. Size	Total Cal.	Carbs GMS	Fat GMS
'High-Life'	12 fl oz	147	13	0.0
'Magnum'	12 fl oz	162	10	0.0
(Milwaukee)				
'Milwaukee's Best'	12 fl oz	133	11	0.0
'Milwaukee's Best Light'	12 fl oz	98	4	0.0
(Natural Light) light	12 fl oz	110	7	0.0
(O'Doul's) nonalcoholic	12 fl oz	70	15	0.0
(Prior) 'Double Dark'	12 fl oz	171	15	0.0
(Rheingold)				
	12 fl oz	148	13	0.0
light	12 fl oz	96	3	0.0
(Rolling Rock)				
light	12 fl oz	104	8	0.0
'Premium'	12 fl oz	145	10	0.0
(Schmidt's)				
	12 fl oz	148	13	0.0
'Classic'	12 fl oz	144	13	0.0
light	12 fl oz	96	3	0.0
(Sharp's) nonalcoholic	12 fl oz	86	10	0.0
BEET				
Fresh				
boiled, drained, whole, approx 2-inch diam	2 med beets	44	10	0.2
boiled, drained, sliced	1/2 cup	37	8	0.2
raw, sliced	1 cup	58	13	0.2
raw, whole, approx 2-inch diam	1 med beet	35	8	0.1
Canned				
cut *(Stokely)*	1/2 cup	40	8	0.0
diced *(S&W)*	1/2 cup	40	9	0.0
diced *(Stokely)*	1/2 cup	35	7	0.0
diced, drained	1 cup	49	11	0.2
Harvard *(Green Giant)*	1/3 cup	60	15	0.0
Harvard *(Stokely)*	1/2 cup	70	18	0.0
Harvard, sliced, w/liquid	1 cup	180	45	0.1
no salt, 'No Salt or Sugar Added' *(Stokely)*	1/2 cup	40	8	0.0
no salt, w/liquid	1 cup	69	16	0.2
pickled *(Freshlike)*	1/2 cup	40	9	0.0
pickled *(Stokely)*	1/2 cup	100	25	0.0
pickled *(Veg-All)*	1/2 cup	100	25	0.0
pickled, crinkle sliced, w/liquid *(Del Monte)*	1/2 cup	80	19	0.0
pickled, sliced, w/liquid	1 cup	148	37	0.2
pickled, sliced, w/red wine vinegar, 'Party' *(S&W)*	1 oz	15	4	0.0
pickled, sliced, w/red wine vinegar, regular *(S&W)*	1/2 cup	70	16	0.0
pickled, whole *(S&W)*	1 oz	15	4	0.0
pickled, whole, extra small *(S&W)*	1/2 cup	70	16	0.0
regular pack, w/liquid	1 cup	69	16	0.2
shredded, drained	1 cup	60	14	0.3
sliced *(A&P)*	1/2 cup	40	9	1.0
sliced *(Featherweight)*	1/2 cup	45	10	0.0
sliced *(Finast)*	1/2 cup	40	9	0.0
sliced *(Green Giant)*	1/2 cup	35	8	0.0
sliced *(Pathmark)*	1/2 cup	45	10	0.0
sliced *(Stokely)*	1/2 cup	40	8	0.0
sliced, no salt added *(Finast)*	1/2 cup	40	9	0.0
sliced, no salt added *(A&P)*	1/2 cup	35	8	1.0
sliced, no salt added *(Green Giant)*	1/2 cup	35	8	0.0
sliced, no salt added *(Pathmark)*	1/2 cup	35	7	0.0
sliced, 'Nutradiet' *(S&W)*	1/2 cup	35	9	0.0

Food Name	Serv. Size	Total Cal.	Carbs GMS	Fat GMS
sliced, drained	1 cup	53	12	0.2
sliced, drained	1 slice	2	1	0.0
sliced, small *(Freshlike)*	1/2 cup	40	9	0.0
sliced, small, tender, 'Premium' *(S&W)*	1/2 cup	40	9	0.0
sliced, water packed, w/o salt *(Freshlike)*	1/2 cup	40	9	0.0
sliced, water packed, w/o sugar or salt *(Freshlike)*	1/2 cup	40	9	0.0
sliced, w/liquid, no salt added *(Del Monte)*	1/2 cup	35	8	0.0
whole *(A&P)*	1/2 cup	40	9	1.0
whole *(Green Giant)*	1/2 cup	35	8	0.0
whole *(IGA)*	1/2 cup	40	9	0.0
whole *(Stokely)*	1/2 cup	40	8	0.0
whole, baby, 'LeSueur' *(Green Giant)*	1/2 cup	35	8	0.0
whole, drained	1 beet	7	2	0.0
whole, drained	1 cup	51	12	0.2
whole, small *(Freshlike)*	1/2 cup	40	9	0.0
Jarred				
pickled *(Stokely)*	1/2 cup	90	22	0.0
pickled, sliced *(Stokely)*	1 oz	25	6	0.0
pickled, whole *(Stokely)*	1 oz	25	6	0.0
BEET GREENS				
boiled, drained, 1-inch pieces	1 cup	39	8	0.3
boiled, drained, 1-inch pieces	1/2 cup	19	4	0.1
raw	1 cup	7	2	0.0
raw	1 med leaf	6	1	0.0
raw, 1-inch pieces	1/2 cup	4	1	0.0
BEET ROOT JUICE *(Biotta)* bottled	6 fl oz	75	16	0.1
BELL PEPPER. See PEPPER, BELL.				
BELLYFISH. See MONKFISH.				
BERRIES. See also individual listings.				
mixed, Oregon, frozen *(Flav-R-Pac)*	4.9 oz	70	16	0.0
BISCOTTI				
chocolate chip, gluten-free *(Ener-G Foods)*	1 serving	122	17	5.1
orange walnut, gluten-free *(Gluten Free Pantry)*	1 serving	110	22	2.5
plain, gluten-free *(Ener-G Foods)*	1 serving	81	11	3.3
BISCUIT				
dough, mixed-grain	1 oz	75	13	1.6
dough, mixed-grain, baked, 2.25-inch diam	1 biscuit	116	21	2.5
dough, plain or buttermilk	1 oz	90	12	3.8
dough, plain or buttermilk, baked	1 oz	98	13	4.2
dough, plain or buttermilk, baked, 2.25-inch diam	1 biscuit	93	13	4.0
dough, plain or buttermilk, less fat	1 oz	73	13	1.3
dough, plain or buttermilk, less fat, baked	1 oz	85	16	1.5
dough, plain or buttermilk, less fat, baked, 2.25-inch diam	1 biscuit	63	12	1.1
(Awrey's)				
2-inch square	1 oz	80	12	3.0
3-inch square	2 oz	160	23	5.0
(Bridgford) frozen	2 oz	180	28	6.0
(Ballard)				
light, oven-ready, 'Extra Lights'	1 piece	50	10	0.0
(Big Country)				
butter	1 biscuit	100	13	4.0
'Butter Tastin"	1 piece	100	14	4.0
buttermilk	1 biscuit	100	14	4.0
Southern style	1 biscuit	100	14	4.0
(1869 Brand)				
baking powder	1 biscuit	100	12	5.0
'Butter Tastin"	1 piece	100	12	5.0

Food Name	Serv. Size	Total Cal.	Carbs GMS	Fat GMS
buttermilk	1 biscuit	100	12	5.0
(Good 'N Buttery)				
fluffy	1 biscuit	90	11	5.0
(Hungry Jack)				
buttermilk, 'Extra Rich'	1 piece	50	9	1.0
flaky	2 biscuits	170	23	7.0
flaky, 'Honey Tastin''	2 biscuits	180	25	7.0
flaky, Southern style	1 biscuit	80	12	4.0
fluffy	2 biscuits	180	23	8.0
(Lite Fluff) buttermilk, ready to bake, Texas style	1 biscuit	90	16	2.5
(Mrs. Wright's)				
butter-flavored, ready to bake, 'Jumbos'	1 biscuit	180	24	9.0
butter-flavored, ready to bake, Texas style	1 biscuit	100	15	3.0
buttermilk, ready to bake, 'Jumbos'	1 biscuit	180	23	9.0
buttermilk, ready to bake, Texas style	1 biscuit	90	16	2.5
(Pillsbury)				
'Big Premium Heat 'n Eat'	2 biscuits	280	32	15.0
butter, 'Grands'	1 biscuit	200	23	10.0
buttermilk, 'Grands'	1 biscuit	200	23	10.0
buttermilk, 'Heat 'n Eat'	2 biscuits	170	27	5.0
buttermilk, light, 'Extra Lights'	3 biscuits	150	29	2.0
cinnamon-raisin	1 biscuit	200	28	8.0
flaky, 'Grands'	1 biscuit	190	23	8.0
home style, 'Grands'	1 biscuit	190	24	9.0
Southern style 'Grands'	1 biscuit	200	23	10.0
w/cinnamon and raisin, 'Grands'	1 biscuit	190	27	7.0
(Roman Meal)				
....	2 biscuits	180	32	3.8
oat bran, w/honey and nuts	1 biscuit	131	20	4.7
white, 'Premium'	1 biscuit	127	19	4.7
(Stilwell) buttermilk, 3-inch diam	1 biscuit	210	30	9.0
(Wonder)	1 piece	80	14	1.0
BISCUIT, TOASTER				
(Northridge) English muffin	1 muffin	80	16	1.0
(Oroweat) 'Australian'	1 biscuit	180	30	5.0
(Oroweat) w/cinnamon and raisin	1 biscuit	200	34	5.0
BISCUIT DOUGH				
buttermilk, artificial flavor, refrigerated *(Pillsbury)*	1 serving	154	30	1.4
BISCUIT MIX				
plain or buttermilk, dry mix	1 cup	548	81	19.7
plain or buttermilk, dry mix	1 oz	121	18	4.4
plain or buttermilk, prepared	1 oz	95	14	3.4
plain or buttermilk, prepared, 3-inch diam	1 biscuit	191	28	6.9
(Arrowhead Mills)	2 oz	100	19	1.0
(Bisquick)	1/2 cup	240	37	8.0
(Bisquick)	1/3 cup	170	25	6.0
(Gold Medal)	1/3 cup	170	26	6.0
(Health Valley) buttermilk, 'Biscuit & Pancake Mix'	1 oz	100	20	1.0
(Kentucky Kernel) all natural, dry mix	1/4 cup	171	28	5.0
(Krusteaz)				
prepared, 2-inch diam	1 biscuit	90	14	3.0
w/cinnamon and raisin, glazed, prepared, 3-inch diam	1 biscuit	200	39	4.0
(Martha White)				
'BixMix' prepared w/2% milk	1 biscuit	90	15	2.0
buttermilk, dry mix	1 serving	171	26	5.9
(Robin Hood) 'Pouch Mix' 0.7 oz mix prepared w/skim milk	1/8 mix	90	14	3.0
(Tone's) buttermilk	1 tsp	1	0	0.0

Food Name	Serv. Size	Total Cal.	Carbs GMS	Fat GMS
BISON/American buffalo				
raw	1 oz	31	0	0.5
ribeye, trimmed to 0-inch fat, raw	1 oz	33	0	0.7
ribeye, trimmed to 0-inch fat, raw	4 oz	131	0	2.7
roasted	3 oz	122	0	2.1
roasted, boneless, yield from 1 lb raw	11.9 oz	486	0	8.2
shoulder, trimmed to 0-inch fat	4 oz	123	0	2.4
shoulder, trimmed to 0-inch fat, raw	1 oz	31	0	0.6
top round, trimmed to 0-inch fat, raw	1 oz	31	0	0.5
top round, trimmed to 0-inch fat, raw	4 oz	124	0	1.8
BITTER GOURD. See BALSAM PEAR.				
BITTER LEMON. See under SOFT DRINKS AND MIXERS.				
BLACK BEAN. See BEAN, BLACK.				
BLACK CHERRY JUICE				
(Knudsen)	8 fl oz	180	43	0.0
(Smucker's) 'Naturally 100%'	8 fl oz	130	31	0.0
BLACK CURRANT. See under CURRANT.				
BLACK PEPPER. See PEPPER, GROUND.				
BLACK TURTLE BEAN. See BEAN, BLACK.				
BLACKBERRIES				
Canned, in heavy syrup, w/liquid	1 cup	236	59	0.4
Fresh, raw	1 cup	75	18	0.6
Frozen				
Marion (Flav-R-Pac)	1 cup	80	19	0.0
unsweetened	18-oz pkg	326	80	2.2
unsweetened	1 cup	97	24	0.6
BLACKBERRY SYRUP. See under SYRUP.				
BLACK-EYED PEAS/cowpeas				
Canned				
(Allens)	1/2 cup	100	18	1.0
Crowder, 'Fresh' (Allens)	1/2 cup	80	15	1.0
Crowder, frozen (Seabrook)	3 oz	130	23	1.0
Crowder, seasoned w/pork, canned (Luck's)	1/2 cup	120	18	3.0
Crowder, Southern, mature seeds, boiled, drained	1 cup	200	36	0.9
Crowder, Southern, mature seeds, w/pork	1 cup	199	40	3.8
immature seeds, drained	1 cup	160	34	0.6
mature (A&P)	7.5 oz	120	20	1.0
mature (Allens)	1/2 cup	105	18	1.0
mature (Green Giant)	1/2 cup	90	18	1.0
mature (Joan of Arc)	1/2 cup	90	18	1.0
packed from fresh shelled (Bush's Best)	1/2 cup	70	16	0.0
packed from soaked dry (Bush's Best)	1/2 cup	70	16	0.0
seasoned w/bacon (Bush's Best)	1/2 cup	90	16	1.0
seasoned w/pork (Luck's)	1/2 cup	130	18	3.0
'Sun-Vista' (S&W)	1/2 cup	70	15	0.0
w/jalapeño peppers (Ranch Style)	1/2 cup	110	19	0.5
w/snaps (Allens)	1/2 cup	100	20	1.0
Dried				
Catjang, mature seeds, boiled, drained	1 cup	200	35	1.2
Catjang, mature seeds, uncooked	1 cup	573	100	3.5
Crowder, Southern, mature seeds, uncooked	1 cup	561	100	2.1
Crowder, Southern, mature seeds, uncooked	1 tbsp	35	6	0.1
immature seeds, uncooked	1 cup	131	27	0.5
mature, boiled (A&P)	1 cup	230	41	1.0
Fresh				
leafy tips, boiled, drained, chopped	1 cup	12	1	0.1
leafy tips, raw, chopped	1 cup	10	2	0.1

Food Name	Serv. Size	Total Cal.	Carbs GMS	Fat GMS
leafy tips, raw, whole	1 med leaf	1	0	0.0
young pods w/seeds, boiled, drained	1 cup	32	7	0.3
young pods w/seeds, raw, chopped	1 cup	41	9	0.3
young pods w/seeds, raw, whole	1 med pod	5	1	0.0
Frozen				
(Flav-R-Pac)	1/2 cup	110	21	1.0
(Freshlike)	3.3 oz	130	23	1.0
(Frosty Acres)	3.3 oz	130	23	1.0
(Pictsweet)	1/2 cup	110	21	1.0
(Seabrook)	3.3 oz	130	23	1.0
(Southern)	3.5 oz	136	24	0.7
(Veg-All)	3.3 oz	130	23	1.0
immature seeds, drained	1 cup	224	40	1.1
immature seeds, unprepared	10-oz pkg	395	71	2.0
immature seeds, unprepared	1 cup	222	40	1.1
BLINTZ				
apple, kosher (Empire Kosher)	2 blintzes	220	36	5.5
blueberry (Golden)	1 crepe	90	18	1.0
blueberry, kosher (Empire Kosher)	2 blintzes	190	36	4.0
cheese, kosher (Empire Kosher)	2 blintzes	200	29	6.0
cheese, low-fat (Golden)	1 crepe	80	13	2.0
cherry (Golden)	1 crepe	95	18	1.0
cherry, kosher (Empire Kosher)	2 blintzes	200	38	4.0
potato, kosher (Empire Kosher)	2 blintzes	190	32	6.0
BLUE CRAB. See under CRAB.				
BLUEBERRIES				
Canned, in heavy syrup, w/liquid	1 cup	225	56	0.8
Fresh				
raw	1 pint	225	57	1.5
raw	50 berries	38	10	0.3
Frozen				
sweetened	10-oz pkg	230	62	0.4
sweetened, thawed	1 cup	186	50	0.3
unsweetened	20-oz pkg	289	69	3.6
unsweetened, unthawed	1 cup	79	19	1.0
(Flav-R-Pac)	1 cup	70	16	0.0
BLUEBERRY JUICE. See also FRUIT DRINK, FRUIT DRINK MIX; FRUIT JUICE BLEND.				
mountain blueberry, organic (Mountain Sun)	8 fl oz	108	27	0.0
BLUEBERRY TOPPING (Flav-R-Pac)	2 tbsp	40	10	0.0
BLUEFIN TUNA. See under TUNA.				
BLUEFISH				
baked, broiled, grilled, or microwaved	3 oz	135	0	4.6
raw	3 oz	105	0	3.6
BOAR, WILD				
raw	1 oz	35	0	0.9
roasted	3 oz	136	0	3.7
roasted, boneless, yield from 1 lb raw	11.9 oz	544	0	14.9
BOBWHITE. See QUAIL.				
BOK CHOY/Chinese cabbage/napa cabbage/pak-choi/pe-tsai				
boiled, drained	1 leaf	2	0	0.0
boiled, drained, shredded	1 cup	20	3	0.3
fresh, shredded (Dole)	1/2 cup	5	1	0.1
raw	1 head	109	18	1.7
raw	1 leaf	2	0	0.0
raw, shredded	1 cup	12	2	0.2
BONITO. See under TUNA.				
BORAGE, raw, 1-inch pieces	1 cup	19	3	0.6

Food Name	Serv. Size	Total Cal.	Carbs GMS	Fat GMS
BORECOLE. See KALE.				
BORLOTTI. See BEAN, CRANBERRY.				
BOYSENBERRIES				
Canned, in heavy syrup	1 cup	225	57	0.3
Frozen				
(Flav-R-Pac)	1 cup	59	20	0.0
unsweetened	10-oz pkg	142	35	0.7
unsweetened	1 cup	66	16	0.3
BOYSENBERRY JUICE (Smucker's) 'Naturally 100%'	8 fl oz	120	30	0.0
BRAMBLE. See RASPBERRY.				
BRATWURST. See under SAUSAGE.				
BRAZIL NUT/paranut				
dried, unblanched, approx 6-8 kernels	1 oz	186	4	18.8
dried, unblanched, shelled, approx 32 kernels	1 cup	918	18	92.7
BREAD				
ALFALFA SPROUT				
(Vermont Bread Company)				
	1 slice	80	15	1.0
'Sandwich'	1 slice	90	17	1.5
APPLE WALNUT (Arnold)	1 slice	64	13	1.3
APPLE HONEY (Brownberry) wheat	1 slice	69	11	1.9
AUSTRIAN (Du Jour) brown and serve	1 oz	70	13	1.0
BARBECUE (Colombo Brand) 'BBQ Loaf'	2 oz	139	24	1.6
BRAN				
(Brownberry)				
'Bran'nola'	1 slice	85	18	1.4
whole, 'Natural'	1 slice	58	12	1.4
w/raisins	1 slice	61	12	1.3
(Earth Grains) 'Gold'N Bran'	1 oz	70	12	1.0
(Oroweat) original, natural, 'Bran'nola'	1 slice	100	19	1.0
(Pepperidge Farm) honey, 1.5-lb loaf	1 slice	90	18	1.0
BROWN				
canned	1 slice	88	19	0.7
canned	1 oz	55	12	0.4
(B&M)				
plain, 1/2-inch slice	1 slice	92	21	0.0
w/raisins, 1/2-inch slice (B&M)	1 slice	94	22	0.0
(Friends)				
plain, 1/2-inch slice	1 slice	92	21	0.0
w/raisins, 1/2-inch slice (Friends)	1 slice	94	22	0.0
(S&W) canned, 'New England'	2 slices	76	17	0.0
BROWN RICE				
(Ener-G Foods)				
gluten free	1 slice	122	20	4.3
gluten free, yeast-free	1 slice	154	25	3.5
(Mystic Lake Dairy) wheat gluten-free	1 slice	155	22	6.0
BUTTERMILK				
(Grant's Farm)	1 slice	70	12	1.0
(Oroweat)	1 slice	100	20	1.0
CINNAMON RAISIN				
(Arizona Original Homestyle) 100% stone ground	1 slice	116	23	0.0
(Arnold)	1 slice	67	13	1.4
(Pepperidge Farm)	1 slice	90	16	2.0
CINNAMON OATMEAL (Oatmeal Goodness)	1 slice	90	15	2.0
CINNAMON SWIRL (Pepperidge Farm)	1 slice	90	15	3.0
DARK (Hollywood)	1 slice	70	13	1.0

Food Name	Serv. Size	Total Cal.	Carbs GMS	Fat GMS
DATE				
(Dromedary) date nut roll	1/2-inch slice	80	13	2.0
(Thomas') date nut loaf.	1 oz	80	15	2.5
EGG				
5 x 3 x 1/2-inch slices	1 slice	115	19	2.4
(Ener-G Foods) gluten-free	1 slice	176	23	6.8
FLAXSEED (Natural Ovens) 'Flax 'N Honey'	1 slice	70	15	0.5
FRENCH				
large slices, approx 5 x 2-1/2 x 1 inch	1 slice	96	18	1.1
medium slices, approx 4-3/4 x 4 x 1/2 inch	1 slice	69	13	0.8
small slices, approx 2-1/2 x 2 x 1/2 inch	1 slice	41	8	0.5
(Colombo Brand)				
extra sour	2 oz	150	27	1.3
sweet, 'French Stick'	2 oz	154	27	1.9
(DiCarlo) 'Parisian'	1 slice	70	13	1.0
(Du Jour) brown and serve	1 oz	70	13	1.0
(Farm Hearth) twin loaves	1 oz	80	15	1.0
(Monterey Baking) high-fiber, low-calorie	1 slice	48	10	0.1
(Pepperidge Farm)				
enriched	1 slice	130	25	1.5
enriched, twin loaves	1 slice	130	26	1.5
'Hearth'	1 oz	75	14	1.0
(Pillsbury)	1 slice	150	28	1.0
GARLIC				
(Campione) frozen	1 serving	101	12	4.7
(Cole's) mini-loaf, ready-to-serve	1.8 oz	180	21	8.0
(Colombo Brand)	2 oz	185	17	10.1
(Mamma Bella)				
frozen	2 slices	150	16	8.0
sliced	2 slices	160	16	9.0
(Marie Callender's) original	1 piece	190	25	8.0
(Pepperidge Farm)				
crusty, Italian	1 serving	186	21	9.6
heat and serve	1.7 oz	170	19	9.0
HAWAIIAN (King's Hawaiian Bread)	2 oz	180	30	4.0
HEALTH (Brownberry) 'Health Nut'	1 slice	71	12	2.6
HONEY BRAN (Pepperidge Farm)	1 slice	90	18	1.0
HONEY NUT (Roman Meal) w/rice bran	1 slice	71	13	1.6
HONEY WHEAT BERRY (Arnold)	1 slice	77	17	1.2
INDIAN FRY				
Navajo, 10.5-inch diam	1 serving	526	85	15.2
Navajo, 5-inch diam	1 serving	296	48	8.6
ITALIAN				
large slices, approx 4-1/2 x 3-1/4 x 3/4 inch	1 slice	81	15	1.1
medium slices	1 slice	54	10	0.7
small slices, approx 3-1/4 x 2-1/2 x 1/2 inch	1 slice	27	5	0.3
(Arnold)				
'Francisco International'	1 slice	72	14	1.1
'Francisco International' sliced thick	1 slice	66	14	0.8
light, 'Bakery'	1 slice	45	10	0.5
(Brownberry) 'Light'	1 slice	44	10	0.5
(Monk's) 'Hi-Fibre'	1 slice	70	13	1.0
(Monterey Baking) twist	1 slice	71	15	0.2
(Pepperidge Farm)				
enriched, brown and serve	1 slice	130	24	2.0
'Hearth'	1 oz	80	14	1.0
(Wonder) 'Family'	1 slice	70	13	1.0

Food Name	Serv. Size	Total Cal.	Carbs GMS	Fat GMS
LIGHT *(Hollywood)*	1 slice	70	13	1.0
MILLET, 'Sunny Millet' *(Natural Ovens)*	1 slice	50	15	0.0
MIXED GRAIN				
7-grain, w/whole grain, large slices	1 slice	80	15	1.2
7-grain, w/whole-grain, medium slices	1 slice	65	12	1.0
(Arizona Original Homestyle) 9-grain, 100% stone-ground	1 slice	94	23	0.0
(Arnold) bran, nutty, 'Bran'nola'	1 slice	85	17	1.6
(Aunt Hattie's) 7-grain	1 slice	100	17	2.0
(Beefsteak) multigrain	1 slice	70	11	1.0
(BreadMill Bakery) 5-grain, organic	1 slice	122	23	1.0
(Brownberry) bran, 'Bran'nola Nutty Grains'	1 slice	85	17	1.6
(Colonial) w/honey, 'Family Recipe'	1 slice	70	14	1.0
(Earth Grains) 12-grain	1 oz	70	13	1.0
(Food for Life) multigrain, w/wheat, rice, and almond, gluten-free	1 slice	120	22	2.5
(Grant's Farm)				
7-grain	1 slice	60	13	1.0
7-grain, 'Light'	1 slice	40	9	1.0
w/honey	1 slice	70	13	1.0
(Healthy Choice)				
multigrain	1 slice	60	12	0.5
7-grain	1 slice	80	18	1.0
(Home Pride) 7-grain	1 slice	70	12	1.0
(Kilpatrick's) w/honey, 'Family Recipe'	1 slice	70	14	1.0
(Monterey Baking)				
9-grain	1 slice	111	23	0.4
9-grain, low salt	1 slice	111	23	0.4
(Natural Ovens)				
7-grain	1 slice	70	15	0.5
whole wheat, flax, millet, and soy, 'Stay Trim'	1 slice	50	15	0.0
(Oroweat)				
9-grain, 'Light'	1 slice	40	10	0.0
12-grain	1 slice	110	20	2.0
(Pepperidge Farm)				
multigrain, granola, w/oat and honey	1 slice	60	12	2.0
7-grain, 'Hearty Slice'	2 slices	180	36	2.0
(Rainbo) w/honey, 'Family Recipe'	1 slice	70	14	1.0
(Roman Meal)				
multigrain, 'Round Top'	1 slice	67	13	0.8
multigrain, sliced, sandwich thin	1 slice	55	11	0.7
multigrain, 'Sun Grain'	1 slice	68	12	1.4
(Rudi's) 'Ancient Grain Bread'	1 slice	85	14	2.0
(Vermont Bread Company) 'Soft 10'	1 piece	90	16	2.0
(Weight Watchers) multigrain	1 slice	40	9	1.0
NUT *(Oroweat)* 'Health Nut'	1 slice	110	20	2.0
OAT				
(Colonial) split top, 'Family Recipe'	1 slice	70	13	1.0
(Earth Grains) w/honey and nuts	1 oz	80	14	2.0
(Kilpatrick's) split top, 'Family Recipe'	1 slice	70	13	1.0
(Oroweat) light, 'Country Oat'	1 slice	40	10	0.0
(Pepperidge Farm)				
hearty, crunchy	1 slice	100	17	2.0
honey granola	1 slice	60	12	2.0
(Rainbo) split top 'Family Recipe'	1 slice	70	13	1.0
OAT BRAN				
	1 slice	71	12	1.3
lower calorie	1 slice	46	9	0.7

Food Name	Serv. Size	Total Cal.	Carbs GMS	Fat GMS
(Awrey's)	1 slice	50	10	0.0
(BreadMill Bakery)				
organic, 'Light'	1 slice	113	22	1.0
w/honey, whole wheat, organic	1 slice	121	23	1.0
(Earth Grains) w/honey	1 oz	80	13	1.0
(Grant's Farm)	1 slice	70	14	1.0
(Monterey Baking)				
....	1 slice	100	18	1.5
low-salt	1 slice	99	16	4.1
(Oatmeal Goodness) 'Light'	1 slice	40	6	1.0
(Oroweat) natural, 'Bran'nola Country'	2 slices	230	39	4.0
(Roman Meal)				
'Split-Top'	1 slice	68	13	0.9
w/honey	1 slice	71	13	1.2
w/honey and nut	1 slice	72	12	1.6
(Vermont Bread Company)				
w/oatmeal, low-sodium	1 slice	70	14	1.0
w/oatmeal, 'Sandwich Bread'	1 slice	100	18	1.5
(Weight Watchers)	1 slice	40	10	1.0
OATMEAL				
....	1 slice	73	13	1.2
lower calorie	1 slice	48	10	0.8
(Arnold) light, 'Bakery'	1 slice	44	10	0.6
(Grant's Farm) w/toasted almonds	1 slice	80	14	1.0
(Hearty Grains) twists	1 serving	80	15	2.0
(Oatmeal Goodness)				
cinnamon	1 slice	90	15	2.0
w/bran	1 slice	90	15	2.0
w/sunflower seeds	1 slice	90	15	2.0
....	1 slice	90	17	1.0
'Light Style'	1 slice	45	9	0.0
1.5 lb. loaf	1 slice	90	17	1.0
'Very Thin'	1 slice	40	8	1.0
OATNUT (Oroweat)	1 slice	100	18	2.0
ORANGE RAISIN (Brownberry)	1 slice	67	13	1.2
PITA				
white, large, 6.5-inch diam	1 pita	165	33	0.7
white, small, 4-inch diam	1 pita	77	16	0.3
whole wheat, large, 6.5-inch diam	1 pita	170	35	1.7
whole wheat, small, 4-inch diam	1 pita	74	15	0.7
(Kangaroo) w/onion, nonfat, sliced, no oils	1 pita	75	15	0.0
(Sahara)				
oat bran	1/2 piece	66	15	0.3
100% whole wheat	1 pita	130	28	1.0
original	1 pita	150	31	1.0
sourdough	1 pita	150	33	0.5
white	1/2 piece	79	16	0.5
white, mini	1 slice	79	16	0.5
whole wheat	1 piece	150	28	2.0
(Vermont Bread Company)	1/2 pita	80	16	0.5
POTATO (Ener-G Foods) gluten-free	1 slice	170	24	5.4
PROTEIN, w/gluten	1 slice	47	8	0.4
PUMPERNICKEL				
regular slices	1 slice	65	12	0.8
snack size	1 slice	18	3	0.2
thick slices, approx 5x4x3/8 inch	1 slice	80	15	1.0
thin slices	1 slice	50	10	0.6

Food Name	Serv. Size	Total Cal.	Carbs GMS	Fat GMS
(Arnold)	1 slice	70	15	0.9
(Pepperidge Farm)				
'Family'	1 slice	80	15	1.0
small, 'Party'	4 slices	60	12	1.0
RAISIN				
large slices	1 slice	88	17	1.4
medium slices	1 slice	71	14	1.1
thin slices	1 slice	63	12	1.0
(BreadMill Bakery) whole wheat, organic	1 slice	120	24	1.0
(Brownberry)				
bran	1 slice	61	12	1.3
cinnamon	1 slice	66	13	1.3
walnut	1 slice	68	11	2.7
(Ener-G Foods)				
gluten-free, egg-free	1 slice	116	20	2.7
gluten-free, w/egg	1 slice	154	32	1.5
(Monk's) cinnamon	1 slice	70	10	2.0
(Northridge) walnut, royal	1 slice	90	16	2.0
(Pepperidge Farm)				
cinnamon swirl	1 slice	90	16	2.0
(Pillsbury) oatmeal, 'Hearty Grain'	1 serving	90	16	2.0
(Vermont Bread Company)				
cinnamon, low-fat, low sodium	1 slice	80	17	0.5
RICE				
(Ener-G Foods)				
gluten-free, 'Papa's Loaf'	1 slice	144	19	5.9
white rice, yeast free, gluten-free	1 slice	147	24	3.1
(French Meadow)				
sourdough, whole grain, yeast-free, organic	1.35 oz	84	17	1.0
RICE BRAN				
	1 slice	66	12	1.2
(Monk's) golden	1 slice	70	14	1.0
(Roman Meal)				
	1 slice	70	12	1.5
w/honey and nuts	1 slice	71	13	1.6
RICE STARCH *(Med Diet)* low-protein	1 slice	155	29	4.0
RYE				
lower calorie, medium slices	1 slice	47	9	0.7
lower calorie, thick slices	1 slice	65	13	0.9
lower calorie, thin slices	1 slice	41	8	0.6
regular, medium slices	1 slice	83	15	1.1
regular, snack size	1 slice	18	3	0.2
regular, thin slices	1 slice	52	10	0.7
(Arnold) w/dill	1 slice	71	14	1.0
(Beefsteak)				
'Hearty'	1 slice	70	13	1.0
'Mild'	1 slice	70	13	1.0
'Soft'	1 slice	70	13	1.0
w/onion	1 slice	70	12	1.0
w/wheat berries	1 slice	70	13	1.0
(Braun's) 'Old Allegheny'	1 slice	70	13	1.0
(Brownberry)				
seedless, natural, sliced thin	1 slice	45	10	0.6
w/caraway, 'Natural'	1 slice	73	15	0.8
(Earth Grains) sliced very thin, 'Light'	1 oz	70	14	1.0
(Food for Life) white, 100% wheat-free, no preservatives	2 slices	217	42	4.0
(Grant's Farm) cracked rye, w/honey	1 slice	70	13	1.0

Food Name	Serv. Size	Total Cal.	Carbs GMS	Fat GMS
(Levy's)				
Jewish, seeded	1 slice	76	16	0.9
Jewish, seedless	1 slice	75	16	0.8
(Mrs. Wright's) Jewish, w/seeds	2 slices	110	20	1.5
(Natural Ovens) mild	1 slice	70	13	0.5
(Oroweat) hearty, 'Light'	1 slice	40	10	0.0
(Pepperidge Farm)				
Dijon	1 slice	50	9	1.0
Dijon, 'Hearty'	1 slice	70	15	1.0
seedless, 'Family'	1 slice	80	16	1.0
small, 'Party'	4 slices	60	12	1.0
w/seeds, 'Family'	1 slice	80	16	1.0
(Vermont Bread Company)				
....	1 slice	70	14	1.0
'Black Russian'	1 slice (1/2")	110	23	0.0
'Sandwich'	1 slice	100	18	1.5
(Weight Watchers)	1 slice	40	10	1.0
(Wonder)	1 slice	70	13	1.0
SOURDOUGH				
(Boudin)	2 slices	130	27	1.0
(DiCarlo)	1 slice	70	12	1.0
(Earth Grains) 'Light'	1 slice	40	9	1.0
(French Meadow) yeast-free, organic	2 oz	132	29	0.9
(Monterey Baking)	1 slice	75	16	0.2
(Rainbo) 'Light'	1 slice	40	9	1.0
SPELT *(French Meadow)* sprouted, yeast-free, organic	1.5 oz	93	18	0.0
SPLIT TOP *(Healthy Choice)*	1 slice	60	12	0.5
SUNFLOWER				
(BreadMill Bakery) w/whole wheat, organic	1 slice	129	21	2.0
(Monk's) w/bran	1 slice	70	12	1.0
SUNFLOWER SESAME *(Vermont Bread Company)*	1 slice	70	14	1.0
SWEET *(Vermont Bread Company)*	1 slice	70	15	0.0
TAPIOCA				
(Ener-G Foods)				
gluten free	1 slice	141	19	6.0
gluten free, thin sliced	1 slice	88	12	3.7
THREE SEED *(Monterey Baking)*	1 slice	100	16	2.5
VIENNA				
(Pepperidge Farm)				
'Light Style'	1 slice	45	10	0.0
sliced thick, 'Hearth'	1 slice	70	13	1.0
WHEAT				
(Arizona Original Homestyle)				
w/honey, 100% stone ground	1 slice	110	23	0.0
(Arnold)				
'Brick Oven'	1 slice	57	11	1.5
light, golden, 'Bakery'	1 slice	44	10	0.5
(Aunt Hattie's)				
buttertop	1 slice	70	13	1.0
w/buttermilk	1 slice	70	12	1.0
(Beefsteak)				
light, 'Hearty'	1 slice	70	11	1.0
'Soft'	1 slice	70	12	1.0
(BreadMill Bakery)				
w/oat bran and honey, all-natural, organic	1 slice	120	23	1.0
w/sunflower, all natural, organic	1 slice	130	1	2.0

Food Name	Serv. Size	Total Cal.	Carbs GMS	Fat GMS
(Brownberry)				
.... 1 slice		74	13	1.8
'Hearth' .... 1 oz		70	14	1.4
'Natural' .... 1 slice		80	17	1.3
w/apple and honey .... 1 slice		69	11	1.9
(Colonial)				
'Family Recipe' .... 1 slice		70	14	1.0
honey buttered, split top .... 1 slice		70	14	1.0
stone ground, 'Family Recipe' .... 1 slice		70	14	1.0
(Country Grain) .... 1 slice		70	12	1.0
(Earth Grains)				
cracked wheat .... 1 oz		70	12	1.0
'Light 35' .... 1 oz		35	8	1.0
sliced very thin .... 1 oz		70	13	1.0
(Fresh and Natural) .... 1 slice		70	13	1.0
(Grant's Farm)				
'Light' .... 1 slice		40	9	1.0
stone ground .... 1 slice		60	12	1.0
(Healthy Choice) honey wheat ... 1 slice		60	12	0.5
(Hearty Grains) cracked wheat, w/honey, twists .... 1 serving		80	14	2.0
(Home Pride)				
butter top wheat .... 1 slice		80	14	1.0
stone ground .... 1 slice		70	12	1.0
(Kamut) stone-ground, yeast-free, organic, frozen .... 1 slice		120	23	0.0
(Kilpatrick's)				
'Family Recipe' .... 1 slice		70	14	1.0
stone ground, 'Family Recipe' .... 1 slice		70	14	1.0
(Mrs. Wright's)				
.... 2 slices		100	18	1.5
crushed wheat, sliced, round top .. 1 slice		70	15	0.5
crushed wheat, sliced, sandwich thin .... 1 slice		60	12	0.5
dark wheat, 'Bran'nola' .... 1 slice		83	18	1.0
(Natural Ovens) cracked wheat .... 1 slice		80	16	0.5
(Oatmeal Goodness)				
w/oatmeal .... 1 slice		90	15	2.0
w/oatmeal, 'Light' .... 1 slice		40	6	1.0
(Pepperidge Farm)				
cracked wheat .... 1 slice		70	13	1.0
'Light Style' .... 1 slice		45	9	0.0
1.5-lb loaf .... 1 slice		90	18	2.0
sprouted .... 1 slice		70	11	2.0
2-lb loaf, 'Family' .... 1 slice		70	13	1.0
w/sesame, 'Hearty' .... 2 slices		190	36	3.0
(Pipin' Hot) thick sliced .... 1 slice		70	12	2.0
(Rainbo)				
'Family Recipe' .... 1 slice		70	14	1.0
honey buttered, split top .... 1 slice		70	14	1.0
'Light' .... 1 slice		40	9	1.0
stone ground, 'Family Recipe' .... 1 slice		70	14	1.0
(Vermont Bread Company)				
low-sodium .... 1 slice		80	15	1.0
sodium-free .... 1 slice		90	15	2.0
sprouted .... 1 slice		70	15	0.5
(Weight Watchers) .... 1 slice		40	9	1.0
(Wonder)				
nonfat, 'Light' .... 1 slice		40	7	1.0
sliced .... 1 slice		80	14	1.0

Food Name	Serv. Size	Total Cal.	Carbs GMS	Fat GMS
sliced, 'Family'	1 slice	80	13	1.0
WHEAT BERRY				
(Arizona Original Homestyle) cracked, stone-ground	1 slice	93	23	0.0
(Arnold) w/honey	1 slice	77	17	1.2
(Earth Grains) w/honey	1 oz	70	12	1.0
(Grant's Farm)	1 slice	70	13	1.0
(Healthy Choice)	1 slice	80	18	1.0
(Oroweat) w/honey	1 slice	90	17	1.0
WHEAT BRAN (Grant's Farm) w/honey	1 slice	70	14	1.0
WHEAT GERM	1 slice	73	14	0.8
WHITE				
medium slices	1 slice	67	12	0.9
medium slices, crust removed	1 slice	32	6	0.4
thick slices	1 slice	80	15	1.1
thin slices	1 slice	53	10	0.7
very thin slices	1 slice	40	7	0.5
(Arnold)				
'Brick Oven'	1 slice	61	11	1.2
'Country White'	1 slice	98	19	1.8
extra fiber, 'Brick Oven'	1 slice	55	12	0.8
'Light Premium'	1 slice	42	10	0.5
(Aunt Hattie's)				
buttertop, 'Homestyle'	1 slice	70	13	1.0
w/buttermilk, 'Homestyle'	1 slice	80	13	1.0
(Beefsteak) 'Robust'	1 slice	70	13	1.0
(Brownberry)				
'Light Premium'	1 slice	42	10	0.5
'Natural'	1 slice	59	11	1.1
(Colonial) honey buttered, split top	1 slice	80	14	1.0
(Earth Grains)				
'Light 35'	1 oz	35	8	1.0
very thin sliced	1 oz	80	14	1.0
(Grant's Farm) 'Light'	1 slice	40	9	1.0
(Holsum)				
enriched, 'Country Style'	1 slice	70	14	1.0
thin sliced	1 slice	70	14	1.0
(Kilpatrick's) honey buttered, split top	1 slice	80	14	1.0
(Monk's)	1 slice	60	10	1.0
(Mrs. Wright's)				
enriched	2 slices	100	20	1.0
sliced, Sandwich style, 'Winners'	1 slice	70	13	1.0
(Northridge) 'Old Fashioned'	1 slice	70	13	1.0
(Pepperidge Farm)				
'Hearty Country'	2 slices	190	38	2.0
sliced, sandwich style	2 slices	130	24	2.0
thin sliced, 1-lb loaf	1 slice	80	14	2.0
'Toasting'	1 slice	90	17	1.0
2-lb loaf, 'Large Family'	1 slice	70	13	1.0
very thin sliced	1 slice	40	8	0.0
(Pipin' Hot) loaf, thick sliced	1 slice	70	12	2.0
(Rainbo)				
honey buttered, split top	1 slice	80	14	1.0
'Light'	1 slice	40	9	1.0
thin sliced, special recipe, 'Iron Kids'	1 slice	60	13	1.0
(Vermont Bread Company)				
'Old Fashioned Sandwich'	1 slice	70	14	1.0
'Soft'	1 piece	80	15	1.0

Food Name	Serv. Size	Total Cal.	Carbs GMS	Fat GMS
(Weight Watchers)	1 slice	40	10	1.0
(Wonder)				
'High-Fiber'	1 slice	40	6	0.0
'Light'	1 slice	40	7	0.0
sliced	1 slice	70	14	1.0
sliced thin	1 slice	50	10	1.0
w/buttermilk	1 slice	70	13	1.0
WHOLE GRAIN				
(Healthy Choice)	1 slice	80	18	1.0
(Natural Ovens)	1 slice	70	13	0.5
WHOLE WHEAT				
	1 slice	69	13	1.2
(Arnold) 100%, stone ground	1 slice	48	10	0.7
(Aunt Hattie's)	1 slice	90	14	2.0
(BreadMill Bakery)				
w/orange, organic	1 slice	130	24	1.0
w/poppyseed, organic	1 slice	120	22	1.0
w/raisin, organic	1 slice	120	24	1.0
(Daily)	1 piece	140	26	0.0
(Earth Grains)	1 oz	70	11	1.0
(Monk's) 100% stone ground	1 slice	70	13	1.0
(Northridge) 100%	1 slice	60	11	1.0
(Oroweat) 100% stone ground	1 slice	60	11	1.0
(Pepperidge Farm)				
thin sliced, 1-lb loaf	1 slice	60	12	1.0
very thin sliced	1 slice	35	7	0.0
(Vermont Bread Company)				
'Sandwich'	1 slice	90	18	1.0
'Soft Whole Wheat'	1 piece	80	15	1.0
sourdough	1 slice	80	16	0.5
(Wonder)				
'High-Fiber'	1 slice	40	6	0.0
'Light'	1 slice	40	7	0.0
100%	1 slice	70	12	1.0
'Soft 100%'	1 slice	70	10	1.0
BREAD, QUICK				
cornbread (Ballard)	1 piece	130	23	2.5
cornbread (Marie Callender's)	1 piece	150	27	3.0
raisin loaf, fat-free, cholesterol-free (Entenmann's)	1 slice	140	33	0.0
BREAD, QUICK, MIX				
APPLE CINNAMON				
(Pillsbury)				
mix only	1/12 pkg	140	30	1.0
prepared w/1/4 cup oil, 1/4 cup egg substitute	1/12 loaf	190	31	6.0
prepared w/water, 1/4 cup oil, 1 egg	1/12 loaf	180	31	6.0
BANANA				
(Keebler) individual, 'Elfin Loaf' prepared w/margarine	1 loaf	186	31	6.0
(Krusteaz) w/nuts, prepared	3/4-inch slice	190	33	6.0
(Pillsbury)				
mix only	1/12 pkg	120	27	1.0
prepared, regular recipe	1/12 loaf	170	27	6.0
prepared w/water, 3 tbsp oil, 1/2 cup egg substitute	1/12 loaf	170	27	6.0
prepared w/water, 3 tbsp oil, 2 eggs	1/12 loaf	170	27	5.0
BLUEBERRY				
(Pillsbury)				
mix only	1/12 pkg	130	29	1.0
nut, prepared	1/12 loaf	150	26	4.0

Food Name	Serv. Size	Total Cal.	Carbs GMS	Fat GMS
prepared, regular recipe	1/12 loaf	150	26	4.0
prepared w/water, 1/4 cup oil, 1 egg	1/12 loaf	180	30	6.0
prepared w/water, 1/4 cup oil, 1/4 cup egg substitute	1/12 loaf	180	30	6.0
CHERRY *(Pillsbury)* prepared, regular recipe	1/12 loaf	180	29	5.0
CORNBREAD				
(Aunt Jemima) 'Easy'	1/3 cup	150	26	4.0
(Ballard)				
mix only	1/16 pkg	120	24	2.0
prepared	1 serving	110	21	1.5
(Dromedary)				
mix only	3 tbsp	100	19	2.0
prepared, 2x2-inch pieces	1 piece	130	20	3.0
(Gluten Free Pantry) gluten-free, prepared	1 serving	130	29	0.0
(Gold Medal)				
white, 'Pouch Mix' prepared w/egg, whole milk	1/6 pan	150	22	5.0
yellow, 'Pouch Mix' prepared w/egg, whole milk	1/6 pan	150	23	5.0
(Hodgson Mill)				
Mexican, w/jalapeño, mix only	1/4 cup	100	21	1.0
and muffin mix, whole-grain cornmeal	1/4 cup	130	28	1.0
(Kentucky Kernel) sweet, all-natural, mix only	1/4 cup	120	24	2.0
(Krusteaz)				
Southern, prepared, 2 x 2-inch pieces	1 piece	140	27	3.0
w/honey, prepared	1/16 loaf	120	21	3.0
(Martha White)				
'Cotton Pickin' prepared w/water	1/6 pan	110	21	2.0
'Cotton Pickin' prepared	1/4 pan	170	31	3.0
Mexican, prepared w/2% milk	1/6 pan	140	24	4.0
w/buttermilk, prepared w/water	1/6 pan	110	21	2.0
yellow, 'Light Crust' prepared	2 oz	140	21	4.0
yellow, prepared w/water	1/6 pan	130	27	2.0
(Pillsbury)				
prepared	1/18 pkg	130	23	2.5
twists, prepared	1 serving	130	17	6.0
(Robin Hood)				
white, 'Pouch Mix' prepared w/egg, whole milk	1/6 pan	150	22	5.0
yellow, 'Pouch Mix' prepared w/egg, whole milk	1/6 pan	150	23	5.0
CRANBERRY				
(Pillsbury)				
mix only	1/12 pkg	140	30	1.0
prepared w/water, 2 tbsp oil, 1 egg	1/12 loaf	160	30	4.0
prepared w/water, 2 tbsp oil 1/4 cup egg substitute	1/12 loaf	170	30	4.0
CRANBERRY-ORANGE				
(Gluten Free Pantry) gluten-free, prepared	1 serving	150	35	0.0
DATE NUT				
(Dromedary)				
mix only	1/12 pkg	166	26	7.0
prepared	1/12 loaf	183	26	8.0
(Pillsbury)				
mix only	1/12 pkg	140	31	1.0
prepared.	1/12 loaf	180	32	4.0
prepared w/water, 1 tbsp oil, 1/4 cup egg substitute	1/12 loaf	160	32	3.0
IRISH SODA *(Gluten Free Pantry)* gluten-free	1 serving	130	28	1.0
NUT				
(Pillsbury)				
mix only	1/12 pkg	150	27	3.0
prepared w/water, 2 tbsp oil, 1 egg	1/12 loaf	170	27	6.0
prepared w/water, 2 tbsp oil, 1/4 cup egg substitute	1/12 loaf	170	28	6.0

Food Name	Serv. Size	Total Cal.	Carbs GMS	Fat GMS
OATMEAL-RAISIN				
(Pillsbury)				
mix only	1/12 pkg	140	30	2.0
prepared w/water, 1/4 cup oil, 1 egg	1/12 loaf	190	30	7.0
prepared w/1/4 cup oil, 1/4 cup egg substitute	1/12 loaf	190	30	7.0
PUMPKIN				
(Pillsbury)				
mix only	1/12 pkg	130	26	1.5
prepared	1/12 loaf	170	27	6.0
BREAD CRUMBS				
Italian, dry, grated *(Tone's)*	1 tsp	8	2	0.1
Italian or plain, whole wheat, organic *(Jaclyn's)*	14 grams	28	13	1.0
Italian style *(Devonsheer)*	1 oz	104	21	1.3
Italian style *(Progresso)*	1/4 cup	110	20	1.5
Italian style *(Progresso)*	2 tbsp	60	11	1.0
Italian style, whole wheat *(Jaclyn's)*	0.5 oz	28	13	1.0
plain *(Contadina)*	1/3 cup	100	19	1.5
plain *(Devonsheer)*	1 oz	108	22	1.4
plain *(Progresso)*	1/4 cup	100	19	1.5
plain *(Progresso)*	2 tbsp	60	11	1.0
plain, dry, grated	1 cup	427	78	5.8
plain, dry, grated	1 oz	112	21	1.5
plain, dry, grated *(Tone's)*	1 tsp	8	2	0.1
seasoned, dry, grated	1 cup	440	84	3.1
seasoned, dry, grated	1 oz	104	20	0.7
BREAD DOUGH				
cracked wheat, unbleached, high-protein, frozen *(Rhodes)*	1 oz	75	15	1.0
French, crusty, refrigerated, prepared, 1-inch slice *(Pillsbury)*	1 slice	60	11	1.0
raisin, unbleached flour, no preservatives, frozen, prepared *(Rhodes)*	1 slice	70	13	1.0
refrigerated *(Roman Meal)*	1 oz	85	13	2.8
wheat, refrigerated, prepared, thick sliced *(Pipin' Hot)*	1 slice	70	12	2.0
white, enriched, frozen *(Bridgford)*	2 oz	150	28	2.0
white, frozen *(Bridgford)*	1 oz	76	14	1.2
white, frozen *(Rhodes)*	1 slice	139	26	2.3
white, frozen *(Rich's)*	2 slices	120	23	1.0
white, refrigerated, prepared, 1-inch slice *(Pipin' Hot)*	1 slice	70	12	2.0
w/honey, frozen *(Bridgford)*	2 oz	150	27	2.0
w/honey, unbleached high-protein flour, frozen *(Rhodes)*	1 slice	125	23	2.0
w/walnuts and honey, frozen *(Bridgford)*	1 oz	76	14	0.9
BREAD MIX				
caraway rye, mix only *(Hodgson Mill)*	1/4 cup	120	22	2.0
caraway rye, gluten-free *(Gluten Free Pantry)*	1 serving	110	23	0.0
cracked wheat, for bread machines *(Pillsbury)*	1/12 pkg	130	25	2.0
European cheese and herb, low-fat, cholesterol-free, mix only *(Hodgson Mill)*	1/4 cup	130	21	2.0
French, country, gluten-free, prepared *(Gluten Free Pantry)*	1 slice	110	25	0.0
Italian, frozen *(Rhodes)*	1 slice	130	23	2.0
9-grain, low-fat, mix only *(Hodgson Mill)*	1/4 cup	130	22	2.0
oatmeal, w/raisin, mix only *(Pillsbury)*	1/12 pkg	140	30	2.0
oatmeal, w/raisin, prepared w/water, 1/4 cup oil, 1 egg *(Pillsbury)*	1/12 pkg	190	30	7.0
oatmeal, w/raisin, prepared w/water, 1/4 cup oil, 1/4 cup egg substitute *(Pillsbury)*	1/12 pkg	190	30	7.0
potato, fat free, cholesterol free, mix only *(Hodgson Mill)*	1/4 cup	120	23	0.0
sandwich, gluten-free, 'Favorite' *(Gluten Free Pantry)*	1 slice	110	24	0.0
tapioca, gluten-free *(Gluten Free Pantry)*	1 serving	110	25	0.0
white, crusty, for bread machines *(Pillsbury)*	1/8 pkg	130	25	2.0

Food Name	Serv. Size	Total Cal.	Carbs GMS	Fat GMS
white, unbleached flour, mix only *(Hodgson Mill)*	1/4 cup	120	22	2.0
whole grain, stone ground, w/honey, mix only *(Hodgson Mill)* . . .	1/4 cup	120	22	2.0
whole wheat, low-fat, cholesterol free, mix only *(Hodgson Mill)* . . .	1/4 cup	120	22	2.0
whole wheat, 100% all natural, stone ground *(Bob's Red Mill)*	1.5 oz	152	28	2.0
BREAD PUDDING				
w/apples, frozen, food service product *(Stouffer's)*	1 oz	42	5	1.6
BREADFRUIT				
Fresh, raw, whole, small fruit	1/4 fruit	99	26	0.2
Frozen, unthawed	1 cup	227	60	0.5
BREADFRUIT SEEDS				
boiled	1 oz	48	9	0.7
raw	1 oz	54	8	1.6
roasted	1 oz	59	11	0.8
BREADNUT TREE SEEDS/Jamaican breadnut				
dried	1 cup	587	127	2.7
dried	1 oz	104	23	0.5
raw, 8–14 seeds	1 oz	62	13	0.3
BREADSTICK				
garlic, frozen *(Cole's)*	1.9 oz	170	27	5.0
garlic, Italian style *(Barbara's Bakery)*	1 oz	120	18	3.0
garlic and sesame *(Angonoa's)*	7 pieces	120	19	3.0
onion *(Stella D'oro)*	1 piece	40	6	1.3
pizza *(Fattorie & Pandea)*	3 pieces	59	10	1.0
pizza *(Stella D'oro)*	1 piece	43	7	1.2
plain *(Angonoa's)*	6 pieces	120	20	2.5
plain *(Stella D'oro)*	1 piece	41	7	1.2
plain, 4.25-inch length	1 breadstick	21	3	0.5
plain, 7-5/8 x 5/8 inch	1 breadstick	41	7	0.9
plain, 9-1/4 x 3/8 inch	1 breadstick	25	4	0.6
plain, dietetic *(Stella D'oro)*	1 piece	46	7	1.4
plain, regular *(Barbara's Bakery)*	1 oz	120	18	3.0
sesame, dietetic *(Stella D'oro)*	1 piece	49	6	2.1
soft *(Pillsbury)*	1 serving	110	18	2.5
sesame *(Fattorie & Pandea)*	3 pieces	65	10	2.0
sesame *(Stella D'oro)*	1 piece	51	6	2.2
sesame, Italian style *(Barbara's Bakery)*	1 oz	120	18	3.0
soft, refrigerated ready-to-bake *(Mrs. Wright's)*	1 stick	100	17	2.5
soft, refrigerated *(Roman Meal)*	1 piece	117	17	3.9
wheat *(Stella D'oro)*	1 piece	42	6	1.4
whole wheat, w/sesame *(Angonoa's)*	5 pieces	130	19	4.0
whole wheat *(Fattorie & Pandea)*	3 pieces	57	10	1.0
BREAKFAST BAR				
(Carnation)				
chocolate chip	1 bar	200	20	11.0
chocolate crunch	1 bar	190	20	10.0
peanut butter chocolate chip	1 bar	200	20	11.0
peanut butter crunch	1 bar	190	20	10.0
BREAKFAST BURRITO. See under BURRITO.				
BREAKFAST DRINK MIX				
(Carnation)				
regular, prepared w/8 fl oz 2% milk	9 oz	250	39	5.0
sugarless, prepared w/8 fl oz 2% milk	9 oz	190	24	5.0
(Ovaltine) traditional flavor, 'Classic'	4 tbsp	80	17	0.0
(Pillsbury)				
chocolate, variety pack, dry mix, 'Instant Breakfast'	1/10 pkg	130	25	0.0
BREAKFAST SANDWICH				
(Great Starts)				
egg, beefsteak, and cheese	4.9 oz	360	27	20.0

Food Name	Serv. Size	Total Cal.	Carbs GMS	Fat GMS
egg, Canadian bacon, cheese	5.2 oz	420	37	22.0
muffin w/egg, Canadian style bacon, cheese	1 pkg	290	25	15.0
muffin w/egg, sausage, cheese	1 pkg	490	36	30.0
sausage, egg, and cheese biscuit	1 entrée	460	37	28.0
(Jimmy Dean)				
biscuit w/egg, bacon, cheese	1 biscuit	300	28	16.0
biscuit w/egg, ham, cheese	1 biscuit	240	26	10.0
biscuit w/egg, sausage, cheese	1 biscuit	390	28	27.0
biscuit w/sausage, frozen	1 pkg	385	23	28.2
biscuit w/sausage, frozen	1 sandwich	192	12	14.1
biscuit w/sausage, frozen	1 serving	385	23	28.2
biscuit w/sausage, microwaveable	2 sandwiches	310	23	20.0
sausage, refrigerated, microwave	1 sandwich	160	10	11.0
(La Choy) ham, egg, and cheese breakfast roll,				
food service product	1 serving	237	22	12.6
(Morningstar Farms)				
vegetarian, 'Breakfast Sandwich' w/muffin, patty,				
cheese, and Scramblers	1 sandwich	280	35	3.0
vegetarian, Scramblers patty sandwich	1 serving	300	29	12.0
(Owens)				
sausage, biscuit, refrigerated, 'Border Breakfasts'	2 oz	210	14	14.0
sausage, egg, and cheese, biscuit, refrigerated,				
'Border Breakfasts'	2.5 oz	250	15	15.0
sausage, smoked, biscuit, refrigerated, 'Border Breakfasts'	2 oz	200	15	6.0
(Red Baron)				
bacon scramble, 'Sunrise Singles'	1 unit	420	34	24.0
(Pierre)				
ham and cheese, wrapped, product 1295, 'Ham-n-Go'	1 piece	236	26	10.6
ham, wrapped, product 1293, 'Ham-n-Go'	1 piece	223	26	8.9
wrapped, 'Link-N-Dog' 'Dine'n w/Pierre'	1 piece	203	20	9.1
wrapped, 'Saus-A-Rage' 'Dine'n w/Pierre'	1 piece	263	26	13.2
(Quick Meal)				
sausage, biscuit	3.7 oz	350	29	22.0
sausage, w/cheese, biscuit	4.3 oz	420	31	27.0
sausage, w/egg and cheese, muffin	5.1 oz	76	5	4.0
sausage, w/egg, biscuit	4.5 oz	350	30	21.0
(Red Baron)				
ham scramble, 'Sunrise Singles'	1 unit	370	34	19.0
(Sunny Fresh)				
biscuit w/ham and cheese, pre-cooked, frozen	1 pkg	29206	3028	1165.4
biscuit w/ham and cheese, pre-cooked, frozen	1 serving	243	25	9.7
egg and cheese biscuit, pre-cooked, frozen	1 pkg	26910	2957	1066.9
egg and cheese biscuit, pre-cooked, frozen	1 serving	224	25	8.9
egg and cheese pocket sandwich, pre-cooked, frozen,				
'Breakfast Stuff-Its'	1 pkg	17605	1760	913.9
egg and cheese pocket sandwich, pre-cooked, frozen,				
'Breakfast Stuff-Its'	1 serving	147	15	7.6
(Red Baron) sausage scramble 'Sunrise Singles'	1 unit	380	34	21.0
(Swanson) egg, sausage & cheese 'Great Starts'	5.5 oz	460	35	28.0
(Weight Watchers) sausage, biscuit	1 biscuit	230	20	11.0

BREAKFAST STRIPS. See under BACON SUBSTITUTE.
BREWER'S YEAST. See under YEAST.
BROAD BEAN. See BEAN, FAVA.
BROCCOLI
Fresh

boiled, drained, chopped	1/2 cup	22	4	0.3
boiled, drained, spears, large, 11-12 inches long	1 spear	78	14	1.0

Food Name	Serv. Size	Total Cal.	Carbs GMS	Fat GMS
boiled, drained, spears, medium, 7.5–8 inches long	1 spear	50	9	0.6
boiled, drained, spears, small, 5 inches long	1 spear	39	7	0.5
raw, bunch	1 medium	170	32	2.1
raw, chopped	1 cup	25	5	0.3
raw, chopped or diced	1/2 cup	12	2	0.2
raw, florets	1 cup	20	4	0.2
raw, florets	1 medium	3	1	0.0
raw, spears, medium *(Dole)*	1 spear	40	4	1.0
raw, spears, medium, 7.5-8 inches long	1 spear	42	8	0.5
raw, spears, small, 5 inches long	1 spear	9	2	0.1
Frozen				
(Flav-R-Pac)	1 cup	25	4	0.0
(Health Valley)	1/2 cup	26	5	0.0
chopped *(A&P)*	3.3 oz	25	5	1.0
chopped *(Birds Eye)*	3.3 oz	25	5	0.0
chopped *(Finast)*	3.3 oz	25	5	0.0
chopped *(Flav-R-Pac)*	3/4 cup	30	5	0.0
chopped *(Frosty Acres)*	3.3 oz	25	5	0.0
chopped *(Seabrook)*	3.3 oz	25	5	0.0
chopped *(Southern)*	3.5 oz	28	4	0.3
chopped, drained	1 cup	52	10	0.2
chopped, no salt added, drained	1 cup	52	10	0.2
chopped, 'Plain Polybag' *(Green Giant)*	3/4 cup	25	4	0.0
chopped, unprepared	1 cup	41	7	0.5
chopped, unprepared	10-oz pkg	74	14	0.8
cuts *(A&P)*	3.3 oz	25	5	1.0
cuts *(Birds Eye)*	3.2 oz	25	5	0.0
cuts *(Flav-R-Pac)*	1 cup	25	4	0.0
cuts *(Frosty Acres)*	3.3 oz	25	5	0.0
cuts *(Pictsweet)*	1 cup	25	4	0.0
cuts *(Seabrook)*	3.3 oz	25	5	0.0
cuts, 'Plain Polybag' *(Green Giant)*	1/2 cup	18	5	0.0
cuts, 'Portion Pack' *(Birds Eye)*	3 oz	20	4	0.0
cuts, 'Singles' *(Stokely)*	3 oz	25	5	1.0
drained	1/2 cup	26	5	0.1
drained	10-oz pkg	70	13	0.3
florets *(C&W)*	3.3 oz	25	5	0.0
florets *(Frosty Acres)*	3.3 oz	30	5	0.0
florets, 'Deluxe' *(Birds Eye)*	3.3 oz	25	5	0.0
florets, 'Select Polybag' *(Green Giant)*	1 1/3 cup	25	4	0.0
Normandy *(Flav-R-Pac)*	3/4 cup	25	4	0.0
Normandy, w/buttery sauce *(Flav-R-Pac)*	1/2 cup	45	7	2.5
spears *(A&P)*	3.3 oz	25	5	1.0
spears *(Birds Eye)*	3.3 oz	25	5	0.0
spears *(Frosty Acres)*	3.3 oz	25	5	0.0
spears *(Seabrook)*	3.3 oz	25	5	0.0
spears *(Southern)*	3.5 oz	30	5	0.2
spears and florets, 'Deluxe' *(Birds Eye)*	3.3 oz	25	5	0.0
spears, 'Select Polybag' *(Green Giant)*	3 oz	25	4	0.0
spears, baby *(Seabrook)*	3.3 oz	30	5	0.0
spears, baby, 'Deluxe' *(Birds Eye)*	3.3 oz	30	5	0.0
spears, mini, *(Green Giant)*	1/5 pkg	18	5	0.0
spears, no salt added, drained	10-oz pkg	70	13	0.3
spears, no salt added, drained	1/2 cup	26	5	0.1
spears, whole, 'Farm Fresh' *(Birds Eye)*	4 oz	30	6	0.0
unprepared	2-lb pkg	263	49	3.1
unprepared	10-oz pkg	82	15	1.0

Food Name	Serv. Size	Total Cal.	Carbs GMS	Fat GMS
BROCCOLI, CHINESE, cooked	1 cup	19	3	0.6
BROCCOLI DISH/ENTRÉE				
(A&P) w/cauliflower, frozen	3.2 oz	25	4	1.0
(Amy's Kitchen)				
pie, w/cheddar cheese, organic	8-oz pie	390	46	18.0
pot pie	1 serving	430	46	22.0
(Birds Eye)				
stir-fry, 'Farm Fresh Mixtures'	1 cup	30	5	0.0
w/baby carrots and water chestnuts, 'Farm Fresh'	4 oz	45	10	0.0
(Flav-R-Pac) cheddar broccoli Normandy, frozen,				
'Grande Classics'	1/2 cup	45	6	2.0
(Frosty Acres) w/cauliflower, 'Swiss Mix'	3 oz	25	5	0.0
(Green Giant)				
'Broccoli Fanfare' 'Valley Combinations'	1/2 cup	80	14	2.0
in cheese flavored sauce	1 pkg	188	25	7.0
in cheese flavored sauce	1 cup	113	15	4.2
in cheese flavored sauce	1 serving	75	10	2.8
w/cauliflower, 'Valley Combinations'	1/2 cup	60	9	2.0
w/red peppers, 'Select'	1/2 cup	25	4	0.0
(Nancy's) broccoli-cheddar quiche, frozen, microwave,				
'French Baked'	1 quiche	490	33	33.0
Pepperidge Farm) w/cheese, in pastry, frozen	1 piece	200	18	16.0
(Stokely)				
w/cauliflower 'Singles'	3 oz	20	4	1.0
w/whole baby carrots, and water chestnuts, 'Singles'	3 oz	30	6	1.0
(Stouffer's)				
and cheese soufflé, frozen, food service product	1 oz	35	2	2.1
au gratin, frozen, food service product	1 oz	27	3	1.3
BROCCOLI DISH/ENTRÉE MIX				
(Pasta Roni) and mushroom noodles entrée, 'Tenderthin'	1 serving	260	28	13.6
(Rice A Roni)				
and cheese rice, 'Fast Cook'	2.5 oz	169	23	6.8
au gratin	2.5 oz	209	27	9.6
au gratin, w/rice, 1/3 less sodium	2.5 oz	181	28	6.2
BROTH. See under SOUP.				
BROWN RICE. See under RICE.				
BROWNIE. See under CAKE, SNACK.				
BRUSSELS SPROUTS				
Fresh				
boiled, drained	1/2 cup	30	7	0.4
boiled, drained, whole	1 medium	8	2	0.1
raw	1 cup	38	8	0.3
raw	1 medium	8	2	0.1
raw *(Dole)*	1/2 cup	19	4	0.1
Frozen				
(A&P)	3.3 oz	35	7	1.0
(Birds Eye)	3.3 oz	35	7	0.0
(Flav-R-Pac)	6 medium	35	5	0.0
(Frosty Acres)	3.3 oz	35	7	0.0
(Pictsweet)	85 grams	35	5	0.0
(Seabrook)	3.3 oz	35	7	0.0
(Southern)	3.5 oz	37	8	0.0
baby *(Seabrook)*	3.3 oz	40	7	0.0
no salt, drained	1 cup	65	13	0.6
petite *(C&W)*	3.2 oz	30	5	0.0
'Plain Polybag' *(Green Giant)*	1/2 cup	25	6	0.0
'Singles' *(Stokely)*	3 oz	35	7	0.0
unprepared	2-lb pkg	372	71	3.7

Food Name	Serv. Size	Total Cal.	Carbs GMS	Fat GMS
unprepared	10-oz pkg	116	22	1.2
w/salt, drained	1 cup	65	13	0.6
BUBBLE GUM. See under CANDY, GUM.				
BUCKWHEAT	1 cup	583	122	5.8
BUCKWHEAT FLOUR. See under FLOUR.				
BUCKWHEAT GROATS, ROASTED/kasha				
cooked	1 cup	155	33	1.0
dry	1 cup	567	123	4.4
(Wolff's Kasha)	3/4 cup	150	35	0.0
BUFFALO. See BISON.				
BULGUR. See also CEREAL, HOT.				
cooked	1 cup	151	34	0.4
cooked	1 tbsp	7	2	0.0
dry	1 cup	479	106	1.9
BULGUR DISH/ENTRÉE MIX				
(Casbah)				
pilaf mix, dry	1 oz	100	21	0.0
tabbouleh, seasoned, prepared	2/3 cup	120	24	0.5
(Fantastic Foods) tabbouleh, seasoned	1/4 cup	120	26	0.5
BULLOCK'S HEART. See CUSTARD APPLE.				
BUN. See also BISCUIT; BUN, FRANKFURTER; BUN, HAMBURGER; BUN, SWEET; CROISSANT; ENGLISH MUFFIN; ROLL.				
hoagie, deli *(Wonder)*	1 serving	260	49	3.5
'Sof-Buns' *(Holsum)*	1 bun	120	23	2.0
spelt, yeast-free, organic *(French Meadow)*	1 bun	160	33	1.4
w/sesame seeds, 'Big BBQ Buns' *(Holsum)*	1 bun	200	38	3.0
BUN, FRANKFURTER				
	1 oz	81	14	1.4
(Arnold)				
	1 bun	100	20	1.8
'New England Style'	1 bun	108	21	2.0
oat bran	1 bun	110	20	2.0
(Aunt Hattie's) potato	1 bun	150	23	4.0
(Country Grain)	1 bun	100	18	1.0
(Mrs. Wright's)				
crushed wheat	1 bun	110	20	1.5
enriched	1 bun	100	19	1.5
(Pepperidge Farm)				
	1 bun	140	24	3.0
Dijon	1 bun	160	23	5.0
(Roman Meal)				
'Original'	1 bun	104	20	1.9
whole-grain	1 bun	120	19	3.0
(Wonder)				
	1 bun	110	21	1.5
footlong Coney	1 bun	220	42	3.0
'Light'	1 bun	80	13	1.0
BUN, HAMBURGER				
	1 oz	81	14	1.4
(Arnold)	1 bun	115	22	2.2
(Aunt Hattie's) potato	1 bun	150	23	4.0
(Mrs. Wright's)				
crushed wheat	1 bun	110	21	1.5
enriched	1 bun	110	21	1.5
enriched, w/sesame	1 bun	110	21	1.5
(Pepperidge Farm)	1 bun	130	22	2.0
(Roman Meal)				
'Original'	1 bun	113	21	1.9

Food Name	Serv. Size	Total Cal.	Carbs GMS	Fat GMS
whole grain .... 1 bun		130	20	3.0
(Wonder)				
.... 1 bun		110	21	1.5
4-inch diam *(Wonder)* .... 1 bun		110	21	1.5
'Light' .... 1 bun		80	13	1.0
BUN, SWEET. See also PASTRY; ROLL, SWEET.				
(Aunt Fanny's)				
honey .... 3 oz		360	42	30.0
honey, apple bear .... 4 oz		460	50	26.0
honey, applesauce-filled .... 1 bun		330	43	17.0
honey, banana creme filled .... 1 bun		350	32	18.0
honey, birdie, jelly-filled .... 4 oz		450	53	24.0
honey, bogie, creme-filled .... 4 oz		460	49	27.0
honey, chocolate creme filled .... 1 bun		350	32	18.0
honey, iced .... 1 bun		350	32	18.0
honey, lemon bear .... 4 oz		440	52	23.0
honey, raspberry-filled .... 1 bun		350	45	17.0
honey, regular .... 1 bun		360	41	20.0
honey, snow bear .... 4 oz		480	60	24.0
honey, vanilla creme filled .... 1 bun		350	32	18.0
(Break Cake)				
apple honey, multi pak, 1.5 oz .... 1 bun		170	20	10.0
honey, 3 oz .... 1 bun		420	38	28.0
honey, multi pak, 2.75 oz .... 1 bun		380	34	24.0
(Entenmann's)				
blueberry cheese, nonfat, no cholesterol .... 1 serving		140	31	0.0
cheese-topped .... 1 bun		240	29	12.0
cinnamon .... 1 bun		230	31	10.0
pineapple cheese, nonfat, no cholesterol .... 1 serving		140	30	0.0
raspberry cheese, nonfat, no cholesterol .... 1 serving		160	36	0.0
(Hostess)				
honey glazed, 'Breakfast Bake Shop' .... 1 piece		360	38	21.0
honey iced, 'Breakfast Bake Shop' .... 1 piece		430	55	22.0
(Morton) honey, microwave .... 1 bun		250	35	10.0
(Pepperidge Farm) cinnamon, frozen, '2/pkg.' .... 1 piece		280	34	14.0
(Rich's)				
cinnamon, frozen, 2.5 oz, *'Ever Fresh'* .... 1 bun		293	38	14.6
honey, frozen, mini, 'Ever Fresh' .... 1.36 oz		133	18	6.6
(Tastykake)				
honey glazed .... 3.25 oz		362	42	20.4
honey iced .... 3.25 oz		348	50	14.9
(Weight Watchers)				
cheese bun, frozen, 'Microwave' .... 1/2 pkg		180	32	4.0
BURBOT				
baked, broiled, grilled, or microwaved .... 3 oz		98	0	0.9
raw .... 3 oz		77	0	0.7
BURDOCK ROOT/gobo				
boiled, drained, sliced, 1-inch pieces .... 1 cup		110	26	0.2
boiled, drained, whole .... 1 med root		146	35	0.2
raw, sliced, 1-inch pieces .... 1 cup		85	20	0.2
raw, whole .... 1 med root		112	27	0.2
BURGER. See under BEEF DINNER/ENTRÉE; BEEF SUBSTITUTE DINNER/ENTRÉE; and individual ground meat listings.				
BURGUNDY. See under WINE.				
BURRITO				
(Amy's Kitchen)				
bean and cheese burrito. .... 1 burrito		280	43	8.0

Food Name	Serv. Size	Total Cal.	Carbs GMS	Fat GMS
bean and rice burrito.	1 burrito	250	44	5.0
bean burrito, w/rice and cheese, organic, frozen, 6 oz	1 burrito	280	43	8.0
breakfast burrito	1 serving	230	38	5.0
(Don Miguel)				
beef, cheese, and green chili	1 burrito	390	53	11.0
chicken, cheese, no beans	1 burrito	410	52	14.0
(Great Starts)				
breakfast burrito, hot and spicy	1 pkg	220	30	7.0
breakfast burrito, w/cheese and chili peppers, 'Original'	1 pkg	200	25	8.0
breakfast burrito, w/eggs, bacon, cheese	1 pkg	250	27	11.0
breakfast, burrito, w/eggs, ham, cheese	1 pkg	210	29	6.0
breakfast, burrito, w/eggs, pepperoni, cheese w/pizza sauce	1 pkg	240	28	9.0
(Healthy Choice)				
beef and bean, 'Quick Meals'	5.2 oz	270	42	7.0
chicken con queso, frozen, 'Quick Meals'	5.4 oz	280	40	8.0
chicken con queso entrée	1 entrée	350	60	6.0
(Homestyle Kitchens) black bean, organic, frozen	1 burrito	190	36	1.5
(Hormel)				
beef, frozen	1 piece	205	31	8.0
cheese, frozen	1 piece	210	32	5.0
chicken and rice, frozen	1 piece	200	32	4.0
chili, hot, frozen	1 piece	240	33	8.0
(Las Campanas)				
bean and cheese, no lard	1 burrito	272	42	7.0
beef and bean, frozen	1 pkg	2964	382	120.8
beef and bean, frozen	1 serving	296	38	12.1
beef and bean, no lard	1 burrito	304	39	12.0
(Maria's)				
bean and cheese, jalapeno	1 burrito	360	54	11.0
beef and bean	1 burrito	420	49	19.0
(Marquez Pimera)				
beef, green chili, and cheese, 'Primera'	1 burrito	330	43	11.0
beef, green chili, and Monterey Jack cheese, frozen	1 pkg	324	40	11.6
(Old El Paso)				
bean and cheese, frozen	1 burrito	330	45	11.0
beef and bean, frozen, 'Festive Dinners'	11 oz	470	72	9.0
beef and bean, hot, frozen	1 burrito	310	41	11.0
beef and bean, medium, frozen	1 burrito	330	41	13.0
beef and bean, mild, frozen	1 burrito	320	42	11.0
packaged, prepared, w/filling	1 burrito	299	36	13.0
(Patio)				
beef and bean, frozen	5 oz	370	43	16.0
beef and bean, frozen, 'Britos'	3.63 oz	250	33	10.0
beef and bean, green chili, frozen	5 oz	330	43	12.0
beef and bean, nacho, frozen, 'Britos'	3.63 oz	270	30	13.0
beef and bean, red chili, frozen	5 oz	340	44	13.0
beef and bean, w/green chili, mild	1 pkg	325	44	11.9
beef and bean, w/green chili, mild	1 serving	325	44	11.9
chicken, spicy, frozen, 'Britos'	3.63 oz	250	33	10.0
frozen	12 oz	517	74	16.0
green chili, frozen, 'Britos'	3.63 oz	250	33	10.0
nacho cheese, frozen, 'Britos'	3.63 oz	250	32	10.0
red chili, frozen, 'Britos'	3.63 oz	240	31	10.0
red hot, frozen, 'Britos'	5 oz	360	43	15.0
(Ruiz)				
beefsteak fajita, 'Supreme'	1 burrito	290	42	9.0
chicken fajita, 'Supreme'	1 burrito	260	50	1.0

Food Name	Serv. Size	Total Cal.	Carbs GMS	Fat GMS
BURRITO FILLING				
beans *(Del Monte)*	1/2 cup	110	20	1.0
'Manwich' *(Hunt's)*	1/4 cup	25	6	0.2
BURRITO SEASONING. See under SEASONING MIX.				
BUSH NUT. See MACADAMIA NUT.				
BUTTER				
light, salted, stick *(Land O'Lakes)* stick	1 tbsp	50	0	6.0
light, salted, whipped *(Land O'Lakes)* whipped	1 tbsp	35	0	4.0
light, unsalted, stick *(Land O'Lakes)*	1 tbsp	50	0	6.0
lightly salted *(Darigold)*	1 tsp	25	0	3.0
lightly salted *(Hotel Bar)*	1 tsp	35	0	4.0
lightly salted *(Kellers)*	1 tsp	35	0	4.0
lightly salted, stick *(Breakstone's)*	1 tbsp	100	0	11.0
lightly salted, whipped *(Breakstone's)*	1 tbsp	70	0	7.0
lightly salted, whipped *(Breakstone's)*	1 tbsp	70	0	7.0
'Quarters' *(Darigold)*	1 tsp	35	0	4.0
salted	1 cup	1628	0.	184.1
salted	1 pat	36	0	4.1
salted	1 stick	813	0	92.0
salted	1 tbsp	102	0	11.5
salted *(Hotel Bar)*	1 tsp	35	0	4.0
salted *(Kellers)*	1 tsp	35	0	4.0
salted, 'Quarters' *(Darigold)*	1 tsp	35	0	4.0
salted, stick *(Land O'Lakes)*	1 tbsp	100	0	11.0
salted, whipped *(Land O'Lakes)*	1 tsp	25	0	3.0
salted, whipped	1 cup	1082	0	122.5
salted, whipped	1 pat	27	0	3.1
salted, whipped	1 stick	542	0	61.3
salted, whipped	1 tbsp	67	0	7.6
unsalted	1 pat	36	0	4.1
unsalted	1 cup	1628	0	184.1
unsalted	1 stick	813	0	92.0
unsalted	1 tbsp	102	0	11.5
unsalted *(Land O'Lakes)*	1 tsp	35	0	4.0
unsalted, sweet, stick *(Breakstone's)*	1 tbsp	100	0	11.0
unsalted, sweet, whipped *(Breakstone's)*	1 tbsp	70	0	7.0
unsalted, whipped *(Darigold)*	1 tsp	25	0	3.0
unsalted, whipped *(Land O'Lakes)*	1 tsp	25	0	3.0
whipped *(Breakstone's)*	1 tbsp	70	0	7.0
whipped *(Darigold)*	1 tsp	25	0	3.0
whipped *(Land O'Lakes)*	1 tsp	25	0	3.0
BUTTER ALTERNATIVE				
(Canola Harvest) canola oil spread	1 tbsp	100	0	11.0
(Fleischmann's) corn oil spread, 60% oil, 'Light'	1 tbsp	80	0	8.0
(I Can't Believe It's Not Butter!)				
buttermilk, no salt	1 tbsp	90	0	10.0
buttermilk, stick	1 tbsp	90	0	10.0
cream, buttermilk, squeezable	1 tbsp	90	0	10.0
light spread, 40% vegetable oil, stick	1 tbsp	50	0	6.0
soft, 70% vegetable oil	1 tbsp	90	0	10.0
whipped	1 tbsp	60	0	7.0
(Land O'Lakes)				
stick, no salt	1 tbsp	90	na	10.0
tub	1 tbsp	80	na	8.0
w/sweet cream, salted, stick	1 tbsp	90	na	10.0
(Mazola) corn oil spread, 40% corn oil, light	1 tbsp	50	0	6.0

Food Name	Serv. Size	Total Cal.	Carbs GMS	Fat GMS
(Spectrum Naturals) canola oil spread, 100% dairy-free, nonhydrogenated .... 1 tbsp		94	0	11.0
BUTTER FLAVORING				
(Butter Buds) fat-free, sprinkles .... 1 tsp		5	2	0.0
(Fry's) .... 1/2 tsp		4	0	0.0
(Molly McButter) fat-free, natural butter flavor, sprinkles .... 1 tsp		5	1	0.0
(Schilling) naturally flavored, 'Best 'O Butter' .... 1/2 tsp		4	1	1.0
BUTTER OIL				
anhydrous .... 1 cup		1796	0	203.9
anhydrous .... 1 tbsp		112	0	12.7
BUTTERBEAN. See BEAN, LIMA.				
BUTTERBUR/fuki				
Canned				
chopped .... 1 cup		4	0	0.2
stalks, whole .... 3 medium		1	0	0.1
Fresh				
raw, chopped .... 1 cup		13	3	0.0
raw, petioles, whole .... 1 medium		1	0	0.0
BUTTERFISH				
baked, broiled, grilled, or microwaved .... 3 oz		159	0	8.7
raw .... 3 oz		124	0	6.8
BUTTERHEAD LETTUCE. See under LETTUCE.				
BUTTERMILK				
cultured *(A&P)* .... 1 cup		90	12	1.0
cultured *(Crowley)* .... 1 cup		110	12	4.0
cultured, low-fat .... 1 quart		396	47	8.6
cultured, low-fat .... 1 cup		99	12	2.2
cultured, low-fat .... 1 fl oz		12	1	0.3
cultured, 1.5%, 'Golden Churn' *(Borden)* .... 1 cup		120	11	4.0
cultured, 1.5% ,'Unsalted' *(Friendship)* .... 1 cup		120	12	4.0
cultured, 2%, *(Knudsen)* .... 1 cup		120	12	5.0
cultured, 'Unsalted' *(Crowley)* .... 1 cup		110	12	4.0
cultured, 'Unsalted' *(Friendship)* .... 1 cup		120	12	4.0
dry .... 1 cup		464	59	6.9
dry .... 1 tbsp		25	3	0.4
dry, blend, cultured *(Saco Foods)* .... 3.5 tbsp		79	11	0.7
BUTTERNUT				
dried .... 1 cup		734	14	68.4
dried .... 1 oz		174	3	16.2
dried .... 1 nutmeat		18	0	1.7
BUTTERNUT SQUASH. See under SQUASH.				
BUTTERSCOTCH. See under CANDY.				
BUTTERSCOTCH TOPPING				
(Kraft) .... 1 tbsp		60	13	1.0
(Smucker's) .... 2 tbsp		140	33	1.0
BUTTON MUSHROOM. See MUSHROOM, WHITE.				

C

Food Name	Serv. Size	Total Cal.	Carbs GMS	Fat GMS
CABBAGE, COMMON				
boiled, drained, shredded .... 1/2 cup		17	3	0.3
boiled, drained, whole, medium, approx 5.75-inch diam .... 1 head		278	56	5.4
raw, chopped .... 1 cup		22	5	0.2
raw, leaf, large leaf .... 1 leaf		8	2	0.1

Food Name	Serv. Size	Total Cal.	Carbs GMS	Fat GMS
raw, leaf, medium leaf	1 leaf	6	1	0.1
raw, leaf, small leaf	1 leaf	4	1	0.0
raw, shredded	1 cup	18	4	0.2
raw, whole, large, approx 7-inch diam	1 head	312	68	3.4
raw, whole, medium head, approx 5.75-inch diam	1 head	227	49	2.5
raw, whole, small head, approx 4.5-inch diam	1 head	179	39	1.9
CABBAGE, DANISH				
raw, shredded	1/2 cup	8	2	0.1
raw, whole, medium	1 head	218	49	1.6
CABBAGE, NAPA. See BOK CHOY.				
CABBAGE, RED				
Canned or jarred				
sweet and sour *(Green Giant)*	1/2 cup	90	21	0.0
sweet and sour *(S&W)*	2 tbsp	15	3	0.0
Fresh				
boiled, drained, leaf	1 leaf	5	1	0.0
boiled, drained, shredded	1/2 cup	16	3	0.1
raw, chopped	1 cup	24	5	0.2
raw, leaf, medium	1 leaf	6	1	0.1
raw, shredded	1 cup	19	4	0.2
raw, whole, large, approx 5.5-inch diam	1 head	306	69	2.9
raw, whole, medium, approx 5-inch diam	1 head	227	51	2.2
raw, whole, small, approx 4 inch diam	1 head	153	35	1.5
CABBAGE, SAVOY				
boiled, drained, shredded	1 cup	35	8	0.1
raw, shredded	1 cup	19	4	0.1
CABBAGE, SKUNK/swamp cabbage/water convolvulus				
boiled, drained, chopped	1 cup	20	4	0.2
raw, chopped	1 cup	11	2	0.1
raw, medium shoot	1 shoot	2	0	0.0
CABBAGE DISH/ENTRÉE				
(Lean Cuisine)				
stuffed cabbage, w/whipped potatoes	1 entrée	220	27	7.0
stuffed cabbage w/meat and tomato sauce, potato	1 pkg	199	26	5.6
(Efficienc)				
stuffed cabbage roll entrée, food service product	1 serving	168	17	6.0
(Stouffer's)				
stuffed cabbage, w/o sauce, frozen, food service product	1 oz	36	3	1.9
stuffed cabbage, w/sauce, frozen, food service product	1 oz	27	3	1.2
CABBAGE TURNIP. See KOHLRABI.				
CAJUN SEASONING. See under MARINADE MIX; SEASONING MIX; SEASONING AND COATING MIX.				
CAKE. See also BREAD, QUICK; CAKE, SNACK; CAKE MIX.				
(Awrey's)				
'Best Wishes' 6-inch diam	1/4 cake	150	18	9.0
'Four-in-One Occasion'	1.3 oz	150	18	8.0
BANANA				
(Entenmann's)				
crunch, fat-free, cholesterol-free	1 slice	140	33	0.0
loaf, fat-free, cholesterol-free	1 slice	150	34	0.0
(Sara Lee) single layer, iced	1/8 cake	170	28	6.0
BLACK FOREST				
(Awrey's) torte	1/14 cake	350	38	21.0
(Sara Lee) two-layer, frozen	1/8 cake	190	28	8.0
BLUEBERRY				
(Entenmann's) crunch, fat-free, cholesterol-free	1 slice	140	32	0.0
BOSTON CREAM PIE				
(Pepperidge Farm)	1 slice	260	42	9.0

Food Name	Serv. Size	Total Cal.	Carbs GMS	Fat GMS
(Weight Watchers) frozen, approx 1/2 pkg	3 oz	160	34	4.0
CARAMEL FUDGE *(Weight Watchers)* à la mode	1 serving	160	29	3.0
CARROT				
(Awrey's) cream cheese iced, three-layer	1/12 cake	390	44	23.0
(Entenmann's) fat-free, cholesterol-free	1 slice	170	40	0.0
(Pepperidge Farm)				
cream cheese iced, frozen, 'Old Fashioned'	1.5 oz	150	19	9.0
'Deluxe'	1 slice	310	39	16.0
(Sara Lee) single layer, iced, frozen	1/8 cake	250	30	13.0
(Stilwell) frozen, 'Oregon Farms'	1/6 cake	280	38	15.0
(Weight Watchers) frozen, 1/2 pkg	3 oz	170	27	5.0
CHEESECAKE				
(Sara Lee)				
cream strawberry, frozen	1/6 cake	222	34	8.0
cream, cherry, frozen	1/6 cake	243	35	8.0
cream, plain, frozen	1/6 cake	230	27	11.0
French, frozen, 'Classics'	1/8 cake	250	23	16.0
strawberry, French, frozen, 'Classics'	1/8 cake	240	28	13.0
(Tofutti) nondairy, frozen, 'Better than Cheesecake'	1/10 cake	160	16	10.0
(Weight Watchers)				
brownie	1 serving	200	33	6.0
frozen	3.9 oz	210	29	7.0
New York style	1 serving	150	21	5.0
strawberry, frozen, 'Sweet Celebrations'	3.9 oz	180	28	4.0
triple chocolate	1 serving	200	32	5.0
triple chocolate, frozen, 'Sweet Celebrations'	1 cake	190	30	4.0
CHERRY *(Weight Watchers)* cherries and cream, frozen	3 oz	190	32	6.0
CHOCOLATE				
(Awrey's)				
double chocolate torte	1/14 cake	340	51	15.0
double chocolate, three-layer	1/12 cake	310	48	14.0
double chocolate, two-layer	1/12 cake	250	38	11.0
German, iced, 2 x 2-inch piece	1 piece	160	19	9.0
German chocolate, three-layer	1/12 cake	350	46	18.0
'Happy Birthday'	1.4 oz	150	18	8.0
milk chocolate, yellow, two-layer	1/12 cake	290	33	17.0
white iced, two-layer	1/12 cake	270	34	15.0
(Entenmann's)				
crunch, fat-free, cholesterol-free	1 slice	130	32	0.0
devil's food, fudge iced	1.2 oz	130	19	5.0
fudge iced, fat-free, cholesterol-free	1 slice	210	51	0.0
loaf, fat-free, cholesterol-free	1 slice	130	30	0.0
(Pepperidge Farm)				
chocolate mousse	1 slice	250	35	10.0
devil's food, layer	1 slice	290	40	14.0
frozen, 'Supreme'	2 7/8 oz	300	37	16.0
fudge layer cake	1 slice	300	38	16.0
fudge stripe layer cake	1 slice	290	38	14.0
German chocolate, layer	1 slice	300	37	16.0
(Sara Lee)				
chocolate mousse, frozen, 'Classics'	1/8 cake	260	23	17.0
double chocolate, three layer, frozen	1/8 cake	220	26	11.0
frozen, 'Free & Light'	1/8 cake	110	26	0.0
(Stilwell) bar cake, frozen	1/6 cake	260	43	9.0
(Weight Watchers)				
devil's food, 'Sweet Rewards'	1 serving	160	36	1.5
double fudge	1 serving	190	36	4.5

Food Name	Serv. Size	Total Cal.	Carbs GMS	Fat GMS
frozen	2.5 oz	180	31	5.0
German chocolate, frozen	2.5 oz	200	31	7.0
CHOCOLATE VANILLA ROLL				
(Ener-G Foods) gluten-free	2 oz	168	28	4.0
CINNAMON *(Pillsbury)* swirl, refrigerated	1/8 pkg	180	22	9.0
CINNAMON APPLE				
(Entenmann's) twist, fat-free, cholesterol-free	1 slice	150	35	0.0
COCONUT				
(Pepperidge Farm) layer	1 slice	300	41	14.0
(Awrey's) yellow, three-layer	1/12 cake	350	40	21.0
COFFEECAKE				
(Awrey's)				
caramel nut	1/12 cake	140	15	8.0
'Long John'	1/12 cake	160	19	8.0
(Entenmann's)				
cheese	1.6 oz	150	20	7.0
cinnamon apple, fat-free, cholesterol-free	1 slice	130	29	0.0
crumb	1.3 oz	160	21	7.0
crumb, cheese-filled	1.4 oz	130	18	6.0
(Pillsbury)				
cinnamon swirl, w/icing	1 serving	230	29	11.0
pecan crumb, w/icing	1 serving	230	29	12.0
(Sara Lee)				
cheese, all butter, frozen	1/8 cake	210	25	11.0
pecan, all butter, frozen	1/8 cake	160	19	8.0
streusel, all butter, frozen	1/8 cake	160	20	7.0
CRUMB				
(Entenmann's)				
apple spice, fat-free, cholesterol-free	1 slice	138	32	0.0
French, all butter	1.6 oz	180	26	8.0
golden, French, fat-free, cholesterol-free	1 slice	140	35	0.0
FRUIT *(Ener-G Foods)* loaf, gluten-free	1 slice	118	22	2.2
FUNNEL *(Funnel Cake Factory)* 5-inch	1 serving	270	31	14.0
GOLDEN				
(Entenmann's)				
fudge iced, fat-free, cholesterol-free	1 slice	220	52	0.0
thick fudge	1.2 oz	130	20	6.0
(Pepperidge Farm) layer	1 slice	290	38	14.0
LEMON				
(Awrey's)				
three-layer	1/12 cake	320	38	19.0
yellow, two-layer	1/12 cake	290	33	17.0
(Pepperidge Farm)				
lemon coconut, frozen, 'Supreme'	3 oz	280	38	13.0
lemon cream, frozen, 'Supreme'	1 5/8 oz	170	21	9.0
LOUISIANA CRUNCH				
(Entenmann's)				
	1.7 oz	180	27	8.0
fat-free, cholesterol-free	1 slice	220	51	0.0
MARBLE *(Entenmann's)* loaf, fat-free, cholesterol-free	1 slice	130	29	0.0
NEAPOLITAN *(Awrey's)* torte	1/14 cake	380	43	22.0
ORANGE *(Awrey's)* three-layer	1/12 cake	320	40	17.0
PEANUT BUTTER *(Awrey's)* torte	1/14 cake	380	44	22.0
PECAN STREUSEL *(Pillsbury)* refrigerated	1/8 pkg	180	21	9.0
PINEAPPLE				
(Entenmann's) crunch	1 oz slice	70	16	0.0
(Pepperidge Farm) pineapple cream, frozen, 'Supreme'	2 oz	190	28	7.0

Food Name	Serv. Size	Total Cal.	Carbs GMS	Fat GMS
PISTACHIO *(Awrey's)* torte	1/12 cake	370	41	22.0
POUND				
(Awrey's) golden	1/14 loaf	130	19	5.0
(Ener-G Foods) gluten-free	1 serving	236	32	9.9
(Entenmann's)				
all butter, loaf	1 oz	110	15	5.0
sour cream, loaf	1 oz	120	14	7.0
(Pepperidge Farm) frozen, 'Old Fashioned Cholesterol-Free'	1 oz	110	13	6.0
(Sara Lee)				
all butter, frozen, 'Family Size Original'	1/15 cake	130	14	7.0
all butter, frozen, 'Original'	1/10 cake	130	14	7.0
all butter, frozen, 1.6 oz	1 piece	200	23	11.0
frozen, 'Free & Light'	1/10 cake	70	17	0.0
RASPBERRY				
(Awrey's) nut	1/16 cake	310	39	16.0
(Entenmann's) twist, fat-free, cholesterol-free	1 slice	140	33	0.0
(Great Cakes) bar, all natural	3 oz	175	35	2.0
SHORTCAKE *(Sara Lee)* strawberry, frozen	1/8 cake	190	26	8.0
SPONGE *(Awrey's)* 2 x 2-inch piece	1 piece	80	11	3.0
STRAWBERRY				
(Awrey's) strawberry supreme torte	1/14 cake	270	38	12.0
(Pepperidge Farm)				
strawberry cream, frozen, 'Supreme'	2 oz	190	30	7.0
strawberry stripe, layer	1 slice	310	47	13.0
VANILLA *(Pepperidge Farm)* layer	1 slice	290	41	13.0
WALNUT *(Awrey's)* torte	1/14 cake	320	38	19.0
YELLOW *(Awrey's)* white iced, 2 x 2-inch piece	1 piece	150	18	9.0
CAKE, SNACK				
(Awrey's) 'Best Wishes, Miniature'	3 oz	320	33	22.0
(Break Cake)				
filled twins, 3 oz	2 cakes	310	53	10.0
filled twins, multi-pak, 1.5 oz	1 cake	150	26	5.0
(Drake's)				
cream filled, 'Sunny Doodle'	1 piece	100	16	3.0
cream filled, 'Ring Ding'	1 piece	100	16	4.0
'Funny Bone'	1.25 oz	150	18	8.0
'Zoinks'	1.25 oz	130	20	5.0
(Erewhon) 'Poppets'	1 oz	110	24	1.0
(Hostess)				
dessert cup	1 piece	90	18	2.0
'Lil' Angels'	1 piece	90	14	2.0
'Snowballs'	1 serving	180	31	5.0
'Suzy Q's'	1 serving	230	35	9.0
'Tiger Tail'	1 piece	240	38	8.0
'Twinkie'	1 serving	150	25	5.0
(Little Debbie)				
'Be My Valentine'	2.5 oz	330	44	17.0
'Caravella'	1.2 oz	200	26	9.0
Christmas tree	1 cake	190	26	10.0
dessert cup	0.79 oz	80	4	1.0
'Doodle Dandies'	2.5 oz	320	44	16.0
'Easter Bunny'	2.5 oz	320	45	15.0
'Tiger Cake'	1 cake	310	44	15.0
(Sunbelt) bar, baked	1.31 oz	130	28	2.0
(Tastykake) 'Tasty Twist'	1 piece	18	3	0.6
ANGEL FOOD *(Break Cake)*	1 oz	70	16	0.0
APPLE				
(Aunt Fanny's) applesauce	2.5 oz	234	40	7.0

Food Name	Serv. Size	Total Cal.	Carbs GMS	Fat GMS
(Awrey's) apple streusel	1 piece	160	18	9.0
(Erewhon) 'Apple Stroodles'	1 oz	90	23	0.0
(Hostess) 'Light'	1 piece	130	29	1.0
(Little Debbie)				
'Apple Delight'	1.25 oz	140	24	4.0
apple spice, 2.2 oz	1 piece	270	41	11.0
(Pepperidge Farm)				
apple spice, frozen, 'Dessert Lights' 4.25 oz	1 piece	170	37	2.0
(Sara Lee) frozen, apple crisp 'Lights' 3 oz	1 piece	150	31	2.0
(Weight Watchers) apple raisin bar	1 bar	70	14	2.0
BANANA				
(Awrey's) iced	1 piece	140	17	8.0
(Break Cake) banana marshmallow pie	1 pie	150	25	5.0
(Hostess) 'Suzy Q's'	1 piece	240	4	9.0
(Little Debbie) banana slices	3 oz	340	54	12.0
(Tastykake) 'Creamie'	1.5 oz	185	25	7.1
BLACK FOREST *(Sara Lee)* frozen, 3.6 oz, 'Lights'	1 piece	170	34	5.0
BOSTON CREAM *(Pepperidge Farm)* frozen, 'Hyannis'	1 piece	230	34	10.0
BROWN RICE TREAT				
(Glenny's)				
98% fat-free, 100% natural	1 pkg	120	28	3.0
caramel, 100% natural	1.25 oz	120	29	0.0
chocolate, 100% natural	1.25 oz	120	28	0.0
BROWNIE				
(Auburn Farms)				
butterscotch, nonfat, 'Jammers'	1 serving	100	22	0.0
cappuccino fudge, nonfat, 'Jammers'	1 serving	90	22	0.0
chocolate fudge, nonfat, 'Jammers'	1 serving	90	22	0.0
butterscotch, nonfat, 'Jammers'	1 brownie	100	22	0.0
cappuccino fudge, nonfat, 'Jammers'	1 brownie	100	22	0.0
chocolate fudge, nonfat, 'Jammers'	1 brownie	90	22	0.0
raspberry fudge, nonfat, 'Jammers'	1 brownie	90	22	0.0
whole wheat fudge	1 serving	90	22	0.0
(Awrey's)				
Dutch chocolate, 'Cake'	1/16 cake	340	40	20.0
fudge nut, iced, 'Sheet Cake' 2.5 oz	1 brownie	300	36	17.0
fudge nut, 'Sheet Cake' 1.25 oz	1 brownie	150	16	9.0
(Break Cake)				
chocolate nut, mini, 0.5 oz	1 brownie	70	9	4.0
fudge, 2.8 oz	1 brownie	370	47	18.0
(Ener-G Foods) gluten free	1 serving	108	16	4.1
(Entenmann's) fudge, cholesterol-free	1 piece	110	27	0.0
(Frito-Lay's) fudge nut, 3 oz	1 brownie	360	56	14.0
(Health Valley) fudge brownie bar, nonfat	1 bar	110	26	0.0
(Hostess) fudge, chocolate iced, lowfat, 'Lights'	1 brownie	140	29	2.6
(Little Debbie)				
fudge	1 brownie	270	39	13.0
low-fat	1 serving	190	39	3.0
twin wrapped	1 pkg	247	39	9.9
(Nestlé)				
chocolate chip, frozen, 'Toll House Ready to Bake'	1.4 oz	150	19	7.0
(Pepperidge Farm) hot fudge, 'Newport'	1 ramekin	400	50	20.0
(Tastykake) fudge walnut, 3 oz	1 brownie	335	53	14.2
(Weight Watchers)				
brownie à la mode	1 serving	190	34	4.0
chocolate, frosted	1 serving	100	22	2.5
chocolate, frozen, 'Sweet Celebrations'	1/3 pkg	100	16	3.0

Food Name	Serv. Size	Total Cal.	Carbs GMS	Fat GMS
mint frosted 'Sweet Celebrations'	1.23 oz	100	18	2.0
peanut butter fudge	1 serving	110	21	2.5
Swiss mocha fudge, 'Sweet Celebrations'	1.23 oz	90	18	2.0
BUTTERSCOTCH *(Tastykake)* 'Krimpets'	1 oz	103	19	2.6
CARAMEL *(Little Debbie)* peanut filled, chocolate coated	1 piece	230	28	12.0
CARROT				
(Break Cake)				
multi pak, 1.2 oz	1 cake	120	20	4.0
3.5 oz	2 cakes	370	64	12.0
(Pepperidge Farm) frozen 'Classic' 2.5 oz	1 piece	260	32	16.0
(Sara Lee)				
frozen, 1.8 oz, 'Deluxe'	1 piece	180	26	7.0
frozen, 2.5 oz, 'Lights'	1 piece	170	30	4.0
CHEESECAKE				
(Pepperidge Farm) strawberry, frozen, 'Manhattan'	1 piece	300	49	9.0
(Sara Lee)				
classic, 2 oz	1 piece	200	16	14.0
French, frozen, 3.2 oz, 'Lights'	1 piece	150	24	4.0
French, strawberry, frozen, 3.5 oz, 'Lights'	1 piece	150	29	2.0
(Weight Watchers)				
brownie, 'Sweet Celebrations'	3.5 oz	200	34	5.0
strawberry, 'Sweet Celebrations'	3.9 oz	180	28	4.0
CHERRY *(Pepperidge Farm)* frozen, supreme, 3.25 oz, 'Dessert Lights'	1 piece	170	38	2.0
CHOCOLATE				
(Aunt Fanny's)				
chocolate fudge	2.5 oz	222	39	6.0
fingers, devil's food	3 oz	288	49	9.0
(Awrey's) one piece	0.8 oz	70	11	3.0
(Break Cake)				
chocolate marshmallow pie	1 pie	150	24	5.0
chocolate marshmallow pie, double-decker	1 pie	360	61	11.0
devil's food marshmallow pie	1 pie	140	25	4.0
rounds, multi pak, 1.3 oz	1 cake	160	24	7.0
rounds, 3.25 oz	2 cakes	390	58	16.0
(Drake's)				
Swiss chocolate roll, cream filled	1.4 oz	170	22	8.0
chocolate mint, cream filled 'Ring Ding'	1.5 oz	190	22	11.0
chocolate roll, cream filled, 'Yodel'	1.1 oz	150	16	9.0
cream filled, 'Devil Dog'	1.5 oz	160	24	6.0
cream filled, 'Ring Ding'	1.5 oz	180	23	10.0
(Hostess)				
'Choco Bliss'	1 piece	200	29	9.0
'Chocodiles'	1 serving	240	33	11.0
'Chocolicious'	1 serving	190	30	7.0
creme filled, 'Ding Dongs'	1 serving	368	45	19.4
vanilla pudding filled, 'Light'	1 piece	130	28	1.0
(Little Debbie)				
	2.5 oz	320	45	14.0
'Be My Valentine'	1 cake	270	39	13.0
'Choco-Cake'	2.17 oz	270	37	13.0
'Choco-Jel'	1.16 oz	150	21	7.0
chocolate fudge, crispy	2.1 oz	260	48	7.0
chocolate fudge, round	2.75 oz	330	55	12.0
chocolate slices	3 oz	320	56	9.0
chocolate twins	2.2 oz	240	41	7.0
(Pepperidge Farm)				
chocolate fudge, frozen, 1.6 oz cake	1 piece	190	24	10.0

Food Name	Serv. Size	Total Cal.	Carbs GMS	Fat GMS
double chocolate, frozen, 2.25 oz, 'Classic'	1 piece	250	31	13.0
double chocolate, frozen, 2.5 oz, 'Lights'	1 piece	150	23	5.0
German chocolate, frozen, 2.25 oz, 'Classic'	1 piece	250	29	13.0
mousse, frozen, 1.5 oz, 'Dessert Lights'	1 piece	190	25	9.0
mousse, frozen, 3 oz serving	1 piece	180	20	9.0
mousse, frozen, 3 oz, 'Lights'	1 piece	170	20	8.0
(Snackwell's)				
devil's food cookie cake, nonfat	1 cookie	50	13	0.0
double fudge cookie cake, nonfat	1 serving	50	12	0.0
frosted fudge cake	1 cake	180	25	10.0
(Tastykake)				
cream filled, 'Krimpets'	1 piece	124	20	4.3
'Creamie'	1.5 oz	168	24	7.6
'Juniors'	3.3 oz	341	57	12.3
'Kandy Kakes'	0.7 oz	78	13	3.1
CHOCOLATE CHIP *(Little Debbie)*	1 cake	290	42	14.0
CINNAMON *(Aunt Fanny's)* twirl	1 oz	110	16	4.0
COCONUT				
(Little Debbie)				
coconut creme cake	1 cake	210	30	10.0
coconut crunch	2 oz	320	35	19.0
(Pepperidge Farm) frozen, 2.25 oz, 'Classic'	1 piece	230	31	11.0
(Tastykake) 'Juniors'	3.3 oz	296	60	6.0
COFFEECAKE				
(Drake's)				
cinnamon crumb	1.33 oz	150	22	6.0
'Jr.'	1.1 oz	140	18	6.0
'Small'	2 oz	220	33	9.0
(Hostess Snack Cake)	1 serving	130	19	5.0
(Little Debbie)				
	2.1 oz	250	39	9.0
apple streusel	1 cake	230	39	7.0
(Sara Lee)				
apple cinnamon, individually wrapped	1 piece	290	40	13.0
butter streusel, individually wrapped	1 piece	230	27	12.0
pecan, individually wrapped	1 piece	280	30	16.0
(Tastykake)				
cream filled, 'Koffee Kake'	1 oz	110	18	4.0
'Koffee Kake Juniors'	2.5 oz	261	44	8.5
(Weight Watchers) cinnamon streusel, 'Microwave'	1/2 pkg	190	28	7.0
CRUMB *(Hostess)*	1 serving	90	19	0.5
CUPCAKE				
(Aunt Fanny's) orange	3 oz	334	54	12.0
(Break Cake)				
chocolate, 3.5 oz	2 cupcakes	350	64	9.0
chocolate, multi-pak, 1.3 oz	1 cupcake	130	24	4.0
white, 1.3 oz	1 cupcake	130	24	3.0
(Hostess)				
chocolate	1 cupcake	180	30	6.0
chocolate, creme-filled, 'Light'	1 cupcake	120	25	2.0
orange	1 serving	160	27	5.0
(Tastykake)				
butter cream, cream filled, 1.1 oz	1 cupcake	118	20	4.2
chocolate, 'Royale'	1 cupcake	171	28	6.6
chocolate, cream filled, 1.1 oz	1 cupcake	118	19	4.2
chocolate, cream filled, 1.1 oz, 'Tastylite'	1 cupcake	100	22	1.3
'Kreme Kup'	0.9 oz	86	15	2.8

Food Name	Serv. Size	Total Cal.	Carbs GMS	Fat GMS
vanilla, cream filled, 'Tastylite'	1 cupcake	100	21	1.5
FRUIT *(Hostess)* 'Fruit Loaf'	1 piece	400	77	9.0
GOLDEN *(Hostess)* creme-filled, 'Twinkies'	1 piece	150	27	5.0
JELLY				
(Little Debbie) jelly roll	2.2 oz	250	43	9.0
(Tastykake) 'Krimpets'	1 oz	85	19	1.0
LEMON				
(Little Debbie) lemon stix	1.5 oz	220	29	10.0
(Pepperidge Farm) frozen, supreme 'Dessert Lights'	1 piece	170	26	5.0
(Sara Lee) frozen, lemon cream 'Lights'	1 piece	180	29	6.0
(Tastykake) 'Juniors'	3.3 oz	306	64	4.0
ORANGE *(Tastykake)* 'Juniors'	3.3 oz	337	61	9.2
PEANUT BUTTER				
(Little Debbie) wafer, 'Peanut Butter Naturals'	1.25 oz	170	19	10.0
(Tastykake) 'Kandy Kakes'	0.7 oz	87	11	4.2
PECAN				
(Aunt Fanny's) twirls	2 twirls	210	33	8.0
(Little Debbie) twins	2 oz	220	34	10.0
(Tastykake) twirls	1 oz	109	17	4.9
POUND				
(Aunt Fanny's)	2.5 oz	260	41	9.0
(Drake's) approx. 1.1 oz	1/10 cake	110	16	5.0
(Sara Lee) frozen, all butter, 1.6 oz	1 piece	200	23	11.0
PUDDING *(Hostess)*	1 piece	170	32	4.0
RASPBERRY				
(Aunt Fanny's) fingers	3 oz	303	53	9.0
(Little Debbie) raspberry angel cake	1 cake	120	28	1.5
(Pepperidge Farm) vanilla swirl, frozen, 'Dessert Lights'	1 piece	160	25	5.0
SHORTCAKE				
(Pepperidge Farm) strawberry, frozen, 'Dessert Lights'	1 piece	170	30	5.0
(Weight Watchers) strawberry à la mode	1 serving	170	33	2.0
SPICE				
(Aunt Fanny's) fingers	3 oz	290	49	9.0
(Little Debbie)	1 cake	300	44	14.0
STRAWBERRY *(Hostess)* 'Twinkies Fruit N Creme'	1.75 oz	160	32	3.0
VANILLA				
(Aunt Fanny's) fingers	3 oz	250	50	9.0
(Little Debbie)	2.6 oz	330	46	16.0
(Pepperidge Farm) fudge swirl, frozen, 'Classic'	1 piece	250	33	11.0
(Tastykake)				
cream filled 'Krimpets'	1.1 oz	116	19	4.1
'Creamie'	1.5 oz	184	25	9.0
YELLOW *(Awrey's)* one piece	0.9 oz	80	12	3.0
CAKE, SNACK, MIX				
APPLE				
(Pillsbury)				
apple streusel bar, deluxe, mix only	1/24 pkg	130	22	4.5
apple streusel bar, deluxe, prepared	1/24 pkg	150	23	6.0
BROWNIE				
regular, mix only	1 oz	123	22	4.2
regular, mix only	21.5-oz pkg	2647	467	90.9
(Betty Crocker)				
caramel, 'Supreme' prepared	1 brownie	110	21	2.0
caramel, 'Supreme' prepared w/1/4 cup oil, 1 egg	1 brownie	120	21	4.0
chocolate chip, 'Supreme' prepared	1 brownie	110	20	3.0
chocolplate chip, 'Supreme' prepared w/1/4 cup oil, 1 egg	1 brownie	130	20	5.0
frosted, 'Supreme' prepared	1 brownie	140	26	3.0

Food Name	Serv. Size	Total Cal.	Carbs GMS	Fat GMS
frosted, 'Supreme' prepared w/1/4 cup oil, 1 egg	1 brownie	160	26	6.0
German chocolate, prepared w/oil, margarine, egg, 2% milk . . .	1 brownie	160	24	7.0
original, 'Supreme' prepared w/1/4 cup oil, 2 eggs	1 brownie	140	22	5.0
party, 'Supreme' prepared	1 brownie	140	26	3.0
party, 'Supreme' prepared w/1/4 cup oil, 1 egg	1 brownie	160	26	6.0
peanut butter candies 'Supreme' mix only	1/24 pkg	120	21	3.0
peanut butter candies 'Supreme' prepared	1/24 pkg	140	21	5.0
(Duncan Hines)				
blonde, prepared	1 piece	160	22	8.0
'Dark 'n Fudgy' prepared	1 piece	170	25	8.0
double fudge, 'Brownies Plus' mix only	1 brownie	120	22	3.0
double fudge, 'Brownies Plus' prepared	1 brownie	150	22	6.0
double fudge, prepared	1 piece	170	29	7.0
fudge, chewy, prepared	1 piece	160	25	7.0
fudge, prepared	1 brownie	130	18	5.0
fudge, mix only	1 brownie	100	18	18.0
'Gourmet Turtle' mix only	1 brownie	160	27	5.0
'Gourmet Turtle' prepared	1 brownie	200	27	9.0
milk chocolate, 'Brownies Plus' prepared	1 brownie	160	20	8.0
milk chocolate, 'Brownies Plus' mix only	1 brownie	120	20	4.0
milk chocolate chunk, prepared	1 piece	170	26	7.0
Mississippi mud, prepared	1 piece	160	26	6.0
peanut butter, 'Brownies Plus'	1 brownie	150	16	8.0
peanut butter, 'Brownies Plus' mix only	1 brownie	120	16	5.0
peanut butter, prepared	1 piece	160	23	8.0
w/walnuts, 'Brownies Plus'	1 brownie	150	19	7.0
w/walnuts 'Brownies Plus' mix only	1 brownie	120	19	4.0
turtle, prepared	1 piece	160	26	6.0
walnut, prepared	1 piece	170	24	8.0
(Estee) prepared, 2-inch square	1 brownie	50	11	2.0
(Finast)				
fudge, 'Ultra Moist'	1/16 pkg	130	20	5.0
w/walnuts, 'Ultra Moist'	11/16 pkg	130	19	6.0
(General Mills)				
caramel 'Supreme' prepared	1 brownie	110	21	2.0
caramel 'Supreme' prepared w/1/4 cup oil, 1 egg	1 brownie	120	21	4.0
chocolate chip, 'Supreme' prepared	1 brownie	110	20	3.0
chocolate chip, 'Supreme' prepared w/1/4 cup oil, 1 egg	1 brownie	130	20	5.0
frosted, 'Supreme' prepared	1 brownie	140	26	3.0
frosted, 'Supreme' prepared w/1/4 cup oil, 1 egg	1 brownie	160	26	6.0
fudge, 'Family Size' prepared as directed	1 brownie	110	22	2.0
fudge, 'Family Size' prepared w/1/4 cup oil, 1 egg	1 brownie	140	22	5.0
fudge, 'Light' prepared	1 brownie	100	21	1.0
fudge, 'Regular Size' prepared	1 brownie	110	23	2.0
fudge, 'Regular Size' prepared w/1/4 cup oil, 1 egg	1 brownie	150	23	6.0
German chocolate, 'Supreme' prepared.	1 brownie	130	24	3.0
German chocolate, prepared w/oil, margarine, egg, 2% milk . . .	1 brownie	160	24	7.0
original, 'Supreme' prepared	1 brownie	120	22	3.0
original, 'Supreme' prepared w/1/4 cup oil, 2 eggs	1 brownie	140	22	5.0
party, 'Supreme' prepared	1 brownie	140	26	3.0
party, 'Supreme' prepared w/1/4 cup oil, 1 egg	1 brownie	160	26	6.0
walnut, 'Supreme' prepared	1 brownie	110	18	4.0
walnut, 'Supreme' prepared w/1/4 cup oil, 1 egg	1 brownie	130	18	6.0
(Gluten Free Pantry) chocolate truffle, gluten-free	1 serving	150	30	2.5
(Gold Medal)				
fudge, prepared	1 brownie	120	24	2.0
fudge, 'Pouch Mix'	1/16 pkg	100	16	4.0

Food Name	Serv. Size	Total Cal.	Carbs GMS	Fat GMS
(Great Additions)				
double chocolate, mix only	1/24 pkg	110	19	3.0
double chocolate, prepared w/1/3 cup oil, 1egg,				
2-inch square	1 brownie	140	19	6.0
double chocolate, prepared w/1/3 cup oil, 2 egg whites,				
2-inch square	1 brownie	130	19	6.0
frosted, 'Funfetti Frosted' mix only	1/24 pkg	100	18	2.0
frosted, 'Funfetti' prepared w/1/3 cup oil, 1 egg,				
2-inch square	1 brownie	160	23	7.0
frosted, 'Funfetti' prepared w/1/3 cup oil, 1 egg white,				
2-inch square	1 brownie	150	23	6.0
walnut, mix only	1/24 pkg	110	16	4.0
walnut, prepared w/water, 1/3c oil 2 egg whites,				
2-inch square	1 brownie	130	16	7.0
walnut, prepared w/water, 1/3 cup oil 1 egg, 2-inch square	1 brownie	140	16	8.0
(Krusteaz) fudge, prepared	1.5 oz mix	190	28	8.0
(Lovin' Lites)				
fudge, mix only	1/24 pkg	100	19	2.0
fudge, prepared w/water, 1 egg	1/24 pkg	100	19	2.0
fudge, prepared w/water, 2 egg whites	1/24 pkg	100	19	2.0
(Martha White) mix only	1 serving	114	23	1.8
(MicroRave)				
frosted	1 brownie	180	27	7.0
'Singles' prepared	1 brownie	250	39	9.0
walnut, 1.1 oz	1 brownie	160	21	7.0
w/hot fudge topping, 'Singles'	1 brownie	340	54	12.0
(Mixed Company) organic, chewy	1/4 cup	150	31	2.0
(Pillsbury)				
caramel fudge chunk, prepared, 2-inch square	1 brownie	170	25	7.0
chocolate chip, deluxe, mix only	1/20 pkg	140	28	3.0
chocolate chip, deluxe, prepared	1/20 pkg	180	28	7.0
cream cheese swirl, mix only	1/20 pkg	140	22	5.0
cream cheese swirl, prepared	1/20 pkg	180	22	9.0
double fudge, 2-inch square	1 brownie	160	24	6.0
fudge, deluxe 'Lovin' Bites'	1 piece	160	29	3.5
fudge, 15-oz pkg, mix only	1/16 pkg	110	21	2.0
fudge, 15-oz, prep	1/16 pkg	150	22	6.0
fudge, mix only	1/9 pkg	130	25	3.0
fudge, prepared	1 brownie	190	25	9.0
fudge, prepared w/1/4 cup oil	1/9 pkg	190	25	9.0
fudge, prepared w/1/2 cup oil, 2 egg whites, 2-inch square	1 brownie	150	20	7.0
fudge, prepared w/water, 1/4 cup oil, 1 egg, 2-inch square	1 brownie	140	21	6.0
fudge, prepared w/water, 1/4 cup oil, 1 egg white,				
2-inch square	1 brownie	140	21	6.0
fudge, 21.5-oz pkg, mix only	1/24 pkg	100	20	2.0
fudge, 21.5-oz, prepared	1/20 pkg	180	25	8.0
fudge, w/fudge frosting, 'Microwave Mix'	1/9 pkg	50	7	2.0
fudge, w/fudge frosting, mix only	1/9 pkg	130	25	3.0
fudge, w/fudge frosting, prepared w/1/4 cup oil, frosting	1/9 pkg	240	32	11.0
fudge deluxe, 'Family Size' 2-inch square	1 brownie	150	20	7.0
fudge deluxe, 2-inch square	1 brownie	150	21	6.0
fudge deluxe, w/walnuts, 2-inch square	1 brownie	150	19	8.0
fudge swirl cookie bar, deluxe, mix only	1/20 pkg	150	25	5.0
fudge swirl cookie bar, deluxe, prepared	1/20 pkg	180	25	8.0
hot fudge, mix	1/24 pkg	130	24	3.5
hot fudge, prepared	1/24 pkg	160	24	7.0
rocky road, fudge, 2-inch square	1 brownie	170	24	8.0

Food Name	Serv. Size	Total Cal.	Carbs GMS	Fat GMS
walnut, mix only	1/18 pkg	140	22	5.0
walnut, prepared	1/18 pkg	180	22	9.0
traditional, mix only	1 serving	132	23	3.6
triple fudge, chunky, 2-inch square	1 brownie	170	25	7.0
(Robin Hood) fudge, 'Pouch Mix'	1/16 pkg	100	16	4.0
(Weight Watchers) fudge, low-fat, 'Sweet Rewards'	1 serving	130	27	2.5
CHEESECAKE				
(Pillsbury)				
lemon, bar, mix only	1/24 pkg	170	20	9.0
lemon, bar, prepared	1/24 pkg	180	20	10.0
CHOCOLATE				
(Pillsbury)				
Oreo bar, deluxe, mix only	1/24 pkg	130	22	4.0
Oreo bar, deluxe, prepared	1/24 pkg	150	22	6.0
CUPCAKE				
(Funfetti)				
chocolate, microwave, mix only	1/9 pkg	100	14	4.0
chocolate, microwave, w/chocolate fudge frosting, prepared	1/9 pkg	160	24	7.0
yellow, microwave, mix only	1/9 pkg	110	17	5.0
yellow, microwave, w/vanilla frosting, prepared	1/9 pkg	180	28	7.0
GINGERBREAD				
(Betty Crocker)				
'Classic' cholesterol-free recipe, prepared	1/9 pkg	210	35	6.0
'Classic' prepared w/1 egg	1/9 pkg	220	35	7.0
(Dromedary) mix only	3 tbsp	100	19	2.0
(Hodgson Mill) whole wheat, mix only	1/4 cup	110	24	0.0
(Pillsbury)				
	1 serving	220	40	5.0
prepared, 3-inch square	1 piece	190	36	4.0
prepared w/water	1/9 pkg	180	32	5.0
(Sweet 'n Low) w/'Sweet 'n Low' mix only	1/6 cake	150	30	3.0
NUT				
(Pillsbury)				
Nutter Butter bar, deluxe, mix only	1/18 pkg	150	26	4.0
Nutter Butter bar, deluxe, prepared	1/18 pkg	180	26	7.0
CAKE DECORATION. See also under FROSTING; TOPPING.				
candies, rainbow mix (Dec-a-Cake)	1 tsp	15	3	0.5
candies, sugar crystals (Dec-a-Cake)	1 tsp	15	3	0.0
CAKE MIX				
ANGEL FOOD				
(Betty Crocker)				
confetti, 'SuperMoist'	1/12 cake	150	34	0.0
one-step white, SuperMoist' prepared	1/12 cake	140	32	0.0
'Traditional' mix only	1/12 mix	130	30	0.0
'Traditional' 'Supermoist' prepared	1/12 cake	130	30	0.0
(Duncan Hines)				
mix only	1/12 mix	140	30	0.0
prepared	1/12 cake	130	30	0.0
(General Mills)				
chocolate, mix only	1/12 mix	150	34	0.0
confetti, mix only	1/12 mix	150	34	0.0
lemon custard, mix only	1/12 mix	150	34	0.0
lemon pudding, mix only	1/12 mix	150	34	0.0
strawberry, mix only	1/12 mix	150	35	0.0
white, one-step, mix only	1/12 mix	150	34	0.0
(Gluten Free Pantry) gluten-free	1 serving	140	32	0.0
(Lovin' Loaf)				
mix only	1/8 pkg	90	20	0.0

Food Name	Serv. Size	Total Cal.	Carbs GMS	Fat GMS
prepared w/water	1/8 pkg	90	20	0.0
(Pillsbury)				
'Moist Supreme' mix only	1/12 pkg	140	31	0.0
prepared	1/12 cake	150	34	0.0
APPLE				
(Betty Crocker)				
apple cinnamon, 'SuperMoist' prepared	1/12 cake	250	36	10.0
apple cinnamon, 'SuperMoist' prepared,				
cholesterol-free recipe	1/12 cake	210	36	6.0
(Gold Medal) applesauce raisin, mix only	1/9 mix	140	28	3.0
(MicroRave)				
apple streusel, prepared	1/12 cake	240	33	11.0
apple streusel, prepared w/cholesterol-free egg product	1/12 cake	210	33	8.0
(Robin Hood) applesauce raisin, mix only	1/9 mix	140	28	3.0
BANANA				
(Duncan Hines)				
'Banana Supreme' prepared	1/12 cake	250	36	11.0
cholesterol-free recipe, prepared	1/12 cake	250	36	10.0
mix only	1/12 pkg	190	36	4.0
(Gold Medal) banana walnut, mix only	1/9 mix	150	27	4.0
(Pillsbury)				
microwave, mix only	1/9 pkg	110	17	5.0
'Moist Supreme' mix only	1/12 pkg	180	35	4.0
'Moist Supreme' prepared	1/12 pkg	260	36	11.0
'Pillsbury Plus' prepared	1/12 cake	260	36	11.0
'Pillsbury Plus' prepared w/water, 1/3 cup oil, 3 eggs	1/12 cake	250	35	11.0
'Pillsbury Plus' prepared w/water, 3 egg whites, 2 tbsp flour	1/12 cake	190	36	4.0
w/vanilla frosting, microwave, 'Snack' prepared	1/9 pkg	170	26	7.0
(Robin Hood) banana walnut, mix only	1/9 mix	150	27	4.0
(Sweet 'n Low) mix only	1/6 cake	150	30	3.0
BLACK FOREST				
(Duncan Hines) mousse,'Tiarra'	1/12 cake	260	33	13.0
(Pillsbury)				
cherry 'Bundt Ring Cake' mix only	1/16 pkg	200	40	4.0
cherry, 'Bundt' prepared	1/16 cake	240	38	8.0
cherry, prepared w/1/2 cup oil, 3 egg whites	1/16 pkg	270	41	12.0
cherry, prepared w/1/2 cup oil, 4 egg whites	1/16 pkg	260	41	11.0
BLUEBERRY				
(Streusel Swirl)				
streusel, mix only	1/16 pkg	210	39	5.0
streusel, prepared w/1/3 cup oil, 3 eggs	1/16 pkg	260	39	11.0
streusel, prepared w/1/3c oil, 4 egg whites	1/16 pkg	250	39	10.0
BOSTON CREAM				
(Betty Crocker)				
'Classic' mix only	1/8 pkg	230	48	4.0
'Classic' prepared w/egg, 2% milk	1/8 pkg	270	50	6.0
(Pillsbury)				
'Bundt' prepared	1/16 cake	270	43	10.0
chocolate éclair, 'Bundt Ring' mix only	1/16 pkg	210	42	4.0
chocolate éclair, prepared w/1/2 cup oil, 4 egg whites	1/16 cake	250	42	9.0
chocolate éclair, prepared w/1/3 cup oil, 3 eggs	1/16 pkg	260	42	10.0
BUTTER BRICKLE				
(Betty Crocker)				
'SuperMoist' prepared	1/12 cake	250	38	10.0
'SuperMoist' prepared w/cholesterol-free egg product	1/12 cake	220	38	6.0
BUTTER PECAN				
(Betty Crocker)				
'SuperMoist' mix only	1/12 mix	180	35	4.0

Food Name	Serv. Size	Total Cal.	Carbs GMS	Fat GMS
'SuperMoist' prepared w/3 eggs, 1/3 cup oil	1/12 cake	250	35	11.0
'SuperMoist' prepared w/oil, cholesterol-free egg product	1/12 cake	220	35	7.0
CARAMEL *(Duncan Hines)* prepared	1/12 cake	250	36	11.0
CARROT				
(Betty Crocker)				
'SuperMoist' mix only	1/12 mix	180	36	3.0
'Supermoist' prepared	1/12 cake	200	42	3.0
'SuperMoist' prepared w/1/3 cup oil, 3 eggs	1/12 cake	250	36	10.0
'SuperMoist' prepared w/1/3 cup oil, egg substitute	1/12 cake	210	36	6.0
(Dromedary) prepared	1/12 cake	232	23	15.0
(Estee) prepared	1/10 cake	100	18	2.0
(Pillsbury)				
carrot 'n spice, 'Pillsbury Plus' prepared	1/12 cake	260	36	11.0
microwave, mix only	1/9 pkg	110	17	5.0
'Moist Supreme' mix only	1/12 pkg	180	35	4.0
'Moist Supreme' prepared	1/12 pkg	260	35	12.0
'Pillsbury Plus' prepared w/1/3 cup oil, 3 eggs	1/12 pkg	260	34	12.0
'Pillsbury Plus' prepared w/water, 3 egg whites, 2 tbsp flour	1/12 pkg	190	35	5.0
'Quick Bread Mix' mix only	1/12 pkg	110	22	1.0
'Quick Bread Mix' prepared	1/12 pkg	140	22	5.0
w/cream cheese frosting, microwave, prepared	1/9 pkg	170	25	7.0
CHEESECAKE				
(Jell-O)				
lemon, no bake, mix only	1 pkg	170	31	3.0
lemon, no bake, prepared, 8-inch cake	1/8 cake	270	36	13.0
New York style, no bake, mix only	1 pkg	180	33	3.0
New York style, no bake, prepared, 8-inch cake	1/8 cake	280	38	12.0
strawberry, no bake, prepared	1/12 cake	340	52	12.0
(Royal)				
lite, 'No-Bake'	1/8 cake	210	23	10.0
real, 'No-Bake'	1/8 cake	280	31	9.0
CHERRY				
(Betty Crocker)				
cherry chip, 'SuperMoist' mix only	1/12 mix	180	37	3.0
cherry chip, 'SuperMoist' prepared w/3 egg whites	1/12 mix	190	37	3.0
(Duncan Hines)				
cherries and cream 'Tiarra'	1/12 cake	250	34	11.0
cherry vanilla, prepared	1/12 cake	250	36	11.0
CHOCOLATE				
(Betty Crocker)				
butter recipe, 'SuperMoist' mix only	1/12 mix	190	35	5.0
butter recipe, 'SuperMoist' prepared w/1/2 cup butter, 3 eggs	1/12 mix	280	35	14.0
chocolate chocolate chip, 'SuperMoist' prepared w/1/3 cup oil, 3 eggs	1/12 mix	260	34	12.0
chocolate chocolate chip, 'SuperMoist' mix only	1/12 mix	190	34	5.0
chocolate fudge, 'SuperMoist' mix only	1/12 mix	180	35	4.0
chocolate fudge, 'SuperMoist' prepared w/1/3 cup oil, 3 eggs	1/12 mix	260	35	12.0
chocolate pudding, 'Classic Dessert' mix only	1/6 pkg	220	44	4.0
chocolate pudding, 'Classic Dessert' prepared w/1 egg	1/6 pkg	230	44	5.0
devil's food 'SuperMoist' 'Light' cholesterol-free recipe, prepared	1/12 mix	180	36	3.0
devil's food 'SuperMoist' 'Light' mix only	1/12 mix	180	36	3.0
devil's food 'SuperMoist' 'Light' prepared w/3 eggs	1/12 mix	200	36	4.0
devil's food, 'SuperMoist' mix only	1/12 mix	190	35	5.0
devil's food, 'SuperMoist' prepared w/1/3 cup oil, 3 eggs	1/12 mix	260	35	12.0
devil's food, 'SuperMoist' prepared w/oil, cholesterol-free egg product	1/12 mix	220	35	7.0

Food Name	Serv. Size	Total Cal.	Carbs GMS	Fat GMS
fudge marble, 'SuperMoist' mix only	1/12 mix	180	36	4.0
fudge marble, 'SuperMoist' prepared w/1/3 cup oil, 3 eggs	1/12 mix	260	36	11.0
fudge marble, 'SuperMoist' prepared w/oil, cholesterol-free egg substitute	1/12 mix	220	36	7.0
German chocolate, 'SuperMoist' cholesterol-free recipe, prepared	1/12 mix	220	35	8.0
German chocolate, 'SuperMoist' mix only	1/12 mix	180	35	4.0
German chocolate, 'SuperMoist' prepared w/1/3 cup oil, 3 eggs	1/12 mix	260	35	12.0
milk chocolate, 'SuperMoist' cholesterol-free recipe, prepared	1/12 mix	210	34	7.0
milk chocolate, 'SuperMoist' mix only	1/12 mix	190	34	5.0
milk chocolate, 'SuperMoist' prepared w/1/3 cup oil, 3 eggs	1/12 mix	260	34	12.0
sour cream, 'SuperMoist' mix only	1/12 mix	180	35	4.0
sour cream, 'SuperMoist' prepared w/egg substitute	1/12 mix	220	35	8.0
sour cream, 'SuperMoist' prepared w/1/3 cup oil, 3 eggs	1/12 mix	260	35	12.0
(Duncan Hines)				
chocolate mousse, Amaretto, 'Tiarra' prepared	1/12 cake	270	29	16.0
chocolate mousse, 'Tiarra' prepared	1/12 cake	270	29	16.0
dark Dutch fudge, prepared	1/12 cake	280	33	15.0
dark Dutch fudge, cholesterol-free recipe, prepared	1/12 cake	270	33	14.0
dark Dutch fudge, mix only	1/12 cake	190	33	5.0
devil's food, cholesterol-free recipe, prepared	1/12 cake	270	33	14.0
devil's food, mix only	1/12 pkg	190	33	5.0
devil's food, prepared	1/12 cake	280	33	15.0
fudge, butter recipe, mix only	1/12 cake	190	34	4.0
fudge, butter recipe, prepared	1/12 cake	320	40	17.0
fudge, butter recipe, prepared w/stick margarine	1/12 cake	270	34	13.0
fudge marble, cholesterol-free recipe, prepared	1/12 cake	250	36	10.0
fudge marble, mix only	1/12 cake	190	36	4.0
fudge marble, prepared	1/12 cake	260	36	11.0
Swiss chocolate, cholesterol-free recipe, prepared	1/12 cake	270	33	14.0
Swiss chocolate, mix only	1/12 pkg	190	33	5.0
Swiss chocolate, prepared	1/12 cake	280	33	15.0
(Estee) prepared	1/10 cake	100	18	2.0
(Finast) devil's food, 'Ultra Moist' prepared	1/12 cake	250	33	11.0
(Gold Medal) mix, chocolate chip fudge, mix only	1/9 mix	150	25	5.0
(Krusteaz) devil's food, 8-inch double cake, prepared	1/12 cake	190	37	2.0
(MicroRave)				
chocolate fudge, w/vanilla frosting, prepared	1/6 cake	310	40	15.0
devil's food, 'Lovin' Lites' mix only	1/12 pkg	160	32	2.0
devil's food, 'Lovin' Lites' prepared w/water, 2 eggs	1/12 pkg	170	32	3.0
devil's food, 'Lovin' Lites' prepared w/water, 3 egg whites	1/12 pkg	160	32	2.0
devil's food, microwave, 'Singles' mix only	1 cake	250	35	10.0
devil's food, w/chocolate frosting, microwave, mix only	1/6 pkg	210	35	7.0
devil's food, w/chocolate frosting, microwave, prepared	1/6 pkg	310	36	17.0
devil's food, w/chocolate frosting, microwave, prepared w/egg substitute	1/6 pkg	240	36	9.0
devil's food, w/chocolate frosting, microwave, 'Singles' prepared	1 cake	450	65	19.0
German chocolate, w/frosting, microwave, mix only	1/6 pkg	230	37	8.0
German chocolate, w/frosting, microwave, prepared	1/6 pkg	320	37	18.0
(Pillsbury)				
butter recipe, 'Moist Supreme' mix only	1/12 pkg	180	33	4.0
butter recipe, 'Moist Supreme' mix only	1/12 pkg	270	33	13.0
butter recipe, 'Pillsbury Plus' mix only	1/12 pkg	170	32	4.0
butter recipe, 'Pillsbury Plus' prepared	1/12 pkg	270	33	13.0

Food Name	Serv. Size	Total Cal.	Carbs GMS	Fat GMS
butter recipe, 'Pillsbury Plus' prepared w/1/2 cup margarine,				
4 egg whites .... 1/12 cake	240	32	12.0
caramel nut, 'Bundt Ring Cake' mix .... 1/16 pkg	180	28	7.0
caramel nut, 'Bundt Ring Cake' prepared .... 1/16 cake	290	28	18.0
caramel, 'Bundt Ring Cake' mix only .... 1/16 pkg	220	43	5.0
caramel, prepared w/1/3 cup oil, 4 egg whites .... 1/16 cake	280	43	12.0
caramel, prepared w/water, 1/2 cup oil, 3 eggs .... 1/16 cake	290	43	13.0
chocolate macaroon, prepared w/1/2c oil, 4 egg whites ...... 1/16 cake	270	37	14.0
chocolate macaroon, 'Bundt Ring Cake' mix only .... 1/16 pkg	210	37	7.0
chocolate macaroon, prepared w/1/2 cup oil, 3 eggs .... 1/16 cake	280	37	14.0
chocolate mousse, 'Bundt Ring Cake' mix only .... 1/16 pkg	180	37	4.0
chocolate mousse, prepared w/1/2 cup oil, 3 eggs .... 1/16 cake	260	37	12.0
chocolate mousse, prepared w/1/2 cup oil, 4 egg whites ..... 1/16 cake	250	37	11.0
dark chocolate, 'Moist Supreme' mix only .... 1/12 pkg	180	34	4.0
dark chocolate, 'Moist Supreme' prepared .... 1/12 cake	250	34	11.0
dark chocolate, 'Pillsbury Plus' prepared w/3 egg whites,				
2 tbsp flour .... 1/12 cake	180	33	5.0
dark chocolate, 'Pillsbury Plus' prepared w/water, 1/3 cup				
oil, 3 eggs .... 1/12 cake	250	32	12.0
devil's food, 'Lovin Lites' prepared .... 1/10 cake	230	41	5.0
devil's food, 'Lovin' Lites' mix only .... 1/10 pkg	210	41	4.5
devil's food, 'Moist Supreme' mix only .... 1/12 pkg	180	33	4.0
devil's food, 'Moist Supreme' prepared .... 1/12 cake	270	33	14.0
devil's food, 'Pillsbury Plus' prepared w/water, 3 egg whites,				
2 tbsp flour .... 1/12 cake	180	33	4.0
double hot fudge, bundt, prepared .... 1/12 cake	280	32	16.0
double supreme, microwave, prepared .... 1/8 cake	330	39	19.0
fudge, 'Tunnel of Fudge' mix only .... 1/16 pkg	210	42	4.0
fudge, 'Tunnel of Fudge' prepared w/3/4c oil, 4 egg whites .... 1/16 cake	300	42	15.0
fudge, 'Tunnel of Fudge' prepared w/3/4 cup oil, 3 eggs ...... 1/16 cake	310	42	16.0
fudge swirl, 'Moist Supreme' mix only .... 1/12 pkg	200	37	4.5
fudge swirl, 'Moist Supreme' prepared .... 1/12 cake	250	37	10.0
fudge swirl, 'Pillsbury Plus' prepared w/1/3 cup oil, 3 eggs .... 1/12 cake	270	36	12.0
fudge swirl, 'Pillsbury Plus' prepared w/water, 3 egg whites,				
2 tbsp flour .... 1/12 cake	200	37	5.0
German chocolate, 'Moist Supreme' mix only .... 1/12 pkg	180	34	4.0
German chocolate, 'Moist Supreme' prepared .... 1/12 cake	250	34	11.0
German chocolate, 'Pillsbury Plus' prepared w/1/3 cup oil,				
3 eggs .... 1/12 cake	250	34	11.0
German chocolate, 'Pillsbury Plus' prepared w/3 egg				
whites, 2 tbsp flour .... 1/12 cake	180	34	4.0
microwave, mix only .... 1/9 pkg	110	16	5.0
microwave, prepared .... 1/8 cake	210	23	13.0
'Pillsbury Plus' prepared .... 1/12 cake	260	34	12.0
'Pillsbury Plus' prepared w/1/2 cup butter, 3 eggs .... 1/12 pkg	250	32	13.0
w/chocolate frosting, microwave, prepared .... 1/8 cake	300	35	17.0
w/chocolate fudge frosting, prepared .... 1/9 cake	160	24	7.0
w/vanilla frosting, microwave, prepared .... 1/8 cake	300	36	17.0
(Robin Hood) mix, chocolate chip fudge, mix only .... 1/9 mix	150	25	5.0
(Sweet 'n Low)				
low-fat, low-sodium, low-cholesterol, microwave,				
prepared 1/10 cake 90	2	40	0.0
mix only .... 1/6 cake	150	30	3.0
CHOCOLATE CHIP				
(Betty Crocker)				
'SuperMoist' mix only .... 1/12 mix	180	35	4.0
'SuperMoist' prepared w/oil, cholesterol-free egg substitute ... 1/12 mix	220	35	8.0

Food Name	Serv. Size	Total Cal.	Carbs GMS	Fat GMS
'SuperMoist' prepared w/1/2 cup oil, 3 eggs	1/12 mix	290	35	15.0
(Gold Medal) golden, mix only	1/9 mix	140	26	4.0
(Pillsbury)				
'Moist Supreme' mix only	1/12 pkg	190	35	5.0
'Moist Supreme' prepared	1/12 cake	240	35	10.0
'Pillsbury Plus' prepared w/1/4 cup oil, 2 eggs	1/12 cake	240	34	10.0
'Pillsbury Plus' w/2 egg whites, 2 tbsp flour	1/12 cake	190	35	5.0
(Robin Hood) golden, mix only	1/9 mix	140	26	4.0
CINNAMON				
(MicroRave)				
pecan, microwave	1/6 cake	290	39	13.0
pecan, microwave, prepared w/cholesterol-free egg product	1/6 cake	240	39	8.0
(Pillsbury)				
streusel, microwave, 'Streusel Swirl' prepared	1/8 cake	240	33	11.0
streusel, 'Streusel Swirl' mix only	1/16 pkg	210	38	5.0
streusel, 'Streusel Swirl' prepared	1/16 cake	260	38	11.0
streusel, 'Streusel Swirl' prepared w/1/3 cup oil, 4 egg whites	1/16 pkg	250	38	10.0
streusel, 'Streusel Swirl' prepared w/water, 1/3 cup oil, 3 eggs	1/16 pkg	260	38	11.0
COFFEECAKE				
(Aunt Jemima) 'easy'	1/3 cup	170	30	5.0
(Pillsbury) apple cinnamon	1/8 cake	240	40	7.0
FRUIT				
(Duncan Hines) tropical fruit, prepared	1/12 cake	250	36	11.0
GOLDEN				
(Betty Crocker) vanilla, 'Supermoist' prepared	1/12 cake	170	35	3.0
(Duncan Hines)				
golden, butter recipe, mix only	1/12 pkg	190	36	4.0
golden, butter recipe, prepared	1/12 cake	320	42	16.0
golden, butter recipe, prepared w/stick margarine	1/12 cake	270	36	13.0
KEY LIME (Duncan Hines) prepared	1/12 cake	250	36	11.0
LEMON				
(Betty Crocker)				
'SuperMoist' mix only	1/12 mix	180	36	4.0
'SuperMoist' prepared w/1/3 cup oil, 3 eggs	1/12 mix	260	37	11.0
'SuperMoist' prepared w/3 tbsp oil, egg substitute	1/12 mix	220	37	7.0
lemon chiffon, 'Classic Dessert' mix only	1/12 pkg	190	36	4.0
lemon chiffon, 'Classic Dessert' w/2 eggs	1/12 pkg	200	36	5.0
lemon pudding, 'Classic Dessert' mix only	1/6 pkg	220	45	4.0
lemon pudding, 'Classic Dessert' prepared w/1 egg	1/6 pkg	230	45	5.0
(Duncan Hines)				
lemon supreme	1/12 cake	260	36	11.0
lemon supreme, cholesterol-free recipe, prepared	1/12 cake	250	36	10.0
lemon supreme, mix only	1/12 cake	190	36	4.0
(Estee)	1/10 cake	100	18	2.0
(MicroRave) w/lemon frosting	1/6 cake	300	37	16.0
(Pillsbury)				
'Moist Supreme' mix only	1/10 pkg	210	42	4.0
'Moist Supreme' prepared	1/10 pkg	300	42	13.0
'Pillsbury Plus' prepared w/1/3 cup oil, 3 eggs	1/12 pkg	240	34	10.0
'Pillsbury Plus' prepared w/water, 3 egg whites, 2 tbsp flour	1/12 pkg	180	35	3.0
'Pillsbury Plus' prepared	1/12 cake	310	43	13.0
bundt, 'Tunnel of Lemon' mix only	1/16 pkg	210	44	4.0
bundt, 'Tunnel of Lemon' prepared	1/16 cake	270	45	9.0
bundt, 'Tunnel of Lemon' prepared w/1/3 cup oil, 3 eggs	1/16 pkg	270	44	9.0

Food Name	Serv. Size	Total Cal.	Carbs GMS	Fat GMS
bundt, 'Tunnel of Lemon' prepared w/1/3 cup oil, 4 egg whites	1/16 pkg	260	44	8.0
double supreme, microwave, prepared	1/8 cake	300	40	15.0
microwave, prepared	1/8 cake	220	23	13.0
w/lemon frosting, microwave, prepared	1/8 cake	300	37	17.0
(Streusel Swirl)				
lemon supreme, mix only	1/16 pkg	200	37	6.0
lemon supreme, prepared	1/16 cake	270	39	11.0
lemon supreme, prepared w/water, 1/3 cup oil, 3 eggs	1/16 pkg	260	37	11.0
lemon supreme, prepared w/water, 1/3c oil, 4 egg whites	1/16 pkg	250	37	10.0
(Sweet 'n Low) mix only	1/6 cake	150	30	3.0
ORANGE				
(Duncan Hines)				
orange supreme, cholesterol-free recipe, prepared	1/12 cake	250	36	10.0
orange supreme, mix only	1/12 cake	190	36	4.0
orange supreme, prepared	1/12 cake	260	36	11.0
PEACH *(Duncan Hines)* prepared	1/12 cake	250	36	11.0
PINEAPPLE				
(Betty Crocker)				
upside down, prepared w/egg substitute	1/9 cake	270	43	10.0
upside down, prepared w/eggs, margarine	1/9 cake	270	43	10.0
supreme, cholesterol-free recipe, prepared	1/12 cake	250	36	10.0
supreme, mix only	1/12 cake	190	36	4.0
supreme, prepared	1/12 cake	260	36	11.0
(Pillsbury)				
crème, bundt, mix only	1/16 pkg	200	42	3.0
crème, bundt, prepared	1/16 cake	260	41	9.0
crème, prepared w/water, 1/2 cup oil, 4 egg whites	1/16 pkg	270	42	10.0
crème, prepared w/water, 1/3 cup oil, 3 eggs	1/16 pkg	280	42	11.0
POUND				
(Betty Crocker) golden 'Classic Dessert' mix only	1/12 pkg	190	28	8.0
(Dromedary)				
mix only	5 tbsp	130	20	5.0
prepared	1/2 inch	150	21	6.0
(Estee) prepared	1/8 cake	120	23	2.5
(Martha White) prepared	1/10 cake	120	19	4.0
RAINBOW CHIP				
(Betty Crocker)				
party cake, 'SuperMoist' mix only	1/12 mix	180	35	4.0
party cake, 'Supermoist' prepared	1/12 cake	220	41	5.0
party cake, 'SuperMoist' prepared w/1/3 cup oil, 3 eggs	1/12 cake	250	35	11.0
RASPBERRY *(Duncan Hines)* prepared	1/12 cake	250	36	11.0
SPICE				
(Betty Crocker)				
'SuperMoist' mix only	1/12 mix	180	36	4.0
'SuperMoist' prepared w/1/3 cup oil, 3 eggs	1/12 cake	260	36	11.0
'SuperMoist' prepared w/3 tbsp oil, cholesterol-free egg product	1/12 cake	220	36	7.0
(Duncan Hines)				
cholesterol-free recipe, prepared	1/12 cake	250	36	10.0
mix only	1/12 cake	190	36	4.0
prepared	1/12 cake	260	36	11.0
(Estee)	1/8 cake	120	23	3.0
(Gluten Free Pantry) gluten-free	1 serving	110	26	0.0
STRAWBERRY				
(Duncan Hines)				
supreme, mix only	1/12 pkg	190	36	4.0

Food Name	Serv. Size	Total Cal.	Carbs GMS	Fat GMS
supreme, prepared	1/12 cake	260	36	11.0
supreme, prepared, cholesterol-free recipe	1/12 cake	250	36	10.0
(Pillsbury)				
'Moist Supreme' mix only	1/12 pkg	180	36	4.0
'Moist Supreme' prepared	1/12 cake	260	36	11.0
cream cheese, 'Bundt Ring Cake' mix only	1/16 pkg	190	34	5.0
cream cheese, 'Bundt RingCake' prepared	1/16 cake	300	34	17.0
'Pillsbury Plus' prepared	1/12 cake	260	36	11.0
'Pillsbury Plus' prepared w/1/3 cup oil & 3 eggs	1/12 pkg	190	36	4.0
SWIRL				
(Betty Crocker)				
party cake, 'SuperMoist' mix only	1/12 mix	190	36	4.0
party cake, 'SuperMoist' prepared, cholesterol-free recipe,	1/12 cake	220	36	7.0
party cake, 'SuperMoist' prepared w/1/3 cup oil, 3 eggs	1/12 cake	260	36	11.0
(Pillsbury)				
white and fudge, 'Moist Supreme' mix only	1/12 pkg	200	37	4.5
white and fudge, 'Moist Supreme' prepared	1/12 pkg	250	37	10.0
white and fudge, 'Pillsbury Plus' mix only	1/12 pkg	190	36	4.0
white and fudge, 'Pillsbury Plus' prepared	1/12 pkg	250	36	10.0
white and fudge, 'Pillsbury Plus' prepared, cholesterol-free recipe	1/12 pkg	200	37	4.0
VANILLA				
(Betty Crocker)				
golden, 'SuperMoist' mix only	1/12 mix	180	36	4.0
golden, 'SuperMoist' prepared w/1/2 cup oil, 3 eggs	1/12 mix	280	36	14.0
golden, 'SuperMoist' prepared w/oil, egg substitute	1/12 mix	220	36	7.0
(Duncan Hines)				
French, mix only	1/12 cake	190	36	4.0
French, prepared	1/12 cake	260	36	11.0
French, prepared, cholesterol-free recipe	1/12 cake	250	36	10.0
(MicroRave) golden	1/6 cake	320	40	17.0
(Pillsbury)				
French, 'Moist Supreme' mix only	1/10 pkg	220	42	5.0
French, 'Moist Supreme' prepared	1/10 pkg	300	42	13.0
French, 'Pillsbury Plus' mix only	1/10 pkg	230	41	6.0
French, 'Pillsbury Plus' prepared	1/10 pkg	320	41	15.0
sunshine, 'Moist Supreme' mix only	1/12 pkg	190	34	5.0
sunshine, 'Moist Supreme' prepared	1/12 cake	260	34	12.0
sunshine, 'Pillsbury Plus'prepared w/3 egg white, 2 tbsp flour	1/12 pkg	190	35	5.0
WHITE				
(Betty Crocker)				
'Light' prepared	1/12 mix	180	37	3.0
'Light' mix only	1/12 mix	180	34	4.0
'Light' prepared w/3 egg whites	1/12 mix	180	37	3.0
sour cream, 'SuperMoist' mix only	1/12 mix	180	36	3.0
sour cream, 'SuperMoist' prepared	1/12 cake	210	41	4.5
sour cream, 'SuperMoist' prepared w/3 egg whites	1/12 mix	180	36	3.0
'SuperMoist' prepared w/1/3 cup oil, 3 eggs	1/12 mix	230	34	10.0
(Duncan Hines)				
cholesterol-free recipe, prepared	1/12 cake	240	36	10.0
mix only	1/12 cake	190	36	4.0
prepared	1/12 cake	240	35	10.0
(Estee)	1/10 cake	100	18	2.0
(Krusteaz) prepared, 8-inch double cake	1/12 cake	190	37	3.0
(Pillsbury)				
'Lovin Lites' mix only	1/10 pkg	210	42	4.0
'Lovin Lites' prepared	1/10 cake	230	42	5.0

Food Name	Serv. Size	Total Cal.	Carbs GMS	Fat GMS
'Moist Supreme' mix only	1/10 pkg	220	41	5.0
'Moist Supreme' prepared	1/10 cake	280	41	11.0
'Pillsbury Plus' mix only	1/12 pkg	170	35	2.0
'Pillsbury Plus' prepared w/water, egg whites	1/12 cake	170	35	2.0
'Pillsbury Plus' prepared w/water, eggs	1/12 cake	180	35	3.0
'Pillsbury Plus' prepared w/1/4 cup oil, 3 egg whites	1/12 cake	220	34	9.0
'Pillsbury Plus' prepared w/water, 3 egg whites, 2 tbsp flour	1/12 cake	190	35	4.0
(Lovin' Loaf)				
mix only	1/12 pkg	170	35	2.0
prepared w/water, 2 eggs	1/12 cake	180	35	3.0
prepared w/water, 3 egg whites	1/12 cake	170	35	2.0
(Sweet 'n Low) lowfat, mix only	1/6 pkg	140	30	3.0
(Weight Watchers) low-fat, 'Sweet Rewards'	1 serving	170	36	2.0
YELLOW				
(Betty Crocker)				
'Supermoist' 'Light' prepared	1/12 cake	180	37	3.0
'Supermoist' 'Light' prepared w/3 eggs	1/12 cake	200	37	4.0
'Supermoist' 'Light' prepared w/egg substitute	1/12 cake	190	37	3.0
'Supermoist' mix only	1/12 mix	180	36	4.0
'Supermoist' prepared w/1/3 cup oil, 3 eggs	1/12 cake	260	36	11.0
'Supermoist' prepared w/3 tbsp oil, egg substitute	1/12 cake	220	36	7.0
(Duncan Hines)				
cholesterol-free recipe, prepared	1/12 cake	250	36	10.0
mix only	1/12 pkg	190	36	4.0
prepared	1/12 cake	260	36	11.0
(Finast) 'Ultra Moist' prepared	1/12 cake	240	34	10.0
(Krusteaz) prepared, 8-inch double cake	1/12 cake	200	36	5.0
(Lovin' Loaf)				
prepared w/water, 2 eggs	1/12 pkg	180	35	3.0
prepared w/water, 3 egg whites	1/12 pkg	170	35	2.0
(MicroRave)				
microwave, 'Singles' prepared	1 cake	260	36	11.0
w/chocolate frosting, microwave, mix only	1/6 pkg	210	36	7.0
w/chocolate frosting, microwave, 'Singles' prepared	1 cake	460	65	20.0
w/chocolate frosting, microwave, prepared w/1 tbsp oil, egg substitute	1/6 pkg	230	36	9.0
yellow, w/chocolate frosting, microwave, prepared w/1/4 cup oil, 1 egg	1/6 pkg	300	36	17.0
(Pillsbury)				
butter recipe, 'Moist Supreme' mix only	1/12 pkg	170	35	3.0
butter recipe, 'Pillsbury Plus' prepared	1/12 cake	260	36	12.0
butter recipe, 'Pillsbury Plus' prepared w/1/2 cup butter, 3 eggs	1/12 cake	260	35	12.0
butter recipe, 'Pillsbury Plus' prepared w/1/2 cup margarine, 4 egg whites	1/12 cake	250	35	11.0
butter recipe, 'SuperMoist' mix only	1/12 mix	170	37	2.0
butter recipe, 'SuperMoist' prepared w/1/2 cup butter, 3 eggs	1/12 mix	260	37	11.0
'Lovin' Lites' mix only	1/10 pkg	220	43	4.0
'Lovin' Lites' prepared	1/10 cake	230	43	5.0
microwave, prepared	1/8 cake	220	23	13.0
'Moist Supreme' mix only	1/12 pkg	180	35	4.0
'Moist Supreme' prepared	1/12 cake	240	35	10.0
'Pillsbury Plus' prepared w/1/3 cup oil, 3 eggs	1/12 cake	260	34	12.0
'Pillsbury Plus' prepared w/water, 3 egg whites, 2 tbsp flour	1/12 cake	190	35	5.0
w/chocolate frosting, microwave, prepared	1/8 cake	300	36	17.0
(Sweet 'n Low)				
low-fat, low-sodium, low-cholesterol, microwave, prepared	1/10 cake	90	16	2.0

Food Name	Serv. Size	Total Cal.	Carbs GMS	Fat GMS
mix only	1/6 pkg	150	30	3.0
(Weight Watchers) less fat 'Sweet Rewards'	1 serving	160	37	1.0

CALABASH GOURD. See GOURD, BOTTLE.

CALAMARI. See SQUID.

CALICO BASS. See SUNFISH.

CALZONE. See under SANDWICH.

CANADIAN BACON. See BACON, CANADIAN STYLE.

CANARY TREE. See PILI NUT.

CANDY. See also CANDY COATING.

Food Name	Serv. Size	Total Cal.	Carbs GMS	Fat GMS
(Boyer) 'Smoothie'	1.6 oz	250	24	15.0
(Brach's) 'Bridge Mix'	1 oz	140	17	7.0
(Estee) 'Estee-ets'	5 pieces	35	4	2.0
(Nestlé) 'Butterfinger' round 'BBs'	10 pieces	125	17	4.9
(Russell Stover) 'Home Fashioned Favorites'	1.4 oz	170	27	7.0
ALMOND				
(Brach's) candy-coated, 'Jordan Almonds'	1 oz	120	23	2.0
(Estee) chocolate covered	2 squares	60	5	4.5
(Featherweight) chocolate covered	1 section	90	6	7.0
(Hershey's) chocolate covered, solitaires, 'Hershey's Golden Collection' 2.8-oz pieces	1 piece	444	37	28.9
(M&M Mars) candy-coated, 'M&M's'	1 oz	150	17	8.0
(Russell Stover) 'Almond Delights'	1.4 oz	210	22	12.0
BUTTERSCOTCH *(Russell Stover)* squares	1.4 oz	180	29	6.5
CANDY BAR				
(Barat)				
chocolate tofu, w/almonds	1 oz	170	13	11.0
chocolate tofu, w/almonds and raisins	1 oz	160	14	11.0
chocolate tofu truffle, w/pralines	1 oz	170	12	11.0
(Cadbury)				
chocolate, w/crisps and honey	1 oz	150	18	7.0
chocolate, w/fruit and nuts	1 oz	150	17	8.0
chocolate, w/roasted almonds	1 oz	150	15	9.0
'Dairy Milk'	1 oz	150	17	8.0
(Carafection)				
'Almond Crunch' date sweetened carob	1 oz	139	17	7.0
'Cashew Coconut Crunch' carob	1 oz	139	17	7.0
'Crispy Crunch' date sweetened carob	1 oz	139	17	7.0
'Mint Honey Graham' carob coated	1 oz	139	17	7.0
'Mint' date sweetened carob	1 oz	139	17	7.0
'Original Honey Graham' carob coated	1 oz	139	17	7.0
'Peanut Crunch' date sweetened, carob	1 oz	139	17	7.0
plain, date sweetened, carob	1 oz	139	17	7.0
(Caroby) carob	4 sections	150	13	9.0
(Cocofection) original	1 oz	155	15	10.0
(Estee)				
chocolate, coconut	2 squares	60	5	4.0
chocolate, dark, deluxe	2 squares	50	6	3.0
chocolate, fruit and nut	2 squares	60	5	4.5
chocolate, milk	2 squares	60	5	4.0
crunch	2 squares	45	4	3.0
mint	2 squares	50	6	3.0
(Fantastic Foods) 'Halvah'	1.5 oz	232	17	10.0
(Fifty 50)				
chocolate, milk, extra thick, w/o sugar	1 section	80	6	6.0
chocolate, milk, mini	4 pieces	90	6	6.0
chocolate, w/almonds, extra thick, w/o sugar	1 section	90	6	6.0
crunch, chocolate, extra thick, w/o sugar	1 section	70	6	5.0

Food Name	Serv. Size	Total Cal.	Carbs GMS	Fat GMS
fruit and nut, chocolate, extra thick, w/o sugar . . . . 1 section		80	6	5.0
(Ghirardelli)				
chocolate, dark, 'Premier Bar' . . . . 1 bar		428	51	28.6
chocolate, dark, w/almonds, 'Premier Bar' . . . . 1 bar		442	45	31.6
chocolate, dark, w/raspberries, 'Premier Bar' . . . . 1 bar		423	52	27.6
(Heath) 'Soft'n Crunchy Bar' 2 pieces . . . . 1.19 oz serving		190	19	12.0
(Hershey's)				
'Almond Joy' 1.7-oz bar . . . . 1 bar		229	29	13.1
'Almond Joy' snack size, 0.7 oz . . . . 1 bar		93	12	5.4
'Caramello' 5-oz bar . . . . 1 bar		673	90	30.8
'Caramello' 1.6-oz bar . . . . 1 bar		213	29	9.8
chocolate, 'Hershey's Milk Chocolate Bar' . . . . 1.55 oz		240	25	14.0
chocolate, snack size, 0.7-oz bar . . . . 1 bar		91	11	4.8
chocolate, w/almonds, 'Hershey's Milk Chocolate				
Bar w/Almonds' . . . . 1.45 oz		230	20	14.0
chocolate almond, 'Golden Collection' . . . . 2.8 oz		448	36	29.7
'Cookies 'N' Mint' . . . . 1 bar		220	26	12.0
'5th Avenue' 2-oz bar . . . . 1 bar		280	38	12.1
'5th Avenue' snack size, 0.6 oz . . . . 1 bar		79	11	3.4
'Kit Kat' 3.375-oz bar . . . . 1 bar		493	61	24.5
'Kit Kat' 2.8-oz bar . . . . 1 bar		401	50	19.9
'Kit Kat' 1.62-oz bar . . . . 1 bar		236	29	11.7
'Kit Kat' 1.5-oz bar . . . . 1 bar		216	27	10.7
'Kit Kat' mini, 0.35-oz bar . . . . 1 bar		51	6	2.5
'Krackel' 7-oz pkg . . . . 1 pkg		982	114	53.1
'Krackel' 2.2-oz bar . . . . 1 bar		329	38	17.8
'Krackel' 1.5-oz bar . . . . 1 bar		218	25	11.8
'Mounds' 1.9-oz bar . . . . 1 bar		253	31	13.3
'Mr. Goodbar' 2.6-oz bar . . . . 1 bar		398	38	25.5
'Mr. Goodbar' 1.75-oz bar . . . . 1 bar		267	25	17.1
'Skor' 1.4-oz bar . . . . 1 bar		217	23	13.3
'Special Dark' extra large, 8 oz . . . . 1 bar		1253	138	73.5
'Special Dark' large, 4-oz bar . . . . 1 bar		624	68	36.6
'Special Dark' 2.8-oz bar . . . . 1 bar		436	48	25.6
'Special Dark' 2.2-oz bar . . . . 1 bar		342	38	20.1
'Special Dark' 1.45-oz bar . . . . 1 bar		226	25	13.3
'Symphony' 1.5-oz bar . . . . 1 bar		232	24	13.8
'Symphony' 2.4-oz bar . . . . 1 bar		371	39	22.0
'Whatchamacallit' 1.7-oz bar . . . . 1 bar		214	29	9.3
(M&M Mars)				
'Bounty' milk chocolate . . . . 1 oz		140	17	7.0
'Dove' dark chocolate . . . . 1 bar		200	22	12.0
'Dove' dark chocolate, miniatures . . . . 4 pieces		130	14	8.0
'Dove' milk chocolate . . . . 1 bar		200	22	12.0
'Dove' milk chocolate, miniatures . . . . 4 pieces		130	14	8.0
'Mars' almond, 1.76-oz bar . . . . 1 bar		234	31	11.5
'Milky Way' 2.15-oz bar . . . . 1 bar		258	44	9.8
'Milky Way' 2.1-oz bar . . . . 1 bar		254	43	9.7
'Milky Way' 2.05-oz bar . . . . 1 bar		245	42	9.3
'Milky Way' 1.9-oz bar . . . . 1 bar		228	39	8.7
'Milky Way' 0.8-oz bar . . . . 1 bar		97	16	3.7
'Milky Way' fun size . . . . 1 bar		76	13	2.9
'Munch' . . . . 1.42 oz		220	19	14.0
'Snickers' king size, 4-oz bar . . . . 1 bar		541	67	27.8
'Snickers' 2-oz bar . . . . 1 bar		273	34	14.0
'Snickers' fun size . . . . 1 bar		72	9	3.7
'3 Musketeers' 2.13-oz bar . . . . 1 bar		250	46	7.7

Food Name	Serv. Size	Total Cal.	Carbs GMS	Fat GMS
'3 Musketeers' 1.813-oz bar	1 bar	212	39	6.6
'3 Musketeers' 0.8-oz bar	1 bar	96	18	3.0
'3 Musketeers' fun size	1 bar	69	13	2.1
'Twix' 11-oz pkg	1 pkg	1557	205	76.1
'Twix' 3.35-oz bar	4 bars	474	62	23.2
'Twix' 2.06-oz bar	2 bars	289	38	14.1
'Twix' 2-oz pkg	1 pkg	284	37	13.9
'Twix' peanut, 9.43-oz pkg	1 pkg	1415	141	85.9
'Twix' peanut, 2.06-oz pkg	1 pkg	307	31	18.7
'Twix' peanut, 1.89-oz pkg	1 pkg	286	28	17.4
'Twix' peanut, 1.77-oz pkg	1 pkg	265	26	16.1
(Natures Warehouse)				
'A-Ok' fruit juice sweetened	1 oz	130	17	6.2
'My O My' fruit juice sweetened	1 oz	103	21	1.4
'No How' peanut butter, fruit juice sweetened	1 oz	140	11	10.0
'Non Stop' fruit juice sweetened	1 oz	122	18	5.0
'Nut Wit' carob caramel and peanuts	1 oz	135	17	6.3
(Necco) 'Sky Bar'	1.5 oz	196	32	7.1
(Nestlé)				
'100 Grand' 1.5-oz bar	1 bar	200	30	7.8
'100 Grand' miniature	1 bar	98	15	3.8
'Aero' regular size	1 bar	210	20	12.0
'Aero' bite size	2 bars	85	10	5.0
'Baby Ruth' 2.28-oz bar	1 bar	313	42	13.8
'Baby Ruth' 2.1-oz bar	1 bar	289	39	12.7
'Baby Ruth' 1.2-oz bar	1 bar	164	22	7.2
'Baby Ruth' miniature	1 bar	101	14	4.4
'Baby Ruth' fun size	1 bar	67	9	3.0
'Butterfinger' king size	1 bar	518	71	20.2
'Butterfinger' 2.16-oz bar	1 bar	293	40	11.4
'Butterfinger' 1.6-oz bar	1 bar	216	30	8.4
'Butterfinger' fun size	1 bar	101	14	3.9
'Butterfinger' bite size	1 bar	34	5	1.3
'Chunky' 1.4-oz bar	1 bar	198	23	11.7
'Chunky' 1.25-oz bar	1 bar	173	20	10.2
'Crunch' 1.55-oz bar	1 bar	230	29	11.6
'Crunch' 1.4-oz bar	1 bar	209	26	10.5
'Crunch' miniature	1 bar	52	7	2.6
'Oh Henry!' 2-oz bar	1 bar	246	37	9.6
(Pay Day) 'Pay Day'	1.85 oz	250	28	12.0
(Russell Stover)				
French chocolate	1 bar	200	20	13.0
mint, French chocolate	1 bar	230	20	15.5
peanut butter	1 bar	290	22	19.0
(Weight Watchers)				
caramel nut	1 bar	130	14	8.0
English toffee crunch	1 bar	120	12	7.0
(Yogafection)				
'Brazil Nut Crunch'	1 oz	180	17	10.0
'Cashew Nut Crunch'	1 oz	180	17	10.0
CARAMEL				
(Allen Wertz)				
	1 piece	37	6	2.0
nougat swirl	1 piece	32	6	1.0
(Brach's) chocolate, 'Milk Maid'	1 oz	110	20	3.0
(Estee)				
chocolate	2 pieces	50	9	2.0

Food Name	Serv. Size	Total Cal.	Carbs GMS	Fat GMS
vanilla	2 pieces	50	9	2.0
(Featherweight)	1 piece	30	5	1.0
(Hershey's)				
in milk chocolate, 1.91-oz pkg 'Rolo'	1 pkg	218	28	10.6
in milk chocolate, 1.74-oz roll 'Rolo'	1 roll	202	26	9.8
in milk chocolate, 0.2-oz pieces 'Rolo'	1 piece	12	2	0.6
(Kraft)	1 piece	30	6	1.0
(Pom Poms) chocolate coated	1 oz	100	15	3.0
(Russell Stover)				
butter cream, squares	1.4 oz	170	26	7.5
marshmallow, milk chocolate, soft-chewy, squares	1.4 oz	190	25	10.0
CHERRY				
(Brach's)				
chocolate cream	1 oz	110	21	2.0
dark chocolate coated	1 oz	110	22	2.0
milk chocolate covered, 'Villa'	1 oz	110	22	2.0
(Russell Stover)				
'Cherry Cordials'	1.4 oz	170	25	7.5
squares	1.4 oz	160	28	5.5
CHOCOLATE				
(Allen Wertz) assortment, 'Gourmet'	11.9 grams	55	9	2.0
(Barat)				
tofu, 'Passionettes'	1 piece	70	6	5.0
tofu pastilles 'Bits'	0.75 oz	120	11	8.0
(Brach's)				
assorted, wrapped	1 oz	110	24	2.0
'Jots'	1 oz	130	21	5.0
milk, 'Stars'	1 oz	150	17	8.0
milk chocolate coated, 'Malted Milk Balls'	1 oz	130	21	5.0
(Callard and Bowser) cream	1 oz	120	22	3.7
(Cocofection) trail mix, premium	1 oz	130	13	9.0
(Featherweight)				
crunch	1 section	80	7	6.0
milk	1 section	80	7	6.0
(Great Cakes) amaretto, confection, 'Buffalo Ball'	1 ball	105	27	3.5
(Hershey's)				
milk, 'Kisses'	6 pieces	150	16	9.0
milk, creamy, w/almonds and toffee chips	0.75 oz	280	26	17.0
w/almonds, 'Kisses w/Almonds'	6 pieces	160	14	10.0
(M&M Mars)				
'M&M's' mini, 5-oz pkg	1 pkg	707	95	33.1
'M&Ms' plain	1 cup	1023	148	44.0
'M&Ms' plain	10 pieces	34	5	1.5
'M&Ms' plain, 1.69-oz pkg	1 pkg	236	34	10.1
'M&Ms' plain, 1.48-oz box	1 box	207	30	8.9
(Nabisco) milk, 'Stars' approx 13 pieces	1 oz	160	19	8.0
(Russell Stover)				
dark and milk mix, 'The Gift Box'	1.4 oz	180	26	8.5
milk, assortment	1.4 oz	190	27	8.5
(Saco Foods)				
'Choc'Oh's'	1.5 oz	111	14	6.6
chunks	3.5 oz	466	67	26.4
(Spangler)				
coated, creme center	1 piece	80	15	2.0
coated, creme center caramel, w/nuts	1 piece	100	11	6.0
coated, creme center cherry, w/nuts	1 piece	110	12	5.0
coated, creme center fudge, w/nuts	1 piece	140	17	6.0

Food Name	Serv. Size	Total Cal.	Carbs GMS	Fat GMS
coated, creme center fudge, w/pecans	1 piece	140	18	7.0
coated, creme center maple, w/nuts	1 piece	110	12	5.0
coated, creme center vanilla, w/nuts	1 piece	110	13	5.0
(Tootsie Roll) chewy roll	1 oz	112	23	2.5
(Whoppers) milk chocolate coated, malted milk balls	1 oz	136	20	6.0
COCONUT				
(Brach's) Neapolitan	1 oz	120	24	2.0
(Sunbelt) chocolate coated 'Macaroo'	2 oz	288	33	16.0
COFFEE				
(Allen Wertz)				
'Coffee Time'	1 piece	20	4	1.0
'Coffee Time' assorted	1 piece	28	5	1.0
'Coffee Time' decaffeinated	1 piece	20	4	1.0
(Brach's)	1 oz	120	25	2.0
FRUIT				
(Bonkers!) chews, all flavors	1 piece	20	5	0.0
(Featherweight)				
berry patch	1 piece	12	3	0.0
drops, all flavors	0.33 oz	30	8	0.0
orchard	1 piece	12	3	0.0
tropical blend	1 piece	12	3	0.0
(Glenny's)				
black cherry, 'Drops'	1 drop	6	1	1.0
lemon, twist of, 'Drops'	1 drop	6	1	1.0
mandarin orange, 'Drops'	1 drop	6	1	1.0
mixed fruit, 'Drops'	1 drop	6	1	1.0
(Hershey's) 'Jujyfruits'	11 pieces	100	25	1.0
(M&M Mars)				
'Skittles' original, bite size	1 cup	830	186	9.0
'Skittles' original, bite size, 4-oz pkg	1 pkg	458	102	4.9
'Skittles' original, bite size, 2.3-oz pkg	1 pkg	263	59	2.8
'Skittles' original, bite size, 2.17-oz pkg	1 pkg	251	56	2.7
'Skittles' original, bite size, 2-oz pkg	1 pkg	231	52	2.5
'Skittles' original, bite size	10 pieces	43	10	0.5
chews, 'Starburst'	1 piece	20	4	0.4
chews, 'Starburst' 2.07-oz pkg	1 pkg	234	50	4.9
chews, 'Starburst' fun size	1 pkg	166	35	3.5
(Rascals) chews, all flavors	1 piece	4	1	0.0
(SweeTARTS) chewy	1 oz	113	25	1.0
FUDGE				
(Kraft) 'Fudgies'	1 piece	35	6	1.0
(Woodys)				
cheese, w/walnuts	1 oz	120	18	4.0
chocolate, w/walnuts	1 oz	120	18	4.0
maple walnut	1 oz	120	19	4.0
mint, w/walnuts	1 oz	120	18	4.0
GUM				
(Beech-Nut)				
candy-coated, 'Beechies'	1 piece	6	2	0.0
cinnamon	1 piece	10	2	0.0
fruit	1 piece	10	2	0.0
peppermint	1 piece	10	2	0.0
spearmint	1 piece	10	2	0.0
(Brach's) balls, 'Gumdinger' all flavors,	1 oz	110	24	2.0
(Bubble Yum)				
bananaberry split	1 piece	25	7	0.0
checkermint	1 piece	25	7	0.0

Food Name	Serv. Size	Total Cal.	Carbs GMS	Fat GMS
cherry	1 piece	25	7	0.0
fruit	1 piece	25	7	0.0
fruit, sugarless	1 piece	20	5	0.0
grape	1 piece	25	7	0.0
grape, sugarless	1 piece	20	5	0.0
Hawaiian punch	1 piece	25	7	0.0
lime, luscious	1 piece	25	7	0.0
peppermint, sugarless	1 piece	20	5	0.0
strawberry stripe	1 piece	25	7	0.0
strawberry, sugarless	1 piece	20	5	0.0
3-flavor, grape, cherry, and fruit	1 piece	25	7	0.0
watermelon, wet 'n wild	1 piece	25	7	0.0
(Bubblicious)				
original	1 piece	25	6	0.0
sugarless	1 piece	5	1	0.0
(Care Free)				
bubble, fruit, sugarless	1 piece	10	2	0.0
bubble, wild cherry, sugarless	1 piece	10	2	0.0
bubble, wintergreen, sugarless	1 piece	10	2	0.0
cinnamon, sugarless	1 piece	8	2	0.0
peppermint, sugarless	1 piece	8	2	0.0
spearmint, sugarless	1 piece	8	2	0.0
(Chewels) all flavors	1 piece	8	2	0.0
(Chiclets)				
	10 pieces	55	15	0.0
candy-coated	1 piece	6	2	0.0
candy-coated, 'Tiny'	1 pkg	8	0	0.0
(Clorets) stick, all flavors	1 piece	9	2	0.0
(Dentyne)				
all flavors	1 piece	6	2	0.0
all flavors, sugarless	1 piece	5	1	0.0
(Extra)				
bubble, classic	1 piece	6	0	0.0
bubble, original	1 piece	7	0	0.0
cinnamon	1 stick	8	0	0.0
peppermint	1 stick	8	0	0.0
spearmint	1 stick	8	0	0.0
winter fresh	1 stick	8	0	0.0
(Freedent)				
cinnamon	1 stick	10	2	0.0
peppermint	1 stick	10	2	0.0
spearmint	1 stick	10	2	0.0
(Freshen-Up) all flavors	1 piece	13	3	0.0
(Fruit Stripe)				
bubble, cherry	1 piece	8	2	0.0
bubble, fruit	1 piece	8	2	0.0
bubble, grape	1 piece	8	2	0.0
bubble, lemon	1 piece	8	2	0.0
cherry	1 piece	10	2	0.0
lemon	1 piece	10	2	0.0
lime	1 piece	10	2	0.0
orange	1 piece	10	2	0.0
(Hubba Bubba)				
all flavors except cola and grape	1 piece	23	6	0.0
cola	1 piece	23	5	0.0
grape, sugar-free	1 piece	13	0	0.0
original, sugar-free	1 piece	14	0	0.0

Food Name	Serv. Size	Total Cal.	Carbs GMS	Fat GMS
(Wrigley's)				
....	1 serving	10	2	0.0
'Big Red'	1 piece	10	2	0.0
'Doublemint'	1 piece	10	2	0.0
'Juicy Fruit'	1 piece	10	2	0.0
'Spearmint'	1 piece	10	2	0.0
GUMDROP				
1-inch diam	1 gumdrop	45	11	0.0
3/4-inch diam	1 gumdrop	16	4	0.0
(Estee)	4 pieces	25	6	0.0
HARD CANDY				
(Brach's)				
butterscotch, 'Disks'	1 oz	110	27	0.0
cinnamon, 'Disks'	1 oz	110	27	0.0
cinnamon, 'Imperials'	1 oz	110	27	0.0
'Cut Rock'	1 oz	110	27	0.0
filled, assorted	1 oz	110	27	0.0
lemon drops	1 oz	110	27	0.0
raspberry filled	1 oz	110	27	0.0
ribbon, crimp	1 oz	110	27	0.0
'Royals'	1 oz	100	20	2.0
'Spicettes'	1 oz	100	26	0.0
sour balls	1 oz	110	27	0.0
(Breath Savers)				
mint-cinnamon	1 piece	8	2	0.0
mint-cinnamon, cores	1 piece	2	1	0.0
peppermint	1 piece	8	2	0.0
peppermint, cores	1 piece	2	1	0.0
spearmint	1 piece	8	2	0.0
spearmint, cores	1 piece	2	1	0.0
wintergreen	1 piece	8	2	0.0
wintergreen, cores	1 piece	2	1	0.0
(Callard and Bowser) butterscotch	1 oz	115	25	1.9
(Ce De) 'Smarties'	1 roll	25	6	0.0
(Certs)				
mini, sugar-free	1 piece	1	0	0.0
mints, sugar-free	1 piece	6	2	0.0
(Clorets)				
clear mint	1 piece	8	2	0.0
pressed mints	1 piece	6	2	0.0
(Estee)	2 pieces	25	6	0.0
(Featherweight)				
butterscotch	1 piece	25	6	0.0
tropical blend, 'Sweet Pretenders'	1 piece	12	3	0.0
(Fruit Juicers)				
mixed berries	1 piece	8	2	0.0
citrus fruits	1 piece	8	2	0.0
fruit punch	1 piece	8	2	0.0
grape	1 piece	8	2	0.0
strawberry	1 piece	8	2	0.0
(Glenny's)				
fruit	1 piece	19	4	1.0
peppermint	1 piece	19	4	1.0
(Jolly Joes)	1 piece	9	2	0.0
(Jolly Rancher)				
apple	1 piece	23	6	0.0
butterscotch	1 piece	25	6	1.0

Food Name	Serv. Size	Total Cal.	Carbs GMS	Fat GMS
cherry	1 piece	23	6	0.0
fire cinnamon	1 piece	23	6	0.0
fruit punch	1 piece	23	6	0.0
grape	1 piece	23	6	0.0
lemon	1 piece	23	6	0.0
orange	1 piece	23	6	0.0
peach	1 piece	23	6	0.0
peppermint	1 piece	23	6	0.0
pink lemonade	1 piece	23	6	0.0
raspberry	1 piece	23	6	0.0
strawberry	1 piece	23	6	0.0
watermelon	1 piece	23	6	0.0
(Jurassic Park)				
jawbreakers, tropical flavors				
jawbreakers, wild cherry, 'Raptor Bites'	13 pieces	60	15	0.0
(Life Savers)				
butter creme mint	1 piece	8	2	0.0
butter rum	1 piece	8	2	0.0
butter rum, 'Holes'	1 piece	2	1	0.0
butterscotch	1 piece	8	2	0.0
'Cin-O-Mon'	1 piece	8	2	0.0
'Cryst-O-Mint'	1 piece	8	2	0.0
fancy fruits	1 piece	8	2	0.0
five flavor	1 piece	8	2	0.0
five flavor, 'Holes'	1 piece	2	1	0.0
'Pep-O-Mint'	1 piece	8	2	0.0
'Pep-O-Mint,' 'Holes'	1 piece	2	1	0.0
root beer flavor	1 piece	8	2	0.0
'Spear-O-Mint'	1 piece	8	2	0.0
sunshine fruits	1 piece	8	2	0.0
sunshine fruits, 'Holes'	1 piece	2	1	0.0
tangerine, 'Holes'	1 piece	2	1	0.0
tropical fruits	1 piece	8	2	0.0
wild cherry	1 piece	8	2	0.0
'Wint-O-Green'	1 piece	8	2	0.0
'Wint-O-Green,' 'Holes'	1 piece	2	1	0.0
(Mike and Ike)		9	2	0.0
(Russell Stover) mixed, sugar-free	3 pieces	70	18	0.0
'Spitters'	13 pieces	60	15	0.0
(Spree) fruit	1 oz	110	26	0.0
(SweeTARTS) fruit	1 oz	110	26	0.0
(Sunmark) jawbreakers, 'Willy Wonka's Everlasting Gobstoppers'	6 pieces	59	15	0.0
HOLIDAY				
(Brach's) holiday mints	1 oz	110	26	1.0
Christmas				
(Brach's)				
bell, chocolate, in foil	1 oz	150	17	8.0
candy cane	1 oz	110	27	0.0
chocolate, assorted	1 oz	110	23	2.0
jellies	1 oz	100	24	0.0
jellies, snowbase	1 oz	100	24	0.0
'Jots'	1 oz	130	21	5.0
mint 'Pearls'	1 oz	110	25	1.0
mint 'Starlight'	1 oz	110	27	0.0
nougat	1 oz	110	24	2.0
ornaments	1 oz	150	17	8.0

Food Name	Serv. Size	Total Cal.	Carbs GMS	Fat GMS
'Perkys'	1 oz	90	23	0.0
Santa, chocolate, in foil	1 oz	140	18	7.0
Santa, marshmallow	1 oz	120	23	3.0
(Just Born)				
snowman, marshmallow, large	1 piece	111	27	0.1
snowman, marshmallow, small	1 piece	37	9	0.1
tree, marshmallow, large	1 piece	111	27	0.1
tree, marshmallow, small	1 piece	37	9	0.1
(Spangler) candy cane	1 piece	60	14	1.0
Easter				
(Brach's)				
assorted, 'Chicks and Rabbits'	1 oz	100	26	0.0
assorted, 'Easter Fun'	1 oz	100	26	0.0
corn	1 oz	100	26	0.0
eggs, 'Hide'n Seek'	1 oz	110	27	0.0
eggs, chocolate malted milk	1 oz	130	21	5.0
eggs, chocolate, in foil	1 oz	150	17	8.0
eggs, creme, chocolate coated buttercream	1 oz	120	22	3.0
eggs, creme, chocolate coated cherry	1 oz	110	23	2.0
eggs, creme, chocolate coated coconut	1 oz	110	22	3.0
eggs, creme, chocolate coated fruit and nut	1 oz	110	23	2.0
eggs, creme, chocolate coated maple	1 oz	110	23	2.0
eggs, creme, chocolate coated vanilla	1 oz	110	23	2.0
eggs, jelly	1 oz	100	24	0.0
eggs, jelly, 'Tiny'	1 oz	100	26	0.0
eggs, jelly, speckled	1 oz	110	27	0.0
eggs, jelly, spiced	1 oz	90	22	0.0
eggs, marshmallow	1 oz	100	25	0.0
eggs, pastel 'Fiesta'	1 oz	120	23	3.0
lollipop, pastels, 'Easter'	1 lollipop	40	10	0.0
mint, 'Starlight'	1 oz	110	27	0.0
nougats,	1 oz	100	24	1.0
rabbits, jel, 'Jube'	1 oz	100	24	0.0
rabbits, marshmallow	1 oz	120	22	3.0
'Robin's Eggs'	1 oz	140	20	6.0
(Cadbury)				
eggs, creme	1.37 oz	190	26	8.0
eggs, creme, mini	1 oz	140	20	7.0
(Just Born) peeps, marshmallow	1 piece	27	7	0.1
Halloween				
(Brach's)				
corn, Indian	1 oz	100	26	0.0
corn, three color	1 oz	100	26	0.0
jelly beans	1 oz	100	26	0.0
lollipops 'Picture Pops'	1 oz	110	27	0.0
'Mellowcremes'	1 oz	100	26	0.0
pumpkin heads, crazy	1 oz	100	24	1.0
pumpkins	1 oz	100	26	0.0
'Scary Cats'	1 oz	100	26	0.0
'Trick or Treat Party Pack'	1 oz	110	27	0.0
witches' teeth	1 oz	100	26	0.0
(Just Born)				
cats, marshmallow	1 piece	28	7	0.1
pumpkins, marshmallow, large	1 piece	111	27	0.1
pumpkins, marshmallow, small	1 piece	14	3	0.1
Valentine's Day				
(Brach's)				
chocolate, 'I Luv U'	1 oz	150	17	8.0

Food Name	Serv. Size	Total Cal.	Carbs GMS	Fat GMS
'Heart Box' 1/2-lb box	1 oz	110	23	2.0
hearts	1 oz	110	23	2.0
hearts, cherry jel 'Jube'	1 oz	100	26	0.0
hearts, cinnamon 'Imperial'	1 oz	110	27	0.0
hearts, 'Conversation' large	1 oz	110	27	0.0
hearts, 'Conversation' small	1 oz	110	27	0.0
hearts, fruity	1 oz	100	24	0.0
hearts, jelly, red	1 oz	100	24	0.0
hearts, 'Sassy Hearts'	1 oz	100	25	0.0
kisses, nougat	1 oz	110	24	2.0
'Love'	1 oz	150	17	8.0
'Mellowcremes'	1 oz	100	26	0.0
'Valentine Heart' 1/3-lb box	1 oz	110	23	2.0
'Valentine Heart' 1-lb box	1 oz	110	23	2.0
JELLIED AND GUMMED				
jellybeans, large	10 pieces	104	26	0.1
jellybeans, small	10 pieces	40	10	0.1
(Brach's)				
cinnamon bears	1 oz	80	21	0.0
'Fruit Bunch'	1 oz	100	24	0.0
gummi bears	1 oz	100	22	0.0
gummi worms	1 oz	100	22	0.0
jelly beans	1 oz	100	26	0.0
jelly nougat	1 oz	100	24	1.0
'Jels' sour cherry	1 oz	100	26	0.0
'Jube'	1 oz	100	24	0.0
jube jels	1 oz	100	24	0.0
mint, assorted	1 oz	100	26	0.0
'Rainbow Bears'	1 oz	100	24	0.0
'Spearmint Leaves'	1 oz	100	24	0.0
spicettes	1 oz	100	26	0.0
(Callard and Bowser) juicy	1 oz	90	23	0.0
(Estee)				
gummi bears	4 pieces	20	4	0.0
ring, 1.25-inch diam	1 piece	39	10	0.0
(Hershey's)				
gummi bears, 'Amazin Fruit' 12 pieces	1 oz	90	21	1.0
gummi bears, tropical, 'Amazin Fruit'	1 oz	90	21	1.0
(Hot Tamales) cinnamon, hot	1 piece	9	2	0.0
(Jurassic Park) gummi dinosaurs, tropical	15 pieces	140	31	0.0
(Just Born)				
eggs, 'Petite'	1 piece	4	1	0.0
'Teenee Beanee Gourmet'	1 piece	4	1	0.0
(Life Savers) 'Gummi Savers'	1 piece	12	3	0.0
(Rodda) eggs	1 piece	7	2	0.0
LEMON *(Russell Stover)* squares	1.4 oz	160	27	5.5
LICORICE				
(Brach's)				
'Red Laces'	1 oz	100	22	0.0
'Twin Twists'	1 oz	100	22	0.0
'Twists'	1 oz	100	22	1.0
(Good and Fruity) candy-coated	1 oz	106	26	0.1
(Hershey's)				
cherry bits, 'Twizzlers'	5 oz pkg	474	110	2.3
cherry bits, 'Twizzlers' 4-oz bag	22 pieces	139	31	1.0
strawberry bits, 'Twizzlers' 2.5-oz pkg	1 pkg	237	55	1.1
LOLLIPOP				
(Brach's) all flavors, 'Pops'	1 oz	110	27	0.0

Food Name	Serv. Size	Total Cal.	Carbs GMS	Fat GMS
(Estee) all flavors	1 lollipop	30	7	0.0
(Fruit Juicers)				
black raspberry	1 lollipop	40	10	0.0
fruit punch	1 lollipop	40	10	0.0
pineapple	1 lollipop	40	10	0.0
strawberry	1 lollipop	40	10	0.0
(Glenny's)				
fruit	1 lollipop	21	5	1.0
Vit-C	1 lollipop	35	8	1.0
(Life Savers)				
assorted	1 lollipop	45	11	0.0
swirled	1 lollipop	45	11	0.0
(Sorbee) assorted fruit flavors	1 lollipop	22	5	0.0
(Spangler)				
all flavors, 'Dum Dums'	1 lollipop	25	6	1.0
all flavors, 'Saf-T-Pops'	1 lollipop	45	11	1.0
bubble gum center, all flavors	1 lollipop	57	14	1.0
(Tootsie Pop)				
all flavors except chocolate	1 oz	111	26	0.6
chocolate	1 oz	110	26	0.6
MARSHMALLOW				
(Boyer) 'Mallow Cup'	2 pieces	224	30	11.0
(Brach's) 'Perkys Circus Peanuts'	1 oz	100	26	0.0
(Campfire) large	2 pieces	40	10	0.0
(FunMallows)				
	1 piece	30	7	0.0
miniature	10 pieces	18	5	0.0
(Just Born) coconut, toasted	1 piece	30	6	0.6
(Spangler) 'Circus Peanuts'	4 pieces	110	26	1.0
MINT				
(Andes) chocolate mint thins, 'Creme de Menthe'	6 pieces	150	16	9.0
(Barat)				
chocolate tofu, 'Bits'	0.75 oz	120	11	8.0
chocolate tofu, after dinner	1 piece	40	4	2.0
(Brach's)				
'Kentucky Mints'	1 oz	110	27	0.0
chocolate covered, thin	1 oz	110	24	2.0
'Coolers/Starlight'	1 oz	110	27	0.0
creme, chocolate covered, regular	1 oz	110	24	2.0
'Creme de Menthe'	1 oz	150	16	9.0
'Dessert Mints' assorted	1 oz	110	27	0.0
'Jots/Pearls'	1 oz	120	25	2.0
parfait	1 oz	150	16	9.0
peppermint, 'Star Brites'	3 pieces	59	15	0.0
peppermint kisses	1 oz	100	24	1.0
straws, filled	1 oz	110	26	1.0
(Featherweight)				
'Cool Blue'	1 piece	25	6	0.0
peppermint swirls	1 piece	20	5	0.0
(Glenny's) gentle, 'Drops'	1 piece	6	1	1.0
(Hershey's)				
'Peppermnt Pattie' large, 1.5 oz	1 piece	165	34	3.0
'Peppermint Pattie' 0.6 oz	1 patty	67	14	1.2
'Peppermint Pattie' 0.5 oz	1 patty	55	11	1.0
(Kraft)				
butter	1 piece	8	2	0.0
party	1 piece	8	2	0.0

Food Name	Serv. Size	Total Cal.	Carbs GMS	Fat GMS
(Mint) 'Meltaway'	1 piece	50	5	3.0
(Nestlé)				
'After Eight'	5 pieces	147	31	5.6
'After Eight'	1 piece	29	6	1.1
(Rowntree) dark chocolate, wafer thin, 'After Eight'	1 piece	35	6	1.0
(Russell Stover) squares	1.4 oz	160	28	5.0
(Saco Foods) 'Mint'Oh's'	1.5 oz	111	14	6.6
(Spangler) dark chocolate coated	1 piece	80	14	2.0
(Velamints)				
all flavors except cocoamint	1 piece	7	2	0.0
cocoamint	1 piece	7	2	0.3
NONPAREILS				
(Brach's) dark chocolate	1 oz	140	20	6.0
(Nestlé) 'Sno-Caps'	1 oz	140	21	6.0
ORANGE				
(Brach's)				
'Orangettes'	1 oz	100	24	0.0
sticks, chocolate coated	1 oz	110	23	2.0
PEANUT				
(Barat) chocolate tofu, dipped, 'Bits'	1 oz	120	8	8.0
(Brach's)				
caramel cluster	1 oz	150	15	8.0
chocolate covered 'Small'	1 oz	140	15	7.0
filled	1 oz	110	25	1.0
French, burnt	1 oz	130	18	5.0
'Jots'	1 oz	140	18	6.0
milk chocolate coated	1 oz	150	15	9.0
milk chocolate, 'Peanut Clusters'	1 oz	150	15	9.0
'Nut Goodies'	1 oz	130	21	4.0
parfait	1 oz	160	14	10.0
(Cocofection) enrobed in chocolate	1 oz	140	10	12.0
(Estee)				
candy-coated	10 pieces	70	8	4.0
chocolate-covered	2 squares	60	5	4.5
(M&M Mars)				
chocolate, candy-coated, 'M&Ms'	1 cup	877	103	44.6
chocolate, candy-coated, 'M&Ms' 1.74-oz pkg	1 pkg	253	30	12.9
chocolate, candy-coated, 'M&Ms' 1.67-oz pkg	1 pkg	243	28	12.3
chocolate, candy-coated, 'M&Ms' fun size pkg	1 pkg	108	13	5.5
chocolate, candy-coated, 'M&Ms'	10 pieces	103	12	5.2
(Nabisco) chocolate covered, approx 14 pieces	1 oz	160	14	9.0
(Nestlé)				
chocolate-covered, 'Goobers' 7-oz pkg	1 pkg	1016	96	66.3
chocolate-covered, 'Goobers'	1/4 cup	210	20	13.7
chocolate-covered, 'Goobers' 1.375-oz pkg	1 pkg	200	19	13.1
chocolate-covered, 'Goobers'	10 pieces	51	5	3.4
(Russell Stover) 'Peanut Delights'	1.4 oz	210	22	12.0
PEANUT BRITTLE				
(Estee)	0.5 oz	60	10	2.0
(Kraft)	1 oz	130	20	5.0
(Sophie Mae)	1.4 oz	170	30	5.0
PEANUT BUTTER				
(Boyer)				
cup	1.6 oz	250	23	15.0
cup, 0.5 oz	1 piece	75	12	7.5
(Brach's) kisses	1 oz	110	22	2.0
(Estee) cup	1 piece	40	3	3.0

Food Name	Serv. Size	Total Cal.	Carbs GMS	Fat GMS
(Hershey's)				
'Reese's Crunchy Peanut Butter Cup'	1.8 oz	280	24	18.0
'Reese's Peanut Butter Cup' individual, 0.6 oz	1 piece	92	9	5.3
'Reese's Peanut Butter Cup' miniature	5 pieces	211	21	12.2
'Reese's Peanut Butter Cup' miniature	1 piece	38	4	2.2
'Reese's Peanut Butter Cup' 2-pack, 1.6 oz	1 pkg	243	25	14.1
'Reese's Pieces'	1/4 cup	231	29	9.9
'Reese's Pieces'	1.6-oz pkg	226	28	9.7
'Reese's Pieces'	50 pieces	191	24	8.2
'Reese's Pieces'	10 pieces	39	5	1.7
(M&M Mars)				
chocolate-covered, 'Kudos'	1.3 oz	200	19	12.0
chocolate-covered cookie, 'PB Max'	1 piece	240	20	15.0
PECAN				
(Russell Stover)				
'Pecan Crowns'	1.4 oz	200	19	13.0
'Pecan Delights'	1.4 oz	220	19	14.5
(Demet's)				
turtles	6-oz pkg	825	99	47.3
turtles	1 piece	82	10	4.7
POWDER CANDY				
(Lik-m-aid Fun Dip)	1 oz	110	26	0.0
(Pixy Stix)	1 oz	100	26	0.0
RAISIN				
(Barat) chocolate tofu, 'Bits'	1 oz	120	14	7.0
(Brach's) chocolate-coated	1 oz	130	20	5.0
(Cocofection) enrobed in chocolate	1 oz	120	20	5.0
(Estee) chocolate-coated	8 pieces	30	5	1.0
(Fruit Source) yogurt-coated, made w/real fruit juice	9 pieces	170	27	7.0
(Harmony) chocolate-coated	44 pieces	160	29	5.0
(Nabisco) chocolate-coated, approx 29 pieces	1 oz	130	21	5.0
(Nestlé)				
chocolate-covered, 'Raisinets'	1.58-oz pkg	185	32	7.2
chocolate-covered, 'Raisinets'	10 pieces	41	7	1.6
TAFFY				
(Beich's)				
all flavors, 'Salt Water Taffy'	1 oz	100	24	1.0
apple flavor chews, 'Laffy Taffy'	2 pieces	110	26	1.0
banana flavor chews, 'Laffy Taffy'	2 pieces	120	26	1.0
cherry flavor chews, 'Laffy Taffy'	2 pieces	110	26	1.0
grape flavor chews, 'Laffy Taffy'	2 pieces	110	26	1.0
passion punch flavor, 'Laffy Taffy'	2 pieces	120	26	1.0
strawberry flavor chews, 'Laffy Taffy'	2 pieces	110	26	1.0
watermelon flavor chews, 'Laffy Taffy'	2 pieces	110	26	1.0
TOFFEE				
(Brach's)	1 oz	110	23	2.0
(Callard and Bowser)	1 oz	135	19	6.5
(Flavor House) peanut butter	1 oz	150	17	7.0
(Heath)				
'Bits O'Brickle'	3 oz	448	50	28.0
English, 'Bits O'Heath'	3.5 oz	520	62	31.0
English, 'Heath Bar'	2 pieces	180	20	11.0
CANDY COATING				
bars, butterscotch, confectioner's coating	1 oz	153	19	8.2
bars, white, confectioner's coating	3 oz	458	50	27.3
chips, butterscotch, confectioner's coating	1 cup	916	114	49.4
chip, white, confectioner's coating	1 cup	916	101	54.6

Food Name	Serv. Size	Total Cal.	Carbs GMS	Fat GMS
CANNELLINI BEAN. See BEAN, CANNELLINI.				
CANOLA OIL				
....	1 cup	1927	0	218.0
....	1 tbsp	124	0	14.0
(Hain)	1 tbsp	120	0	14.0
(Kroger)	1 tbsp	122	0	13.6
(Smart Beat)	1 tbsp	117	0	13.6
(Wesson)	1 tbsp	122	0	13.6
(Westbrae Naturals)	1 tbsp	100	0	11.0
cholesterol-free, no sodium *(Country Pure)*	1 tbsp	120	0	14.0
'Food Service' *(Wesson)*	1 tbsp	122	0	13.6
'Heart Beat' *(Nucoa)*	1 tbsp	120	0	14.0
100% pure pressed *(Loriva')*	1 tbsp	120	0	14.0
pure pressed, organic, lowest in saturated fat *(Spectrum Naturals)*	1 tbsp	120	0	14.0
CANTALOUPE. See MELON, CANTALOUPE.				
CAPERS				
canned, drained	1 tbsp	2	0	0.1
canned, drained *(Progresso)*	1 tsp	0	0	0.0
canned, non-pareilles *(Reese)*	1 tsp	0	0	0.0
CAPPUCCINO. See under COFFEE, FLAVORED.				
CARAMBOLA. See STAR FRUIT.				
CARAMEL. See under CANDY.				
CARAMEL TOPPING				
(Kraft)	2 tbsp	120	28	0.0
(Mrs. Richardson's)				
....	2 tbsp	130	28	2.0
nonfat	2 tbsp	130	31	0.0
(Smucker's)				
hot	2 tbsp	150	28	4.0
'Special Recipe'	2 tbsp	160	33	3.0
CARAWAY SEED				
....	1 tbsp	22	3	1.0
....	1 tsp	7	1	0.3
(Spice Islands)	1 tsp	8	1	0.4
(Tone's)	1 tsp	7	1	0.3
dried *(McCormick/Schilling)*	1 tsp	14	1	0.8
whole seeds *(Durkee)*	1 tsp	9	0	0.0
whole seeds *(Laurel Leaf)* whole seeds	1 tsp	9	0	0.0
CARDAMOM				
ground	1 tbsp	18	4	0.4
ground	1 tsp	6	1	0.1
ground *(Tone's)*	1 tsp	6	1	0.1
ground, fresh *(Durkee)*	1 tsp	7	0	0.0
ground, fresh *(Laurel Leaf)*	1 tsp	7	0	0.0
whole *(McCormick/Schilling)*	1 tsp	7	2	0.0
whole *(Spice Islands)*	1 tsp	6	1	0.1
CARDONI. See CARDOON.				
CARDOON/cardoni				
boiled, drained	4 oz	25	6.0	0.1
raw, shredded	1 cup	36	9.0	0.2
CARIBOU				
raw	1 oz	36	0	1.0
roasted	3 oz	142	0	3.8
CARISSA/Natal plum				
Fresh				
raw, sliced	1 cup	93	20	1.9

Food Name	Serv. Size	Total Cal.	Carbs GMS	Fat GMS
raw, whole, peeled and seeded	1 fruit	12	3	0.3
CAROB CHIPS, unsweetened *(Sunspire)*	1 oz	133	15	6.0
CAROB FLAVOR DRINK				
mix, powder	1 tbsp	45	11	0.0
mix, powder, prepared w/milk	8 fl oz	195	23	8.2
CAROB FLOUR. See under FLOUR.				
CARP				
baked, broiled, grilled, or microwaved	3 oz	138	0	6.1
raw	3 oz	108	0	4.8
CARROT				
Canned				
(A&P)	1/2 cup	30	6	1.0
(Stokely)	1/2 cup	35	7	0.0
baby, petite, whole *(Stokely)*	4.5 oz	30	5	0.0
baby, whole *(Allens)*	1/2 cup	30	6	1.0
baby, whole, 'LeSueur' *(Green Giant)*	1/2 cup	35	8	0.0
crinkle sliced *(Freshlike)*	1/2 cup	30	6	0.0
crinkle sliced *(Stokely)*	1/2 cup	35	7	0.0
crinkle sliced *(Veg-All)*	1/2 cup	30	6	0.0
diced *(Allens)*	1/2 cup	30	5	1.0
diced, 'Fancy' *(S&W)*	1/2 cup	30	7	0.0
diced, w/liquid *(Del Monte)*	1/2 cup	30	7	0.0
mashed, no salt added, drained	1 cup	57	13	0.4
no salt added *(A&P)*	1/2 cup	25	6	1.0
no salt or sugar added *(Stokely)*	1/2 cup	35	7	0.0
regular pack, mashed, drained	1 cup	57	13	0.4
regular pack, sliced, drained	1 cup	37	8	0.3
regular pack, sliced, drained	1 slice	1	0	0.0
regular pack, sliced, w//liquid	1/2 cup	28	7	0.2
sliced *(Featherweight)*	1/2 cup	30	6	0.0
sliced *(Finast)*	1/2 cup	35	8	0.0
sliced *(Green Giant)*	1/2 cup	25	6	6.0
sliced *(IGA)*	1/2 cup	30	6	0.0
sliced *(Pathmark)*	1/2 cup	35	7	0.0
sliced, no salt added, drained	1 cup	37	8	0.3
sliced, no salt added, drained	1 slice	1	0	0.0
sliced, no salt added, w/liquid	1/2 cup	28	7	0.2
sliced, large *(Allens)*	1/2 cup	30	7	1.0
sliced, medium *(Allens)*	1/2 cup	30	7	1.0
sliced, Nutradiet *(S&W)*	1/2 cup	30	7	0.0
sliced, small *(Allens)*	1/2 cup	30	7	1.0
sliced no salt added *(Finast)*	1/2 cup	35	8	0.0
sliced no salt added *(Pathmark)*	1/2 cup	35	8	0.0
sliced, water packed, no salt *(Freshlike)*	1/2 cup	30	6	0.0
Fresh				
baby, raw, large	1 carrot	6	1	0.1
baby, raw, medium	1 carrot	4	1	0.1
boiled, drained, sliced	1/2 cup	35	8	0.1
boiled, drained, whole, medium	1 carrot	21	5	0.1
raw, chopped	1 cup	55	13	0.2
raw, cut, 3-inch strips	1 strip	3	1	0.0
raw, cut, strips or slices	1 cup	52	12	0.2
raw, grated	1 cup	47	11	0.2
raw, shredded	1/2 cup	24	5.6	0.1
raw, whole, medium *(Dole)*	1 carrot	40	8.0	1.0
raw, whole, large, 7.25–8.5-inch long	1 carrot	31	7	0.1
raw, whole, small, 5.5-inch long	1 carrot	22	5	0.1

Food Name	Serv. Size	Total Cal.	Carbs GMS	Fat GMS
Frozen				
(A&P)	3.3 oz	40	9	1.0
(Seabrook)	3.3 oz	40	9	0.0
baby, cut, 'Select Polybag' (Green Giant)	3/4 cup	30	7	0.0
baby, whole (C&W)	2/3 cup	35	7	0.0
baby, whole (Flav-R-Pac)	2/3 cup	35	6	0.0
baby, whole, 'Deluxe' (Birds Eye)	3.3 oz	40	9	0.0
baby, whole, 'Harvest Fresh' (Green Giant)	1/2 cup	18	5	0.0
baby, whole, 'Select' (Green Giant)	1/2 cup	20	7	0.0
baby, whole, 'Singles' (Stokely)	3 oz	35	8	0.0
Parisienne, 'Deluxe' (Birds Eye)	2.6 oz	30	7	0.0
sliced (Birds Eye)	3.2 oz	35	8	0.0
sliced (Flav-R-Pac)	2/3 cup	35	6	0.0
sliced (Frosty Acres)	3.3 oz	40	9	0.0
sliced, drained	1 cup	53	12	0.2
sliced, no salt, drained	1 cup	53	12	0.2
sliced, unprepared	10-oz pkg	111	26	0.6
sliced, unprepared	1/2 cup	25	6	0.1
small, round, European style, 'Parisienne' (C&W)	2/3 cup	40	10	0.0
whole (Southern)	3.5 oz	42	9	0.2
CARROT CHIPS				
(Hain)				
	1 oz	150	16	9.0
barbecue	1 oz	140	16	8.0
no salt added	1 oz	150	16	7.0
CARROT DISH				
(Birds Eye)				
w/sweet peas, pearl onions, 'Deluxe'	3.3 oz	50	10	0.0
(Flav-R-Pac)				
baby, orange glazed, 'Grande Classics'	1/2 cup	60	14	1.5
baby, whole, w/buttery sauce	1/2 cup	45	9	2.0
shoestring, frozen	1 cup	35	6	0.0
CARROT JUICE				
Canned or bottled				
	1 cup	94	22	0.4
	1 fl oz	12	3	0.0
(Biotta)	6 fl oz	51	11	0.1
(Hain)	6 fl oz	80	17	0.0
(Hollywood)	6 fl oz	80	17	0.0
CASABA MELON. See MELON, CASABA.				
CASHEW/heart nut				
(Beer Nuts)	1 oz	170	8	13.0
(Frito-Lay's)	1 oz	170	9	14.0
halves (Fisher)	1 oz	160	8	13.0
halves, lightly salted (Eagle)	1 oz	180	8	14.0
lightly salted (Eagle)	1 oz	190	8	14.0
pieces (Fisher)	1 oz	170	8	14.0
salted, whole (Guy's)	1 oz	170	5	14.0
salted (Pathmark)	1 oz	170	9	13.0
salted, 'No Frills' (Pathmark)	1 oz	170	8	13.0
salted (Planters)	1 oz	160	9	13.0
unsalted, natural (Flanigan Farms)	1/4 cup	160	9	13.0
whole (Fisher)	1 oz	160	8	13.0
Dry roasted				
halves and whole, saltd	1 cup	786	45	63.5
halves and whole, unsalted	1 cup	786	45	63.5
lightly salted (Planters)	1 oz	160	9	13.0

Food Name	Serv. Size	Total Cal.	Carbs GMS	Fat GMS
salted	1 oz	163	9	13.1
unsalted	1 oz	163	9	13.1
unsalted	1 tbsp	49	3	4.0
unsalted *(Planters)*	1 oz	160	9	13.0
Honey roasted				
(Eagle)	1 oz	180	9	14.0
(Planters)	1 oz	170	11	12.0
halves *(Eagle)*	1 oz	180	9	14.0
halves *(Fisher)*	1 oz	150	7	13.0
whole *(Fisher)*	1 oz	150	7	13.0
w/peanuts *(Planters)*	1 oz	170	9	12.0
Oil roasted				
halves, salted *(Fisher)*	1/4 cup	170	8	15.0
halves, salted *(Planters)*	1 oz	170	8	14.0
halves, salted *(Planters)*	1 oz	170	8	14.0
halves, unsalted *(Planters)*	1 oz	170	8	14.0
halves and whole, salted	1 cup	749	37	62.7
halves and whole, unsalted	1 cup	749	37	62.7
lightly salted *(Planters)*	1 oz	160	8	14.0
salted *(Flavor House)*	1 oz	180	3	16.0
salted *(Pathmark)*	1 oz	170	8	14.0
salted, approx 18 kernels	1 oz	163	8	13.7
salted, 'Fancy' *(Planters)*	1 oz	170	8	14.0
salted, 'No Frills' *(Pathmark)*	1 oz	170	8	14.0
unsalted, approx 18 kernels	1 oz	163	8	13.7
w/almonds *(Fisher)*	1 oz	170	6	15.0
whole *(Fisher)*	1/4 cup	170	8	15.0
CASHEW BUTTER				
creamy, roasted fresh, no salt added *(Roaster Fresh)*	1 oz	165	9	14.0
gourmet *(Roaster Fresh)*	1 oz	165	9	14.0
peanut date *(Maranatha Natural)*	2 tbsp	190	8	14.0
peanut date, 'Natural' *(Westbrae)*	2 tbsp	200	8	15.0
raw *(Hain)*	2 tbsp	190	8	15.0
raw, 'Natural' *(Westbrae)*	2 tbsp	300	8	28.0
raw, unsalted *(Hain)*	2 tbsp	210	8	19.0
roasted *(Maranatha Natural)*	2 tbsp	190	10	14.0
roasted, 'Natural' *(Westbrae)*	2 tbsp	190	8	17.0
roasted, organic *(Maranatha Natural)*	2 tbsp	210	8	16.0
salted	1 oz	166	8	14.0
salted	1 tbsp	94	4	7.9
toasted *(Hain)*	2 tbsp	210	7	17.0
unsalted	1 oz	166	8	14.0
unsalted	1 tbsp	94	4	7.9
unsalted, 'Fancy' *(Planters)*	1 oz	170	8	14.0
CASSAVA/manioc/yuca				
raw, chopped or sliced	1 cup	330	78	0.6
raw, whole	1 root	653	155	1.1
CATFISH, CHANNEL				
Fresh				
breaded, fried	3 oz	195	7	11.3
farmed, baked, broiled, grilled, or microwaved	3 oz	129	0	6.8
farmed, raw	3 oz	115	0	6.5
wild, baked, broiled, grilled, or microwaved	3 oz	89	0	2.4
wild, raw	3 oz	81	0	2.4
Frozen, fillets *(Delta Pride)*	4 oz	132	5	4.9

CATFISH, OCEAN. See WOLF FISH.

Food Name	Serv. Size	Total Cal.	Carbs GMS	Fat GMS
CATSUP/ketchup				
....	1 cup	250	65	0.9
....	1 tbsp	16	4	0.1
....	1 pkt	6	2	0.0
low-salt	1 cup	250	65	0.9
low-salt	1 tbsp	16	4	0.1
low-salt	1 pkt	6	2	0.0
(Del Monte)				
....	1/4 cup	60	16	0.0
....	1 tbsp	15	4	0.0
'No Salt Added'	1/4 cup	60	16	0.0
(Estee)	1 tbsp	6	0	0.0
(Featherweight)	1 tbsp	6	1	0.0
(Hain)				
'Natural'	1 tbsp	16	4	0.0
'Natural No Salt Added'	1 tbsp	16	4	0.0
(Healthy Choice)	0.5 oz	9	2	0.1
(Heinz)				
hot	1 tbsp	16	4	0.0
light	1 tbsp	10	3	0.0
regular	1 tbsp	16	4	0.0
w/onions	1 tbsp	19	0	0.0
(Hunt's)				
....	1 tbsp	16	4	0.1
bulk packaged, food service product	1 tbsp	16	4	0.1
no salt added	1 tbsp	16	3	0.1
packets, food service product	1 pkt	10	2	0.1
(Life) 'All Natural'	1 tbsp	17	4	0.0
(Millina's Finest)				
organic	1 oz	17	4	0.1
organic, fruit juice sweetened	1 tbsp	25	6	0.0
(Smucker's)	1 tsp	8	2	0.0
(Snider's)	1 tbsp	16	4	0.1
(Stokely)	1 tbsp	20	5	0.0
(Weight Watchers)	2 tsp	8	2	0.0
(Westbrae)				
fruit sweetened	1 tbsp	12	2	0.0
fruit sweetened, no salt....................	1 tbsp	12	2	0.0
unsweetened	1 tbsp	5	1	0.0
unsweetened 'Unketchup'	1 tbsp	8	1	0.0
CAULIFLOWER				
Canned or jarred				
pickled, 'Hot & Spicy' *(Vlasic)*	1 oz	4	1	0.0
sweet *(Vlasic)*	1 oz	35	9	0.0
Fresh				
green, cooked..............................	1/5 head	29	6	0.3
green, raw, chopped	1 cup	20	4	0.2
green, raw, florets	1 floret	8	2	0.1
green, raw, whole, large, approx 6-7 inch diam	1 head	158	31	1.5
green, raw, whole, medium, approx 5-6 inch diam	1 head	134	26	1.3
green, raw, whole, small, approx 4-inch diam	1 head	101	20	1.0
white, boiled, drained, florets	3 florets	12	2	0.2
white, boiled, drained, 1-inch pieces	1/2 cup	14	3	0.3
white, raw, chopped	1 cup	25	5	0.2
white, raw, florets	1 floret	3	1	0.0
white, raw, whole, large, approx 6-7 inch diam	1 head	210	44	1.8
white, raw, whole, medium, approx 5-6 inch diam	1 head	144	30	1.2

Food Name	Serv. Size	Total Cal.	Carbs GMS	Fat GMS
white, raw, whole, small, approx 4-inch diam	1 head	66	14	0.6
Frozen				
(A&P)	3.3 oz	25	5	1.0
(Birds Eye)	3.3 oz	25	5	0.0
(Finast)	3.3 oz	25	5	0.0
(Flav-R-Pac)	4 pieces	20	3	0.0
(Frosty Acres)	3.3 oz	25	5	0.0
(Kohl's)	3 oz	20	4	1.0
(Seabrook)	3.3 oz	25	5	0.0
(Southern)	3.5 oz	26	5	0.2
cuts (Green Giant)	1/2 cup	12	3	0.0
cuts, no salt, drained, 1-inch pieces	1 cup	34	7	0.4
cuts, unprepared, 1-inch pieces	1/2 cup	16	3	0.2
cuts, w/salt, drained, 1-inch pieces	1 cup	34	7	0.4
florets, 'Plain Polybag' (Green Giant)	1/2 cup	12	3	0.0
'Singles' (Stokely)	3 oz	20	4	0.0
unprepared	10-oz pkg	68	13	0.8
CAULIFLOWER DISH				
(Green Giant) w/cheese flavored sauce	1/2 cup	60	8	2.5
CAVATELLI. See under PASTA; DISH/ENTRÉE.				
CAVIAR				
black or red, granular	1 oz	71	1	5.1
black or red, granular	1 tbsp	40	1	2.9
CAYENNE. See under PEPPER, GROUND.				
CECI. See CHICKPEA.				
CELERIAC				
boiled, drained, chopped	1 cup	42	9	0.3
raw, chopped	1 cup	66	14	0.5
CELERY				
boiled, drained, diced	1 cup	27	6	0.2
boiled, drained, whole	2 stalks	14	3	0.1
raw, cut, approx 4-inch strips	1 cup	20	5	0.2
raw, cut, approx 4-inch strips	1 strip	1	0	0.0
raw, diced	1 cup	19	4	0.2
raw, diced	1 tbsp	1	0	0.0
raw, whole, large, 11-12 inches long	1 stalk	10	2	0.1
raw, whole, medium, 7.5–8 inches long	1 stalk	6	1	0.1
raw, whole, small, approx 5 inches long	1 stalk	3	1	0.0
CELERY FLAKES (Tone's)	1 tsp	9	1	0.5
CELERY ROOT JUICE, bottled (Biotta)	6 fl oz	67	13	0.2
CELERY SALT (Tone's)	1 tsp	6	1	0.4
CELERY SEED				
	1 tbsp	25	3	1.6
	1 tsp	8	1	0.5
(McCormick/Schilling)	1 tsp	7	1	0.4
(Spice Islands)	1 tsp	11	1	0.5
(Tone's)	1 tsp	9	1	0.5
whole seeds (Durkee)	1 tsp	9	0	0.0
whole seeds (Laurel Leaf)	1 tsp	9	0	0.0
CELLOPHANE NOODLES. See under NOODLE.				
CELTUCE, fresh, raw	1 med leaf	1	0	0.0
CEREAL, HOT				
(Krusteaz)				
'Ala'	1/4 cup	150	33	0.0
'Zoom'	1/3 cup	120	24	0.0
(Malt-O-Meal)				
'Maple Brown Sugar' 30% formulation, prepared, w/2% milk	1 oz	160	28	3.0

Food Name	Serv. Size	Total Cal.	Carbs GMS	Fat GMS
'Maple Brown Sugar' 30% formulation, unprepared	1 oz	100	22	0.0
(Quaker) plus fiber, prepared w/1/2 cup nonfat milk	1/2 cup	170	27	2.5
BARLEY				
(Erewhon) organic	1 oz	110	22	1.0
(Quaker) Scotch, quick	1/3 cup	170	37	1.0
BRAN				
(Breadshop) oat, rice, corn, 'Triple Bran' unprepared	1 oz	100	15	2.0
(H-O Brand) 'Super Bran' unprepared	1/3 cup	110	18	2.0
BULGUR				
(Arrowhead Mills)	2 oz	200	43	1.0
(Hodgson Mill) w/soy grits, unprepared	1/4 cup	120	24	1.0
CORN GRITS. See GRITS.				
FARINA				
(H-O Brand) instant, unprepared	1 pkt	110	22	0.0
(Krusteaz)	1 oz	100	22	0.0
(Pillsbury)				
prepared w/water, 1/8 tsp salt	2/3 cup	80	18	0.0
unprepared	1/12 pkg	80	18	0.0
(Quaker)	1/4 cup	154	33	0.4
GRANOLA				
(Breadshop)				
almond raisin, nectarsweet	1 oz	120	18	4.0
'Blueberry 'N Cream' nectarsweet	1 oz	115	19	3.0
'California Orange Crunch' honeysweet	1 oz	130	18	5.0
'Cinnapple Spice' honeysweet	1 oz	125	19	4.5
'Crunchy Oat Bran' nectarsweet	1 oz	120	18	5.0
'Golden Maple Nut' honeysweet	1 oz	130	17	5.0
'Golden Maple Nut'	1/2 cup	230	32	9.5
'Gone Nuts!' nectarsweet	1 oz	125	17	5.0
honey apple blueberry, honeysweet	1 oz	125	18	5.0
'Honey Gone Nuts!' honeysweet	1 oz	130	18	5.5
'New England Supernatural'	1/2 cup	220	31	9.0
orange almond	1/2 cup	240	35	8.5
orange almond, nectarsweet	1 oz	120	18	4.0
'Oregon Blueberry Crunch' honeysweet	1 oz	125	18	5.0
'Peaches 'N Cream' nectarsweet	1 oz	115	19	3.0
raspberries and cream, w/organic oats	1/2 cup	220	34	7.5
'Raspberry 'N Cream' nectarsweet	1 oz	115	19	3.0
'Strawberry 'N Cream' nectarsweet	1 oz	110	16	4.0
'Supernatural New England' honeysweet	1 oz	130	18	5.0
'Supernatural' honeysweet	1 oz	100	18	5.0
(Ener-G Foods) gluten-free	1 cup	436	47	26.8
(Erewhon)				
apple, spiced	1 oz	130	17	6.0
honey almond	1 oz	130	17	6.0
maple	1 oz	130	17	5.0
'Sunflower Crunch'	1 oz	130	18	4.0
w/bran, '#9'	1 oz	130	17	6.0
w/dates and nuts	1 oz	130	17	6.0
(Golden Temple)				
apple cinnamon, low-fat	1/2 cup	190	39	2.0
blueberry	1 oz	132	19	5.0
blueberry, coconut-free	1 oz	131	19	4.5
blueberry, wild	1/2 cup	230	33	9.0
cashew almond	1 oz	129	19	3.5
cinnamon apple raisin	1 oz	125	20	3.5
coconut almond	1 oz	145	18	3.5

Food Name	Serv. Size	Total Cal.	Carbs GMS	Fat GMS
fruit and nut	1 oz	129	19	4.5
golden	1 oz	138	19	6.0
Hawaiian	1 oz	126	19	4.0
high-protein	1 oz	124	19	3.5
honey almond	1 oz	130	20	3.5
honey blueberry apple	1 oz	128	20	3.5
'Lite & Crunchy'	1/2 cup	220	33	8.0
maple almond	1 oz	129	20	3.5
'Natural Delite'	1 oz	128	20	3.5
oat bran, w/berries	1 oz	120	20	3.5
oat bran, w/raisins and almonds	1 oz	119	19	3.5
orange almond	1 oz	133	19	4.0
'Rainforest Granola'	1/2 cup	240	33	10.0
raisin apricot date	1 oz	127	20	3.5
'Super Nutty'	1 oz	135	19	5.0
'Super Nutty'	1/2 cup	230	33	9.0
'Sweet Home Farm' low-fat	1 oz	110	22	2.0
(Health Valley)				
date and almond, nonfat	1 oz	90	21	0.0
raisin cinnamon, nonfat	1 oz	90	21	0.0
raspberry, nonfat	1 oz	140	35	0.0
tropical fruit, nonfat	1 oz	90	21	0.0
(Stone-Buhr) apple, no preservatives, no added sugar	1/3 cup	130	31	1.0
GRITS. See GRITS.				
MULTIGRAIN				
(Arrowhead Mills)				
four grain, unprepared	1 oz	94	18	1.0
seven grain, unprepared	1 oz	100	17	1.0
(Pritikin) hearty, microwave, prepared	1 pkt	190	38	2.0
(Quaker)				
prepared w/1/2 cup nonfat milk	1/2 cup	170	30	1.5
unprepared	1/2 cup	133	29	1.0
(Roman Meal)				
oats, wheat, and other grains, prepared w/water	1 cup	170	34	1.9
oats, wheat, and other grains, prepared w/water	3/4 cup	128	26	1.4
oats, wheat, and other grains, unprepared	1 cup	340	69	4.0
oats, wheat, and other grains, unprepared	1/4 cup	85	17	1.0
wheat w/other grains, plain, prepared w/water	1 cup	147	33	1.0
wheat w/other grains, plain, prepared w/water	3/4 cup	110	25	0.7
wheat w/other grains, unprepared	1 cup	299	67	2.0
wheat w/other grains, unprepared	1/3 cup	100	22	0.7
wheat w/other grains, unprepared	1 tbsp	19	4	0.1
w/apple cinnamon, prepared	2/3 cup	112	24	2.8
OAT BRAN				
(Arrowhead Mills) unprepared	1 oz	110	17	1.0
(Breadshop)				
'Oat Bran Muesli' unprepared	1 oz	100	20	2.0
100% pure 'Oat Bran' unprepared	1 oz	100	17	2.0
(Erewhon) w/toasted wheat germ *(Erewhon)*	1 oz	115	18	2.0
(Health Valley)				
apple/cinnamon, 'Natural' unprepared	1/4 cup	100	19	1.0
raisin, nonfat	1 oz	100	19	1.0
(Hodgson Mill) low-fat, cholesterol-free, unprepared	1/4 cup	120	23	3.0
(Malt-O-Meal)				
'Plus 40% Oat Bran' prepared, w/1/2 cup nonfat milk	1.3 oz	170	31	2.0
'Plus 40% Oat Bran' prepared, w/1/2 cup 2% milk	1.3 oz	190	31	4.0
'Plus 40% Oat Bran' unprepared	1.3 oz	130	25	2.0

Food Name	Serv. Size	Total Cal.	Carbs GMS	Fat GMS
(Mother's)				
prepared w/o salt	2/3 cup	92	17	2.0
prepared w/1/2 cup whole milk, w/o salt	1 oz	180	22	7.0
unprepared	1/3 cup	92	17	2.1
(Quaker) 'Mother's' unprepared	1/2 cup	146	25	3.2
(3-Minute Brand)				
'Quick' unprepared	1 oz	100	18	2.0
'Regular' unprepared	1 oz	90	17	2.0
(Wholesome 'N Hearty)				
apple cinnamon, unprepared	1 pkt	130	30	2.0
honey, unprepared	1 pkt	110	26	2.0
regular, unprepared	1 oz	100	18	2.0
OATMEAL AND OATS				
(Arrowhead Mills)				
apple, date, and almond, unprepared	1 oz	130	23	3.0
apple spice, unprepared	1 oz	130	23	2.0
cinnamon, raisin, almond, unprepared	1 oz	140	23	3.0
instant, unprepared	1 oz	100	18	2.0
(Erewhon)				
apple cinnamon, instant	1.25 oz	145	25	3.0
apple cinnamon, 100% natural, instant.	1 pkt	130	24	2.0
apple raicin, instant	1.3 oz	150	27	3.0
apple raisin, 100% natural, instant.	1 pkt	150	27	3.0
maple spice, instant	1.2 oz	140	24	3.0
maple spice, 100% natural, instant	1 pkt	130	25	2.0
w/oat bran, instant	1.25 oz	125	23	3.0
w/raisins, dates, and walnuts, instant	1.2 oz	130	24	3.0
(General Mills)				
apple and cinnamon, instant, unprepared	1.5 oz	150	32	2.0
cinnamon raisin, unprepared	1.8 oz	170	38	2.0
(H-O Brand)				
apple and bran w/fiber, instant, unprepared	1 pkt	130	26	2.0
apple and cinnamon, instant, unprepared	1 pkt	130	26	2.0
'Gourmet' unprepared	1/3 cup	100	18	2.0
instant, unprepared	1 pkt	110	18	2.0
instant, unprepared	1/2 cup	130	22	2.0
maple brown sugar, unprepared	1 pkt	160	32	2.0
'Quick' unprepared	1/2 cup	130	23	2.0
raisin and bran, w/fiber, instant, unprepared	1 pkt	150	32	2.0
ralsins and spice, instant, unprepared	1 pkt	150	32	2.0
sweet'n mellow, instant, unprepared	1 pkt	150	30	2.0
w/fiber, instant, unprepared	1 pkt	110	18	2.0
w/fiber, instant, unprepared	1/3 cup	100	15	2.0
(Maypo)				
maple flavored, 'Vermont Style' unprepared	1 oz	105	20	1.0
'Maypo' prepared w/water, salt	1 cup	170	32	2.4
'Maypo' prepared w/water, salt	3/4 cup	128	24	1.8
'Maypo' prepared w/water, no salt added	1 cup	170	32	2.4
'Maypo' prepared w/water, no salt added	3/4 cup	128	24	1.8
'Maypo' prepared w/water, no salt added	1 tbsp	11	2	0.1
'Maypo' '30 Second' unprepared	1 oz	100	19	1.0
'Maypo' unprepared	1 cup	362	68	5.0
'Maypo' unprepared	1/2 cup	181	34	2.5
(Mother's)				
instant, prepared w/1/2 cup whole milk	1 oz	190	24	6.0
instant, unprepared	1 oz	110	18	2.0

Food Name	Serv. Size	Total Cal.	Carbs GMS	Fat GMS
(Oatmeal Swirlers)				
cherry, unprepared	1.7 oz	150	33	2.0
cinnamon spice, unprepared	1.6 oz	160	35	2.0
maple brown sugar, unprepared	1.6 oz	160	35	2.0
milk chocolate, unprepared	1.7 oz	170	37	2.0
apple and cinnamon, instant, unprepared	1.7 oz	160	34	2.0
strawberry, unprepared	1.6 oz	150	32	2.0
(Quaker)				
apple spice, microwave, 'Quick 'n Hearty'	1 pkt	166	35	2.0
apples and cinnamon, instant, unprepared	1 pkt	130	26	1.5
apples and spice, instant, 'Extra' unprepared	1 pkt	133	27	1.9
brown sugar cinnamon, microwave, 'Quick 'n Hearty'	1 pkt	155	31	2.2
cinnamon and spice, instant, unprepared	1 pkt	164	35	2.1
cinnamon double raisin, microwave, 'Quick 'n Hearty'	1 pkt	169	35	2.2
cinnamon graham, instant, 'Kids' Choice' unprepared	1 pkt	140	29	2.0
cinnamon graham cookie, instant, 'Kids Choice'	1 pkt	190	35	2.0
cinnamon toast, instant, unprepared	1 pkt	130	27	2.0
'Cinnamagic' instant, unprepared	1 pkt	144	30	2.0
'Extra' unprepared	1 pkt	95	18	2.0
fruit punch flavor, instant, 'Power Rangers' unprepared	1 pkt	149	31	2.0
fruit and cream, instant, unprepared	1 pkt	135	26	2.5
fruit and cream blueberry, instant, unprepared	1 pkt	130	27	2.5
honey bran, microwave, 'Quick 'n Hearty'	1 pkt	151	31	2.1
honey nut, instant, unprepared	1 pkt	130	25	3.0
instant, unprepared	1 pkt	94	18	2.0
low-salt, instant, unprepared	1 pkt	103	19	2.0
maple and brown sugar, instant, prepared w/water	1 pkt	153	31	1.8
maple and brown sugar, instant, 'Kids' Choice' unprepared	1 pkt	140	31	2.0
maple and brown sugar, instant, unprepared	1 pkt	152	32	2.1
'Old Fashioned' prepared	2/3 cup	99	19	2.0
'Old Fashioned' unprepared	1/3 cup	99	19	2.0
peaches and cream, instant, unprepared	1 pkt	129	26	2.2
plus fiber, instant, unprepared	1/2 cup	130	21	2.5
'Quick' prepared	2/3 cup	99	19	2.0
'Quick' unprepared	1/3 cup	99	19	2.0
radical raspberry, instant, 'Kids' Choice' unprepared	1 pkt	150	28	3.0
raisin bran, plus fiber, instant, unprepared	1 pkt	190	34	2.0
raisins and cinnamon, instant, 'Extra' unpreparedd	1 pkt	129	27	1.9
raisins and spice, instant, unprepared	1 pkt	149	32	2.0
raisins, dates, and walnuts, instant, unprepared	1 pkt	141	25	3.8
regular flavor, instant	1 pkt	94	18	2.0
regular flavor, microwave, 'Quick 'n Hearty'	1 pkt	106	19	2.1
strawberries and cream, instant, unprepared	1 pkt	129	27	2.0
strawberries and stuff, instant, 'Kids' Choice' unprepared	1 pkt	140	30	2.0
unprepared	1/3 cup	99	19	2.0
w/apples and cinnamon, instant, prepared w/water	1 pkt	125	26	1.4
w/apples and cinnamon, instant, unprepared	1 pkt	128	27	1.5
(Ralston)				
prepared w/water, salt	1 cup	134	28	0.8
prepared w/water, salt	3/4 cup	101	21	0.6
(3-Minute Brand)				
'Old Fashioned' unprepared	1 oz	100	18	2.0
'Quick' unprepared	1 oz	100	18	2.0
raisin, unprepared	1 oz	100	18	2.0
raisin, w/oat bran, unprepared	1 oz	100	18	2.0
(Total)				
instant, unprepared	1.2 oz	110	22	2.0

Food Name	Serv. Size	Total Cal.	Carbs GMS	Fat GMS
maple brown sugar, unprepared .... 1.6 oz	160	34	2.0
'Quick' unprepared .... 1 oz	90	18	2.0
(Under Cover Bears) plain, instant, prepared w/water .... 1 pkt	71	12	1.2
RICE			
(Arrowhead Mills)			
brown, 'Rise and Shine' unprepared .... 1.5 oz	160	35	1.0
(Cream of Rice)			
cream of, prepared w/water, no salt .... 1 cup	127	28	0.2
cream of, prepared w/water, no salt .... 3/4 cup	95	21	0.2
cream of, prepared w/water, no salt .... 1 tbsp	8	2	0.0
cream of, prepared w/water, salt .... 1 cup	127	28	0.2
cream of, prepared w/water, salt .... 3/4 cup	95	21	0.2
cream of, unprepared .... 1 cup	640	143	0.9
cream of, unprepared .... 1 tbsp	38	8	0.1
(Erewhon)			
brown, cream of, organic .... 1 oz	110	23	1.0
(Lundberg Family)			
almond-date, 'Hot'n Creamy' prepared .... 1 oz	110	24	1.0
organic, 'Hot'n Creamy' prepared .... 1 oz	110	23	1.0
RYE			
(Breadshop) 'Rye Date Muesli' unprepared .... 1 oz	100	19	2.0
(Roman Meal) cream of, unprepared .... 1/3 cup	110	27	1.0
WHEAT			
(Ancient Harvest) whole-grain, steam rolled .... 1/3 cup	105	23	1.0
(Arrowhead Mills)			
'Bear Mush' unprepared .... 1 oz	100	21	0.0
cracked wheat, unprepared .... 2 oz	180	40	1.0
(Cream of Wheat)			
cream of, apple, banana and maple flavored, instant, 'Mix 'N Eat' prepared .... 1 pkt	132	29	0.5
cream of, apple, banana and maple flavored, instant, 'Mix 'N Eat' unprepared .... 1 pkt	132	29	0.4
cream of, apple and cinnamon, 'Mix'n Eat' unprepared .... 1 oz	130	29	0.0
cream of, brown sugar cinnamon, 'Mix'n Eat' unprepared .... 1 oz	130	29	0.0
cream of, instant, prepared w/water, no salt .... 1 cup	121	26	0.2
cream of, instant, prepared w/water, no salt .... 3/4 cup	116	24	0.4
cream of, instant, prepared w/water, salt .... 1 serving	96	20	0.2
cream of, instant, prepared w/water, salt .... 1 cup	154	32	0.5
cream of, instant, prepared w/water, salt .... 3/4 cup	116	24	0.4
cream of, instant, prepared w/water, salt .... 1 tbsp	10	2	0.0
cream of, instant, unprepared .... 1 cup	651	134	2.5
cream of, instant, unprepared .... 1 tbsp	42	9	0.2
cream of, maple brown sugar, 'Mix'n Eat' unprepared .... 1 oz	130	29	0.0
cream of, original, 'Mix'n Eat' unprepared .... 1 oz	100	21	0.0
cream of, plain, instant, 'Mix 'N Eat' prepared .... 1 pkt	102	21	0.3
cream of, plain, instant, 'Mix 'N Eat' unprepared .... 1 pkt	102	21	0.3
cream of, quick, prepared w/water .... 1 cup	129	27	0.5
cream of, quick, prepared w/water .... 3/4 cup	97	20	0.4
cream of, quick, prepared w/water .... 1 tbsp	8	2	0.0
cream of, quick, prepared w/water, salt .... 1 cup	129	27	0.5
cream of, quick, prepared w/water, salt .... 3/4 cup	97	20	0.4
cream of, quick, unprepared .... 1 cup	635	132	2.3
cream of, quick, unprepared .... 1 tbsp	40	8	0.1
cream of, regular, prepared w/water, no salt .... 1 cup	133	28	0.5
cream of, regular, prepared w/water, no salt .... 3/4 cup	100	21	0.4
cream of, regular, prepared w/water, no salt .... 1 tbsp	8	2	0.0
cream of, regular, prepared w/water, salt .... 1 cup	133	28	0.5

Food Name	Serv. Size	Total Cal.	Carbs GMS	Fat GMS
cream of, regular, prepared w/water, salt	3/4 cup	100	21	0.4
cream of, regular, unprepared	1 cup	640	132	2.6
cream of, regular, unprepared	1 tbsp	39	8	0.2
(General Mills)				
'Wheat Hearts' prepared, w/3/4 cup nonfat milk	3/4 cup	170	29	1.0
'Wheat Hearts' unprepared	1 oz	110	21	1.0
(Wheat Hearts) unprepared	1 oz	110	21	1.0
(H-O Brand) wheat farina, cream of, unprepared	3 tbsp	120	26	0.0
(Hodgson Mill) cracked, coarse milled, unprepared	1/4 cup	110	26	1.0
(Malt-O-Meal)				
and barley, chocolate, prepared, w/1/2 cup 2% milk	1 oz	160	28	3.0
and barley, chocolate, unprepared	1 cup	607	128	1.5
and barley, chocolate, unprepared	1 oz	100	22	0.0
and barley, plain or chocolate, prepared w/water	1 cup	122	26	0.2
and barley, plain or chocolate, prepared w/water	3/4 cup	92	19	0.2
and barley, plain or chocolate, prepared w/water	1 tbsp	8	2	0.0
and barley, plain or chocolate, prepared w/water, salt	1 cup	122	26	0.2
and barley, plain or chocolate, prepared w/water, salt	3/4 cup	92	19	0.2
and barley, plain, unprepared	1 cup	607	128	1.5
and barley, plain, unprepared	1 tbsp	38	8	0.1
(Maltex)				
and barley, unprepared	1 oz	105	21	1.0
'Maltex' prepared w/water, no salt	1 cup	179	40	1.0
'Maltex' prepared w/water, no salt	3/4 cup	135	30	0.7
'Maltex' prepared w/water, no salt	1 tbsp	11	2	0.1
'Maltex' prepared w/water, salt	1 cup	179	40	1.0
'Maltex' prepared w/water, salt	3/4 cup	135	30	0.7
'Maltex' unprepared	1 cup	532	117	3.2
'Maltex' unprepared	1/4 cup	134	29	0.8
(Mother's)				
whole wheat, prepared, w/1/2 cup whole milk	1 oz	180	26	5.0
whole wheat, unprepared	1/3 cup	92	21	0.6
(Nabisco)				
cream of, apple cinnamon, prepared	1 serving	114	25	0.3
cream of, apple cinnamon, unprepreed	1 oz	108	24	0.3
cream of, enriched w/iron, quick, prepared	1 cup	78	16	0.3
cream of, enriched w/iron, quick, unprepared	1 cup	629	127	2.1
cream of, enriched w/iron, unprepared	1 oz	105	21	0.4
(Ralston)				
100% wheat, prepared	1/2 cup	160	31	1.0
'Ralston' prepared w/water, no salt	1 cup	134	28	0.8
'Ralston' prepared w/water, no salt	3/4 cup	101	21	0.6
'Ralston' prepared w/water, no salt	1 tbsp	8	2	0.0
'Ralston' unprepared	1 cup	402	85	2.5
'Ralston' unprepared	1/4 cup	102	22	0.6
(Roman Meal)				
w/dates, raisins, almonds, unprepared	1/3 cup	140	26	3.0
w/honey, coconut, almond	1/3 cup	150	21	6.0
w/rye, bran, flax, unprepared	1/3 cup	116	25	1.7
(Wheatena)				
wheat, unprepared	1 oz	100	21	1.0
'Wheatena' prepared w/water, no salt	1 cup	136	29	1.2
'Wheatena' prepared w/water, no salt	3/4 cup	102	21	0.9
'Wheatena' prepared w/water, salt	1 cup	136	29	1.2
'Wheatena' prepared w/water, salt	3/4 cup	102	21	0.9
'Wheatena' unprepared	1 cup	503	107	4.1
'Wheatena' unprepared	1/4 cup	125	26	1.0

Food Name	Serv. Size	Total Cal.	Carbs GMS	Fat GMS
CEREAL, READY-TO-EAT				
(Arrowhead Mills)				
bran flakes	1 oz	100	21	1.0
buckwheat groats, brown	2 oz	190	41	1.0
buckwheat groats, white	2 oz	190	41	1.0
corn flakes	1 oz	100	25	0.0
corn flakes, organic	1 cup	130	30	0.0
'Maple Corns'	1 oz	100	23	1.0
'Maple Corns' organic	1 cup	190	43	3.0
multigrain, organic	1 cup	140	29	1.5
'Nature-O's' organic	1 cup	130	24	2.0
oat bran flakes	1 oz	100	19	2.0
oat flakes	2 oz	220	39	4.0
oat groats	2 oz	220	38	4.0
puffed corn	0.5 oz	50	11	0.0
puffed rice	0.5 oz	50	12	0.0
puffed wheat	0.5 oz	50	11	0.0
wheat flakes	2 oz	210	42	1.0
(Barbara's Bakery)				
raisin bran	1 oz	170	36	1.0
'Shredded Spoonfuls' natural, 97% fat-free	3/4 cup	120	23	1.5
'Shredded Wheat'	2 biscuits	140	31	1.0
(Breadshop)				
'Almond Raisin' nectarsweet premium	1 oz	120	18	4.0
'Blueberry 'N Cream' nectarsweet gourmet	1 oz	115	19	3.0
'California Orange Crunch' honeysweet premium	1 oz	130	18	5.0
'Cinnapple Spice' honeysweet premium	1 oz	125	19	4.5
'Crunchy Oat Bran' nectarsweet gourmet	1 oz	120	18	5.0
'Golden Maple Nut' honeysweet premium	1 oz	130	17	5.0
'Gone Nuts!' nectarsweet premium	1 oz	125	17	5.0
'Honey Apple Blueberry' honeysweet premium	1 oz	125	18	5.0
'Honey Gone Nuts!' honeysweet premium	1 oz	130	18	5.5
'Orange Almond' nectarsweet premium	1 oz	120	18	4.0
'Oregon Blueberry Crunch' honeysweet gourmet	1 oz	125	18	5.0
'Peaches 'N Cream' nectarsweet gourmet	1 oz	115	19	3.0
'Raspberry 'N Cream' nectarsweet gourmet	1 oz	115	19	3.0
'Strawberry 'N Cream' nectarsweet gourmet	1 oz	110	16	4.0
'Supernatural' honeysweet gourmet	1 oz	100	18	5.0
'Supernatural New England' honeysweet gourmet	1 oz	130	18	5.0
(Eden Foods) 'Puffed Rice' five-flavor	30 puffs	110	24	0.0
(Erewhon)				
'Aztec' natural, nonfat	1 cup	110	26	0.0
'Banana-O's' organic, natural	3/4 cup	110	26	0.0
'Brown Rice' crispy	1 oz	110	24	1.0
brown rice, crispy, low-sodium	1 oz	110	24	1.0
brown rice, crispy, nonfat	1 cup	110	25	0.0
corn flakes, natural, no sweeteners	3/4 cup	100	22	1.0
'Crisp Rice' brown, natural	1 cup	110	25	0.0
'Fruit 'N Wheat'	1 oz	100	21	1.0
'Galaxy Grahams' natural, organic	3/4 cup	100	23	0.5
kamut flakes	3/4 cup	90	18	0.0
'Poppets' natural, organic	1 cup	120	25	1.0
raisin bran	1 oz	100	22	0.0
raisin bran, high-fiber, low-fat, low-sodium	1 cup	170	40	1.0
'Raisin Grahams' natural, nonfat, low-sodium	3/4 cup	100	23	0.0
'Right Start'	1 oz	90	24	0.0
'Right Start w/Raisins'	1 oz	90	22	0.0

Food Name	Serv. Size	Total Cal.	Carbs GMS	Fat GMS
'Wheat Flakes'	1 oz	110	22	0.0
'Super O's'	1 oz	110	24	0.0
(General Mills)				
'Addam's Family'	1 oz	110	25	1.0
'Basic 4'	1 cup	201	42	2.8
'Batman Returns'	1 oz	110	26	0.0
'Berry Berry Kix'	3/4 cup	120	26	1.2
'Body Buddies'	1 cup	115	26	0.9
'Boo Berry'	1 cup	116	27	0.5
'Bunuelitos'	1 oz	120	25	2.0
'Cheerios'	1 cup	110	23	1.8
'Cheerios' apple cinnamon	3/4 cup	118	25	1.6
'Cheerios' apple cinnamon, breakfast pack	1-oz box	120	24	2.0
'Cheerios' honey nut	1 cup	115	24	1.2
'Cheerios' multigrain	1 cup	112	24	1.1
'Cheerios Plus' multigrain	1 cup	108	24	1.1
'Cheerios-To-Go' apple cinnamon	1 pouch	110	22	2.0
'Cheerios-To-Go' honey nut	1 pouch	110	23	1.0
'Cheerios-To-Go'	1 pouch	80	15	2.0
'Chex' corn	1 cup	113	26	0.4
'Chex' honey nut	3/4 cup	117	26	0.7
'Chex' multi-bran	1 cup	165	41	1.2
'Chex' rice	1.25 cup	117	27	0.2
'Chex' wheat	1 cup	104	24	0.7
'Cinnamon Streusel' Betty Crocker	3/4 cup	120	25	1.3
'Cinnamon Toast Crunch'	3/4 cup	124	24	3.0
'Cocoa Puffs'	1 cup	119	27	0.9
'Cookie-Crisp'	1 cup	120	26	1.1
'Corn Flakes'	1 cup	98	22	0.1
'Count Chocula'	1 cup	117	26	0.9
'Country Corn Flakes'	1 cup	114	26	0.5
'Crispy Wheats 'N Raisins'	1 cup	191	44	0.8
'Crunchy Bran'	3/4 cup	90	23	0.9
'Dutch Apple' Betty Crocker	1 cup	219	46	2.0
'Fiber One'	1/2 cup	62	24	0.8
'Fingos' cinnamon	1 oz	110	22	3.0
'Fingos' honey toasted oat	1 oz	110	21	3.0
'40% Bran Flakes'	1 cup	159	39	0.7
'Frankenberry'	1 cup	117	27	0.5
'Golden Grahams'	3/4 cup	116	26	1.1
'Hidden Treasures' fruit juice added	3/4 cup	120	25	2.0
'Honey Almond Delight'	1 oz	110	23	2.0
'Honey Frosted Wheaties'	3/4 cup	110	26	0.3
'Honey Nut Clusters'	1 cup	213	43	3.5
'Kaboom'	1.25 cup	118	24	1.1
'Kix'	1 1/3 cup	114	26	0.6
'Lucky Charms'	1 cup	116	25	1.1
'Muesli' apple almond	1.45 oz	150	31	2.0
'Muesli' banana walnut	1.45 oz	150	30	3.0
'Muesli' cranberry walnut	1.45 oz	150	30	3.0
'Muesli' date almond	1.45 oz	140	32	2.0
'Muesli' peach pecan	1.45 oz	150	30	3.0
'Muesli' raspberry almond	1.45 oz	150	30	3.0
'Nature Valley Granola' cinnamon and raisin	3/4 cup	235	38	7.7
'Nature Valley Granola' fruit, low-fat	2/3 cup	212	44	3.0
'Nature Valley Granola' fruit and nut	2/3 cup	253	34	11.2
'Nature Valley Granola' fruit and nut	1/3 cup	130	19	5.0

Food Name	Serv. Size	Total Cal.	Carbs GMS	Fat GMS
'Nature Valley Granola' toasted oats	3/4 cup	248	36	9.7
'Nature Valley Granola' toasted oats	1/3 cup	130	20	5.0
'Oatmeal Crisp w/Almonds'	1 cup	219	42	4.6
'Oatmeal Crisp w/Apples'	1 cup	205	46	1.8
'Oatmeal Raisin Crisp'	1 cup	204	44	2.4
'Raisin Bran'	1 cup	178	46	0.3
'Raisin Bran'	1-1/3 oz box	120	31	0.2
'Raisin Nut Bran'	1 cup	209	41	4.4
'Reese's Peanut Butter Puffs'	3/4 cup	129	23	3.2
'Ripple Crisp'	1 oz	110	24	1.0
'Ripple Crisp' honey bran	1 oz	100	24	1.0
'S'Mores Grahams'	3/4 cup	117	26	1.2
'Sprinkle Spangles' corn puffs w/sprinkles	1 oz	110	25	1.0
'Sugar Frosted Flakes'	1 cup	149	34	0.5
'Sun Crunchers'	1 cup	216	44	3.2
'Sunflakes' multigrain	1 oz	100	24	1.0
'Team Cheerios'	1 cup	113	25	1.1
'Teenage Mutant Ninja Turtles'	1 oz	110	26	0.0
'Total'	3/4 cup	105	24	0.7
'Total Corn Flakes'	1 1/3 cup	112	26	0.5
'Total Raisin Bran'	1 cup	178	43	1.0
'Triples'	1 cup	116	25	1.0
'Trix'	1 cup	122	26	1.7
'Urkel-O's'	1 oz	110	25	1.0
'Wheaties'	1 cup	110	24	0.9
'Wheaties' honey gold'	3/4 cup	100	25	1.0
(Glenny's)				
'Maple Frosted Corn' mini puffs	1 oz	109	20	0.5
'Oat Mini Puffs'	1 oz	108	22	0.5
'Oat Mini Puffs' no salt, no sugar	1 oz	108	22	0.5
'Rice Mini Puffs'	1 oz	109	20	0.5
(Golden Temple)				
'Almond Raisin' low-fat	1 oz	110	22	1.5
'Apple Cinnamon' low-fat	1 oz	110	22	1.5
'Cashew Almond Granola'	1 oz	129	19	3.5
'Cinnamon & Spice Crunch' psyllium and chia seed	1 oz	132	20	4.5
'Cinnamon Granola' apple and raisin	1 oz	125	20	3.5
'Coconut Almond Granola'	1 oz	145	18	7.0
'Fruit 'N Nut Granola'	1 oz	129	19	4.5
'Golden Granola'	1 oz	138	19	6.0
'Hawaiian Granola'	1 oz	126	19	4.0
'Hazelnut Boysenberry' organic oats	1 oz	135	19	5.5
'High-Protein Granola'	1 oz	124	19	3.5
'Honey Almond Granola'	1 oz	130	20	3.5
'Honey Blueberry Granola' apple	1 oz	128	20	3.5
'Lite 'N Crunchy Granola'	1 oz	129	19	4.5
'Lite Muesli'	1 oz	102	20	1.0
'Maple Almond Granola'	1 oz	129	20	3.5
'Natural Blueberry Granola'	1 oz	132	19	5.0
'Natural Blueberry Granola' coconut-free	1 oz	131	19	4.5
'Natural Delite Granola'	1 oz	128	20	3.5
'Natural Foods' almond and raisin, lowfat	1 oz	110	22	1.0
'Natural Foods' apple and cinnamon, lowfat	1 oz	110	22	1.0
'Natural Foods' strawberry and raspberry, lowfat	1 oz	111	22	1.0
'Oat Bran Almond'	1 oz	120	20	3.5
'Oat Bran Apple'	1 oz	112	19	3.5
'Oat Bran Granola' berries	1 oz	120	20	3.5

Food Name	Serv. Size	Total Cal.	Carbs GMS	Fat GMS
'Oat Bran Granola' raisins and almonds	1 oz	119	19	3.5
'Oat Bran Muesli' dates and almonds	1 oz	108	21	1.5
'Oat Bran Muesli' raisins and hazelnut	1 oz	102	20	1.5
'Oat Bran Oregonberry'	1 oz	116	20	3.5
'100% Natural Almond'	1 oz	123	18	4.0
'100% Natural Apple/Cinnamon'	1 oz	120	18	4.0
'100% Natural Oat Bran'	1 oz	70	19	2.5
'100% Natural Raisin/Almond'	1 oz	120	19	4.0
'Orange Almond Granola'	1 oz	133	19	4.0
'Raisin Granola' apricot and dates	1 oz	127	20	3.5
'Six-Grain Crisp' fruit and flaxseed	1 oz	118	20	3.5
'Super Nutty Granola'	1 oz	135	19	5.0
'Sweet Home Farm Almond'	1 oz	123	18	4.0
'Sweet Home Farm Granola' lowfat	1 oz	110	22	2.0
'Sweet Home Farm Muesli' crunchy, lowfat	1 oz	105	21	2.0
'Sweet Home Farm Raisin'	1 oz	120	19	4.0
'Swiss Style Muesli'	1 oz	105	19	1.5
'35% Fruit Muesli'	1 oz	97	19	1.0
(Health Valley)				
'Almond Flavor O's' fat-free	1 oz	90	19	0.0
granola, date and almond flavor, nonfat	1 oz	90	21	0.0
granola, raisin cinnamon, nonfat	1 oz	90	21	0.0
granola, tropical fruit, nonfat	1 oz	90	21	0.0
'High-Fiber O's, nonfat'	1 oz	90	19	0.0
'100% Organic Blue Corn Flakes'	1 oz	90	19	1.0
'Organic Amaranth Flakes'	1 oz	90	20	0.0
'Sprouts 7' bananas and Hawaiian fruit, nonfat	1 oz	90	16	0.0
'Sprouts 7' raisins, nonfat	1 oz	90	16	0.0
(Heartland)				
'Heartland Natural' plain	1 cup	499	79	17.7
'Heartland Natural, plain	1 oz	123	19	4.4
'Heartland Natural' w/coconut	1 cup	463	71	17.1
'Heartland Natural' w/coconut	1 oz	125	19	4.6
'Heartland Natural' w/raisins	1 cup	468	76	15.6
(Honeybran)				
'Honeybran'	1 cup	119	29	0.7
'Honeybran'	1 oz	97	23	0.6
(Kashi)				
'Multigrain' medley	1 oz	100	20	1.0
'Puffed' honey, no refined sugars, no added oils	2 oz	120	25	1.0
'Puffed' sodium-free	2 oz	70	19	1.0
(Kellogg's)				
'All-Bran'	1/2 cup	79	23	0.9
'All-Bran Bran Buds'	1/3 cup	83	24	0.7
'All-Bran' w/extra fiber	1/2 cup	53	23	0.9
'Apple Jacks'	1 cup	116	27	0.4
'Apple Raisin Crisp'	1 cup	185	47	0.5
'Bran Flakes'	3/4 cup	95	23	0.6
'Cinnamon Mini Buns'	3/4 cup	115	27	0.6
'Cocoa Frosted Flakes'	3/4 cup	120	28	0.5
'Cocoa Krispies'	3/4 cup	120	27	0.8
'Common Sense Oat Bran Flakes'	3/4 cup	109	23	1.2
'Corn Flakes'	1 cup	102	24	0.2
'Corn Pops'	1 cup	118	28	0.2
'Cracklin' Oat Bran'	3/4 cup	225	40	7.0
'Crispix'	1 cup	108	25	0.3
'Double Dip Crunch'	3/4 cup	115	27	0.1

Food Name	Serv. Size	Total Cal.	Carbs GMS	Fat GMS
'Fiberwise'	1 oz	90	23	1.0
'Froot Loops'	1 cup	117	26	0.9
'Frosted Bran'	3/4 cup	101	25	0.3
'Frosted Flakes'	3/4 cup	119	28	0.2
'Frosted Krispies'	3/4 cup	113	27	0.2
'Frosted Mini-Wheats' bite size	1 cup	187	45	0.9
'Frosted Mini-Wheats' regular	1 cup	173	42	0.8
'Fruity Marshmallow Krispies'	3/4 cup	113	27	0.1
granola, w/o raisins, low-fat	1/2 cup	213	44	3.2
granola, w/raisins, low-fat	2/3 cup	202	44	2.8
'Healthy Choice Almond Crunch with Raisins'	1 cup	198	43	2.6
'Healthy Choice Multigrain' clusters w/raisins and almonds	1 1/4 cup	200	44	2.0
'Healthy Choice Multigrain' flakes w/brown sugar	1 cup	110	26	0.0
'Healthy Choice Multigrain' flakes	1 cup	104	25	0.4
'Healthy Choice Multigrain' squares w/honey	1 1/4 cup	190	45	1.0
'Healthy Choice Toasted Brown Sugar Squares'	1.25 cup	189	45	1.0
'Honey Crunch Corn Flakes'	3/4 cup	115	26	0.9
'Just Right' fruit and nut	1 cup	193	44	1.6
'Just Right' w/crunchy nuggets	1 cup	204	46	1.5
'Kenmei Rice Bran'	3/4 cup	110	24	1.0
'Mini-Wheats' apple cinnamon	3/4 cup	182	44	1.0
'Mini-Wheats' blueberry	3/4 cup	182	44	1.0
'Mini-Wheats' raisin	3/4 cup	187	43	1.5
'Mini-Wheats' strawberry	1 cup	187	43	1.3
'Mueslix' apple and orange crunch	3/4 cup	211	41	5.0
'Mueslix' raisin and almond crunch, w/dates	2/3 cup	200	40	3.2
'Nut & Honey Crunch'	1.25 cup	223	46	2.5
'Nutri-Grain Raisin Bran'	1 cup	130	31	1.0
'Nutri-Grain Wheat'	3/4 cup	101	24	1.0
'Oatbake Honey Bran'	1/3 cup	110	21	3.0
'Oatbake Raisin Nut'	1 oz	110	21	3.0
'Pop Tarts Crunch' cinnamon, brown sugar, frosted	3/4 cup	120	26	1.0
'Pop-Tarts Crunch' strawberry, frosted	3/4 cup	118	27	0.8
'Product 19'	1 cup	110	25	0.4
'Raisin Bran'	1 cup	186	47	1.5
'Razzle Dazzle Rice Krispies'	3/4 cup	108	25	0.3
'Rice Krispies'	1.25 cup	124	29	0.4
'Rice Krispies' apple cinnamon	3/4 cup	112	27	0.1
'Rice Krispies Treats'	3/4 cup	120	26	1.6
'Smacks'	3/4 cup	103	24	0.5
'Smart Start'	1 cup	183	43	0.7
'Special K'	1 cup	115	22	0.3
'Temptations' French vanilla almond	3/4 cup	119	25	1.6
'Temptations' honey roasted pecan	1 cup	122	24	2.3
'Whole Grain Shredded Wheat'	1 oz	90	23	0.0
(Kolln) 'Oat Bran Crunch'	1 oz	100	20	2.0
(Krusteaz)				
'Corn Flakes'	1 oz	110	24	1.0
'Crisp Rice'	1 oz	110	25	0.0
'Fruit Whirls'	1 oz	110	25	1.0
'Honey Nut O's'	1 oz	110	23	1.0
'Raisin Bran'	3/4 cup	120	30	1.0
'Sugar Frosted Flakes'	1 oz	110	26	0.0
'Toasted Oats'	1 oz	110	22	1.0
(Lundberg Family) 'Crunchies' brown rice	1 cup	171	38	0.8
(Malt-O-Meal)				
'Apple & Cinnamon Toasted Oat'	1 oz	110	22	2.0

Food Name	Serv. Size	Total Cal.	Carbs GMS	Fat GMS
'Berry Colossal Crunch'	3/4 cup	120	26	1.7
'Bran Flakes'	1 oz	90	23	1.0
'Colossal Crunch'	3/4 cup	120	26	1.7
'Corn Bursts'	1 cup	118	29	0.1
'Corn Flakes'	1 oz	110	25	0.0
'Crisp 'N' Crackling Rice'	1 oz	110	25	0.0
'Crispy Rice'	1 cup	125	29	0.4
'Fruit & Frosted O's' multigrain	1 oz	110	25	1.0
'Honey & Nut Toasted Oat'	1 oz	110	23	1.0
'Marshmallow Mateys'	1 cup	115	25	1.0
'Puffed Rice'	0.5 oz	50	12	0.0
'Puffed Wheat'	0.5 oz	50	10	0.0
'Raisin Bran Flakes'	1.4 oz	130	30	2.0
'Sugar Frosted Flakes'	1 oz	110	26	0.0
'Sugar Puffs'	1 oz	110	25	0.0
'Sweetened Puffed Wheat'	1 oz	110	25	0.0
'Toasted Oats'	1 oz	110	20	2.0
'Toasty O's'	1 cup	112	22	1.8
'Tootie Fruities'	1 cup	125	28	1.0
(Nabisco)				
'Fruit Wheats' apple	1 oz	90	23	0.0
'Team Flakes'	1 oz	110	24	1.0
(Nature Valley) See under General Mills.				
(Nature's Path) 'Heritage O's'	1 cup	165	34	1.0
(Perky's) 'Rice' nutty	1/2 cup	210	47	1.5
(Post)				
'Alpha-Bits' w/marshmallows	1 cup	115	25	1.0
'Banana Nut Crunch'	1 cup	249	44	6.1
'Blueberry Morning'	1.25 cup	211	43	2.5
'Bran Flakes'	3/4 cup	96	24	0.7
'C.W. Post Hearty Granola'	1 oz	130	21	4.0
'Cocoa Pebbles'	3/4 cup	115	25	1.2
'Dino Pebbles'	1 oz	110	25	1.0
'Frosted Alpha-Bits'	1 cup	130	27	1.3
'Frosted Shredded Wheat' bite size	1 cup	183	44	1.0
'Fruit & Fibre' tropical fruit	1.25 oz	120	27	3.0
'Fruit & Fibre' w/dates, raisins and walnuts	1 cup	212	42	3.1
'Fruity Pebbles'	3/4 cup	108	24	1.1
'Golden Crisp'	3/4 cup	107	25	0.4
'Grape-Nuts'	1/2 cup	208	47	1.1
'Grape-Nuts Flakes'	3/4 cup	106	24	0.8
'Great Grains' crunchy pecan	2/3 cup	216	38	6.3
'Great Grains' double pecan	1 oz	120	20	3.0
'Great Grains' raisin, date, and pecan	2/3 cup	204	40	4.5
'Honey Bunches Of Oats'	3/4 cup	118	25	1.6
'Honey Bunches Of Oats' w/almonds	3/4 cup	126	24	2.6
'Honeycomb'	1 1/3 cup	115	26	0.6
'Oat Flakes'	1 oz	110	21	1.0
'100% Bran'	1/3 cup	83	23	0.6
'Oreo O's'	3/4 cup	112	22	2.4
'Raisin Bran'	1 cup	187	46	1.1
'Raisin Grape-Nuts'	1 oz	100	23	0.0
'Shredded Wheat' original	2 biscuits	156	38	0.6
'Shredded Wheat' spoon size	1 cup	167	41	0.5
'Shredded Wheat N Bran' original	1.25 cup	197	47	0.8
'Smurf-Magic Berries'	1 oz	120	26	1.0
'Toasties' corn flakes	1 cup	101	24	0.0

Food Name	Serv. Size	Total Cal.	Carbs GMS	Fat GMS
'Waffle Crisp'	1 cup	129	24	2.9
(Quaker)				
'Apple Zaps'	3/4 cup	118	27	1.0
'Cap'n Crunch'	3/4 cup	107	23	1.4
'Cap'n Crunch's Crunchberries'	3/4 cup	104	22	1.3
'Cap'n Crunch's Peanut Butter Crunch'	3/4 cup	112	22	2.3
'Cinnamon Life'	1 cup	190	40	1.7
'Cinnamon Oatmeal Squares'	1 cup	232	47	2.6
'Cocoa Blasts'	1 cup	129	29	1.2
'Corn Blasts'	1 cup	133	28	1.9
'Frosted Flakers'	3/4 cup	117	28	0.2
'Fruitangy Oh!s'	1 cup	122	27	1.1
'Honey Graham Oh!'	3/4 cup	112	23	1.9
'King Vitaman'	1.25 cup	120	26	1.1
'Kretschmer Honey Crunch Wheat Germ'	1 2/3 tbsp	52	8	1.1
'Marshmallow Safari'	3/4 cup	119	25	1.5
'Oat Bran'	1.25 cup	213	41	2.9
'Oat Life, Plain'	3/4 cup	121	25	1.3
'Oatmeal Squares'	1 cup	216	43	2.6
'100% Natural,' oats, honey, and raisins	1/2 cup	218	36	7.3
'100% Natural,' oats and honey'	1/2 cup	213	33	7.9
'100% Natural,' whole grain w/raisins, lowfat	1/2 cup	195	40	2.7
'Puffed Rice'	1 cup	54	12	0.1
'Puffed Wheat'	1.25 cup	55	11	0.3
'Quisp'	1 cup	109	23	1.5
'Sun Country Granola' w/almonds'	1/2 cup	266	38	10.3
'Sun Country Granola' w/raisins and dates	1/2 cup	135	22	4.2
'Toasted Oatmeal' honey nut	1 cup	191	39	2.7
'Toasted Oatmeal' original	1 oz	100	22	1.0
(Rainforest Flake)				
flakes w/cashews, Brazil nuts, and raisins	4 oz	230	35	8.0
'Honey Nut Clusters' lowfat	4 oz	210	45	1.5
(Ralston Purina) See under *(General Mills)*.				
(Rice Krinkles)				
'Frosted Rice Krinkles'	1 cup	173	41	0.1
'Frosted Rice Krinkles' single serving box	0.75 oz	82	19	0.0
(Stone-Buhr)				
'Cereal Mates' 4-grain	1/3 cup	140	31	1.5
'Cereal Mates' 7-grain	1/3 cup	140	31	2.0
(Sunbelt)				
granola, banana almond	1 oz	130	20	4.0
granola, fruit and nut	1 oz	120	19	5.0
(US Mills) 'Uncle Sam'	1 oz	110	20	1.0
(Wonder)				
'Apple Cinnamon Corn Flakes'	1 oz	110	25	0.0
'Crunch Graham Oat Rings'	1 oz	110	24	1.0
'Honey Nut Crispy Rice'	1 oz	110	25	1.0

CEREAL BAR. See GRANOLA/CEREAL BAR.

CEREAL GRAIN BEVERAGE. See COFFEE SUBSTITUTE.

CEREAL SNACK. See also GRANOLA/CEREAL BAR.

(Barbara's Bakery)				
chocolate chip, 'Grrr-nola Treat'	1 serving	80	15	2.0
peanut butter and jelly, 'Grrr-nola Treat'	1 serving	80	14	3.0
(General Mills)				
'Cheerios-to-Go' apple cinnamon	1 pouch	110	22	2.0
'Cheerios-to-Go' honey nut	1 pouch	110	23	1.0
'Cheerios-to-Go' plain	1 pouch	80	15	2.0

Food Name	Serv. Size	Total Cal.	Carbs GMS	Fat GMS
'Fingos' cinnamon	1 oz	110	22	3.0
'Fingos' honey toasted oat	1 oz	110	21	3.0
(Natural Nectar)				
granola, almond butter crunch 'Nectar Nuggets'	1 cup	120	11	7.0
granola, almond cappuccino crunch 'Nectar Nuggets'	1 cup	110	14	5.0
granola, coconut almond crunch, 'Nectar Nuggets'	1 cup	110	15	5.0
granola, peanut butter crunch, 'Nectar Nuggets'	1 cup	120	11	7.0
(Nature Valley)				
granola, apple-cinnamon, 'Granola Bites'	1 pouch	170	25	7.0
granola, honey nut, 'Granola Bites'	1 pkg	170	24	8.0
granola, variety pack, 'Granola Bites'	1 pkg	170	24	8.0
(Nature's Choice)				
granola, chocolate chip, 'Grrr-Nola Treats'	0.75 oz	80	15	2.0
granola, cinnamon toast, 'Grrr-Nola Treats'	0.75 oz	80	15	2.0
granola, peanut butter and jelly, 'Grrr-Nola Treats'	0.75 oz	80	14	3.0
granola, tutti-frutti, 'Grrr-Nola Treats'	0.75 oz	75	15	2.0
CHARD. See SWISS CHARD.				
CHAYOTE				
Fresh				
boiled, drained, chopped, 1-inch pieces	1 cup	38	8	0.8
raw, chopped, 1-inch pieces	1 cup	25	6	0.2
raw, whole, 5.75-inches	1 chayote	39	9	0.3
CHEDDARWURST. See under SAUSAGE, CHEESE.				
CHEESE. See also CHEESE FOOD; CHEESE PRODUCT; CHEESE SPREAD; CHEESE SUBSTITUTE.				
AMERICAN				
pasteurized, process	1 oz	106	0	8.9
pasteurized process, w/disodium phosphate added	1 oz	106	0	8.9
(Borden)				
processed, 'Light'	1-1/3 slices	70	1	4.0
processed, 'Loaf'	1 oz	110	1	9.0
processed, nonfat, low-cholesterol	1 oz	40	4	0.0
processed, 'Slices'	1 oz	110	1	9.0
processed, slices, 'Premium'	1 oz	110	1	9.0
(Dorman's)				
processed	1 oz	110	1	9.0
processed, low-sodium, 'Loaf'	1 oz	110	1	9.0
(Healthy Choice)				
white, singles	1 slice	40	2	1.0
yellow, singles	1 slice	40	2	1.0
(Healthy Favorites) processed	2/3 oz	45	2	2.0
(Hoffman's) processed	1 oz	110	1	9.0
(Kraft)				
processed, 'Deluxe Loaf'	1 oz	110	1	9.0
processed, 'Deluxe Slices'	1 oz	110	1	9.0
(Land O'Lakes)				
processed	1 oz	110	1	9.0
processed, sharp	1 oz	100	1	9.0
(Old English)				
processed, sharp, 'Loaf'	1 oz	110	1	9.0
processed, sharp, 'Slices'	1 oz	110	1	9.0
(Sargento) hot pepper, pasteurized process	1 oz	106	0	8.9
(Smart Beat) fat-free	1 slice	25	3	0.0
(Weight Watchers) low-fat	1 slice	30	2	0.0
ASIAGO *(Frigo)* natural, wheel	1 oz	110	1	9.0
BABYBEL				
(Laughing Cow)				
natural	1 oz	91	0	7.0

Food Name	Serv. Size	Total Cal.	Carbs GMS	Fat GMS
natural, mini	3/4 oz	74	0	6.0
BEL PAESE				
(Bel Paese)				
'Domestic Traditional'	1 oz	101	1	8.0
'Imported'	1 oz	90	0	7.4
'Lite'	1 oz	76	1	5.0
primavera, 'Lite'	1 oz	68	2	4.0
BLUE				
	1 oz	100	1	8.1
(Dorman's)				
natural, 'Castello 70%'	1 oz	134	0	12.3
natural, 'Danablu 50%'	1 oz	100	0	8.2
natural, 'Danablu 60%'	1 oz	108	0	9.7
natural, 'Saga 70%'	1 oz	134	0	12.3
(Frigo) natural	1 oz	100	1	8.0
(Hickory Farms) natural, 'Domestic'	1 oz	101	1	8.3
(Kraft) natural	1 oz	100	1	9.0
(Sargento)				
crumbled	1/4 cup	100	1	8.0
natural	1 oz	100	1	8.0
BONBEL				
(Laughing Cow)				
mini	3/4 oz	74	0	6.0
natural	1 oz	100	0	8.0
BONBINO *(Laughing Cow)* natural	1 oz	103	0	9.0
BRICK				
	1 oz	105	1	8.4
(Dorman's) natural	1 oz	110	1	8.0
(Kraft) natural	1 oz	110	0	9.0
(Land O'Lakes) natural	1 oz	110	1	8.0
BRIE				
	1 oz	95	0	7.8
(Dorman's) natural	1 oz	81	0	6.6
(Sargento) natural	1 oz	100	0	8.0
BURGER *(Sargento)* natural	1 oz	110	1	9.0
BUTTERNIP *(Hickory Farms)* natural	1 oz	110	1	9.4
CAJUN *(Sargento)*	1 oz	110	0	9.0
CALJACK *(Churny)*	1 oz	100	1	8.0
CAMEMBERT				
	1 cup	737	1	59.7
(Dorman's)				
'45%'	1 oz	82	0	6.3
'50%'	1 oz	89	0	7.3
(Hickory Farms)	1 oz	90	0	7.0
(Sargento)	1 oz	90	0	7.0
CHEDDAR				
	1 oz	114	0	9.4
low-fat	1 oz	49	1	2.0
low-salt	1 oz	113	1	9.2
(Alpine Lace)				
'Cheddar Flavored'	1 oz	100	1	8.0
milk, natural, shredded, 'Ched-R-Lo'	1 oz	80	1	5.0
(Alta Dena)				
mild, natural	1 oz	110	1	9.0
sharp, natural	1 oz	110	1	9.0
(Axelrod)				
extra sharp	1 oz	110	1	9.0

Food Name	Serv. Size	Total Cal.	Carbs GMS	Fat GMS
sharp	1 oz	110	1	9.0
(Boar's Head) sharp sliced	1 oz	110	1	9.0
(Darigold)	1 oz	110	1	9.0
(Dorman's)				
	1 oz	110	1	9.0
'Chedda-Delite'	1 oz	90	1	7.0
cheddar Jack, low-salt	1 oz	80	1	5.0
less fat, 'Low Sodium'	1 oz	80	1	5.0
low-salt, low-fat	1 oz	80	1	5.0
w/Monterey Jack, 'Chedda-Jack'	1 oz	90	1	7.0
(Featherweight) 'Low Sodium'	1 oz	110	1	9.0
(Frigo)				
	1 oz	110	1	9.0
low-fat	1 oz	20	1	1.0
(Golden Balance)				
mild, natural, shredded 'Natural Shreds'	1 oz	90	1	6.0
sharp, natural, shredded 'Natural Shreds'	1 oz	90	1	6.0
(Healthy Choice)				
low-fat, 'Fancy Shreds'	1/4 cup	50	1	1.5
mild, natural, 'Fancy Shreds'	1 oz	70	0	4.0
(Hickory Farms)				
	1 oz	110	1	9.0
raw milk, 'Light Choice Low Sodium'	1 oz	114	0	8.0
(Hoffman's) super sharp, processed	1 oz	110	2	8.0
(Kraft)				
mild, natural	1 oz	110	1	9.0
mild, natural, low-fat, made w/2% milk	1 oz	90	1	6.0
mild, natural, shredded 'Light Naturals'	1 oz	80	1	5.0
sharp, less fat, 'Light Naturals'	1 oz	80	1	5.0
sharp, low-fat, natural, made w/2% milk	1 oz	90	1	6.0
sharp, natural, made w/2% milk, 'Cracker Barrel'	1 oz	90	1	6.0
sharp, white, light, 'Cracker Barrel'	1 oz	80	1	5.0
(Land O'Lakes)				
natural	1 oz	110	1	9.0
natural, 'Chedarella'	1 oz	100	1	8.0
(Laughing Cow)				
	1 oz	110	0	9.0
'Reduced Mini'	3/4 oz	45	0	2.5
(Sargento)				
	1 oz	110	0	9.0
mild, fancy, shredded, 'Preferred Light'	1/4 cup	70	1	4.5
mild, light, 'Mootown Snackers'	1 piece	60	1	4.0
mild, shredded, 'Classic Supreme'	1/4 cup	110	1	9.0
mild or sharp, 'Mootown Snackers'	1 piece	100	1	8.0
'New York'	1 oz	110	0	9.0
sliced	1 slice	110	1	9.0
(Smart Beat) sharp, nonfat	1 slice	25	3	0.0
(Stilwell) cheddar, frozen 'Bumpers'	1 piece	60	6	3.0
(Weight Watchers)				
mild, 'Natural'	1 oz	80	1	5.0
mild, shredded, 'Natural'	1 oz	80	1	5.0
sharp, 'Natural'	1 oz	80	1	5.0
CHESHIRE	1 oz	110	1	8.7
CHUTTER (Hickory Farms) 'Cold Pack'	1 oz	87	3	5.8
COLBY				
	1 oz	112	1	9.1
low-fat	1 oz	49	1	2.0

Food Name	Serv. Size	Total Cal.	Carbs GMS	Fat GMS
low-salt	1 oz	113	1	9.2
(Alpine Lace) 'Colby-Lo'	1 oz	80	1	5.0
(Dorman's)	1 oz	110	1	9.0
(Hickory Farms)				
'Light Choice Low Sodium'	1 oz	100	1	6.0
'Longhorn'	1 oz	112	1	8.6
low-fat, calcium-enriched 'Light Choice'	1 oz	100	1	8.0
(Kraft)				
	1 oz	110	1	9.0
made w/2% milk, natural	1 oz	80	0	6.0
w/Monterey Jack, less fat, 'Light Naturals'	1 oz	80	1	5.0
w/Monterey Jack, natural, shredded, 'Light Naturals'	1 oz	80	1	5.0
(Land O'Lakes) natural	1 oz	110	1	9.0
(Sargento)				
	1 oz	110	1	9.0
Jack	1 oz	110	1	9.0
Jack, 'Mootown Snackers'	1 piece	90	1	8.0
Jack, shredded, 'Fancy Supreme'	1/4 cup	110	1	9.0
sliced	1 slice	110	0	9.0
(Weight Watchers) 'Natural'	1 oz	80	1	5.0
COTTAGE CHEESE				
creamed, not packed	1 cup	217	6	9.5
dry, large or small curd, not packed	1 cup	123	3	0.6
nonfat, dry, large or small curd	4 oz	96	2	0.5
(Bison)				
chive, creamed	1/2 cup	120	4	5.0
creamed, low-fat, 1% milk fat	1/2 cup	90	4	2.0
creamed, 4% milk fat	1/2 cup	120	4	5.0
garden salad, creamed	1/2 cup	110	4	4.0
w/pineapple, creamed	1/2 cup	140	18	4.0
(Borden)				
creamed, 4% milk fat	1/2 cup	120	4	5.0
creamed, 4% milk fat, unsalted	1/2 cup	120	4	5.0
dry curd, unsalted	1/2 cup	80	3	1.0
(Breakstone's)				
creamed	4 oz	110	3	5.0
creamed, low-fat, 2% milk fat	4 oz	100	4	2.0
dry curd, nonfat, unsalted	4 oz	90	6	0.0
(Carnation)				
large curd, 4% milk fat	1/2 cup	115	4	5.0
low-fat, 1.5% milk fat, 'Slender'	1/2 cup	90	4	2.0
small curd, 4% milk fat	1/2 cup	115	4	5.0
w/pineapple, 4% milk fat,	1/2 cup	130	12	5.0
(Crowley)				
calcium-fortified, creamed, low-fat, 1% milk fat	1/2 cup	90	4	1.0
creamed, 4% milk fat	1/2 cup	120	4	5.0
creamed, low-fat, 1% milk fat	1/2 cup	90	4	1.0
no salt added, creamed, low-fat, 1% milk fat	1/2 cup	90	4	1.0
w/peaches, creamed, 4% milk fat	1/2 cup	140	17	3.0
w/pineapple, creamed, 4% milk fat	1/2 cup	140	15	4.0
w/pineapple, creamed, low-fat, 1% milk fat	1/2 cup	110	15	1.0
(Darigold)				
creamed, 4% milk fat	4 oz	120	4	4.2
dry curd, unsalted	4 oz	80	3	1.0
'Trim' creamed, low-fat, 2% milk fat	4 oz	100	4	3.2
(Friendship)				
'California Style' creamed, 4% milk fat	1/2 cup	120	4	5.0

Food Name	Serv. Size	Total Cal.	Carbs GMS	Fat GMS
creamed, low-fat, 1% milk fat	1/2 cup	90	4	1.0
lactose-reduced, creamed, low-fat, 1% milk fat	1/2 cup	90	4	1.0
no salt added, creamed, low-fat, 1% milk fat	1/2 cup	90	4	1.0
pot style, large curd, creamed, low-fat, 2% milk fat	1/2 cup	100	4	2.0
w/pineapple, creamed, 4% milk fat	1/2 cup	140	15	4.0
w/pineapple, creamed, low-fat, 1% milk fat	1/2 cup	110	15	1.0
(Knudsen)				
creamed, 4% milk fat	4 oz	120	4	5.0
low-fat, 2% milk fat	4 oz	100	4	2.0
nonfat	1/2 cup	80	4	0.0
nonfat	4 oz	70	3	0.0
small curd, creamed, 4% milk fat	4 oz	120	4	5.0
w/fruit cocktail low-fat, 2% milk fat	4 oz	130	16	2.0
w/mandarin orange, low-fat, 2% milk fat	4 oz	110	11	2.0
w/peach, low-fat, 2% milk fat	6 oz	170	19	2.0
w/pear, low-fat, 2% milk fat	4 oz	110	12	2.0
w/pineapple, creamed, 4% milk fat	4 oz	140	14	5.0
w/pineapple, low-fat, 2% milk fat	6 oz	170	18	2.0
w/spiced apple, low-fat, 2% milk fat	6 oz	180	20	2.0
w/strawberry, low-fat, 2% milk fat	6 oz	170	19	2.0
(Light n' Lively)				
garden salad, low-fat, 1% milk fat	4 oz	80	5	2.0
low-fat, 1% milk fat	4 oz	80	4	2.0
nonfat	4 oz	90	7	0.0
w/peach and pineapple, low-fat	4 oz	100	12	1.0
(Lite-Line) creamed, low-fat 1.5% milk fat	1/2 cup	90	4	2.0
(Lucerne)				
no added salt	1/2 cup	80	4	1.0
nonfat	1/2 cup	70	4	0.0
(Sealtest) low-fat, 2% milk fat	4 oz	100	4	2.0
(Weight Watchers)				
creamed, low-fat, 1% milk fat	1/2 cup	90	4	1.0
creamed, low-fat, 2% milk fat	1/2 cup	100	4	2.0
CREAM CHEESE				
	1 cup	810	6	80.9
	3-oz pkg	297	2	29.6
	1 oz	99	1	9.9
	1 tbsp	51	0	5.1
whipped	1 tbsp	35	0	3.5
(Alta Dena) pasteurized	1 oz	100	2	10.0
(Crowley)	1 oz	110	1	9.0
(Darigold)	1 oz	99	1	9.9
(Dorman's)				
'65%'	1 oz	90	1	8.4
'70%'	1 oz	102	1	9.9
(Friendship) soft	1 oz	103	1	10.0
(Healthy Choice) plain, nonfat	2 tbsp	25	2	0.0
(Healthy Favorites)	1 oz	60	2	5.0
(Philadelphia Brand)				
	1 oz	100	1	10.0
brick	1 oz	100	1	10.0
light, soft	2 tbsp	70	2	5.0
nonfat, 'Free'	1 oz	25	1	0.0
pasteurized process, 'Light'	1 oz	60	2	5.0
soft	2 tbsp	100	1	10.0
strawberry, soft	2 tbsp	110	5	9.0
whipped	2 tbsp	70	1	7.0

Food Name	Serv. Size	Total Cal.	Carbs GMS	Fat GMS
w/chives	1 oz	90	1	9.0
w/chives, brick	1 oz	90	1	9.0
w/chives, whipped	2 tbsp	70	1	6.0
w/chives and onion, soft	2 tbsp	110	2	10.0
w/herb and garlic, soft	1 oz	100	2	9.0
w/olive and pimiento, nonfat	1 oz	90	2	8.0
w/olive and pimiento, soft	1 oz	90	2	8.0
w/onion, whipped	1 oz	90	2	8.0
w/pimiento	1 oz	90	1	9.0
w/pineapple, soft	2 tbsp	100	4	9.0
w/salmon, soft	2 tbsp	100	1	9.0
w/smoked salmon, whipped	2 tbsp	70	1	6.0
(Stilwell) frozen, 'Bumpers'	1 piece	60	5	3.0
(Temp-Tee) whipped	1 oz	100	1	10.0
CREMA DANIA (Dorman's) 'Crema Dania 70%'	1 oz	134	0	12.3
DANBO				
(Dorman's)				
45%	1 oz	98	0	7.5
20%	1 oz	62	0	2.8
EDAM				
	1 oz	101	0	7.9
(Dorman's)				
	1 oz	100	1	8.0
45%	1 oz	91	0	7.0
(Hickory Farms) 'Domestic'	1 oz	100	1	8.4
(Kaukauna)	1 oz	100	1	8.0
(Kraft)	1 oz	90	0	7.0
(Land O'Lakes) natural	1 oz	100	1	8.0
(Laughing Cow)	1 oz	100	0	8.0
(May-Bud)	1 oz	100	0	8.0
(Sargento)	1 oz	100	0	8.0
FARMER				
(Friendship)				
	1/2 cup	160	4	12.0
'No Salt Added'	1/2 cup	160	4	12.0
(Hickory Farms)				
	1 oz	90	1	7.0
'Light Choice'	1 oz	90	1	7.0
(Kaukauna)	1 oz	100	1	8.0
(May-Bud)	1 oz	90	1	7.0
(Sargento)	1 oz	100	1	8.0
FETA				
	1 oz	75	1	6.0
(Churny) 'Natural'	1 oz	75	1	6.5
(Dorman's) 45%	1 oz	91	0	7.3
(Sargento)	1 oz	80	1	6.0
FONTINA				
	1 oz	110	0	8.8
(Sargento)	1 oz	110	0	9.0
GJETOST				
	1 oz	132	12	8.4
(Sargento)	1 oz	130	12	8.0
GOAT				
hard	1 oz	128	1	10.1
semisoft	1 oz	103	1	8.5
soft	1 oz	76	0	6.0
GOUDA				
	1 oz	101	1	7.8

Food Name	Serv. Size	Total Cal.	Carbs GMS	Fat GMS
(Dorman's)	1 oz	100	1	8.0
(Kaukauna)				
	1 oz	100	1	8.0
w/caraway seed	1 oz	100	1	8.0
w/hickory smoke flavor	1 oz	100	1	8.0
(Kraft)	1 oz	110	0	9.0
(Land O'Lakes) natural	1 oz	100	1	8.0
(Laughing Cow)				
	1 oz	110	0	9.0
mini	3/4 oz	80	0	6.4
(May-Bud)	1 oz	100	1	8.0
(Sargento)	1 oz	100	1	8.0
GRUYERE	1 oz	117	0	9.2
HAVARTI				
(Casino)	1 oz	120	0	11.0
(Dorman's)				
45%	1 oz	91	0	7.0
60%	1 oz	118	0	10.6
(Hickory Farms) 'Danish Special'	1 oz	117	0	10.5
(Sargento)	1 oz	120	0	11.0
HORSERADISH (Kaukauna) hearty, cold pack 'Cup'	1 oz	100	3	7.0
HOT PEPPER (Hickory Farms)	1 oz	106	1	8.9
ITALIAN STYLE				
(Sargento)				
grated	1 oz	110	1	8.0
6-cheese blend, 'Recipe Blend'	1/4 cup	90	0	7.0
JACK. See MONTEREY JACK.				
JARLSBERG				
(Hickory Farms)	1 oz	100	1	7.0
(Norseland)	1 oz	97	1	7.0
(Sargento) sliced	1 slice	120	1	9.0
LIMBURGER				
	1 cup	438	1	36.5
(Mohawk Valley) natural 'Little Gem'	1 oz	90	0	8.0
(Sargento)	1 oz	90	0	8.0
MASCARPONE (Galbani) 'Imported'	1 oz	128	1	13.1
MEXICAN STYLE				
(Healthy Choice) fancy shreds	1/4 cup	50	1	1.5
(Sargento) 4-cheese blend, 'Recipe Blend'	1/4 cup	110	1	9.0
(Velveeta) mild, pasteurized process, shredded	1/4 cup	120	3	9.0
MONTEREY JACK				
	1 oz	106	0	8.6
(Alpine Lace)				
'Monti-Jack-Lo'	1 oz	80	1	5.0
natural, milk cheese 'Monti-Jack-Lo'	1 oz	80	1	5.0
(Alta Dena)				
natural	1 oz	100	1	8.0
natural, w/jalapeño peppers	1 oz	100	1	8.0
(Axelrod)				
	1 oz	100	1	8.0
w/jalapeño pepper	1 oz	100	1	8.0
(Darigold)	1 oz	110	1	8.0
(Dorman's)				
	1 oz	100	1	8.0
less fat, 'Low Sodium'	1 oz	80	1	5.0
low-salt	1 oz	80	1	5.0
'Slim Jack'	1 oz	90	1	7.0

Food Name	Serv. Size	Total Cal.	Carbs GMS	Fat GMS
(Hickory Farms) 'Light Choice Low Sodium'	1 oz	110	0	8.0
(Kaukauna)	1 oz	110	1	9.0
(Kraft)				
	1 oz	110	0	9.0
natural, low-fat, made w/2% milk	1 oz	80	1	6.0
natural, w/jalapeño peppers	1 oz	110	1	9.0
w/caraway	1 oz	100	1	8.0
w/peppers, less fat, 'Light Naturals'	1 oz	80	1	5.0
(Land O'Lakes)				
natural	1 oz	110	1	9.0
natural, hot pepper	1 oz	110	1	9.0
processed, 'Jalapeño Jack'	1 oz	90	1	8.0
(May-Bud)	1 oz	110	0	9.0
(Sargento)				
	1 oz	110	0	9.0
shredded	1/4 cup	100	0	9.0
sliced	1 slice	100	0	9.0
(Weight Watchers) 'Natural'	1 oz	80	1	5.0
MOZZARELLA				
part skim	1 oz	72	1	4.5
part skim, low-moisture	1 oz	79	1	4.9
part skim, low-moisture, diced	1 cup	370	4	22.6
part skim, low moisture, shredded	1 cup	316	4	19.3
whole milk	1 oz	80	1	6.1
whole milk, low moisture	1 oz	90	1	7.0
whole milk, low-moisture, shredded	1 cup	315	2	24.2
(Alpine Lace)				
natural, shredded	1 oz	70	1	5.0
natural, sliced	1 oz	70	1	5.0
part skim, low-moisture	1 oz	70	1	5.0
(Crowley)				
part skim	1 oz	70	1	4.0
whole milk	1 oz	90	1	7.0
(Dorman's)				
	1 oz	90	1	6.0
less fat, 'Low Sodium'	1 oz	80	1	4.0
low-salt	1 oz	80	1	4.0
part skim, low-moisture, 'Low Sodium'	1 oz	80	1	5.0
(Frigo)				
part skim, low-moisture	1 oz	80	1	5.0
part skim, low-moisture, less fat	1 oz	60	1	3.0
whole milk, low-moisture	1 oz	90	1	7.0
(Healthy Choice)				
ball	1 oz	45	1	0.0
fat-free, shredded	1 oz	40	1	0.0
low-fat, fancy, shredded	1/4 cup	50	1	1.5
natural, fat-free, chunk	1 oz	40	1	0.0
string	1 oz	50	1	1.5
(Hickory Farms)				
	1 oz	72	1	4.5
low-salt, 'Light Choice Low Sodium'	1 oz	80	1	5.0
(Kraft)				
	1 oz	90	1	7.0
less fat, 'Light Naturals'	1 oz	80	1	4.0
natural, low-fat, made w/2% milk	1/3 cup	80	1	5.0
part skim, low-moisture	1 oz	80	1	5.0
part skim, w/jalapeño pepper	1 oz	80	1	5.0

Food Name	Serv. Size	Total Cal.	Carbs GMS	Fat GMS
(Land O'Lakes) natural, low moisture, part skim	1 oz	80	1	5.0
(Polly-O)				
fresh 'Fior di Latte'	1 oz	80	1	6.0
grated	1 oz	130	1	10.0
'Lite'	1 oz	70	1	4.0
part skim	1 oz	80	1	5.0
whole milk	1 oz	90	1	6.0
(Sargento)				
light, sliced, 'Preferred Light'	1 slice	90	0	5.0
part skim, low-moisture	1 oz	80	1	5.0
shredded, 'Classic Supreme'	1/4 cup	80	1	6.0
shredded, 'Preferred Light'	1/4 cup	70	1	3.0
sliced	1 slice	130	2	9.0
whole milk	1 oz	90	1	7.0
(Weight Watchers)				
'Natural'	1 oz	70	1	4.0
shredded, 'Natural'	1 oz	80	1	4.0
MUENSTER				
	1 oz	104	0	8.5
(Alpine Lace)				
	1 oz	100	1	8.0
low-salt, natural, sliced 'Low Sodium'	1 oz	100	1	9.0
(Dorman's)				
	1 oz	110	0	9.0
50%	1 oz	100	0	8.2
less fat, 'Low Sodium'	1 oz	80	0	5.0
low-salt	1 oz	80	0	5.0
low-salt, 'Low Sodium'	1 oz	110	0	9.0
(Hickory Farms)				
	1 oz	100	0	8.5
low-salt, 'Light Choice Low Sodium'	1 oz	110	0	9.0
(Kaukauna)	1 oz	110	1	9.0
(Land O'Lakes) natural	1 oz	100	1	9.0
(Sargento) sliced	1 slice	100	1	9.0
NACHO *(Sargento)* shredded, 'Fancy Supreme'	1/4 cup	110	1	9.0
NEUFCHATEL CHEESE				
	3-oz pkg	221	2	19.9
	1 oz	74	1	6.6
(Hickory Farms)				
chocolate	1 oz	110	8	8.0
date nut, rum	1 oz	100	4	8.0
orange	1 oz	100	4	8.0
peach	1 oz	90	3	8.0
pineapple	1 oz	90	2	8.0
strawberry	1 oz	90	3	8.0
(Kaukauna)				
garlic and herbs	1 oz	80	1	7.0
vegetable, garden	1 oz	80	1	7.0
(Philadelphia Brand)				
	1 oz	70	1	6.0
'Light'	1 oz	80	1	7.0
NEW HOLLAND				
(Hickory Farms) w/herbs, 'Light Choice'	1 oz	90	1	8.0
PARMESAN				
grated	1 cup	456	4	30.0
grated	1 oz	129	1	8.5
grated	1 tbsp	23	0	1.5

Food Name	Serv. Size	Total Cal.	Carbs GMS	Fat GMS
hard	1 oz	111	1	7.3
shredded	1 tbsp	21	0	1.4
(Churny) 'Natural'	1 oz	110	1	7.0
(Frigo)				
fresh, grated	1 oz	110	1	7.0
grated	1 oz	130	1	9.0
wheel	1 oz	110	1	7.0
w/Romano cheese, grated	1 oz	130	1	9.0
(Hickory Farms)	1 oz	110	1	7.0
(Kraft)				
	1 oz	100	1	7.0
grated	1 oz	130	1	9.0
(Polly-O) grated	1 oz	130	1	9.0
(Progresso) grated	1 tbsp	23	1	2.0
(Sargento)				
fresh	1 oz	110	1	7.0
grated	1 oz	130	2	9.0
shredded, 'Fancy Supreme'	1/4 cup	110	1	7.0
w/Romano, grated	1 oz	110	1	7.0
w/Romano, shredded, 'Fancy Supreme'	1/4 cup	110	1	7.0
PARMESANO REGGIANO *(Galbani)* 'Imported'	1 oz	105	1	7.1
PIZZA				
(Frigo)				
low-fat, shredded	1 oz	65	1	3.0
shredded	1 oz	90	1	7.0
(Healthy Choice) low-fat, fancy, shredded	1/4 cup	50	1	1.5
(Precious) mozzarella cheddar, natural, shredded	1 oz	95	1	7.0
(Sargento)				
double cheese, shredded, 'Fancy Supreme'	1/4 cup	90	1	6.0
shredded, 'Classic Supreme'	1/4 cup	90	0	6.0
PORT DU SALUT	1 oz	100	0	8.0
PORT WINE *(Hickory Farms)* natural	1 oz	97	2	6.9
POT *(Sargento)*	1 oz	25	1	0.2
PROVOLONE				
	1 oz	100	1	7.5
(Alpine Lace) 'Provo-Lo'	1 oz	70	1	5.0
(Dorman's)				
	1 oz	90	1	7.0
low-salt	1 oz	80	1	4.0
(Frigo)				
	1 oz	100	1	7.0
smoked	1 oz	100	1	7.0
(Hickory Farms) low-salt, 'Light Choice Low Sodium'	1 oz	90	1	7.0
(Kraft)	1 oz	100	1	7.0
(Land O'Lakes) natural	1 oz	100	1	8.0
(Sargento) sliced	1 slice	100	0	8.0
PUB *(Hickory Farms)*	1 oz	94	2	6.9
QUESO ANEJO				
Mexican	1 oz	106	1	8.5
Mexican, crumbled	1 cup	492	6	39.6
QUESO ASEDERO				
Mexican	1 oz	101	1	8.0
Mexican, diced	1 cup	470	4	37.3
Mexican, shredded	1 cup	402	3	31.9
QUESO BLANCO *(Sargento)*	1 oz	100	0	9.0
QUESO CHIHUAHUA				
Mexican	1 oz	106	2	8.4

Food Name	Serv. Size	Total Cal.	Carbs GMS	Fat GMS
Mexican, diced	1 cup	494	7	39.2
Mexican, shredded	1 cup	423	6	33.5
QUESO DE PAPA *(Sargento)*	1 oz	110	0	9.0
QUESO DE TACO *(Hickory Farms)*	1 oz	106	1	8.9
RICOTTA				
part skim	1 cup	340	13	19.5
part skim	1 oz	39	1	2.2
whole milk	1 cup	428	7	31.9
(Breakstone's) whole milk	4 oz	200	6	15.0
(Crowley)				
part skim	2 oz	80	3	4.0
whole milk	2 oz	100	3	7.0
(Frigo)				
low-fat	1/4 cup	64	3	1.9
nonfat	1/4 cup	48	2	0.4
nonfat, 'Truly Lite'	1 oz	20	2	0.0
part skim	1 oz	45	1	3.0
whole milk	1 oz	50	1	4.0
(Gardenia) low-fat	1/4 cup	65	2	2.8
(Polly-O)				
light, 'Lite'	2 oz	80	3	4.0
part skim	2 oz	90	2	6.0
whole milk	2 oz	100	2	7.0
(Precious) low-fat, natural	1 oz	40	2	2.0
(Sargento)				
	1 oz	40	1	3.0
light	1/4 cup	60	3	2.5
old fashioned	1/4 cup	90	3	6.0
part skim	1/4 cup	80	2	5.0
ROMANO				
	1 oz	110	1	7.6
(Frigo)				
grated	1 oz	130	1	9.0
wedge	1 oz	110	1	8.0
(Kraft) grated	1 oz	130	1	9.0
(Hickory Farms) loaf	1 oz	110	1	8.0
(Kraft) 'Natural'	1 oz	100	1	7.0
(Polly-O) grated	1 oz	130	1	10.0
(Progresso) grated	1 tbsp	23	1	2.0
(Sargento)	1 oz	110	1	8.0
ROQUEFORT	1 oz	105	1	8.7
SMOKED				
(Hickory Farms) 'Light Choice Smoky Lyte'	1 oz	80	1	6.0
(Hoffman's) sharp, processed	1 oz	110	1	9.0
(Sargento) 'Smokestick'	1 oz	100	1	7.0
SOY. See under CHEESE SUBSTITUTE.				
STRING				
(Frigo)	1 oz	80	1	5.0
(Kraft) low moisture	1 oz	80	1	5.0
(Polly-O)	1 oz slice	90	2	6.0
(Sargento)				
	1 oz	80	1	5.0
light, 'Mootown Snackers'	1 piece	60	1	3.0
smoked	1 oz	80	1	5.0
SWISS				
	1 oz	107	1	7.8
diced	1 cup	496	4	36.2

Food Name	Serv. Size	Total Cal.	Carbs GMS	Fat GMS
pasteurized process, w/disodium phosphate added	1 oz	95	1	7.1
shredded	1 cup	406	4	29.6
(Alpine Lace)				
light, 'Swiss-Lo'	1 oz	100	1	7.0
natural, milk, sliced, 'Swiss-Lo'	1 oz	90	1	6.0
(Boar's Head)				
'Domestic'	1 oz	110	1	8.0
no salt added	1 oz	100	1	8.0
(Borden)				
processed	1 oz	100	1	8.0
processed, fat-free, low cholesterol	1 oz	40	4	0.0
(Casino)	1 oz	110	1	8.0
(Dorman's)				
	1 oz	100	0	8.0
less fat	1 oz	90	0	5.0
low-fat, low-sodium	1 oz	90	0	5.0
no salt added	1 oz	100	0	8.0
no salt added, 'Deli Light'	1 oz	100	0	8.0
smoked	1 oz	100	1	7.0
(Healthy Favorites) less fat, natural, sliced	1 oz	80	1	4.0
(Hickory Farms)				
creamy, 'Cold Pack'	1 oz	92	3	7.2
'Domestic'	1 oz	110	1	7.8
light, 'Light Choice Lorraine'	1 oz	100	0	7.8
low-salt, 'Light Choice Low Sodium'	1 oz	100	0	8.0
(Hoffman's) w/cheddar, smoky	1 oz	110	1	8.0
(Kraft)				
	1 oz	110	1	8.0
aged	1 oz	110	1	8.0
light, 'Light Naturals'	1 oz	90	1	5.0
low-salt, '75% Very Low Sodium'	1 oz	110	1	8.0
natural, baby, 'Cracker Barrel'	1 oz	110	0	9.0
natural, less fat, 'Light Naturals'	1 oz	90	1	5.0
processed, 'Deluxe'	1 oz	90	1	7.0
processed, 'Light'	1 oz	70	2	3.0
(Land O'Lakes) natural	1 oz	110	1	8.0
(Sargento)				
'Finland'	1 oz	110	1	8.0
light, thin sliced, 'Preferred Light'	1 slice	80	1	4.0
mild, wafer thin sliced	1 slice	110	0	9.0
shredded, 'Fancy Supreme'	1/4 cup	110	0	8.0
sliced	1 slice	80	0	6.0
(Weight Watchers)				
'Natural'	1 oz	90	1	5.0
nonfat	1 slice	30	2	0.0
TACO				
(Frigo) shredded	1 oz	110	1	9.0
(Kraft) shredded	1 oz	110	1	9.0
(Sargento)				
	1 oz	110	1	9.0
shredded, 'Classic Supreme'	1/4 cup	110	1	9.0
shredded, 'Preferred Light'	1/4 cup	70	1	4.5
TALEGGIO *(Tal-Fino)* natural, 'Brand Imported'	1 oz	89	0	7.4
TILSIT				
	1 oz	96	1	7.4
(Sargento)	1 oz	100	1	7.0
TYBO				
(Dorman's) 45%	1 oz	98	0	7.5

Food Name	Serv. Size	Total Cal.	Carbs GMS	Fat GMS
(Sargento) red wax	1 oz	100	0	7.0
VERMONT *(Churny)*	1 oz	110	1	9.0
CHEESE-BALL				
cheddar, sharp, w/almonds *(Kaukauna)*	1 oz	100	3	7.0
cheddar, w/almonds and bacon *(Kaukauna)*	1 oz	100	3	7.0
green onion flavor, w/almonds *(Kaukauna)*	1 oz	100	3	7.0
Port wine, w/almonds *(Kaukauna)*	1 oz	100	3	7.0
CHEESE DISH/ENTRÉE				
(Snow's) Welsh rarebit, canned	1/2 cup	170	10	11.0
(Stouffer's)				
Swiss cheese strata, frozen, food service product	4 oz	176	10	11.2
Welsh rarebit	1/4 cup	120	5	9.0
CHEESE FLAVORED SEASONING				
(Molly McButter)	1/2 tsp	4	1	0.1
CHEESE FLAVORED SNACK				
(Barbara's Bakery)				
cheese flavored puffs, tangy triple cheese, 'Pinta Puffs'	1 oz	70	10	2.0
cheese puff bakes *(Barbara's Bakery)*	1 1/2 cup	160	13	11.0
(Bearitos)				
cheddar flavored puffs, light	1 oz	120	20	4.0
cheddar flavored puffs, original	1 oz	160	14	10.0
(Cheetos)				
cheddar valley	1 oz	160	16	9.0
cheese flavored puffs	1 oz	160	15	10.0
cheese flavored puffs, balls	1 oz	150	15	10.0
cheese flavored puffs, crunchy	1 oz	160	15	10.0
cheese flavored puffs, curls	1 oz	150	15	10.0
cheese flavored puffs, flamin' hot	1 oz	160	15	10.0
cheese flavored puffs, jumbo	1 oz	160	13	10.0
light, approx 38 pieces	1 oz	140	19	6.0
paws, approx 16 pieces	1 oz	160	15	10.0
(Eagle)				
cheese crunch, 'Cheegles'	1 cup	160	15	10.0
cheese flavored balls, 'Cheegles'	2 1/2 cups	160	15	10.0
cheese flavored balls, less fat, 'Cheegles'	2 1/2 cups	150	18	6.0
'Shamu Shapes'	1 cup	160	15	10.0
(Flavor Tree)				
cheese flavored sticks, cheddar	1/4 cup	129	12	8.1
(Health Valley)				
cheese flavored puffs, baked, w/organic corn, 'Cheddar Lite'	0.25 oz	40	4	2.0
cheese flavored puffs, nonfat	1 cup	73	15	0.0
cheese flavored puffs, w/chili, nonfat	1 oz	100	21	0.0
(Keebler)				
zesty cheddar, 'RC Ricers'	1 oz	140	17	8.0
(Planters)				
cheese flavored balls, 'Cheez Balls'	1 oz	160	14	11.0
cheese flavored balls, nacho, 'Cheez Balls'	1 oz	160	15	10.0
cheese flavored curls, 'Cheez Curls'	1 oz	160	14	11.0
cheese flavored curls, nacho, 'Cheez Curls'	1 oz	160	15	10.0
(Ralston)				
cheddar snacks, 'Stop & Shop'	18 crackers	150	20	7.0
(Weight Watchers)				
cheese curls	1 serving	70	10	2.5
(Wise)				
cheese flavored puffs, baked, 'Cheez Doodles'	1 oz	150	16	9.0
cheese flavored spirals, nacho cheese	1 oz	160	16	10.0
'Cheez Waffies'	1 oz	140	14	8.0

Food Name	Serv. Size	Total Cal.	Carbs GMS	Fat GMS
cheese flavored twists, nacho cheese, crispy	1 oz	160	16	10.0
fried, crunchy, 'Cheez Doodles'	1 oz	160	16	10.0
CHEESE FOOD. See also CHEESE PRODUCT.				
(Kraft)				
nonfat, processed, singles, 'Free'	1 oz	45	4	0.0
pasteurized process, shredded, 'Velveeta'	1/4 cup	130	3	9.0
shredded, 'Velveeta'	1 oz	100	3	7.0
(Land O'Lakes)				
processed	1 oz	90	2	6.0
processed, slices	3/4 oz	70	2	5.0
(Nippy)	1 oz	90	2	7.0
AMERICAN				
(Borden)				
processed, sharp, 'Singles'	1 oz	90	2	7.0
processed, 'Singles'	1 oz	90	3	7.0
processed, 'Slices'	1 oz	100	2	7.0
(Darigold) processed	1 oz	80	2	6.0
(Hoffman's) processed, colored	1 oz	100	3	7.0
(Kraft)				
processed, grated	1 oz	130	8	7.0
processed, 'Light'	1 oz	70	2	4.0
processed, 'Singles'	1 oz	90	2	7.0
processed, white, 'Singles'	1 oz	90	2	7.0
(Land O'Lakes) processed, w/Swiss cheese	1 oz	100	1	8.0
BACON				
(Hoffman's) 'Chees'N Bacon'	1 oz	90	3	6.0
(Kraft)				
'Chees'N Bacon'	1 oz	90	2	7.0
'Cracker Barrel'	1 oz	90	3	7.0
CARAWAY *(Hoffman's)* 'Swisson Rye'	1 oz	90	2	7.0
CHEDDAR				
(Alpine Lace) nonfat	1 oz	45	2	0.0
(Kaukauna)				
extra sharp, cold pack, 'Cup'	1 oz	100	3	7.0
nacho, processed, cold pack 'Cup'	1 oz	100	3	7.0
sharp, 'Lite'	1 oz	70	5	4.0
sharp, cold pack, 'Cup'	1 oz	100	3	7.0
sharp, cup, 'Lite 50'	1 oz	70	5	3.0
smoky, 'Lite'	1 oz	70	5	4.0
w/bacon and horseradish, cold pack, 'Cup'	1 oz	100	3	7.0
(Kraft)				
extra sharp, processed, 'Cracker Barrel'	1 oz	90	3	7.0
sharp, processed, 'Cracker Barrel'	1 oz	100	4	7.0
sharp, 'Singles'	1 oz	100	1	8.0
(Land O'Lakes)				
extra sharp, processed	1 oz	100	1	9.0
'La Chedda'	1 oz	90	2	7.0
processed, w/bacon	1 oz	110	1	9.0
(Wispride) sharp, cold pack	1 oz	100	2	7.0
GARLIC *(Kraft)* pasteurized process	1 oz	90	2	7.0
ITALIAN HERB *(Land O'Lakes)* processed	1 oz	90	2	7.0
JALAPEÑO				
(Hoffman's)	1 oz	90	2	7.0
(Kraft)				
pasteurized process	1 oz	90	2	7.0
'Singles'	1 oz	90	2	7.0
(Land O'Lakes)				
. . . .	1 oz	90	2	7.0

Food Name	Serv. Size	Total Cal.	Carbs GMS	Fat GMS
processed	1 oz	90	2	7.0
MEXICAN				
(Kraft)				
hot, pasteurized process, shredded, 'Velveeta'	1/4 cup	130	3	9.0
hot, shredded, 'Velveeta'	1 oz	100	3	7.0
mild, shredded, 'Velveeta'	1 oz	100	3	7.0
ONION				
(Hoffman's) 'Chees'N Onion'	1 oz	100	3	7.0
(Land O'Lakes) processed	1 oz	90	2	7.0
PEPPERONI *(Land O'Lakes)* processed	1 oz	90	1	7.0
PIMIENTO				
(Kraft)				
'Singles'	1 oz	90	2	7.0
processed, 'Deluxe'	1 oz	100	1	8.0
PORT WINE				
(Kaukauna)				
cold pack, 'Cup'	1 oz	100	3	7.0
cup, 'Lite 50'	1 oz	70	5	3.0
(Wispride) cold pack	1 oz	100	3	7.0
SALAMI				
(Hoffman's) 'Chees'N Salami'	1 oz	90	3	6.0
(Land O'Lakes) processed	1 oz	90	2	7.0
SMOKY *(Kaukauna)* cold pack 'Cup'	1 oz	100	3	7.0
SWISS				
(Borden) processed, slices 'Singles'	1 oz	100	2	7.0
(Kaukauna)				
almond, cup, 'Lite 50'	1 oz	70	5	3.0
country, cold pack 'Cup'	1 oz	100	3	7.0
country, 'Lite'	1 oz	70	5	4.0
(Kraft)				
fat-free, singles, 'Free'	1 oz	45	4	0.0
singles	1 oz	90	2	7.0
(Velveeta)	1 oz	100	3	7.0
CHEESE-LOG				
CHEDDAR				
(Kraft)				
sharp, w/almonds, 'Cracker Barrel'	1 oz	90	4	6.0
smoky, w/almonds, 'Cracker Barrel'	1 oz	90	4	6.0
(Kaukauna)				
white, sharp, w/green onion	1 oz	100	3	7.0
white, sharp hickory smoke	1 oz	100	3	7.0
(Sargento)				
Port wine	1 oz	100	3	7.0
sharp	1 oz	100	3	7.0
SWISS				
(Kaukauna) w/almonds	1 oz	100	3	7.0
(Sargento) w/almonds	1 oz	90	2	7.0
CHEESE NUGGET, mozzarella, breaded, frozen, 'Cheese Hot Bites' *(Banquet)*	2.63 oz	240	16	13.0
CHEESE NUT				
(Kraft)				
cheddar, sharp, 'Cracker Barrel'	1 oz	100	4	7.0
Port wine, 'Cracker Barrel'	1 oz	90	4	6.0
(Kaukauna) sharp, w/bell and jalapeño peppers	1 oz	100	3	7.0
CHEESE PRODUCT				
(Borden) 'Singles' processed, slices, fat-free	1 oz	40	4	0.0
(Kraft)				
'Cheez Whiz' light, pasteurized process	2 tbsp	75	6	3.3

Food Name	Serv. Size	Total Cal.	Carbs GMS	Fat GMS
'Cheez Whiz' pasteurized process	2 tbsp	91	3	6.9
'Velveeta' less fat, pasteurized process	1 oz	62	3	3.0
(Lite-Line) slices, processed, fat-free	1 slice	25	3	0.0
(Lunch Wagon) sandwich slices, processed	1 oz	90	2	7.0
AMERICAN FLAVOR				
(Alpine Lace) processed	1 oz	90	2	7.0
(Borden) processed, 'Light'	1 oz	70	1	5.0
(Harvest Moon) processed	1 oz	70	2	4.0
(Kraft)				
pasteurized process	1 slice	31	2	0.2
processed, 'Light Singles'	1 oz	70	2	4.0
white, processed, 'Light Singles'	1 oz	70	2	4.0
(Light n' Lively) white, processed, 'Singles'	1 oz	70	2	4.0
(Lite-Line)				
processed	1 oz	50	1	2.0
processed, reduced sodium	1 oz	70	2	4.0
processed, 'Sodium Lite'	1 oz	70	2	4.0
CHEDDAR FLAVOR				
(Kraft)				
sharp, processed, 'Free'	1 oz	45	4	0.0
sharp, processed, 'Light'	1 oz	70	2	4.0
sharp, processed, 'Singles'	1 oz	100	1	8.0
(Light n' Lively) sharp, processed, 'Singles'	1 oz	70	2	4.0
(Lite-Line)				
mild, processed	1 oz	50	1	2.0
sharp, processed	1 oz	50	1	2.0
sharp, processed, slices	1 slice	35	1	2.0
(Spreadery)				
medium, processed	1 oz	70	3	4.0
sharp, processed	1 oz	70	3	4.0
Vermont white, processed	1 oz	70	3	4.0
CREAM CHEESE FLAVOR				
(Philadelphia Brand) processed, 'Light'	1 oz	60	2	5.0
MEXICAN FLAVOR				
(Spreadery) mild, w/jalapeños, processed	1 oz	70	3	4.0
MOZZARELLA FLAVOR				
(Alpine Lace) nonfat	1 oz	45	2	0.0
(Lite-Line) processed	1 oz	50	1	2.0
MUENSTER FLAVOR (Lite-Line) processed	1 oz	50	1	2.0
NACHO FLAVOR (Spreadery) processed	1 oz	70	3	4.0
NEUFCHATEL				
(Spreadery)				
French onion, processed	1 oz	70	2	6.0
garden vegetable, processed	1 oz	70	2	6.0
garlic and herb, processed	1 oz	70	1	6.0
ranch, classic, processed	1 oz	70	1	7.0
strawberry, processed	1 oz	70	1	5.0
PORT WINE FLAVOR (Spreadery) processed	1 oz	70	3	4.0
SWISS FLAVOR				
(Kraft) processed, slices, 'Free Singles'	1 oz	45	4	0.0
(Light n' Lively) processed, 'Singles'	1 oz	70	2	3.0
(Lite-Line) processed	1 oz	50	1	2.0
CHEESE SPREAD				
(Kraft)				
'Velveeta'	1 oz	80	3	6.0
'Velveeta' pasteurized process	1 oz	85	3	6.2
'Velveeta' slices	1 oz	90	3	6.0

Food Name	Serv. Size	Total Cal.	Carbs GMS	Fat GMS
(Land O'Lakes) processed, 'Golden Velvet'	1 oz	80	2	6.0
(Laughing Cow) 'Cheezbits'	1/6 oz	13	0	1.0
(Micro Melt)	1 oz	80	2	6.0
AMERICAN				
(Easy Cheese) pasteurized process	2 tbsp	100	2	7.0
(Kraft) processed	1 oz	80	2	6.0
(Nabisco) 'Easy Cheese American'	1 oz	80	2	6.0
(Sargento)				
sharp, processed, 'Cracker Snacks'	1 oz	110	1	9.0
w/pimento, processed, 'Cracker Snacks'	1 oz	110	1	9.0
BACON				
(Kraft)	1 oz	80	1	7.0
(Squeez-A-Snak)	1 oz	80	1	7.0
BLUE *(Roka)*	1 oz	70	2	6.0
BRICK 'Cracker Snacks' *(Sargento)*	1 oz	100	1	9.0
CHEDDAR				
(Kraft)				
extra sharp, 'Cracker Barrel'	2 tbsp	80	1	8.0
sharp, and cream cheese, 'Cracker Barrel'	2 tbsp	80	1	8.0
(Nabisco)				
'Easy Cheese Cheddar'	1 oz	80	2	6.0
'Easy Cheese Cheddar 'n Bacon'	1 oz	80	2	6.0
'Easy Cheese Sharp Cheddar'	1 oz	80	2	6.0
(Old English) sharp	1 oz	80	1	7.0
(Squeez-A-Snak) sharp	1 oz	80	1	7.0
(Weight Watchers) sharp, 'Cup'	1 oz	70	7	3.0
GARLIC *(Squeez-A-Snak)*	1 oz	80	1	7.0
HICKORY SMOKE *(Squeez-A-Snak)*	1 oz	80	1	7.0
JALAPEÑO				
(Kraft)				
	1 oz	70	3	5.0
loaf	1 oz	80	2	6.0
(Squeez-A-Snak)	1 oz	80	1	6.0
LIMBURGER *(Mohawk Valley)*	1 oz	70	0	6.0
MEXICAN *(Velveeta)* mild	1 oz	80	3	6.0
NACHO *(Nabisco)* 'Easy Cheese Nacho'	1 oz	80	2	6.0
OLIVE *(Kraft)* olives and pimiento	1 oz	60	2	5.0
PIMIENTO				
(Kraft)	1 oz	70	3	5.0
'Velveeta' *(Kraft)*	1 oz	80	3	6.0
PINEAPPLE *(Kraft)*	1 oz	70	4	5.0
PORT WINE 'Cup' *(Weight Watchers)*	1 oz	70	7	3.0
GARLIC				
(Alouette) and spices	1 oz	95	2	9.0
(Rondel) w/herbs, soft, 'Lite'	1 oz	70	2	6.0
HERB				
(Alouette) and garlic, soft, 'Light'	1 oz	60	2	4.5
(Rondel) soft, 'Fines Herbes'	1 oz	90	2	8.0
HORSERADISH *(Alouette)* and chive	1 oz	85	1	8.0
LIMBURGER *(Mohawk Valley)*	1 oz	70	0	6.0
MEXICAN				
(Kraft)				
hot, 'Velveeta'	1 oz	80	3	6.0
mild, 'Velveeta'	1 oz	80	3	6.0
ONION *(Alouette)* French	1 oz	95	2	9.0
PIMENTO				
(Kraft)				
	1 oz	70	3	5.0

Food Name	Serv. Size	Total Cal.	Carbs GMS	Fat GMS
'Velveeta'	1 oz	80	3	6.0
PINEAPPLE (Kraft)	1 oz	70	4	5.0
PORT WINE (Weight Watchers) 'Cup'	1 oz	70	7	3.0
SALMON (Alouette)	1 oz	70	2	6.0
SPINACH (Alouette) creamy	1 oz	90	2	8.0
SWISS (Sargento) 'Cracker Snacks'	1 oz	100	1	7.0
VEGETABLE				
(Alouette) spring, soft, 'Light'	1 oz	60	1	4.5
(Rondel) garden, soft	1 oz	90	3	8.0
CHEESE STICK				
CHEDDAR				
(Farm Rich) breaded, frozen	3 oz	300	19	21.0
(Flavor Tree) snack	1/4 cup	129	12	8.1
(Stilwell) battered, frozen	1 piece	80	8	4.0
PEPPER				
(Farm Rich) hot, breaded, frozen	3 oz	260	20	17.0
(Stilwell) jalapeño, breaded, frozen	1 piece	70	8	3.0
MOZZARELLA				
(Farm Rich) breaded, frozen	3 oz	240	19	13.0
(Frigo) string, natural, 'Truly Lite'	0.83 oz	50	1	2.0
(Stilwell)				
baby, battered, frozen	3 pieces	80	8	4.0
battered, frozen	1 piece	80	7	5.0
premium, battered, frozen	1 piece	100	9	5.0
PROVOLONE				
(Farm Rich) provolone, breaded, frozen	3 oz	270	22	16.0
CHEESE SUBSTITUTE. See also CHEESE FOOD; CHEESE PRODUCT.				
(Cheeztwin)	1 oz	90	3	6.0
(Fisher) 'Sandwich-Mate'	1 oz	90	3	6.0
(Lite-Line) low-cholesterol	1 oz	90	2	7.0
(Nucoa) 'Heart Beat'	1 1/2 slices	50	2	2.0
AMERICAN STYLE				
(Delicia)				
	1 oz	80	1	6.0
hickory smoked	1 oz	80	0	6.0
w/caraway	1 oz	80	1	6.0
w/hot pepper	1 oz	80	1	6.0
w/salami	1 oz	80	1	6.0
(Formagg) lactose-free, singles	3/4 oz	70	1	5.0
(Golden Image)	1 oz	90	2	6.0
CHEDDAR STYLE				
(Fisher) shredded, 'Ched-O-Mate'	1 oz	90	1	7.0
(Formagg) fancy, shredded	1 oz	70	1	5.0
(Frigo)	1 oz	90	1	7.0
(Golden Image) mild	1 oz	110	0	9.0
(Nu Tofu)				
	1 oz	70	1	4.0
low salt	1 oz	70	1	4.0
nonfat	1 oz	40	2	0.0
(Rella Good)				
California style, 'AlmondRella'	1 oz	50	1	1.4
California style, 'Zero-Fat Rella'	1 oz	45	3	0.0
mild, 'TofuRella'	1 oz	80	1	5.0
mild, slices, 'TofuRella'	0.75-oz slice	60	1	4.0
(Sargento)				
	1 oz	90	1	6.0
shredded, 'Fancy Supreme'	1/4 cup	90	2	7.0

Food Name	Serv. Size	Total Cal.	Carbs GMS	Fat GMS
(Savoldi)	1 oz	90	1	6.0
(Soya Kaas)	1 oz	79	2	5.4
COLBY STYLE				
(Golden Image)	1 oz	110	1	9.0
(Delicia) Longhorn style	1 oz	80	1	6.0
(Dorman's) 'LoChol'	1 oz	90	1	6.0
CREAM CHEESE STYLE				
(Soya Kaas)	1 oz	90	0	9.4
(Tofutti) 'Better Than Cheese'	1 tbsp	40	1	4.0
(Weight Watchers)	1 oz	35	1	2.0
GARLIC HERB				
(Rella Good)				
'AlmondRella'	1 oz	60	3	3.0
'TofuRella'	1 oz	80	2	5.0
ITALIAN STYLE				
(Rella Good) 'VeganRella'	1 oz	60	7	3.0
(Weight Watchers) Italian topping, grated, nonfat	1 tbsp	20	2	0.0
JACK				
(Nu Tofu)				
. . . .	1 oz	70	2	4.0
nonfat	1 oz	40	2	0.0
(Rella Good) 'TofuRella'	1 oz	80	2	5.0
JALAPEÑO				
(Rella Good)				
jack, 'Zero-FatRella'	1 oz	45	3	0.0
'TofuRella'	1 oz	80	2	5.0
'Zero-FatRella'	1 oz	40	3	0.0
(Soya Kaas) 'Jalapeño Mexi Kaas'	1 oz	77	0	5.3
MEXICAN (Rella Good) 'VeganRella'	1 oz	60	7	3.0
MOZZARELLA STYLE				
(Fisher) shredded, 'Pizza-Mate'	1 oz	90	1	7.0
(Frigo)	1 oz	90	1	7.0
(Nu Tofu)				
. . . .	1 oz	70	2	4.0
low sodium	1 oz	70	2	4.0
nonfat	1 oz	40	2	0.0
(Rella Good)				
'AlmondRella'	1 oz	60	3	3.0
slices	0.75-oz slice	60	1	4.0
'TofuRella'	1 oz	80	2	5.0
'Zero-Fat Rella'	1 oz	40	3	0.0
(Sargento)				
. . . .	1 oz	80	1	6.0
'Classic Supreme'	1/4 cup	80	1	6.0
(Savoldi)	1 oz	80	1	6.0
(Soya Kaas)	1 oz	78	2	5.6
MUENSTER STYLE 'LoChol' (Dorman's)	1 oz	100	1	7.0
PARMESAN STYLE (Soyco) grated	1 tbsp	23	1	0.8
SWISS STYLE				
(Dorman's) 'LoChol'	1 oz	100	1	7.0
(Formagg) lactose-free, singles	3/4 oz	70	1	5.0
CHEESE TOPPING (Tone's) cheddar, w/bacon	1 tsp	10	1	1.0
CHERIMOYA. See CUSTARD APPLE.				
CHERRY				
SOUR				
Canned				
red, in extra heavy syrup, w/liquid	1 cup	298	76	0.2

Food Name	Serv. Size	Total Cal.	Carbs GMS	Fat GMS
red, in heavy syrup, w/liquid	1 cup	233	60	0.3
red, in light syrup, w/liquid	1 cup	189	49	0.3
red, in water, w/liquid	1 cup	88	22	0.2
Fresh				
red, raw	1 cup	52	13	0.3
red, raw, pitted	1 cup	78	19	0.5
Frozen				
red, unsweetened	18-oz pkg	235	56	2.2
red, unsweetened, unthawed	1 cup	71	17	0.7
SWEET				
Canned				
pitted, in extra heavy syrup w/liquid	1 cup	266	68	0.4
pitted, in heavy syrup, w/liquid	1 cup	210	54	0.4
pitted, in juice, w/liquid	1 cup	135	35	0.1
pitted, in light syrup, w/liquid	1 cup	169	44	0.4
pitted, in water, w/liquid	1 cup	114	29	0.3
Fresh				
raw	1 cup	84	19	1.1
raw, medium	1 cherry	5	1	0.1
raw, pitted	1 cup	104	24	1.4
Frozen				
	10-oz pkg	253	64	0.4
thawed	1 cup	231	58	0.3

CHERRY JUICE. See also BLACK CHERRY JUICE; FRUIT DRINK; FRUIT JUICE DRINK; FRUIT JUICE DRINK MIX.

Food Name	Serv. Size	Total Cal.	Carbs GMS	Fat GMS
Canned, bottled, or boxed				
(Dole) blend 'Pure & Light Mountain Cherry'	6 fl oz	87	22	0.1
(Juicy Juice)	6 fl oz	90	22	0.0
(Knudsen & Sons) tart	8 fl oz	125	30	0.0
(Mountain Sun) organic, 'Mountain Cherry'	8 fl oz	109	27	0.0
(Santa Cruz Natural) organic, 'Cruz'	8 fl oz	125	29	1.0
(Welch's) 'Orchard'	6 fl oz	180	45	0.0
Frozen				
(Welch's) concentrate, 'Welchade'	2 fl oz	130	31	0.0

CHERRY PEPPER. See PEPPER, CHERRY.
CHERRY, SURINAM. See PITANGA.
CHERVIL

Food Name	Serv. Size	Total Cal.	Carbs GMS	Fat GMS
dried	1 tbsp	4	1	0.1
dried	1 tsp	1	0	0.0
dried (McCormick/Schilling)	1 tsp	2	0	0.0
dried (Tone's)	1 tsp	1	0	0.1

CHESTNUT, CHINESE

Food Name	Serv. Size	Total Cal.	Carbs GMS	Fat GMS
boiled or steamed	1 oz	43	9.6	0.2
dried	1 oz	103	22.6	0.5
raw	1 oz	64	13.9	0.3
raw, in shell	1 lb	852	187.0	4.2
roasted	1 oz	68	14.9	0.3

CHESTNUT, EUROPEAN/Italian chestnut/sweet chestnut

Food Name	Serv. Size	Total Cal.	Carbs GMS	Fat GMS
boiled or steamed, shelled	1 oz	37	7.9	0.4
dried, in shell	1 lb	1357	280.5	16.1
dried, shelled, peeled	1 oz	105	22.3	1.1
dried, shelled, unpeeled	1 oz	106	22.0	1.3
raw, in shell	1 lb	714	152.8	7.6
raw, shelled, peeled	1 oz	56	12.5	0.4
raw, shelled, unpeeled	1 cup	309	66.0	3.3
raw, shelled, unpeeled	1 oz	60	12.9	0.6
roasted, in shell	1 lb	700	151.3	6.3

Food Name	Serv. Size	Total Cal.	Carbs GMS	Fat GMS
roasted, in shell	1 cup	350	75.7	3.2
roasted, in shell	1 oz	70	15.0	0.6
roasted, shelled	1 oz	70	15.0	0.6
roasted, shelled, approx 17 nuts	1 cup	350	75.7	3.2
CHESTNUT, ITALIAN. See CHESTNUT, EUROPEAN.				
CHESTNUT, JAPANESE				
boiled or steamed	1 oz	16	3.6	0.1
dried, in shell	1 lb	1078	243.7	3.7
dried, shelled	1 oz	102	23.1	0.4
dried, shelled	1 cup	558	126.2	1.9
raw, in shell	1 lb	462	104.5	1.6
raw, shelled	1 oz	44	9.9	0.2
roasted	1 oz	57	12.8	0.2
CHESTNUT, SWEET. See CHESTNUT, EUROPEAN.				
CHESTNUT FLOUR. See under FLOUR.				
CHEWING GUM. See under CANDY, GUM.				
CHIA SEEDS, dried	1 oz	134	13.6	7.4
CHICKEN				
AVERAGE OF ALL PARTS				
Fresh				
capon, meat and skin, raw	1 lb	1056	0.0	76.8
capon, meat and skin, raw	1 oz	66	0.0	4.8
capon, meat and skin, roasted	4 oz	260	0.0	13.2
roaster, meat and skin, raw	1 lb	976	0.0	72.0
roaster, meat and skin, raw	1 oz	61	0.0	4.5
roaster, meat and skin, roasted	4 oz	253	0.0	15.2
stewing, meat and skin, raw	1 oz	73	0.0	5.8
stewing, meat and skin, stewed	4 oz	323	0.0	21.4
BACK				
Fresh				
broiler/fryer, meat and skin, flour-coated, fried	4 oz	375	7.4	23.5
broiler/fryer, meat and skin, raw	1 oz	90	0.0	8.1
broiler/fryer, meat and skin, roasted	4 oz	340	0.0	23.8
broiler/fryer, meat and skin, stewed	4 oz	293	0.0	20.6
broiler/fryer, meat only, raw	1 lb	624	0.0	28.8
broiler/fryer, meat only, raw	1 oz	39	0.0	1.7
broiler/fryer, meat only, roasted	4 oz	271	0.0	14.9
broiler/fryer, meat only, stewed	4 oz	237	0.0	12.7
BREAST				
Canned				
chunk *(Hormel)*	6.75 oz	350	0	20.0
Fresh				
broiler/fryer, meat and skin, batter-dipped, fried	4 oz	295	10.2	15.0
broiler/fryer, meat and skin, flour-coated, fried	4 oz	252	1.9	10.1
broiler/fryer, meat and skin, raw	1 lb	784	0.0	41.6
broiler/fryer, meat and skin, raw	1 oz	49	0.0	2.6
broiler/fryer, meat and skin, roasted	4 oz	223	0.0	8.8
broiler/fryer, meat and skin, stewed	4 oz	209	0.0	8.4
broiler/fryer, meat only, raw	1 lb	496	0.0	6.4
broiler/fryer, meat only, raw	1 oz	31	0.0	0.4
broiler/fryer, meat only, roasted	4 oz	187	0.0	4.0
broiler/fryer, meat only, stewed	4 oz	171	0.0	3.4
Frozen or refrigerated				
Breast				
baked, 'Classic' *(Carving Board)*	1 slice	40	1	0.5
boneless, barbecue marinated, frozen *(Tyson)*	3.75 oz	120	5	3.0
boneless, butter garlic marinated *(Tyson)*	3.75 oz	160	3	7.0

Food Name	Serv. Size	Total Cal.	Carbs GMS	Fat GMS
boneless, Italian marinated, frozen *(Tyson)*	3.75 oz	130	6	2.0
boneless, teriyaki marinated, frozen *(Tyson)*	3.75 oz	130	6	2.0
broiler/fryer, baked *(Tyson)*	3 oz	116	0	1.5
fillet, barbecue, boneless, frozen *(Tyson)*	3 oz	110	6	3.0
fillet, boneless, grilled *(Tyson)*	2.75 oz	100	4	3.0
fillet, boneless, skinless, raw *(Delightful Farms)*	1 med breast	140	0	1.5
fillet, lemon-pepper breast, boneless, frozen *(Tyson)*	2.75 oz	100	4	3.0
grilled *(Carving Board)*	1 slice	40	1	0.5
half, roasted, w/skin *(Tyson)*	1 med piece	250	1	13.0
hickory smoked, nonfat *(Tyson)*	1 slice	35	1	0.0
honey flavor, nonfat *(Tyson)*	1 slice	35	2	0.0
mesquite flavor, roasted, nonfat *(Tyson)*	1 slice	35	1	0.0
peppered, roasted, nonfat *(Tyson)*	1 slice	35	1	0.0
roasted, nonfat *(Tyson)*	1 slice	35	1	0.0
split, skinless, raw *(Hudson)*	1 med breast	140	0	1.5
split, w/skin, raw *(Hudson)*	1 med breast	270	0	14.0
w/rib meat, boneless, skinless, raw *(Hudson)*	1 med breast	140	0	1.5
CHUNK				
Canned				
(Featherweight)	3 oz	90	0	3.0
(Swanson)	1 cup	360	8	12.0
DARK MEAT				
Canned, chunk *(Hormel)*	6.75 oz	327	0	18.0
Fresh				
broiler/fryer, meat and skin, batter-dipped, fried	4 oz	338	10.6	21.1
broiler/fryer, meat and skin, flour-coated, fried	4 oz	323	4.6	19.2
broiler/fryer, meat and skin, raw	1 oz	67	0.0	5.2
broiler/fryer, meat and skin, roasted	4 oz	287	0.0	17.9
broiler/fryer, meat and skin, stewed	4 oz	264	0.0	16.6
broiler/fryer, meat only, fried, chopped or diced	1 cup	335	3.6	16.3
broiler/fryer, meat only, raw	1 oz	35	0.0	1.2
broiler/fryer, meat only, roasted	1 cup	287	0.0	13.6
broiler/fryer, meat only, roasted	4 oz	232	0.0	11.0
broiler/fryer, meat only, roasted, chopped or diced	1 cup	286	0.0	13.6
broiler/fryer, meat only, stewed	1 cup	269	0.0	12.6
broiler/fryer, meat only, stewed	4 oz	218	0.0	10.2
broiler/fryer, meat only, stewed, chopped or diced	1 cup	269	0.0	12.6
roaster, meat only, raw	1 oz	32	0.0	1.0
roaster, meat only, roasted	4 oz	202	0.0	9.9
stewing, meat only, raw	1 oz	45	0.0	2.3
stewing, meat only, stewed	1 cup	361	0.0	21.4
stewing, meat only, stewed	4 oz	293	0.0	17.3
DRUMSTICK				
Fresh				
broiler/fryer, meat and skin, batter-dipped, fried	4 oz	304	9.4	17.9
broiler/fryer, meat and skin, flour-coated, fried	4 oz	278	1.8	15.6
broiler/fryer, meat and skin, raw	1 lb	736	0.0	40.0
broiler/fryer, meat and skin, raw	1 oz	46	0.0	2.5
broiler/fryer, meat and skin, roasted	4 oz	245	0.0	12.6
broiler/fryer, meat and skin, stewed	4 oz	231	0.0	12.1
broiler/fryer, meat only, raw	1 lb	544	0.0	16.0
broiler/fryer, meat only, raw	1 oz	34	0.0	1.0
broiler/fryer, meat only, roasted	4 oz	195	0.0	6.4
broiler/fryer, meat only, stewed	4 oz	192	0.0	6.5
DRUMSTICK AND WING				
Frozen				
drumette and wing portions, raw *(Delightful Farms)*	4 sections	150	0	10.0

Food Name	Serv. Size	Total Cal.	Carbs GMS	Fat GMS
GIBLETS				
Fresh				
all classes, fried	1 cup	402	6.3	19.5
all classes, simmered	1 cup	228	1.4	6.9
broiler/fryer, fried, chopped or diced	1 cup	402	6	19.5
broiler/fryer, raw	2.6 oz	93	1	3.4
broiler/fryer, simmered, chopped or diced	1 cup	228	1	6.9
capon, raw	1 lb	592	6.4	24.0
capon, raw	1 oz	37	0.4	1.5
capon, simmered	1 cup	238	1.1	7.8
capon, simmered	4 oz	186	0.9	6.1
roaster, simmered	1 Cup	239	1.3	7.6
stewing, raw	1 lb	560	8.0	20.8
stewing, raw	1 oz	35	0.5	1.3
stewing, simmered	1 cup	281	0.2	13.5
GIZZARD				
Fresh				
all classes, simmered	1 cup	222	1.6	5.3
broiler-fryer, raw, approx 1.3 oz	1 medium	44	0.2	1.6
broiler-fryer, simmered, approx .8 oz	1 medium	34	0.3	0.8
roaster, raw	1 medium	44	0	1.6
roaster, simmered	1 medium	11	0	0.3
roaster, simmered, chopped or diced	1 cup	222	2	5.3
HEART				
Fresh				
all classes, simmered	1 cup	268	0.2	11.5
broiler-fryer, raw, 1 heart	2 oz	9	<.1	0.6
broiler-fryer, simmered	4 oz	210	0.1	9.0
roaster, raw	1 medium	9	0	0.6
roaster, simmered, chopped or diced	1 cup	268	0	11.5
LEG				
Fresh				
broiler/fryer, meat and skin, batter-dipped, fried	4 oz	310	9.9	18.3
broiler/fryer, meat and skin, flour-coated, fried	4 oz	285	2.8	16.2
broiler/fryer, meat and skin, raw	1 lb	848	0.0	54.4
broiler/fryer, meat and skin, raw	1 oz	53	0.0	3.4
broiler/fryer, stewed	4 oz	249	0.0	14.7
broiler/fryer, meat only, raw	1 lb	544	0.0	17.6
broiler/fryer, meat only, raw	1 oz	34	0.0	1.1
broiler/fryer, meat only, roasted	4 oz	217	0.0	9.6
broiler/fryer, meat only, stewed	4 oz	210	0.0	9.1
Frozen or refrigerated				
broiler/fryer, baked *(Tyson)*	3 oz	131	0	3.8
raw *(Delightful Farms)*	1 med drumstick	200	0	11.0
w/skin *(Hudson)*	2 med drumsticks	230	0	12.0
LIGHT MEAT				
Fresh				
broiler/fryer, meat and skin, batter-dipped, fried	4 oz	312	10.7	17.4
broiler/fryer, meat and skin, flour-coated, fried	4 oz	279	2.1	13.7
broiler/fryer, meat and skin, raw	1 oz	53	0.0	3.1
broiler/fryer, meat and skin, roasted	4 oz	252	0.0	12.3
broiler/fryer, meat and skin, stewed	4 oz	228	0.0	11.3
broiler/fryer, meat only, fried	8 oz	269	0.6	7.8
broiler/fryer, meat only, raw	1 oz	32	0.0	0.5
broiler/fryer, meat only, roasted	1 cup	242	0.0	6.3
broiler/fryer, meat only, roasted	4 oz	196	0.0	5.1
broiler/fryer, meat only, roasted, chopped or diced	1 cup	242	0.0	6.3

Food Name	Serv. Size	Total Cal.	Carbs GMS	Fat GMS
broiler/fryer, meat only, stewed, chopped or diced	1 cup	223	0.0	5.6
broiler/fryer, meat only, stewed	4 oz	180	0.0	4.5
roaster, meat only, raw	1 oz	31	0.0	0.5
roaster, meat only, roasted	4 oz	174	0.0	4.6
roaster, meat only, roasted, chopped or diced	1 cup	214	0.0	5.7
stewing, meat only, raw	1 oz	39	0.0	1.2
stewing, meat only, stewed	1 cup	298	0.0	11.2
stewing, meat only, stewed	4 oz	242	0.0	9.0
LIVER				
Fresh				
all classes, simmered	1 cup	220	1.2	7.6
broiler-fryer, chopped, simmered	1 cup	219	1.2	7.6
broiler-fryer, raw, approx 1.1 oz	1 liver	40	1.1	1.2
broiler-fryer, simmered	4 oz	178	1.0	6.2
NECK				
Fresh				
broiler/fryer, meat and skin, batter-dipped, fried	4 oz	374	9.9	26.7
broiler/fryer, meat and skin, flour-coated, fried	4 oz	376	4.8	26.8
broiler/fryer, meat and skin, raw	1 lb	1344	0.0	118.4
broiler/fryer, meat and skin, raw	1 oz	84	0.0	7.4
broiler/fryer, meat and skin, simmered	4 oz	280	0.0	20.5
broiler/fryer, meat only, raw	1 lb	704	0.0	40.0
broilor/fryer, meat only, raw	1 oz	44	0.0	2.5
broiler/fryer, meat only, simmered	4 oz	203	0.0	9.3
SKIN				
Fresh				
broiler/fryer, batter-dipped, fried	1 oz	112	6.6	8.2
broiler/fryer, roasted	1 oz	129	0.0	11.5
broiler/fryer, stewed	1 oz	103	0.0	9.4
THIGH				
Fresh				
broiler/fryer, meat and skin, batter-dipped, fried	4 oz	314	10.3	18.7
broiler/fryer, meat and skin, flour-coated, fried	4 oz	297	3.6	17.0
broiler/fryer, meat and skin, raw	1 lb	960	0.0	68.8
broiler/fryer, meat and skin, raw	1 oz	60	0.0	4.3
broiler/fryer, meat and skin, roasted	4 oz	280	0.0	17.6
broiler/fryer, meat and skin, stewed	4 oz	263	0.0	16.7
broiler/fryer, meat only, raw	1 lb	544	0.0	17.6
broiler/fryer, meat only, raw	1 oz	34	0.0	1.1
broiler/fryer, meat only, roasted	4 oz	237	0.0	12.3
broiler/fryer, meat only, stewed	4 oz	221	0.0	11.1
Frozen or refrigerated				
boneless, skinless, raw *(Hudson)*	1 med thigh	100	0	3.0
broiler/fryer, baked *(Tyson)*	3 oz	152	0	6.7
roasted, w/skin *(Tyson)*	1 med piece	270	1	19.0
w/skin, raw *(Hudson)*	1 med thigh	230	0	17.0
THIGH AND DRUMSTICK				
Frozen, 'Plump and Juicy' *(Swanson)*	3.25 oz	290	17	18.0
WHITE AND DARK MEAT				
Canned				
(Swanson)	2.5 oz	100	0	4.0
chunk *(Hormel)*	6.75 oz	340	0	20.0
chunk, unsalted *(Hormel)*	6.75 oz	330	0	18.0
cooked, in water, 96% fat-free *(Valley Fresh)*	2 oz	80	0	2.0
puréed *(bryan foods)*	1/3 cup	120	0	7.0
WHITE MEAT				
Canned				
(Swanson)	2.5 oz	100	0	4.0

Food Name	Serv. Size	Total Cal.	Carbs GMS	Fat GMS
chunk, cooked, in water, 98% fat-free *(Valley Fresh)*	2 oz	70	0	1.0
chunk, premium *(Swanson)*	3 oz	80	1	1.0
WHOLE				
Frozen or refrigerated				
barbecue *(Empire Kosher)*	5 oz	280	1	17.0
broiler/fryer, baked *(Tyson)*	3 oz	134	0	4.1
roasted, w/skin *(Tyson)*	3 oz	180	1	12.0
WING				
Fresh				
broiler/fryer, meat and skin, batter-dipped, fried	4 oz	367	12.4	24.7
broiler/fryer, meat and skin, flour-coated, fried	4 oz	364	2.7	25.1
broiler/fryer, meat and skin, raw	1 lb	1008	0.0	72.0
broiler/fryer, meat and skin, raw	1 oz	63	0.0	4.5
broiler/fryer, meat and skin, roasted	4 oz	329	0.0	22.1
broiler/fryer, meat and skin, stewed	4 oz	282	0.0	19.1
broiler/fryer, meat only, raw	1 lb	576	0.0	16.0
broiler/fryer, meat only, raw	1 oz	36	0.0	1.0
broiler/fryer, meat only, roasted	4 oz	230	0.0	9.2
broiler/fryer, meat only, stewed	4 oz	205	0.0	8.1
Frozen or refrigerated				
w/skin *(Hudson)*	3 med wings	280	0	20.0
broiler/fryer, baked *(Tyson)*	3 oz	147	0	5.6

CHICKEN DINNER/ENTRÉE. See also BURRITO; CHICKEN DINNER/ENTRÉE MIX; CHILI; CHIMICHANGA; ENCHILADA; FAJITA; LUNCH COMBINATION, PACKAGED; RAVIOLI DISH ENTRÉE; SANDWICH; TORTELLINI DISH ENTRÉE.

Food Name	Serv. Size	Total Cal.	Carbs GMS	Fat GMS
(Armour)				
à la king, frozen, 'Classics Lite'	11.25 oz	290	38	7.0
Burgundy, frozen, 'Classics Lite'	10 oz	210	25	2.0
glazed, frozen, 'Classics'	10.75 oz	300	24	16.0
Marsala, frozen, 'Classics Lite'	10.5 oz	250	27	7.0
mesquite, frozen, 'Classics'	9.5 oz	370	42	16.0
Oriental, 'Classics Lite'	10 oz	180	24	1.0
parmigiana, frozen, 'Classics'	11.5 oz	370	27	19.0
sweet and sour, frozen, 'Classics Lite'	11 oz	240	39	2.0
w/noodles, frozen, 'Classics'	11 oz	230	23	7.0
w/wine and mushroom sauce, frozen, 'Classics'	10.75 oz	280	24	11.0
(Banquet)				
à la king, frozen, 'Cookin' Bags'	4 oz	110	9	5.0
and dumplings, w/gravy	1 entrée	270	35	9.0
breast patty, fried, w/biscuit, frozen, 'Southern'	4 oz	320	37	14.0
chow mein, w/egg roll	1 entrée	210	28	7.0
drumsticks, frozen, 'Drumsnackers' 'Platters'	7 oz	430	49	19.0
fingers, barbecue	1 entrée	340	36	16.0
fried, 'Original'	1 entrée	470	35	27.0
fried, white meat	1 entrée	480	40	28.0
fried, white meat, frozen, 'Extra Helping'	16 oz	570	70	28.0
fried, white meat, hot 'n spicy, frozen, 'Platter'	9 oz	430	21	22.0
fried, w/mashed potatoes and corn, seasoned sauce	1 entrée	470	35	27.0
grilled	1 entrée	330	37	13.0
hot'n spicy, frozen, 'Snack'n'	3.75 oz	140	8	9.0
nugget meal, frozen	1 meal	410	38	21.0
nuggets, fried	1 entrée	430	42	23.0
nuggets, hot'n spicy, w/barbecue sauce	4.5 oz	360	23	21.0
nuggets, sweet and sour, 'Extra Helping'	10 oz	650	64	34.0
nuggets, sweet and sour, w/sauce, 'Microwave'	4.5 oz	360	22	21.0
nuggets, w/BBQ sauce, 'Extra Helping'	10 oz	640	56	36.0
nuggets, w/BBQ sauce, frozen, 'Southern'	4.5 oz	370	20	23.0

Food Name	Serv. Size	Total Cal.	Carbs GMS	Fat GMS
Oriental, w/egg rolls	1 entrée	260	36	9.0
parmigiana	1 entrée	320	29	18.0
patty, frozen, 'Platters'	7.5 oz	380	34	21.0
pie, frozen	7 oz	550	39	36.0
pie, frozen, 'Supreme Microwave'	7 oz	430	30	28.0
pot pie, frozen	1 serving	382	36	22.0
primavera, w/vegetable, frozen, 'Cookin' Bags'	4 oz	100	14	2.0
primavera, w/vegetable, frozen, 'Family Entrees'	7 oz	140	18	3.0
Southern fried	1 entrée	560	40	33.0
sweet and sour, frozen, 'Cookin' Bags'	4 oz	130	22	2.0
w/dumplings, frozen	10 oz	430	34	24.0
(Barber Foods)				
cordon bleu, w/cheese and ham, frozen	1 pkg	697	30	41.5
cordon bleu, w/cheese and ham, frozen	1 serving	344	15	20.5
w/broccoli and cheese stuffing, frozen	1 pkg	527	12	34.7
w/broccoli and cheese stuffing, frozen	1 serving	260	6	17.1
(Budget Gourmet)				
and egg noodles, w/broccoli, frozen	10 oz	450	31	26.0
au gratin, 'Light'	1 entrée	250	26	8.0
breast, herbed, frozen, 'Special Selections	1 entrée	300	34	8.0
breast, honey mustard	1 entrée	310	45	6.0
breast, honey mustard, 'Light & Healthy'	1 dinner	310	46	6.0
breast, orange glazed	1 entrée	280	51	3.0
breast, orange glazed, 'Light'	1 entrée	300	56	2.0
cacciatore, frozen	11 oz	300	27	13.0
French, light, w/vegetables, potato, sauce	1 serving	179	9	5.6
French recipe, 'Light'	1 entrée	200	19	8.0
frozen, w/egg noodles, frozen	1 entrée	410	30	23.0
herbed, w/fettuccini	1 entrée	260	29	8.0
Italian style, frozen, 'Special Selections'	1 entrée	280	44	7.0
Mandarin, w/vegetables, frozen, 'Special Selections'	1 entrée	250	37	5.0
Marsala, frozen	10 oz	250	37	5.0
Mexican, frozen	12.8 oz	510	70	15.0
Oriental, w/vegetables	1 entrée	290	43	8.0
Oriental, w/vegetables, 'Light & Healthy'	9 oz	280	44	6.0
Oriental, w/vegetables and rice, frozen, 'Special Selections'	1 entrée	290	42	9.0
roasted, frozen	11.2 oz	280	34	7.0
roasted, w/herb gravy	1 entrée	260	34	8.0
sweet and sour, w/rice	10 oz	350	53	7.0
Szechuan, spicy, w/vegetable, frozen, 'Special Selections'	1 entrée	300	41	9.0
teriyaki, frozen	12 oz	360	44	12.0
teriyaki, w/Oriental style vegetables, frozen, 'Light and Healthy'	1 entrée	317	52	3.7
w/fettuccini	1 entrée	380	33	19.0
w/rigatoni, broccoli 'Special Selections'	1 entrée	310	46	6.0
white meat, w/Chinese style vegetables, rice	1 entrée	250	39	7.0
white meat, w/Italian style vegetables, rice	1 entrée	250	39	7.0
(Celentano)				
breaded, w/pasta marinara w/cheese	10 oz tray	390	36	19.0
parmigiana, frozen	9 oz	330	15	20.0
primavera, frozen	11.5 oz	270	18	10.0
(Chicken By George)				
Cajun, boneless, skinless	1 med breast	120	2	4.0
Cajun, packaged	5 oz	180	4	8.0
Caribbean grill, packaged	5 oz	200	10	6.0
Italian bleu cheese, packaged	5 oz	180	2	8.0
lemon herb, boneless, skinless, raw	1 med breast	120	3	3.0
lemon herb, packaged	5 oz	170	6	6.0

Food Name	Serv. Size	Total Cal.	Carbs GMS	Fat GMS
lemon oregano, packaged	5 oz	160	4	4.0
mesquite barbecue, packaged	5 oz	170	6	6.0
mustard dill, packaged	5 oz	180	3	7.0
roasted, packaged	5 oz	150	2	4.0
teriyaki, breast, boneless, skinless, raw	1 med breast	130	6	3.0
tomato herb, w/basil, packaged,	5 oz	190	7	7.0
(Chun King)				
chow mein, frozen	13 oz	370	53	6.0
imperial, frozen	13 oz	300	54	1.0
sweet and sour, w/vegetables, fruit, and sauce, canned	1 pkg	802	154	8.6
sweet and sour, w/vegetables, fruit, and sauce, canned	1 serving	165	32	1.8
walnut, crunchy, frozen	13 oz	310	49	5.0
(Contadina) parmigiana, frozen, food service product	1 oz	43	3	2.3
(Country Pride) primavera, sticks, frozen	3 oz	240	16	15.0
(Dining Lite)				
à la king, frozen	9 oz	240	30	7.0
and noodles, frozen	9 oz	240	28	7.0
chow mein, frozen	9 oz	180	31	2.0
glazed, frozen	9 oz	220	30	4.0
(Dinty Moore)				
and dumplings, microwave cup	1 cup	100	12	3.0
stew, microwave cup	7.5 oz	260	15	18.0
w/dumplings, microwave cup	7.5 oz	166	17	5.0
w/gravy and mashed potatoes, packaged	1 bowl	220	24	4.0
w/noodles, 'Micro Meal'	1 bowl	260	26	8.0
(Empire Kosher)				
breast, battered and breaded, fried, kosher	3 oz	170	3	8.0
cutlets, battered and breaded, fried, kosher	1 med cutlet	200	11	9.0
nuggets, battered and breaded, fried, kosher	5 nuggets	200	9	13.0
nuggets, kosher	5 nuggets	180	12	9.0
pie, kosher	1 pie	440	41	21.0
(Featherweight)				
stew, w/wild rice, canned	7.5 oz	140	23	1.0
w/dumplings, canned	7.5 oz	160	18	5.0
(Freezer Queen)				
à la king, frozen, 'Cook-In-Pouch'	4 oz	70	6	1.0
à la king, w/rice, frozen, 'Single Serve'	9 oz	270	37	5.0
cacciatore, frozen, 'Single Serve'	9 oz	270	33	6.0
croquettes, breaded, 'Family Suppers'	7 oz	240	20	12.0
nuggets, frozen, 'Deluxe Family Suppers'	3 oz	270	15	17.0
nuggets, platter, frozen	6 oz	410	36	23.0
patty, frozen, 'Platter'	7.5 oz	360	33	17.0
primavera, sliced, w/gravy, 'Cook-In-Pouch'	5 oz	80	6	3.0
sweet and sour, w/rice, frozen, 'Single Serve'	9 oz	300	48	4.0
(Green Giant) and broccoli, frozen, 'Entrées'	9.5 oz	340	28	15.0
(Healthy Choice)				
à l'orange, frozen	9 oz	260	38	2.0
and broccoli, 'Hearty Handfuls'	1 entrée	320	51	5.0
and mushrooms, 'Hearty Handfuls'	1 entrée	310	49	5.0
broccoli Alfredo	1 entrée	300	34	7.0
cacciatore	1 entrée	340	52	5.0
cacciatore, in sauce, w/vegetables	1 serving	266	36	4.0
Cantonese	1 entrée	280	34	6.0
chow mein, lowfat, low-cholesterol, frozen	9 oz	240	29	5.0
country breaded	1 entrée	350	51	9.0
country glazed	1 entrée	230	30	4.0
country herb	1 entrée	320	44	8.0

Food Name	Serv. Size	Total Cal.	Carbs GMS	Fat GMS
Dijon	1 entrée	270	33	5.0
divan, w/pasta, frozen	11.5 oz	300	41	4.0
entrée	1 entrée	250	31	6.0
Francesca	1 entrée	330	46	6.0
garlic, 'Hearty Handfuls'	1 entrée	330	53	5.0
glazed, frozen	8.5 oz	220	27	3.0
grilled, Sonoma	1 entrée	230	30	4.0
grilled, Southwestern	1 entrée	260	30	6.0
grilled, w/mashed potatoes	1 entrée	170	18	3.5
herb roasted, frozen	11 oz	380	56	7.0
honey mustard	1 entrée	290	38	6.0
Mandarin	1 entrée	280	44	2.5
Marsala, w/vegetables	1 entrée	240	32	4.0
mesquite barbecue	1 entrée	310	48	5.0
mesquite barbecue, w/rice, vegetable, apple raisin cobbler	1 serving	310	48	5.0
Mexican, low-fat, low-cholesterol, frozen	12.5 oz	340	51	5.0
Milano, garlic	1 entrée	260	34	6.0
Oriental, frozen	11.25 oz	200	32	1.0
parmigiana	1 entrée	330	46	8.0
picante	1 entrée	250	30	7.0
roasted	1 entrée	230	25	5.0
roasted, frozen	1 serving	290	39	4.0
'Salsa Chicken Dinner' frozen	1 serving	240	36	2.0
sesame	1 entrée	250	38	4.0
Shanghai, sesame	1 entrée	360	54	7.0
stir-fry, w/vermicelli, frozen, 'Extra Portion'	12 oz	300	42	5.0
sweet and sour	1 entrée	360	53	7.0
sweet and sour, frozen	11.5 oz	280	52	2.0
teriyaki	1 entrée	270	37	6.0
teriyaki, w/rice, vegetable, apple cherry compote	1 serving	268	37	5.6
(Heinz) stew, w/dumplings, canned	7.5 oz	210	22	9.0
(Hormel) loaf, canned	2 oz	130	0	10.0
(Hot Bites)				
breast tenders, boneless	2.25 oz	150	12	6.0
breast tenders, boneless, 'Microwave'	4 oz	260	24	10.0
drumsticks, frozen, 'Drumsnackers'	2.63 oz	220	13	15.0
nuggets, fried, frozen, 'Southern'	2.63 oz	220	13	14.0
nuggets, frozen	2.63 oz	210	11	14.0
nuggets, hot'n spicy, frozen	2.63 oz	250	10	19.0
nuggets, w/cheddar, frozen	2.63 oz	250	11	18.0
sticks, primavera, frozen	2.63 oz	220	11	15.0
(Kid Cuisine)				
fried, frozen 'Mega Meal'	10.8 oz	720	53	41.0
fried, frozen	7.25 oz	420	41	22.0
fried, white meat, w/potato, corn, chocolate pudding, frozen	1 meal	440	48	20.0
nuggets, frozen	6.25 oz	400	46	19.0
nuggets, frozen, 'Mega Meal'	8.4 oz	470	51	20.0
nuggets, w/macaroni and cheese, corn, pudding, 'Cosmic'	1 serving	524	53	26.7
nuggets, w/macaroni, corn, chocolate pudding	1 meal	360	46	13.0
(La Choy)				
almond, w/rice, vegetable, 'Fresh and Lite'	9.75 oz	270	40	8.0
chow mein, canned	1 cup	80	6	3.5
chow mein, canned, 'Bi-Pack'	3/4 cup	80	8	3.0
chow mein, canned, food service product	1 cup	91	11	3.6
chow mein, frozen, food service product	1 cup	133	19	3.1
imperial, w/rice, frozen, 'Fresh and Lite'	11 oz	260	45	6.0
Oriental, canned, 'Bi-Pack'	3/4 cup	240	47	2.0

Food Name	Serv. Size	Total Cal.	Carbs GMS	Fat GMS
Oriental, spicy, frozen, 'Fresh and Lite'	9.75 oz	270	52	4.0
Oriental, w/noodles, canned, 'Bi-Pack'	9 oz	160	23	3.8
sweet and sour, canned	3/4 cup	240	47	2.0
sweet and sour, canned, 'Dinner Classics'	1/4 pkg	120	29	1.0
sweet and sour, packaged, 'Dinner Classics'	3/4 cup	310	30	6.0
sweet and sour, w/noodles, frozen	1 cup	256	49	3.1
sweet and sour, w/rice, vegetables, frozen 'Fresh & Lite'	10 oz	260	50	3.0
Szechwan, spicy, bi-pack	1 cup	98	11	2.6
(Le Menu)				
à la king, w/seasoned rice, frozen, 'LightStyle'	8.25 oz	240	29	5.0
breast, glazed, frozen, 'LightStyle'	10 oz	230	25	3.0
breast, roasted, w/herbs, rice, and vegetable	7.75 oz	260	29	6.0
cordon bleu, frozen	11 oz	460	47	20.0
Dijon, w/pasta and vegetables, 'LightStyle'	8.5 oz	240	21	7.0
herb roasted, frozen, 'LightStyle'	10 oz	240	18	7.0
in wine sauce, frozen	10 oz	280	27	7.0
Kiev, frozen	8 oz	530	24	39.0
Oriental, à la king, frozen	10.25 oz	330	29	13.0
parmigiana, frozen	11.75 oz	410	31	20.0
sweet and sour, frozen	11.25 oz	400	41	18.0
sweet and sour, frozen, 'LightStyle'	10 oz	250	29	7.0
(Lean Cuisine)				
'Fiesta' frozen	8.5 oz	240	30	5.0
à l'orange	1 entrée	260	40	2.5
à l'orange, in sauce, w/broccoli and rice	1 serving	268	39	1.8
and vegetables, w/vermicelli	1 pkg	252	32	5.6
and vegetables, w/vermicelli, frozen	11.75 oz	240	30	5.0
baked	1 entrée	230	31	4.0
baked, w/whipped potatoes	1 entrée	250	30	6.0
barbecue, w/rice pilaf, frozen	8.75 oz	260	32	6.0
barbecue, w/sauce, 'Hearty Portions'	1 entrée	380	58	6.0
breaded, baked, w/potato and vegetable, frozen	8 oz	200	21	5.0
cacciatore, w/vermicelli, frozen	10 7/8 oz	280	31	7.0
Calypso, frozen, 'Café Classics'	1 pkg	280	42	6.0
carbonara	1 entrée	280	33	8.0
chow mein	1 entrée	220	33	5.0
chow mein, w/rice, frozen	9 oz	240	34	5.0
classica, frozen, food service product	1 oz	23	2	0.8
fiesta, w/rice and vegetables	1 entrée	260	35	5.0
Florentine, 'Hearty Portions'	1 entrée	420	61	9.0
glazed	1 entrée	240	25	6.0
glazed, frozen, food service product	1 oz	26	1	1.1
glazed, w/vegetable rice, frozen	8.5 oz	250	24	7.0
grilled, and penne pasta, 'Hearty Portions'	1 entrée	380	52	8.0
grilled, w/salsa, frozen, 'Café Classics'	1 pkg	240	32	6.0
herb roasted	1 entrée	210	27	5.0
herb roasted, 'Café Classics'	1 entrée	210	25	5.0
honey mustard, 'Café Classics'	1 entrée	270	39	5.0
honey mustard, frozen	7.5 oz	230	30	4.0
honey roasted	1 entrée	290	46	6.0
in peanut sauce	1 entrée	290	35	6.0
Italienne, frozen, food service product	1 oz	20	1	0.9
medallions, w/creamy cheese sauce	1 entrée	260	31	8.0
Marsala, w/vegetables, frozen	8-1/8 oz	180	13	4.0
Mediterranean, frozen, 'Café Classics'	1 pkg	260	36	4.0
Mexicali style, frozen, food service product	1 oz	20	2	0.7
Oriental	1 entrée	250	30	6.0

Food Name	Serv. Size	Total Cal.	Carbs GMS	Fat GMS
Oriental, glazed, 'Hearty Portions'	1 entrée	410	69	6.0
Oriental, w/vermicelli, frozen	9 oz	280	31	7.0
Parmesan	1 entrée	220	27	5.0
Parmesan, 'Café Classics'	1 entrée	240	25	7.0
piccata	1 entrée	270	41	6.0
picatta, frozen, 'Café Classics'	1 pkg	290	45	6.0
pie	1 entrée	320	39	10.0
pie, 100% white meat, frozen	1 pkg	310	32	10.0
primavera, frozen, food service product	1 oz	16	1	0.7
roasted, w/herbs, frozen, 'Café Classics'	1 pkg	210	25	5.0
roasted, w/mushrooms, 'Hearty Portions'	1 entrée	380	57	7.0
sweet and sour, frozen, food service product	1 oz	22	3	0.5
sweet and sour, w/rice, frozen	9 oz	280	39	6.0
tenderloins, in herb sauce, frozen	9.5 oz	240	19	5.0
tenderloins, in peanut sauce, frozen	9 oz	290	33	7.0
w/bow tie pasta, frozen, 'Café Classics'	1 pkg	270	34	6.0
w/rice and vegetables	1 entrée	240	24	6.0
(Libby's)				
chow mein, microwave cup	7.75 oz	130	19	4.0
w/pasta spirals, microwave cup, 'Diner'	7.75 oz	120	16	3.0
(Lloyds) breast fillet, roasted, barbecue, w/sauce	1 fillet	140	12	3.0
(Luck's)				
and dumplings, microwave bowl	1 serving	150	21	1.0
and rice, microwaveable bowl	1 serving	140	19	1.0
Brunswick stew, microwave bowl	1 serving	130	23	0.0
thighs and wings, w/dumplings, in sauce	1 cup	340	23	20.0
w/dumplings, canned	7.25 oz	240	18	11.0
(Lunch Bucket)				
w/beans and rice, micro cup, 'Light'n Healthy'	7.5 oz	170	28	3.0
w/dumplings, microwave lunch cup	7.5 oz	140	25	2.0
(Lunch Express)				
Alfredo	1 entrée	373	33	18.5
chow mein	1 entrée	260	43	4.0
Mandarin	1 entrée	270	41	6.0
Oriental	1 entrée	370	55	12.0
stir-fry, w/rice and vegetables, frozen	1 entrée	270	40	7.4
w/vegetables and rice	1 entrée	340	45	11.0
(Manor House) fried, assorted pieces	3 oz	270	13	18.0
(Marie Callender's)				
and noodles	13 oz	520	42	30.0
and noodles, escalloped, frozen	1 pkg	629	61	33.6
and noodles, escalloped, frozen	1 cup	397	38	21.2
and noodles, escalloped, frozen	1 serving	292	28	15.6
chicken and dumplings	1 cup	250	22	12.0
cordon bleu	13 oz	590	58	25.0
country fried, w/gravy	16 oz	620	63	30.0
grilled, in mushroom sauce	14 oz	480	54	15.0
grilled, w/rice pilaf	11.7 oz	360	38	14.0
herb roasted, w/mashed potatoes	14 oz	670	32	31.0
Marsala	14 oz	450	42	17.0
parmigiana, breaded	16 oz	620	63	27.0
pot pie	1 pie	600	53	37.0
pot pie, au gratin	1 pie	690	50	46.0
pot pie, frozen	1 pkg	999	88	61.1
pot pie, frozen	1 serving	501	44	30.6
pot pie, w/broccoli	1 pie	670	54	43.0
sweet and sour	14 oz	530	86	9.0

Food Name	Serv. Size	Total Cal.	Carbs GMS	Fat GMS
(Michelina's)				
primavera, w/spirals, 'Lean 'n Tasty'	1 entrée	250	32	7.0
teriyaki, w/rice 'Lean 'n Tasty'	1 entrée	290	65	3.0
(Mrs. Paterson's) pie, hand held pie, frozen, 'Aussie Pie'	1 serving	434	40	24.0
(Mountain House) stew, freeze-dried, prepared	1 cup	230	30	8.0
(Myers)				
à la king, frozen	3.5 oz	137	6	9.0
and noodles, frozen	3.5 oz	136	9	8.0
creamed, frozen	3.5 oz	151	5	10.0
croquettes, frozen	3.5 oz	168	10	7.0
frozen, à la gratin, frozen	3.5 oz	129	9	7.0
pie, frozen	3.5 oz	129	10	7.0
(Pierre)				
barbecue, frozen, 'Chix-B-Q' product 9845	1 piece	137	6	5.8
breaded, frozen, 'Two-Fers' product 1870	1 piece	92	4	6.5
breast, breaded, frozen, cooked, product 1881	1 piece	95	3	6.6
breast patty, fillet-shaped, flame-broiled, 'Caboose' product 9863	1 piece	121	3	5.4
breast patty, fillet-shaped, flame-broiled, product 9820	1 piece	157	4	6.0
breast patty, fillet-shaped, flame-broiled, product 9916	1 piece	152	4	6.3
breast patty, mesquite, fillet-shaped, flame-broiled, product 9816	1 piece	149	1	7.4
nuggets, breaded, frozen, product 3800	1 piece	47	2	3.3
patty, breaded, frozen, product 1915	1 piece	185	7	13.1
patty, cutlet-shaped, flame-broiled, frozen, product 9835	1 piece	145	4	6.2
patty, cutlet-shaped, honey mustard, flame-broiled, frozen, product 9852	1 piece	167	8	7.1
patty, cutlet-shaped, mesquite, flame-broiled, frozen, product 9805	1 piece	138	1	6.3
patty, cutlet-shaped, rotisserie style, flame-broiled, frozen, product 9878	1 piece	133	2	5.7
patty, cutlet-shaped, teriyaki sauce, flame-broiled, frozen, product 9829	1 piece	165	7	6.7
patty, fillet-shaped, flame-broiled, frozen, product 9840	1 piece	123	3	5.8
(Pilgrim's Pride)				
Cajun style, frozen	3 oz	241	9	17.0
primavera, frozen	3 oz	183	8	10.4
(Pillsbury)				
casserole, frozen, 'Microwave Classic'	1 pkg	400	30	22.0
w/cheese, casserole, 'Microwave Classic'	1 pkg	480	33	29.0
(Redi-Serve) nuggets, white meat, breaded and cooked	6 nibblers	270	17	16.0
(Rice A Roni)				
w/mushrooms, rice	2.5 oz	203	29	7.9
w/vegetable rice	2.5 oz	164	29	4.0
(Right Course)				
primavera, sesame, frozen	10 oz	320	34	9.0
tenderloins, barbecue, w/sauce, frozen	8.75 oz	270	35	6.0
tenderloins, in peanut sauce, frozen	9.25 oz	330	32	10.0
(Shanghai) stir-fry, frozen	10.3 oz	190	19	3.0
(Shelton's)				
pie, white flour	1 serving	230	18	10.0
pie, whole wheat	1 serving	230	18	10.0
(Smart Ones)				
à l'orange, frozen	8 oz	190	34	1.0
chow mein	1 entrée	200	34	2.0
chow mein, frozen	9 oz	170	27	1.0
fiesta	1 entrée	220	38	2.0

Food Name	Serv. Size	Total Cal.	Carbs GMS	Fat GMS
Francais, w/garlic vegetables, frozen	8.5 oz	150	18	1.0
grilled, glazed, w/sauce, frozen	8 oz	130	17	1.0
honey mustard	1 entrée	200	33	2.0
honey mustard, w/sauce, frozen	7.5 oz	140	20	1.0
Marsala	1 entrée	150	22	2.0
Mexican, w/Spanish rice, frozen, 'Fiesta'	8 oz	210	37	1.0
Mexican style, w/rice, frozen, 'Monterey'	1 pkg	410	35	20.0
Mirabella	1 entrée	170	26	2.0
picatta	1 entrée	190	34	2.0
Szechwan style, spicy, w/vegetables	1 entrée	220	39	2.0
(Stouffer's)				
à la king	1 entrée	320	43	10.0
à la king, w/rice, frozen	9.5-oz pkg	270	38	5.0
and dumplings, frozen, food service product	1 oz	39	3	2.3
and noodles, escalloped	1 entrée	450	32	28.0
and noodles, escalloped, frozen	1 entrée	365	4	31.4
and noodles, escalloped, frozen, food service product	1 oz	42	3	2.5
and noodles, 'Homestyle'	1 entrée	300	25	13.0
and vegetables, w/cream sauce, frozen	1 oz	31	2	2.0
baked, w/mashed potatoes, 'Homestyle'	1 entrée	270	19	12.0
chow mein, w/rice, frozen	10 3/4 oz pkg	250	39	5.0
creamed	1 entrée	280	8	20.0
creamed, frozen, food service product	1 oz	46	1	3.7
divan, frozen.	8-oz pkg	220	11	10.0
fried, w/mashed potatoes, 'Homestyle'	1 entrée	330	29	16.0
grilled, homestyle, w/BBQ sauce, frozen	7 5/8 oz	210	14	7.0
Monterey, w/Mexican rice, homestyle, food service product	1 entrée	410	35	20.0
noodle, homestyle, frozen, food service product	1 oz	31	2	1.6
parmigiana, w/pasta Alfredo, homestyle, frozen	9 7/8 oz	360	24	15.0
parmigiana, w/spaghetti, 'Homestyle'	1 entrée	320	30	10.0
pie, frozen	1 entrée	572	37	37.1
tenders, breaded, w/potatoes, homestyle	8 3/8 oz	430	46	18.0
w/dumplings, in broth, frozen, food service product	1 oz	26	2	1.1
(Swanson)				
à la king, canned	1 cup	320	17	22.0
à la king, canned	5.25 oz	190	9	12.0
and dumplings, canned	1 cup	260	22	13.0
boneless, 'Hungry Man'	1 entrée	630	80	22.0
cacciatore, frozen, 'Homestyle Recipe'	10.95 oz	260	33	8.0
fried, barbecue flavored, frozen	10 oz	540	61	22.0
fried, dark meat	1 entrée	580	54	30.0
fried, dark meat, 'Hungry Man'	1 entrée	780	74	39.0
fried, mostly white meat, 'Hungry Man'	1 entrée	800	79	39.0
fried, white meat	1 entrée	630	62	31.0
grilled, white meat, w/garlic sauce, almonds	10 oz	310	39	9.0
nibbles, frozen, 'Homestyle Recipe'	4.25 oz	340	29	20.0
nibbles, 'Plump and Juicy'	3.25 oz	300	19	19.0
nuggets, 'Plump and Juicy'	3 oz	230	14	14.0
nuggets, fried	1 entrée	590	71	25.0
nuggets, frozen	8.75 oz	470	47	23.0
parmigiana, frozen, 'Budget'	10 oz	300	35	15.0
pie, frozen, 'Homestyle Recipe'	8 oz	410	41	21.0
pot pie	1 pie	410	43	22.0
pot pie, 'Hungry Man'	1 pie	650	64	35.0
stew, canned	1 cup	180	17	8.0
(Sweet Sue)				
and dumplings, canned	1 pkg	620	65	21.1

Food Name	Serv. Size	Total Cal.	Carbs GMS	Fat GMS
chicken and dumplings, canned	1 serving	218	23	7.4
(Swift)				
cordon bleu, frozen, 'International'	6 oz	360	23	17.0
Kiev, frozen, 'International'	6 oz	420	22	24.0
(Top Shelf)				
à la king, packaged	10 oz	360	49	10.0
Acapulco, packaged	1 serving	390	41	13.0
cacciatore, packaged	10 oz	210	25	3.0
glazed, packaged	10 oz	170	19	2.0
sweet and sour, packaged	1 serving	270	41	1.0
w/Spanish rice, packaged	10 oz	400	38	15.0
(Tyson)				
à l'orange, 'Gourmet Selection' frozen	9.5 oz	300	36	8.0
barbecue, frozen	12.5 oz	400	56	8.0
barbecue, glazed, frozen, 'Yosemite Sam'	7.38 oz	230	28	8.0
barbecue, w/potato and vegetable medley	1 entrée	560	73	21.0
blackened, w/Spanish rice and corn	1 entrée	260	36	5.0
breast patty, breaded	1 piece	80	9	0.0
breast patty, breaded, Southern fried	1 entrée	180	8	12.0
chunks, frozen, 'Chick'n Chunks'	2.6 oz	220	11	15.0
chunks, frozen, 'Looney Tunes Bugs Bunny'	7.7 oz	290	31	11.0
chunks, Southern fried 'Chick'n Chunks'	2.6 oz	220	11	15.0
cordon bleu, wholesale club item, 'Mini Cordon Bleu'	1 piece	90	5	4.0
cordon bleu, wholesale club item, frozen	7 oz	480	28	22.0
divan, w/candied carrots and pasta	1 entrée	370	38	15.0
drummettes, frozen, 'Tazmanian Devil'	8 oz	310	31	14.0
drumsticks, roasted, w/skin	3 med pieces	330	1	18.0
Francais, frozen, 'Gourmet Selection'	9.5 oz	280	20	14.0
fried, w/mashed potatoes, gravy, corn	1 entrée	360	30	15.0
glazed, w/sauce 'Gourmet Selections'	9.25 oz	240	29	4.0
grilled, w/corn O'Brien and ranch beans	1 entrée	230	30	4.0
grilled, w/Italian style w/pasta and vegetable medley	1 entrée	190	19	3.5
'Herb Chicken Meal' frozen	13.75 oz	340	43	4.0
honey Dijon, w/pasta and peas	1 entrée	340	49	7.0
'Honey Mustard Chicken Meal' frozen	13.75 oz	390	52	6.0
honey roasted, frozen, 'Gourmet Selections'	9 oz	220	23	4.0
Italian, grilled, 'Gourmet Selections'	9 oz	210	19	3.0
'Italian Style Chicken Meal' frozen	13.75 oz	310	38	4.0
Kiev, w/rice pilaf, broccoli, carrots	1 entrée	440	36	25.0
'Looney Tunes Road Runner' frozen	6.7 oz	300	42	11.0
marinara, frozen	13.75 oz	340	37	7.0
Marsala, w/carrots and red potatoes	1 entrée	180	19	5.0
mesquite breast tenders, boneless, frozen	2.75 oz	110	4	3.0
mesquite, w/barbecue sauce, corn, potato	1 entrée	321	45	7.8
mesquite, w/corn, pea, and au gratin	1 entrée	320	44	8.0
'Mesquite Chicken Meal' frozen	13.25 oz	330	38	5.0
nuggets, frozen, 'Microwave'	3.5 oz	220	11	15.0
Oriental, breast strips, boneless, frozen	2.75 oz	110	6	3.0
Oriental, frozen, 'Gourmet Selection'	10.25 oz	270	32	7.0
parmigiana, frozen, 'Gourmet Selection'	11.25 oz	380	37	17.0
picatta, w/broccoli and parslied potatoes	1 entrée	190	18	6.0
pie, premium, frozen	9 oz	390	36	20.0
pie, white meat, premium, frozen	9 oz	400	33	20.0
primavera	1 entrée	350	48	6.0
roasted, frozen, 'Gourmet Selections'	9 oz	200	21	2.0
roasted, w/garlic sauce, pasta, vegetable	1 entrée	214	22	6.7
'Salsa Chicken Meal' frozen	13.75 oz	370	52	6.0

Food Name	Serv. Size	Total Cal.	Carbs GMS	Fat GMS
sesame, frozen, 'Healthy Portions'	13.5 oz	390	58	5.0
stir-fry, w/vegetable, frozen, wholesale club item	3.5 oz	130	13	5.0
supreme, frozen, 'Gourmet Selections'	9 oz	230	23	6.0
sweet and sour, frozen, 'Gourmet Selection'	11 oz	420	50	15.0
tabasco barbecue	1 entrée	260	37	7.0
tenders, frozen 'Microwave'	3.5 oz	230	19	11.0
w/cheddar, boneless, 'Chick'n Cheddar'	2.6 oz	220	11	15.0
wholesale club item, 'Classic Colonial'	3.5 oz	180	11	9.0
wings, hot, wholesale club item, frozen 'Wings of Fire'	3.5 oz	220	2	12.0
wings, teriyaki style	4 pieces	190	2	12.0
(Ultra Slim-Fast)				
and vegetables	12 oz	290	45	3.0
chow mein	12 oz	320	43	6.0
in mushroom sauce	12 oz	280	30	6.0
mesquite	12 oz	350	61	1.0
sweet and sour, frozen	12 oz	330	57	2.0
(Weaver)				
'Honey Batter Tenders' frozen	3 oz	220	14	12.0
'Italian Rondolet' frozen	2.6 oz	190	11	11.0
'Original Rondolet' frozen	3 oz	190	13	10.0
'Premium Tenders' frozen	3 oz	170	11	9.0
assorted pieces, frozen, 'Crispy Dutch Frye'	3.6 oz	290	16	18.0
breast, frozen 'Crispy Dutch Frye'	4.5 oz	350	17	22.0
crispy, light, skinless, frozen	2.9 oz	170	9	9.0
croquettes, frozen	2 pieces	280	22	16.0
frozen, 'Cheese Rondolet'	2.6 oz	190	12	11.0
mini drums, herb and spice, frozen	3 oz	200	13	11.0
mini-drums, crispy, frozen	3 oz	210	13	12.0
(Weight Watchers)				
barbecue glazed	1 entrée	230	33	2.5
barbecue, glazed, w/vegetables, frozen, 'Ultimate 200'	7 oz	200	22	6.0
barbecue, w/sauce, mixed vegetables, frozen, 'Ultimate 200'	1 serving	217	26	4.4
cordon bleu	1 entrée	230	31	4.5
cordon bleu, w/vegetables, frozen, 'Ultimate 200'	7.7 oz	170	15	5.0
divan, w/baked potato, frozen	11.25 oz	280	38	7.0
glazed	1 entrée	240	29	6.0
grilled, glazed, frozen, 'Ultimate 200'	7.5 oz	150	17	2.0
grilled, w/Spanish rice, frozen, 'Suiza'	8.6 oz	220	18	7.0
Hunan, w/vegetables, frozen, 'Stir Fry'	9 oz	160	21	2.0
imperial, frozen, 'Ultimate 200'	8.5 oz	200	25	3.0
Kiev, w/vegetables, rice, frozen, 'Ultimate 200'	7 oz	190	22	5.0
orange glazed, w/rice, frozen, 'Stir Fry'	9 oz	170	25	2.0
parmigiana	1 entrée	310	39	7.0
patty, Southern baked, w/vegetables, frozen, 'Ultimate 200'	6.3 oz	170	10	7.0
Polynesian, frozen, 'Stir Fry'	9 oz	190	34	1.0
sesame, w/lo mein noodles, frozen, 'Stir Fry'	9 oz	200	23	4.0
teriyaki, frozen, 'Ultimate 200'	7.6 oz	150	7	4.0
teriyaki, w/spring vegetables, frozen, 'Stir Fry'	9 oz	140	16	3.0
w/Spanish rice, frozen 'TexMex'	8.3 oz	250	33	5.0
(Wonderbites)				
barbecue, flame-broiled, frozen, 'Dippers'	1 piece	41	2	1.7
breast, flame-broiled, frozen, 'Dippers'	1 piece	35	1	1.5
Buffalo flavored, flame-broiled, frozen, 'Dippers'	1 piece	33	1	1.5
chili salsa, breaded, frozen, 'Dippers'	1 piece	69	3	4.8
flame-broiled, frozen, 'Dippers'	1 piece	35	1	1.5
honey mustard, flame-broiled, frozen, 'Dippers'	1 piece	40	2	1.6
Italian, flame-broiled, frozen, 'Dippers'	1 piece	33	0	1.4

Food Name	Serv. Size	Total Cal.	Carbs GMS	Fat GMS
rotisserie style, flame-broiled, frozen, 'Dippers' product 9896 .... 1 piece		34	0	1.4
teriyaki, flame broiled, frozen, 'Dippers' product 3727 .... 1 piece		45	2	2.3
teriyaki, flame broiled, frozen, 'Dippers' product 3827 .... 1 piece		45	2	2.4
teriyaki, flame-broiled, frozen, 'Dippers' product 9879 .... 1 piece		41	2	1.7
(Yu Sing)				
lo mein, frozen .... 1 container		230	35	5.0
sweet and sour, w/rice .... 1 container		300	50	6.0
w/almonds, w/rice, frozen .... 1 container		250	33	8.0
CHICKEN DINNER/ENTRÉE MIX				
(Chicken Helper)				
cheesy broccoli, 'Skillet' dry .... 1/5 pkg		160	32	2.0
cheesy broccoli, 'Skillet' prepared .... 7 oz		310	34	9.0
stir-fry, 'Skillet' mix only .... 1/5 pkg		170	36	1.0
stir-fry, 'Skillet' prepared .... 7 oz		370	36	14.0
creamy, 'Skillet' mix only .... 1/5 pkg		170	26	5.0
creamy, 'Skillet' prepared .... 8.25 oz		330	29	13.0
fettuccini Alfredo, 'Skillet' mix only .... 1/5 pkg		160	25	4.0
fettuccini Alfredo, 'Skillet' prepared .... 7.5 oz		320	27	12.0
creamy mushroom, 'Skillet' mix only .... 1/5 pkg		170	28	4.0
creamy mushroom, 'Skillet' prepared .... 8 oz		320	31	11.0
(Lipton)				
barbecue, 'Microeasy' mix only .... 1/4 pkg		110	24	1.0
barbecue, 'Microeasy' prepared .... 1/4 pkg		220	24	6.0
country style, 'Microeasy' mix only .... 1/4 pkg		80	15	1.0
country style, 'Microeasy' prepared .... 1/4 pkg		190	15	6.0
(Skillet Chicken Helper) stir-fried .... 1/4 cup		140	30	0.5
CHICKEN FAT				
.... 1 cup		1846	0.0	204.6
.... 1 oz		178	0.0	19.3
.... 1 tbsp		115	0.0	12.8
kosher, retail rendered (Empire Kosher) .... 1 tbsp		120	1	13.0
CHICKEN SALAD SPREAD				
(Libby's) 'Spreadables' .... 1 pkg		329	23	21.3
(Libby's) 'Spreadables' .... 1/3 cup		140	7	9.0
(Libby's) 'Spreadables' .... 1 serving		171	12	11.1
CHICKEN SEASONING. See under SEASONING MIX.				
CHICKEN SEASONING AND COATING MIX. See under SEASONING AND COATING MIX.				
CHICKEN SPREAD				
(Hormel) canned .... 0.5 oz		30	0	2.0
(Underwood) canned, chunky .... 2 1/8 oz		150	2	9.0
(Underwood) canned, 'Light' .... 2 1/8 oz		80	2	3.0
(Underwood) canned, smoky .... 2 1/8 oz		150	10	8.0
CHICKEN SUBSTITUTE				
(Heartline)				
vegetarian, 'Chicken Fillet Style' .... 2 oz		176	9	7.0
vegetarian, lite, 'Chicken Fillet Style' .... 0.5 oz		22	1	0.0
(Morningstar Farms)				
nuggets, vegetarian, 'Chik Nuggets' .... 4 nuggets		160	17	4.0
nuggets, vegetarian, homestyle, frozen, 'Country Crisps' .... 3 oz		250	18	16.0
nuggets, vegetarian, zesty, frozen, 'Country Crisps' .... 3 oz		280	17	19.0
patty, vegetarian, 'Chik Patty' .... 1 patty		177	15	9.8
patty, vegetarian, frozen, 'Country Crisps' .... 2.5 oz		220	13	15.0
vegetarian, 'Meatless Chicken' .... 1 patty		170	13	10.0
(Worthington)				
chicken style, vegetarian .... 1 slice		86	1	4.6
diced, vegetarian, 'Diced Chik' .... 1/4 cup drained		40	1	0.0
diced, vegetarian, frozen, 5-lb pkg 'Meatless Chicken' .... 1/4 cup		50	2	0.0

Food Name	Serv. Size	Total Cal.	Carbs GMS	Fat GMS
nuggets, vegetarian, 'Chik Stiks'	1 serving	111	3	7.3
pie, vegetarian, frozen	8 oz	380	43	20.0
roll, vegetarian, 4-lb pkg, 'Meatless Chicken'	3/8-inch slice	80	1	4.5
roll, vegetarian, frozen, 'Meatless Chicken'	2.5 oz	150	4	10.0
sliced, vegetarian, 'Chic-Ketts'	2 3/8-inch slices	120	2	7.0
sliced, vegetarian, 'Sliced Chik'	3 slices	70	2	0.5
slices, vegetarian, 8-oz pkg, 'Meatless Chicken'	2 slices	80	1	4.5
slices, vegetarian, frozen, 'Meatless Chicken' 2 oz	2 slices	130	3	9.0
vegetarian, 'Chic-Ketts'	1 slice	121	2	6.5
vegetarian, diced, canned drained	1/4 cup	90	2	8.0
vegetarian, diced, frozen, 'Meatless Chicken'	1/2 cup	190	5	13.0
vegetarian, frozen, 'Crispy Chik'	3 oz	280	17	19.0
vegetarian, sliced, canned, drained, 2.1 oz	2 slices	90	2	8.0

CHICKEN SUBSTITUTE DINNER/ENTRÉE
(Loma Linda)

croquette, loaf, or patty, vegetarian, dry mix, 'Chicken Supreme'	1/3 cup	90	6	1.0
fried chicken style, vegetarian, 'Fried Chik'n with Gravy'	2 pieces	160	4	10.0
nuggets, vegetarian, 'Meatless Chik-Nuggets'	5 pieces	240	13	16.0

(Morningstar Farms)

wings, vegetarian, 'Meat-Free Buffalo Wings'	5 nuggets	200	16	9.0

(Worthington)

croquettes, vegetarian, 'Golden Croquettes'	4 pieces	210	14	10.0
drumsticks, vegetarian, 'Chik Stiks'	1 piece	110	3	7.0
fried chicken style, vegetarian, 'FriChik'	2 pieces	120	1	8.0
fried chicken style, vegetarian, low-fat, 'Low Fat FriChik'	2 pieces	80	21	1.0
patties, vegetarian, lightly breaded, seasoned, 'Crispy Chik Patties'	1 pattie	150	15	6.0

CHICKPEA/ceci/garbanzo
Canned

	1 cup	286	54	2.7
(A&P)	1/2 cup	100	17	1.0
(Allens)	1/2 cup	110	18	1.0
(Bush's Best)	1/2 cup	80	21	0.0
(Finast)	8 oz	210	35	3.0
(Green Giant)	1/2 cup	90	18	2.0
(Old El Paso)	1/2 cup	190	16	1.0
(Progresso)	1/2 cup	110	22	1.0
'Nutradiet' *(S&W)*	1/2 cup	100	19	1.0
dry beans in brine *(Green Giant)*	1/2 cup	110	18	1.5
50% less salt *(Green Giant)*	1/2 cup	90	18	2.0
50% less salt *(Joan of Arc)*	1/2 cup	90	18	2.0
large 'Lite 50% Less Salt' *(S&W)*	1/2 cup	110	21	1.0
organic, no salt added *(Eden Foods)*	1/2 cup	90	17	1.0
organic, w/liquid *(Eden Foods)*	1/2 cup	110	17	2.0

Fresh

mature seed, boiled	1 cup	269	45	4.2
mature seed, raw	1 cup	728	121	12.1
mature seed, raw	1 tbsp	46	8	0.8
raw *(Arrowhead Mills)*	2 oz	200	35	3.0
Jarred, organically grown *(Eden Foods)*	1/2 cup	110	20	1.0

CHICKPEA FLOUR. See under FLOUR.
CHICORY

trimmed	1 oz	7	1.3	0.1
trimmed, chopped	1/2 cup	21	4.2	0.3
untrimmed	1 lb	87	17.5	1.1

CHICORY, WITLOOF

raw	1/2 cup	8	1.8	0.0

Food Name	Serv. Size	Total Cal.	Carbs GMS	Fat GMS
raw, medium, approx 2.1 oz	1 head	9	2.1	0.1
trimmed	1 oz	4	0.9	<.1
untrimmed	1 lb	61	12.9	0.4
CHICORY ROOT				
raw, medium, approx 2.6 oz	1 root	44	10.5	0.1
raw, 1-inch pieces	1/2 cup	33	7.9	0.1
trimmed	1 oz	21	5.0	0.1
untrimmed	1 lb	272	65.1	0.7
CHILE PEPPER. See PEPPER, CHILI.				
CHILI				
(Armour)				
hot, w/beans, canned	7.5 oz	390	27	26.0
w/beans, canned	7.5 oz	390	27	26.0
w/beans, canned, 'Premium Lite'	7.5 oz	260	27	10.0
w/beans, microwave	7.5 oz	300	26	14.0
w/o beans, canned	7.5 oz	390	14	31.0
(Bearitos)				
black bean, low-fat, 'Premium'	1 cup	150	20	1.0
original, lowfat, 'Premium'	1 cup	190	36	1.0
spicy, lowfat, 'Premium'	1 cup	190	36	1.0
(Chef Boyardee)				
beef, w/beans, canned	7.5 oz	330	30	17.0
'Chili Mac' canned	7.5 oz	230	26	11.0
(Chili Bowl) homestyle	1 cup	680	12	59.0
(Cimmaron)				
beef, w/beans, canned	7.5 oz	230	21	9.0
chicken, w/beans, canned	7.5 oz	180	22	5.0
(Dennison's)				
chunky, w/beans, canned	7.5 oz	310	28	14.0
hot, w/beans, 15-oz can	7.5 oz	310	26	16.0
w/beans, 15-oz can	7.5 oz	310	27	15.0
'Cook-Off' w/beans, canned	7.5 oz	340	25	19.0
w/o beans, 15-oz can	7.5 oz	300	15	19.0
(El Rio)				
con carne, w/o beans, canned	1 pkg	497	26	32.7
con carne, w/o beans, canned	1 serving	305	16	20.1
(Estee) w/beans, canned	7.5 oz	370	27	20.0
(Featherweight) w/beans, canned	7.5 oz	280	29	10.0
(Gebhardt)				
hot, w/beans, canned	1 cup	470	47	27.0
hot, w/beans, canned	4 oz	189	9	14.2
longhorn, w/beans	1 cup	450	32	31.4
plain	1 cup	412	15	30.4
plain, w/o beans	1 cup	530	20	41.0
vegetarian, canned	4 oz	219	7	17.1
w/beans	1 cup	322	32	14.9
(Hain)				
w/chicken, canned	7.5 oz	130	19	2.0
spicy Tempeh, vegetarian, canned	7.5 oz	160	24	4.0
vegetarian, spicy, canned	7.5 oz	160	29	1.0
vegetarian, spicy, canned, 'Reduced Sodium'	7.5 oz	170	31	1.0
(Health Valley)				
three-bean, vegetarian, mild, fat-free	5 oz	90	12	0.0
w/beans, vegetarian, mild, canned, 'No Salt Added'	4 oz	130	16	3.0
w/beans, vegetarian, spicy, canned, 'No Salt Added'	4 oz	130	16	3.0
w/black beans, vegetarian, mild, fat-free	5 oz	140	23	0.0
w/black beans, vegetarian, spicy, canned	5 oz	70	9	0.0

Food Name	Serv. Size	Total Cal.	Carbs GMS	Fat GMS
w/lentils, vegetarian, mild, 'No Salt Added'	4 oz	130	16	3.0
w/lentils, vegetarian, mild, canned	4 oz	130	16	3.0
(Heinz)				
'Chili Con Carne' canned	7.75 oz	350	27	21.0
'Chili Mac' canned	7.5 oz	250	26	12.0
hot, w/beans, canned	7.75 oz	330	30	16.0
(Hormel)				
'Chili Mac' microwave	7.5 oz	192	18	9.0
chunky, w/beans, canned	7.5 oz	290	25	14.0
hot, w/beans, 15-oz can	7.5 oz	310	24	16.0
hot, w/beans, microwave	7.38 oz	250	24	11.0
hot, w/o beans, 15-oz can	7.5 oz	370	12	28.0
microwave	1 cup	220	27	6.0
turkey, w/beans, canned	1 cup	203	26	2.8
vegetarian, w/beans, canned	1 cup	205	38	0.7
w/beans, canned	1 cup	240	34	4.4
w/beans, 15-oz can	7.5 oz	310	23	17.0
w/beans, 40-oz can	8 oz	320	25	17.0
w/beans, microwave	7.5 oz	250	23	11.0
w/o beans, canned	10.5 oz	540	19	41.0
w/o beans, canned	1 cup	194	18	6.6
w/o beans, 15-oz can	7.5 oz	370	12	28.0
w/o beans, microwave	7.38 oz	290	15	17.0
(Just Rite)				
hot, w/beans, hot, canned	4 oz	195	16	10.0
vegetarian, w/beans, canned	4.55 oz	190	15	13.3
w/beans, canned	4 oz	200	16	11.0
w/o beans, canned	4 oz	180	9	11.0
(Lean Cuisine) 3-bean, frozen, food service product	1/2 cup	80	12	2.0
(Legume) chicken style, vegetarian	1 cup	160	29	1.0
(Libby's)				
w/beans, 15-oz can	7.5 oz	270	25	13.0
w/beans, microwave, 'Diner'	7.75 oz	280	29	12.0
w/o beans, canned	7.5 oz	390	11	30.0
(Luck's) hot, w/pinto beans	1/2 cup	120	20	1.0
(Lunch Bucket) w/beans, microwave	7.5 oz	300	26	14.0
(Marie Callender's) w/cornbread	1 cup	350	45	13.0
(Michelina's) black bean, 'Lean 'n Tasty'	1 entrée	400	77	5.0
(Mountain House)				
w/beans, freeze-dried, prepared	1 cup	390	38	16.0
w/beef, freeze-dried, prepared	1 cup	250	31	8.0
(Nalley's)				
chunky, w/o beans, canned, 'Big Chunk'	7.5 oz	270	14	16.0
con carne, w/beans, canned	1 serving	281	12	8.0
hot jalapeño, w/beans, canned	7.5 oz	260	29	10.0
hot, w/beans, canned	7.5 oz	280	30	10.0
w/beans	7.5 oz	260	27	9.0
w/beans, canned, 'Thick'	7.5 oz	260	29	9.0
(Natural Touch)				
vegetarian, 'Low Fat Vegetarian Chili'	1 cup	170	21	1.0
vegetarian, spicy, canned	2/3 cup	230	19	12.0
(Nestlé)				
spicy, w/beans, canned, 'Chef Mate'	1 cup	423	33	24.7
w/beans, canned 'Chef Mate'	1 cup	412	29	25.0
w/o beans, canned, 'Chef Mate'	1 cup	430	18	31.6
(Norpac) w/beans, vegetarian, lowfat. 'Soup Supreme'	1 cup	130	27	1.0
(Old El Paso)	1 serving	249	22	10.3

Food Name	Serv. Size	Total Cal.	Carbs GMS	Fat GMS
(Open Range)				
vegetarian, plain, canned	4.41 oz	176	9	12.8
vegetarian, w/beans, canned	4.5 oz	136	13	8.0
w/beans, food service product	1 cup	281	25	16.0
w/o beans, food service product	1 cup	353	19	25.6
(Right Course) vegetarian, frozen	9.75 oz	280	45	7.0
(Shelton's)				
chicken, mild or spicy	1 cup	210	26	3.0
turkey, mild or spicy	1 cup	210	26	4.0
(Stagg)				
chicken, w/beans, canned	7.5 oz	200	21	6.0
chicken, w/beans, canned, 'Ranch House'	7.5 oz	210	26	5.0
country, w/beans, canned	7.5 oz	270	25	12.0
w/beans, canned, 'Chunkero'	1 cup	330	28	15.0
w/beans, canned, 'Classic'	1 cup	324	29	16.3
w/beans, canned, 'Country'	1 cup	319	29	15.8
w/beans, canned, 'Dynamite'	1 cup	333	31	15.4
w/beans, canned, 'Laredo'	7.5 oz	260	22	12.0
w/beans, canned, 'Ranchhouse'	1 cup	284	32	8.9
w/beans, canned, 'Silverado'	1 cup	227	33	2.8
w/o beans, canned, 'Steak House'	7.5 oz	300	17	19.0
(Stouffer's)				
con carne, w/beans, frozen	8.75 oz	280	28	10.0
con carne, w/beans, frozen, food service product	4 oz	128	12	4.8
w/beans	1 entrée	270	29	10.0
(Swanson) con carne, frozen, 'Homestyle Recipe'	8.25 oz	270	26	10.0
(Top Shelf) con carne suprema, packaged	1 serving	320	30	12.0
(Tyson) chicken, frozen, wholesale club item	3.5 oz	105	11	3.0
(Van Camp's)				
w/beans, canned	1 cup	352	21	23.2
w/franks, w/o beans, canned, 'ChileeWeenee'	1 cup	309	28	15.7
w/o beans, canned	1 cup	412	12	33.5
(Wolf Brand)				
extra spicy, w/beans, canned	7.75 oz	324	21	20.6
extra spicy, w/o beans, canned	7.5 oz	363	15	24.9
w/beans, canned	8 oz	345	22	22.0
w/o beans, canned	8 oz	387	16	26.6
w/o beans, canned, 'Chili-Mac'	7.75 oz	317	23	19.9
(Worthington)				
vegetarian, 'Chili'	1 cup	290	21	15.0
vegetarian, 'Low Fat Chili'	1 cup	170	21	1.0
CHILI BEANS. See BEANS, CHILI.				
CHILI MIX				
(Gebhardt) 'Chili Quik' mix only	1.5 oz pkt	82	17	1.1
(Mountain House)				
w/beans, freeze-dried, prepared	1 cup	390	38	16.0
w/beef, freeze-dried, 'Chili Mac' prepared	1 cup	250	31	8.0
(Old El Paso)				
'Chili con Carne' prepared	1 cup	162	8	7.0
w/beans, prepared	1 cup	217	17	10.0
CHILI PEPPER. See PEPPER, CHILI. See also under PEPPER, GROUND.				
CHILI POWDER. See under SEASONING MIX.				
CHILI SEASONING. See under SEASONING MIX.				
CHIMICHANGA				
(Banquet)	1 entrée	500	56	24.0
(Fiesta Cafe) beef and bean, frozen	1 serving	422	56	11.6
(Marquez) shredded beef 'Primera'	1 chimichanga	380	42	17.0

Food Name	Serv. Size	Total Cal.	Carbs GMS	Fat GMS
(Old El Paso)				
bean and cheese, frozen	1 pkg	380	40	19.0
beef, frozen	1 piece	370	34	21.0
beef and cheese, frozen, 'Festive Dinners'	11 oz	510	53	23.0
beef and pork, frozen	1 pkg	340	35	16.0
beef, frozen, 'Festive Dinners'	11 oz	540	65	21.0
chicken, frozen	1 piece	360	33	20.0
CHINESE APPLE. See POMEGRANATE.				
CHINESE BROCCOLI. See BROCCOLI, CHINESE.				
CHINESE CABBAGE. See BOK CHOY.				
CHINESE DATE				
dried	1 oz	81	20.1	0.3
raw, seeded	1 oz	22	5.7	0.1
raw, w/seeds	1 lb	331	85.3	0.8
CHINESE FUNGUS/Jew's ear/pepeao				
approx 0.2 oz	1 piece	2	0.4	(tr)
dried	1 cup	72	19	0.1
sliced	1/2 cup	13	3.3	(tr)
trimmed	1 oz	7	1.9	na
untrimmed	1 lb	111	30.0	0.2
CHINESE GOOSEBERRY. See KIWI FRUIT.				
CHINESE JUJUBE. See JUJUBE, CHINESE.				
CHINESE NOODLE. See under NOODLE.				
CHINESE PARSLEY LEAF. See CORIANDER LEAF.				
CHINESE PARSLEY SEED. See CORIANDER SEED.				
CHINESE PEA PODS. See PEAS, SNOW.				
CHINESE PEAR. See ASIAN PEAR.				
CHINESE RADISH. See DAIKON.				
CHINESE WATERMELON. See GOURD, WHITE.				
CHINESE YAM. See JICAMA.				
CHIVES				
Fresh				
raw	1 oz	7	1.1	0.2
raw, chopped	1 tbsp	1	0.1	0.0
raw, chopped	1 tsp	0	0.0	0.0
Dried *(McCormick/Schilling)*	1 tsp	1	0	0.0
Freeze-dried				
	1/4 cup	2	0.5	0.0
	1 tbsp	1	0.1	0.0
(McCormick/Schilling)	1 tsp	1	0	0.0
(Tone's)	1 tsp	1	0	0.0
CHOCOLATE. See CHOCOLATE, BAKING. See also under CANDY.				
CHOCOLATE, BAKING				
Bars				
bittersweet *(Ghirardelli)*	1 bar	551	63	39.3
dark, dark *(Ghirardelli)*	1 bar	570	68	38.0
semisweet *(Baker's)*	1/2 bar	70	8	4.5
semisweet *(Ghirardelli)*	1 bar	555	66	38.1
semisweet *(Nestlé)*	1 oz	160	16	9.0
semisweet, 'Premium' *(Hershey's)*	1 oz	140	16	8.0
unsweetened *(Baker's)*	1/2 bar	70	4	7.0
unsweetened *(Ghirardelli)*	1 serving	571	33	59.9
unsweetened *(Hershey's)*	1 oz	190	7	16.0
unsweetened *(Nestlé)*	1 oz	180	9	14.0
unsweetened, 'Premium' *(Hershey's)*	1 oz	190	7	16.0
white *(Baker's)*	1/2 bar	80	8	4.5

Food Name	Serv. Size	Total Cal.	Carbs GMS	Fat GMS
white, classic *(Ghirardelli)*	1 bar	627	66	39.5
white, 'Premier' *(Nestlé)*	1 oz	150	18	9.0
Chips				
less fat *(Hershey's)*	1 tbsp	60	10	3.5
milk chocolate *(Baker's)*	1/2 oz	70	9	4.0
milk chocolate *(Hershey's)*	1/4 cup	220	27	12.0
milk chocolate *(Hershey's)*	1 oz	150	27	12.0
milk chocolate *(Hershey's)*	1 tbsp	79	9	4.2
chips, milk chocolate, 'Big Chips' *(Baker's)*	1/4 cup	240	30	13.0
milk chocolate, 'Mini Baking Bits' *(M&M Mars)*	1 oz	142	20	6.6
mint chocolate *(Hershey's)*	1.5 oz	230	28	12.0
semisweet *(Baker's)*	1/2 oz	60	9	3.5
semisweet *(Hershey's)*	1.5 oz	220	27	12.0
semisweet, 'Big Chips' *(Baker's)*	1/4 cup	220	31	13.0
semisweet, mini, approx 1/4 cup *(Hershey's)*	1.5 oz	220	26	12.0
semisweet, 'Mini Baking Bits' *(M&M Mars)*	1 oz	146	18	7.4
white *(Hershey's)*	1.5 oz	240	25	14.0
Chunks				
milk chocolate *(Hershey's)*	12 pieces	160	16	9.0
semisweet *(Hershey's)*	1 oz	140	15	8.0
semisweet *(Saco Foods)*	12-oz bag	466	67	26.5
white, 'Premier Treasures' *(Nestlé)*	1 oz	160	15	10.0
Liquid, unsweetened, premelted, 'Choco Bake' *(Nestlé)*	1 oz	190	7	16.0
Shreds *(Tone's)*	1 tsp	21	2	1.4
Squares, Mexican	1 square	85	15	3.1
CHOCOLATE FLAVORED DRINK. See also CHOCOLATE MILK.				
(Frostee) canned	8 fl oz	200	30	8.0
(Yoo-Hoo)	9 fl oz	140	27	1.0
CHOCOLATE FLAVORED DRINK MIX				
(Butterfinger) Butterfinger flavored, w/vitamins A and D, prepared w/2% milk	8 fl oz	200	30	5.0
(Hershey's)				
'Hershey's Genuine' prepared	8 fl oz	150	28	2.0
'Hershey's Chocolate Milk Mix' mix only	3 heaping tsp	90	22	1.0
(Nestlé)				
chocolate raspberry truffle, prepared.	8 fl oz	180	23	2.0
classic chocolate chip, prepared.	8 fl oz	180	24	2.0
classic chocolate chip, mix only	1.13 oz	90	12	2.0
creamy milk chocolate, prepared.	8 fl oz	180	24	2.0
creamy milk chocolate, mix only	1.13 oz	90	12	2.0
dark chocolate fudge, mix only	1.13 oz	90	11	2.0
'Quik' prepared w/1 cup skim milk	8 fl oz	170	31	1.0
'Quik' prepared w/1 cup whole milk	8 fl oz	230	31	9.0
sugar-free, 'Quik' prepared w/1 cup 2% milk	8 fl oz	140	15	5.0
sugar-free, 'Quik' dry, mix only	1 heaping tsp	18	3	1.0
(Swiss Miss) 'Chocolate Milk Maker'	0.67 oz	73	17	0.3
(Weight Watchers) chocolate fudge shake mix	1 serving	80	12	1.0
CHOCOLATE MILK				
1% fat	1 quart	630	104	10.0
1% fat	1 cup	158	26	2.5
2% fat	1 quart	715	104	20.0
2% fat	1 cup	179	26	5.0
2% fat	1 fl oz	22	3	0.6
2% fat, vitamin A and D enriched *(Lucerne)*	1 cup	200	29	5.0
2% low-fat *(Darigold)*	1 cup	190	28	5.0
2% low-fat *(Hershey's)*	1 cup	190	29	5.0
2% low-fat, 'Dutch Brand' *(Borden)*	1 cup	180	25	5.0

Food Name	Serv. Size	Total Cal.	Carbs GMS	Fat GMS
3.5% fat *(Hershey's)*	1 cup	210	28	8.0
whole	1 quart	834	103	33.9
whole	1 cup	208	26	8.5
whole	1 fl oz	26	3	1.1
whole, ready to drink, 'Quik' *(Nestlé)*	1 cup	230	31	9.0
whole, vitamin D added *(Meadow Gold)*	1 cup	210	25	8.0
CHOCOLATE TOPPING. See also DESSERT TOPPING; FUDGE TOPPING.				
(Kraft)	2 tbsp	110	26	0.0
(Mrs. Richardson's)				
fudge, dark	2 tbsp	130	19	6.0
fudge, dark, microwaveable	2 tbsp	130	19	6.0
(Nestlé)				
milk, w/almonds, 'Candytops'	1.25 oz	230	14	18.0
milk, w/crisps, 'Crunch Candytops'	2 tbsp	220	16	17.0
white, w/almonds, 'Candytops'	1.25 oz	230	12	19.0
(Smucker's)				
dark, 'Special Recipe'	2 tbsp	130	31	1.0
fudge, 'Magic Shell'	2 tbsp	190	16	15.0
fudge, milk, Swiss	2 tbsp	140	31	1.0
'Magic Shell'	2 tbsp	190	16	15.0
nut, 'Magic Shell'	2 tbsp	200	25	16.0
CHOP SUEY SEASONING. See under SEASONING MIX.				
CHORIZO. See under SAUSAGE.				
CHOW MEIN SEASONING. See under SEASONING MIX.				
CHRYSANTEMUM LEAVES				
raw, whole	1 leaf	4	1	0.1
raw, chopped	1 cup	12	2	0.3
CHRYSANTHEMUM GARLAND				
boiled, drained, 1-inch pieces	1 cup	20	4	0.1
raw, 1-inch pieces	1 cup	5	1	0.0
raw, whole, approx 8.75-inch long	1 stem	3	1	0.0
CHUB/cisco				
raw	3 oz	83	0	1.6
smoked	3 oz	150	0	10.1
smoked	1 oz	50	0	3.4
CHURRO. See under PASTRY.				
CIDER				
APPLE				
(Alpine) spiced	8 fl oz	80	21	0.0
(Indian Summer) canned or bottled	6 fl oz	80	20	1.0
(Knudsen) and spice	8 fl oz	110	28	0.0
(Krusteaz) spiced	8 fl oz	16	4	0.0
(Lucky Leaf)				
canned or bottled	6 fl oz	90	21	0.0
sparkling, canned or bottled	6 fl oz	80	18	0.0
(Musselman's) canned or bottled	6 fl oz	90	21	0.0
(Tree Top) canned or frozen, prepared	6 fl oz	90	22	0.0
APPLE CHERRY *(Indian Summer)*	6 fl oz	100	25	1.0
APPLE CINNAMON *(Indian Summer)* canned or bottled	6 fl oz	90	21	1.0
APPLE CRANBERRY *(Indian Summer)*	6 fl oz	100	24	1.0
CHERRY				
(Knudsen)				
	8 fl oz	100	24	0.0
blend	8 fl oz	130	33	0.0
CIDER MIX				
APPLE				
spiced, instant *(Alpine)*	1 pouch	80	19	0.0

Food Name	Serv. Size	Total Cal.	Carbs GMS	Fat GMS
spiced, instant, sugar-free *(Alpine)*	1 pouch	15	4	0.0
(Swiss Miss)	0.78 oz	84	20	0.3
CILANTRO LEAF				
dried *(McCormick/Schilling)*	1 tsp	2	0	0.0
dried *(Tone's)*	1 tsp	2	0	0.1
raw, chopped	1 cup	11	2	0.2
raw, minced	1 tsp	0	0	0.0
CILANTRO SEED *(Spice Islands)*	1 tsp	6	1	0.3
CINNAMON				
ground	1 tbsp	18	5	0.2
ground	1 tsp	6	2	0.1
ground *(McCormick/Schilling)*	1 tsp	6	1	0.0
ground *(Spice Islands)*	1 tsp	6	1	0.1
ground *(Tone's)*	1 tsp	6	2	0.1
ground, fresh *(Durkee)*	1 tsp	8	0	0.0
ground, fresh *(Laurel Leaf)*	1 tsp	8	0	0.0
CISCO, RAW. See CHUB.				
CITRONELLA. See LEMONGRASS.				
CLAM				
Canned				
baby *(S&W)*	1/4 cup	50	2	1.5
baby, smoked *(S&W)*	2 oz	130	2	10.0
baby, smoked, in cottonseed oil *(Crown Prince)*	1/3 cup	90	2	5.0
chopped *(Gorton's)*	1/2 can	70	4	1.0
chopped *(Progresso)*	1/2 cup	70	2	1.0
chopped *(S&W)*	1/4 cup	20	1	0.0
chopped, w/liquid *(Doxsee)*	6.5 oz	100	8	1.0
chopped, w/liquid *(Orleans)*	6.5 oz	100	8	1.0
minced *(Gorton's)*	1/2 can	70	4	1.0
minced *(Progresso)*	1/2 cup	70	2	1.0
minced *(S&W)*	1/4 cup	20	1	0.0
minced, in clam juice *(Gorton's)*	1/4 cup	20	1	0.0
minced, w/liquid *(Doxsee)*	6.5 oz	100	8	1.0
minced, w/liquid *(Orleans)*	6.5 oz	100	8	1.0
mixed species, drained	1 cup	237	8	3.1
mixed species, drained	3 oz	126	4	1.7
Fresh				
mixed species, boiled or steamed	3 oz	126	4	1.7
mixed species, boiled or steamed, small	20 clams	281	10	3.7
mixed species, breaded, fried	3 oz	172	9	9.5
mixed species, breaded, fried, small	20 clams	380	19	21.0
mixed species, raw	3 oz	63	2	0.8
mixed species, raw, large	9 clams	133	5	1.7
mixed species, raw, large	1 clam	15	1	0.2
mixed species, raw, medium	1 clam	11	0	0.1
mixed species, raw, small	1 clam	7	0	0.1
CLAM DISH/ENTRÉE				
(Gorton's) 'Crunchy Clam Strips' microwave, 5.8-oz pkg	1/2 pkg	270	20	17.0
(Matlaw's) stuffed, New England style	2 clams	180	21	8.0
CLAM JUICE				
(Doxsee)	3 fl oz	4	0	0.0
(S&W)	9.6 fl oz	0	0	0.0
(Snow's)	3 fl oz	4	0	0.0
all natural *(Reese)*	1 tbsp	0	0	0.0
CLAM-TOMATO JUICE				
canned	5.5-oz can	80	18	0.3
canned	1 fl oz	14	3	0.1

Food Name	Serv. Size	Total Cal.	Carbs GMS	Fat GMS
CLARIFIED BUTTER. See GHEE.				
CLOUD EAR FUNGUS				
dried	1 cup	80	20	0.2
dried, whole	1 medium	13	3	0.0
CLOVES				
ground	1 tbsp	21	4	1.3
ground	1 tsp	7	1	0.4
ground (McCormick/Schilling)	1 tsp	5	1	0.3
ground (Spice Islands)	1 tsp	7	1	0.2
ground (Tone's)	1 tsp	7	1	0.4
ground, fresh (Durkee)	1 tsp	9	0	0.0
ground, fresh (Laurel Leaf)	1 tsp	9	0	0.0
COATING MIX. See SEASONING AND COATING MIX.				
COBBLER				
Fresh				
(Awrey's)				
apple, deep dish	1/8 cobbler	320	48	14.0
blueberry, deep dish	1/8 pie	310	45	14.0
Frozen				
(Pet-Ritz)				
apple, 4.33-oz pkg	1/6 pkg	290	50	9.0
blackberry, 4.33-oz pkg	1/6 pkg	250	39	10.0
blueberry, 4.33-oz pkg	1/6 pkg	370	50	12.0
cherry, 4.33-oz pkg	1/6 pkg	280	46	10.0
peach, 4.33-oz pkg	1/6 pkg	260	46	10.0
strawberry, 4.33-oz pkg	1/6 pkg	290	50	9.0
(Stilwell)				
apple, 'Deli'	1/8 cobbler	240	39	9.0
apple, light, 'Deli Lite'	1/8 cobbler	140	22	4.5
apple, 'Thrifty House'	1/22 cobbler	290	45	11.0
apricot	1/8 cobbler	240	39	9.0
berry, 'Festival of Berry'	1/8 cobbler	250	42	9.0
berry, light, 'Festival of Berry-Lite'	1/8 cobbler	140	22	4.5
blackberry, 'Deli'	1/8 cobbler	250	39	9.0
blackberry, light, 'Deli Lite'	1/8 cobbler	150	24	4.5
blackberry, 'Thrifty House'	1/22 cobbler	320	46	14.0
blueberry	1/18 cobbler	270	42	10.0
cherry, 'Deli'	1/8 cobbler	250	39	9.0
cherry, light, 'Deli Lite'	1/8 cobbler	150	24	4.5
cherry, 'Thrifty House'	1/22 cobbler	330	47	14.0
peach, 'Deli'	1/8 cobbler	240	38	9.0
peach, light, 'Deli Lite'	1/8 cobbler	140	22	4.5
peach, 'Thrifty House'	1/22 cobbler	300	43	12.0
pecan	1/6 cobbler	440	66	17.0
strawberry	1/8 cobbler	260	41	9.0
COBNUT. See HAZELNUT.				
COCA-COLA. See under SOFT DRINKS AND MIXERS.				
COCKTAIL. See also COCKTAIL MIX; LIQUEUR; SHERRY; VERMOUTH; WINE.				
DAIQUIRI				
canned	6.8 fl oz	259	32	0.0
canned	1 fl oz	38	5	0.0
PIÑA COLADA				
canned	6.8 fl oz	526	61	16.9
canned	1 fl oz	77	9	2.5
TEQUILA SUNRISE				
canned	6.8 fl oz	232	24	0.2
canned	1 fl oz	34	4	0.0

Food Name	Serv. Size	Total Cal.	Carbs GMS	Fat GMS
TOM COLLINS .... 1 fl oz		16	0.4	0.0
WHISKEY SOUR				
canned .... 6.8 fl oz		249	28	0.0
canned .... 1 fl oz		37	4	0.0
COCKTAIL MIX				
BLOODY MARY				
(Holland House) bottled 'Smooth 'N' Spicy' .... 1 fl oz		3	1	0.0
(Mr. & Mrs. T)				
bottled .... 4.5 fl oz		20	4	0.0
bottled, rich and spicy .... 4.5 fl oz		30	6	0.0
(V8) .... 8 fl oz		49	9	0.0
DAIQUIRI				
(Bacardi)				
banana, frozen, prepared w/rum .... 7 fl oz		210	35	1.0
banana, frozen, prepared w/water .... 7 fl oz		150	35	1.0
lime, shelf-stable, prepared w/rum .... 7 fl oz		210	33	0.0
lime, shelf-stable, prepared w/water .... 7 fl oz		130	33	0.0
peach, frozen, prepared w/rum .... 7 fl oz		200	33	0.0
peach, frozen, prepared w/water .... 7 fl oz		130	33	0.0
strawberry, frozen, prepared w/rum .... 7 fl oz		200	34	0.0
strawberry, frozen, prepared w/water .... 7 fl oz		140	34	0.0
strawberry, shelf-stable, prepared w/rum .... 7 fl oz		200	31	0.0
strawberry, shelf-stable, prepared w/water .... 7 fl oz		130	31	0.0
(Holland House)				
bottled .... 1 fl oz		36	9	0.0
instant, dry .... 0.56 oz		65	16	0.0
prepared w/liquor .... 3.5 fl oz		177	18	0.0
raspberry, bottled .... 1 fl oz		30	7	0.0
strawberry, bottled .... 1 fl oz		31	7	0.0
GRENADINE SYRUP *(Roses)* .... 1 fl oz		65	16	0.0
MAI TAI				
(Holland House)				
bottled .... 1 fl oz		32	8	0.0
instant, dry .... 0.56 oz		64	16	0.0
MANHATTAN *(Holland House)* bottled .... 1 fl oz		28	7	0.0
MARGARITA				
(Bacardi)				
frozen, prepared w/rum .... 7 fl oz		160	24	0.0
frozen, prepared w/water .... 7 fl oz		90	24	0.0
shelf stable, prepared w/rum .... 7 fl oz		210	33	0.0
shelf stable, prepared w/water .... 7 fl oz		130	33	0.0
(Holland House)				
bottled .... 1 fl oz		27	6	0.0
instant, dry .... 0.5 oz		57	14	0.0
strawberry, bottled .... 1 fl oz		31	7	0.0
strawberry, instant, dry .... 0.56 oz		66	16	0.0
(Mr. & Mrs. T)				
bottled .... 3 fl oz		80	20	1.0
strawberry, bottled .... 3.5 fl oz		100	24	1.0
OLD-FASHIONED DRINK *(Holland House)* bottled .... 1 fl oz		33	8	0.0
PIÑA COLADA				
(Bacardi)				
frozen, prepared w/rum .... 7 fl oz		260	37	6.0
frozen, prepared w/water .... 7 fl oz		200	37	6.0
shelf-stable, prepared w/rum .... 7 fl oz		240	36	2.0
shelf-stable, prepared w/water .... 7 fl oz		170	36	2.0

Food Name	Serv. Size	Total Cal.	Carbs GMS	Fat GMS
(Holland House)				
bottled	1 fl oz	33	8	0.0
instant, dry	0.56 oz	82	12	3.0
(Mr. & Mrs. T) bottled	4 fl oz	150	39	1.0
RUM RUNNER				
(Bacardi)				
shelf-stable, prepared w/rum	7 fl oz	210	33	0.0
shelf-stable, prepared w/water	7 fl oz	140	33	0.0
STRAWBERRY COLADA				
(Bacardi)				
shelf-stable, prepared w/rum	7 fl oz	230	34	1.0
shelf-stable, prepared w/water	7 fl oz	150	34	1.0
SWEET AND SOUR DRINK				
(Holland House) liquid	1 fl oz	34	8	0.0
(Mr. & Mrs. T) bottled	3 fl oz	70	17	1.0
TOM COLLINS				
(Holland House)				
bottled	1 fl oz	47	11	0.0
instant, dry	0.56 oz	65	16	0.0
WHISKEY SOUR				
bottled	1 fl oz	26	7	0.0
bottled, w/added potassium and sodium	1 fl oz	27	7	0.0
instant, dry	1 pkt	64	16	0.0
(Bar-Tender's) powder, prepared w/whiskey	3.5 fl oz	177	18	0.0
(Holland House)				
bottled	1 fl oz	37	9	0.0
instant, dry	0.56 oz	64	16	0.0
COCKTAIL ONIONS. See under ONION.				
COCOA				
baking, 'Premium' *(Saco Foods)*	1 tbsp	15	4	0.9
100% *(Nestlé)*	1 oz	80	5	5.0
powder *(Bensdorp)*	1 oz	130	8	7.0
powder *(Nestlé)*	1.5 oz	180	21	6.0
unsweetened, European style *(Hershey's)*	1 cup	332	45	8.0
unsweetened, European style *(Hershey's)*	1 tbsp	19	3	0.5
unsweetened, powder	1 cup	197	47	11.8
unsweetened, powder	1 tbsp	12	3	0.7
unsweetened, processed w/alkali, powder	1 cup	191	47	11.3
unsweetened, processed w/alkali, powder	1 tbsp	12	3	0.7
COCOA, HOT, MIX				
(Alba '66)				
milk chocolate flavor, mix only	0.68 oz	60	10	0.0
milk chocolate flavor, w/marshmallows, mix only	0.68 oz	60	10	0.0
w/aspartame, mix only	1 pkt	61	11	0.6
(Carnation)				
chocolate fudge flavor, mix only	1 pkt	110	24	1.3
mocha flavor, 'Sugar-free' mix only	1 pkt	50	9	0.3
rich, mix only	1 pkt	112	24	1.1
'70-Calorie' mix only	1 pkt	70	16	0.3
sugarless, mix only	1 pkt	55	8	0.4
w/marshmallows, mix only	1 pkt	112	24	1.0
(Featherweight)				
mix only	0.44 oz	50	8	1.0
(Finast)				
regular, prepared	6 fl oz	110	24	1.0
w/mini marshmallows, prepared	6 fl oz	110	24	1.0

Food Name	Serv. Size	Total Cal.	Carbs GMS	Fat GMS
(Hills Bros)				
regular, mix only	2 tbsp	110	23	1.0
'Sugar-free' mix only	3 tbsp	60	9	2.0
(Land O'Lakes)				
chocolate and mint 'Cocoa Classics' mix only	1 pkt	160	24	5.0
chocolate and raspberry, 'Cocoa Classics' mix only	1 pkt	160	25	5.0
chocolate cinnamon, mix only	1.25 oz pkt	160	25	5.0
chocolate mint, mix only	1.25-oz pkt	160	25	5.0
chocolate raspberry, mix only	1.25-oz pkt	160	25	5.0
chocolate supreme, 'Cocoa Classics' mix only	1.25-oz pkt	160	25	5.0
(Pathmark)				
chocolate flavor, mix only	1 oz	110	24	1.0
w/mini marshmallows, mix only	1 oz	110	24	1.0
(Saco Foods)				
milk chocolate flavor, mix only	1 oz	110	24	1.0
sugar-free, sweetened w/NutraSweet, mix only	1 pkt	50	9	1.0
(Swiss Miss)				
Amaretto creme flavor, mix only	1.25 oz	150	29	3.0
Bavarian chocolate, mix only	1 oz	110	20	3.0
chocolate Bavarian mint, mix only	1.23 oz	142	28	2.3
chocolate flavor, mix only	1 oz	110	24	1.0
chocolate flavor, 'Sugar-free' mix only	0.5 oz	50	9	1.0
chocolate praline and crème, mix only	1.23 oz	142	29	2.3
diet, mix only	0.26 oz	20	3	1.0
double rich chocolate flavor, mix only	1 oz	110	24	1.0
fat-free, mix only	1 serving	50	9	0.3
light, mix only	0.75 oz	74	17	0.5
'Marshmallow Lovers' 'Hot Cocoa Mix' mix only	1.2 oz	132	24	1.5
milk chocolate, 'Hot Cocoa Mix' mix only	1.2 oz	133	29	1.5
milk chocolate, sugar-free, mix only	1 serving	49	10	0.2
milk chocolate, w/marshmallows, 'Hot Cocoa Mix' mix only	1.2 oz	132	29	1.5
milk chocolate flavor, mix only	1-oz pkt	110	20	3.0
sugar free, mix only	1 serving	51	11	0.6
vending machine product, 'Hot Cocoa Mix'	1.34 oz	146	32	1.7
w/aspartame, w/added calcium or phosphorus, w/o added salt or vitamin A, mix only	1 pkt	48	9	0.5
w/aspartame, w/added salt and vitamin A, w/o added calcium or phosphorus, mix only	1 pkt	48	9	0.5
w/mini marshmallows, 'Sugar-Free' mix only	0.5-oz pkt	50	9	1.0
(Weight Watchers) rich milk flavor, w/marshmallows, mix only	1 pkt	60	10	0.0
COCOA BUTTER OIL				
	1 cup	1927	0	218.0
	1 tbsp	120	0	13.6
COCONUT				
Dried				
meat, creamed	1 oz	194	6	19.6
meat, sweetened, flaked, canned	1 cup	341	32	24.4
meat, sweetened, flaked, canned	4 oz	505	47	36.1
meat, sweetened, flaked, packaged	1 cup	351	35	23.8
meat, sweetened, flaked, packaged	1 oz	134	13	9.1
meat, sweetened, flaked, packaged, 'Snowflake' *(Finast)*	1 oz	137	12	9.0
meat, sweetened, shredded	1 cup	466	44	33.0
meat, sweetened, shredded	7-oz pkg	997	95	70.6
meat, sweetened, shredded, 'Angel Flake' *(Baker's)*	2 tbsp	70	6	5.0
meat, sweetened, shredded, canned, 'Angel Flake' *(Baker's)*	2 tbsp	70	6	6.0
meat, sweetened, shredded, premium *(Baker's)*	2 tbsp	70	6	5.0
meat, sweetened, toasted	1 oz	168	13	13.3

Food Name	Serv. Size	Total Cal.	Carbs GMS	Fat GMS
meat, sweetened, toasted, flaked, packaged *(Baker's)*	1/3 cup	200	17	17.0
meat, unsweetened	1 oz	187	7	18.3
Fresh				
mature kernel, in shell	1 lb	834	35.9	79.0
mature kernel, shelled	1 oz	100	4.3	9.5
mature kernel, shelled, grated, packed	1 cup	460	19.8	43.5
meat, raw, shredded	1 cup	283	12.2	26.8
meat, raw, 2 x 2 x 1/2-inch pieces	1 piece	159	7	15.1
meat, raw, whole, medium	1 coconut	1405	60	133.0
COCONUT CREAM				
Canned				
liquid expressed from grated meat	1 cup	568	25	52.5
liquid expressed from grated meat	1 tbsp	36	2	3.4
sweetened *(Coco Lopez)*	2 tbsp	120	20	5.0
Fresh				
liquid expressed from grated meat, raw	1 cup	792	16	83.2
liquid expressed from grated meat, raw	1 tbsp	50	1	5.2
COCONUT MILK				
Canned				
liquid expressed from grated meat and water	1 cup	445	6	48.2
liquid expressed from grated meat and water	1 tbsp	30	0	3.2
Fresh				
liquid expressed from grated meat and water, raw	1 cup	552	13	57.2
liquid expressed from grated meat and water, raw	1 tbsp	35	1	3.6
Frozen				
liquid expressed from grated meat and water	1 cup	485	13	49.9
liquid expressed from grated meat and water	1 tbsp	30	1	3.1
COCONUT OIL				
	1 cup	1879	0	218.0
	1 tbsp	117	0	13.6
(Hain)	1 tbsp	120	0	14.0
COCONUT WATER				
liquid from coconuts	1 cup	46	9	0.5
liquid from coconuts	1 tbsp	3	1	0.0
COD				
Frozen				
(Booth) fillet, 'Individually Wrapped'	4 oz	90	0	1.0
(Finast) fillet, skinless	4 oz	80	0	1.0
(SeaPak) fillet	4 oz	90	0	1.0
(Van de Kamp's) fillet, light	1 piece	250	20	11.0
(Van de Kamp's) fillet, natural	4 oz	90	0	1.0
ALASKAN/sablefish/skil				
Fresh				
baked, broiled, grilled, or microwaved	3 oz	213	0	16.7
raw	3 oz	166	0	13.0
smoked	3 oz	218	0	17.1
ATLANTIC				
Canned, w/liquid	3 oz	89	0	0.7
Dried/salted				
	1 oz	82	0	0.7
	3 oz	247	0	2.0
Fresh				
baked, broiled, grilled, or microwaved	3 oz	89	0	0.7
raw	3 oz	70	0	0.6
PACIFIC				
baked, broiled, grilled, or microwaved	3 oz	89	0	0.7
raw	3 oz	70	0	0.5

Food Name	Serv. Size	Total Cal.	Carbs GMS	Fat GMS
COD DISH/ENTRÉE				
(Gorton's) cod cakes, canned .... 4 oz		100	16	0.5
(Booth)				
fillet, au gratin, frozen .... 9.5 oz		280	18	11.0
fillet, Florentine, frozen .... 9.5 oz		244	29	6.0
fillet, w/lemon butter sauce and rice, frozen .... 9.5 oz		567	27	38.0
fillet, w/mushroom sauce and rice, frozen .... 9.5 oz		280	19	11.0
COD LIVER OIL. See under FISH OIL.				
COFFEE				
Brewed				
decaffeinated, prepared w/tap water .... 6 fl oz		4	1	0.0
regular, prepared w/distilled water .... 6 fl oz		4	1	0.0
regular, prepared w/tap water .... 6 fl oz		4	1	0.0
Instant				
regular, powder, mix only .... 1 rounded tsp		4	1	0.0
regular, powder, mix only .... 1 tsp		2	0	0.0
regular, powder, prepared .... 6 fl oz		4	1	0.0
w/chicory, powder, prepared .... 6 fl oz		7	1	0.0
(Brim) decaffeinated mix only .... 1 tsp		4	1	0.0
(Kava) regular, powder, mix only .... 1 tsp		2	1	0.0
(Nescafé)				
decaffeinated, 'Decaf' prepared .... 8 fl oz		4	1	1.0
regular, prepared .... 8 fl oz		4	1	1.0
regular, 'Brava' prepared .... 8 fl oz		4	1	1.0
regular, 'Classic' prepared .... 8 fl oz		4	1	1.0
regular, 'Silka' prepared .... 8 fl oz		4	1	1.0
w/chicory, 'Mountain Blend' prepared .... 8 fl oz		6	1	1.0
(Sanka)				
decaffeinated, mix only .... 1 tsp		4	1	0.0
decaffeinated, prepared .... 8 fl oz		3	1	0.0
(Sunrise) w/chicory, prepared .... 8 fl oz		6	1	1.0
(Taster's Choice)				
dark roast, decaffeinated, freeze-dried, 'Maragor' prepared ...... 8 fl oz		4	1	1.0
dark roast, freeze-dried, 'Maragor' prepared .... 8 fl oz		4	1	1.0
decaffeinated, freeze-dried, 'Original' prepared .... 8 fl oz		4	1	1.0
regular, freeze-dried, 'Colombian Select' prepared .... 8 fl oz		4	1	1.0
regular, freeze-dried, 'Original' prepared .... 8 fl oz		4	1	1.0
(Yuban) regular, mix only .... 1 tsp		4	1	0.0
FLAVORED				
Instant				
(General Foods)				
Belgian café, 'International Coffees' mix only .... 1-1/3 tbsp		70	12	2.0
café Amaretto, mix only .... 1-1/3 tbsp		60	8	3.5
café Francais, 'International Coffees' mix only .... 1-1/3 tbsp		60	7	3.5
café Francais, 'International Coffees' prepared .... 6 fl oz		62	7	3.5
café Francais, sugar-free, 'International Coffees' prepared ...... 6 fl oz		35	3	2.0
café Vienna, 'International Coffees' mix only .... 1-1/3 tbsp		70	11	2.5
café Vienna, sugar-free, 'International Coffees' mix only ..... 1-1/3 tbsp		30	3	1.5
cappuccino, Italian, mix only .... 1-1/3 tbsp		50	10	1.5
cappuccino, sugar-free, mix only .... 1-1/3 tbsp		30	3	1.5
double Dutch chocolate, 'International Coffees,' prepared .... 6 fl oz		50	8	2.0
Dutch chocolate mint, 'International Coffees' prepared .... 6 fl oz		50	8	2.0
French vanilla, sugarless, 'International Coffees' mix only .... 1-1/3 tbsp		35	4	2.0
French vanilla, sugarless, 'International Coffees' prepared ...... 8 fl oz		25	5	0.0
Irish crème café, 'International Coffees' prepared .... 6 fl oz		50	8	2.0
Kahlua café, mix only .... 1-1/3 tbsp		60	10	2.0
Suisse mocha, 'International Coffees' mix only .... 1-1/3 tbsp		60	8	2.5

Food Name	Serv. Size	Total Cal.	Carbs GMS	Fat GMS
Suisse mocha, decaffeinated, 'International Coffees' mix only	1 1/3 tbsp	60	8	3.0
Suisse mocha, decaffeinated, sugar-free, 'International Coffees' mix only	1 1/3 tbsp	30	4	1.5
Suisse mocha, sugar-free, 'International Coffees' mix only	1 1/3 tbsp	30	4	2.0
Suisse mocha, sugar-free, 'International Coffees' prepared	8 fl oz	25	5	0.0
Viennese chocolate, 'International Coffees' mix only	1 1/3 tbsp	60	10	2.0
(Hills Bros)				
café Vienna, 'Cafe Coffees' prepared	6 fl oz	60	9	2.0
Capri orange, 'Cafe Coffees' prepared	6 fl oz	60	9	2.0
Swiss mocha, 'Cafe Coffees' prepared	6 fl oz	60	8	2.0
Swiss mocha, sugarless, 'Cafe Coffees' prepared	6 fl oz	40	5	2.0
(Maxwell House)				
'Cinnamon Hot Cappuccino' prepared	6 fl oz	60	11	1.0
'Coffee Hot Cappuccino' prepared	6 fl oz	60	12	1.0
'Mocha Hot Cappuccino' prepared	6 fl oz	70	12	2.0
(MJB)				
mocha, banana nut, sugar-free, prepared	6 fl oz	39	5	1.8
mocha, cherry, prepared	6 fl oz	53	10	1.4
mocha, fudge, sugar-free, prepared	6 fl oz	39	5	1.8
mocha, mint, prepared	6 fl oz	53	10	1.3
mocha, mint, sugar-free, prepared	6 fl oz	37	6	1.3
mocha, prepared	6 fl oz	52	10	1.3
mocha, vanilla, sugar-free, prepared	6 fl oz	39	5	1.7
(Superior) cappuccino, mix only	1 serving	90	13	3.0
Ready to drink				
(Cappio)				
cappuccino, cinnamon, iced	8 fl oz	130	25	3.0
cappuccino, coffee flavored, iced	8 fl oz	120	23	3.0
cappuccino, mocha, iced	8 fl oz	130	25	2.0
cappuccino, vanilla, iced	8 fl oz	130	25	2.0
COFFEE SUBSTITUTE				
cereal grain beverage, mix only	1 tsp	8	2	0.1
cereal grain beverage, prepared w/milk	6 fl oz	120	10	6.1
cereal grain beverage, prepared w/water	6 fl oz	9	2	0.0
(Cafix)				
all natural, 100% caffeine-free	1.5 grams	6	1	0.0
(Inka)				
grain beverage, caffeine-free, instant, 'Naturalis' mix only *(Inka)*	1 tsp	0	1	1.0
(Kaffree Roma)				
cereal grain beverage, coffee flavor, prepared	8 fl oz	6	1	0.0
(Pero)				
cereal grain beverage, caffeine-free, mix only	1 serving	4	1	0.0
cereal grain beverage, caffeine-free, prepared	5 fl oz	4	1	0.0
(Pionier)				
cereal grain beverage, coffee flavor, mix only	1 serving	6	1	0.0
(Postum)				
cereal grain beverage, coffee flavor, 'Instant' prepared	6 fl oz	12	3	0.0
COLE. See KALE.				
COLESLAW				
fresh	1/2 cup	41	7	1.6
fresh	1 tbsp	6	1	0.2
COLESLAW DRESSING. See under SALAD DRESSING.				
COLEWORT. See KALE.				
COLLARDS				
Canned				
chopped *(Allens)*	1/2 cup	20	2	1.0

Food Name	Serv. Size	Total Cal.	Carbs GMS	Fat GMS
chopped, greens *(Bush's Best)*	1/2 cup	30	5	0.0
seasoned w/pork *(Luck's)*	1 cup	60	5	3.0
Fresh				
boiled, drained, chopped	1 cup	49	9	0.7
raw, chopped	1 cup	11	2	0.2
Frozen				
chopped *(Flav-R-Pac)*	1/2 cup	30	2	0.0
chopped *(Seabrook)*	3.3 oz	25	4	0.0
chopped *(Southern)*	3.5 oz	30	5	0.4
chopped, unprepared	3-lb pkg	449	88	5.0
chopped, unprepared	10-oz pkg	94	18	1.1
no salt added, chopped, drained	1 cup	61	12	0.7
COLLINS MIXER. See under SOFT DRINKS AND MIXERS.				
COLORADO PINYON. See PINE NUT.				
COOKIE				
(Archway)				
'Aunt Bea's Pound Cake' 'Home Style'	1 serving	105	16	4.1
hermits, 'Home Style'	1 serving	95	17	2.7
'Select Assortment'	1 piece	50	7	2.0
windmill, old fashioned, 'Home Style'	1 serving	91	14	3.5
(Break Cake)				
'Hermit'	1 cookie	230	38	7.0
'Striper Wafer'	1 wafer	190	23	10.0
(Carr's) 'Hob-Nobs'	1 piece	72	10	3.2
(Featherweight) double	1 piece	45	6	2.0
(Frookie) 'Trolls'	11 cookies	60	10	2.0
(Glenny's) 'Nookie'	1.5 oz	180	18	12.0
(Lu)				
'Crokine'	2 cookies	35	7	0.0
'Little Schoolboy'	1 cookie	70	8	4.0
'Marie Lu'	1 cookie	50	8	2.0
'Marie Lu' mini	5 cookies	50	8	2.0
'Pims'	2 cookies	95	18	2.0
wafer, creme filled	3 cookies	110	11	7.0
(Made 'em Myself) ready-to-decorate	0.25 oz piece	45	7	2.0
(Mother's)				
dinosaur, original, mini	7 cookies	60	9	1.0
wafer, checkerboard	5 cookies	85	13	4.0
(Nabisco) wafer, striped, 'Cookies, 'N Fudge'	1 piece	70	8	4.0
(Oven Lovin')				
candy	1 cookie	70	10	3.0
w/Reese's Pieces	1 cookie	70	9	3.0
(Stella D'oro)				
'Angel Bars'	1 piece	76	7	4.7
'Angel Wings'	1 piece	74	7	4.7
'Angelica Goodies'	1 piece	106	16	4.0
'Como Delight'	1 piece	145	18	7.2
'Holiday Trinkets'	1 piece	38	5	1.9
'Hostess' assorted	1 piece	42	6	2.0
'Lady Stella' assorted	1 piece	42	6	2.0
'Love Cookies'	1 piece	106	13	5.2
'Royal Nuggets'	1 piece	2	0	0.1
ALMOND				
(Ener-G Foods)				
amaretti, gluten-free	1 serving	141	14	4.7
butter, gluten-free	2 cookies	119	13	6.1
French, gluten-free	1 serving	104	17	3.6

Food Name	Serv. Size	Total Cal.	Carbs GMS	Fat GMS
macaroon, gluten-free	1 serving	109	16	4.1
(Mother's) shortbread	2 cookies	120	13	7.0
(Natures Warehouse) butter	2 cookies	122	19	4.1
(Stella D'oro)				
'Breakfast Treats'	1 cookie	101	15	3.6
'Chinese Dessert'	1 cookie	169	20	8.9
toast, 'Mandel'	1 piece	58	10	1.4
AMARANTH				
(Hansa) whole grain, biscuit, organic	1 cookie	120	22	3.0
(Health Valley)	1 cookie	90	12	3.0
ANIMAL CRACKERS				
(Barbara's Bakery) vanilla	1 oz	145	18	7.0
(Barnum's)	12 cookies	141	23	4.0
(Finast)	5 cookies	120	22	3.0
(Frookie) cinnamon, 'Animal Frackers'	6 cookies	60	9	2.0
(Glenny's) peanut butter, 'Noah 'N Friends Animal Cookies'	0.5 oz	65	9	3.0
(Grandma's) candied	5 cookies	140	20	6.0
(Keebler)	5 cookies	70	11	2.0
(Mother's) circus animals	4 cookies	110	14	6.0
(Ralston)	12 cookies	130	22	3.0
(Sunshine)	14 cookies	140	24	4.0
ANISE				
(Biscotti Thins) fat- and cholesterol-free, low-sodium	5 cookies	80	20	0.0
(Stella D'oro)				
'Anisette Sponge'	1 piece	51	10	0.8
'Anisette Toast'	1 piece	46	9	0.6
'Anisette Toast Jumbo'	1 piece	109	23	1.0
APPLE				
(Archway) cinnamon 'Home Style'	1 serving	106	17	3.7
(Bakery Wagon)				
oatmeal, filled	1 cookie	90	14	4.0
w/cinnamon	1 cookie	100	17	3.0
w/walnuts and raisins	1 cookie	100	17	3.0
(Estee) w/cinnamon, 'Snack Crisps'	0.66 oz	80	15	2.0
(Frookie)				
'Fruitins'	1 cookie	60	12	1.0
w/spice, nonfat	1 cookie	50	11	0.0
(Great Cakes)	4.5 oz	260	40	6.0
(Health Valley)				
raspberry, nonfat	2 cookies	67	16	0.0
spice, nonfat	1 serving	33	8	0.0
w/cinnamon, nonfat 'Mini Fruit Centers'	3 cookies	75	17	0.0
w/raisin, nonfat, 'Fruit Chunks'	3 cookies	85	19	0.0
(Healthy Times) organic, 'Hugga Bears'	1 oz	120	17	3.0
(Nabisco) nonfat, 'Newton's'	2 cookies	100	24	0.0
(Natures Warehouse) cinnamon	1 bar	54	10	1.0
(Stella D'oro)				
bar, Dutch	1 piece	112	19	3.3
pastry, dietetic	1 piece	86	13	3.3
(Sunshine) low-fat, 'Golden Fruit'	1 serving	70	15	1.0
(Weight Watchers) fruit-filled	1 cookie	80	21	1.0
APPLE RAISIN				
(Archway)				
'Apple n' Raisin'	1 piece	120	20	3.0
filled, 'Home Style'	1 serving	100	16	3.5
gourmet, 'Home Style'	1 serving	111	17	4.2

Food Name	Serv. Size	Total Cal.	Carbs GMS	Fat GMS
(Health Valley)				
almond, 'Fancy Fruit Chunks'	2 pieces	90	14	4.0
apple, nonfat, 'Fruit Chunks'	3 cookies	85	19	0.0
delight, nonfat	1 serving	33	8	0.0
nonfat, 'Fruit Centers'	1 cookie	80	17	0.0
nonfat, jumbo	1 serving	80	19	0.0
(Pepperidge Farm) raspberry, 'Zurich'	1 piece	60	10	2.0
ARROWROOT *(Nabisco)* 'National Arrowroot'	1 oz	130	21	4.0
BANANA				
(Break Cake) creme	1 cookie	240	37	9.0
(Frookie) nonfat	1 cookie	45	10	0.0
(Health Valley) spice, nonfat	2 cookies	67	16	0.0
(Natures Warehouse)				
all natural, nonfat	1 cookie	75	17	0.4
wheat-free, nonfat	1 cookie	80	19	0.0
BLUEBERRY *(Great Cakes)*	4.5 oz	260	40	6.0
BRAN *(Archway)* w/raisin	1 piece	100	18	3.0
BROWNIE				
(Break Cake) creme	1 cookie	240	38	8.0
(Eagle) chocolate fudge, 'Gourmet'	1 cookie	330	42	16.0
(Pepperidge Farm)				
chocolate nut, 'Old Fashioned'	2 pieces	110	11	7.0
cream sandwich, 'Capri'	1 piece	80	10	5.0
BUTTER				
(Barbara's Bakery) pecan, bites, 'Small Indulgences'	1 oz	140	16	8.0
(Delicious) frosted, made w/Land O'Lakes butter	1 cookie	88	11	5.0
(Fifty 50)				
fructose-sweetened	4 cookies	160	20	8.0
fructose-sweetened, low-sodium	1 cookie	40	5	2.0
(Hansa) biscuit, whole-grain, organic	1 cookie	130	24	3.5
(Keebler)				
chocolate coated, 'Baby Bear'	3 pieces	70	10	2.0
chocolate coated, 'E.L. Fudge'	2 pieces	80	10	4.0
(Lu) 'Petit Beurre'	1 cookie	40	7	1.0
(Mother's)	5 cookies	140	20	6.0
CARAMEL				
(Barbara's Bakery) apple minis, nonfat	6 cookies	110	24	0.0
(FFV) patties	2 pieces	150	20	7.0
(Little Debbie) bar	1 bar	160	22	8.0
(Natures Warehouse)				
crisp, all natural, nonfat	1 cookie	80	19	0.0
wheat-free, crisp, nonfat	1 cookie	80	19	0.0
(Snackwell's) 'Caramel Delights'	1 serving	69	13	2.0
CAROB				
(Great Cakes) w/cherry)	4.5 oz	280	40	8.0
(Heaven Scent) fudge, wheat-free	1 cookie	70	15	1.0
(Jennies) macaroon, gluten- and lactose-free	1 cookie	310	41	15.0
(Natures Warehouse) fudge	2 cookies	116	21	3.1
(Westbrae) 'Rice Malt Snap'	1 oz	140	18	7.0
CARROT				
(Archway) cake, gourmet, 'Home Style'	1 serving	120	18	5.0
(Pepperidge Farm) w/walnut, lowfat, soft, 'Wholesome Choice'	1 cookie	60	11	1.0
CHERRY				
(Archway) filled, 'Home Style'	1 serving	100	16	3.5
(Natures Warehouse)				
all natural, nonfat	1 cookie	72	17	0.4
wheat-free, nonfat	1 cookie	80	18	0.5

Food Name	Serv. Size	Total Cal.	Carbs GMS	Fat GMS
CHOCOLATE				
(Archway)				
devil's food, nonfat, 'Home Style'	1 serving	68	16	0.2
mud pie, 'Home Style'	1 serving	107	15	4.9
(Auburn Farms)				
chewy, nonfat	2 cookies	80	19	0.5
w/mint, nonfat	2 cookies	90	20	0.0
(Barbara's Bakery)				
double chocolate, minis, nonfat	6 cookies	100	23	0.0
w/raspberry, 'Cookies & Creme'	2 cookies	120	18	5.0
(Betty Crocker) w/peanut butter creme, 'Dunkaroos'	1 tray	140	15	8.0
(Biscotti Thins) fat- and cholesterol-free, low sodium	5 cookies	80	20	0.0
(Break Cake) wafer	4 wafers	200	30	9.0
(Cookietree) fudge, nonfat	1 cookie	120	27	0.0
(Delicious) wafer	1 wafer	34	2	2.0
(Drake's)	2 pieces	130	19	5.0
(Ener-G Foods)				
nut, gluten-free	1 serving	102	12	4.5
walnut, gluten-free	1 serving	109	11	6.8
(Estee) 'Snack Crisps'	0.66 oz	80	15	2.0
(FFV) devil's food, 'Trolley Cakes' 2 oz serving	2 pieces	120	25	2.0
(Frookie)				
'Animal Frackers'	6 cookies	60	9	2.0
'Funky Monkeys'	8 cookies	60	10	2.0
(Grandma's) cookie bits	1 oz	140	19	6.0
(Health Valley) fudge, nonfat	2 cookies	70	17	0.0
(Heaven Scent) wheat-free	1 cookie	71	15	1.0
(Keebler) devil's food, fat free, 'Elfin Delights'	1 serving	70	14	0.0
(Lu)				
'Chocolatiers'	2 cookies	85	10	4.0
dipped, 'Chocolatiers'	2 cookies	105	12	6.0
(M&M Mars) fudge, and crunchy, 'Twix'	1 bar	100	11	6.0
(Nabisco)				
'Pure Chocolate Middles'	0.5 oz piece	80	9	5.0
cake, 'Mallomars'	1 piece	60	8	3.0
devil's food, cakes	1 piece	70	15	1.0
w/peanut butter, 'Ideal Bars'	0.5 oz piece	90	10	5.0
(Snackwell's) devil's food	1 serving	49	12	0.2
(Stella D'oro)				
'Castelets'	1 piece	64	9	2.8
'Margherite'	1 piece	72	10	3.1
(Tastykake) 'Soft, 'n Chewy'	1.4 oz	171	26	7.0
(Weight Watchers)	3 cookies	80	13	3.0
CHOCOLATE CHIP				
(Almost Home)	0.5 oz piece	60	8	3.0
(Archway)				
	1 piece	50	7	3.0
and toffee, gourmet, 'Home Style'	1 serving	131	18	6.1
drop, 'Home Style'	1 serving	101	15	3.7
ice box, 'Home Style'	1 serving	117	15	5.7
no sugar, 'Home Style'	1 serving	108	16	5.3
rocky road, gourmet, 'Home Style'	1 serving	127	18	5.9
rocky road, sugarless, 'Home Style'	1 serving	101	15	4.9
(Barbara's Bakery) crisp, 'Small Indulgences'	1 oz	140	18	7.0
(Break Cake)	5 cookies	140	20	6.0
(Drake's)	2 pieces	140	18	6.0
(Duncan Hines) milk chocolate	2 pieces	110	15	5.0

Food Name	Serv. Size	Total Cal.	Carbs GMS	Fat GMS
(Eagle)				
....	1 cookie	190	26	8.0
peanut butter, 'Gourmet'	1 cookie	360	39	20.0
(Ener-G Foods) potato, gluten-free	1 serving	91	12	3.9
(Entenmann's)	3 cookies	140	19	7.0
(Estee)	3 cookies	110	13	5.0
(Featherweight)	1 piece	45	6	2.0
(Fifty 50) fructose sweetened	1 cookie	35	4	2.0
(Finast)	1 oz	90	18	7.0
(Frookie)				
Mandarin	1 cookie	45	7	2.0
mint	1 cookie	45	7	2.0
(Grandma's)				
'Big Cookies'	1 serving	200	28	9.0
'Rich'N Chewy'	3 cookies	140	20	6.0
(Keebler)				
bakery crisp, 'Chips Deluxe'	1 cookie	60	7	3.0
chewy, 'Elfin Delights'	1 cookie	65	11	2.0
'Chips Deluxe'	1 piece	80	10	4.0
'Coconut Chocolate Drop'	1 cookie	80	10	5.0
food service product, 'Old Fashioned'	1 serving	80	10	4.0
less fat, 'Chips Deluxe'	1 serving	70	11	3.0
rainbow chips 'Chips Deluxe'	1 piece	80	11	3.0
regular, enriched, 'Rich, 'n Chips'	1 large	67	9	3.2
'Soft Batch'	1 serving	80	10	3.5
(Mother's)				
....	1 cookie	70	10	3.0
angel	2 cookies	120	14	8.0
(Nabisco)				
'Chips Ahoy'	1 cookie	68	9	3.2
chunky, 'Chips Ahoy!'	0.5 oz piece	90	10	5.0
chunky, 'Chips Ahoy!'	1 serving	80	11	4.0
mini, 'Chips Ahoy!'	0.5 oz	70	9	3.0
mini, 'Chips Ahoy!'	1 cookie	11	1	0.5
pecan, 'Selections' 'Chips Ahoy!'	0.5 oz piece	100	10	6.0
'Rockers' 'Chips Ahoy!'	1 cookie	60	8	3.0
walnut, 'Selections' 'Chips Ahoy!'	0.5 oz piece	100	9	6.0
walnut, w/white fudge chunks 'Chips Ahoy!'	1 cookie	90	11	5.0
(Oven Lovin')	1 cookie	70	9	3.0
(Pepperidge Farm)				
'Family Request'	2 cookies	90	15	5.0
'Old Fashioned'	2 pieces	100	12	5.0
w/pecan, regular, enriched	1 cookie	58	8	2.7
(Pillsbury)	1 serving	130	17	6.0
(Snackwell's) less fat	13 cookies	130	22	3.5
(Soft Batch)	1 piece	80	10	4.0
(Tastykake)				
bar	1 piece	193	28	8.4
'Soft 'n Chewy'	1.4 oz	174	26	7.3
CHOCOLATE CHOCOLATE CHIP				
(Lady J.) 100% natural	1 cookie	120	15	7.0
(Natures Warehouse)	2 cookies	130	16	6.1
(Pillsbury) 'Pillsbury's Best'	1 cookie	70	9	3.0
CINNAMON				
(Archway) honey hearts, nonfat, 'Home Style'	1 serving	106	25	0.2
(Biscotti Thins) fat- and cholesterol-free, low sodium	5 cookies	80	20	0.0
(Natures Warehouse) w/nuts	2 cookies	113	19	3.6

Food Name	Serv. Size	Total Cal.	Carbs GMS	Fat GMS
COCOA				
(Archway) Dutch, 'Home Style'	1 serving	98	17	3.3
(Barbara's Bakery) mocha, minis, nonfat	6 cookies	100	23	0.0
(Westbrae)				
'Rice Malt Snap'	1 oz	140	17	7.0
w/cocoa chip, 'Rice Malt Snap'	1 oz	130	18	7.0
COCONUT				
(Archway) macaroon, 'Home Style'	1 serving	106	12	6.1
(Break Cake) macaroon	2 cookies	270	34	14.0
(Drake's)	2 pieces	130	20	5.0
(Estee)	3 cookies	110	14	5.0
(Fifty 50) fructose-sweetened	4 cookies	160	18	10.0
(Glenny's) w/almonds and raisins, 'Nookie Bar'	1.15 oz	138	18	3.0
(Jennies) macaroon, gluten- and lactose-free	1 cookie	270	34	14.0
(Mother's)				
'Cocadas'	4 cookies	120	17	6.0
macaroon	1 cookie	80	8	5.0
(Mrs. Denson's) macaroon, quinoa	2 cookies	150	14	12.0
(Pepperidge Farm) chocolate-filled, 'Tahiti'	1 piece	90	9	6.0
(Stella D'oro)				
dietetic	1 piece	52	7	2.4
macaroon	1 piece	60	7	3.4
COFFEE-FLAVORED				
(Barbara's Bakery) cake crunch, 'Small Indulgences'	1 oz	130	18	6.0
(Pepperidge Farm) chocolate, praline-filled, 'Cappuccino'	1 piece	50	6	3.0
CRANBERRY				
(Frookie) orange, nonfat	1 cookie	45	10	0.0
(Nabisco) nonfat, 'Newton's'	2 cookies	100	23	0.0
(Pepperidge Farm) honey, soft, 'Wholesome Choice'	1 cookie	60	11	2.0
(Sunshine) low-fat, 'Golden Fruit'	1 serving	70	15	1.0
CREAM				
(Break Cake)				
'Chips & Creme'	1 cookie	140	21	6.0
devil's food creme	1 cookie	130	20	5.0
w/raisins	1 cookie	140	22	5.0
(Delicious) mini	1 wafer	24	3	1.0
(Eagle)				
lemon	6 sandwiches	260	37	11.0
vanilla	6 sandwiches	260	37	11.0
DATE				
(Ener-G Foods) gluten-free	1 serving	76	13	2.3
(Health Valley)				
almond, 'Fruit Jumbos'	1 cookie	70	10	3.0
delight	1 serving	33	8	0.0
granola, nonfat	2 cookies	67	16	0.0
w/pecan, 'Fancy Fruit Chunks'	2 pieces	90	15	4.0
(Lady J.)				
w/almond, 100% natural	1 cookie	120	14	6.0
w/pecan, 100% natural	1 cookie	110	16	5.0
(Pepperidge Farm) w/pecan, 'Kitchen Hearth'	2 pieces	110	15	5.0
EGG BISCUIT				
(Estee) 'Original Sandwich'	1 cookie	45	6	2.0
(FFV)				
'Kreem Pilot Bread'	1 piece	60	9	2.0
'Royal Dainty' 7 oz serving	2 pieces	120	14	6.0
'T.C. Rounds' 1 oz serving	2 pieces	160	20	8.0
'Tango' 1.2 oz serving	2 pieces	160	26	5.0

Food Name	Serv. Size	Total Cal.	Carbs GMS	Fat GMS
(Stella D'oro)				
'Anginetti'	1 piece	31	5	1.0
dietetic	1 piece	43	7	1.1
dietetic, 'Kitchen'	1 piece	8	1	0.5
'Jumbo'	1 piece	47	9	0.7
'Roman'	1 piece	137	20	5.0
sugared	1 piece	75	14	1.4
FIG				
(Estee) bar	2 cookies	90	21	1.0
(FFV)				
w/vanilla, bar	1 piece	70	12	1.0
whole wheat, bar	1 piece	70	11	2.0
(Figaroo) bar	1 cookie	150	30	3.1
(Frookie)				
'Fruitins'	1 cookie	60	12	1.0
nonfat, 'Fruitins'	2 cookies	90	21	0.0
(Keebler) bar	1 piece	60	11	2.0
(Little Debbie) snack squares, 'Figaroos'	1 cookie	150	31	3.5
(Mother's)				
bar	2 cookies	110	23	2.0
whole wheat	2 cookies	120	25	2.0
(Nabisco)				
'Newton's'	2 cookies	110	20	2.5
nonfat, 'Newton's'	2 cookies	100	22	0.0
(Natures Warehouse)				
fruit juice sweetened	1 bar	70	12	1.5
wheat-free, bar	1 oz	98	19	2.0
wheat-free, fruit juice sweetened	1 bar	54	10	1.0
whole wheat, bar	1 oz	98	19	2.0
w/apple and cinnamon, bar, wheat-free	1 oz	98	19	2.0
w/raspberry, bar, wheat-free	1 oz	98	19	2.0
(Stella D'oro) pastry, dietetic	1 piece	89	13	3.7
(Weight Watchers) filled	1 serving	70	16	0.0
FORTUNE				
(La Choy) food service product	1 serving	112	26	0.2
(Umeya)	30 grams	110	24	0.0
FRUIT				
(Archway) and honey, bar, 'Home Style'	1 serving	103	18	3.3
(Bakery Wagon) honey, bar	1 cookie	100	16	3.0
(Barbara's Bakery) w/nuts	1 oz	140	18	6.0
(Hansa) whole grain, organic, biscuit, 'Fruit, 'n Nut'	1 cookie	120	20	3.5
(Health Valley)				
'Fruit & Fitness'	5 pieces	200	40	6.0
Hawaiian, nonfat	1 serving	33	8	0.0
tropical, 'Fancy Fruit Chunks'	2 pieces	80	13	3.0
tropical, 'Fruit Jumbos'	1 piece	70	10	2.0
tropical, nonfat, 'Fruit Centers'	1 cookie	80	17	0.0
(Nabisco) chewy, nonfat, "Newton's"	2 cookies	100	22	0.0
(Stella D'oro) slices	1 piece	60	9	2.2
FUDGE				
(Almost Home) w/chocolate chips	0.5 oz piece	70	9	3.0
(Eagle) w/chocolate chips	1 cookie	260	36	11.0
(Estee)	1 cookie	30	4	1.0
(Grandma's)				
'Big Cookies'	2 pieces	350	54	13.0
w/chocolate chips, 'Big Cookies'	1 serving	190	28	7.0
(Mother's) wafer, 'Flaky Flix'	2 cookies	130	14	9.0

Food Name	Serv. Size	Total Cal.	Carbs GMS	Fat GMS
(Nabisco)				
middles	0.5 oz piece	80	9	5.0
mini bites, 'Little Fudgies' 'Chips Ahoy!'	1 oz	230	27	12.0
snaps	4 pieces	70	11	2.0
wafer, 'Famous Wafers'	5 pieces	70	11	2.0
w/caramel and peanuts, 'Heyday Bars'	0.75 oz	110	13	6.0
(Stella D'oro) 'Swiss'	1 piece	68	9	3.4
(Tastykake) bar	1.8 oz	205	35	6.8
GINGER				
(Archway)				
snap, 54 per package	1 piece	35	6	1.0
snap, 80 per package	1 piece	25	4	1.0
snap, iced, 'Home Style'	1 serving	172	26	7.0
snap, less fat, 'Home Style'	1 serving	136	25	3.6
(Break Cake) snap	5 cookies	130	20	5.0
(Delicious) snap	0.5 oz	64	11	1.7
(Eagle) 'Gourmet'	1 cookie	240	49	3.5
(Ener-G Foods) gluten-free	1 serving	75	12	2.7
(FFV) boys	1.25 oz pkg	150	26	5.0
(Frookie) spice	1 cookie	45	7	2.0
(Little Debbie)	1 cookie	90	15	3.0
(Sunshine) snap	5 pieces	100	16	3.0
(Westbrae) 'Rice Malt Snap'	1 oz	130	20	5.0
GRAHAM				
(Betty Crocker)				
cinnamon, w/vanilla frosting, 'Dunkaroos'	1 serving	130	21	4.5
w/chocolate frosting, 'Dunkaroos'	1 tray	130	19	5.0
w/vanilla frosting, 'Dunkaroos'	1 tray	130	21	5.0
(Carafection)				
honey, carob coated, 'Original'	1 oz	139	17	7.0
mint honey, carob coated	1 oz	139	17	7.0
(Carr's) wheat and honey, 'Home Wheat Graham'	1 piece	74	11	3.3
(Delicious)				
w/cinnamon	0.5 oz	60	11	2.0
w/honey	0.5 oz	60	11	2.0
(Eagle) peanut butter	6 sandwiches	250	36	10.0
(Health Valley)				
amaranth, nonfat	8 pieces	100	23	0.0
honey, 'Fancy'	7 pieces	130	21	5.0
oat bran, nonfat	1 serving	13	3	0.0
(Honey Grahams) honey	4 pieces	70	12	2.0
(Keebler)				
	4 crackers	70	12	2.0
chocolate, 'Selects'	4 cookies	60	9	3.0
chocolate, 'Selects'	4 crackers	60	9	3.0
chocolate, 'Thin Bits'	12 pieces	70	9	3.0
cinnamon, 'Alpha Grahams'	6 pieces	70	10	2.0
cinnamon, 'Cinnamon Crisp'	4 pieces	70	11	2.0
cinnamon, fudge covered, 'Deluxe'	2 pieces	90	11	4.0
cinnamon, 'Thin Bits'	12 pieces	70	10	3.0
honey nut, 'Selects'	4 cookies	60	9	3.0
(Mi-Del) 100% whole wheat	1 cracker	60	12	1.5
(Mother's)				
cinnamon, dinosaurs	1 cookie	80	12	3.0
cinnamon, dinosaurs, mini's	7 cookies	70	9	2.0
dinosaurs, original	1 cookie	70	12	2.0

Food Name	Serv. Size	Total Cal.	Carbs GMS	Fat GMS
(Nabisco)				
....	1 serving	119	21	2.8
....	2 pieces	60	11	1.0
apple cinnamon,'Honey Maid Graham Bites'	11 crackers	60	11	2.0
brown sugar, 'Honey Maid Graham Bites'	11 crackers	60	11	2.0
'Bugs Bunny'	0.5 oz	60	11	2.0
chocolate...	11 pieces	60	10	2.0
chocolate, 'Bugs Bunny'	0.5 oz	60	10	2.0
chocolate, w/vanilla creme, 'Bearwichs' 'Teddy Grahams'	4 pieces	70	10	3.0
'Chocolate Grahams'	0.5 oz piece	150	17	7.0
cinnamon, 'Bearwichs' 'Teddy Grahams'	0.5 oz	70	10	3.0
cinnamon, 'Bugs Bunny'	0.5 oz	60	11	2.0
cinnamon, 'Honey Maid'	2 pieces	60	12	1.0
cinnamon, w/fudge, 'Cookies'N Fudge'	1 piece	45	6	2.0
honey, 'Honey Maid'	2 pieces	60	11	1.0
honey vanilla	11 pieces	60	10	2.0
oat bran, w/honey, 'Graham Bites' 'Honey Maid'	0.5 oz	60	11	2.0
vanilla and honey, 'Bearwichs' 'Teddy Grahams'	4 pieces	70	10	3.0
(Pepperidge Farm)				
cinnamon, 'Goldfish'	1 oz	130	19	7.0
'Goldfish'	1 oz	140	18	7.0
honey hazelnut, 'Old Fashioned'	2 pieces	110	15	6.0
(Regal)	2 crackers	140	19	7.0
(Rokeach)..	8 crackers	120	21	3.0
(Sunshine)				
cinnamon	1 piece	70	11	3.0
'Grahamy Bears'	9 crackers	130	21	5.0
GRANOLA				
(Health Valley) 'Healthy'	3 cookies	75	17	0.0
(Incredibites)				
w/chocolate filling	1 pouch	170	24	7.0
w/peanut butter	1 pouch	170	23	8.0
w/vanilla creme	1 pouch	170	24	7.0
HONEY				
(Health Valley)				
w/cinnamon, crisp, 'Honey Jumbos'	1 piece	70	10	2.0
w/oat bran, fancy, 'Honey Jumbos'	1 piece	70	10	2.0
w/peanut butter, crisp, 'Honey Jumbos'	1 piece	70	10	2.0
JELLY *(Delicious)* jelly top	0.8 oz	112	14	5.3
LEMON				
(Archway)				
drop, 'Home Style'	1 serving	93	15	3.3
frosty, 'Home Style'	1 serving	112	17	4.4
nuggets, nonfat, 'Home Style'	1 serving	115	27	0.2
snap, 'Home Style'	1 serving	152	20	7.3
(Cookietree) poppyseed, nonfat	1 cookie	130	28	0.0
(Estee)				
....	3 cookies	100	14	5.0
'Snack Crisps'	0.66 oz	80	15	2.0
(Featherweight)	1 piece	45	6	2.0
(Westbrae) 'Rice Malt Snap'	1 oz	130	20	6.0
MACADAMIA				
(Eagle) w/coconut, 'Gourmet Cookie'	1 cookie	330	42	16.0
(Pepperidge Farm) 'Special Collection'	1 piece	70	8	4.0
MARSHMALLOW				
(Nabisco)				
cake, chocolate-coated, 'Mallomars'	0.5-oz piece	60	9	3.0

Food Name	Serv. Size	Total Cal.	Carbs GMS	Fat GMS
cake, chocolate-coated, 'Pinwheels' .... 1 piece		130	20	5.0
(Suddenly S'Mores) fudge graham .... 0.75-oz piece		100	15	4.0
MINT				
(Girl Scout) thin .... 4 cookies		160	20	9.0
(Little Debbie) creme, wafers .... 1 wafer		150	18	9.0
(Snackwell's) creme .... 1 serving		108	19	3.6
(Soft Batch) .... 1 piece		80	10	4.0
MOLASSES				
(Archway)				
.... 1 piece		100	18	2.0
dark, 'Home Style' .... 1 serving		115	20	3.4
iced, 'Home Style' .... 1 serving		114	20	3.6
old fashioned, 'Home Style' .... 1 serving		105	18	3.0
3.5- 4-inch diam .... 1 cookie		138	24	4.1
(Bakery Wagon) iced .... 1 cookie		100	17	4.0
(Little Debbie) .... 1 cookie		86	15	2.6
(Nabisco) 'Pantry' .... 0.5 oz piece		80	13	3.0
MUESLI (Carr's) .... 1 piece		84	11	4.1
OAT BRAN				
(Awrey's) w/raisins .... 1 piece		100	14	4.0
(Frookie) muffin cookie .... 1 cookie		45	7	2.0
(Health Valley)				
animal cookies ..,.,.................................. 7 pieces		110	20	4.0
w/fruit and nuts .... 2 pieces		110	17	4.0
w/fruit, 'Oat Bran Fruit Jumbos' .... 1 piece		70	10	2.0
w/raisins, 'Fancy Fruit Chunks' .... 2 pieces		90	15	3.0
(Natures Warehouse)				
w/chocolate chips .... 2 cookies		139	17	6.0
wheat-free .... 2 cookies		129	16	6.2
OATMEAL				
(Almost Home) w/raisins .... 0.5 oz piece		70	10	3.0
(Archway)				
.... 1 piece		110	19	3.0
apple-filled .... 1 piece		90	18	1.0
apple-filled, 'Home Style' .... 1 serving		99	16	3.2
date-filled .... 1 piece		100	18	2.0
date-filled, 'Home Style' .... 1 serving		99	17	3.1
golden, gourmet, 'Ruth's' 'Home Style' .... 1 serving		122	18	5.0
'Home Style' .... 1 serving		106	17	3.8
iced .... 1 piece		140	22	5.0
pecan, gourmet, 'Home Style' .... 1 serving		134	16	6.8
raisin, 'Home Style' .... 1 serving		107	17	3.5
raisin, nonfat, 'Home Style' .... 1 serving		106	24	0.5
raspberry, nonfat, 'Home Style' .... 1 serving		109	25	0.5
'Ruth's Golden' .... 1 piece		120	20	4.0
sugar-free, 'Home Style' .... 1 serving		106	16	5.0
w/raisins .... 1 piece		50	7	2.0
(Auburn Farms) raisin, nonfat, 'Jammers' .... 2 cookies		80	19	0.5
(Bakers Bonus) .... 0.5 oz piece		80	12	3.0
(Bakery Wagon)				
date-filled .... 1 cookie		90	15	3.0
soft .... 1 cookie		100	15	5.0
w/chocolate chunks.................................... 1 cookie		100	17	3.0
w/walnuts and raisins .... 1 cookie		100	16	4.0
(Barbara's Bakery)				
raisin, minis, nonfat .... 6 cookies		110	24	0.0
w/raisins.. 1 oz		100	19	2.0

Food Name	Serv. Size	Total Cal.	Carbs GMS	Fat GMS
(Break Cake)				
....	5 cookies	140	20	6.0
w/creme	1 cookie	140	21	5.0
(Cookietree) raisin, nonfat	1 cookie	120	27	0.0
(Drake's)	2 pieces	120	19	4.0
(Duncan Hines) w/raisins	2 pieces	110	15	5.0
(Eagle)				
creme pie	1 cookie	310	46	12.0
fudge stripe, creme pie	1 cookie	310	47	12.0
'Gourmet Oatmeal Raisin Cookie'	1 cookie	330	40	17.0
iced	1 cookie	170	28	5.0
w/raisins	3 cookies	100	14	4.0
(Fifty 50) hearty, fructose sweetened	1 cookie	35	5	1.0
(Frookie)				
7-grain	1 cookie	45	7	2.0
w/raisins	1 cookie	45	7	2.0
w/raisins, nonfat	1 cookie	50	11	0.0
(Glenny's) wheat-free, 'Noah, 'N Friends Animal'	0.5 oz	65	10	2.0
(Grandma's)				
raisin, 'Big Cookies'	1 serving	180	30	6.0
w/apple and spice, 'Big Cookies'	2 pieces	330	51	12.0
(Health Valley)				
raisin, nonfat	1 serving	33	8	0.0
w/raisins and cinnamon, nonfat, 'Fruit Chunks' ...	3 cookies	85	19	0.0
w/raisins, nonfat	3 cookies	80	18	0.0
(Keebler)				
caramel, oatmeal, w/apple, 'Elfin Delights'	1 cookie	65	12	2.0
food service product, 'Old Fashioned'	1 serving	80	10	3.5
raisin, 'Soft Batch'	1 serving	70	10	3.0
w/caramel and apple, 50% less fat, 'Elfin Delights' ...	1 cookie	70	13	1.5
(Little Debbie)	2.75 oz	340	52	12.0
(Magic Middles) chocolate-filled	1 piece	80	8	5.0
(Mother's)				
....	1 cookie	60	8	3.0
iced	1 cookie	70	10	3.0
w/chocolate chips	1 cookie	70	10	3.0
w/walnuts and chocolate chips	1 cookie	70	9	3.0
(Nabisco) w/chocolate chips, 'Selections' 'Chips Ahoy!'	0.5 oz piece	90	10	5.0
(Natures Warehouse) w/raisins	2 cookies	135	17	6.4
(Pepperidge Farm)				
'Family Request'	2 cookies	90	13	4.0
w/chocolate chunks, 'Dakota'	1 piece	110	15	6.0
(Raisin Ruckus)				
w/chocolate-covered raisins	1 cookie	70	11	3.0
w/raisins, chewy	1 cookie	70	10	3.0
(Snackwell's) oatmeal w/raisins, less fat	2 cookies	110	20	2.5
(Weight Watchers) spice	3 cookies	80	13	2.0
(Westbrae) 'Rice Malt Snap'	1 oz	130	19	5.0
ORANGE				
(Archway) frosty, 'Home Style'	1 serving	113	17	4.6
(Biscotti Thins) fat and cholesterol free, low sodium	5 cookies	80	20	0.0
(Ener-G Foods) almond, gluten-free	1 cookie	74	9	3.7
(Health Valley) pineapple, nonfat, 'Mini Fruit Centers'	3 cookies	75	17	0.0
(Lady J.) pineapple, 100% natural	1 cookie	100	16	4.0
PEACH				
(FFV)				
apricot, whole wheat, bar	1 piece	70	11	2.0

Food Name	Serv. Size	Total Cal.	Carbs GMS	Fat GMS
apricot, w/vanilla, bar	1 piece	70	14	1.0
(Great Cakes)	4.5 oz	260	40	6.0
(Health Valley) apricot, nonfat	2 cookies	70	19	0.0
(Stella D'oro)				
apricot, pastry	1 piece	93	14	3.8
apricot, pastry, dietetic	1 piece	87	12	3.7
PEANUT				
(Archway) jumble, 'Home Style'	1 serving	116	13	6.2
(Cookietree) crunchy, nonfat	1 cookie	130	28	0.0
(Health Valley) chunky, 'Fancy Peanut Chunks'	2 pieces	100	14	3.0
(Nabisco) creme, 'Nutter Butter Patties'	0.5 oz	80	8	4.0
PEANUT BUTTER				
(Archway)				
gourmet, old fashioned, 'Home Style'	1 serving	117	14	5.9
'Home Style'	1 serving	101	12	5.1
(Auburn Farms) nonfat, natural, 'P'nutty crisp'	2 cookies	90	19	0.0
(Bakery Wagon) w/oatmeal	1 cookie	110	12	7.0
(Break Cake)				
	1 cookie	140	18	7.0
wafer, w/peanut butter	1 wafer	180	24	9.0
(Delicious) made w/Skippy peanut butter	1 cookie	80	7	5.0
(Eagle) bar	1 bar	170	19	10.0
(Ener-G Foods) gluten-free	1 serving	94	11	4.6
(Featherweight)	1 piece	40	5	2.0
(Fiber Classic)	1 serving	220	36	9.0
(Fifty 50) fructose-sweetened	1 cookie	40	5	2.0
(Grandma's)				
'Big Cookies'	1 serving	200	24	10.0
cookie bits	1 oz	140	19	6.0
(Keebler) food service product, 'Old Fashioned'	1 serving	80	9	4.5
(Little Debbie)				
bar	1 bar	270	32	15.0
wafer, w/peanut butter, chocolate covered	1 serving	312	31	18.7
(Natures Warehouse)				
	2 cookies	128	18	6.1
w/chocolate chips,	2 cookies	139	14	8.5
(Pepperidge Farm) w/chocolate chunks, 'Cheyenne'	1 piece	110	13	6.0
(Planters) crispy, 'P.B. Crisps'	1 oz	140	17	7.0
(Soft Batch)				
w/chocolate chips	1 piece	80	9	5.0
w/nuts	1 piece	80	9	4.0
PECAN				
(Archway)				
crunch	1 piece	60	8	3.0
iced, 'Home Style'	1 serving	120	15	6.3
(FFV) praline	1 piece	40	10	2.0
(Keebler)				
shortbread, less fat, 'Sandies'	1 serving	70	10	3.0
shortbread, rich, 'Sandies'	1 serving	80	9	5.0
(Pepperidge Farm)				
chunk, 'Chesapeake'	1 piece	120	14	7.0
chunk, 'Special Collection'	1 piece	70	8	4.0
PRUNE (Stella D'oro) pastry, dietetic	1 piece	95	15	3.4
RAISIN				
(Almost Home)	0.5 oz piece	70	10	3.0
(Archway)	1 piece	100	18	3.0
(Entenmann's) nonfat	2 pieces	80	17	0.0

Food Name	Serv. Size	Total Cal.	Carbs GMS	Fat GMS
(Featherweight)	1 piece	45	6	2.0
(Grandma's) soft, 'Big Cookies'	2 pieces	320	54	10.0
(Health Valley)				
jumbo, nonfat	1 serving	80	19	0.0
w/nuts, 'Fruit Jumbos'	1 piece	70	10	3.0
(Keebler) iced, bar	1 piece	80	11	4.0
(Mother's) iced	1 cookie	80	11	4.0
(Pepperidge Farm)				
'Old Fashioned'	2 pieces	110	15	5.0
'Santa Fe'	1 piece	100	16	4.0
w/bran, 'Kitchen Hearth'	2 pieces	110	13	5.0
(Soft Batch)	1 piece	70	10	3.0
(Stella D'oro) 'Golden Bars'	1 piece	109	16	4.3
(Sunshine)				
....	2 pieces	110	16	5.0
'Golden Fruit'	1 serving	80	15	1.5
(Tastykake)				
bar	1.8 oz	212	32	8.3
'Soft'n Chewy'	1.4 oz	161	27	5.4
(Weight Watchers) w/spice	3 cookies	80	13	2.0
RASPBERRY				
(Archway) filled, 'Home Style'	1 serving	101	16	3.5
(Bakery Wagon) filled	1 cookie	90	16	3.0
(Frookie) nonfat, 'Fruitins'	2 cookies	90	21	0.0
(Great Cakes)	4.5 oz	260	40	6.0
(Health Valley)				
center, nonfat	1 serving	70	18	0.0
jumbo, nonfat	1 serving	80	19	0.0
(Nabisco) nonfat, 'Newton's'	2 cookies	100	23	0.0
(Natural Nectar) swirl, 'Incredible Edible Novelties'	1 cookie	220	33	8.0
(Natures Warehouse)				
all natural, nonfat	1 cookie	80	19	0.0
wheat-free, nonfat	1 cookie	80	19	0.0
(Pepperidge Farm)				
filled, 'Chantilly'	1 piece	80	14	2.0
filled, w/chocolate, 'Chantilly'	1 piece	90	14	3.0
tart, lowfat, 'Wholesome Choice'	1 cookie	60	11	1.0
(Weight Watchers) filled	1 serving	70	16	0.0
SANDWICH				
(Break Cake) apple	1 cookie	90	15	3.0
(Delicious) peanut butter, w/jelly, 'Skippy & Welchs'	1 cookie	120	15	6.0
(Ener-G Foods) lemon, gluten-free	1 serving	194	30	8.2
(Estee)				
chocolate	1 cookie	50	7	2.0
original	2 cookies	110	17	4.0
vanilla	2 cookies	110	17	4.0
w/peanut butter	1 cookie	50	5	3.0
(FFV)				
mint	2 pieces	160	22	7.0
w/peanut butter	2 pieces	170	21	8.0
(Frookie)				
chocolate, 'Frookwich'	1 cookie	50	7	2.0
chocolate, w/vanilla filling, 'Frookwich'	1 cookie	50	7	2.0
lemon, 'Frookwich'	1 cookie	50	7	2.0
vanilla, 'Frookwich'	1 cookie	50	7	2.0
w/peanut butter, 'Frookwich'	1 cookie	50	7	2.0
(Great Cakes) peanut butter, w/jelly	4.5 oz	280	40	8.0

Food Name	Serv. Size	Total Cal.	Carbs GMS	Fat GMS
(Keebler)				
butter flavor, w/fudge creme, 'E.L. Fudge'	3 cookies	170	24	8.0
chocolate, 'E.L. Fudge'	1 cookie	70	9	3.0
chocolate, w/chocolate filling, 'E.L. Fudge'	1 cookie	60	8	3.0
chocolate, w/fudge creme, 'Elfin Delights'	1 cookie	55	10	2.0
chocolate, w/fudge creme, 50% less fat, 'Elfin Delights'	3 cookies	150	27	3.5
chocolate, w/peanut butter, 'E.L. Fudge'	1 cookie	50	7	3.0
chocolate, w/vanilla creme, 'E.L. Fudge'	3 cookies	170	23	8.0
chocolate, w/vanilla creme, 50% less fat, 'Elfin Delights'	3 cookies	150	26	3.5
chocolate-filled sandwich creme, 50% less fat, 'Elfin Delights'	3 cookies	150	27	3.5
fudge 'E.L. Fudge'	3 cookies	160	23	7.0
fudge, food service product	1 serving	80	12	3.5
less fat, 'Elfin Delights'	2 cookies	110	19	2.5
praline cream, 'Sandies'	1 cookie	80	9	6.0
vanilla, French, 'Classic Collection'	1 serving	80	12	3.5
vanilla, French, food service product	1 serving	80	12	3.5
(Little Debbie) chocolate	1.8 oz	250	35	12.0
(Mother's)				
duplex	2 cookies	105	15	5.0
English tea	1 cookie	100	14	4.0
fudge, double	2 cookies	100	15	4.0
taffy	1 cookie	100	12	6.0
w/peanut butter, 'Gaucho'	1 cookie	90	12	5.0
(Nabisco)				
chocolate, w/creme filling, 'Big Stuf Oreo'	0.25-oz piece	200	27	9.0
chocolate, w/creme filling, 'Oreo'	1 oz	140	20	6.0
peanut butter, 'Nutter Butter'	0.5-oz piece	70	9	3.0
vanilla, w/creme, 'Cameo'	0.5-oz piece	70	10	3.0
vanilla, w/vanilla creme, 'Cameo'	0.5-oz piece	70	10	3.0
vanilla, w/vanilla creme, 'Cookie Break'	1 piece	50	7	2.0
vanilla, w/vanilla creme, 'Giggles'	2 cookies	60	8	3.0
(Pepperidge Farm)				
butter, chocolate filled, 'Brussels'	2 cookies	110	13	5.0
butter, chocolate filled, 'Double Chocolate Milano'	2 cookies	150	18	8.0
butter, chocolate filled, 'Hazelnut Milano'	2 cookies	130	15	8.0
butter, chocolate filled, 'Lido'	1 cookie	90	10	5.0
butter, chocolate filled, 'Milano'	2 cookies	120	15	6.0
butter, chocolate filled, 'Orleans'	2 cookies	120	14	8.0
butter, chocolate mint filled, 'Brussels Mint'	2 cookies	130	17	7.0
butter, chocolate mint filled, 'Mint Milano'	2 cookies	150	17	7.0
butter, chocolate orange filled, 'Orange Milano'	2 cookies	150	17	7.0
(Pitter Patter) peanut butter, cream filled	1 cookie	90	12	4.0
(Tastykake) shortbread, w/vanilla creme	0.4 oz	55	6	3.0
SESAME				
(Glenny's) bite size, 'Nookie'	0.5 oz	60	6	4.0
(Stella D'oro)				
dietetic, 'Regina'	1 piece	41	5	2.0
'Regina'	1 piece	48	6	2.2
SHORTBREAD				
(Archway) sugarless, 'Home Style'	1 serving	107	16	5.4
(Break Cake)	5 cookies	140	19	6.0
(Ener-G Foods) lemon, gluten-free	1 serving	110	16	5.0
(FFV) country style	1 piece	70	9	4.0
(Keebler)				
fudge-covered, 'Toffee Toppers'	2 cookies	60	10	4.0
pecan, bite size, 'Sandies'	4 cookies	90	9	5.0

Food Name	Serv. Size	Total Cal.	Carbs GMS	Fat GMS
pecan, 'Sandies'	1 piece	80	9	5.0
toffee, "Sandies'	2 cookies	130	16	7.0
w/toffee pieces, 'Sandies'	1 cookie	70	8	4.0
(Magic Middles) w/chocolate center	1 piece	80	9	5.0
(Mother's) striped	2 cookies	100	14	5.0
(Nabisco)				
fudge-striped, 'Cookies, 'n Fudge'	0.5 oz piece	60	7	3.0
pecan, supreme, low-cholesterol	1 cookie	80	9	5.0
(Pepperidge Farm) pecan, 'Old Fashioned'	1 piece	70	7	5.0
SPICE				
(Stella D'oro) drops, 'Pfeffernusse'	1 piece	35	7	0.8
(Westbrae) 5-spice wafer	4 1/2 wafers	40	8	0.0
STRAWBERRY				
(Archway) filled, 'Home Style'	1 serving	100	16	3.5
(Health Valley) nonfat, 'Mini Fruit Centers'	3 cookies	75	17	0.0
(Healthy Times) organic, 'Hugga Bears'	1 oz	120	17	3.0
(Little Debbie) fruits	1 cookie	130	33	0.0
(Nabisco) nonfat, 'Newton's'	2 cookies	100	23	0.0
(Natural Nectar) swirl, 'Incredible Edible Novelties'	1 cookie	220	33	8.0
(Suddenly S'Mores)	0.75-oz piece	100	15	4.0
SUGAR				
(Almost Home) 'Old Fashioned'	0.5 oz piece	70	10	3.0
(Archway)				
'Home Style'	1 serving	98	17	3.1
nonfat, 'Home Style'	1 serving	71	17	0.2
(Cookietree) butter, 'Thaw & Serve'	1 cookie	120	18	4.5
(Ener-G Foods) crisp, gluten-free	1 serving	93	14	3.1
(Keebler) food service product, 'Old Fashioned'	1 serving	80	10	4.0
(Mother's)	1 cookie	70	8	4.0
(Pepperidge Farm) cinnamon, 'Family Request'	2 cookies	80	12	4.0
SUGAR WAFER				
(Break Cake) strawberry	4 wafers	220	28	11.0
(Delicious)				
chocolate, w/strawberry creme	1 wafer	35	3	2.0
lemon	1 wafer	35	4	2.0
strawberry	1 wafer	35	4	2.0
vanilla w/strawberry	1 wafer	35	4	2.0
(Estee)				
chocolate, w/chocolate creme	4 wafers	90	11	5.0
strawberry	3 wafers	100	14	5.0
vanilla	3 wafers	100	14	5.0
w/vanilla creme	4 wafers	90	12	4.0
(Featherweight)				
chocolate, w/chocolate creme	1 piece	20	3	1.0
peanut butter	1 piece	25	3	1.0
w/strawberry cream	1 piece	20	3	1.0
w/vanilla creme	1 piece	20	3	1.0
(Fifty 50)				
chocolate, cream filled, sugarless	1 wafer	35	4	2.0
w/vanilla creme filled, sugarless	1 wafer	35	4	2.0
(Tastykake) vanilla	10 pieces	34	4	1.9
TEA BISCUIT (Nabisco) 'Social Tea'	0.5 oz	60	11	2.0
TOFFEE				
(Delicious) w/Heath English toffee	1 cookie	90	10	5.0
(Nabisco) Heath chunk, 'Selections' 'Chips Ahoy!'	1 piece	90	5	5.0
(Pepperidge Farm) 'Old Fashioned'	2 pieces	100	12	5.0
TOFU (Health Valley) 'The Great Tofu Cookie'	2 pieces	90	16	3.0

Food Name	Serv. Size	Total Cal.	Carbs GMS	Fat GMS
VANILLA				
(Archway) wafer	1 piece	30	6	1.0
(Biscotti Thins) fat- and cholesterol-free, low sodium	5 cookies	80	20	0.0
(Break Cake) wafer	4 wafers	220	28	11.0
(Delicious) wafer	1 wafer	35	4	2.0
(Estee)	3 cookies	100	14	5.0
(Featherweight)	1 piece	45	6	2.0
(FFV) wafer	8 cookies	130	19	5.0
(Fiber Classic) 'Original'	1 serving	210	37	8.0
(Frookie) 'Funky Monkeys'	8 cookies	60	10	2.0
(Glenny's) 'Noah, 'N Friends Animal Cookies'	0.5 oz	65	10	2.0
(Keebler)				
wafer, 'Keebler Golden'	1 serving	147	22	6.0
wafer, golden, 30% less fat	8 wafers	130	25	3.5
(Mother's) wafer, 'Flaky Flix'	2 cookies	115	18	5.0
(Nabisco)				
wafer, 'Nilla Wafers'	3 1/2 cookies	60	11	2.0
wafer, w/cinnamon, 'Nilla Wafers'	3 1/2 cookies	60	11	2.0
(Pepperidge Farm)				
chocolate nut coated, 'Geneva'	2 pieces	130	14	6.0
chocolate-coated, 'Orleans'	3 pieces	90	11	6.0
chocolate-laced, 'Pirouettes'	2 pieces	70	8	4.0
'Goldfish'	1 oz	140	19	7.0
'Pirouettes'	2 pieces	70	9	4.0
(Stella D'oro)				
'Castelets'	1 piece	72	10	3.1
'Margherite'	1 piece	72	11	2.8
VANILLA CHIP (Mrs. Denson's) macaroon	2 cookies	150	14	11.0
WALNUT				
(Archway) black, ice box, 'Home Style'	1 serving	119	15	6.2
(Mother's) w/fudge	1 cookie	70	8	4.0
(Soft Batch)	1 piece	80	10	4.0
WHOLE WHEAT (Lu) w/cinnamon, 'Marie Lu'	1 cookie	45	8	1.0
COOKIE CRUMB TOPPING				
(Nabisco) 'Oreo Crunchies'	1 serving	52	8	2.4
COOKIE CRUMBS				
graham cracker (Sunshine)	3 tbsp	80	13	2.0
graham cracker, food service product (Keebler)	1 cup	550	81	23.0
'Nilla' (Nabisco)	2 tbsp	70	13	2.5
'Oreo' (Nabisco)	2 tbsp	80	13	3.0
COOKIE DOUGH				
(Pillsbury)				
dinosaurs, ready to bake, prepared	2 cookies	120	17	5.0
holiday, ready to bake, prepared	2 cookies	130	16	7.0
teddy bears, ready to bake, prepared	2 cookies	120	18	5.0
CANDY (Pillsbury) ready to bake	1 oz	130	18	6.0
CHOCOLATE CHIP				
(Mrs. Goodcookie) gourmet, ready to bake, prepared	2 cookies	120	15	6.0
(Nestlé) ready to bake	2 tbsp	150	23	6.0
(Pillsbury)				
	1 serving	127	18	5.7
ready to bake, prepared	1 cookie	70	9	3.0
(Toll House)				
double chips	1.2 oz	150	19	7.0
ready to bake	1.2 oz	150	20	7.0
w/nuts, ready to bake	1.2 oz	160	19	8.0
CHOCOLATE CHOCOLATE CHIP (Nestlé)	2 tbsp	150	21	6.0

Food Name	Serv. Size	Total Cal.	Carbs GMS	Fat GMS
OATMEAL				
(Nestlé) w/Raisinets	2 tbsp	150	22	6.0
(Pillsbury)				
w/chocolate chips, ready to bake	1 oz	120	16	6.0
w/raisins, prepared	1 cookie	60	9	3.0
(Toll House) w/raisins, ready to bake	1.2 oz	130	21	5.0
PEANUT BUTTER *(Pillsbury)* prepared	1 cookie	70	9	3.0
COOKIE MIX				
(Krusteaz) 'Deluxe' prepared	1 cookie	120	16	5.0
CHOCOLATE CHIP				
(Big Batch) prepared	2 cookies	120	16	6.0
(Duncan Hines) prepared	2 cookies	130	20	5.0
(Estee) prepared	2 cookies	90	13	4.0
(Finast) prepared	2 cookies	110	16	5.0
(Gluten-Free Pantry) gluten-free, prepared	1 serving	60	12	1.0
(Pillsbury)				
bar, 'Chips Ahoy' mix only	1/18 pkg	140	26	4.0
bar, 'Chips Ahoy' prepared	1/18 pkg	180	26	7.0
(Sweet 'n Low) low-fat, w/'Sweet 'n Low, prepared	4 cookies	120	22	2.5
DATE *(Betty Crocker)* bar, prepared	1 serving	150	23	6.0
OATMEAL *(Duncan Hines)* w/raisins, prepared	2 cookies	130	18	6.0
PEANUT BUTTER *(Duncan Hines)* prepared	2 cookies	140	15	7.0
SUGAR				
(Duncan Hines) golden, prepared	2 cookies	130	17	6.0
(Gluten-free Pantry) gluten-free, prepared	1 serving	130	31	0.0
COOKING OIL. See individual listings.				
COOKING SPRAY				
(Canola Harvest) Canola, nonstick	0.25 grams	0	0	0.0
(I Can't Believe It's Not Butter)	1 spray	0	0	0.0
(Mazola)				
corn oil	2.5-sec spray	6	0	1.0
corn oil	1 tsp	2	0	0.2
(Pam)				
	1 serving	0	0	0.0
butter-flavored	1 serving	0	0	0.0
olive oil	1 serving	0	0	0.0
(Town House) Canola oil	0.25 grams	0	0	0.0
(Weight Watchers)				
	1-sec spray	2	0	1.0
butter flavor, 'Buttery Spray'	1 spray	2	0	1.0
Canola oil	0.33 grams	2	0	1.0
(Wesson)				
	0.25 grams	2	0	0.3
lite	0.27 grams	1	0	1.0
COOKING WINE. See WINE, COOKING.				
CORIANDER LEAF/Chinese parsley leaf				
dried	1 tbsp	5	1	0.1
dried	1 tsp	2	0	0.0
dried *(Tone's)*	1 tsp	2	0	0.1
fresh, raw, chopped	1/4 cup	1	0	0.0
fresh, raw, whole, med plants	9 plants	4	1	0.1
CORIANDER SEED/Chinese parsley seed				
round *(McCormick/Schilling)*	1 tsp	7	1	0.4
whole	1 tbsp	15	3	0.9
whole	1 tsp	5	1	0.3
whole *(Durkee)* whole seeds	1 tsp	8	0	0.0
whole *(Laurel Leaf)* whole seeds	1 tsp	8	0	0.0

Food Name	Serv. Size	Total Cal.	Carbs GMS	Fat GMS
whole *(McCormick/Schilling)*	1 tsp	12	2	0.4
whole *(Spice Islands)*	1 tsp	6	1	0.3

CORN. See also CORN DISH/ENTRÉE.

Canned

(Del Monte)	1/2 cup	90	22	1.0
'Crisp 'N Sweet' *(Freshlike)*	1/2 cup	80	18	1.0
'Crisp 'N Sweet' *(Stokely)*	1/2 cup	80	13	1.5
'Delicorn' *(Green Giant)*	1/2 cup	80	19	1.0
50% less sodium, 'Niblets' *(Green Giant)*	1/3 cup	60	14	0.0
in brine, w/liquid *(Green Giant)*	1/2 cup	70	18	0.0
kernels, extra sweet, 'Niblets' *(Green Giant)*	1/3 cup	50	10	0.5
kernels, 'Niblets' *(Green Giant)*	1/2 cup	80	20	0.0
kernels, w/liquid *(A&P)*	1/2 cup	80	20	1.0
kernels, w/liquid *(Featherweight)*	1/2 cup	80	16	1.0
kernels, w/liquid *(Finast)*	1/2 cup	90	20	1.0
kernels, w/liquid *(Green Giant)*	1/2 cup	80	18	0.0
kernels, w/liquid, 50% less salt, no sugar *(Green Giant)*	1/2 cup	50	11	1.0
kernels, w/liquid, 'No Frills' *(Pathmark)*	1 cup	160	38	1.0
kernels, w/liquid, 'No Salt Added' *(A&P)*	1/2 cup	80	18	1.0
kernels, w/liquid, 'No Salt Added' *(Finast)*	1/2 cup	80	19	1.0
kernels, w/liquid, 'No Salt Added' *(Pathmark)*	1/2 cup	70	16	1.0
kernels, w/liquid, 'Nutradiet' *(S&W)*	1/2 cup	80	15	1.0
no salt or sugar added, 'Niblets' *(Green Giant)*	1/2 cup	80	18	1.0
sweet *(TenderSweet)*	1/2 cup	100	20	1.0
sweet, select *(Green Giant)*	1/2 cup	60	15	1.0
vacuum pack, w/liquid, 'No Salt Added' *(Del Monte)*	1/2 cup	90	22	1.0
Dried, approx 4 oz prepared *(John Cope's)*	1 oz	101	21	1.2
Freeze-Dried, prepared *(Mountain House)*	1/2 cup	90	18	1.0

Frozen

(Health Valley)	1/2 cup	76	17	0.0
kernels *(Finast)*	3.3 oz	80	20	1.0
kernels, cut *(Frosty Acres)*	3.3 oz	80	20	1.0
kernels, cut *(Seabrook)*	3.3 oz	80	20	1.0
kernels, cut *(Southern)*	3.5 oz	98	21	0.7
kernels, cut, petite, 'Deluxe' *(Birds Eye)*	2.6 oz	70	16	1.0
kernels, cut, 'Portion Pack' *(Birds Eye)*	3 oz	70	18	1.0
kernels, cut, 'Portion Pack' *(Birds Eye)*	3 oz	70	18	1.0
kernels, cut, 'Singles' *(Stokely)*	3 oz	75	18	1.0
kernels, cut, whole *(Flav-R-Pac)*	2/3 cup	80	19	1.0
on the cob, half ears. 'Sweet Select' *(Green Giant)*	2 half-ears	90	19	2.0
kernels, harvest fresh, 'Niblets' *(Green Giant)*	1/2 cup	80	17	1.0
kernels, 'Niblets' *(Green Giant)*	1/2 cup	90	19	1.0
kernels, plain polybag, 'Nibblers' *(Green Giant)*	1 ear	70	14	0.5
kernels, plain polybag, 'Niblets' *(Green Giant)*	1/2 cup	90	19	1.0
kernels, supersweet, 'Niblets' *(Green Giant)*	1/2 cup	60	13	1.0
kernels, 'Sweet' *(Birds Eye)*	3.3 oz	80	20	1.0
kernels, 'Tender Sweet Deluxe' *(Birds Eye)*	3.3 oz	80	20	1.0
on the cob *(A&P)*	1 ear	120	28	1.0
on the cob *(Birds Eye)*	1 ear	120	29	1.0
on the cob *(Frosty Acres)*	1 ear	120	29	1.0
on the cob *(Ore-Ida)*	1 ear	180	39	2.0
on the cob, baby, 'Deluxe' *(Birds Eye)*	2.6 oz	25	4	0.0
on the cob, 'Big Ears' *(Birds Eye)*	1 ear	160	37	1.0
on the cob, 'Cob Treats' *(A&P)*	2 ears	130	28	1.0
on the cob, 5-inch ear *(Seabrook)*	1 ear	120	29	1.0
on the cob, 5-inch ear *(Southern)*	1 ear	140	30	1.0
on the cob, 'Little Ears' *(Birds Eye)*	2 ears	130	30	1.0

Food Name	Serv. Size	Total Cal.	Carbs GMS	Fat GMS
on the cob, miniature, 'Mini-Gold' *(Ore-Ida)*	2 ears	180	39	2.0
on the cob, mini-cob *(Superior Pride)*	1 ear	80	18	1.0
on the cob, mini-cob *(Trader Joe's)*	1/2 cup	90	20	0.5
on the cob, 'Niblet Ears' *(Green Giant)*	1 ear	120	27	1.0
on the cob, 'One Serving' *(Green Giant)*	2 half-ears	120	26	1.0
on the cob, 'Plain Polybag' *(Green Giant)*	1 ear	120	22	2.0
on the cob, 6-ear pkg, 'Nibblers' *(Green Giant)*	2 ears	120	27	1.0
on the cob, supersweet, 'Nibblers' *(Green Giant)*	2 ears	90	19	2.0
on the cob, supersweet, 'Niblet Ears' *(Green Giant)*	1 ear	90	19	2.0
on the cob, sweet, no salt added, mini-cob *(TenderSweet)*	1/2 cup	80	19	1.0
on the cob, sweet, unprepared, med ears	1 ear	123	29	1.0
on the cob, 'Sweet Select' *(Green Giant)*	1 ear	90	19	2.0
sweet *(Birds Eye)*	3.3 oz	80	20	1.0
sweet, petite, 'Early Harvest' *(C&W)*	2/3 cup	80	19	1.0
sweet, select, 'Plain Polybag' *(Green Giant)*	1/2 cup	60	13	1.0
sweet, tender, 'Deluxe' *(Birds Eye)*	3.3 oz	80	20	1.0
GOLD AND WHITE, canned *(Stokely)*	1/2 cup	60	10	1.5
GOLDEN				
Canned				
(Pathmark)	1/2 cup	90	19	1.0
(Stokely)	1/2 cup	90	20	0.0
50% less salt *(Green Giant)*	1/2 cup	70	16	1.0
kernels *(Veg-All)*	1/2 cup	80	19	1.0
kernels, sweet *(Green Giant)*	1/2 cup	70	18	0.0
kernels, sweet, 50% less salt *(Green Giant)*	1/2 cup	70	16	1.0
kernels, vacuum packed *(Freshlike)*	1/2 cup	100	22	1.0
kernels, vacuum packed *(Veg-All)*	1/2 cup	100	22	1.0
kernels, water pack, w/o salt *(Freshlike)*	1/2 cup	80	19	1.0
kernels, water pack, w/o sugar, salt *(Freshlike)*	1/2 cup	80	19	1.0
no salt added *(Del Monte)*	1/2 cup	80	18	1.0
no salt or sugar added *(Green Giant)*	1/2 cup	80	18	1.0
no salt or sugar added *(Stokely)*	1/2 cup	80	16	0.0
'Pantry Express' *(Green Giant)*	1/2 cup	80	18	1.0
vacuum-packed *(Green Giant)*	1/2 cup	80	20	0.0
vacuum-packed *(Stokely)*	1/2 cup	90	22	0.0
w/liquid *(Del Monte)*	1/2 cup	70	17	1.0
WHITE				
Canned				
(Green Giant)	1/2 cup	80	20	0.0
(Stokely)	1/2 cup	90	21	0.0
kernels, sweet, drained	1 cup	133	30	1.6
kernels, sweet, no salt, vacuum pack	1/2 cup	83	20	0.5
kernels, sweet, no salt, w/liquid	1/2 cup	82	20	0.6
kernels, sweet, w/liquid	1/2 cup	82	20	0.6
sweet, vacuum packed	1/2 cup	83	20	0.5
vacuum-packed *(A&P)*	1/2 cup	100	25	1.0
vacuum-packed *(Finast)*	4 oz	90	20	1.0
vacuum-packed *(Green Giant)*	1/2 cup	80	20	0.0
vacuum-packed *(Pathmark)*	1/2 cup	120	25	1.0
vacuum-packed, 'Niblets' *(Green Giant)*	1/2 cup	80	16	1.0
w/liquid *(Del Monte)*	1/2 cup	70	16	0.0
young, tender, 'Premium' *(S&W)*	1/2 cup	90	20	1.0
Fresh				
kernels, sweet, boiled, drained	1/2 cup	76	18	0.6
kernels, sweet, raw	1 cup	132	29	1.8
on the cob, sweet, large ears, 7.75 to 9 inches	1 ear	123	27	1.7
on the cob, sweet, med ears, 6.75 to 7.5 inches	1 ear	83	19	1.0

Food Name	Serv. Size	Total Cal.	Carbs GMS	Fat GMS
on the cob, sweet, small ears, 5.5 to 6.5 inches	1 ear	63	14	0.9
Frozen				
(Green Giant)	1/2 cup	90	19	1.0
(Seabrook)	3.3 oz	80	19	1.0
kernels, sweet, boiled, drained	1/2 cup	66	16	0.4
kernels, sweet, boiled, drained	10-oz pkg	227	56	1.2
kernels, sweet, unprepared	1/2 cup	72	17	0.6
kernels, sweet, unprepared	10-oz pkg	250	59	2.2
on the cob, sweet, unprepared, med ears	1 ear	123	29	1.0
petite, 'Early Harvest' *(C&W)*	2/3 cup	80	19	1.0
shoepeg, 'Harvest Fresh' *(Green Giant)*	1/2 cup	90	19	1.0
shoepeg, 'Select' *(Green Giant)*	1/2 cup	90	19	1.0
YELLOW				
Canned				
kernels, sweet, drained	12-oz can	171	39	2.1
kernels, sweet, drained	1 cup	133	30	1.6
kernels, sweet, regular pack, w/liquid	1/2 cup	82	20	0.6
sweet, no salt, vacuum-packed	1/2 cup	83	20	0.5
sweet, no salt, w/liquid	1/2 cup	82	20	0.6
Fresh				
baby, sweet, whole, boiled, drained	1 ear	9	2	0.1
kernels, sweet, boiled, drained	1/2 cup	76	18	0.6
kernels, sweet, raw	1 cup	132	29	1.8
on the cob, large ears, 7.75 to 9 inches	1 ear	123	27	1.7
on the cob, medium ears, 6.75 to 7.5 inches	1 ear	77	17	1.1
on the cob, small ears, 5.5 to 6.5 inches	1 ear	63	14	0.9
Frozen				
kernels, sweet, boiled, drained	10-oz pkg	227	56	1.2
kernels, sweet, unprepared	10-oz pkg	250	59	2.2
kernels, sweet, unprepared	1/2 cup	72	17	0.6
CORN, CREAMED. See under CORN DISH/ENTRÉE.				
CORN BRAN, crude	1 cup	170	65	0.7
CORN CAKE				
apple cinnamon flavor *(Roman Meal)*	1 cake	49	11	1.0
caramel flavor, nonfat *(Roman Meal)*	1 cake	50	11	0.0
caramel flavored *(Quaker)*	1 serving	50	12	0.0
cheddar flavor *(Roman Meal)*	1 cake	43	9	1.0
natural butter flavor, nonfat *(Roman Meal)*	1 cake	40	8	0.0
popcorn, butter flavor *(Chico-San)*	1 cake	40	8	0.0
popcorn, caramel *(Chico-San)*	1 cake	50	10	0.0
popcorn, lightly salted *(Chico-San)*	1 cake	40	8	0.0
popcorn, white cheddar cheese *(Chico-San)*	1 cake	50	9	1.0
popped, butter flavor *(Quaker)*	1 cake	35	7	0.0
white cheddar, mild *(Quaker)*	1 serving	40	8	0.0
white cheddar flavor, nonfat *(Roman Meal)*	1 cake	45	9	0.0
CORN CHIPS AND SNACKS. See also TORTILLA CHIPS.				
(Arrowhead Mills)				
chips, blue corn, 'Corn Curls'	1 oz	120	22	2.0
chips, blue corn, unsalted, 'Corn Curls'	1 oz	120	22	2.0
chips, yellow, 'Corn Chips'	0.75 oz	90	18	1.0
chips, yellow, w/cheese, 'Corn Chips'	0.75 oz	90	15	2.0
(Azteca) chips, 'Unsalted'	1 oz	140	18	7.0
(Bachman)				
chips	1 oz	160	15	10.0
chips, barbecue	1 oz	150	17	9.0
(Barbara's Bakery)				
chips, blue corn	15 chips	140	16	7.0

Food Name	Serv. Size	Total Cal.	Carbs GMS	Fat GMS
chips, blue corn, no salt added	15 chips	140	16	7.0
chips, chipotle chili, 'Potilla'	1 oz	140	18	8.0
chips, 'Potilla'	1 oz	140	18	8.0
chips, salsa, 'Pinta Puffs'	1 oz	70	10	2.0
(Corn Snackers)				
chips	0.5-oz pkg	60	10	2.0
chips, nacho cheese	0.5-oz pkg	60	10	2.0
(Cornuts)				
nuggets, toasted, barbecue	1 oz	124	20	4.1
nuggets, toasted, chili picante	1 oz	120	22	4.0
nuggets, toasted, nacho	1 oz	124	20	4.0
nuggets, toasted, plain	1 oz	124	21	4.0
nuggets, toasted, ranch	1 oz	120	20	4.0
nuggets, toasted, unsalted	1 oz	120	19	4.0
(Dipsy Doodles) chips, rippled, 'Rippled Corn Chips'	1 oz	160	15	10.0
(Doritos)				
chips, 'Nacho Cheesier'	1 oz	140	17	7.0
chips, '3-D's'	1 oz	140	18	6.0
(Featherweight)				
chips, 'Low-Salt'	1 oz	170	15	11.0
puffs, cheese, low-salt 'Cheese Curls'	1 oz	150	16	9.0
(Fritos)				
chips, 'Bar-B-Q'	34 pieces	150	16	9.0
chips, barbecue, 'Rowdy Rustlers'	34 chips	150	17	9.0
chips, chili cheese flavor	34 chips	160	15	10.0
chips, 'Dip Size'	13 pieces	150	17	9.0
chips, nacho cheese, 'Non-Stop'	34 chips	150	16	9.0
chips, original	34 pieces	150	16	9.0
chips, 'Wild N' Mild'	32 chips	160	16	9.0
nuggets, toasted	1.38 oz	170	29	5.0
(Harry's)				
chips, bean 'Garden Vegetable Chips'	1 oz	144	17	7.0
chips, bean, mild, 'Garden Vegetable Chips'	1 oz	144	17	7.0
chips, bean, wild, 'Garden Vegetable Chips'	1 oz	141	18	6.0
chips, beet-garlic, 'Garden Vegetable Chips'	1 oz	134	20	5.0
chips, bell pepper, 'Garden Vegetable Chips'	1 oz	140	19	6.0
chips, blue corn, garlic 'Garden Vegetable Chips'	1 oz	129	21	4.0
chips, carrot caraway 'Garden Vegetable Chips'	1 oz	131	20	4.0
chips, vegetable, 'Garden Vegetable Chips'	1 oz	141	18	7.0
(Health Valley)				
chips	1 oz	160	13	11.0
chips, 'No Salt Added'	1 oz	160	13	11.0
puffs, caramel, nonfat, orignal	1 cup	110	24	0.0
puffs, caramel corn, peanut flavor	1 oz	100	21	0.0
puffs, cheddar cheese	1 oz	160	15	10.0
(Jax)				
puffs, cheese 'Crunchy'	1 oz	160	14	11.0
puffs, cheese, 'Baked'	1 oz	140	17	7.0
(Maine Coast)				
chips, corn-dulse-kelp-onion-garlic, organic	1 oz	146	17	6.6
(Peddlers)				
chips, bean 'Offbeat Originals'	1 oz	144	17	7.0
chips, bean, mild, 'Offbeat Originals'	1 oz	144	17	7.0
chips, bean, wild, 'Offbeat Originals'	1 oz	141	18	6.0
chips, beet-garlic 'Offbeat Originals'	1 oz	134	20	5.0
chips, bell pepper 'Offbeat Originals'	1 oz	140	19	6.0
chips, blue corn, garlic 'Offbeat Originals'	1 oz	129	21	4.0

Food Name	Serv. Size	Total Cal.	Carbs GMS	Fat GMS
chips, carrot caraway 'Offbeat Originals'	1 oz	131	20	4.0
chips, vegetable, 'Offbeat Originals'	1 oz	141	18	7.0
(Planters) chips	1 oz	160	15	10.0
(Skinny Snacks)				
chips, barbecue	1 cup	60	12	1.0
chips, nacho flavor	1 cup	60	12	1.0
chips, no salt	1 cup	60	12	1.0
chips, salted	1 cup	60	12	1.0
chips, sour cream and onion	1 cup	65	12	1.0
(Snyder's)				
chips	1 oz	160	14	11.0
(Tio Sancho) nachos	0.5 oz	70	1	5.7
(Ultra Slim Fast) curls, cheese, 'Great Tasting'	1 oz	110	20	3.0
(Wise)				
corn chips	1 oz	160	15	10.0
chips, ridged	1 oz	160	15	10.0
crunchies	1 oz	160	15	10.0
puffs, cheese, fried, 'Cheez Doodles Corn Puffs'	1 oz	160	15	10.0
puffs, cheese, baked, 'Cheez Doodles Corn Puffs'	1 oz	150	17	8.0
spirals	1 oz	160	15	10.0
twists	1 oz	160	15	10.0
CORN DISH/ENTRÉE				
(A&P)				
cream style, canned	1/2 cup	100	25	1.0
kernels, cream style, frozen	3.3 oz	80	18	1.0
(Del Monte)				
cream style, no salt added, canned	1/2 cup	90	20	1.0
golden, cream style, canned	1/2 cup	80	18	1.0
golden, cream style, no salt added, canned	1/2 cup	80	20	1.0
(Diamond A) sweet, cream style, canned	1 cup	245	50	1.0
(Finast) cream style, canned	1/2 cup	105	25	1.0
(Flav-R-Pac)				
cream style, frozen	1/2 cup	130	24	3.0
w/buttery sauce, frozen	1/2 cup	130	24	3.0
(Freshlike)				
and peppers, vacuum packed	1/2 cup	90	23	1.0
golden, cream style, canned	1/2 cup	110	25	1.0
golden, cream style, no salt added, canned	1/2 cup	110	25	1.0
(Green Giant)				
cream style, canned	1/2 cup	100	24	1.0
cream style, canned	1/2 cup	110	23	1.0
w/peppers, canned, 'Mexicorn'	1/2 cup	80	19	1.0
(IGA) golden, sweet, cream style, canned	1/2 cup	70	16	1.0
(Pathmark)				
cream style, canned, 'No Frills'	1 cup	210	51	1.0
golden, cream style, canned	1/2 cup	100	25	1.0
(S&W)				
cream style, canned	1/2 cup	100	24	1.0
cream style, canned, 'Nutradiet'	1/2 cup	100	21	1.0
cream style, no starch added, canned, 'Premium Homestyle'	1/2 cup	120	24	1.0
cream style, starch added, canned, 'Premium Homestyle'	1/2 cup	105	25	1.0
(Stokely)				
gold and white, cream style, canned	1/2 cup	100	23	0.0
gold and white, w/red peppers, canned	1/2 cup	60	10	1.5
white, cream style, canned	1/2 cup	100	21	1.0
(Stouffer's)				
pudding, frozen, food service product	1 oz	38	5	1.7

Food Name	Serv. Size	Total Cal.	Carbs GMS	Fat GMS
soufflé	1/2 cup	170	21	7.0
(Veg-All)				
golden, cream style, canned	1/2 cup	110	25	1.0
w/peppers, vacuum packed	1/2 cup	90	23	1.0
CORN DOG. See under FRANKFURTER.				
CORN FLOUR. See under FLOUR. See also CORNMEAL.				
CORN OIL				
(Hain)	1 tbsp	120	0	14.0
(Kroger)	1 tbsp	122	0	13.6
(Mazola)	1 tbsp	120	0	14.0
(Wesson)	1 tbsp	122	0	13.6
'No Frills' *(Pathmark)*	1 tbsp	130	0	14.0
pure pressed, organic *(Spectrum)*	1 tbsp	120	0	14.0
CORN SYRUP				
dark	1 cup	925	251	0.0
dark	1 tbsp	56	15	0.0
dark *(Karo)*	1 tbsp	60	15	0.0
high-fructose	1 cup	871	236	0.0
high-fructose	1 tbsp	53	14	0.0
light	1 cup	925	251	0.0
light	1 tbsp	56	15	0.0
light *(Karo)*	1 tbsp	60	15	0.0
table blend, w/sugar	1 cup	1008	265	0.0
table blend, w/sugar	1 tbsp	64	17	0.0
CORNBREAD. See under BREAD, QUICK.				
CORNBREAD MIX. See under BREAD, QUICK, MIX.				
CORNED BEEF. See BEEF, CORNED.				
CORNED BEEF HASH. See under HASH.				
CORNISH GAME HEN				
meat and skin, raw	1/2 medium	336	0	23.6
meat and skin, roasted	1/2 medium	335	0	23.5
meat only, raw	1/2 medium	139	0	4.0
meat only, roasted	1/2 medium	147	0	4.3
(Tyson)				
meat and skin, frozen	3.5 oz	250	1	15.0
meat only, frozen	3.5 oz	240	0	14.0
CORNISH GAME HEN DINNER/ENTRÉE				
(Tyson) w/wild rice, wholesale club item	3.5 oz	190	6	11.0
CORNMEAL				
organic, stone ground, gluten free *(Hodgson Mill)*	1/4 cup	100	22	1.0
whole-grain, high-lysine *(Arrowhead Mills)*	2 oz	210	43	2.0
whole-grain, stone-ground *(Hodgson Mill)*	1/4 cup	100	22	1.0
BLUE				
(Arrowhead Mills)	1/4 cup	120	27	1.0
whole-grain *(Arrowhead Mills)*	2 oz	210	41	3.0
WHITE				
Regular				
(Albers)	1 oz	100	22	1.0
bolted *(Aunt Jemima)*	1/6 cup	99	21	0.7
enriched *(Aunt Jemima)*	3 tbsp	102	22	0.5
enriched, degermed	1 cup	505	107	2.3
unenriched, degermed	1 cup	505	107	2.3
whole-grain	1 cup	442	94	4.4
whole-grain, stone-ground *(Hodgson Mill)*	1/4 cup	100	22	1.0
Self-rising				
(Aunt Jemima)	1/6 cup	98	21	0.5
bolted, plain, enriched	1 cup	407	86	4.1

Food Name	Serv. Size	Total Cal.	Carbs GMS	Fat GMS
bolted, w/wheat flour added, enriched	1 cup	592	125	4.8
buttermilk *(Aunt Jemima)*	3 tbsp	101	20	1.1
enriched, degermed	1 cup	490	103	2.4
YELLOW				
Regular				
(Albers)	1 oz	100	22	1.0
bolted *(Tone's)*	1 tsp	9	2	0.1
degermed, unenriched	1 cup	505	107	2.3
enriched *(Aunt Jemima)*	3 tbsp	102	22	0.5
enriched, degermed	1 cup	505	107	2.3
whole-grain	1 cup	442	94	4.4
whole-grain *(Arrowhead Mills)*	2 oz	210	43	2.0
whole-grain *(Arrowhead Mills)*	2 oz	210	43	2.0
Self-rising				
(Aunt Jemima)	3 tbsp	100	21	1.0
bolted, plain, enriched	1 cup	407	86	4.1
bolted, w/wheat flour added, enriched	1 cup	592	125	4.8
enriched, degermed	1 cup	490	103	2.4
whole-grain *(Hodgson Mill)*	1/4 cup	90	21	1.0
CORNSTARCH				
	1 cup	488	117	0.1
(Argo)	1 tbsp	30	7	0.0
(Cream)	1 tbsp	29	7	0.0
(Kingsford)	1 tbsp	30	7	0.0
(Tone's)	1 tsp	10	2	0.1
100% pure *(Hodgson Mill)*	2 tsp	35	9	0.0
COTTAGE CHEESE. See under CHEESE.				
COTTONSEED FLOUR. See under FLOUR.				
COTTONSEED KERNELS				
roasted	1 cup	754	33	54.1
roasted	1 tbsp	51	2	3.6
COTTONSEED MEAL, partially defatted	1 oz	104	11	1.4
COTTONSEED OIL				
	1 cup	1927	0	218.0
	1 tbsp	120	0	13.6
(Wesson)	1 tbsp	122	0	13.6
w/sesame oil, seasoned, 'Mongolian Fire Oil' *(House of Tsang)*	1 tsp	45	0	5.0
COUSCOUS				
cooked	1 cup	176	36	0.3
savory, prepared *(Fantastic Foods)*	2/3 cup	160	33	0.7
uncooked	1 cup	591	123	0.8
uncooked	1 oz	96	20	0.1
uncooked *(Near East)*	1.25 oz	120	26	0.0
uncooked 'Elegant Grains' *(Fantastic Foods)*	1/4 cup	210	43	0.0
whole wheat, prepared w/2 tbsp salted butter *(Fantastic Foods)*	1/2 cup	111	20	2.0
whole wheat, uncooked, 'Elegant Grains' *(Fantastic Foods)*	1/4 cup	210	45	1.0
COUSCOUS DISH/ENTRÉE				
pilaf, cooked *(Casbah)*	3/4 cup	220	40	0.5
pilaf, savory, prepared w/2 tbsp salted butter *(Quick Pilaf)*	1/2 cup	124	19	3.0
pilaf, savory, prepared w/o additional ingredients *(Quick Pilaf)*	1/2 cup	94	19	0.0
pilaf, uncooked *(Casbah)*	28 grams	100	20	0.0
w/lentils, cooked *(Fantastic Foods)*	1 serving	220	47	1.0
w/lentils, uncooked *(Fantastic Foods)*	2.3 oz	220	47	1.0
CRAB				
ALASKA KING				
boiled, poached, or steamed	1 med leg	130	0	2.1
boiled, poached, or steamed	3 oz	82	0	1.3

Food Name	Serv. Size	Total Cal.	Carbs GMS	Fat GMS
raw	1 med leg	144	0	1.0
raw	3 oz	71	0	0.5
BLUE				
Canned				
	1 cup	134	0	1.7
	3 oz	84	0	1.0
	1 oz	28	0	0.3
drained	6.5-oz can	124	0	1.5
Fresh				
boiled, poached, or steamed	3 oz	87	0	1.5
boiled, poached, or steamed, flakes and pieces	1 cup	120	0	2.1
boiled, poached, or steamed, pieces	1 cup	138	0	2.4
boiled, poached, or steamed, w/o shell	1 oz	29	0	0.5
raw	1 med crab	18	0	0.2
raw	3 oz	74	0	0.9
DUNGENESS				
Canned *(S&W)*	1/3 cup	80	0	1.0
Fresh				
boiled, poached, or steamed	1 med crab	140	1	1.6
boiled, poached, or steamed	3 oz	94	1	1.1
raw	1 med crab	140	1	1.6
raw	3 oz	73	1	0.8
MIXED SPECIES				
15% leg meat, canned *(Crown Prince)*	1/2 can	50	1	0.0
white meat, canned *(Crown Prince)*	1/2 can	50	0	0.0
QUEEN				
boiled, poached, or steamed	3 oz	98	0	1.3
raw	3 oz	77	0	1.0
SNOW				
frozen *(Wakefield)*	3 oz	60	0	1.0
raw, Opilio, clusters *(Peter Pan Seafoods)*	3.5 oz	91	0	1.2
raw, Opilio, scored, 'Snap 'n' Eat' *(Peter Pan Seafoods)*	3.5 oz	91	0	1.2
SOFTSHELL				
boiled	4 oz	116	0.0	2.0
boiled, approx 4.75 oz	1 cup	138	0.0	2.4
poached	4 oz	116	0.0	2.0
poached, approx 4.75 oz	1 cup	138	0.0	2.4
raw	1 lb	395	0.2	4.9
raw	1 oz	25	<.1	0.3
raw, approx 0.7 oz	1 crab	18	<.1	0.2
steamed	4 oz	116	0.0	2.0
steamed, approx 4.75 oz	1 cup	138	0.0	2.4
CRAB ENTRÉE/DINNER *(Wakefield)*				
w/shrimp, frozen	3 oz	60	0	1.0
CRAB SUBSTITUTE				
Alaska King style, made from surimi	3 oz	87	9	1.1
made from surimi	1 oz	28	2	0.3
made from surimi	3 oz	84	6	0.8
(Icicle Brand)	3.5 oz	99	11	0.1
(Peter Pan Seafoods)				
leg style, made from surimi and 10% crab, 'Classic Seablends'	3.5 oz	85	0	0.4
leg style, made from surimi, 'Standard Seablends'	3.5 oz	88	0	0.4
salad style made from surimi and 10% crab, 'Classic Seablends Combo'	3.5 oz	85	0	0.4
salad style, made from surimi 'Standard Seablends Combo'	3.5 oz	88	0	0.4
(Trader Joe's) made from surimi	1/2 cup	80	14	1.0
CRABAPPLE, raw, sliced	1 cup	84	22	0.3

Food Name	Serv. Size	Total Cal.	Carbs GMS	Fat GMS
CRACKER				
(Adrienne's)				
lahvosh, 'Classic Island'	7 crackers	140	21	4.0
lahvosh, onion	4 crackers	66	10	1.9
lahvosh, 10-grain	4 crackers	59	10	1.6
(Ak-Mak) wheat, 100% stone ground, w/sesame	5 crackers	116	19	2.3
(American Classic)				
butter flavor	4 crackers	70	9	3.0
cracked wheat	4 crackers	70	8	4.0
golden, w/sesame	4 crackers	70	9	3.0
onion, minced	4 crackers	70	10	3.0
toasted poppy	4 crackers	70	9	3.0
(Auburn Farms)				
onion, 7-grain, nonfat, bite size	0.5 oz	60	12	0.0
7-grain, bite size	1 oz	120	24	0.0
vegetable, 7-grain, nonfat, bite size	1 oz	120	24	0.0
(Barbara's Bakery)				
'Wheatines' less salt	1 serving	50	10	1.5
'Wheatines' unsalted tops	0.5 oz	60	9	2.0
'Wheatines' sesame, less salt	1 serving	50	10	1.5
'Wheatines,' w/pepper	1 serving	50	10	1.5
'Wheatine' bits	0.5 oz	60	9	2.0
(Breton)				
low-sodium	3 crackers	70	8	3.0
sesame	3 crackers	80	9	3.5
(Cabaret)	3 crackers	70	9	3.5
(Carr's)				
'Monterey' savory wheat	3 crackers	70	9	2.5
'Monterey' hearty wheat	3 crackers	60	9	2.0
'Monterey' sesame and onion	3 crackers	70	9	3.0
'Monterey' roasted vegetable	3 crackers	60	10	2.0
'Table Water'	5 crackers	70	13	1.5
'Table Water' w/toasted sesame seeds	5 crackers	70	13	1.5
'Table Water' w/cracked pepper	5 crackers	70	13	1.5
'Table Water' w/roasted garlic and herbs	5 crackers	70	13	1.5
(Cheddar Wedges) cheese flavor, bite size	31 pieces	70	9	3.0
(Cheez-It)				
cheese flavor	12 crackers	70	7	4.0
hot and spicy	12 crackers	70	8	4.0
low-salt	12 crackers	70	7	4.0
party mix	1/2 cup	140	19	5.0
white cheddar	12 crackers	76	9	4.0
(Club Partners) garlic bread flavor	4 crackers	60	10	2.0
(Crackups)				
cheddar	0.5 oz	70	10	3.0
salsa	0.5 oz	70	9	3.0
(Crisp & Light)				
'Crackerbread'	1 slice	17	3	1.0
'Crackerbread' salt-free	1 slice	17	3	1.0
(Dandy) soup and oyster, 5 oz serving	20 crackers	60	10	2.0
(Dar-Vida)				
crispbread, regular	1 cracker	20	4	1.0
crispbread, sesame	1 cracker	22	4	1.0
sesame, 'Crispbread'	1 cracker	22	4	1.0
(Delicious)				
bacon flavor	0.5 oz	70	10	3.0
bite size	0.5 oz	70	9	3.0

Food Name	Serv. Size	Total Cal.	Carbs GMS	Fat GMS
cheese flavor, 'Big'	25 crackers	140	19	6.0
'Crackerdiles'	0.5 oz	70	9	3.0
garden vegetable	0.5 oz	70	10	3.0
garlic 'Discos'	0.5 oz	78	6	5.0
low-sodium, bite size	0.5 oz	70	9	3.0
nacho cheese	0.5 oz	89	8	5.0
onion, 'Discos'	0.5 oz	76	7	5.0
pumpernickel	0.5 oz	70	9	3.0
'Regency'	0.5 oz	70	9	3.0
'Snackers'	0.5 oz	70	9	3.0
sour cream, w/onion, 'Discos'	0.5 oz	79	6	5.0
sourdough	0.5 oz	70	9	3.0
'Wheat On'	0.5 oz	68	8	3.0
wheat wafer, w/sesame	0.5 oz	80	9	4.0
'Wheatstone'	0.5 oz	70	9	3.0
(Devonsheer)				
Melba toast, honey bran	1 cracker	16	3	0.4
Melba toast, honey bran, 'Rounds'	0.5 oz	52	10	0.9
Melba toast, plain	1 cracker	16	3	0.4
Melba toast, plain, 'Rounds'	0.5 oz	53	11	0.6
Melba toast, plain, 'Unsalted'	1 cracker	16	3	0.4
Melba toast, plain, 'Unsalted Rounds'	0.5 oz	52	11	0.6
Melba toast, rye	1 cracker	16	3	0.4
Melba toast, rye, 'Rounds'	0.5 oz	53	11	0.6
Melba toast, rye, 'Unsalted'	1 cracker	16	3	0.4
Melba toast, sesame	1 cracker	16	3	0.5
Melba toast, sesame, 'Rounds'	0.5 oz	57	9	1.8
Melba toast, w/onion, 'Rounds'	0.5 oz	51	11	0.6
Melba toast, w/vegetable	1 cracker	16	3	0.4
Melba toast, whole wheat	1 cracker	16	3	0.4
Melba toast, whole wheat, unsalted	1 cracker	16	3	0.4
(Distinctive)				
cracked wheat	3 crackers	100	14	4.0
'English Water Biscuit'	4 crackers	70	13	1.0
sesame	4 crackers	80	12	4.0
thins	4 crackers	70	10	3.0
toasted wheat	4 crackers	80	12	3.0
wheat	4 crackers	100	13	5.0
(Eagle)				
'Cheese on Cheese'	6 crackers	210	24	11.0
peanut butter and cheese sandwich	6 crackers	230	25	12.0
peanut butter on toast	6 crackers	210	23	10.0
wheat, w/cheddar cheese	6 crackers	200	24	10.0
(Eden Foods)				
nori maki	15 crackers	110	24	0.0
rice, brown	5 crackers	120	22	2.0
(Escort) butter flavor	3 crackers	70	9	4.0
(Estee)				
Melba toast, wheat, '6-calorie'	1 cracker	6	1	1.0
Melba toast, wheat, 'Snax'	1 oz	100	22	1.0
saltine, unsalted	4 crackers	60	9	2.0
ranch flavor 'Snack Crisps'	0.66 oz	80	13	2.0
(Euphrates)				
wheat	1 cracker	19	3	0.8
wheat, low-salt	1 cracker	19	3	0.8
(Featherweight) low-salt	2 pieces	30	5	1.0

Food Name	Serv. Size	Total Cal.	Carbs GMS	Fat GMS
(FFV)				
'Schooners'	0.5 oz	60	10	2.0
sesame, 'Crisp'	1 cracker	60	10	2.0
soda, 'Ocean Crisps'	1 cracker	60	10	2.0
stoned wheat	4 crackers	60	10	2.0
wafer, w/sesame, 'Crisp'	4 crackers	60	9	2.0
wheat, 'Crispy Wafer'	6 crackers	70	9	3.0
(FiberRich) bran	1 cracker	18	6	1.0
(Finast)				
snack	12 crackers	70	9	3.0
wheat, 'Snacks'	7 crackers	70	9	3.0
(Finn Crisp)				
crispbread, dark	2 crackers	38	9	1.0
crispbread, light, 'Hi-Fiber'	1 cracker	35	8	1.0
crispbread, regular	2 crackers	38	9	1.0
crispbread, rye, original, 'Hi-Fiber'	1 cracker	40	10	0.0
crispbread, w/caraway	2 slices	38	9	1.0
(Flavor Tree)				
sesame chips	1/4 cup	163	11	9.2
sesame sticks	1/4 cup	133	11	9.1
sesame sticks, no salt	1/4 cup	131	13	8.1
(Frito-Lay's)				
cheddar	0.5 oz	70	8	4.0
cheese-filled	1.5 oz	210	24	10.0
Italian, zesty	0.5 oz	70	9	3.0
peanut butter, bar	1.75 oz	270	30	16.0
peanut butter filled	6 crackers	210	24	10.0
(Frookie)				
garlic, w/herbs, nonfat, 'Gourmet'	4 crackers	35	7	0.0
pepper, nonfat, 'Gourmet'	4 crackers	35	7	0.0
water, nonfat, 'Gourmet'	4 crackers	35	7	0.0
whole wheat, nonfat, 'Gourmet'	4 crackers	35	7	0.0
(Garden Crisps) vegetables	15 crackers	130	22	3.5
(Grand Union) cheese flavor, 'Big'	25 crackers	140	19	6.0
(Hain)				
cheese flavor	1 oz	130	17	6.0
onion flavor	1 oz	130	17	6.0
onion flavor, no salt added	1 oz	130	17	6.0
'Rich'	1 oz	130	18	5.0
'Rich' no salt added	1 oz	130	18	5.0
rye	1 oz	120	19	4.0
rye, no salt added	1 oz	120	19	4.0
sesame	1 oz	140	16	7.0
sesame, no salt added	1 oz	140	16	7.0
sour cream, w/chive	1 oz	130	15	6.0
sour cream, w/chive, no salt added	1 oz	130	15	6.0
sourdough	0.5 oz	65	9	3.0
sourdough, low-salt	1 oz	130	18	5.0
vegetable, no salt added	1 oz	130	10	5.0
(Health Valley)				
cheese, organic, nonfat	0.5 oz	40	9	0.0
cheese, whole wheat, nonfat	5 crackers	50	11	0.0
herb, organic, nonfat	0.5 oz	40	9	0.0
onion, organic, nonfat	0.5 oz	40	9	0.0
rice bran	7 crackers	130	19	4.0
7-grain, stoned wheat	13 crackers	120	17	5.0
7-grain, stoned wheat, no salt added	13 crackers	120	17	5.0

Food Name	Serv. Size	Total Cal.	Carbs GMS	Fat GMS
7-grain, w/vegetable, organic	0.5 oz	40	9	0.0
stoned wheat	13 crackers	120	17	6.0
stoned wheat, no salt added	13 crackers	120	17	6.0
stoned wheat, w/herbs, no salt added	13 crackers	120	17	6.0
stoned wheat, w/sesame	13 crackers	130	16	6.0
stoned wheat, w/sessame, no salt added	13 crackers	130	17	6.0
whole wheat, nonfat	5 crackers	50	11	0.0
whole wheat, w/herbs, nonfat	5 crackers	50	11	0.0
whole wheat, w/onions, nonfat	5 crackers	50	11	0.0
whole wheat, w/vegetables, nonfat	5 crackers	50	11	0.0
(Kraft)				
'Handi-Snacks' bacon flavor, w/cheese	1 pkg	130	8	9.0
'Handi-Snacks' peanut butter and cheese sandwich	1 pkg	190	11	14.0
(Hickory Farms)				
cracked wheat wafers	8 crackers	100	17	3.0
'Old Fashioned' *(Hickory Farms)*	10 pieces	90	16	3.0
'Rounds O' Rye' barbecue flavor	1 oz	153	13	10.6
'Rounds O' Rye' garlic	1 oz	147	15	8.9
'Rounds O' Rye' natural	1 oz	156	12	10.9
'Rounds O'Rye' sour cream	1 oz	155	13	10.7
rye wafers	8 crackers	90	17	2.0
rye wafers, salt-free	8 crackers	90	18	1.0
stoned wheat wafers, salt-free	8 crackers	100	18	2.0
'Wheat Mill Wafers' salt-free	4 crackers	50	9	1.0
(Kavli)				
Norwegian crispbread, thick	1 slice	35	8	0.3
Norwegian crispbread, thin	2 slices	40	8	0.3
(Keebler)				
cheese, sandwich, w/peanut butter	2 crackers	70	9	3.0
'Club' low-salt	4 crackers	60	9	3.0
'Hi Ho'	5 crackers	70	10	2.5
'Krispy' saltine	5 crackers	60	11	1.0
'Krispy' saltine, mild cheddar	5 crackers	60	10	2.0
'Krispy' saltine, unsalted tops	5 crackers	60	11	1.0
peanut butter and toast sandwich	2 crackers	70	9	3.0
sesame breadstix, food service product	2 pieces	26	4	0.8
'Toasteds' bacon flavor	4 crackers	60	8	3.0
'Toasteds' buttercrisp	4 crackers	60	8	3.0
'Toasteds' cheddar, juniors	8 pieces	80	8	4.0
'Toasteds' onion flavor	4 crackers	60	9	3.0
'Toasteds' rye	4 crackers	60	8	3.0
'Toasteds' sesame	4 crackers	60	8	3.0
'Town House'	4 crackers	70	8	4.0
'Town House' 50% less fat	5 crackers	70	11	2.0
'Town House' food service product	2 crackers	35	4	2.0
'Town House' low-salt	4 crackers	70	8	4.0
'Town House' sandwich, cheddar	1 cracker	70	6	4.0
'Waldorf' no salt, food service product	2 crackers	30	5	1.0
wheat, sandwich, w/American cheese	1 cracker	70	7	4.0
wheats, whole grain, food service product	2 crackers	35	5	1.5
'Wheatables'	12 crackers	70	9	3.0
'Wheatables' low-salt	1 cracker	5	1	0.2
'Wheatables' reduced-fat	29 crackers	130	21	3.5
'Zesta' saltine	5 crackers	60	10	2.0
'Zesta' saltine, 50% less salt	5 crackers	60	11	2.0
'Zesta' saltine, food service product	2 crackers	25	4	1.0
'Zesta' saltine, low-salt	5 crackers	60	10	2.0

Food Name	Serv. Size	Total Cal.	Carbs GMS	Fat GMS
'Zesta' saltine, nonfat	5 crackers	50	11	0.0
'Zesta' saltine, unsalted tops	5 crackers	60	10	2.0
'Zesta' saltine, unsalted tops, food service product	2 crackers	25	4	1.0
'Zesta' saltine, wheat	5 crackers	60	10	2.0
(Lite 'N Krispy)				
rice sticks	6 sticks	40	8	0.5
rice sticks, no salt	6 sticks	40	8	0.5
(Little Debbie) wheat, w/cheddar cheese	1 serving	140	15	8.0
(M&M Mars)				
'Combos' cheese flavor	1.8 oz	240	34	10.0
'Combos' peanut butter	1.8 oz	240	30	10.0
(Manischewitz)				
'Tam Tams'	10 crackers	147	17	8.0
'Tam Tams' no salt	10 crackers	138	18	7.0
'Garlic Tams'	10 crackers	153	19	8.0
matzo, American	1 matzo	115	22	1.9
matzo, board, 'Daily Unsalted'	1 oz	110	24	0.3
matzo, board, 'Passover'	1.1 oz	129	27	0.4
matzo, board, thin	0.9 oz	100	21	0.3
matzo, dietetic, thin	0.8 oz	91	19	0.4
matzo, egg and onion, board	1 oz	112	23	1.0
matzo, egg, board, 'Passover'	1.2 oz	132	27	2.0
matzo, egg, miniature, 'Passover'	10 crackers	108	20	2.0
matzo, miniature	10 crackers	90	20	1.0
matzo, tea, thin	1 matzo	100	22	0.3
matzo, whole wheat, w/bran, board	1 oz	110	21	0.6
'Onion Tams'	10 crackers	150	18	8.0
'Wheat Tams'	10 crackers	150	18	8.0
(McCrakens)				
cheddar, tangy	1 oz	140	18	8.0
country butter flavor	1 oz	140	18	8.0
sour cream w/chive flavor	1 oz	140	18	8.0
wheat, toasted	1 oz	140	18	8.0
(Meal Mates)				
bread wafer, w/sesame	3 crackers	70	9	3.0
crispbread, w/sesame	3 crackers	70	9	3.0
(Musso's) garlic toast, w/cheese	3 pieces	70	11	2.5
(Nabisco)				
bacon-flavored	15 crackers	160	19	8.0
'Bran Thins' *(Nabisco)*	7 crackers	60	9	3.0
cheese, sandwich, w/peanut butter	4 pieces	130	15	7.0
'Cheese Nips'	13 pieces	70	9	3.0
'Chicken in a Biskit'	7 pieces	80	8	5.0
'Crown Pilot'	1 cracker	70	13	1.5
'Harvest Crisps' oat	6 crackers	60	10	2.0
'Harvest Crisps' rice	6 crackers	60	11	2.0
'Harvest Wheat'	4 crackers	60	8	3.0
'Harvest Wheat' low-salt	1 cracker	14	2	0.6
'Oat Thins'	18 crackers	140	20	6.0
'Oysterettes' soup and oyster	18 crackers	60	10	1.0
'Premium' saltine, low salt	5 crackers	60	10	1.0
'Premium' saltine, multigrain	5 crackers	60	10	1.5
'Premium' saltine, original	5 crackers	59	10	1.4
'Premium' saltine, unsalted tops	5 crackers	60	10	1.5
'Premium' saltine, wheat	4 crackers	60	10	2.0
'Ritz'	4 crackers	70	9	4.0
'Ritz' low-salt	5 crackers	80	10	4.0

Food Name	Serv. Size	Total Cal.	Carbs GMS	Fat GMS
'Ritz' wheat	1 cracker	14	2	0.6
'Ritz' wheat, low salt	1 cracker	14	2	0.6
'Ritz' whole wheat	5 crackers	70	9	3.0
'Ritz Bits' cheese flavor	22 pieces	70	8	4.0
'Ritz Bits Sandwiches' w/peanut butter	12 crackers	80	8	4.0
'Ritz Bits Sandwiches' w/cheese	6 crackers	80	7	5.0
'Royal Lunch' milk biscuit	1 cracker	60	10	2.0
'Royal Lunch' soda	0.5 oz	60	17	3.0
Swiss cheese, 'Naturally Flavored'	7 crackers	70	9	3.0
'Toast Sandwich' w/peanut butter	4 pieces	130	15	7.0
'Triscuit' wheat	10 bits	44	7	1.7
'Triscuit' wheat, low-salt	3 crackers	60	10	2.0
'Triscuit Bits'	15 pieces	60	10	3.0
'Triscuit Bits' wheat	8 crackers	60	10	2.0
'Twigs' cheese	1 cracker	10	1	0.5
'Uneeda Biscuits' no salt tops	2 crackers	60	10	2.0
'Waverly Wafer'	4 crackers	70	10	3.0
'Waverly Wafer' low-salt	4 crackers	70	10	3.0
'Wheat Thins'	16 crackers	140	19	6.0
'Wheat Thins'	7 crackers	70	9	4.0
'Wheat Thins' less fat	18 crackers	120	21	4.0
'Wheat Thins' low-salt	1 cracker	14	2	0.6
'Wheat Thins' multigrain	17 crackers	130	21	4.0
'Wheatsworth'	1 cracker	14	2	0.6
'Wheatsworth' low-salt	1 cracker	14	2	0.6
(Nature's Path)				
unleavened bread, carrot raisin, flourless, sprouted, organic	2 oz	130	22	1.0
unleavened bread, millet-rice, flourless, sprouted, organic	2 oz	140	23	1.0
unleavened bread, rye, w/carrot and raisin, organic	1 slice	120	26	0.0
unleavened bread, salt-free, organic, 'Sun Seed'	1 slice	160	29	2.0
unleavened bread, w/apple and spice, organic	1 slice	130	9	0.0
unleavened bread, w/fruit and nuts, organic	1 slice	140	27	0.0
unleavened bread, whole rye, flourless, sprouted, organic	2 oz	140	23	1.0
unleavened bread, whole wheat, flourless, sprouted, organic	2 oz	140	23	1.0
(North Castles) soda, 'English'	1 cracker	10	3	0.0
(Old London)				
Melba toast, bacon, 'Rounds'	0.5 oz	53	10	1.0
Melba toast, garlic, 'Rounds'	0.5 oz	56	10	1.2
Melba toast, pumpernickel	0.5 oz	54	11	0.6
Melba toast, rye	0.5 oz	52	11	0.7
Melba toast, rye, 'Rounds'	0.5 oz	52	11	0.7
Melba toast, sesame	0.5 oz	55	9	1.8
Melba toast, sesame, 'Rounds'	0.5 oz	56	9	1.8
Melba toast, sesame, unsalted	0.5 oz	55	9	1.8
Melba toast, wheat	0.5 oz	51	11	0.7
Melba toast, white	0.5 oz	51	10	0.6
Melba toast, white, 'Rounds'	0.5 oz	48	10	0.6
Melba toast, white, unsalted	0.5 oz	51	11	0.6
Melba toast, whole grain	0.5 oz	52	10	0.9
Melba toast, whole grain, 'Rounds'	0.5 oz	54	10	1.2
Melba toast, whole grain, unsalted	0.5 oz	53	10	1.0
(Orchard Crisps)				
apple cinnamon	0.5 oz	60	11	2.0
banana walnut *(Orchard Crisps)*	0.5 oz	60	11	2.0
(OTC) soup and oyster	1 cracker	25	4	1.0
(Pacific Grain)				
barbecue, baked, 94% fat-free	30 grams	120	25	1.5

Food Name	Serv. Size	Total Cal.	Carbs GMS	Fat GMS
potato, 100% natural, baked, 94% fat-free,	30 grams	120	26	0.5
potato, au gratin flavored, baked, 94% nonfat	1 oz	120	24	2.0
sour cream, w/chive, baked, 94% fat-free	30 grams	120	24	2.0
(Pepperidge Farm)				
'Flutters'	0.75 oz	100	15	4.0
'Flutters' garden herb	0.75 oz	100	14	4.0
'Flutters' golden, w/sesame	0.75 oz	110	13	5.0
'Flutters' toasted wheat	0.75 oz	110	13	5.0
'Goldfish' cheddar	1 oz	120	19	4.0
'Goldfish' cheddar, original	1 oz	130	18	5.0
'Goldfish' Parmesan cheese	1 oz	120	19	4.0
'Goldfish' pizza	1 oz	130	19	5.0
'Goldfish Snack' honey nut, w/roasted cashews and almonds	1/2 cup	180	20	9.0
'Goldfish Snack' w/roasted peanuts	1/2 cup	170	21	8.0
'Goldfish Thins' cheddar	4 crackers	50	8	2.0
'Guppies' cheddar	12 pieces	40	5	2.0
'Snack Sticks'	8 crackers	130	19	5.0
'Snack Sticks' pumpernickel	8 crackers	140	20	6.0
'Snack Sticks' sesame	8 crackers	140	19	5.0
(Premier Japan)				
rice, sembei, 'Fire & Spice'	4 crackers	50	10	1.0
rice sembei, w/sesame, wheat-free, lowfat	4 crackers	60	10	1.0
(Ralston)				
'Oat Bran Krisps'	0.5 oz	60	9	3.0
'Oat Krisp'	0.5 oz	50	7	2.0
vegetable	17 crackers	150	19	7.0
vegetable, less fat	21 crackers	120	23	3.0
wheat, w/sesame, 'Jacquet'	8 crackers	140	18	6.0
(Red Oval Farms)				
stoned wheat, w/toasted sesame, mini	19 crackers	140	21	4.0
(Rokeach)				
cheese flavor	1 oz	140	16	8.0
saltine	10 pieces	120	20	3.0
snack	9 crackers	130	19	5.0
(Roman Meal)				
wheat, w/onion, baked	6 crackers	70	9	3.0
wheat, w/sesame, baked	6 crackers	70	9	3.0
whole wheat, baked	6 crackers	70	9	3.0
whole wheat, rye and bran, baked	6 crackers	70	9	3.0
(RyKrisp)				
'Rykrisp Twindividuals' 2 triple pieces.	0.5 oz	45	11	1.0
crispbread, original	2 crackers	60	8	0.0
crispbread, rye, triple cracker	1 wafer	92	21	0.3
crispbread, rye, w/sesame, 2 triple pieces	0.5 oz	50	10	2.0
crispbread, seasoned	2 crackers	60	10	1.5
crispbread, sesame	2 crackers	60	11	1.5
(Ryvita)				
crispbread, dark rye	1 cracker	26	6	1.0
crispbread, high-fiber, 'Crisp Bread'	1 cracker	23	4	1.0
crispbread, high-fiber, 'Snackbread'	1 cracker	14	3	1.0
crispbread, light	1 cracker	26	6	1.0
crispbread, rye, light	1 cracker	26	6	1.0
crispbread, rye, dark	1 cracker	26	6	1.0
crispbread, rye, w/sesame	1 cracker	31	5	1.0
wheat, 'Original Snackbroad'	1 cracker	20	4	1.0
(Snackwell's)				
cheese, zesty	1 serving	129	23	3.0

Food Name	Serv. Size	Total Cal.	Carbs GMS	Fat GMS
cracked pepper	7 crackers	61	10	1.6
French onion	1 serving	128	23	3.0
golden, reduced fat	6 crackers	60	11	1.0
Italian ranch	1 serving	128	23	3.0
salsa, snack	1 serving	128	23	3.0
wheat	1 serving	62	12	1.5
wheat, nonfat	5 crackers	60	12	0.0
wheat thins, baked	1 serving	136	20	5.8
(Spicer's)				
diet, natural, for weight control	1 oz	100	11	4.0
w/onion, for weight control	1 oz	100	12	4.0
wheat, barbecue, for weight control	1 oz	100	12	5.0
(Stop & Shop) cheese flavor, 'Big'	25 crackers	140	19	6.0
(Sunshine)				
heart shaped	1 cracker	9	1	0.4
soup and oyster	16 crackers	60	11	1.0
wheat	8 crackers	70	9	4.0
wheat, heart shaped	1 cracker	9	1	0.4
(Valley Bakery)	8 crackers	110	21	1.0
'Janet Saghatelian's Hearts'	8 crackers	110	21	1.0
lahvosh, 5-inch rounds	1.2 oz	140	26	1.5
lahvosh, 5-inch wheat rounds	1.2 oz	130	26	1.5
lahvosh, hearts	1 oz	110	21	1.0
lahvosh, 'Sweet-heart Crispies'	1 oz	120	22	2.5
lahvosh, 3-inch rounds	1 oz	110	21	1.0
lahvosh, 3-inch wheat rounds	1 oz	110	20	1.0
lahvosh, 2-inch rounds	1 oz	110	21	1.0
rounds, hors d'oeurvre size	1 cracker	28	6	0.3
rounds, snack size	2 crackers	130	26	1.0
w/sesame seed, original, Armenian	1 slice	190	37	2.0
(Vivant) vegetable	3 crackers	70	9	3.0
(Wasa)				
crispbread, 'Extra Crisp'	1 cracker	25	5	0.0
crispbread, cinnamon toast	1 slice	60	11	1.0
crispbread, corn, original, gluten- and wheat-free	1 slice	40	7	1.0
crispbread, light, 'Crisp 'N Light'	1 cracker	25	5	0.0
crispbread, multigrain, original	1 slice	45	8	0.0
crispbread, rye	1 crispbread	37	8	0.1
crispbread, rye, fiber	1 slice	30	4	1.0
crispbread, rye, golden	1 cracker	35	7	0.0
crispbread, rye, hearty	1 slice	45	9	0.0
crispbread, rye, light	1 slice	25	5	0.0
crispbread, rye, organic, salt-free	1 slice	25	7	0.0
crispbread, rye, original	1 slice	30	7	0.0
crispbread, sesame, savory	1 cracker	30	4	1.0
crispbread, sourdough rye, light, 'Crisp 'N Light'	3 pieces	60	12	0.0
crispbread, sourdough rye, original	1 slice	35	7	0.0
crispbread, sourdough, crisp	3 pieces	50	11	0.0
crispbread, wheat, light, 'Crisp 'N Light'	2 crackers	50	10	0.0
crispbread, wheat, toasted, original	1 slice	50	8	1.5
crispbread, wheat, w/sesame	1 cracker	50	8	2.0
crispbread, whole wheat	1 slice	30	4	1.0
crispbread, whole wheat, original	1 slice	50	11	0.5
(Weight Watchers)				
crispbread, garlic flavor	2 crackers	30	7	0.0
crispbread, harvest rice	2 crackers	30	7	0.0

Food Name	Serv. Size	Total Cal.	Carbs GMS	Fat GMS
(Westbrae)				
no salt, wafer	4-1/2 wafers	40	8	0.0
onion garlic, wafer	4-1/2 wafers	40	8	0.0
tamari, wafer	4-1/2 wafers	40	8	0.0
w/sesame, wafer	4-1/2 wafers	40	8	0.0
(Wheat Krisp) wheat	0.5 oz	50	11	1.0
(Zings)				
cracker chips, cheddar, baked	0.5 oz	70	9	3.0
cracker chips, ranch flavor, baked	0.5 oz	70	9	3.0
CRACKER CRUMBS				
'Ritz' *(Nabisco)*	1/3 cup	140	17	7.0
'Premium' *(Nabisco)*	1/4 cup	100	23	0.0
CRACKER MEAL				
	1 cup	440	93	2.0
	1 oz	109	23	0.5
(Golden Dipt)	1 oz	100	22	0.0
(Nabisco)	1/4 cup	110	24	0.0
extra fine, food service product *(Keebler)*	4 tbsp	130	23	0.0
matzo *(Manischewitz)*	1/2 cup	243	54	0.3
matzo, 'Daily' *(Manischewitz)*	1 cup	514	109	1.4
matzo, 'Farfel' *(Manischewitz)*	1 cup	280	60	0.8
CRANBERRY				
Fresh				
raw, chopped	1 cup	54	14	0.2
raw, whole	1 cup	47	12	0.2
CRANBERRY BEAN. See BEAN, CRANBERRY.				
CRANBERRY JUICE				
(J. Hungerford) 100% juice	9.03 fl oz	133	33	0.0
(Knudsen)				
	8 fl oz	60	14	0.0
'Just Cranberry'	8 fl oz	40	10	0.0
'Yankee'	8 fl oz	120	30	0.0
(Lucky Leaf)	6 fl oz	110	26	0.0
(Ocean Spray) 'Crantastic'	6 fl oz	100	26	0.0
(Santa Cruz Natural) organic, 'Sparkling'	8 fl oz	90	22	1.0
CRANBERRY JUICE COCKTAIL. See under FRUIT JUICE DRINK.				
CRANBERRY SAUCE				
Canned				
(A&P)	2 oz	100	25	1.0
(Knudsen)	1 oz	30	8	1.0
jellied *(Finast)*	2 oz	90	22	0.0
jellied *(Ocean Spray)*	2 oz	80	22	0.0
jellied *(Pathmark)*	2 oz	90	22	0.0
jellied *(S&W)*	1/4 cup	100	26	0.0
jellied, 'Old Fashioned' *(S&W)*	1/2 cup	90	22	0.0
sweetened, 1/2-inch slices	1 slice	86	22	0.1
sweetened	1 cup	418	108	0.4
whole berry *(Finast)*	2 oz	90	22	0.0
whole berry *(Ocean Spray)*	2 oz	80	21	0.0
whole berry *(S&W)*	1/4 cup	100	26	0.0
whole berry, 'Old Fashioned' *(S&W)*	1/2 cup	90	22	0.0
CRAPPIE. See SUNFISH.				
CRAYFISH				
mixed species, farmed, cooked	3 oz	74	0	1.1
mixed species, farmed, raw	3 oz	61	0	0.8
mixed species, wild, cooked	3 oz	70	0	1.0
mixed species, wild, raw	3 oz	65	0	0.8

Food Name	Serv. Size	Total Cal.	Carbs GMS	Fat GMS
CRAYFISH DINNER/ENTRÉE				
(Cajun Cookin') crayfish etouffee, frozen	12 oz	390	51	10.0
CREAM				
half and half	1 cup	315	10	27.8
half and half	1 fl oz	39	1	3.5
half and half	1 tbsp	20	1	1.7
half and half *(Crowley)*	1 fl oz	35	1	3.0
half and half *(Darigold)*	8 fl oz	310	11	27.0
half and half *(Knudsen)*	4 fl oz	150	5	13.0
half and half *(Rockview)*	2 tbsp	35	0	3.0
Hawaiian macadamia flavored *(International Delight)*	1 tbsp	30	7	0.0
heavy, whipping	8 fl oz	821	7	88.1
heavy, whipping	1 fl oz	103	1	11.0
heavy, whipping	1 tbsp	52	0	5.5
heavy, whipping *(Crowley)*	1 oz	110	1	11.0
heavy, whipping *(Darigold)*	1 cup	790	8	81.0
heavy, whipping, 'Classic' *(Darigold)*	1 cup	858	7	90.0
heavy, whipping, ultra-pasteurized *(Darigold)*	1 cup	790	8	81.0
light	1 cup	469	9	46.3
light	1 fl oz	59	1	5.8
light	1 tbsp	29	1	2.9
light, whipping	1 cup	699	7	73.9
light, whipping	1 tbsp	44	0	4.6
CREAM CHEESE. See under CHEESE.				
CREAM OF TARTAR				
. . . .	1 tsp	8	2	0.0
. . . .	1/2 tsp	4	1	0.0
(Tone's)	1 tsp	2	1	0.0
CREAM SUBSTITUTE				
Liquid				
(Carnation)				
butter rum flavored, nondairy, nonfat	1 tbsp	25	6	0.0
French vanilla flavored, nondairy, nonfat	1 tbsp	25	6	0.0
Irish cream flavored, nondairy, nonfat	1 tbsp	25	6	0.0
(Coffee-Mate)				
. . . .	1 tbsp	16	2	1.0
French vanilla flavored, nondairy	1 tbsp	40	5	2.0
mocha almond flavored, nondairy	2 tsp	60	9	3.0
nondairy, 'Amaretto'	1 tbsp	40	5	2.0
nondairy, 'Cinnamon Creme'	1 tbsp	40	5	2.0
nondairy, 'Hazelnut'	1 tbsp	40	5	2.0
nondairy, 'Irish Creme'	1 tbsp	40	5	2.0
nondairy, fat-free	1 tbsp	10	2	0.0
nondairy, light	1 tbsp	10	1	0.5
(Crowley) nondairy	0.5 fl oz	16	1	1.0
(Finast) nondairy, frozen	0.5 fl oz	20	2	2.0
(International Delight)				
Amaretto flavored, nondairy	1 tbsp	45	7	1.5
Hawaiian macadamia flavored, dairy	1 tbsp	30	7	0.0
Irish cream flavored, nondairy	1 tbsp	45	7	1.5
(Lucerne) nondairy, 100% milk-free	0.5 fl oz	16	1	2.0
(Mocha Mix)				
nondairy	1 tbsp	20	1	1.5
nondairy, lite	1 tbsp	10	1	1.0
(Rich's)				
nondairy, frozen, 'Coffee Rich'	0.5 fl oz	20	2	2.0
nondairy, frozen, 'Farm Rich'	0.5 fl oz	20	1	2.0

Food Name	Serv. Size	Total Cal.	Carbs GMS	Fat GMS
nondairy, frozen, 'Poly Rich'	0.5 fl oz	20	2	1.0
(Saco Foods) nondairy, 'Kwik Kream'	1 tbsp	10	2	1.0
(Westbrae) nondairy	1 tbsp	10	2	1.0
(WestSoy) nondairy, lite, all natural	1 tbsp	10	2	1.0
Powder				
(Coffee-Mate)				
nondairy	1 tsp	10	1	1.0
nondairy, 'Amaretto'	2 tsp	60	9	3.0
nondairy, 'Hazelnut'	2 tsp	60	0	3.0
nondairy, 'Irish Creme'	2 tsp	60	9	3.0
nondairy, light	1 tsp	10	2	0.0
nondairy, nonfat	1 tsp	10	2	0.0
(Cremora) nondairy	1 tsp	10	1	1.0
(Diehl) nondairy	1 tsp	10	1	1.0
(IGA) nondairy	1 tsp	10	2	1.0
(Pathmark) nondairy, 'No Frills'	1 tsp	10	1	0.0
CREAM TOPPING				
(Birds Eye)				
chocolate, nondairy, frozen, 'Cool Whip'	1 tbsp	12	1	1.0
extra creamy, nondairy, frozen, 'Cool Whip Dairy Recipe'	1 tbsp	14	1	1.0
nondairy, frozen, 'Cool Whip Lite'	1 tbsp	8	1	1.0
nondairy, frozen, 'Cool Whip'	1 tbsp	12	1	1.0
(Crowley)				
whipped, pressurized can	1 tbsp	20	1	1.0
whipping, heavy	1 oz	110	1	11.0
(Darigold)				
whipping, heavy	1 cup	790	8	81.0
whipping, heavy, 'Classic'	1 cup	858	7	90.0
whipping, heavy, ultra-pasteurized	1 cup	790	8	81.0
(Estee) nondairy, prewhipped	1 tbsp	4	1	1.0
(Kraft)				
frozen, whipped, 'Real Cream'	1/4 cup	30	2	2.0
nondairy, frozen, 'Whipped Topping'	1/4 cup	35	2	3.0
(La Creme) frozen, whipped	1 tbsp	16	1	1.0
(Pet) nondairy, frozen, 'Whip'	1 tbsp	14	1	1.0
(Rich's)				
nondairy, pressurized can, 'Richwhip'	0.25 oz	20	1	2.0
nondairy, prewhipped, 'Richwhip'	1 tbsp	12	1	1.0
(Saco Foods)				
chocolate, dark, 'Dolci Frutta Con Cioccolatta'	1 serving	111	14	6.6
white, 'Dolci Frutta Crema Bianca'	1 serving	112	12	6.0
CREAM TOPPING MIX				
(D-Zerta) prepared	1 tbsp	8	0	1.0
(Dream Whip)				
mix only.	1 tbsp	6	1	0.0
prepared w/whole milk	1 tbsp	10	1	0.0
(Featherweight) prepared	1 tbsp	4	0	0.0
(Rich's) mix only, 'Richwhip'	0.25 oz	20	1	2.0
CREOLE SEASONING. See under SEASONING MIX.				
CREPE MIX (Krusteaz) prepared, 7-inch diam	2 crepes	80	14	1.0
CRIMINI MUSHROOM. See MUSHROOM, CRIMINI.				
CROAKER, ATLANTIC				
breaded, fried	3 oz	188	6	10.8
raw	3 oz	88	0	2.7
CROISSANT				
(Awrey's)				
butter	1 oz	100	10	6.0

Food Name	Serv. Size	Total Cal.	Carbs GMS	Fat GMS
margarine	1.25 oz	120	13	7.0
wheat	2.5 oz	240	24	14.0
(Pepperidge Farm)				
butter, petite, frozen	1 piece	140	13	7.0
'Sandwich Quartet'	1 croissant	170	22	7.0
(Sara Lee) butter, petite, frozen	1 croissant	120	13	6.0

CROOKNECK SQUASH. See SQUASH, CROOKNECK. Also see under SQUASH, SUMMER.

CROUTONS

Food Name	Serv. Size	Total Cal.	Carbs GMS	Fat GMS
(Brownberry)				
Caesar salad flavored	0.5 oz	62	8	2.6
cheddar cheese flavored	0.5 oz	63	8	2.8
onion and garlic flavored	0.5 oz	60	9	2.2
seasoned	1/2 oz	59	9	2.2
toasted	0.5 oz	56	10	1.4
(Ener-G Foods)				
Italian, gluten free	1 cup	241	31	12.5
onion and garlic, gluten free	1 cup	147	37	0.4
plain, gluten free	1 cup	125	17	7.0
(Fresh Gourmet)				
Caesar flavor	4 croutons	30	4	1.0
cheese and garlic flavor, homestyle	4 croutons	30	4	1.0
herb seasoned	4 croutons	30	5	1.0
(Hidden Valley Ranch)				
parmesan, Italian style, 'Salad Crispins'	1 serving	30	5	0.9
(Just Off Melrose)				
cheese and garlic	3 croutons	25	3	1.5
garlic	3 croutons	30	3	2.0
sun-dried tomato and basil	3 croutons	30	3	2.0
(Other Fine Foods) whole grain, all natural	1 oz	110	15	4.0
(Pepperidge Farm)				
cheddar and romano	9 croutons	30	4	1.0
cheese and garlic	9 croutons	35	4	1.5
onion and garlic	9 pieces	30	5	1.0
seasoned	9 croutons	35	4	1.5
seasoned, classic style	1 serving	33	4	1.3
sour cream and chive	0.5 oz	70	9	3.0
(Reese) Caesar salad flavored	0.5 oz	60	9	2.0
(Rothbury Farms)				
onion flavor poppy toast, nonfat	9 grams	35	7	0.0
seasoned, French style, nonfat	7 grams	25	5	0.0
seasoned, nonfat	7 grams	25	5	0.0

CROWDER PEA. See under BLACK-EYED PEAS.

CRUMPET

Food Name	Serv. Size	Total Cal.	Carbs GMS	Fat GMS
(Wolferman's)				
blueberry, low-fat, cholesterol-free	1 crumpet	90	21	1.0
brown sugar-cinnamon, lowfat	1 crumpet	110	21	2.0
raspberry, low-fat, cholesterol-free	1 crumpet	90	20	1.0

CUCUMBER

Fresh

Food Name	Serv. Size	Total Cal.	Carbs GMS	Fat GMS
peeled, raw, chopped	1 cup	16	3	0.2
peeled, raw, sliced	1 cup	14	3	0.2
peeled, raw, sticks, 4-inches	1 stick	1	0	0.0
peeled, raw, whole, large, 8.25 inches	1 cucumber	34	7	0.4
peeled, raw, whole, small 6-3/8 inches	1 cucumber	19	4	0.3
w/peel, raw, whole, large, 8.25 inches	1 cucumber	39	8	0.4
w/peel, raw, sliced	1/2 cup	7	1	0.1

Food Name	Serv. Size	Total Cal.	Carbs GMS	Fat GMS
CUMIN SEED				
ground *(McCormick/Schilling)*	1 tsp	11	1	0.4
whole	1 tbsp	22	3	1.3
whole	1 tsp	8	1	0.5
whole *(Durkee)*	1 tsp	10	0	0.0
whole *(Laurel Leaf)*	1 tsp	10	0	0.0
whole *(McCormick/Schilling)*	1 tsp	16	2	0.8
whole *(Spice Islands)*	1 tsp	7	1	0.4
whole *(Tone's)*	1 tsp	7	1	0.4
CUPU ASSU OIL				
	1 cup	1927	0	218.0
	1 tbsp	120	0	13.6
CURRANT				
BLACK/European currant, raw	1 cup	71	17	0.5
RED OR WHITE, raw	1 cup	63	15	0.2
ZANTE				
dried	1 cup	408	107	0.4
dried *(Sun-Maid)*	1/4 cup	130	31	0.0
dried *(S&W)*	1/4 cup	130	31	0.0
CURRY POWDER. See under SEASONING MIX.				
CUSK/torsk/tusk				
baked, broiled, grilled, or microwaved	3 oz	95	0	0.7
raw	3 oz	74	0	0.6
CUSTARD APPLE/bullock's heart/cherimoya				
Fresh, raw, skin and seeds removed	1 fruit	514	131	2.2
CUTTLEFISH				
mixed species, cooked	3 oz	134	1	1.2
mixed species, raw	3 oz	67	1	0.6

D

Food Name	Serv. Size	Total Cal.	Carbs GMS	Fat GMS
DAIKON/Chinese radish/Oriental radish				
boiled, drained	4 oz	19	3.9	0.3
boiled, drained, sliced	1 cup	25	5	0.4
boiled, drained, sliced	1/2 cup	13	2.5	0.2
dried	1 cup	314	74	0.8
dried	1/2 cup	157	36.8	0.4
dried	1 oz	77	18.0	0.2
raw, trimmed	1 oz	5	1.2	<.1
raw, trimmed *(Frieda's)*	1 lb	86	19.1	0.5
raw, trimmed *(Frieda's)*	1 oz	5	1.2	<.1
raw, trimmed, sliced	1/2 cup	8	1.8	<.1
raw, untrimmed	1 lb	65	14.7	0.4
raw, whole, approx 7 inches long, 2 1/4 inch diam	1 daikon	62	13.9	0.3
DAIQUIRI. See under COCKTAIL; COCKTAIL MIX.				
DANDELION GREENS				
boiled, drained, chopped	1 cup	35	7	0.6
raw, chopped	1 cup	25	5	0.4
DANISH CABBAGE. See CABBAGE, DANISH.				
DANISH PASTRY. See under PASTRY; PASTRY, TOASTER.				
DASHEEN				
cooked	4 oz	161	39.2	0.1
cooked, sliced	1/2 cup	94	22.8	0.1
raw, sliced	1/2 cup	56	13.8	0.1

Food Name	Serv. Size	Total Cal.	Carbs GMS	Fat GMS
raw, trimmed	1 oz	30	7.5	0.1
raw, untrimmed	1 lb	419	103.2	0.8
DASHEEN LEAF				
raw	1/2 cup	6	0.9	0.1
raw, trimmed	1 oz	12	1.9	0.2
raw, untrimmed	1 lb	115	18.3	2.0
steamed	1/2 cup	18	3.0	0.3
steamed	4 oz	27	4.6	0.5
DASHEEN SHOOTS				
cooked	4 oz	16	3.6	0.1
cooked, sliced	1/2 cup	10	2.2	0.1
raw, sliced	1/2 cup	5	1.0	<.1
raw, trimmed	1 oz	3	0.7	<.1
raw, untrimmed	1 lb	45	9.3	0.4
DATE				
Domestic, natural and dry				
	1 lb	1123	300.1	1.8
chopped	1/2 cup	245	65.4	0.4
pitted	1 oz	78	20.8	0.1
pitted *(Dole)*	1/2 cup	280	62.0	0.0
pitted, whole, approx 10 dates	2.9 oz	228	61.0	0.4
Imported, pitted				
(Amport Foods)				
chopped	1.5 oz	135	36.0	0.0
whole	1.5 oz	135	36.0	0.0
(Bordo)				
	2 oz	204	47.2	1.2
diced	2 oz	203	47.5	1.1
(Dromedary)				
chopped	1/4 cup	130	31.0	0.0
whole, approx 5 dates	1 oz	100	23.0	0.0
DATE, INDIAN. See TAMARIND.				
DEER				
raw	1 lb	544	0.0	11.0
raw	1 oz	34	0.0	0.7
roasted	3 oz	134	0.0	2.7
DESSERT TOPPING				
(Nestlé)				
'Butterfinger'	1 cup	835	114	32.5
'Butterfinger'	2 tbsp	120	16	4.7
'Crunch'	2 tbsp	125	16	6.3
crunchy, 'Buncha Crunch'	1 serving	103	13	5.1
crunchy, 'Buncha Crunch'	2 lb pkg	4671	598	230.7
crunchy, 'Buncha Crunch'	2 tbsp	103	13	5.1
'Rainbow Morsel'	1 pkt	68	10	2.7
'Rainbow Morsel'	1 serving	68	10	2.7
'Rainbow Morsel'	3 lb pkg	6628	1008	263.8
(Snack Pack)				
chocolate fudge	3.88 oz	166	25	6.3
chocolate, w/dinosaurs	3.84 oz	163	26	5.8
milk chocolate sprinkles	3.88 oz	178	28	6.3
vanilla chocolate sprinkles	3.88 oz	166	26	6.1
DIET BAR. See under SPORTS AND DIET/NUTRITION BARS.				
DIET DRINK. See under SPORTS AND DIET/NUTRITION DRINKS.				
DILL SEASONING. See under SEASONING MIX.				
DILL SEED				
whole	1 tbsp	20	4	1.0

Food Name	Serv. Size	Total Cal.	Carbs GMS	Fat GMS
whole	1 tsp	6	1	0.3
whole *(Durkee)*	1 tsp	9	0	0.0
whole *(Laurel Leaf)*	1 tsp	9	0	0.0
whole *(McCormick/Schilling)*	1 tsp	13	2	0.4
whole *(Spice Islands)*	1 tsp	9	1	0.4
whole *(Tone's)*	1 tsp	6	1	0.3
DILL WEED				
dried	1 tbsp	8	2	0.1
dried	1 tsp	3	1	0.0
dried *(McCormick/Schilling)*	1 tsp	4	0	0.0
dried *(Tone's)*	1 tsp	3	1	0.1
fresh, sprigs	1 cup sprigs	4	1	0.1
fresh, sprigs	5 med sprigs	0	0	0.0
DINNER ROLL. See under ROLL.				
DIP				
ACAPULCO *(Ortega)* nonfat	1 oz	8	2	0.0
AVOCADO				
(Kraft)	2 tbsp	60	4	4.0
(Rod's Dips)	2 tbsp	110	2	11.0
BACON AND HORSERADISH				
(Breakstone's)	2 tbsp	70	2	6.0
(Kraft)				
	2 tbsp	60	3	5.0
'Premium'	2 tbsp	50	2	5.0
(Sealtest)	2 tbsp	70	2	6.0
BACON AND ONION				
(Breakstone's) 'Gourmet'	2 tbsp	70	2	6.0
(Kraft) 'Premium'	2 tbsp	60	2	5.0
BEAN				
(Bearitos)				
black bean, vegetarian, organic, fat-free	1 oz	24	4	0.0
vegetarian, organic, fat-free	1 oz	25	5	0.0
(Chi-Chi's) 'Fiesta'	1 oz	30	4	1.0
(Eagle)				
black bean	2 tbsp	35	5	1.0
mild	2 tbsp	40	5	1.5
(Frito-Lay's)				
	2 tbsp	40	6	1.0
hot	2 tbsp	40	5	1.0
(Garden of Eden)				
Baja black bean, organic	2 tbsp	25	5	0.0
chipotle red bean, organic	2 tbsp	25	5	0.0
(Guiltless Gourmet)				
barbecue, mild, nonfat	2 tbsp	23	4	0.0
barbecue, spicy, nonfat	2 tbsp	35	6	0.0
black bean, barbecue, nonfat	2 tbsp	35	6	0.0
black bean, spicy, nonfat	2 tbsp	30	5	0.0
mild, nonfat	2 tbsp	23	4	0.0
pinto bean, barbecue, mild	2 tbsp	27	5	0.0
pinto bean, barbecue, spicy	2 tbsp	40	7	0.0
pinto bean, mild	2 tbsp	27	5	0.0
pinto bean, spicy, nonfat	2 tbsp	35	6	0.0
(Hain)				
hot	4 tbsp	70	10	1.0
Mexican	4 tbsp	60	9	1.0
w/onion	4 tbsp	70	10	1.0

Food Name	Serv. Size	Total Cal.	Carbs GMS	Fat GMS
(Mi Ranchito)				
low-fat	2 tbsp	30	8	1.0
spicy, low-fat	2 tbsp	27	7	1.0
(Old El Paso) black bean	2 tbsp	20	4	0.0
(Tostitos) black, medium, nonfat	2 tbsp	30	6	0.0
BLUE CHEESE				
(Kraft) 'Premium'	2 tbsp	50	2	4.0
(Litehouse)				
and dressing, refrigerated, 'Lite'	1 tbsp	33	1	3.0
and dressing, refrigerated, 'Original'	1 tbsp	77	0	8.0
country, and dressing, refrigerated	1 tbsp	76	0	8.0
CAESAR *(Litehouse)* and dressing, refrigerated	1 tbsp	57	0	6.0
CHEESE				
(Chi-Chi's) 'Fiesta'	1 oz	41	3	3.0
(Frito-Lay's) cheddar, mild	2 tbsp	60	3	4.0
(Kraft) nacho, 'Premium'	2 tbsp	55	2	4.0
(Guiltless Gourmet)				
queso, mild	2 tbsp	20	5	0.0
queso, spicy	2 tbsp	20	5	0.0
CHEESE AND SALSA				
(Eagle) medium	2 tbsp	40	3	3.0
(Old El Paso) mild or medium	2 tbsp	40	3	3.0
CHILI *(La Victoria)*	1 tbsp	6	1	1.0
CLAM				
(Breakstone's)				
	2 tbsp	50	2	4.0
'Gourmet Chesapeake'	2 tbsp	50	2	4.0
(Kraft)	2 tbsp	60	3	4.0
(Sealtest)	2 tbsp	50	2	4.0
CUCUMBER *(Kraft)* creamy, 'Premium'	2 tbsp	50	2	4.0
CUCUMBER AND ONION				
(Breakstone's)	2 tbsp	50	2	4.0
(Sealtest)	2 tbsp	50	2	4.0
DILL *(Nasoya)* creamy, 'Vegi-Dip'	1 oz	60	4	4.0
GARLIC				
(Life) and dressing, w/tofu, 'All Natural'	1 tbsp	70	1	7.1
(Nasoya) and herb, 'Vegi-Dip'	1 oz	50	6	2.0
GREEN ONION, *(Kraft)*	2 tbsp	60	4	4.0
GUACAMOLE				
(Kraft)	2 tbsp	50	3	4.0
(Lucerne)	2 tbsp	80	1	8.0
(Rod's Dips)	2 tbsp	80	1	8.0
HONEY MUSTARD *(Litehouse)* and dressing, refrigerated	1 tbsp	67	2	7.0
ITALIAN *(Litehouse)* creamy, and dressing, refrigerated	1 tbsp	60	0	6.0
JALAPEÑO				
(Breakstone's) cheddar, 'Gourmet'	2 tbsp	70	2	6.0
(Frito-Lay's)				
and cheddar cheese	2 tbsp	50	4	4.0
bean	1 oz	30	4	1.0
(Hain) bean, medium	4 tbsp	70	10	1.0
(Kraft)	2 tbsp	60	3	4.0
(Old El Paso) bean, nonfat	1 tbsp	14	2	0.0
(Price's) nacho	1 oz	80	2	7.1
(Wise) bean, nonfat	2 tbsp	25	5	0.0
MUSHROOM *(Breakstone's)* and herb, 'Gourmet'	2 tbsp	50	2	4.0
NACHO *(Guiltless Gourmet)* spicy, nonfat	2 tbsp	25	5	0.0

Food Name	Serv. Size	Total Cal.	Carbs GMS	Fat GMS
ONION				
(Bison) French	1 oz	60	2	5.0
(Breakstone's)				
French	2 tbsp	50	2	5.0
toasted, 'Gourmet'	2 tbsp	50	2	5.0
(Frito-Lay's) French	2 tbsp	60	4	5.0
(Heluva Good) French, real sour cream	2 tbsp	50	2	5.0
(Kraft)				
creamy, 'Premium'	2 tbsp	45	2	4.0
French	2 tbsp	60	4	4.0
French, 'Premium'	2 tbsp	45	2	4.0
(Lucerne) French	2 tbsp	70	2	6.0
(Nasoya) French, 'Vegi-Dip'	1 oz	50	4	3.0
(Rod's Dips)				
French	2 tbsp	70	2	6.0
French, nonfat	2 tbsp	25	3	0.0
French, w/bacon	2 tbsp	70	2	6.0
(Sealtest) French	2 tbsp	50	2	5.0
PEPPERCORN *(Litehouse)* and dressing, refrigerated	1 tbsp	67	0	7.0
PICANTE				
(Frito-Lay's) nonfat	1 oz	10	3	0.0
(Tostitos) medium	1 tbsp	8	2	0.0
(Wise) nonfat	2 tbsp	12	3	0.0
POPPYSEED *(Litehouse)* and dressing, refrigerated	1 tbsp	65	3	6.0
RANCH				
(Heluva Good) real sour cream	2 tbsp	60	2	5.0
(Litehouse)				
and dressing, refrigerated	1 tbsp	59	1	6.0
and dressing, refrigerated, 'Lite'	1 tbsp	35	1	3.0
country, and dressing, refrigerated	1 tbsp	61	1	7.0
jalapeño, and dressing, refrigerated	1 tbsp	60	1	6.0
refrigerated, 'Veggie Dip'	1 tbsp	60	1	7.0
(Lucerne)	2 tbsp	110	2	11.0
(Rod's Dips)				
nonfat	2 tbsp	25	3	0.0
w/bacon	2 tbsp	110	2	11.0
SALSA				
(Eagle)				
medium	2 tbsp	10	2	0.0
mild	2 tbsp	10	2	0.0
(Pace)				
medium, 'Chunky'	2 tbsp	4	1	1.0
mild, 'Chunky'	2 tbsp	4	1	1.0
SOUR CREAM AND CHIVES				
(Litehouse) vinaigrette, and dressing, refrigerated	1 tbsp	63	1	7.0
TACO				
(Hain) and sauce	4 tbsp	25	5	1.0
(Wise) nonfat	2 tbsp	12	3	0.0
THOUSAND ISLAND				
(Litehouse) and dressing, refrigerated	1 tbsp	65	1	7.0
VEGETABLE *(Marzetti)* and dressing	1 tbsp	88	1	10.0
DIP MIX				
onion and chive *(Knorr)*	1/20 pkg	5	1	0.0
sour cream *(Durkee)*	2 tsp	25	4	0.5
nacho cheese, 'Microwave Snacks' *(Tio Sancho)*	3.5 oz	247	2	20.0

DISHCLOTH GOURD. See GOURD, DISHCLOTH.

Food Name	Serv. Size	Total Cal.	Carbs GMS	Fat GMS
DOCK				
Fresh				
boiled, drained, chopped	3.5 oz	20	2.9	0.6
boiled, drained, chopped	4 oz	23	3.3	0.7
raw, chopped	1 cup	29	4	0.9
raw, chopped	1/2 cup	15	2.1	0.5
raw, trimmed	1 oz	6	0.9	0.2
raw, untrimmed	1 lb	70	10.2	2.2
DOLPHIN FISH. See MAHI MAHI.				
DOUGHNUT				
(Awrey's)				
crunch	1 doughnut	600	65	34.0
plain	1 doughnut	490	48	30.0
sugared	1 doughnut	610	68	35.0
(Break Cake)				
chocolate, gem	1 doughnut	70	7	4.0
chocolate, 1 oz	1 doughnut	130	14	8.0
cinnamon, gem	1 doughnut	60	8	3.0
cinnamon, 1 oz	1 doughnut	120	15	6.0
dunkin stix, 3 oz	2 stix	420	43	27.0
powdered sugar, gem	1 doughnut	60	8	3.0
powdered sugar, 1 oz	1 doughnut	120	16	5.0
(Ener-G Foods) pumpkin, gluten-free	1 serving	128	18	5.9
(Entenmann's)				
crumb-topped	1 doughnut	260	34	12.0
devil's food crumb	1 doughnut	250	34	12.0
frosted, rich	1 doughnut	280	27	18.0
(Hostess)				
cinnamon, 'Breakfast Bake Shop Donette Gems'	1 doughnut	60	7	3.0
cinnamon, 'Breakfast Bake Shop Family Pack'	1 doughnut	120	14	6.0
cinnamon, 'Breakfast Bake Shop Pantry'	1 doughnut	190	24	10.0
cinnamon, apple-filled, mini	1 doughnut	70	10	3.0
crumb, 'Breakfast Bake Shop'	1 doughnut	160	16	10.0
frosted, 'Breakfast Bake Shop Donette Gems'	1 doughnut	80	8	5.0
frosted, 'Breakfast Bake Shop' 1.5 oz	1 doughnut	190	20	12.0
frosted, 'O's'	1 doughnut	260	32	14.0
glazed, 'Breakfast Bake Shop Old Fashioned'	1 doughnut	250	33	12.0
glazed, whirl, 'Breakfast Bake Shop'	1 doughnut	190	27	7.0
honey wheat, 'Breakfast Bake Shop'	1 doughnut	250	32	12.0
'Krunch'	1 doughnut	110	16	4.0
plain, 'Breakfast Bake Shop Donette Gems'	1 doughnut	60	6	3.0
plain, 'Breakfast Bake Shop Family Pack'	1 doughnut	120	13	6.0
plain, 'Breakfast Bake Shop Old Fashioned'	1 doughnut	170	21	9.0
plain, 'Breakfast Bake Shop Pantry'	1 doughnut	190	21	11.0
plain, 'O's'	1 doughnut	230	34	10.0
powdered sugar, 'Breakfast Bake Shop Pantry'	1 doughnut	190	24	10.0
powdered sugar, mini	1 doughnut	60	7	3.0
strawberry-filled, frosted, mini	1 doughnut	80	10	4.0
strawberry-filled, powdered sugar, mini	1 doughnut	70	10	3.0
(Rich's)				
glazed, frozen, 1.2 oz, 'Ever Fresh'	1 doughnut	141	17	7.0
jelly, frozen, 2.17 oz, 'Ever Fresh'	1 doughnut	213	26	9.5
(Tastykake)				
cinnamon, mini	1 doughnut	48	6	2.4
cinnamon, 1.6 oz	1 doughnut	179	25	8.2
frosted, rich, mini	1 doughnut	61	8	3.2
frosted, rich, 2 oz	1 doughnut	258	28	16.0

Food Name	Serv. Size	Total Cal.	Carbs GMS	Fat GMS
honey wheat, mini	1 doughnut	40	7	1.2
honey wheat, mini	1 doughnut	40	7	1.2
honey wheat, 2 oz	1 doughnut	209	33	7.5
orange glazed, 2 oz	1 doughnut	219	32	9.1
plain, 1.6 oz	1 doughnut	185	22	10.1
powdered sugar, mini	1 doughnut	42	7	1.3
powdered sugar, 1.6 oz	1 doughnut	188	24	8.6
DOUGHNUT HOLES (Ener-G Foods) gluten free	1 serving	17	2	0.6

DRAGON'S EYE. See LONGAN.
DREAM WHIP. See under TOPPING.
DRESSING. See SALAD DRESSING; STUFFING.
DRUM, FRESHWATER
Fresh

baked, broiled, grilled, or microwaved	3 oz	130	0	5.4
raw	3 oz	101	0	4.2

DUCK
AVERAGE OF ALL PARTS
Domestic

meat and skin, cooked	10 oz	1159	0	112.9
meat and skin, roasted, chopped or diced	1 cup	472	0	39.7
meat only, raw	4.8 oz	181	0	8.2
meat only, roasted, chopped or diced	1 cup	281	0	15.7
Wild, meat and skin, raw	8.3 oz	504	0	36.3

BREAST
Domestic

meat and skin, roasted	3 oz	172	0	9.2
meat only, broiled	3 oz	119	0	2.1
meat only, broiled, chopped or diced	1 cup	244	0	4.3
Wild, meat only, raw	3 oz	102	0	3.5

LEG
Domestic

meat and skin, braised, chopped or diced	1 cup	310	0	10.4
meat and skin, roasted	3 oz	184	0	9.7
meat only, braised	3 oz	151	0	5.1
LIVER, domestic, raw	1 oz	39	1.0	1.3

DUCK FAT

	1 cup	1846	0	204.6
	1 tbsp	115	0	12.8

DULSE. See under SEA VEGETABLE.
DUMPLING

(Creamette) egg noodle, w/pasteurized eggs	2 oz	220	40	3.0
(Stilwell) apple dumpling, w/3 tbsp sauce	1 dumpling	390	59	15.0

DUNGENESS CRAB. See under CRAB.
DURIAN

raw or frozen, chopped or diced	1 cup	357	66	13.0
raw or frozen, whole	1 medium	885	163	32.1

E

Food Name	Serv. Size	Total Cal.	Carbs GMS	Fat GMS
ÉCLAIR. See under PASTRY.				
EEL				
mixed species, baked, broiled, grilled, or microwaved	3 oz	201	0	12.7
mixed species, baked, broiled, grilled, or microwaved, 1-inch cubes	1 piece	40	0	2.5

Food Name	Serv. Size	Total Cal.	Carbs GMS	Fat GMS
mixed species, raw	3 oz	156	0	9.9
EGG				
CHICKEN				
Dried				
white, flakes, glucose-reduced	1/2 lb	797	9	0.1
white, powdered, 100% egg whites *(Nutra/Balance)*	1 tbsp	30	1	0.0
white, stabilized, glucose-reduced, flakes	1 oz	100	1.2	<.1
white, stabilized, glucose-reduced, powder	1 cup	402	4.8	<.1
white, stabilized, glucose-reduced, powder	1 oz	107	1.3	<.1
whole	1 tbsp	30	0	2.0
whole, powder, glucose-reduced	1 tbsp	53	1	0.0
whole, powder, glucose-reduced, sifted	1 cup	402	5	0.0
whole, sifted	1 cup	505	4	34.8
whole, stabilized, glucose-reduced	1 tbsp	31	0	2.2
whole, stabilized, glucose-reduced, sifted	1 cup	523	2	37.4
yolk, powdered	1 tbsp	27	0	2.2
yolk, powdered, sifted	1 cup	446	2	37.4
Fresh				
white, raw	1 cup	122	2.5	0.0
white, raw	1 oz	14	0.3	0.0
white, raw, large	1 white	17	0.3	0.0
whole, cooked, omelet	1 tbsp	23	0	1.7
whole, cooked, omelet-style, large	1 egg	93	1	7.0
whole, fried, large	1 egg	92	1	6.9
whole, hard-boiled	1 tbsp	13	0	0.9
whole, hard-boiled, chopped	1 cup	211	2	14.4
whole, hard-boiled, large	1 egg	78	1	5.3
whole, poached, large	1 egg	75	1	5.0
whole, raw	1 cup	362	3	24.3
whole, raw, brown, grade AA *(Lucerne)*	1 egg	70	1	4.5
whole, raw, extra large	1 egg	86	1	5.8
whole, raw, extra large, grade AA *(Lucerne)*	1 egg	80	1	5.0
whole, raw, jumbo	1 egg	97	1	6.5
whole, raw, jumbo, grade A *(Lucerne)*	1 egg	90	1	5.0
whole, raw, large	1 egg	75	1	5.0
whole, raw, medium	1 egg	66	1	4.4
whole, raw, medium, grade AA *(Lucerne)*	1 egg	70	1	4.0
whole, raw, small	1 egg	55	0	3.7
whole, scrambled	1 cup	365	5	26.9
whole, scrambled	1 tbsp	23	0	1.7
whole, scrambled, large	1 egg	101	1	7.4
yolk, raw	1 cup	870	4	75.0
yolk, raw, large	1 yolk	59	0	5.1
Frozen				
diced *(Sunny Fresh)*	1 serving	80	1	5.0
liquid, 'Country Gold' *(Sunny Fresh)*	1/2 cup	130	2	9.0
whole	1/2 lb	688	3	58.1
whole, raw, sugared	1/2 lb	697	25	51.6
Pickled *(Penrose)* approx 2 oz	1 egg	80	1	5.0
DUCK				
whole, fresh, raw	1 large	130	1.0	9.6
whole, fresh, raw	1 oz	52	0.4	3.9
GOOSE				
whole, fresh, raw	1 large	267	1.9	19.1
whole, fresh, raw	1 oz	52	0.4	3.8
QUAIL				
whole, fresh, raw	1 oz	45	0.1	3.1

Food Name	Serv. Size	Total Cal.	Carbs GMS	Fat GMS
whole, fresh, raw	1 large	14	0.0	1.0
TURKEY				
whole, fresh, raw	1 large	135	0.9	9.4
whole, fresh, raw	1 oz	48	0.3	3.4
EGG DISH/MEAL				
(Aunt Jemima)				
scrambled, w/cheddar cheese and fried potatoes	5.9 oz	250	22	13.0
scrambled, w/sausages and hash browns, frozen	5.7 oz	290	14	20.0
scrambled, w/sausages and pancakes, frozen	5.2 oz	270	21	14.0
(Downyflake)				
scrambled, w/ham and hash browns, frozen	6.25 oz	360	17	26.0
scrambled, w/ham and pecan twirl, frozen	6.25 oz	470	40	28.0
scrambled, w/hash browns and sausage link	6.25 oz	420	17	34.0
scrambled, w/sausages and pecan twirl, frozen	6.25 oz	510	39	33.0
(Great Starts) scrambled, w/home fried potatoes	1 pkg	200	15	12.0
(Healthy Choice)				
omelet, turkey sausage, on English muffin, frozen	1 serving	210	30	4.0
omelet, Western style, on English muffin, frozen	1 serving	200	29	3.0
(Mountain House)				
omelet, cheese, freeze-dried, prepared	1/2 pkg	180	8	9.0
w/bacon, freeze-dried, prepared	1/2 pkg	170	7	10.0
w/bacon, precooked, , freeze-dried, prepared	1/2 pkg	180	3	12.0
w/butter, freeze-dried, prepared	1/2 pkg	160	8	8.0
(Sunny Fresh)				
scrambled, precooked	2 oz	90	2	5.0
scrambled, squares	1 serving	60	1	3.5
(Swanson)				
omelet w/cheese sauce, w/ham, 'Great Starts'	7 oz	390	15	29.0
scrambled, w/bacon and home fries	5.6 oz	340	16	26.0
scrambled, w/cheese and cinnamon pancakes	3.4 oz	290	14	23.0
scrambled, w/sausages and hash browns, frozen	6.5 oz	430	19	34.0
w/mini oat bran muffins, reduced cholesterol.	4.75 oz	250	27	12.0
(Weight Watchers)				
ham and cheese omelet, 'Handy'	1 serving	220	30	5.0
omelet sandwich, 'Classic'	1 sandwich	220	26	5.0
omelet sandwich, 'Garden'	3.60 oz	210	28	6.0
EGG DISH/MEAL MIX				
(LaChoy)				
egg foo yung, w/3 oz sauce, 'Dinner Classics' prepared	2 patties	170	20	7.0
egg foo yung, packaged, 'Dinner Classics'	1/4 pkg	85	19	1.0
EGG ROLL				
(Chun King)				
chicken, mini	6 egg rolls	210	25	9.0
pork and shrimp, mini	6 egg rolls	210	27	9.0
shrimp, mini	6 egg rolls	190	28	6.0
(La Choy)				
pork, spicy, frozen, food service product	1 roll	196	23	9.4
shrimp, frozen, food service product	1 roll	187	26	7.1
vegetable, food service product	1 roll	174	28	5.1
(Worthington) vegetarian	1 serving	181	20	8.5
EGG ROLL WRAPPER				
(Azumaya) square	2 wraps	130	26	0.0
(Azumaya) wonton	5 wraps	100	21	0.0
(Nasoya)	1 piece	23	5	0.0
EGG SUBSTITUTE				
(Best of Egg) 99% egg white product	1/4 cup	30	1	0.0
(Ener-G Foods) egg-free, gluten-free	1 1/2 tsp	15	4	0.0

Food Name	Serv. Size	Total Cal.	Carbs GMS	Fat GMS
(Fantastic Foods) dry, 'Tofu Scrambler'	2 1/2 tbsp	60	12	0.5
(Featherweight)	2 eggs	120	2	8.0
(Fleischmann's)				
cheese omelet mix, 'Egg Beaters'	1/2 cup	110	2	5.0
'Egg Beaters'	1/4 cup	30	1	0.0
vegetable omelet mix, 'Egg Beaters'	1/2 cup	50	5	0.0
(Healthy Choice) 'Cholesterol-Free Egg Product'	1/4 cup	30	1	1.0
(Morningstar Farms)				
vegetarian, 'Better 'N Eggs'	1/4 cup	23	0	0.3
vegetarian, 'Scramblers'	1/4 cup	37	2	0.4
(Nu Laid) nonfat, cholesterol-free	1/4 cup	30	1	0.0
(Second Nature)				
cholesterol-free, real egg product	1/4 cup	60	3	2.0
nonfat, real egg product	1/4 cup	40	3	0.0
(Tofu Scrambler)				
mix, prepared w/tofu	1/2 cup	98	7	5.0
mix, prepared w/tofu, 3 tbsp salt	1/2 cup	158	7	12.0
(Tofutti)				
frozen, 'Egg Watchers'	2 oz	50	2	2.0
nonfat, 'Egg Watchers'	1/4 cup	30	1	0.0
(Wonder Slim)				
for cooking, baking, and salad dressing	1/4 cup	45	9	1.0
nonfat, no animal or dairy products	1/4 cup	35	8	0.0
EGG SUBSTITUTE DISH/MEAL				
(Morningstar Farms)				
frozen, w/hash browns and links 'Scramblers'	7 oz	360	22	23.0
frozen, w/pancakes and links 'Scramblers'	6.8 oz	380	33	19.0
EGG WHITE STABILIZER *(Tone's)*	1 tsp	12	3	0.0
EGGNOG				
Canned				
(Borden) nonalcoholic	1/2 cup	160	16	9.0
Refrigerated				
(Crowley) nonalcoholic	6 fl oz	270	34	13.0
(Darigold) nonalcoholic	8 fl oz	350	43	17.0
(Darigold) nonalcoholic 'Classic'	8 fl oz	390	48	17.0
(Lucerne)	1/2 cup	170	19	9.0
EGGPLANT/aubergine				
Fresh				
boiled, drained, cubed	1 cup	28	7	0.2
raw, cubed	1 cup	21	5	0.1
raw, whole, approx 1.25 lb, peeled	1 eggplant	119	28	0.8
raw, whole, approx 1.25 lb, unpeeled	1 eggplant	142	33	1.0
Frozen				
cutlets *(Celentano)*	3/4 cup	330	23	23.0
cutlets, breaded *(Bernardi)*	1/2 cup	180	17	11.0
rollettes *(Celentano)*	11 oz	320	36	14.0
rollettes, 'Great Choice' *(Celentano)*	10-oz tray	330	39	15.0
rollettes, 'Selects' *(Celentano)*	10-oz tray	360	27	23.0
EGGPLANT DISH/ENTRÉE				
(Celentano) Parmigiana	10-oz tray	420	30	27.0
(Progresso) appetizer, canned, 'Caponata'	2 tbsp	30	2	2.0
ELDERBERRY				
Fresh				
raw	1 lb	329	83.5	2.3
raw	1 oz	21	5.2	0.1
raw	1 cup	106	26.7	0.7

Food Name	Serv. Size	Total Cal.	Carbs GMS	Fat GMS
ELK				
raw	1 lb	504	0.0	6.6
raw	1 oz	31	0.0	0.4
roasted	3 oz	124	0.0	1.6
roasted	4 oz	166	0.0	2.2
roasted, diced, approx 4.9 oz	1 cup	204	0.0	2.7
ENCHILADA/ENCHILADA ENTRÉE				
(Amy's Kitchen)				
black bean and vegetable	1 serving	130	20	4.0
cheese	1 serving	210	16	9.0
(Banquet)				
	1 entrée	360	55	11.0
chicken	1 entrée	350	54	10.0
beef, frozen	12 oz	500	72	15.0
beef, w/chili and gravy, 'Family Entrées'	7 oz	270	28	13.0
cheese	1 entrée	360	56	10.0
cheese, frozen	12 oz	550	71	19.0
(Gebhardt)				
	2 enchiladas	310	20	24.0
	5.71 oz	258	20	19.1
beef	1 serving	129	10	9.6
(Healthy Choice)				
beef, frozen, 13.4 oz	1 serving	370	66	5.0
chicken, frozen, 9.5 oz	1 serving	310	44	9.0
chicken, frozen, 13.4 oz	1 serving	340	61	5.0
chicken, suprema	1 entrée	300	46	7.0
chicken, suprema, w/green sauce, rice, corn, apple raspberry	1 serving	298	46	6.7
chicken, Suiza	1 entrée	280	43	4.0
(Hormel)				
beef, frozen	1 piece	140	17	5.0
cheese, frozen	1 piece	151	18	6.0
(Le Menu) chicken, frozen, 'Light Style'	8 oz	280	32	8.0
(Legume) w/organic tofu, vegetarian	1 serving	270	36	8.0
(Lean Cuisine)				
beef and bean, frozen	9.25 oz	240	32	6.0
chicken enchilada Suiza	1 entrée	280	48	5.0
chicken enchilada Suiza, w/sour cream sauce, rice	1 serving	298	52	4.8
(Legume) vegetable, w/tofu and sauce, frozen	11 oz	270	36	8.0
(Old El Paso)				
beef, frozen	1 pkg	210	16	13.0
beef, frozen, 'Festive Dinners'	11 oz	390	56	8.0
cheese, frozen	1 pkg	250	24	12.0
cheese, frozen, 'Festive Dinners'	11 oz	590	51	31.0
chicken, frozen	1 pkg	220	20	12.0
chicken, frozen, 'Festive Dinners'	11 oz	460	54	18.0
chicken, w/sour cream sauce, frozen	1 pkg	280	18	19.0
(Patio)				
beef, frozen	13.25 oz	520	59	24.0
cheese, frozen	12.25 oz	380	59	10.0
(Soypreme) tofu, organic, all-natural, frozen	11 oz	370	45	11.0
(Stouffer's)				
cheese, frozen, 1 pkg.	9.75 oz	490	33	29.0
cheese, w/Mexican rice	1 entrée	370	48	14.0
chicken, frozen, 1 pkg.	10 oz	490	31	31.0
chicken enchanadas, frozen, food service product	1 oz	46	4	2.7
chicken enchilada, w/Mexican rice, Monterey Jack sauce	1 serving	376	48	14.7
chicken enchiladas, w/Mexican rice	1 entrée	370	45	14.0

Food Name	Serv. Size	Total Cal.	Carbs GMS	Fat GMS
(Tio Sancho) 'Dinner Kit'	1 shell	80	11	3.5
(Ultimate 200) beef, Ranchero, frozen	9.12 oz	190	18	5.0
(Van de Kamp's)				
beef, frozen, 'Mexican Dinner'	1/2 pkg	200	27	7.0
beef, frozen, 'Mexican Entrées Family Pack'	1/4 pkg	150	19	5.0
beef, frozen, 'Mexican Entrées'	1 pkg	270	30	12.0
beef, shredded, frozen, 'Mexican Entrées'	1 pkg	360	40	14.0
cheese, frozen, 'Mexican Dinner'	1/2 pkg	220	26	9.0
cheese, frozen, 'Mexican Entrées'	1 pkg	300	31	15.0
cheese, frozen, 'Mexican Entrées Family Pack'	1/4 pkg	200	19	10.0
chicken, frozen, 'Mexican Entrées'	1 pkg	260	27	11.0
ranchero, frozen, 'Mexican Entrées'	1/2 pkg	260	26	12.0
Suiza, frozen, 'Mexican Entrées'	1 pkg	230	23	10.0
(Weight Watchers)				
chicken, nacho Grande, frozen 'Mexican Style'	9 oz	280	38	8.0
chicken, Suiza, frozen	9 oz	230	25	7.0
chicken enchiladas, nacho grande	1 entrée	290	42	8.0
chicken enchiladas Suiza	1 entrée	270	33	9.0
chicken enchilada Suiza, w/sour cream sauce and cheese	1 serving	283	33	9.7

ENCHILADA SEASONING. See under SEASONING MIX.

ENDIVE

raw, chopped	1/2 cup	4	1	0.1
raw, whole, approx 1.3 lb	1 head	87	17	1.0

ENERGY BAR. See under SPORTS AND DIET/NUTRITION BARS.

ENGLISH MUFFIN

(Earth Grains)				
oat bran, 12-oz pkg.	1 muffin	120	24	1.0
plain, 12 oz pkg.	1 muffin	120	25	1.0
sourdough, 12-oz pkg.	1 muffin	120	25	1.0
w/raisins, 14-oz pkg	1 muffin	160	33	2.0
w/raisins, 15-oz pkg, 'Sun Maid'.	1 muffin	160	34	1.0
wheat berry, 14-oz pkg.	1 muffin	140	28	1.0
whole wheat, 14-oz pkg.	1 muffin	130	26	1.0
whole wheat, 15-oz pkg.	1 muffin	140	28	2.0
(Ener-G Foods) gluten-free	1 serving	203	37	3.9
(Hi Fiber)				
multigrain	1 muffin	120	23	1.0
plain	1 muffin	110	21	1.0
w/cinnamon and raisins	1 muffin	110	21	1.0
(Oatmeal Goodness)				
oatmeal, w/cinnamon and raisins	1 muffin	140	26	2.0
oatmeal, w/honey	1 muffin	140	26	2.0
(Organic Grains)				
7-grain, sprouted, organic	1 muffin	140	29	2.0
w/cinnamon and raisins, organic	1 muffin	170	33	1.0
(Oroweat)				
extra crisp	1 muffin	130	26	1.0
'Health Nut'	1 muffin	170	29	4.0
sourdough	1 muffin	140	27	1.0
(Pepperidge Farm)				
plain	1 muffin	140	27	1.0
sourdough	1 muffin	135	27	1.0
w/cinnamon and apple	1 muffin	140	27	1.0
w/cinnamon and raisins	1 muffin	150	29	2.0
w/cinnamon chips	1 muffin	160	28	3.0
(Roman Meal)				
honey nut, w/oat bran, refrigerated	1/2 muffin	81	15	1.3

Food Name	Serv. Size	Total Cal.	Carbs GMS	Fat GMS
'Original'	1 muffin	146	29	1.8
plain, refrigerated	1/2 muffin	71	14	0.5
(Thomas')				
honey wheat	1 serving	110	24	1.0
oat bran	1 serving	120	26	1.0
plain	1 muffin	130	25	1.3
plain, sandwich size	1 serving	190	38	2.0
raisin	1 serving	140	31	1.0
rye	1 muffin	120	27	1.0
sourdough	1 serving	120	25	1.0
sourdough, sandwich size	1 muffin	200	41	2.0
w/onion, sandwich size	1 muffin	180	40	1.5
wheat, sandwich size	1 serving	180	39	1.5
(Wonder) plain	1 serving	130	25	1.0
ENOKI. See MUSHROOM, ENOKI.				
ENSURE. See under MEDICAL NUTRITIONALS.				
EPAZOTE				
fresh, raw, whole sprigs	1 medium	1	0	0.0
fresh, raw, chopped	1 tbsp	0	0	0.0
EPPAW, raw	1 cup	150	32	1.8
EUROPEAN CHESTNUT. See CHESTNUT, EUROPEAN.				
EUROPEAN CURRANT. See under CURRANT.				

F

Food Name	Serv. Size	Total Cal.	Carbs GMS	Fat GMS
FAJITA/FAJITA ENTRÉE				
(Healthy Choice)				
beef, frozen	7 oz	210	26	4.0
chicken, fiesta	1 entrée	260	36	4.0
chicken, frozen	7 oz	200	25	3.0
(Wonderbites)				
beef, flame-broiled, 'Dippers'	1 piece	33	1	1.5
beef, flame-broiled, frozen, product 9971	1 piece	51	1	3.6
(Chicken By George) refrigerated	5 oz	170	2	6.0
FAJITA MIX				
(Hudson) beef, meal kit, prepared	1 fajita	220	22	9.0
(Tyson)				
chicken, kit, frozen	1 pkg	915	123	23.2
chicken, kit, frozen	1 serving	129	17	3.3
kit	4 oz	80	2	2.0
kit, wholesale club item	3.5 oz	160	18	5.0
FAJITA SEASONING. See under SEASONING MIX.				
FALAFEL MIX				
(Casbah) mix only	1.5 oz	160	20	3.0
(Fantastic Foods) prepared	1/2 cup	250	42	4.0
FARINA. See under CEREAL, HOT.				
FAT SUBSTITUTE				
(Wonder Slim) for cooking, baking, and salad dressing	1/4 cup	45	9	1.0
(Rokeach) 'Neutral Nyafat'	1 tbsp	99	0	11.0
FATHEAD. See SHEEPSHEAD.				
FAVA BEAN. See BEAN, FAVA.				
FEIJOA				
raw, puréed	1 cup	119	26	1.9
raw, whole, trimmed	1 medium	25	5	0.4

Food Name	Serv. Size	Total Cal.	Carbs GMS	Fat GMS
FENNEL/finnochio				
fresh, raw *(Frieda of California)*	1 oz	4	1	0.1
fresh, raw, sliced	1 cup	27	6	0.2
fresh, raw, whole, bulb	1 medium	73	17	0.5
FENNEL SEED				
whole	1 tbsp	20	3	0.9
whole	1 tsp	7	1	0.3
whole *(Durkee)*	1 tsp	7	0	0.0
whole *(Laurel Leaf)*	1 tsp	7	0	0.0
whole *(McCormick/Schilling)*	1 tsp	14	2	0.8
whole *(Spice Islands)*	1 tsp	8	1	0.2
whole *(Tone"s)*	1 tsp	7	1	0.3
FENUGREEK SEED				
whole	1 tbsp	36	6	0.7
whole	1 tsp	12	2	0.2
FETTUCCINE. See under PASTA.				
FETTUCCINE DISH/ENTRÉE. See under PASTA DISH/ENTRÉE.				
FIELD PEAS. See PEAS, FIELD.				
FIG				
Canned				
in extra heavy syrup, w//liquid	1 cup	279	73	0.3
in heavy syrup, w/liquid	1 cup	228	59	0.3
in heavy syrup, w/liquid	1 medium	25	6	0.0
in light syrup, w/liquid	1 cup	174	45	0.3
in light syrup, w/liquid	1 medium	19	5	0.0
in water, w/liquid	1 cup	131	35	0.2
in water, wliquids	1 medium	14	4	0.0
Dried				
raw, chopped	1 cup	507	130	2.3
raw, whole	1 medium	48	12	0.2
stewed	1 cup	280	71	1.3
Fresh				
raw, large, approx 2.5-inch diam.	1 fig	47	12	0.2
raw, medium, approx 2.25-inch diam	1 fig	37	10	0.1
raw, small, approx 1.5-inch diam	1 fig	30	8	0.1
FILBERT. See HAZELNUT.				
FILBERT BUTTER *(Maranatha Natural)* roasted	2 tbsp	180	6	16.0
FILO DOUGH. See PHYLLO DOUGH.				
FINNIAN HADDIE. See under HADDOCK.				
FINNOCHIO. See FENNEL.				
FIREWEED LEAVES				
raw, chopped	1 cup	24	4	0.6
raw, whole	1 med plant	23	4	0.6
FISH. See individual listings.				
FISH AND CHIPS. See under FISH DINNER/ENTRÉE.				
FISH DINNER/ENTRÉE				
(Banquet)				
fillet	1 entrée	290	33	13.0
frozen, 'Platters'	8.75 oz	450	33	22.0
(Fisher Boy)				
batter-dipped, crispy, frozen	1 fillet	170	15	9.0
batter-dipped, crunchy, 'Portions'	1 portion	110	10	6.0
sticks, crunchy, frozen	5 sticks	230	19	11.0
(Gorton's)				
breaded, garlic and herb, frozen	2 fillets	250	20	14.0
breaded, hot and spicy, frozen	2 fillets	270	19	17.0
in herb sauce, frozen	1 pkg	190	3	8.0

Food Name	Serv. Size	Total Cal.	Carbs GMS	Fat GMS
sticks, mini, breaded, frozen	9 sticks	190	14	11.0
(Healthy Choice) lemon pepper	1 entrée	320	50	7.0
(Kid Cuisine) nuggets, frozen	7 oz	320	33	15.0
(Lean Cuisine)				
baked	1 entrée	270	36	6.0
fillet, divan, frozen	10 3/8 oz	210	13	5.0
fillet, Florentine, frozen	9 5/8 oz	220	13	7.0
(Morton) frozen	9.75 oz	370	46	13.0
(Mrs. Paul's)				
Dijon, frozen, 'Light'	8.75 oz	200	17	5.0
fillet, Florentine, frozen, 'Light'	8 oz	220	10	8.0
Mornay, frozen, 'Light'	9 oz	230	12	10.0
(Stouffer's) fillet, w/macaroni and cheese, 'Homestyle'	1 entrée	430	37	21.0
(Swanson)				
fish 'n chips, battered and fried	1 entrée	490	59	20.0
w/fries, frozen, 'Home Style Recipe'	6.5 oz	340	37	16.0
(Tyson) sticks, , frozen 'Looney Tunes Sylvester'	7.5 oz	290	36	11.0
(Van de Kamp's)				
breaded, baked, 97% fat-free, frozen, 'Crisp and Healthy'	2 fillets	150	18	3.0
fillet, baked, breaded, frozen, microwaveable	2 fillets	150	18	3.0
fillet, battered, frozen	1 serving	180	12	11.0
fillet, breaded	2 pieces	280	18	18.0
fillet, breaded, baked, frozen, 'Crisp and Healthy'	2 pieces	150	18	3.0
fillet, breaded, frozen, 'Snack Pack'	2 pieces	220	13	10.0
fillet, crispy, frozen, microwave	1 piece	140	9	9.0
fillet, large, crispy, frozen, microwave	1 piece	290	21	17.0
nuggets, battered, frozen	4 pieces	130	8	9.0
sticks, battered, frozen	4 pieces	160	12	9.0
sticks, breaded, baked, frozen, 'Crisp and Healthy'	4 pieces	120	17	2.0
sticks, breaded, frozen 'snack Pack'	4 pieces	170	13	10.0
sticks, breaded, frozen 'Value Pack'	4 pieces	170	13	10.0
sticks, breaded, frozen	4 pieces	200	15	12.0
sticks, crispy, frozen, microwave	3 pieces	130	11	7.0
sticks, mini, breaded, frozen, 'Crisp and Healthy'	10 sticks	180	14	10.0
(Wakefield)				
gems, fancy style, frozen	4 oz	80	11	1.0
gems, salad style, frozen	3 oz	70	8	1.0
(Weight Watchers) oven-baked, w/vegetable medley, frozen, 'Ultimate 200'	6.64 oz	120	10	2.0

FISH BATTER SEASONING MIX. See under SEASONING AND COATING MIX.

FISH OIL

COD LIVER

Food Name	Serv. Size	Total Cal.	Carbs GMS	Fat GMS
	1 cup	1966	0.0	218.0
	1 tbsp	123	0.0	13.6
(Hain)				
cherry	1 tbsp	120	0	14.0
mint	1 tbsp	120	0	14.0
regular	1 tbsp	120	0	14.0
HERRING				
	1 cup	1966	0	218.0
	1 tbsp	123	0	13.6
MENHADEN				
	1 cup	1966	0	218.0
	1 tbsp	123	0	13.6
fully hydrogenated	1 cup	1849	0	205.0
fully hydrogenated	1 tbsp	113	0	12.5

Food Name	Serv. Size	Total Cal.	Carbs GMS	Fat GMS
SALMON				
.... 1 cup	1966	0	218.0
.... 1 tbsp	123	0	13.6
SARDINE				
.... 1 cup	1966	0	218.0
sardine .... 1 tbsp	123	0	13.6
FISH PASTE CAKE				
Japanese, block, steamed, 'Kamoboko' .... 4 oz	111	11.0	1.0
Japanese, stick, grilled, 'Chikuwa' .... 4 oz	143	15.3	2.4
FISH SEASONING. See under SEASONING MIX; SEASONING AND COATING MIX.				
FISH STICKS. See under FISH DINNER/ENTRÉE.				
FISH SUBSTITUTE DINNER/ENTRÉE				
(Worthington) vegetarian, 'Fillets' .... 2 pieces	180	8	10.0
(Loma Linda) vegetarian, 'Ocean Platter' dry mix .... 1/3 cup	90	8	1.0
FIVE-SPICE SEASONING. See under SEASONING MIX.				
FLAN MIX. See under PUDDING MIX.				
FLATFISH. See FLOUNDER; HALIBUT; SOLE.				
FLAX OIL				
organic *(Spectrum Naturals)* .... 1 tbsp	120	0.0	14.0
organic, cinnamon flavored *(Spectrum Naturals)* .... 1 tbsp	120	0.0	14.0
FLAXSEED				
.... 1 cup	763	53	52.7
.... 1 tbsp	59	4	4.1
(Arrowhead Mills) .... 1 oz	140	11	10.0
FLORIDA POMPANO. See POMPANO, FLORIDA.				
FLOUNDER				
Fresh				
baked, broiled, grilled, or microwaved .... 3 oz	99	0.0	1.3
raw .... 3 oz	77	0.0	1.0
Frozen				
(Finast) .... 4 oz	90	0	1.0
(SeaPak) .... 4 oz	90	0	1.0
Atlantic *(Booth)* .... 4 oz	90	0	1.0
fillet *(Van de Kamp"s)* .... 1 serving	110	0	2.0
fillet, 'Light' *(Van de Kamp's)* .... 1 piece	260	21	12.0
'Natural' *(Van de Kamp's)* .... 4 oz	100	0	2.0
FLOUNDER DINNER/ENTRÉE				
(Gorton's) stuffed, 'Microwave Entrees' .... 1 pkg	350	21	18.0
FLOUR. See also individual listings.				
ACORN, full-fat .... 1 oz	142	15	8.6
AMARANTH *(Arrowhead Mills)* .... 1/4 cup	110	19	1.5
ARROWROOT. .... 1 cup	457	113	0.1
BARLEY				
.... 1 cup	511	110	2.4
(Arrowhead Mills) .... 2 oz	200	35	1.0
(Arrowhead Mills) .... 1.4 cup	75	19	0.5
BARLEY MALT. .... 1 cup	585	127	3.0
BUCKWHEAT				
100% stone ground *(Hodgson Mill)* .... 1/3 cup	160	33	1.0
whole-grain *(Arrowhead Mills)* .... 2 oz	190	41	1.0
whole-groat .... 1 cup	402	85	3.7
CAROB				
.... 1 cup	229	92	0.7
.... 1 tbsp	18	7	0.1
CHESTNUT .... 100 gm	362	76.2	3.7
CHICKPEA				
(Arrowhead Mills) .... 2 oz	200	35	3.0

Food Name	Serv. Size	Total Cal.	Carbs GMS	Fat GMS
besan	1 cup	339	53	6.2
CORN. See also CORNMEAL.				
masa, enriched	1 cup	416	87	4.3
masa harina, enriched *(Quaker)*	1/4 cup	110	25	1.0
masa harina de maiz *(Quaker)*	1/3 cup	137	27	1.5
masa trigo *(Quaker)*	1/3 cup	149	25	4.0
white, masa harina *(Tone's)*	1 tsp	8	2	0.1
white, whole grain	1 cup	422	90	4.5
yellow, degermed, unenriched	1 cup	473	104	1.8
yellow, enriched	1 cup	416	87	4.3
yellow, whole grain	1 cup	422	90	4.5
COTTONSEED				
low-fat	1 oz	94	10	0.4
partially defatted	1 cup	337	38	5.8
partially defatted	1 tbsp	18	2	0.3
GARBANZO *(Arrowhead Mills)* toasted	1/4 cup	90	15	1.0
GRAHAM				
(Hodgson Mill) whole wheat, organic	1/4 cup	100	22	1.0
(Hodgson Mill) whole grain, stone ground, organic	1/4 cup	100	22	1.0
KAMUT *(Arrowhead Mills)*	1/4 cup	110	25	0.5
MILLET *(Arrowhead Mills)*	1/4 cup	110	26	1.0
MUSTARD *(McCormick/Schilling)* ground	1 tsp	12	0	0.8
OAT				
(Arrowhead Mills)	1/3 cup	120	20	2.0
blend *(Gold Medal)*	1 cup	390	81	3.0
OAT BRAN				
blend, all natural *(Hodgson Mill)*	1/4 cup	110	24	1.0
all-natural *(Hodgson Mill)*	1/4 cup	110	23	2.0
organic, wheat-free *(Hodgson Mill)*	1/4 cup	110	24	1.0
PEANUT				
defatted	1 cup	196	21	0.3
defatted	1 oz	93	10	0.2
low-fat	1 cup	257	19	13.1
low-fat	1 oz	121	9	6.2
POTATO				
	1 cup	571	133	0.5
gluten-free *(Ener-G Foods)*	1 cup	527	136	1.4
QUINOA				
whole-grain, gluten-free *(Ancient Harvest)*	1/4 cup	132	24	2.0
whole-grain, gluten-free *(Quinoa)*	1/4 cup	132	24	2.0
RICE				
(Featherweight)	1 cup	500	113	1.0
brown	1 cup	574	121	4.4
brown *(Arrowhead Mills)*	2 oz	200	44	1.0
brown, whole-grain, stone ground *(Hodgson Mill)*	1/4 cup	110	23	1.0
sweet, gluten-free *(Ener-G Foods)*	1 cup	406	91	1.1
white	1 cup	578	127	2.2
RICE STARCH				
gluten-free *(Ener-G Foods)*	1 cup	263	69	0.0
RYE				
(Krusteaz)	1 cup	351	73	2.0
'Bohemian Style' *(Pillsbury)*	1/4 cup	100	22	0.0
medium *(Pillsbury)*	1/4 cup	100	22	0.0
stone-ground *(Robin Hood)*	1 cup	360	86	2.0
dark	1 cup	415	88	3.4
light	1 cup	374	82	1.4
medium	1 cup	361	79	1.8

Food Name	Serv. Size	Total Cal.	Carbs GMS	Fat GMS
organic *(Hodgson Mill)*	1/4 cup	90	22	1.0
whole-grain *(Arrowhead Mills)*	2 oz	190	39	1.0
whole-grain, stone-ground *(Hodgson Mill)*	1/4 cup	90	22	1.0
SESAME				
high-fat	1 oz	149	8	10.5
low-fat	1 oz	94	10	0.5
partially defatted	1 oz	108	10	3.4
SOY				
(Arrowhead Mills)	2 oz	250	18	11.0
defatted	1 tbsp	20	2	0.1
defatted, stirred	1 cup	329	38	1.2
full-fat	1 tbsp	23	2	1.1
full-fat, roasted, stirred	1 cup	366	30	17.3
full-fat, stirred	1 cup	375	29	18.6
gluten-free *(Hodgson Mill)*	1/4 cup	80	9	0.0
gluten-free, organic *(Hodgson Mill)*	1/4 cup	110	9	5.0
low-fat	1 tbsp	20	2	0.4
low-fat, stirred	1 cup	327	33	5.9
organic *(Hodgson Mill)*	1/4 cup	110	9	5.0
SPELT				
(Arrowhead Mills)	1/4 cup	100	24	0.5
wheat-free, oragnic, raw *(Hodgson Mill)*	1/4 cup	115	22	1.0
SUNFLOWER SEED				
partially defatted	1 cup	209	23	1.0
partially defatted	1 tbsp	13	1	0.1
TAPIOCA, cassava flour, gluten-free *(Ener-G Foods)*	1 cup	313	100	0.0
TEFF, whole-grain *(Arrowhead Mills)*	2 oz	200	41	1.0
TRITICALE, whole-grain	1 cup	439	95	2.4
WHEAT				
Semolina				
golden, and extra fancy durum *(Hodgson Mill)*	1/4 cup	110	22	1.0
pasta flour, unbleached *(Bob's Red Mill)*	1/4 cup	150	31	0.5
White				
all-purpose *(Ballard)*	1 cup	400	87	1.0
all-purpose *(Ceresota)*	4 oz	390	83	1.0
all-purpose *(Gold Medal)*	1 cup	400	87	1.0
all-purpose *(Heckers)*	4 oz	390	83	1.0
all-purpose *(Red Band)*	1 cup	390	85	1.0
all-purpose *(Robin Hood)*	1 cup	400	85	1.0
all-purpose *(White Deer)*	1 cup	400	87	1.0
all-purpose, bleached *(Pillsbury)*	1/4 cup	100	23	0.0
all-purpose, bleached, 'Pillsbury's Best' *(Pillsbury)*	1 cup	400	87	1.0
all-purpose, unbleached *(Gold Medal)*	1 cup	400	87	1.0
all-purpose, unbleached *(Hodgson Mill)*	1/4 cup	100	23	0.0
all-purpose, unbleached *(Pillsbury)*	1/4 cup	100	21	0.0
all-purpose, unbleached *(Robin Hood)*	1 cup	400	85	1.0
all-purpose, unbleached, 'Pillsbury's Best' *(Pillsbury)*	1 cup	400	86	1.0
bread *(Hodgson Mill)*	1/4 cup	100	22	0.0
bread *(Pillsbury)*	1/4 cup	100	22	0.0
bread, 'Better for Bread' *(Gold Medal)*	1 cup	400	83	1.0
bread, high-protein, high-gluten *(Hodgson Mill)*	1/4 cup	100	22	0.0
bread, 'Pillsbury's Best' *(Pillsbury)*	1 cup	400	83	2.0
bread, enriched	1 cup	495	99	2.3
cake, enriched	1 cup	496	107	1.2
'Drifted Snow *(Red Band)*	1 cup	400	87	1.0
enriched bleached	1 cup	455	95	1.2
enriched, unbleached	1 cup	455	95	1.2

Food Name	Serv. Size	Total Cal.	Carbs GMS	Fat GMS
'La Pina' *(Red Band)*	1 cup	400	87	1.0
organic, unbleached, *(Hodgson Mill)*	1/4 cup	100	23	0.0
self-rising *(Rallard)*	1 cup	380	84	1.0
self-rising *(Gold Medal)*	1 cup	380	83	1.0
self-rising *(Red Band)*	1 cup	380	83	1.0
self-rising, bleached *(Pillsbury)*	1/4 cup	100	22	0.0
self-rising, bleached, 'Pillsbury's Best' *(Pillsbury)*	1 cup	380	84	1.0
self-rising, enriched *(Aunt Jemima)*	1/4 cup	109	24	0.3
self-rising, unbleached, 'Pillsbury's Best' *(Pillsbury)*	1 cup	380	84	1.0
self-rising, unbleached *(Pillsbury)*	1/4 cup	100	22	0.0
shake and blend *(Pillsbury)*	1/4 cup	100	23	0.0
'Softasilk' *(Red Band)*	1/4 cup	100	23	0.0
tortilla, enriched	1 cup	450	75	11.8
unbleached *(Arrowhead Mills)*	2 oz	200	53	1.0
unbleached *(Gold Medal)*	1 cup	400	87	1.0
unbleached *(Robin Hood)*	1 cup	400	85	1.0
unbleached *(Stone-Buhr)*	1 cup	400	87	1.0
unenriched	1 cup	455	95	1.2
'Wondra' *(Red Band)*	1 cup	400	87	1.0
White and whole wheat				
50/50 blend *(Hodgson Mill)*	1/4 cup	100	21	1.0
whole grain, blend *(Gold Medal)*	1 cup	380	84	2.0
whole wheat blend *(Gold Medal)*	1 cup	380	84	2.0
Whole wheat				
	1 cup	407	87	2.2
(Gold Medal)	1 cup	350	78	2.0
(Krusteaz)	1 cup	450	90	2.0
(Pillsbury)	1/4 cup	120	22	1.0
100% hard white wheat *(Hodgson Mill)*	1/4 cup	100	21	1.0
pastry, organic *(Hodgson Mill)*	1/4 cup	110	22	1.0
pastry, stone-ground *(Hodgson Mill)*	1/4 cup	110	22	1.0
pastry, whole-grain *(Arrowhead Mills)*	2 oz	180	41	1.0
whole-grain, stone-ground *(Arrowhead Mills)*	2 oz	200	40	1.0
whole-grain *(Ceresota)*	4 oz	400	80	2.0
whole-grain *(Gold Medal)*	1 cup	350	78	2.0
whole-grain *(Heckers)*	4 oz	400	80	2.0
whole-grain, 'Pillsbury's Best' *(Pillsbury)*	1 cup	400	80	2.0
WHEAT AND RYE				
'Bohemian Style' *(Pillsbury)*	1 cup	400	86	1.0
'Pillsbury's Best' *(Pillsbury)*	1 cup	400	83	2.0
FRANKFURTER				
(Armour)				
beef, 25% less sodium	1 frank	180	2	16.0
jumbo, 25% less sodium	1 frank	160	2	14.0
(Ball Park)				
beef, pork, and chicken, 'Lite'	1 frank	140	1	12.0
light	1 serving	110	4	8.0
mini-franks on a bun	1 pkg	180	15	10.0
nonfat	1 serving	40	4	0.0
(Boar's Head)				
beef	1 oz	80	1	7.0
pork and beef	1 oz	80	1	7.0
(Butcher Boy Meats) turkey	1 serving	134	3	10.2
(Butterball)				
nonfat	1 frank	45	4	0.0
turkey	1 frank	140	2	11.0

Food Name	Serv. Size	Total Cal.	Carbs GMS	Fat GMS
(Eckrich)				
beef, 'Bunsize'	1 frank	190	2	17.0
beef, 1 lb pkg	1 frank	150	2	14.0
'Bun Size'	1 frank	190	2	17.0
cheesefurter	1 frank	180	2	16.0
'Jumbo Lean Supreme'	1 frank	140	2	12.0
1-lb pkg	1 frank	160	2	14.0
(Empire Kosher)				
chicken, kosher	1 frank	100	46	23.0
turkey, kosher	1 frank	90	1	6.0
(Health Valley)				
chicken, 'Weiners'	1 frank	96	1	8.0
turkey, 'Weiners'	1 frank	96	1	8.0
(Healthy Choice)				
beef, w/natural smoke flavor, low-fat	1 frank	60	5	1.5
turkey, pork, and beef, lowfat, bun size	1 frank	60	6	1.5
(Healthy Favorites)				
turkey and beef, 97% fat-free	1 frank	60	2	1.5
w/turkey	2 oz	57	2	1.6
(Hebrew National) beef	1 frank	149	1	14.0
(Hillshire Farm)				
beef, bun size	1 serving	180	2	16.0
cheesefurter, 'Bun Size Wieners'	2 oz	180	2	16.0
hot, 'Hot Franks'	2 oz	190	2	16.0
(Hormel)				
batter-wrapped, frozen, 'Corn Dogs'	1 piece	220	21	12.0
batter-wrapped, frozen, 'Tater Dogs'	1 piece	210	15	14.0
beef, 1-lb pkg	1 frank	140	1	13.0
beef, 12-oz pkg	1 frank	100	1	10.0
beef, smoked, 'Wranglers'	1 frank	170	2	15.0
chili, 'Frank 'n Stuff'	1 frank	165	2	15.0
'Light & Lean 97'	1.6 oz	45	2	1.0
meat, 1-lb pkg	1 frank	140	1	13.0
meat, 12-oz pkg	1 frank	110	1	10.0
'Mexicali Dogs'	5 oz	400	41	21.0
smoked, 'Range Brand Wranglers'	1 frank	170	1	16.0
smoked, w/cheese 'Wranglers'	1 frank	180	1	16.0
'Wrangler'	1 frank	162	1	14.4
(Hygrade) chicken, 'Grillmaster'	1 frank	130	3	11.0
(JM)				
10 per lb	1 frank	140	1	13.0
beef	1 frank	100	1	9.0
beef, 'Jumbo'	1 frank	180	2	16.0
beef, 10 per lb	1 frank	140	1	13.0
cheesefurter, 'Cheese Franks'	1.6 oz	140	2	13.0
'German Brand'	1 frank	160	1	14.0
'Jumbo'	1 frank	190	2	17.0
1 frank	1.2 oz	110	1	10.0
w/cheese, 'German Brand' 1 frank	2 oz	160	2	14.0
(Kahn's)				
beef	1 frank	140	2	13.0
beef, 'Bun Size Franks'	1 frank	190	3	17.0
beef, 'Jumbo'	1 frank	190	3	18.0
beef, smoked, 'Bun Size Beef Smokey'	1 frank	190	2	17.0
beef, w/cheddar cheddar, 'Beef n' Cheddar'	1 frank	180	2	16.0
'Bun Size Frank'	1 frank	190	2	17.0
'Cheese Wiener'	1 frank	150	1	13.0

Food Name	Serv. Size	Total Cal.	Carbs GMS	Fat GMS
'Jumbo'	1 frank	190	2	17.0
smoked, 'Big Red Smokey'	1 frank	170	2	14.0
smoked, 'Bun Size Smokey'	1 frank	180	2	15.0
'Wieners'	1 frank	140	1	13.0
(King Kold) beef	2 oz	173	1	16.3
(Loma Linda)				
vegetarian, canned, 'Big Franks'	1 pkg	1315	17	78.7
vegetarian, canned, 'Big Franks'	1 link	118	2	7.1
(Longacre)				
chicken	1 oz	63	1	5.0
turkey	1 oz	66	0	6.0
(Louis Rich)				
cheese	1 frank	90	2	7.0
turkey	1 frank	101	1	8.2
turkey, w/cheese	1 frank	109	1	8.9
turkey and chicken	1 frank	85	2	6.1
turkey and chicken, bun size	1 frank	110	3	8.0
turkey and chicken, w/cheese	1 frank	90	2	6.5
(Morningstar Farms)				
corn dog, vegetarian, 'Meat-Free Corn Dogs'	1 corn dog	150	22	4.0
corn dog, vegetarian, 'Meat-Free Mini Corn Dogs'	1 corn dog	150	21	4.5
hot dog, vegetarian, 'Veggie Dogs'	1 frank	80	6	0.5
vegetarian, 'Deli Franks'	1 serving	109	3	6.5
(Mr. Turkey)				
turkey, 10 per lb	1 frank	106	1	8.9
turkey, w/cheese	1 frank	109	1	9.1
(Natural Touch) vegetarian	1 frank	99	2	5.5
(OHSE)				
beef	1 oz	85	1	8.0
chicken, beef, and pork	1 oz	85	1	8.0
'Wieners'	1 oz	90	1	8.0
(Oscar Mayer)				
bacon and cheddar cheese, 'Hot Dogs'	1 frank	137	1	12.0
beef, deli-style, 'Big & Juicy'	1 frank	230	1	22.0
beef, 'Franks'	1 frank	181	1	16.7
beef, 'Light Franks'	1 frank	131	1	11.1
beef, original, 'Big & Juicy'	1 frank	240	1	22.0
beef, quarter pound, 'Big & Juicy'	1 frank	350	2	33.0
beef, w/cheddar, 'Franks'	1 frank	163	1	14.3
beef, w/garlic, 'Big & Juicy'	2.7 oz	239	0	22.5
fat free	1 frank	35	2	0.0
light	1 frank	110	2	8.0
pork and turkey	1 frank	150	1	13.0
pork, turkey, and beef, light	1 frank	111	2	8.5
turkey, w/cheese	1 frank	143	1	12.9
wiener, hot and spicy, 'Big & Juicy'	1 wiener	220	1	20.0
wiener, original, 'Big & Juicy'	1 wiener	240	1	22.0
wiener, smokie link, 'Big & Juicy'	1 wiener	220	1	19.0
(Pilgrim's Pride)				
1-lb pkg	1 frank	118	1	8.8
12- oz pkg	1 frank	88	1	6.6
(Quick Meal) w/chili and cheese	4.5 oz	340	25	20.0
(Smart Dog) vegetarian, fat-free, 'Lightlife'	1.5 oz	40	1	0.0
(State Fair) beef, batter-wrapped, on a stick, 'Corn Dogs'	2.67 oz	210	24	10.0
(Tyson)				
chicken	1 frank	115	1	10.0
chicken, batter-wrapped, 'Corn Dogs'	3.5 oz	280	28	14.0

Food Name	Serv. Size	Total Cal.	Carbs GMS	Fat GMS
w/cheese	1 frank	145	1	11.0
(White Wave SoyFood) vegetarian, 'Healthy'	1.5 oz	120	5	8.0
(Worthington) vegetarian, 'Leanies'	1 serving	106	2	7.8
FRENCH ARTICHOKE. See under ARTICHOKE.				
FRENCH BEAN. See BEAN, FRENCH.				
FRENCH TOAST				
(Aunt Jemima)				
cinnamon, frozen	1 slice	240	35	7.0
homestyle, frozen	1 slice	240	35	7.0
original, frozen	3 oz	166	27	4.4
sticks, and syrup, frozen, 'Homestyle'	5.2 oz	400	48	20.0
wedges, and sausages, frozen, 'Homestyle'	5.3 oz	360	40	17.0
(Downyflake)				
frozen	1 slice	130	22	3.0
frozen, 'Extra Thick'	1 slice	150	11	9.0
Texas style, w/sausage, frozen	4.25 oz	400	37	24.0
(Farm Rich)				
sticks, apple cinnamon	3 oz	310	39	15.0
sticks, blueberry	3 oz	310	37	14.0
sticks, original	3 oz	300	37	15.0
(French Toast Boat) cinnamon	1 piece	224	28	11.1
(Krusteaz)				
cinnamon swirl, w/sausage, frozen	1 pkg	415	38	23.2
cinnamon swirl, frozen	2 slices	270	46	5.0
regular, frozen	2 slices	250	38	6.0
(Morningstar Farms)				
vegetarian, cinnamon swirl, w/patties, frozen	6.5 oz	380	37	15.0
(Pierre) cinnamon, wedge, product 1847	1 piece	118	16	5.1
(Stilwell) sticks, frozen, 'Qwik-Krisp'	5 pieces	400	46	21.0
(Sunny Fresh)				
bagel, w/maple syrup, frozen	1 pkg	15196	1678	426.4
bagel, w/maple syrup, frozen	1 serving	190	21	5.3
cinnamon swirl, frozen	1 serving	190	26	7.0
(Swanson)				
cinnamon swirl, w/sausage, frozen, 'Great Starts'	5.5 oz	390	37	21.0
mini, w/sausage, frozen, 'Great Starts'	2.5 oz	190	22	9.0
oatmeal, w/lite links, frozen, 'Great Starts'	4.65 oz	310	35	13.0
sticks, w/syrup, 'Great Starts'	1 pkg	320	50	10.0
w/sausage, 'Great Starts'	1 pkg	410	33	26.0
w/sausage, frozen, 'Great Starts'	1 entree	410	33	26.0
FRESHWATER BASS. See BASS, FRESHWATER.				
FRIED RICE SEASONING. See under SEASONING MIX.				
FRITTER				
corn, frozen *(Mrs. Paul's)*	2 pieces	240	35	9.0
apple, frozen *(Mrs. Paul's)*	2 pieces	240	35	9.0
FROG				
legs, raw	3.5 oz	73	0.0	0.3
legs, raw	1 oz	21	0.0	<1.0
FROGFISH. See MONKFISH.				
FROSTING				
(Betty Crocker)				
Amaretto almond, 'Creamy Deluxe'	1/12 can	160	27	6.0
butter pecan 'Creamy Deluxe'	1/12 tub	170	26	7.0
chocolate, light, 'Creamy Deluxe'	1/12 tub	130	28	2.0
chocolate, w/dinosaurs, 'Creamy Deluxe Party'	1/12 tub	160	24	7.0
chocolate, w/red gel 'Creamy Deluxe Party'	1/12 tub	160	24	7.0
chocolate, w/turbo racers, 'Creamy Deluxe Party'	1/12 tub	160	24	7.0

Food Name	Serv. Size	Total Cal.	Carbs GMS	Fat GMS
chocolate chip, 'Creamy Deluxe'	1/12 tub	170	27	7.0
chocolate chip, 'Creamy Deluxe Party'	1/12 can	160	24	7.0
chocolate coconut almond, 'Creamy Deluxe'	1/12 can	100	21	8.0
double chocolate chip, 'Creamy Deluxe'	1/12 can	170	24	8.0
Dutch fudge, dark, 'Creamy Deluxe'	1/12 tub	160	22	7.0
milk chocolate 'Creamy Deluxe Light'	1/12 tub	140	29	2.0
rocky road, 'Creamy Deluxe'	1/12 can	150	20	8.0
vanilla, 'Creamy Deluxe Light'	1/12 tub	140	30	2.0
vanilla, w/blue gel, 'Creamy Deluxe Party'	1/12 tub	160	27	6.0
vanilla, w/teddy bears, 'Creamy Deluxe Party'	1/12 tub	160	27	6.0
(Duncan Hines)				
chocolate	1/12 can	160	24	7.0
cream cheese	1/12 can	160	24	8.0
cream cheese, 'Homestyle'	1/12 can	160	26	6.0
dark chocolate 'Homestyle'	1/12 can	160	25	6.0
Dutch fudge	1/12 can	160	24	7.0
lemon	1/24 tub	60	9	3.0
milk chocolate	1/12 can	160	24	7.0
milk chocolate, 'Homestyle'	1/12 can	160	25	6.0
vanilla	1/12 can	160	24	7.0
vanilla, 'Homestyle'	1/12 can	160	26	6.0
wild chorry	1 tbsp	140	22	5.0
(Finast) milk	1/12 can	160	25	6.0
(Pathmark)				
chocolate, creamy	1/12 can	160	25	6.0
fudge, creamy	1/12 can	160	25	7.0
white, creamy	1/12 can	160	25	6.0
(Pillsbury)				
butter fudge, 'Frosting Supreme'	1/12 pkg	140	22	6.0
candy, creamy, 'Creamy Supreme'	2 tbsp	150	22	7.0
candy, creamy, 'Frosting Supreme'	2 tbsp	150	22	7.0
caramel pecan, 'Frosting Supreme'	1/12 pkg	150	20	8.0
chocolate, 'Creamy Supreme'	2 tbsp	140	21	6.0
chocolate, 'Frost It Hot'	1/8 cake	50	12	0.0
chocolate, 'Frosting Supreme'	2 tbsp	140	21	6.0
chocolate, 'Funfetti, Creamy Supreme'	2 tbsp	140	22	6.0
chocolate, dark, 'Creamy Supreme'	2 tbsp	130	20	6.0
chocolate, dark, 'Frosting Supreme'	2 tbsp	130	20	7.0
chocolate, double Dutch, 'Frosting Supreme'	1/12 can	140	22	6.0
chocolate chip, 'Frosting Supreme'	1/12 can	150	27	5.0
chocolate fudge, 'Funfetti' 'Frosting Supreme'	1/12 pkg	140	23	6.0
chocolate fudge, 'Frosting Supreme'	1/12 pkg	150	22	6.0
chocolate fudge, 'Lovin Lites'	1/12 pkg	130	28	2.0
chocolate fudge, lowfat, 'Creamy Supreme'	2 tbsp	140	26	3.5
coconut almond, 'Frosting Supreme'	1/12 can	150	17	9.0
coconut pecan, 'Frosting Supreme'	1/12 can	160	17	10.0
cream cheese, 'Frosting Supreme'	1/12 can	160	26	6.0
decorator, all flavors except chocolate	1 tbsp	70	12	2.0
decorator, chocolate	1 tbsp	60	11	2.0
fudge, 'Frosting Supreme'	1/12 can	150	24	6.0
lemon, 'Frosting Supreme'	1/12 can	160	26	6.0
milk, 'Frosting Supreme'	1/12 can	150	23	6.0
milk chocolate, 'Creamy Supreme'	2 tbsp	140	21	6.0
milk chocolate, 'Frosting Supreme'	1/12 pkg	150	23	6.0
milk chocolate, 'Lovin' Lites'	2 tbsp	130	25	3.0
milk chocolate, w/fudge glaze, 'Creamy Supreme'	2 tbsp	140	22	6.0
milk chocolate, w/fudge swirl, 'Frosting Supreme'	1/12 pkg	150	23	6.0

Food Name	Serv. Size	Total Cal.	Carbs GMS	Fat GMS
mint, 'Frosting Supreme'	1/12 can	150	24	7.0
mocha, 'Frosting Supreme'	1/12 can	150	24	6.0
Oreo, 'Frosting Supreme'	2 tbsp	150	23	6.0
sour cream vanilla, 'Frosting Supreme'	1/12 can	160	27	6.0
strawberry, 'Frosting Supreme'	1/12 can	160	26	6.0
vanilla	1/8 cake	120	19	5.0
vanilla, 'Creamy Supreme'	2 tbsp	150	23	6.0
vanilla, 'Frosting Supreme'	1/12 can	160	26	6.0
vanilla, 'Funfetti'	2 tbsp	150	25	6.0
vanilla, 'Funfetti Pink'	2 tbsp	150	24	6.0
vanilla, 'Lovin Lites'	1/12 pkg	130	29	2.0
vanilla, French, 'Creamy Supreme'	2 tbsp	150	25	6.0
vanilla, French, 'Frosting Supreme'	2 tbsp	160	26	6.0
vanilla, pink and white, 'Frosting Supreme'	1/12 can	150	24	6.0
vanilla, w/fudge glaze, 'Creamy Supreme'	2 tbsp	150	25	6.0
vanilla, w/fudge swirl, 'Frosting Supreme'	1/12 pkg	150	25	6.0
white, fluffy	1/12 can	60	15	0.0
white, fluffy, 'Frost It Hot'	1/8 cake	50	12	0.0
(Weight Watchers)				
chocolate, less fat, 'Sweet Rewards'	2 tbsp	120	24	2.5
milk chocolate, less fat, 'Sweet Rewards'	2 tbsp	120	24	2.5
vanilla, 'less fat, Sweet Rewards'	2 tbsp	120	26	2.0
FROSTING MIX				
(Betty Crocker)				
cherry, creamy, prepared w/margarine	1/12 pkg	180	31	6.0
chocolate fudge, creamy, prepared w/1/4 cup butter	1/12 mix	180	30	6.0
chocolate fudge, creamy, prepared w/1/4 cup margarine	1/12 mix	180	30	6.0
chocolate fudge, sour cream, creamy, prepared w/margarine	1/12 pkg	180	30	6.0
coconut pecan, creamy, mix only	1/12 mix	110	19	4.0
coconut pecan, creamy, prepared w/butter, 2% milk	1/12 mix	150	19	8.0
coconut pecan, creamy, prepared w/margarine, skim milk	1/12 mix	150	19	8.0
milk chocolate, creamy, prepared w/margarine	1/12 pkg	170	29	5.0
rainbow chip, creamy, prepared w/margarine	1/12 pkg	190	32	7.0
vanilla, creamy, mix only	1/12 mix	150	32	2.0
vanilla, creamy, prepared w/1/4 cup butter	1/12 mix	170	32	5.0
vanilla, creamy, prepared w/1/4 cup margarine	1/12 mix	170	32	5.0
white, sour cream, creamy, prepared w/margarine	1/12 pkg	170	31	5.0
(Sweet 'n Low)				
chocolate fudge, low sodium w/'Sweet 'N Low'	3 tbsp	140	16	8.0
white, low-sodium w/Sweet 'N Low	3 tbsp	120	16	8.0
FRUCTOSE				
(Estee)	1 tsp	16	4	0.0
(Featherweight)	1 tsp	12	3	0.0
crystalline, pure *(Esculent)*	1 tsp	15	4	0.0
crystalline, pure *(Fifty 50)*	1 tsp	15	4	0.0
crystalline, pure *(Healthy Edge)*	1 tsp	15	4	0.0
liquid *(Sweet Lite)*	1 tsp	20	6	0.0
packet *(Estee)*	1 pkt	12	3	0.0
FRUIT, MIXED				
(Flav-R-Pac)				
frozen	2/3 cup	60	14	0.0
melons, mixed, frozen	3/4 cup	40	10	0.0
w/pineapple, frozen	2/3 cup	60	15	0.0
FRUIT AND NUT MIX				
(Eden Foods)	1 oz	160	10	10.0
(Estee)	14 pieces	70	6	5.0

Food Name	Serv. Size	Total Cal.	Carbs GMS	Fat GMS
(Fisher)				
'California Style'	1/4 cup	140	16	8.0
classic	1/4 cup	150	11	11.0
(Planters)				
'Caribbean Crunch'	1 oz	150	14	10.0
'Fruit 'n Nut'	1 oz	150	13	9.0
FRUIT BAR. See also FRUIT BAR, FROZEN.				
APPLE				
(Health Valley)				
nonfat	1 bar	140	35	0.0
nonfat, 'Bakes'	1 bar	70	18	0.0
APPLE RAISIN *(Weight Watchers)*	1 bar	70	14	2.0
APRICOT, nonfat *(Health Valley)*	1 bar	140	35	0.0
BLUEBERRY, nonfat *(Parnasa)*	1 bar	120	28	0.0
CRANBERRY, natural *(Hearty Balance)*	1 bar	150	30	0.5
DATE				
(Health Valley)				
	1 bar	140	34	0.0
nonfat, 'Bakes'	1 bar	70	18	0.0
RAISIN				
(Health Valley)				
nonfat	1 bar	140	35	0.0
nonfat, 'Bakes'	1 bar	70	18	0.0
RASPBERRY *(Parnasa)* nonfat	1 bar	120	29	0.0
FRUIT BAR, FROZEN				
(Dole)				
blueberry and cream, 'Fruit & Cream'	1 bar	90	19	1.4
cherry, 'Fresh Lites'	1 bar	25	6	1.0
chocolate, banana, and cream, 'Fruit & Cream'	1 bar	175	22	9.0
chocolate, strawberry, and cream, 'Fruit & Cream'	1 bar	140	23	8.0
grape, nonfat, no sugar added	1 bar	25	6	0.0
grape, 'SunTops'	1 bar	40	9	1.0
lemon, 'Fresh Lites'	1 bar	25	6	1.0
lemonade, 'SunTops'	1 bar	40	9	1.0
orange, tropical, 'SunTops'	1 bar	40	9	1.0
peach and cream, 'Fruit & Cream'	1 bar	90	19	1.4
piña colada, 'Fruit 'n Juice'	1 bar	90	16	3.0
pineapple, 'Fruit & Juice'	1 bar	70	17	0.1
pineapple-orange, 'Fresh Lites'	1 bar	25	6	1.0
punch, 'SunTops'	1 bar	40	9	1.0
raspberry, 'Fresh Lites'	1 bar	25	6	1.0
raspberry, 'Fruit & Juice'	1 bar	70	16	0.1
raspberry, nonfat, no sugar added	1 bar	25	6	0.0
raspberry and cream, 'Fruit & Cream'	1 bar	90	20	1.4
strawberry, 'Fruit n' Juice'	1 bar	70	16	0.1
strawberry, nonfat, no sugar added	1 bar	25	6	0.0
strawberry and cream, 'Fruit & Cream'	1 bar	90	19	1.4
(Fruit a Freeze)				
banana, all natural	1 bar	99	16	4.0
strawberry, all-natural	1 bar	100	18	3.0
(Minute Maid) all flavors, nonfat, 'Fruit Juicee'	1 bar	60	14	0.0
(Natural Nectar)				
lemony lime, juice snack, all natural, nonfat	1 bar	70	17	0.0
strawberry nectar, juice snack	1 bar	70	16	1.0
'Tropical Delight' juice snack, all-natural, nonfat,	1 bar	70	16	0.0
(Sunkist)				
coconut	1 bar	170	15	10.0

Food Name	Serv. Size	Total Cal.	Carbs GMS	Fat GMS
lemonade, nonfat	1 bar	90	24	0.0
orange, nonfat, 'Juice Bar'	1 bar	100	25	0.0
strawberry and cream	1 bar	90	19	1.0
wildberry, nonfat	1 bar	140	33	0.0
FRUIT COCKTAIL *(Hunt's)*	1/2 cup	90	23	0.0
FRUIT DESSERT MIX				
apple-cinnamon, w/Nutrasweet *(Sans Sucre de Paris)*	1/4 cup	60	14	0.0
piña colada, w/Nutrasweet *(Sans Sucre de Paris)*	1/4 cup	70	12	1.5
FRUIT DRINK. See also CIDER; FRUIT DRINK MIX; FRUIT JUICE BLEND; FRUIT JUICE DRINK.				
(A&P)				
cranberry apple	6 fl oz	130	32	0.0
grape	6 fl oz	100	25	1.0
lemonade, frozen, prepared	8 fl oz	110	28	1.0
lemonade, pink, frozen, prepared	8 fl oz	110	28	1.0
raspberry, w/cranberry	6 fl oz	110	27	1.0
(Awake) orange, frozen concentrate, prepared	6 fl oz	80	20	0.0
(Bama)				
fruit punch	8.45 fl oz	130	32	0.0
grape	8.45 fl oz	120	29	0.0
orange	8.45 fl oz	120	29	0.0
(Bel-Air) lemonade, pink, concentrate, prepared	6 fl oz	110	27	0.0
(Bright & Early)				
'Bright & Early Fruit Punch' prepared	6 fl oz	90	22	0.0
grape, 'Bright & Early Grape'	6 fl oz	100	24	0.0
orange, 'Bright & Early Orange'	6 fl oz	90	21	0.0
pineapple, 'Bright & Early Pineapple'	6 fl oz	90	23	0.0
(Castle Crest)				
fruit punch, artificially flavored	8 fl oz	120	31	0.0
grape flavored	8 fl oz	120	31	0.0
lemonade drink, artificially flavored	8 fl oz	120	31	0.0
(Crowley)				
fruit punch	8 fl oz	130	32	0.0
grape	8 fl oz	130	32	0.0
lemon	8 fl oz	130	32	0.0
orange	8 fl oz	130	32	0.0
(Del Monte)				
pineapple, w/grapefruit	6 fl oz	90	24	0.0
pineapple, w/pink grapefruit	6 fl oz	90	24	0.0
pineapple-orange	6 fl oz	90	24	0.0
(Finast)				
cranberry grape	6 fl oz	103	26	0.0
raspberry, w/cranberry	6 fl oz	110	27	0.0
(Five Alive)				
berry citrus drink	6 fl oz	90	22	0.0
tropical citrus	6 fl oz	90	21	0.0
(Flav-R-Pac) lemonade	8 fl oz	110	27	0.0
(Frostee) strawberry-flavored	8 fl oz	180	27	7.0
(Fruit Corners) soda pop snacks "soda Licious"	1 pouch	100	22	1.0
(Hawaiian Punch)				
fruit punch, red, 'Fruit Juicy Lite'	6 fl oz	60	15	0.0
fruit punch, red, 'Fruit Juicy'	6 fl oz	90	22	0.0
fruit punch, tropical	6 fl oz	90	22	0.0
fruit punch, tropical, wild fruit	6 fl oz	90	23	0.0
fruit punch cocktail, island fruit	6 fl oz	90	22	0.0
orange	6 fl oz	100	24	0.0
'Very Berry'	6 fl oz	90	22	0.0

Food Name	Serv. Size	Total Cal.	Carbs GMS	Fat GMS
(Hi-C)				
'Boppin' Berry'	6 fl oz	90	23	0.0
'Candy Apple Cooler'	6 fl oz	94	23	0.1
cherry, aseptic box	6 fl oz	100	24	0.0
'Double Fruit Cooler'	6 fl oz	93	23	0.1
'Ecto Cooler'	6 fl oz	95	23	0.1
'Fruity Bubble Gum'	6 fl oz	90	22	0.0
grape	6 fl oz	90	23	0.0
'Hula Cooler'	6 fl oz	97	24	0.1
'Hula Punch'	6 fl oz	87	21	0.1
'Jammin' Apple Drink' aseptic box	6 fl oz	90	23	0.0
lemonade	8.45 fl oz	109	27	0.1
orange	6 fl oz	95	23	0.1
peach	6 fl oz	100	24	0.0
'Stompin' Banana Berry'	6 fl oz	90	22	0.0
wild berry	6 fl oz	92	23	0.1
(J. Hungerford)				
fruit punch, 20% plus juice	9.03 fl oz	43	11	0.0
grape, 20% plus juice	9.03 fl oz	41	11	0.0
lemon, 20% plus juice	9.03 fl oz	41	11	0.0
lemonade, pink, 20% plus juice	9.03 fl oz	41	11	0.0
orange, 20% plus juice	9.03 fl oz	41	11	0.0
punch juice	9.03 fl oz	133	33	0.0
(Juicy Juice)				
fruit punch	6 fl oz	100	23	0.0
tropical	6 fl oz	100	24	0.0
(Kern's)				
apple-strawberry nectar, canned or bottled	6 fl oz	110	26	0.0
apricot-mango nectar	11.5 fl oz	220	53	0.0
apricot nectar, canned or bottled	6 fl oz	110	27	0.0
apricot-pineapple nectar	11.5 fl oz	220	53	0.0
banana-pineapple nectar	11.5 fl oz	220	52	0.0
coconut-pineapple nectar, can or bottle	6 fl oz	140	26	4.0
(Knudsen)				
apricot nectar	8 fl oz	105	24	0.0
blueberry nectar	8 fl oz	135	34	0.0
boysenberry nectar	8 fl oz	110	33	0.0
calamansi punch, 'Rain Forest'	8 fl oz	115	27	0.0
cherry lemonade	8 fl oz	120	29	0.0
coconut nectar	8 fl oz	140	26	5.0
guanabana punch, 'Rain Forest'	8 fl oz	125	29	0.0
hibiscus cooler	8 fl oz	95	24	0.0
lime cactus cooler blend *(Knudsen)*	8 fl oz	120	29	0.0
lemonade, 'Natural'	8 fl oz	100	26	0.0
lime, tropical	8 fl oz	130	32	0.0
papaya, concentrate	1.5 fl oz	90	22	0.0
passionfruit, tropical	8 fl oz	80	20	0.0
rainforest punch, cupu assu	8 fl oz	110	25	0.0
rainforest punch, fruit juice sweetened	8 fl oz	120	29	0.0
raspberry float	8 fl oz	130	31	0.0
raspberry lemonade	8 fl oz	110	28	0.0
strawberry lemonade	8 fl oz	90	21	0.0
tropical punch	8 fl oz	120	29	0.0
(Kool-Aid)				
cherry, 'Koolers'	8.45 fl oz	140	38	0.0
grape, 'Koolers'	8.45 fl oz	140	35	0.0
grape-berry, 'Kool-Aid Splash'	1 serving	116	31	0.0

Food Name	Serv. Size	Total Cal.	Carbs GMS	Fat GMS
'Great Bluedini' 'Koolers'	8.45 fl oz	110	29	0.0
mountain berry punch, 'Koolers'	8.45 fl oz	140	37	0.0
rainbow punch, 'Koolers'	8.45 fl oz	130	36	0.0
'Rock-A-Dile Red' 'Koolers'	8.45 fl oz	130	34	0.0
tropical punch, 'Koolers'	8.45 fl oz	130	35	0.0
tropical, 'Kool-Aid Burst'	1 serving	90	24	0.0
(Lemonade Chillers) 'Key Lime'	8 fl oz	110	26	0.0
(Libby's)				
apricot nectar	5.5 fl oz	105	25	0.0
banana nectar.	8 fl oz	132	33	0.0
banana nectar	6 fl oz	110	26	0.0
(Minute Maid)				
apple punch, prepared	6 fl oz	90	23	0.0
berry punch	6 fl oz	90	23	0.0
berry punch, frozen concentrate, prepared.	6 fl oz	90	23	0.0
cranberry lemonade	6 fl oz	90	23	0.0
cranberry lemonade, frozen, concentrate, prepared	6 fl oz	90	22	0.0
lemonade, country style	6 fl oz	80	21	0.0
lemonade, country style, frozen concentrate, prepared	6 fl oz	90	22	0.0
lemonade, pink	6 fl oz	80	21	0.0
lemonade, pink, frozen concentrate, prepared	6 fl oz	90	22	0.0
limeade, frozen concentrate, prepared	6 fl oz	70	19	0.0
orange punch	6 fl oz	80	20	0.0
raspberry lemonade	6 fl oz	90	23	0.0
raspberry lemonade, frozen concentrate, prepared	6 fl oz	90	22	0.0
tropical punch	6 fl oz	90	22	0.0
(Mott's)				
apple cranberry	10 fl oz	176	44	0.0
apple raspberry drink	10 fl oz	158	40	0.0
punch	9.5 fl oz	161	40	0.0
grape-apple	10 fl oz	167	42	0.0
(Mountain Sun)				
cherry lemonade, organic	8 fl oz	101	25	0.0
lemonade, organic	8 fl oz	110	27	0.0
(Natural Choice)				
apple cranberry, 5% juice, vitamin C added	1 cup	120	30	0.0
(Nestlé) strawberry-flavored, ready to drink, 'Quik'	1 cup	230	31	9.0
(Ocean Spray)				
'Cran-Apple'	6 fl oz	120	31	0.0
'Cran-Apple Low-calorie'	6 fl oz	35	9	0.0
cranberry, citrus 'Refreshers'	6 fl oz	100	26	0.0
'Cran-Grape'	6 fl oz	120	31	0.0
'Cranicot'	6 fl oz	120	29	0.0
'Cran-Blueberry'	6 fl oz	120	31	0.0
'Cran-Raspberry' low-calorie	6 fl oz	40	9	0.0
'Cran-Raspberry'	6 fl oz	110	27	0.0
'Cran-Strawberry'	6 fl oz	110	27	0.0
guava-passionfruit, Hawaiian, 'Mauna La'i'	6 fl oz	100	25	0.0
lemonade drink, w/cranberry juice	8 fl oz	110	26	0.0
orangecranberry, 'Refreshers'	6 fl oz	100	26	0.0
peach, citrus, 'Refreshers'	6 fl oz	90	23	0.0
(Orange Julius)				
piña colada flavored	16 fl oz	300	71	1.0
raspberry cream supreme	16 fl oz	510	76	23.0
strawberry, regular	16 fl oz	340	82	1.0
tropical cream supreme	16 fl oz	510	67	25.0

Food Name	Serv. Size	Total Cal.	Carbs GMS	Fat GMS
(Orlando Sun)				
pineapple-orange-banana	8 fl oz	110	29	0.0
strawberry guava	8 fl oz	110	29	0.0
(P&Q) cranberry apple	6 fl oz	130	32	0.0
(Pathmark)				
cranberry-apple	6 fl oz	130	32	0.0
cranberry-grape	6 fl oz	103	26	0.0
fruit punch	6 fl oz	90	22	0.0
grape	6 fl oz	90	22	0.0
guava-passionfruit, Hawaiian, 'Hawaii'	6 fl oz	100	25	0.0
orange, 'No Frills Sodium-free'	6 fl oz	80	22	0.0
pineapple, w/grapefruit	6 fl oz	80	21	0.0
raspberry, w/cranberry	6 fl oz	110	27	0.0
raspberry, w/cranberry, 'Sodium-free'	6 fl oz	110	27	0.0
(Red Cheek) apple punch drink	6 fl oz	113	28	0.0
(S&W)				
apricot nectar, canned or bottled	8 fl oz	140	35	0.0
apricot nectar, canned or bottled	5.5 fl oz	100	24	0.0
apricot-pineapple nectar	4 fl oz	35	12	0.0
(Santa Cruz Natural)				
apricot nectar, certified organic	8 fl oz	150	38	0.0
berry nectar, organic	8 fl oz	90	22	1.0
cherry lemonade, dark, sweet, organic	8 fl oz	60	20	1.0
cranberry guava nectar, certified organic	8 fl oz	110	24	0.0
lemonade, certified organic	8 fl oz	120	29	0.0
lemonade, organic	8 fl oz	60	21	1.0
lemonade, organic, 'Sparkling'	8 fl oz	85	20	1.0
limeade, organic, 'Sparkling'	8 fl oz	60	23	1.0
orangeade, organic	8 fl oz	90	22	1.0
orangeade, organic, 'Sparkling'	8 fl oz	90	24	1.0
organic, 'Kauai Punch'	8 fl oz	120	28	1.0
raspberry lemonade, organic	8 fl oz	60	20	1.0
raspberry lemonade, organic, 'Sparkling'	8 fl oz	85	20	1.0
red raspberry, organic, 'Cruz'	8 fl oz	120	28	1.0
strawberry lemonade, organic	8 fl oz	60	20	1.0
tropical punch, organic	8 fl oz	110	26	1.0
(Shasta) lemonade	12 fl oz	146	39	0.0
(Squeezit)				
'Berry B. Wild'	6.75 fl oz	120	29	0.0
'Chucklin' Cherry'	1 serving	110	28	0.0
'Grumpy Grape'	1 serving	110	28	0.0
'Mean Green Puncher'	6.75 fl oz	100	25	0.0
orange fruit, 'Smarty Arty'	1 serving	110	27	0.0
'Rockin Red Puncher'	6.75 fl oz	110	28	0.0
'Silly Billy Strawberry'	6.75 fl oz	90	23	0.0
strawberry	1 serving	110	29	0.0
(Sunkist)				
lemonade	8 fl oz	141	36	0.0
lemonade, frozen, prepared	8 fl oz	92	24	0.0
(Sunny Delight) orange, 'California Style'	8 fl oz	130	31	0.0
(Tang)				
berry blend drink, 'Fruit Box'	8.45 fl oz	140	36	0.0
orange, tropical, 'Fruit Box'	8.45 fl oz	150	37	0.0
strawberry-flavored	8.45 fl oz	120	32	0.0
(10-K)				
apple	8 fl oz	60	15	0.0
fruit punch	8 fl oz	60	15	0.0

Food Name	Serv. Size	Total Cal.	Carbs GMS	Fat GMS
grape, 'Clear'	8 fl oz	60	15	0.0
lemonade, pink	8 fl oz	60	15	0.0
lemon-lime	8 fl oz	60	15	0.0
orange	8 fl oz	60	15	0.0
strawberry	8 fl oz	60	15	0.0
(Thick & Easy)				
apple, honey consistency	1/2 cup	70	17	0.0
cranberry, honey consistency	1/2 cup	70	17	0.0
cranberry, nectar consistency	1/2 cup	60	15	0.0
orange, honey consistency	1/2 cup	60	16	0.0
orange, nectar consistency	1/2 cup	60	15	0.0
(Tree Top) fruit punch, 100%	8 fl oz	119	30	0.0
(Tropicana)				
apple, 'Single Serve'	10 fl oz	175	43	0.0
berry, 'Berries & Berries'	6 fl oz	90	23	1.0
cranberry raspberry, w/strawberry	8 fl oz	120	31	0.0
cranberry raspberry, w/strawberry, light	8 fl oz	45	11	0.0
fruit punch, 'Single Serve'	10 fl oz	148	37	0.0
grape	6 fl oz	90	22	1.0
lemonade, 'Single Serve'	8 fl oz	120	30	0.0
orange, 'Single Serve'	10 fl oz	132	33	0.0
pineapple, w/grapefruit	6 fl oz	100	24	1.0
(Veryfine)				
fruit punch, '100% Juice Punch'	8 fl oz	122	30	0.0
grape	8 fl oz	130	34	0.0
guava-strawberry, 'Refresher'	8 fl oz	120	30	0.0
lemonade	8 fl oz	120	30	0.0
lemon-lime	8 fl oz	120	30	0.0
orange	8 fl oz	130	33	0.0
papaya punch	8 fl oz	120	30	0.0
pineapple-orange	8 fl oz	130	32	0.0
(Welch's)				
cranberry-apple cocktail, frozen, prepared	6 fl oz	120	30	0.0
cranberry-grape cocktail, frozen, prepared	6 fl oz	110	27	0.0
fruit punch cocktail, 'Orchard Fruit Harvest Punch'	10 fl oz	180	45	0.0
raspberry cocktail, 'Orchard' *(Welch's)*	10 fl oz	160	40	0.0
(Wyler's)				
fruit punch, tropical, 'Fruit Slush'	4 fl oz	157	39	0.0
'Fruit Tea Punch'	12 fl oz	118	30	0.0
grape, 'Fruit Slush'	4 fl oz	157	39	0.0
lemonade	6 fl oz	64	17	0.0
lemonade, pink, 'Fruit Slush'	4 fl oz	157	39	0.0
orange, 'Fruit Slush'	4 fl oz	157	39	0.0
FRUIT DRINK MIX				
(Continental Mills) apple flavored, instant, powdered	1 pouch	83	21	0.0
(Country Time)				
lemonade, pink, sugar-free, w/vitamin C, mix only	1/8 cap/tub	5	2	0.0
lemonade, w/vitamin C, mix only	1/8 cap/tub	64	18	0.2
lemonade drink, pink, prepared	8 fl oz	80	20	0.0
lemonade drink, pink, sugar-free, prepared	8 fl oz	4	0	0.0
lemonade drink, pink, sugar-sweetened, prepared	8 fl oz	80	20	0.0
lemonade drink, pink, w/NutraSweet, prepared	8 fl oz	4	0	0.0
lemonade drink, prepared	8 fl oz	80	20	0.0
lemonade punch, prepared	8 fl oz	80	20	0.0
lemonade punch, sugar-sweetened, prepared	8 fl oz	80	20	0.0
(Crystal Light)				
berry blend, sugar-free, prepared	8 fl oz	4	0	0.0
cherry, cranberry, low-calorie, sugarless	1/8 pkt	5	0	0.0

Food Name	Serv. Size	Total Cal.	Carbs GMS	Fat GMS
fruit punch, sugar-free, prepared	8 fl oz	4	0	0.0
lemonade drink, low-calorie, prepared	8 fl oz	5	0	0.0
lemonade drink, mix only	1 serving	5	0	0.0
lemonade drink, sugar-free, prepared	8 fl oz	4	0	0.0
lemonade drink, w/NutraSweet, prepared	8 fl oz	4	0	0.0
lemon-lime, mix only	1 serving	5	0	0.0
lemon-lime, sugar-free, prepared	8 fl oz	4	0	0.0
(Finast)				
cherry, prepared	8 fl oz	80	21	0.0
grape, prepared	8 fl oz	80	21	0.0
lemonade drink, prepared	8 fl oz	80	20	0.0
orange, breakfast, prepared	8 fl oz	80	20	0.0
(Kool-Aid)				
berry blend, sugar-free, w/NutraSweet, mix, prepared	8 fl oz	4	0	0.0
berry blue, mix, prepared w/sugar	8 fl oz	100	25	0.0
berry blue, mix, sugar-sweetened, prepared	8 fl oz	80	21	0.0
berry blue, mix, unsweetened, prepared	8 fl oz	2	0	0.0
black cherry, prepared w/sugar	8 fl oz	100	25	0.0
black cherry, unsweetened, prepared	8 fl oz	2	0	0.0
cherry, sugar-free, prepared	8 fl oz	4	0	0.0
cherry, sugar-sweetened, prepared	8 fl oz	80	20	0.0
cherry, unsweetened, prepared	8 fl oz	2	0	0.0
cherry, w/aspartame and vitamin C, sugarless	1/8 envelope	3	1	0.0
grape, sugar-free, prepared	8 fl oz	4	0	0.0
grape, sugar-sweetened	8 fl oz	80	25	0.0
grape, unsweetened	8 fl oz	2	0	0.0
'Great Bluedini' prepared w/sugar	8 fl oz	100	25	0.0
'Great Bluedini' sugar-free, prepared	8 fl oz	4	0	0.0
'Great Bluedini' unsweetened, prepared	8 fl oz	2	0	0.0
'Incrediberry' sugar-free, mix only	1/8 envelope	5	0	0.0
lemonade drink, pink, prepared w/sugar	8 fl oz	100	25	0.0
lemonade drink, pink, unsweetened, prepared	8 fl oz	2	0	0.0
lemonade drink, w/NutraSweet, prepared	8 fl oz	4	0	0.0
lemonade drink, sugar-sweetened, prepared	8 fl oz	80	20	0.0
lemon-lime, prepared w/sugar	8 fl oz	100	25	0.0
lemon-lime, unsweetened, prepared	8 fl oz	2	0	0.0
mountain berry punch, prepared w/sugar	8 fl oz	100	25	0.0
mountain berry punch, sugar-free, prepared	8 fl oz	4	0	0.0
mountain berry punch, sugar-sweetened, prepared	8 fl oz	80	20	0.0
mountain berry punch, unsweetened, prepared	8 fl oz	2	0	0.0
orange, prepared w/sugar	8 fl oz	100	25	0.0
orange, sugar-free, prepared	8 fl oz	4	0	0.0
orange, sugar-sweetened, prepared	8 fl oz	80	20	0.0
orange, unsweetened, prepared	8 fl oz	2	0	0.0
'Purplesaurus Rex' prepared w/sugar	8 fl oz	100	25	0.0
'Purplesaurus Rex' sugar-free, prepared	8 fl oz	4	0	0.0
'Purplesaurus Rex' unsweetened, prepared	8 fl oz	2	0	0.0
rainbow punch, prepared w/sugar	8 fl oz	100	25	0.0
rainbow punch, sugar-sweetened, prepared	8 fl oz	80	21	0.0
rainbow punch, unsweetened, prepared	8 fl oz	2	0	0.0
raspberry punch, prepared w/sugar	8 fl oz	100	25	0.0
raspberry punch, sugar-sweetened, prepared	8 fl oz	80	20	0.0
raspberry punch, unsweetened, prepared	8 fl oz	2	0	0.0
'Rock-A-Dile Red' prepared w/sugar	8 fl oz	100	25	0.0
'Rock-A-Dile Red' sugar-free, prepared	8 fl oz	4	0	0.0
'Rock-A-Dile Red' unsweetened, prepared	8 fl oz	2	0	0.0
'Sharkleberry Fin' prepared w/sugar	8 fl oz	100	25	0.0
'Sharkleberry Fin' sugar-free, prepared	8 fl oz	4	0	0.0

Food Name	Serv. Size	Total Cal.	Carbs GMS	Fat GMS
'Sharkleberry Fin' sugar-sweetened, prepared	8 fl oz	80	21	0.0
'Sharkleberry Fin' unsweetened, prepared	8 fl oz	2	0	0.0
strawberry punch, prepared w/sugar	8 fl oz	100	25	0.0
strawberry punch, sugar-sweetened, prepared	8 fl oz	80	20	0.0
strawberry punch, unsweetened, prepared	8 fl oz	2	0	0.0
strawberry-flavored, prepared	8 fl oz	100	25	0.0
strawberry-flavored, presweetened, prepared	8 fl oz	80	20	0.0
'Surfin' Berry' prepared w/sugar	8 fl oz	100	25	0.0
'Surfin' Berry' sugar-free, prepared	8 fl oz	4	0	0.0
'Surfin' Berry' unsweetened, prepared	8 fl oz	2	0	0.0
tropical punch, sugar-sweetened, mix only	1 serving	64	16	0.0
tropical punch, sugar-sweetened, prepared	8 fl oz	80	21	0.0
tropical punch, unsweetened, mix only	1 serving	1	0	0.0
tropical punch, unsweetened, prepared	8 fl oz	2	0	0.0
(Kroger)				
lemonade drink, light, diet, 15% vitamin C, mix only	1/8 pkt	5	1	0.0
lemonade drink, sugar, 10% vitamin C, no preservatives, mix only	1 1/2 tbsp	65	16	0.0
lemon-lime, light, diet, 15% vitamin C	1/8 pkt	6	2	0.0
(Minute Maid)				
grape punch, chilled	6 fl oz	90	23	0.0
grape punch, frozen concentrate, prepared.	6 fl oz	90	23	0.0
(Nestlé)				
strawberry-flavored, 'Quik' mix only	0.75 oz	80	21	0.0
strawberry-flavored, 'Quik' prepared w/skim milk	8 fl oz	160	32	0.0
strawberry-flavored, 'Quik' prepared wwhole milk	8 fl oz	220	32	8.0
(Pathmark)				
cherry, 'No Frills' prepared	8 fl oz	90	22	0.0
fruit punch, 'No Frills' prepared	8 fl oz	90	22	0.0
grape, 'No Frills Sodium-free' prepared	6 fl oz	80	22	0.0
grape, 'No Frills' prepared	8 fl oz	90	22	0.0
lemon, 'No Frills' prepared	8 fl oz	90	20	0.0
orange, breakfast, 'No Frills' prepared	4 fl oz	60	15	0.0
mango flavor, prepared	6 fl oz	80	20	0.0
(Tang)				
orange, mix only	2 tbsp	100	24	0.0
orange, prepared	8 fl oz	90	23	0.0
orange, sugar-free, 'Breakfast Beverage Crystals' prepared	6 fl oz	6	1	0.0
orange, sugar-free, prepared	6 fl oz	6	1	0.0
orange-flavored, mix only	2 tbsp	92	25	0.0
orange-flavored, prepared	8 fl oz	92	25	0.0
orange-flavored, sugarless, prepared	8 fl oz	5	2	0.0
orange, 'Breakfast Beverage Crystals' prepared	6 fl oz	90	22	0.0
(Welch's) grape, frozen concentrate, 'Welchade'	2 fl oz	130	31	0.0
(Wyler's)				
cherry, 'Fruit Slush' prepared	4 fl oz	157	39	0.0
fruit punch, tropical, 'Crystals' prepared	8 fl oz	85	21	0.1
lemonade drink, 'Crystals' prepared.	8 fl oz	92	20	1.5
strawberry-flavored, 'Crystals' prepared	8 fl oz	85	21	0.3
FRUIT JUICE BLEND. See also CIDER; FRUIT DRINK; FRUIT JUICE DRINK.				
AMBROSIA *(Knudsen)*	8 fl oz	110	27	0.0
APPLE APRICOT *(Knudsen)*	8 fl oz	120	30	0.0
APPLE BANANA *(Knudsen)*	8 fl oz	120	30	0.0
APPLE BLACKBERRY				
(Knudsen)	8 fl oz	100	24	0.0
organic *(Santa Cruz Natural)*	8 fl oz	120	29	1.0
APPLE BOYSENBERRY				
organic *(Santa Cruz Natural)*	8 fl oz	120	29	1.0

Food Name	Serv. Size	Total Cal.	Carbs GMS	Fat GMS
(Knudsen)	8 fl oz	120	30	0.0
APPLE CARROT 100% pure juice *(Vruit)*	8.45 fl oz	120	28	0.0
APPLE CHERRY				
'Breakfast Cocktail' *(Musselman's)*	6 fl oz	100	26	0.0
'Naturally 100%' *(Red Cheek)*	6 fl oz	113	28	0.0
100% juice 'Junior' *(McCain)*	4.2 fl oz	50	13	0.0
APPLE CITRUS, canned or frozen *(Tree Top)*	6 fl oz	90	22	0.0
APPLE CRANBERRY				
(Apple & Eve)	6 fl oz	80	19	0.0
(Knudsen)	8 fl oz	120	30	0.0
(Lucky Leaf)	6 fl oz	130	32	0.0
(Mott's)	6 fl oz	83	24	0.0
(Santa Cruz Natural) organic	8 fl oz	115	28	1.0
(Smucker's) 'Naturally 100%'	8 fl oz	120	32	0.0
(Tree Top) canned or frozen	6 fl oz	100	25	0.0
(Veryfine) cocktail	8 fl oz	130	33	0.0
APPLE CRANBERRY RASPBERRY *(Ultra Slim Fast)*	8 fl oz	153	32	1.0
APPLE GRAPE CHERRY				
(Welch's) frozen, 'Orchard Cocktail'	6 fl oz	90	22	0.0
(Welch's) 'Orchard Cocktails-In-A-Box'	8.45 fl oz	150	38	0.0
APPLE GRAPE				
(Juicy Juice)	6 fl oz	90	22	0.0
(Mott's)	6 fl oz	86	23	0.0
(Musselman's) 'Breakfast Cocktail'	6 fl oz	110	28	0.0
(Red Cheek)	6 fl oz	109	27	0.0
(Tree Top) 100%	8 fl oz	130	32	0.0
(Welch's) 'Orchard Cocktail'	6 fl oz	110	27	0.0
APPLE GRAPE RASPBERRY				
(Welch's) 'Orchard Cocktail' frozen, prepared	6 fl oz	90	22	0.0
(Welch's) 'Orchard Cocktails-In-A-Box'	8.45 fl oz	140	35	0.0
APPLE ORANGE PINEAPPLE				
(Welch's) 'Orchard Tropical Cocktails'	6 fl oz	100	25	0.0
APPLE PEACH *(Knudsen)*	8 fl oz	120	30	0.0
APPLE PEAR *(Tree Top)* 100%	8 fl oz	120	29	0.0
APPLE RASPBERRY				
(Knudsen)	8 fl oz	120	30	0.0
(Mott's)	6 fl oz	83	22	0.0
(Red Cheek)	6 fl oz	113	28	0.0
(Santa Cruz Natural) organic	8 fl oz	120	29	1.0
(Tree Top) 100%	8 fl oz	116	28	0.0
(Veryfine) cocktail	8 fl oz	110	27	0.0
APPLE STRAWBERRY				
(Knudsen)	8 fl oz	120	30	0.0
(Santa Cruz Natural) organic	8 fl oz	120	29	1.0
APPLE WHITE GRAPE				
(Welch's) cocktail, frozen 'No Sugar Added'	6 fl oz	40	10	0.0
BERRY				
(Juicy Juice) bottled	6 fl oz	90	22	0.0
CRANBERRY BLUEBERRY				
(Knudsen)	8 fl oz	115	36	0.0
CRANBERRY RASPBERRY				
(Knudsen)	8 fl oz	140	36	0.0
(Welch's) light, frozen, prepared	6 fl oz	40	10	0.0
GRAPE *(Juicy Juice)* juice blend	6 fl oz	100	25	0.0
GUAVA CRANBERRY				
(Santa Cruz Natural) organic 'Cruz'	8 fl oz	130	30	1.0
HIBISCUS CRANBERRY *(Knudsen)*	8 fl oz	120	30	0.0
LEMON GINGER *(Santa Cruz Natural)* organic 'Cruz'	8 fl oz	125	29	1.0

Food Name	Serv. Size	Total Cal.	Carbs GMS	Fat GMS
MANGO PEACH *(Knudsen)*	8 fl oz	120	30	0.0
ORANGE *(Minute Maid)* blend, 'Juices To Go'	6 fl oz	90	22	0.0
ORANGE APRICOT *(Musselman's)* 'Breakfast Cocktail'	6 fl oz	90	21	0.0
ORANGE BANANA *(Smucker's)* 'Naturally 100%'	8 fl oz	120	30	0.0
ORANGE CRANBERRY *(Santa Cruz Natural)* organic 'Cruz'	8 fl oz	125	29	1.0
ORANGE GRAPEFRUIT				
(Kraft) chilled, 'Pure 100%'	6 fl oz	80	19	0.0
(Tropicana) ruby red, 'Pure Premium'	8 fl oz	120	28	0.0
ORANGE KIWI PASSIONFRUIT				
(Tropicana) 100% pure	6 fl oz	80	17	1.0
(Tropicana) 'Pure Premium'	8 fl oz	100	26	0.0
ORANGE MANGO				
(Knudsen)	8 fl oz	120	30	0.0
(Tropicana) 'Twister'	6 fl oz	90	21	1.0
ORANGE PASSIONFRUIT *(Tropicana)* 'Twister'	6 fl oz	80	19	1.0
ORANGE PEACH *(Tropicana Twister)*	8 fl oz	120	31	0.0
ORANGE PEACH MANGO				
(Tropicana) 100% pure	6 fl oz	80	19	1.0
(Tropicana) 'Pure Premium'	8 fl oz	110	28	0.0
ORANGE PINEAPPLE				
(Kraft) 'Pure 100%'	6 fl oz	80	19	0.0
(Musselman's) 'Breakfast Cocktail'	6 fl oz	90	23	0.0
(Tropicana) 100% pure	6 fl oz	80	19	1.0
(Tropicana) 'Pure Premium'	8 fl oz	110	27	0.0
(Ultra Slim Fast)	8 fl oz	153	33	1.0
ORANGE STRAWBERRY BANANA				
(Tropicana) 100% pure	6 fl oz	80	18	1.0
(Ultra Slim Fast)	8 fl oz	153	33	1.0
PAPAYA LIME *(Knudsen)*	8 fl oz	115	29	0.0
PASSIONFRUIT RASPBERRY *(Knudsen)*	8 fl oz	130	32	0.0
PINEAPPLE COCONUT *(Knudsen)*	8 fl oz	130	32	0.0
PINEAPPLE GRAPEFRUIT				
(Dole) frozen, prepared	6 fl oz	90	22	0.0
(Dole) w/pink grapefruit	6 fl oz	101	25	0.1
PINEAPPLE ORANGE				
(Dole)	6 fl oz	90	22	0.0
(Dole) w/banana	6 fl oz	100	23	0.0
(Dole) w/guava	6 fl oz	100	21	0.0
(Minute Maid)	6 fl oz	90	23	0.0
PINEAPPLE PASSIONFRUIT *(Dole)* w/banana	6 fl oz	100	21	0.0
RASPBERRY				
(Apple & Eve) w/cranberry	6 fl oz	90	21	0.0
(Dole) blend, 'Pure & Light Country Raspberry'	6 fl oz	87	24	0.2
(Knudsen) blend, 'Razzleberry'	8 fl oz	90	21	0.0
RASPBERRY PEACH *(Knudsen)*	8 fl oz	120	31	0.0
STRAWBERRY BANANA *(Knudsen)*	8 fl oz	120	30	0.0
STRAWBERRY GUAVA *(Knudsen)*	8 fl oz	105	26	0.0
TOMATO-BEEF COCKTAIL *(Beefamato)*	6 fl oz	80	19	0.0
TOMATO-CHILE COCKTAIL *(Snap-E-Tom)*	6 fl oz	40	8	0.0
TOMATO-CLAM COCKTAIL *(Clamato)*	6 fl oz	96	23	0.0
FRUIT JUICE DRINK				
(A&P)				
cranberry juice cocktail, bottled	6 fl oz	100	26	1.0
(Capri Sun)				
fruit punch	1 serving	100	26	0.0
'Pacific Cooler'	1 serving	100	26	0.0
Maui punch	1 serving	100	27	0.0

Food Name	Serv. Size	Total Cal.	Carbs GMS	Fat GMS
wild cherry	1 serving	110	30	0.0
(Citrus Hill)				
grapefruit, 'Plus Calcium'	6 fl oz	70	19	1.0
orange, 'Lite Premium'	6 fl oz	60	14	1.0
(Clinical Resource)				
orange	8 fl oz	180	36	0.0
peach	8 fl oz	180	36	0.0
wild berry	8 fl oz	180	36	0.0
(Del Monte) apricot nectar	6 fl oz	100	26	0.0
(Hi-C)				
cherry	8.45 fl oz	141	35	0.1
grape	6 fl oz	96	24	0.1
(IGA) pink grapefruit	6 fl oz	80	20	0.0
(J. Hungerford)				
cranberry juice cocktail	9.03 fl oz	141	36	0.0
cranberry juice cocktail, 50% juice	9.03 fl oz	134	35	0.1
fruit punch, 50% juice	9.03 fl oz	107	27	0.0
fruit punch, 100% juice	9.03 fl oz	116	30	0.0
grape, 50% juice	9.03 fl oz	135	34	0.0
grapefruit, 50% juice	9.03 fl oz	109	27	0.0
pineapple, 50% juice	9.03 fl oz	123	31	0.0
(Kern's)				
guava nectar	11.5 fl oz	216	55	0.0
mango nectar	11.5 fl oz	216	52	0.0
mango-orange nectar	8 fl oz	140	35	0.0
orange-banana nectar	6 fl oz	110	25	0.0
orange-guava nectar	8 fl oz	150	36	0.0
papaya nectar	11.5 fl oz	210	51	0.0
peach nectar	11.5 fl oz	210	52	0.0
peach-passionfruit nectar	11.5 fl oz	220	53	0.0
pear nectar	11.5 fl oz	220	54	0.0
pineapple-orange-passionfruit nectar	8 fl oz	146	33	0.0
strawberry nectar	6 fl oz	110	28	0.0
strawberry-banana nectar	8 fl oz	150	36	0.0
tropical nectar	11.5 fl oz	210	48	0.0
(Knudsen)				
breakfast juice, natural	8 fl oz	110	27	0.0
breakfast juice, natural, concentrate, prepared	8 fl oz	110	27	0.0
kiwi nectar	8 fl oz	60	14	0.0
orange juice float	8 fl oz	140	33	0.0
papaya nectar	8 fl oz	130	34	0.0
peach nectar	8 fl oz	120	30	0.0
pineapple juice float	8 fl oz	130	31	0.0
raspberry nectar, concentrate, prepared	8 fl oz	120	30	0.0
red raspberry nectar	8 fl oz	120	30	0.0
strawberry juice float	8 fl oz	130	32	0.0
strawberry nectar	8 fl oz	120	30	0.0
(Kool-Aid) orange, 'Koolers'	8.45 fl oz	110	30	0.0
(Libby's)				
guanabana nectar	8 fl oz	147	35	0.0
guava nectar	8 fl oz	153	38	0.0
mango nectar	6 fl oz	110	26	0.0
papaya nectar	6 fl oz	110	28	0.0
peach nectar	6 fl oz	100	24	0.0
pineapple nectar	6 fl oz	110	27	0.0
strawberry nectar	6 fl oz	110	27	0.0
(Minute Maid) pink grapefruit, 'Juices To Go'	6 fl oz	80	20	0.0

Food Name	Serv. Size	Total Cal.	Carbs GMS	Fat GMS
(Mott's) orange	10 fl oz	144	35	0.0
(Musselman's) w/grapefruit juice, 'Breakfast Cocktail'	6 fl oz	90	22	0.0
(Ocean Spray)				
cranberry juice cocktail, bottled	6 fl oz	110	26	0.0
cranberry juice cocktail, bottled, 'Low-calorie'	6 fl oz	40	9	0.0
cranberry juice drink, citrus, 'Refreshers'	6 fl oz	100	26	0.0
pink grapefruit	6 fl oz	80	20	0.0
orange juice cocktail	6 fl oz	100	25	0.0
pineapple cocktail, w/grapefruit juice	6 fl oz	110	26	0.0
(Orange Julius) orange	16 fl oz	265	66	1.0
(P&Q) cranberry juice cocktail, bottled	6 fl oz	100	24	1.0
(Pathmark)				
cranberry juice cocktail, bottled, 'No Frills'	6 fl oz	100	26	0.0
pink grapefruit	6 fl oz	80	20	0.0
(Santa Cruz Natural)				
papaya nectar, certified organic	8 fl oz	110	28	0.0
red raspberry nectar, certified organic	8 fl oz	100	26	0.0
strawberry-guava nectar, certified organic	8 fl oz	100	24	0.0
(Snapple)				
'Apple Crisp' *(Snapple)*	10 fl oz	140	36	0.0
'Cranberry Royale'	10 fl oz	150	37	0.0
'Passion Supreme'	10 fl oz	160	39	0.0
(Sunkist)				
cranberry juice cocktail, bottled	6 fl oz	110	28	0.1
cranberry juice cocktail, frozen, prepared	6 fl oz	110	28	0.1
grape, frozen, prepared	6 fl oz	69	17	0.1
(Tang)				
cherry, 'Fruit Box'	8.45 fl oz	130	34	0.0
grape, 'Fruit Box'	8.45 fl oz	130	34	0.0
mixed fruit, 'Fruit Box'	8.45 fl oz	140	36	0.0
orange, 'Fruit Box'	8.45 fl oz	130	32	0.0
strawberry, 'Fruit Box'	8.45 fl oz	120	32	0.0
(TreeSweet) pink grapefruit 'Lite'	6 fl oz	40	10	0.0
(Tropic Isle) fruit punch, vitamin-enriched	6 fl oz	90	22	0.0
(Tropicana)				
apple raspberry blackberry drink, 'Twister'	8 fl oz	130	31	0.0
cranberry juice drink, 'Season's Best' 'Medley'	10 fl oz	140	35	0.0
cranberry juice drink, 'Season's Best' 'Medley'	8 fl oz	120	29	0.0
'Cranberry Orchard Juice Sparkler'	8 fl oz	120	30	0.0
grapefruit, 'Juice Sparkler'	8 fl oz	110	26	0.0
pink grapefruit, 'Twister'	8 fl oz	110	28	0.0
grapefruit, ruby red w/cranberry, 'Twister'	8 fl oz	120	30	0.0
Mandarin orange-papaya, 'Twister'	6 fl oz	90	21	1.0
orange-cranberry, 'Twister'	8 fl oz	130	32	0.0
orange-cranberry, light, 'Twister'	8 fl oz	30	7	0.0
orange-raspberry, 'Twister'	6 fl oz	80	20	1.0
orange-raspberry, light, 'Twister'	8 fl oz	35	9	0.0
orange-strawberry-banana, 'Twister'	8 fl oz	130	32	0.0
orange-strawberry-banana, light, 'Twister'	8 fl oz	35	9	0.0
orange-strawberry-guava, 'Twister'	8 fl oz	120	29	0.0
pineapple, w/grapefruit juice, 'Twister'	8 fl oz	125	32	0.0
pineapple-grapefruit, 'Twister'	8 fl oz	120	29	0.0
pineapple-grapefruit, light, 'Twister'	8 fl oz	35	9	0.0
'Season's Best' 'Medley'	8 fl oz	130	32	0.0
wild berry, 'Juice Sparkler'	8 fl oz	110	27	0.0
(Veryfine)				
apple cherry berry	8 fl oz	130	33	0.0

Food Name	Serv. Size	Total Cal.	Carbs GMS	Fat GMS
cranberry juice cocktail, bottled .... 8 fl oz	160	40	0.0
'Passionfruit Refresher' w/orange, tropical .... 8 fl oz	110	26	0.0
pink grapefruit .... 8 fl oz	120	29	0.0
(Welch's)			
cranberry juice cocktail, frozen, diluted as directed .... 6 fl oz	100	26	0.0
cranberry juice cocktail, no sugar added, frozen, prepared ...... 6 fl oz	40	10	0.0
cranberry juice cocktail, w/raspberry, frozen, prepared .... 6 fl oz	110	28	0.0
cranberry juice cocktail, w/blueberry, frozen, prepared .... 6 fl oz	110	27	0.0
cranberry juice cocktail, lite, frozen, prepared .... 6 fl oz	40	10	0.0
grape juice cocktail, no sugar added, frozen concentrate,			
prepared .... 6 fl oz	40	10	0.0
grape juice cocktail, 'Orchard Cocktails-In-A-Box' .... 8.45 fl oz	150	38	0.0
grape juice cocktail, 'Orchard' .... 6 fl oz	110	27	0.0
orange juice cocktail, 'Orchard' .... 10 fl oz	150	37	0.0
'Orchard Harvest Blend Cocktails-In-A-Box' .... 8.45 fl oz	150	38	0.0
'Orchard Harvest Blend' frozen, prepared .... 6 fl oz	110	27	0.0
passionfruit cocktail, 'Orchard Tropical Cocktails-In-A-Box' .... 8.45 fl oz	140	34	0.0
passionfruit cocktail, 'Orchard Tropicals' frozen, prepared .... 6 fl oz	100	25	0.0
pineapple cocktail, w/banana, 'Orchard Tropicals' .... 6 fl oz	100	24	0.0
pineapple cocktail, w/banana, 'Orchard Tropicals' .... 8.45 fl oz	140	34	0.0
(Wyler's)			
grapefruit, 'Fruit Slush' .... 4 fl oz	157	39	0.0
strawberry, 'Fruit Slush' .... 4 fl oz	157	39	0.0

FRUIT ROLL. See FRUIT SNACK.

FRUIT SNACK

Food Name	Serv. Size	Total Cal.	Carbs GMS	Fat GMS
(Betty Crocker)			
all flavors, 'Berry Bears' .... 1 pouch	100	22	1.0
all flavors, 'Fruit Roll-Ups Peel-Outs' .... 1 roll	50	12	1.0
assorted flavors, 'Bugs Bunny & Friends' 1 pouch 90	1	30	0.0
assorted flavors, 'Tasmanian Devil' .... 1 pouch	90	21	1.0
berry fruit roll-up, w/vitamin C .... 2 rolls	104	24	1.0
blueberry, 'Wild Blue' 'Garfield & Friends' .... 1 roll	50	12	1.0
cherry, 'Fruit by the Foot' .... 1 roll	80	17	2.0
cherry, 'Fruit Roll-Ups' .... 0.5-oz roll	50	12	1.0
crazy colors, 'Fruit Roll-Ups' .... 0.5-oz roll	50	12	1.0
grape, 'Fruit by the Foot' .... 1 roll	80	17	2.0
grape, 'Fruit Roll-Ups' .... 0.5-oz roll	50	12	1.0
grape, 'Gushin Grape Gushers' .... 1 pouch	90	21	1.0
raspberry, 'Fruit Roll-Ups' .... 0.5-oz roll	50	12	1.0
strawberry, 'Fruit by the Foot' .... 1 roll	80	17	2.0
strawberry, 'Fruit Roll-Ups' .... 0.5-oz roll	50	12	1.0
strawberry, 'Gushers' .... 1 pouch	90	21	1.0
wild cherry, 'Gushers' .... 1 pouch	90	21	1.0
(Farley)			
assorted flavors, 'Dinosaurs' .... 1 oz	90	22	1.0
assorted flavors, 'Teenage Mutant Ninja Turtles' .... 1 oz	90	22	1.0
assorted flavors, 'Trolls' .... 1 oz	90	22	1.0
w/vitamins A, C, and E .... 1 pouch	89	21	0.0
(Flavor Tree)			
apple roll .... 1 piece	75	19	0.0
apricot roll .... 1 piece	76	18	0.5
assorted flavors, 'Fruit Circus Fruit Bears' .... 1.05 oz	117	25	1.6
cherry roll .... 1 piece	75	18	0.1
grape roll .... 1 piece	76	19	0.1
raspberry roll .... 1 piece	75	18	0.1
strawberry roll .... 1 piece	74	18	0.1
(Fruit Parade)			
assorted flavors, 'Chip 'N Dale Rescue Rangers' .... 1 pouch	100	22	1.0

Food Name	Serv. Size	Total Cal.	Carbs GMS	Fat GMS
assorted flavors, 'Darkwing Duck'	1 pouch	100	22	1.0
assorted flavors, 'Tale Spin'	1 pouch	100	22	1.0
(Rokeach) compote	4 oz	120	31	1.0
(Stretch Island)				
'Berry Blackberry' 100% fruit	1 oz	90	24	0.0
'Chunky Cherry' 100% fruit	1 oz	90	24	0.0
'Great Grape' 100% fruit	1 oz	90	24	0.0
'Rave Raspberry' 100% fruit	1 oz	90	24	0.0
apple, 100% fruit, 'Snappy Apple'	1 oz	90	25	0.0
apricot, 'Tangy Apricot' 100% fruit	1 oz	90	23	0.0
(Sunkist)				
assorted flavors, 'Fun Fruits Fantastic Fruit'	1 pouch	100	22	1.4
assorted flavors, all shapes, 'Fun Fruits'	1 pouch	100	22	1.4
berry, 'Fun Fruits Berry Bunch'	1 pouch	100	22	1.4
cherry, 'Fun Fruits'	1 pouch	100	22	1.4
grape, 'Fun Fruits'	1 pouch	100	22	1.4
orange, 'Fun Fruits'	1 pouch	100	22	1.4
strawberry roll, w/vitamins A, C, and E	1 roll	72	17	0.2
strawberry, 'Fun Fruits'	1 pouch	100	22	1.4
strawberry, yogurt-coated, 'Creme Supremes'	1 pouch	114	20	3.6
(Sun-Maid) raisin, muscat, seeded	1/2 cup	270	67	1.0
(Weight Watchers)				
apple	1 pouch	50	13	1.0
apple chips	0.75 oz	70	19	0.0
cinnamon flavor	1 pouch	50	13	1.0
peach	0.5 oz	50	13	1.0
strawberry	1 pouch	50	13	1.0
FRUIT SPREAD. See also JAM AND PRESERVES.				
(Fifty 50)				
apple, no sugar added	1 tsp	2	1	0.0
grape, no sugar added	1 tsp	2	1	0.0
grape spread, no sugar added, contains phenylalanine	1 tbsp	10	3	0.0
orange marmalade, no sugar added	1 tsp	2	1	0.0
raspberry, no sugar added	1 tsp	2	1	0.0
strawberry, no sugar added	1 tsp	2	1	0.0
(Knott's Berry Farm)				
apricot-pineapple	1 tsp	16	4	0.0
apricot-pineapple, 'Light'	1 tsp	8	2	0.0
apricot-pineapple, portion pack	0.5 oz	35	9	0.0
blackberry	1 tsp	16	4	0.0
blackberry, 'Light'	1 tsp	8	2	0.0
blackberry, portion pack	0.5 oz	35	9	0.0
boysenberry	1 tsp	16	4	0.0
boysenberry, 'Light'	1 tsp	8	2	0.0
boysenberry, portion pack	0.5 oz	35	9	0.0
orange marmalade	1 tsp	16	4	0.0
orange marmalade, 'Light'	1 tsp	8	2	0.0
orange marmalade, portion pack	0.5 oz	35	9	0.0
red raspberry	1 tsp	16	4	0.0
red raspberry, 'Light'	1 tsp	8	2	0.0
red raspberry, portion pack	0.5 oz	35	9	0.0
strawberry, 'Light'	1 tsp	8	2	0.0
(Knudsen)				
calamansi, 'Tropical Rainforest'	2 tsp	35	8	0.0
guanabana, 'Tropical Rainforest'	2 tsp	35	8	0.0
(Polaner)				
apricot, 'All Fruit Spreadable Fruit'	1 tsp	14	4	0.0

Food Name	Serv. Size	Total Cal.	Carbs GMS	Fat GMS
black cherry, 'All Fruit Spreadable Fruit'	1 tsp	14	4	0.0
blueberry, 'All Fruit Spreadable Fruit'	1 tsp	14	4	0.0
grape, 'All Fruit Spreadable Fruit'	1 tsp	14	4	0.0
orange, 'All Fruit Spreadable Fruit'	1 tsp	14	4	0.0
raspberry, seedless, 'All Fruit Spreadable Fruit'	1 tsp	14	4	0.0
strawberry, 'All Fruit Spreadable Fruit'	1 tsp	14	4	0.0
(Smucker's)				
all flavors, 'Homestyle'	1 tsp	15	3	0.0
all flavors, 'Slenderella'	1 tsp	7	2	0.0
apricot, low-sugar	1 tsp	8	2	0.0
apricot, 'Simply Fruit'	1 tsp	16	4	0.0
black raspberry, 'Simply Fruit'	1 tsp	16	4	0.0
blackberry, low-sugar	1 tsp	8	2	0.0
blackberry, 'Simply Fruit'	1 tsp	16	4	0.0
blueberry, 'Simply Fruit'	1 tsp	16	4	0.0
boysenberry, low-sugar	1 tsp	8	2	0.0
concord grape, low-sugar	1 tsp	8	2	0.0
grape, 'Imitation'	1 tsp	2	1	0.0
grape, 'Simply Fruit'	1 tsp	16	4	0.0
orange marmalade, low-sugar	1 tsp	8	2	0.0
orange marmalade, 'Simply Fruit'	1 tsp	16	4	0.0
peach, 'Simply Fruit'	1 tsp	16	4	0.0
red raspberry, low-sugar	1 tsp	8	2	0.0
red raspberry, 'Simply Fruit'	1 tsp	16	4	0.0
strawberry, 'Imitation'	1 tsp	2	1	0.0
strawberry, low-sugar	1 tsp	8	2	0.0
strawberry, 'Simply Fruit'	1 tsp	16	4	0.0
(Weight Watchers)				
grape	1 tsp	8	2	0.0
raspberry	1 tsp	8	2	0.0
strawberry	1 tsp	8	2	0.0
FRUIT TOPPING, pourable, 'Fruit 'n Maple' *(Knudsen)*	1 oz	105	26	0.0
FUDGE. See under CANDY.				
FUDGE TOPPING. See also CHOCOLATE TOPPING.				
(Kraft) hot	2 tbsp	140	24	4.5
(Mrs. Richardson's)				
caramel, microwavable	2 tbsp	130	28	2.0
hot	2 tbsp	140	20	7.0
hot, microwaveable	2 tbsp	140	20	7.0
(Smucker's)				
	2 tbsp	130	31	1.0
hot	2 tbsp	110	18	4.0
hot, 'Light'	2 tbsp	70	19	0.0
hot, 'Special Recipe'	2 tbsp	150	23	5.0
'Magic Shell'	2 tbsp	190	16	15.0
FUKI. See BUTTERBUR.				

G

Food Name	Serv. Size	Total Cal.	Carbs GMS	Fat GMS
GARBANZO BEAN. See CHICKPEA.				
GARDEN CRESS				
boiled, drained	1 cup	31	5	0.8
boiled, drained	1/2 cup	16	3	0.4
raw	1 cup	16	3	0.3

Food Name	Serv. Size	Total Cal.	Carbs GMS	Fat GMS
GARLIC AND HERB SEASONING. See under SEASONING MIX.				
GARLIC				
Fresh				
raw, chopped .... 1 cup		203	45	0.7
raw, chopped .... 1 tsp		4	1	0.0
raw, whole .... 1 med clove		4	1	0.0
raw, whole .... 3 med cloves		13	3	0.0
Jarred				
crushed *(Gilroy)* .... 1 tsp		8	2	0.0
dehydrated *(Basic American)* .... 1 oz		86	22	0.1
minced *(Gilroy)* .... 1 tsp		23	2	1.0
GARLIC BREAD. See under BREAD.				
GARLIC OIL *(Hain)* .... 1 tbsp		120	0	14.0
GARLIC POWDER				
.... 1 tbsp		28	6	0.1
.... 1 tsp		9	2	0.0
(Lawry's) .... 1/4 tsp		0	1	0.0
(McCormick/Schilling) .... 1 tsp		10	2	0.0
(Spice Islands) .... 1 tsp		5	1	0.0
(Tone's) .... 1 tsp		9	2	0.1
fresh ground *(Durkee)* .... 1 tsp		10	0	0.0
fresh ground *(Laurel Leaf)* .... 1 tsp		10	0	0.0
w/parsley *(Lawry's)* .... 1 tsp		12	2	0.9
GARLIC SALT. See under SEASONING MIX.				
GARLIC TABLETS *(Shaklee)* .... 2 tablets		5	1	0.0
GATORADE. See under SPORTS AND DIET/NUTRITION DRINKS.				
GEFILTE FISH				
(Mother's)				
in jelled broth, 'Old Fashioned' 24-oz jar .... 1 ball		70	5	1.0
in jelled broth, 'Old Fashioned' 12-oz jar .... 1 ball		54	4	0.8
in jelled broth, 'Old World' .... 1 ball		70	7	1.0
in jelled broth, 'Unsalted' .... 1 ball		45	2	1.0
in liquid, 'Old Fashioned' 24- or 31-oz jar .... 1 ball		70	7	1.0
in liquid, 'Old Fashioned' 12-oz' .... 1 ball		54	5	0.8
sweet, 'Old World' .... 1 ball		54	5	0.8
(Rokeach)				
hors d'oeuvres .... 8 balls		60	4	1.0
in jelled broth, 'Old Vienna' 31-oz jar .... 3 oz		81	9	1.0
in jelled broth, 'Old Vienna' 24-oz jar .... 2.6 oz		70	8	1.0
in jelled broth, 'Old Vienna' 12-oz jar .... 2 oz		54	6	1.0
in jelled broth, 'Redi-Jelled' .... 2 oz		46	3	1.0
in natural broth, 24-oz pkg .... 4 oz		60	4	1.0
WHITEFISH				
(Mother's)				
in jelled broth, 12-oz jar .... 1 ball		46	3	0.8
in liquid, 12-oz pkg .... 1 ball		54	5	0.8
WHITEFISH AND PIKE				
(Mother's)				
in jelled broth .... 1 ball		60	4	1.0
in jelled broth, 'Old World' .... 1 ball		54	5	0.8
in liquid .... 1 ball		70	7	1.0
(Rokeach) in jelled broth .... 2 oz		46	3	1.0
GELATIN, unflavored *(Knox)* .... 1 pkt		25	0	0.0
GELATIN DESSERT				
(Estee) all flavors .... 1/2 cup		8	1	0.0
(Jell-O)				
'Berry Blue' .... 3.5 oz		80	18	0.0

Food Name	Serv. Size	Total Cal.	Carbs GMS	Fat GMS
cherry	3.5 oz	80	18	0.0
cherry, sugar-free	1 snack	10	0	0.0
orange, sugar-free	1 snack	10	0	0.0
raspberry, sugar-free	1 snack	10	0	0.0
strawberry	3.5 oz	80	18	0.0
strawberry, sugar-free	1 snack	10	0	0.0
GELATIN DESSERT MIX				
(D-Zerta) all flavors, except strawberry, low-calorie, prepared	1/2 cup	8	0	0.0
(Featherweight) all flavors, except lemon, prepared	1/2 cup	10	1	0.0
APPLE (Royal) prepared	1/2 cup	80	19	0.0
BANANA (Ener-G Foods) low-fat, gluten free, prepared	1/2 cup	249	62	0.0
BLACK RASPBERRY (Jell-O) prepared	1/2 cup	80	19	0.0
BLACKBERRY (Royal) prepared	1/2 cup	80	19	0.0
CHERRY				
(Jell-O) sugar-free, prepared	1/2 cup	8	0	0.0
(Royal)				
prepared	1/2 cup	80	19	0.0
sugar-free, mix only	1 serving	8	1	0.0
CHOCOLATE (Ener-G Foods) prepared	1/2 cup	231	56	0.6
GRAPE				
(Jell-O) Concord, prepared	1/2 cup	80	19	0.0
(Royal) Concord, prepared	1/2 cup	80	19	0.0
LEMON				
(Ener-G Foods) prepared	1/2 cup	246	63	0.0
(Featherweight) prepared	1/2 cup	10	1	0.0
(Jell-O) sugar-free, prepared	1/2 cup	10	0	0.0
(Royal) prepared	1/2 cup	80	19	0.0
LEMON-LIME (Royal) prepared	1/2 cup	80	19	0.0
LIME				
(Jell-O) sugar-free, prepared	1/2 cup	8	0	0.0
(Royal)				
prepared	1/2 cup	80	19	0.0
sugar-free, mix only	1 serving	8	1	0.0
MIXED BERRY (Royal) prepared	1/2 cup	80	19	0.0
MIXED FRUIT				
(Jell-O) sugar-free, prepared	1/2 cup	10	0	0.0
(Royal) 'Fruit Punch' prepared	1/2 cup	80	19	0.0
ORANGE				
(Ener-G Foods) prepared	1/2 cup	242	60	0.0
(Jell-O) sugar-free, prepared	1/2 cup	8	0	0.0
(Royal)				
prepared	1/2 cup	80	19	0.0
sugar-free, mix only	1 serving	10	1	0.0
ORANGE-PINEAPPLE (Jell-O) prepared	1/2 cup	80	19	0.0
PEACH (Royal) prepared	1/2 cup	80	19	0.0
PINEAPPLE (Royal) mix only	1 serving	80	19	0.0
RASPBERRY				
(Ener-G Foods) low-fat, prepared	1/2 cup	248	62	0.0
(Jell-O) sugar-free, prepared	1/2 cup	8	0	0.0
(Royal)				
prepared	1/2 cup	80	19	0.0
sugar-free, mix only	1 serving	8	1	0.0
STRAWBERRY				
(D-Zerta) low-calorie, prepared	1/2 cup	10	0	0.0
(Jell-O) sugar-free, prepared	1/2 cup	10	0	0.0
(Royal)				
prepared	1/2 cup	80	19	0.0

Food Name	Serv. Size	Total Cal.	Carbs GMS	Fat GMS
sugar-free, mix only	1 serving	8	1	0.0
STRAWBERRY-BANANA				
(Jell-O) sugar-free, prepared	1/2 cup	10	0	0.0
(Royal)				
prepared	1/2 cup	80	19	0.0
sugar-free, mix only	1 serving	8	1	0.0
STRAWBERRY-ORANGE *(Royal)* mix only	1 serving	80	19	0.0
TROPICAL FRUIT *(Royal)* mix only	1 serving	80	19	0.0
WATERMELON *(Jell-O)* sugar-free, prepared	1/2 cup	10	0	0.0
GHEE/clarified butter	1 oz	249	0.0	28.4
GIN				
80 proof	1 fl oz	64	0	0.0
86 proof	1 fl oz	70	0	0.0
90 proof	1 fl oz	73	0	0.0
94 proof	1 fl oz	76	0	0.0
100 proof	1 fl oz	82	0	0.0
GINGER				
Dried				
ground	1 tbsp	19	4	0.3
ground	1 tsp	6	1	0.1
ground *(Durkee)*	1 tsp	7	0	0.0
ground *(Laurel Leaf)*	1 tsp	7	0	0.0
ground *(McCormick/Schilling)*	1 tsp	7	2	0.0
ground *(Spice Islands)*	1 tsp	6	1	0.1
ground *(Tone's)*	1 tsp	6	1	0.1
Fresh				
raw, minced	1 tsp	1	0	0.0
raw, sliced, 1-inch diam.	1/4 cup	17	4	0.2
Pickled *(Eden Foods)*	1 tbsp	15	3	0.0
GINGERBREAD MIX. See under CAKE, SNACK, MIX.				
GINKGO NUT				
Canned				
approx 78 kernels	1 cup	172	34	2.5
approx 14 kernels	1 oz	31	6	0.5
Dried	1 oz	99	21	0.6
Fresh, raw	1 oz	52	11	0.5
GLOBE ARTICHOKE. See under ARTICHOKE.				
GLUTEN. See WHEAT GLUTEN.				
GLUTINOUS RICE. See under RICE.				
GNOCCHI, RAW. See under POTATO DISH/ENTRÉE.				
GOA BEAN. See BEAN, WINGED.				
GOAT				
raw	1 oz	31	0	0.7
roasted	3 oz	122	0	2.6
GOATFISH				
raw	1 lb	435	0.0	4.5
raw	1 oz	27	0.0	0.3
GOAT'S MILK. See under MILK.				
GOBO. See BURDOCK ROOT.				
GOOSE.				
AVERAGE OF ALL PARTS				
meat and skin, raw	1 oz	105	0.0	9.5
meat and skin, roasted	4 oz	346	0.0	24.9
meat only, raw	1 oz	46	0.0	2.0
meat only, roasted	4 oz	270	0.0	14.4
GIBLETS, raw	3.5 oz	156	0.6	7.0
GIZZARD, raw	3.5 oz	139	0.0	5.3

Food Name	Serv. Size	Total Cal.	Carbs GMS	Fat GMS
LIVER. See also PÂTÉ.				
raw	1 med liver	125	6	4.0
GOOSE FAT				
	1 cup	1846	0	204.6
	1 tbsp	115	0	12.8
GOOSEBERRY				
Canned, in light syrup, w/liquid	1 cup	184	47	0.5
Fresh, raw	1 cup	66	15	0.9
GOOSEFISH. See MONKFISH.				
GORDITA, low-fat *(La Tortilla)*	1 serving	150	29	2.5
GOURD, BOTTLE/calabash gourd/white-flowered gourd				
boiled, drained, cubed	1 cup	22	5	0.0
raw, cubed	1/2 cup	8	2	0.0
raw, whole	1 gourd	108	26	0.2
GOURD, CALABASH. See GOURD, BOTTLE.				
GOURD, DISHCLOTH/loofah gourd/rag gourd/sponge gourd/towelgourd/vegetable sponge				
boiled, drained, chopped, 1-inch pieces	1 cup	100	26	0.6
boiled, drained, sliced, 1-inch slices	1/2 cup	50	13	0.3
raw, chopped, 1-inch pieces	1 cup	19	4	0.2
raw, whole	1 medium	36	8	0.4
GOURD, LOOFAH. See GOURD, DISHCLOTH.				
GOURD, RAG. See GOURD, DISHCLOTH.				
GOURD, SPONGE. See GOURD, DISHCLOTH.				
GOURD, WAX				
boiled, drained, cubed	1 cup	23	5	0.3
raw, cubed	1 cup	17	4	0.3
raw, whole	1 medium	741	171	11.4
GOURD, WHITE/Chinese watermelon/tunka				
boiled, drained	4 oz	15	3.4	0.2
boiled, drained, cubed	1/2 cup	11	2.6	0.2
raw, cubed	1 cup	17	4.0	0.3
raw, trimmed	1 oz	4	0.9	0.1
raw, untrimmed	1 lb	42	9.7	0.6
GOURD, WHITE-FLOWERED. See GOURD, BOTTLE.				
GOVERNOR PLUM, trimmed	1 oz	31	8.4	0.0
GRAHAM CRACKER. See under COOKIE.				
GRAHAM CRACKER CRUMBS. See under COOKIE CRUMBS.				
GRAHAM FLOUR, ORGANIC. See under FLOUR.				
GRAIN CAKE				
(Great Cakes)				
w/summer fruits, 'Nature Cake'	4 oz	250	45	3.5
w/tropical fruits, 'Nature Cake'	4 oz	245	47	2.5
carob, 'Nature Cake'	4 oz	255	45	5.0
w/raspberry, 'Nature Cake'	4 oz	235	47	2.5
GRANADILLA. See PASSIONFRUIT.				
GRANOLA. See under CEREAL, HOT; CEREAL, READY-TO-EAT.				
GRANOLA/CEREAL BAR				
(Barbara's Bakery)				
apple-filled, nonfat	1 bar	110	27	0.0
blueberry-filled, nonfat	1 bar	110	27	0.0
carob chip, no cholesterol	1 bar	80	16	2.0
cinnamon and oats	1 bar	260	31	15.0
cinnamon-raisin, no cholesterol	1 bar	80	16	2.0
coconut-almond	1 bar	290	23	20.0
oats and honey, no cholesterol	1 bar	80	15	2.0
peanut butter	1 bar	260	28	15.0
peanut butter, no cholesterol	1 bar	80	14	3.0

Food Name	Serv. Size	Total Cal.	Carbs GMS	Fat GMS
raspberry-filled, nonfat	1 bar	110	27	0.0
strawberry-filled, nonfat	1 bar	110	27	0.0
(Bear Valley)				
carob-cocoa, food bar, 'Pemmican'	3.75 oz	440	68	12.0
coconut almond, 'Meal Pack'	3.75 oz	400	56	12.0
fruit and nut, 'Pemmican'	3.75 oz	420	59	13.0
sesame lemon, 'Meal Pack'	3.75 oz	410	57	13.0
(Ener-G Foods) gluten-free	1 serving	335	29	21.3
(Glenny's)				
'Bee Pollen Sunrise'	1.5 oz	190	22	8.0
'Ginseng Sunrise'	1.5 oz	160	24	7.0
'Spirulina Sunrise'	1.5 oz	140	21	5.0
almond, toasted, w/oat bran, 'Brown Rice Treats'	1 bar	200	34	5.0
carob mint, w/oat bran, 'Brown Rice Treats'	1 bar	180	37	2.0
cinnamon and raisin, 'Brown Rice Treats'	1.75 oz	170	38	1.0
coconut almandine ,'Moist & Chewy'	1.5 oz	190	22	10.0
oatmeal raisin, 'Moist & Chewy'	1.5 oz	160	30	3.0
peanut and raisin, 'Brown Rice Treats'	2 oz	210	39	5.0
peanut snack, 'Moist & Chewy'	1.5 oz	180	24	7.0
raisin bran, 'Brown Rice Treats'	1.75 oz	170	38	1.0
rice, plain and fancy, 'Brown Rice Treats'	1.25 oz	120	28	1.0
sunflower, 'Moist & Chewy'	1.5 oz	180	24	7.0
(Golden Temple)				
cashew almond, 'Wha Guru Chew Bar'	1 bar	164	15	11.0
peanut cashew, 'Wha Guru Chew Bar'	1 bar	167	14	11.0
sesame almond, 'Wha Guru Chew Bar'	1 bar	160	15	10.0
(Health Valley)				
blueberry apple, nonfat	1 bar	140	33	0.0
blueberry, nonfat	1 bar	140	35	0.0
chocolate chip, nonfat	1 bar	140	35	0.0
date-almond, nonfat	1 bar	140	35	0.0
raisin, nonfat	1 bar	140	35	0.0
strawberry, nonfat	1 bar	140	35	0.0
(Hershey's)				
chocolate chip, chocolate coated	1.2-oz bar	170	22	8.0
cocoa creme, chocolate-coated	1.2-oz bar	180	22	9.0
cookies and creme, chocolate-coated	1.2-oz bar	170	22	8.0
peanut butter, chocolate-coated	1.2-oz bar	180	19	10.0
(Kellogg's)				
almond and brown sugar, low-fat, crunchy	1 bar	80	16	1.5
apple spice, crunchy, low-fat	1 bar	80	16	1.5
raspberry-filled 'Common Sense Smart Start'	1 bar	170	28	6.0
(M&M Mars)				
chocolate chip, 'Kudos'	1 bar	180	21	9.0
chocolate chunk, 'Simply Kudos'	1 bar	100	13	4.0
fudge, nutty, 'Kudos'	1 bar	190	19	11.0
honey nut, 'Simply Kudos'	1 bar	100	13	4.0
oatmeal raisin, 'Simply Kudos'	1 bar	90	13	4.0
peanut butter, chocolate coated, 'Kudos'	1.3-oz bar	190	18	12.0
(Nature Valley)				
chocolate chip, crunchy	2 bars	210	32	9.0
cinnamon	2 bars	180	29	6.0
oat bran-honey graham	0.8-oz bar	110	16	4.0
oats and honey	2 bars	180	29	6.0
peanut butter	2 bars	190	28	6.0
(Nature's Choice)				
carob chip	0.75-oz bar	90	15	3.0

Food Name	Serv. Size	Total Cal.	Carbs GMS	Fat GMS
cinnamon-raisin	0.75-oz bar	90	15	3.0
oats 'n honey	0.75-oz bar	90	15	3.0
peanut butter	0.75-oz bar	90	14	3.0
(Nutri-Grain)				
blueberry, 'Smart Start'	1.5-oz bar	180	26	8.0
corn, mixed berry-filled, 'Smart Start'	1 bar	170	27	7.0
raisin bran, 'Smart Start'	1.5-oz bar	160	28	5.0
Rice Krispies, w/almonds, 'Smart Start'	1-oz bar	130	18	6.0
strawberry, 'Smart Start'	1.5-oz bar	180	26	8.0
(Quaker)				
apple berry, chewy	1-oz bar	120	20	4.0
Butterfinger, chewy	1 bar	160	29	4.0
caramel apple, chewy low-fat	1 bar	120	21	3.5
caramel nut, 'Granola Dipps'	1-oz bar	148	21	6.4
chocolate chip, 'Chewy'	1 bar	128	19	4.7
chocolate chip, 'Granola Dipps'	1-oz bar	139	19	6.3
chocolate chunk, low-fat, chewy	1 bar	110	22	2.0
chocolate fudge 'Granola Dipps'	1-oz bar	160	20	7.9
crunch, chewy	1 bar	160	28	5.0
honey and oats, 'Chewy'	1-oz bar	125	19	4.4
nut and raisin, chunky, 'Chewy'	1-oz bar	131	17	5.8
peanut butter chocolate chip, 'Chewy'	1-oz bar	131	17	5.7
peanut butter chocolate chip, 'Granola Dipps'	1 bar	174	17	10.0
peanut butter, 'Chewy'	1-oz bar	128	18	4.9
peanut butter, 'Granola Dipps'	1-oz bar	170	19	9.1
raisin cinnamon, 'Chewy'	1-oz bar	128	19	5.0
S'mores, 'Chewy'	1-oz bar	126	20	4.4
trail mix, 'Chewy'	1 oz	130	18	5.0
(Sunbelt)				
apple bar, baked	1.31 oz	130	28	2.0
chocolate chip, chewy	1.25 oz	150	23	7.0
chocolate chip, fudge-dipped, chewy	1.5 oz	210	26	10.0
oats and honey, chewy	1-oz bar	130	18	5.0
oats and honey, fudge-dipped, chewy	1.38-oz bar	190	24	10.0
w/almonds, chewy	1-oz bar	120	18	6.0
w/chocolate chips, chewy	1.75-oz bar	220	32	9.0
w/peanuts, fudge-dipped, chewy	1.38-oz bar	190	24	10.0
w/peanuts, fudge-dipped, chewy	1.5-oz bar	200	24	12.0
w/peanuts, fudge-dipped, chewy	2.25-oz bar	300	36	18.0
w/raisins, chewy	1.25-oz bar	150	24	6.0
w/raisins, fudge-dipped, chewy	1.5-oz bar	200	24	12.0

GRANOLA SNACK. See under CEREAL SNACK. Also see GRANOLA/CEREAL BAR.

GRAPE

AMERICAN (Concord, Delaware, Niagara)
Fresh

Food Name	Serv. Size	Total Cal.	Carbs GMS	Fat GMS
(Dole)	1.5 cup	85	24.0	0.0
slipskin, peeled and seeded	1 oz	18	4.9	0.1
slipskin, trimmed	10 medium	15	4.1	0.1
slipskin, untrimmed	1 lb	165	45.1	0.9
slipskin, untrimmed	1 cup	58	15.8	0.3

EUROPEAN (Muskat, Tokay, Thompson)
Canned

Food Name	Serv. Size	Total Cal.	Carbs GMS	Fat GMS
Thompson, seedless, in heavy syrup, w/liquid	1 cup	187	50	0.3
Thompson, seedless, in water, w/liquid	1 cup	98	25	0.3

Fresh

Food Name	Serv. Size	Total Cal.	Carbs GMS	Fat GMS
adherent skin, w/seeds	1/2 cup	57	14.2	0.5
adherent skin, w/seeds	1 oz	20	5.0	0.2

Food Name	Serv. Size	Total Cal.	Carbs GMS	Fat GMS
adherent skin, w/o seeds	1/2 cup	57	14.2	0.5
adherent skin, w/o seeds	1 oz	20	5.0	0.2
adherent skin, w/o seeds, approx 1.75 oz	10 medium	36	8.9	0.3

GRAPE DRINK. See under FRUIT DRINK; FRUIT JUICE BLEND; FRUIT JUICE DRINK.

GRAPE JUICE
Canned, bottled, or boxed

(Flav-R-Pac)	1 cup	130	33	0.0
(IGA) unsweetened	6 fl oz	120	30	0.0
(J. Hungerford)				
100% juice	9.03 fl oz	155	39	0.0
regular	9.03 fl oz	160	40	0.0
(Juicy Juice)	6 fl oz	90	22	0.0
(Knudsen)				
	8 fl oz	150	37	0.0
Concord	8 fl oz	130	32	0.0
(Kraft) 'Pure 100% Unsweetened'	6 fl oz	104	25	0.0
(Lucky Leaf)	6 fl oz	130	32	0.0
(Minute Maid)	6 fl oz	100	24	1.0
(Pathmark)				
'No Frills'	6 fl oz	113	27	0.0
unsweetened	6 fl oz	120	30	0.0
(S&W) Concord, unsweetened	6 fl oz	100	25	0.0
(Sippin' Pak)	8.45 fl oz	130	32	0.0
(Squeezit 100) 100% natural, 'Caped Grape'	6.75 fl oz	100	24	0.0
(Tree Top) 100%	8 fl oz	160	38	0.0
(Tropicana) 'Season's Best'	8 fl oz	160	39	0.0
(Veryfine) '100%'	8 fl oz	153	37	0.0
(Welch's)				
purple	6 fl oz	120	30	0.0
red	6 fl oz	120	30	0.0
red, sparkling	6 fl oz	128	30	0.0
white	6 fl oz	120	30	0.0
white, sparkling	6 fl oz	120	30	0.0

Refrigerated or frozen

(Minute Maid)	6 fl oz	90	24	0.0
(Sunkist) concentrate, prepared	6 fl oz	69	17	0.1
(Welch's)				
purple, concentrate, prepared	6 fl oz	100	25	0.0
white, concentrate, prepared	6 fl oz	100	25	0.0

GRAPE LEAVES

raw	1 cup	13	2	0.3
raw, whole	1 medium	3	1	0.1
whole (Reese)	1 leaf	5	0	0.0

GRAPEFRUIT
PINK
Fresh

Arizona, sections, w/juice	1 cup	85	22	0.2
Arizona, whole, approx 3.75-inch diam	1/2 fruit	46	12	0.1
California, sections, w/juice	1 cup	85	22	0.2
California, whole, approx 3.75-inch diam	1/2 fruit	46	12	0.1
Florida, sections, w/juice	1 cup	69	17	0.2
Florida, whole, approx 3.75-inch diam	1/2 fruit	37	9	0.1
whole, approx 4.5-inch diam	1/2 fruit	53	13	0.2
whole, approx 4-inch diam	1/2 fruit	41	10	0.1
whole, approx 3.5-inch diam	1/2 fruit	32	8	0.1

RED
Fresh

Arizona, sections, w/juice	1 cup	85	22	0.2

Food Name	Serv. Size	Total Cal.	Carbs GMS	Fat GMS
Arizona, whole, approx 3.75-inch diam	1/2 fruit	46	12	0.1
California, sections, w/juice	1 cup	85	22	0.2
California, whole, approx 3.75-inch diam	1/2 fruit	46	12	0.1
Florida, sections, w/juice	1 cup	69	17	0.2
Florida, whole, approx 3.75-inch diam	1/2 fruit	37	9	0.1
whole, approx 4.5-inch diam	1/2 fruit	53	13	0.2
whole, approx 4-inch diam	1/2 fruit	41	10	0.1
whole, approx 3.5-inch diam	1/2 fruit	32	8	0.1
WHITE				
Canned				
sections, in juice, w/liquid	1 cup	92	23	0.2
sections, in light syrup, w/liquid	1 cup	152	39	0.3
sections, in water, w/liquid	1 cup	88	22	0.2
Fresh				
California, sections, w/juice	1 cup	85	21	0.2
California, whole, approx 3.75-inch diam	1/2 fruit	44	11	0.1
Florida, sections, w/juice	1 cup	74	19	0.2
Florida, whole, approx 3.75-inch diam	1/2 fruit	38	10	0.1
whole, approx 4.5-inch diam	1/2 fruit	53	13	0.2
whole, approx 4-inch diam	1/2 fruit	41	10	0.1
whole, approx 3.5-inch diam	1/2 fruit	32	8	0.1
GRAPEFRUIT JUICE				
Canned, bottled, or boxed				
(Del Monte)	6 fl oz	70	17	0.0
(Florida's Natural) ruby red, not from concentrate	8 fl oz	100	24	0.0
(J. Hungerford)				
100% juice	9.03 fl oz	98	24	0.0
regular	9.03 fl oz	120	30	0.0
(Knudsen) pink	8 fl oz	100	23	0.0
(Kraft)	6 fl oz	70	16	0.0
(Libby's)	6 fl oz	70	17	0.0
(Minute Maid) 'Juices To Go'	6 fl oz	70	17	0.0
(Mott's)	10 fl oz	124	30	0.0
(Ocean Spray)				
	6 fl oz	70	16	0.0
'Pink Premium'	6 fl oz	60	15	0.0
'Ruby Red'	6 fl oz	100	24	0.0
(S&W)	6 fl oz	80	18	0.0
(Stokely)	6 fl oz	76	18	1.0
(Sunkist) 'Fresh Squeezed'	8 fl oz	96	23	0.2
(Tree Top) 100%	8 fl oz	104	24	0.0
(TreeSweet)				
pink	6 fl oz	72	17	0.0
regular	6 fl oz	72	17	0.0
(Tropicana)				
100% pure	6 fl oz	70	14	1.0
golden, 'Pure Premium'	8 fl oz	90	23	0.0
'Ruby Red' 100% pure	6 fl oz	70	14	1.0
ruby red, 'Pure Premium'	8 fl oz	100	23	0.0
'Season's Best'	8 fl oz	90	22	0.0
'100%'	8 fl oz	101	23	0.0
Refrigerated or frozen				
(A&P) concentrate, prepared	6 fl oz	80	18	1.0
(Del Monte)	6 fl oz	70	17	0.0
(Kraft)	6 fl oz	70	16	0.0
(Minute Maid) concentrate, prepared	6 fl oz	80	18	0.0
(Ocean Spray)	6 fl oz	70	16	0.0

Food Name	Serv. Size	Total Cal.	Carbs GMS	Fat GMS
(S&W)	6 fl oz	80	18	0.0
(Stokely)	6 fl oz	76	18	1.0
(Sunkist) concentrate, prepared	6 fl oz	56	13	0.2
(TreeSweet)				
	6 fl oz	72	17	0.0
concentrate, prepared	6 fl oz	78	18	0.0
(Veryfine) '100%'	8 fl oz	101	23	0.0
GRAPESEED OIL				
	1 cup	1927	0	218.0
	1 tbsp	120	0	13.6
GRAVY				
AU JUS				
(Franco-American)	1/4 cup	10	2	0.5
(Heinz) 'HomeStyle'	1/4 cup	18	2	1.0
BEEF				
(Franco-American)	1/4 cup	30	3	1.5
(Heinz) nonfat	1/4 cup	15	3	0.0
(Hormel) w/chunky beef. 'Great Beginnings'	5 oz	136	7	7.0
(Pepperidge Farm)				
hearty	1 jar	146	21	2.4
hearty	1 serving	26	4	0.4
98% fat-free	1/4 cup	25	4	1.0
BROWN				
(Heinz)				
'HomeStyle'	1/4 cup	25	3	1.0
savory, 'HomeStyle'	1/4 cup	24	3	0.8
w/onions, 'HomeStyle'	1/4 cup	25	3	1.0
(La Choy)	1/4 cup	275	66	0.0
(McCormick/Schilling)	1/3 cup	30	5	1.0
(Pillsbury)	1/4 cup	10	3	0.0
CHICKEN				
(Franco-American)				
	1/4 cup	40	3	3.0
giblet	1/4 cup	30	3	2.0
(Heinz)				
classic, homestyle	1/4 cup	30	3	1.5
'HomeStyle'	1/4 cup	35	3	2.0
w/mushrooms and onions, 'HomeStyle'	1/4 cup	35	3	2.0
(Hormel) w/chunky chicken, 'Great Beginnings'	5 oz	147	5	8.0
(Pepperidge Farm) golden, 98% fat-free	2 oz	25	3	1.0
(Pillsbury) chicken style	1/4 cup	20	4	0.0
COUNTRY *(Heinz)* homestyle, 'Blue Ribbon'	1/4 cup	25	4	1.0
CREAM *(Franco-American)*	2 oz	35	4	2.0
HOMESTYLE *(Pillsbury)*	1/4 cup	10	3	0.0
MUSHROOM				
(Franco-American) creamy	1/4 cup	20	4	1.0
(Heinz) 'HomeStyle'	1/4 cup	25	3	1.0
PORK				
(Franco-American) golden	1/4 cup	45	3	4.0
(Heinz) 'HomeStyle'	1/4 cup	25	3	1.0
(Hormel) w/chunky pork, 'Great Beginnings'	5 oz	140	5	8.0
SAUSAGE				
(Nestlé)				
country, 'Chef-Mate'	1 pkg	4614	187	369.1
country, 'Chef-Mate'	1/4 cup	96	4	7.7
TURKEY				
(Franco-American)	1/4 cup	25	3	1.0

Food Name	Serv. Size	Total Cal.	Carbs GMS	Fat GMS
(Heinz)				
'HomeStyle'	1/4 cup	25	3	1.0
nonfat	1/4 cup	15	3	0.0
roasted, homestyle	1/4 cup	25	3	1.0
(Hormel) w/chunky turkey, 'Great Beginnings'	5 oz	138	7	8.0
(Pepperidge Farm) seasoned, 98% fat-free	2 oz	25	4	1.0
GRAVY MIX				
AU JUS				
(Custom Foods)				
base, 'Red Label' mix only	16-oz pkg	867	104	18.2
base, 'Red Label' mix only	1 serving	19	2	0.4
instant, 'Superb' mix only	4-oz pkg	334	45	6.8
instant, 'Superb' mix only	1 serving	20	3	0.4
(French's) mix, prepared	1/4 cup	10	2	0.0
(Lawry's) mix, prepared	1 cup	84	11	1.6
(McCormick/Schilling) mix, prepared	1/4 cup	20	4	0.3
(Nestlé)				
'Trio' mix only	7-oz pkg	554	115	9.9
'Trio' mix only	1 tsp	8	2	0.1
(Tone's) mix only	1 tsp	10	1	0.5
BEEF				
(Custom Foods)				
instant, 'Superb' mix only	1 serving	25	4	0.6
instant, 'Superb' mix only	16-oz pkg	1675	277	43.0
(McCormick/Schilling) and herb, mix only	2 tsp	30	3	1.0
BISCUIT				
(Custom Foods)				
old-fashioned, 'Superb' mix only	1 pkg	3366	369	190.6
old-fashioned, 'Superb' mix only	1 serving	48	5	2.7
BROWN				
(Crown Colony) mix only	2 tbsp	15	3	0.0
(Custom Foods)				
instant, 'Superb' mix only	1 pkg	1725	271	53.8
instant, 'Superb' mix only	1 serving	25	4	0.8
(French's) prepared	1/4 cup	20	4	1.0
(Hain) mix only	1/4 cup	16	3	0.0
(Lawry's) prepared	1 cup	94	17	1.4
(Loma Linda) vegetarian, 'Gravy Quik' mix only	1 tbsp	20	4	0.2
(McCormick/Schilling)				
'Lite' prepared	1/4 cup	10	2	1.0
mix only	1 pkg	91	14	3.0
prepared	1/4 cup	23	4	0.8
(Nestlé)				
'Trio' mix only	16-oz pkg	1839	262	67.0
'Trio' mix only	1 tbsp	24	3	0.9
'Trio Supreme' mix only	16-oz pkg	1843	262	68.0
'Trio Supreme' mix only	1 tbsp	24	3	0.9
(Pillsbury)				
mix only	2 tsp	10	3	0.0
prepared w/water	1/4 cup	16	3	0.0
(Tone's) mix only	1 tsp	10	2	0.2
(Weight Watchers)				
prepared	1/4 cup	10	2	0.0
w/mushrooms, prepared	1/4 cup	10	2	0.0
w/onions, prepared	1/4 cup	10	2	0.0
CHICKEN				
(Custom Foods)				
instant, 'Superb' mix only	16-oz pkg	1793	257	64.6

Food Name	Serv. Size	Total Cal.	Carbs GMS	Fat GMS
instant, 'Superb' mix only	1 serving	26	4	1.0
(French's) prepared w/water	1/4 cup	25	4	1.0
(Lawry's) prepared w/water	1 cup	99	16	2.8
(Loma Linda) 'Gravy Quik'	1 tbsp	19	3	0.1
(McCormick/Schilling) prepared w/water	1/4 cup	22	4	0.4
(Nestlé)				
'Trio' mix only	1 pkg	2596	405	75.6
'Trio' mix only	1 tbsp	32	5	0.9
'Trio Supreme' mix only	1 pkg	2291	357	67.2
'Trio Supreme' mix only	1 tbsp	32	5	0.9
(Pillsbury)				
mix only	2 tsp	20	4	0.0
prepared w/water	1/4 cup	25	4	1.0
(Tone's) mix only	1 tsp	11	2	0.2
(Weight Watchers) prepared	1/4 cup	10	2	0.0
COUNTRY				
(Custom Foods)				
'Superb' mix only	1 pkg	3271	364	177.3
'Superb' mix only	1 serving	47	5	2.5
(Loma Linda) 'Gravy Quik'	1 tbsp	22	4	0.6
(Nestlé)				
'Trio' mix only	1 pkg	2702	405	95.3
'Trio' mix only	1 tbsp	35	5	1.2
(Tone's) mix only	1 tsp	12	2	0.5
(Williams) low-fat, low-cholesterol	0.33 oz	40	5	2.0
HOMESTYLE				
(French's) prepared	1/4 cup	20	4	1.0
(McCormick/Schilling) prepared	1/4 cup	24	4	0.8
(Pillsbury)				
mix only	2 tsp	10	3	0.0
prepared w/water, 1/4 cup 2% milk	1/4 cup	25	4	1.0
HERB *(McCormick/Schilling)* prepared	1/4 cup	20	3	0.5
MUSHROOM				
(French's) prepared w/water	1/4 cup	20	3	1.0
(Loma Linda) 'Gravy Quik' mix only	1 tbsp	16	3	0.3
(McCormick/Schilling) mix only	1/4 cup	19	3	0.5
ONION				
(French's) prepared w/water	1/4 cup	25	4	1.0
(Loma Linda) 'Gravy Quik' mix only	1 tbsp	18	3	0.0
(McCormick/Schilling) mix only	2 tsp	20	3	0.5
PORK				
(Custom Foods)				
instant, 'Superb' mix only	16-oz pkg	1648	294	35.8
instant, 'Superb' mix only	1 serving	24	4	0.5
(French's) prepared w/water	1/4 cup	20	4	1.0
(McCormick/Schilling) prepared w/water	1/4 cup	20	4	0.6
SOUTHERN				
(Nestlé)				
'Trio' mix only	1 pkg	1770	223	93.7
'Trio' mix only	1 serving	48	6	2.5
TURKEY				
(Custom Foods)				
instant, 'Superb' mix only	16-oz pkg	1857	261	66.6
instant, 'Superb' mix only	1 serving	27	4	1.0
(Lawry's) prepared w/water	1 cup	102	13	4.1
(McCormick/Schilling) prepared w/water	1/4 cup	22	4	0.5

Food Name	Serv. Size	Total Cal.	Carbs GMS	Fat GMS
(Nestlé)				
'Trio' mix only .... 1 pkg		2053	409	24.6
'Trio' mix only .... 1 serving		29	6	0.3

GREAT NORTHERN BEAN. See BEAN, GREAT NORTHERN.
GREEK SEASONING MIX. See under SEASONING MIX.
GREEN BEAN. See BEAN, FRENCH; BEAN, GREEN; BEAN DISH/ENTRÉE.
GREEN ONION. See SCALLION.
GREEN PEAS. See PEAS, GREEN.
GREEN PEPPER. See PEPPER, BELL.
GREEN PEPPER DISH/ENTRÉE. See PEPPER, BELL, DISH/ENTRÉE.
GREEN TURTLE. See TURTLE, GREEN.
GREENLAND HALIBUT. See under HALIBUT.
GRENADINE SYRUP. See under COCKTAIL MIX.

GRITS
CORN
Instant

Food Name	Serv. Size	Total Cal.	Carbs GMS	Fat GMS
(Quaker)				
butter flavor .... 1 pkt		101	21	1.4
cheddar cheese flavor .... 1 pkt		102	21	1.6
plain .... 1 cup		159	37	0.5
plain .... 1 pkt		06	22	0.3
w/imitation bacon bits .... 1 pkt		94	21	0.5
w/imitation ham bits .... 1 pkt		92	20	0.5
w/sausage bits .... 1 serving		100	21	1.0
Quick-cooking				
white, enriched, cooked w/water, w/o salt .... 1 cup		145	31	0.5
white, enriched, cooked w/water, w/o salt .... 3/4 cup		109	24	0.4
white, unenriched, cooked w/water, w/o salt .... 1 cup		145	31	0.5
white, unenriched, cooked w/water, w/o salt .... 3/4 cup		109	24	0.4
white, unenriched, dry .... 1 cup		579	124	1.9
white, unenriched, dry .... 1 tbsp		36	8	0.1
yellow, enriched, cooked w/water, w/o salt .... 1 cup		145	31	0.5
yellow, enriched, cooked w/water, w/o salt .... 3/4 cup		109	24	0.4
yellow, enriched, dry .... 1 cup		579	124	1.9
yellow, enriched, dry .... 1 tbsp		36	8	0.1
yellow, unenriched, cooked w/water, w/o salt .... 1 cup		145	31	0.5
yellow, unenriched, cooked w/water, w/o salt .... 3/4 cup		109	24	0.4
yellow, unenriched, dry .... 1 cup		579	124	1.9
yellow, unenriched, dry .... 1 tbsp		36	8	0.1
(Arrowhead Mills)				
white, dry .... 2 oz		200	43	1.0
yellow, dry .... 2 oz		200	44	1.0
(Aunt Jemima) white, enriched, dry .... 3 tbsp		101	22	0.2
(Quick) yellow, enriched, dry .... 3 tbsp		101	22	0.2
(Tone's) yellow, enriched, dry .... 1 tsp		12	3	0.1
HOMINY				
Canned				
(Allens)				
golden .... 1/2 cup		80	16	1.0
Mexican .... 1/2 cup		80	16	1.0
white .... 1/2 cup		70	16	1.0
(Bush's Best)				
golden .... 1/2 cup		45	11	0.0
white .... 1/2 cup		45	11	0.0
(Juanita's) Mexican style .... 1/2 cup		60	10	0.5
(S&W)				
golden, 'Sun-Vista' .... 1/2 cup		70	19	0.0

Food Name	Serv. Size	Total Cal.	Carbs GMS	Fat GMS
white	1/2 cup	65	18	0.5
white, 'Sun-Vista'	1/2 cup	65	18	0.5
(Van Camp's)				
golden	1 cup	128	28	0.6
golden, w/red and green peppers	1 cup	129	29	0.5
white	1 cup	138	30	0.7
Instant				
(Albers) 'Hominy Quick Grits'	1/2 cup	150	33	0.0
(Aunt Jemima) white, enriched, 'Quick'	3 tbsp	101	22	0.2
(Quaker) w/real cheddar cheese flavor	1 pkt	104	22	1.0
Quick-cooking				
(Aunt Jemima) white, enriched, 'Regular'	3 tbsp	101	22	0.2
(Quaker)				
white	1/4 cup	130	29	0.5
yellow	1/3 cup	133	30	0.5
GROUND HUSK TOMATO. See TOMATILLO.				
GROUPER				
mixed species, baked, broiled, grilled, or microwaved	3 oz	100	0	1.1
mixed species, raw	3 oz	78	0	0.9
GUACAMOLE. See under DIP.				
GUACAMOLE SEASONING. See under SEASONING MIX.				
GUANABANA/soursop				
raw, trimmed	1/2 cup	75	18.9	0.3
raw, untrimmed	1 lb	202	51.2	0.9
raw, whole, approx 2.1 lb	1 medium	416	105.3	1.9
GUAVA				
raw, chopped	1 cup	84	20	1.0
raw, whole, trimmed	1 medium	46	11	0.5
GUAVA, STRAWBERRY				
raw, chopped	1 cup	168	42	1.5
raw, whole, trimmed	1 medium	4	1	0.0
GUAVA JUICE				
Frozen *(Welch's)* 'Orchard Tropicals' prepared.	6 fl oz	100	25	0.0
GUINEA HEN				
giblets, raw	3.5 oz	157	1.2	7.0
meat and skin, raw	1 lb	567	0.0	23.2
meat only, raw	1 oz	31	0.0	0.7
GUM. See under CANDY.				
GUMBO FILE POWDER. See under SEASONING MIX.				

H

Food Name	Serv. Size	Total Cal.	Carbs GMS	Fat GMS
HADDOCK				
Fresh				
baked, broiled, grilled, or microwaved	3 oz	95	0	0.8
raw	3 oz	74	0	0.6
Frozen				
fillet, 'Fishmarket Fresh' *(Gorton's)*	5 oz	110	0	1.0
fillet *(SeaPak)*	4 oz	90	0	1.0
fillet *(Van de Kamp's)*	4 oz	90	0	1.0
Smoked				
fillet	3 oz	99	0	0.8
fillet, boneless	1 oz	33	0	0.3

Food Name	Serv. Size	Total Cal.	Carbs GMS	Fat GMS
finnian haddie	4 oz	132	0.0	1.1

HADDOCK, NORWAY. See OCEAN PERCH, ATLANTIC.

HADDOCK DINNER/ENTRÉE

(Van de Kamp's)

fillet, battered, frozen	2 pieces	250	19	15.0
fillet, breaded, frozen	2 pieces	270	19	16.0
fillet, light, frozen	1 piece	240	21	11.0

HAKE, SILVER. See WHITING.

HALIBUT

ATLANTIC

Fresh

baked, broiled, grilled, or microwaved	4 oz	159	0.0	3.3
baked, broiled, grilled, or microwaved	3 oz	119	0.0	2.5
raw	1 lb	497	0.0	10.4
raw	3 oz	94	0.0	2.0
raw	1 oz	31	0.0	0.6
Frozen, steaks *(SeaPak)*	6-oz pkg	160	0	1.0

GREENLAND

baked, broiled, grilled, or microwaved	3 oz	203	0.0	15.1
raw	1 lb	845	0.0	62.8
raw	3 oz	158	0.0	11.8
raw	1 oz	53	0.0	3.9

PACIFIC

Fresh

baked, broiled, grilled, or microwaved	4 oz	159	0.0	3.3
baked, broiled, grilled, or microwaved	3 oz	119	0.0	2.5
raw	1 lb	497	0.0	10.4
raw	3 oz	94	0.0	2.0
raw	1 oz	31	0.0	0.6

Frozen

fillet, boneless, skinless, raw *(Peter Pan Seafoods)*	3.5 oz	110	0	2.3
loin steaks, raw *(Peter Pan Seafoods)*	3.5 oz	110	0	2.3
steaks, standard cut, raw *(Peter Pan Seafoods)*	3.5 oz	110	0	2.3
steaks *(SeaPak)*	6 oz pkg	160	0	1.0

HALIBUT DINNER/ENTRÉE

(Van de Kamp's) fillet, battered, frozen	2 pieces	150	16	6.0

HAM. See also HAM SUBSTITUTE; PORK. Also see under LUNCHEON MEAT.

CANNED

chopped	1 oz	68	0.1	5.3
chopped	0.75-oz slice	50	0.1	4.0
cured, extra lean, approx 4% fat, baked	3 oz	116	0.4	4.2
cured, extra lean, approx 4% fat, unheated	1 oz	34	0.0	1.3
cured, extra lean and regular, baked	3 oz	142	0.4	7.2
cured, extra lean and regular, unheated	1 oz	41	0.0	2.1
cured, regular, approx 13% fat, baked	3 oz	192	0.4	12.9
cured, regular, approx 13% fat, unheated	1 oz	54	0.0	3.7
(Armour) chopped	3 oz	190	1	14.0
(Black Label) 3-lb can	4 oz	140	0	7.0
(Chi-Chi's) 'Black Label'	1 oz	37	2	1.0
(EXL)				
	4 oz	120	0	4.0
'Deli Ham' 10-lb can	4 oz	130	0	6.0
(Holiday Glaze) '3-lb can'	4 oz	130	2	4.0
(Hormel)				
'Bone-In'	4 oz	210	1	15.0
chopped, 12-oz can	2 oz	120	0	9.0
chunk	2.5 oz	110	1	7.0

Food Name	Serv. Size	Total Cal.	Carbs GMS	Fat GMS
'Cure/81'	4 oz	160	0	8.0
'Curemaster'	4 oz	140	1	5.0
'Light & Lean 97'	2 oz	60	1	2.0
patty	1 patty	180	0	16.0
patty, w/cheese	1 patty	190	0	18.0
roll	4 oz	170	0	10.0
spiced	3 oz	240	1	21.0
(JM) '95% Fat-Free'	2 oz	60	1	2.0
(Light & Lean) 'No bone'	2 oz	60	0	2.0
(Oscar Mayer) 'Jubilee'	1 oz	29	0	0.9
(Rath) hickory smoked, 'Black Hawk'	2 oz	60	1	2.0
(Swift) patty, 'Premium Brown 'N Serve'	1 patty	130	1	13.0

CURED
(NOTE: TRIMMED = Lean; separable fat removed. UNTRIMMED = Separable fat not removed.)

Food Name	Serv. Size	Total Cal.	Carbs GMS	Fat GMS
Bone in, Boston butt, trimmed				
medium fat, chopped, roasted	1 cup	340	0.0	19.3
medium fat, roasted	9.8 oz	678	0.0	38.5
Bone in, whole				
honey glazed, 'Traditional' (Carving Board)	1 slice	50	1	1.5
trimmed, fully cooked, baked	3 oz	133	0.0	4.7
trimmed, fully cooked, unheated	1 oz	42	0.0	1.6
smoked (Carving Board)	1 slice	45	0	1.5
untrimmed, fully cooked, baked	3 oz	207	0.0	14.2
untrimmed, fully cooked, unheated	1 oz	70	0.0	5.3
water added, baked (Carving Board)	1 slice	50	1	1.5
Boneless				
breakfast, 'Light AM' (Healthy Deli)	1 oz	27	1	0.6
'Breakfast Ham' (Oscar Mayer)	1.5 oz slice	47	1	1.5
center slice, country-style, trimmed, unheated	4 oz	220	0	9.4
center slice, country style, untrimmed, heated	4 oz	229	0	14.6
extra lean, approx 5% fat, baked	3 oz	123	1.3	4.7
extra lean, approx 5% fat, baked, chopped	1 cup	203	2	7.7
extra lean, approx 5% fat, unheated	1 oz	37	0.3	1.4
extra lean and regular, baked	3 oz	140	0.4	6.5
extra lean and regular, baked, chopped	1 cup	231	1	10.7
extra lean and regular, unheated	1 oz	46	0.7	2.4
extra lean and regular, unheated, chopped	1 cup	227	3	11.7
extra lean and regular, unheated, 4 x 6 1/4 inch slice	1 slice	46	0.7	2.4
mini (JM)	3 oz	90	0	3.0
regular, approx 11% fat, baked	3 oz	151	0.0	7.7
regular, approx 11% fat, baked, chopped	1 cup	249	0	12.6
regular, approx 11% fat, unheated	1 oz	52	0.9	3.0
steak, dinner sliced (Oscar Mayer)	1 piece	60	0	2.0
steak, unheated	2 oz	69	0.0	2.4
whole (JM)	3 oz	140	0	8.0
w/natural juices, 'EZ Cut' (JM)	2 oz	70	1	3.0
Patty, raw	1 oz	89	0	8.0
Puréed (Bryan Foods)	1/3 cup	160	0	12.0

HAM DINNER/ENTRÉE

Food Name	Serv. Size	Total Cal.	Carbs GMS	Fat GMS
(Armour) steak, frozen, 'Classics'	10.75 oz	270	36	7.0
(Banquet) frozen, 'Platters'	10 oz	400	43	17.0
(Cook's)				
hickory-smoked, honey, spiral-sliced	3 oz	150	2	10.0
hickory-smoked, honey, w/glaze, spiral-sliced,	3 oz	160	4	10.0
(Hormel) 96% nonfat, water added, cooked, 'Curemaster'	3 oz	80	0	3.0
(Le Menu) steak, frozen	10 oz	300	31	11.0

Food Name	Serv. Size	Total Cal.	Carbs GMS	Fat GMS
(Louis Rich) dinner slices, baked, 98% fat-free	1 slice	80	1	1.5
(Marie Callender's) steak, honey-smoked, w/macaroni and cheese	14 oz	490	63	13.0
(Morton) frozen	10 oz	290	49	4.0
(Pillsbury) casserole, w/cheese, 'Microwave Classic'	1 pkg	470	34	29.0
(Stouffer's) w/asparagus	1 entrée	520	32	36.0
(Swanson) w/scalloped potatoes, 'Homestyle Recipe'	9 oz	300	26	13.0
(West Virginia) boneless, no water added, cooked	3 oz	110	1	4.0
HAM SPREAD				
(Libby's) salad, 'Spreadables'	1/3 cup	110	8	4.5
(Hormel)				
deviled	1 oz	76	1	6.0
deviled	1 tbsp	35	0	3.0
(Underwood)				
deviled	2 1/8 oz	220	1	19.0
deviled, 'Light'	2 1/8 oz	120	1	8.0
deviled, smoked	2 1/8 oz	190	1	18.0
HAM SUBSTITUTE				
(Worthington) meatless, vegetarian, 'Wham'.	1 slice	82	1	5.2
HAMBURG PARSLEY. See PARSLEY ROOT.				
HAMBURGER. See under BEEF; BEEF DINNER/ENTRÉE. See also HAMBURGER ENTRÉE MIX.				
HAMBURGER BUN. See BUN, HAMBURGER.				
HAMBURGER ENTRÉE MIX				
(Hamburger Helper)				
beef noodle, mix only	1/5 pkg	140	26	2.0
beef noodle, prepared	1 cup	320	26	15.0
beef pasta, prepared	1 cup	270	26	10.0
beef Romanoff, prepared	1 cup	280	27	10.0
beef taco, prepared	1 cup	310	31	11.0
beef teriyaki, mix only	1/5 pkg	180	38	1.0
beef teriyaki, prepared	1 cup	360	38	14.0
cheddar 'n bacon meal, mix only	2/3 cup	170	25	5.0
cheddar 'n bacon meal, prepared	1 cup	350	28	16.0
cheeseburger macaroni meal, mix only	1/3 cup	180	30	4.0
cheeseburger macaroni meal, prepared	1 cup	360	33	15.0
cheesy Italian meal, mix only	1/2 cup	150	26	3.0
cheesy Italian meal, prepared	1 cup	330	29	14.0
chili macaroni meal, mix only	1/3 cup	140	30	1.0
chili macaroni meal, prepared	1 cup	290	30	10.0
chili tomato meal, mix only	1/5 pkg	150	31	1.0
chili tomato meal, prepared	1 cup	330	31	14.0
chili w/beans meal, mix only	1/4 pkg	130	25	1.0
chili w/beans meal, prepared	1 1/4 cup	350	25	17.0
creamy Stroganoff, prepared w/whole milk	1 cup	390	30	20.0
creamy Stroganoff, prepared	1 cup	320	30	13.0
hamburger hash meal, mix only	1/5 pkg	140	27	2.0
hamburger hash meal, prepared	1 cup	320	27	15.0
hamburger stew meal, mix only	1/5 pkg	120	25	1.0
hamburger stew meal, prepared	1 cup	300	25	14.0
lasagna meal, mix only	2/3 cup	140	30	1.0
lasagna meal, prepared	1 cup	280	30	10.0
meat loaf meal, mix only	1 1/2 tbsp	50	10	0.5
mushroom and wild rice meal, mix only	1/5 pkg	180	34	3.0
mushroom and wild rice meal, prepared	1 cup	380	37	16.0
nacho cheese meal, mix only	1/2 cup	160	28	2.5
nacho cheese meal, prepared	1 cup	320	30	14.0

Food Name	Serv. Size	Total Cal.	Carbs GMS	Fat GMS
pizza dish meal, mix only	1/5 pkg	180	37	1.0
pizza dish meal, prepared	1 cup	360	37	14.0
pizza pasta w/cheese topping, mix only	1/2 cup	150	30	1.5
pizza pasta w/cheese topping, prepared	1 cup	290	31	10.0
pizzabake, mix only	1 serving	140	28	1.5
pizzabake, prepared	1 serving	270	28	10.0
potato Stroganoff meal, mix only	2/3 cup	120	24	2.0
potato Stroganoff meal, prepared	1 cup	270	25	12.0
potatoes au gratin meal, mix only	2/3 cup	120	23	2.5
potatoes au gratin meal, prepared	1 cup	290	24	14.0
rice Oriental meal, mix only	1/4 cup	160	35	0.5
rice Oriental meal, prepared	1 cup	310	35	10.0
sloppy Joe meal, mix only	1/6 pkg	180	33	3.0
sloppy Joe meal, prepared	5 oz	340	33	15.0
spaghetti meal, mix only	1/2 cup	150	29	1.0
spaghetti meal, prepared	1 cup	300	29	11.0
Stroganoff meal, mix only	1/5 pkg	190	30	5.0
Stroganoff meal, prepared	2/3 cup	160	27	3.0
taco meal, 'Tacobake' mix only	1/6 pkg	170	31	4.0
taco meal, 'Tacobake' prepared	5.75 oz	320	31	15.0
tamale pie meal, mix only	1/5 pkg	200	39	3.0
tamale pie meal, prepared	1 cup	380	39	16.0
three cheese meal mix, prepared	1/5 pkg	400	32	20.0
three cheese meal, mix only	1/5 pkg	210	30	7.0
zesty Italian meal, mix only	1/3 cup	160	34	1.0
zesty Italian meal, prepared	1 cup	320	34	11.0

HAMBURGER RELISH. See under RELISH.
HAMBURGER SUBSTITUTE. See under BEEF SUBSTITUTE DINNER/ENTRÉE.
HARD ROLL. See under ROLL.
HARICOTS. See BEAN, FRENCH.
HASH
CORNED BEEF
(Armour)

canned	1 pkg	897	22	71.0
canned	1 serving	498	12	39.4
(Hormel) canned	1 cup	387	22	24.2
(Libby's)				
	1 cup	470	25	35.0
	1/4 cup	120	0	7.0
(Nestlé)				
'Chef Mate'	1 pkg	5823	348	363.7
'Chef Mate'	1 cup	486	29	30.3
ROAST BEEF				
(Libby's)	1 cup	460	23	33.0
(Hormel) canned	1 cup	385	23	23.6

HAWAIIAN YAM. See under YAM.
HAWS/hawthorn tree fruit, scarlet, w/skin, raw ... 3.5 oz   87   20.8   0.7
HAZELNUT/cobnut/filbert

dried	1 oz	178	5	17.2
dried	10 medium	88	2	8.5
dried, blanched	1 oz	178	5	17.3
dried, chopped	1 cup	722	19	69.9
dried, ground	1 cup	471	13	45.6
dried, whole	1 cup	848	23	82.0
dry-roasted, no salt added	1 oz	183	5	17.7
natural, unsalted *(Flanigan Farms)*	1/4 cup	180	4	18.0

Food Name	Serv. Size	Total Cal.	Carbs GMS	Fat GMS
natural, whole *(Oregon Hazelnuts)*	1/2 cup	396	12	36.8
HAZELNUT BUTTER				
creamy, roasted fresh, no salt added *(Roaster Fresh)*	1 oz	188	5	19.0
HAZELNUT OIL				
	1 cup	1927	0	218.0
	1 tbsp	120	0	13.6
(International Collection)	1 tbsp	120	0	14.0
HAZELNUT SPREAD				
w/milk and cocoa, 'Nutella' *(Ferrero)*	1 tbsp	80	9	5.0
HEAD CHEESE. See under SAUSAGE.				
HEART NUT. See CASHEW.				
HEARTS OF PALM. See under PALM.				
HERB SEASONING MIX. See under SEASONING MIX.				
HERBAL TEA. See under TEA.				
HERRING				
ATLANTIC				
fillet, baked, broiled, grilled, or microwaved	3 oz	173	0	9.9
fillet, kippered, large, approx 7 x 2.25 x 1/4 inch	1 fillet	141	0	8.0
fillet, kippered, medium, approx 5 x 1.75 x 1/4 inch	1 fillet	87	0	4.9
fillet, kippered, small, approx 2-3/8 x 1-3/8 x 1/4 inch	1 fillet	43	0	2.5
fillet, kippered, boneless	1 oz	62	0	3.5
fillet, kippered, smoked, salt added *(Crown Prince)*	1/4 cup	110	0	8.0
fillet, kippered, w/naturally smoked wood flavoring *(Beach Cliff)*	3.3 oz	220	1	17.0
pickled	1 cup	367	13	25.2
pickled, approx 1.75 x 7/8 x 1/2 inch	1 piece	39	1	2.7
pickled, boneless	1 oz	74	3	5.1
raw	3 oz	134	0	7.7
raw, boneless	1 oz	45	0	2.6
snacks, kippered, w/smoke flavoring, drained *(Beach Cliff)*	3.3 oz	220	1	17.0
steaks, in soybean oil, drained *(Beach Cliff)*	3 oz	240	0	20.0
steaks, in water, drained *(Beach Cliff)*	3 oz	230	1	18.0
steaks, w/mustard, drained *(Beach Cliff)*	3 oz	227	4	18.0
steaks, w/tomato, drained *(Beach Cliff)*	3 oz	210	0	17.0
PACIFIC				
baked, broiled, grilled, or miocrowaved	3 oz	213	0	15.1
raw	3 oz	166	0	11.8
HERRING OIL. See under FISH OIL.				
HICKORY NUT				
dried	1 cup	788	22	77.2
dried	1 oz	186	5	18.2
dried	1 medium	20	1	1.9
HIRITAKE. See MUSHROOM, OYSTER.				
HIZIKI. See under SEA VEGETABLE.				
HOG PLUM. See JOBO.				
HOMINY. See under GRITS.				
HON SHIMEJI. See MUSHROOM, JAPANESE HONEY.				
HONEY				
(Golden Blossom)	1 tbsp	60	16	0.0
(Knott's Berry Farm)	1 tbsp	60	17	0.0
(Sioux)	1 tbsp	60	16	0.0
mesquite, desert, 100%, raw, wild, unblended *(Trader Joe's)*	1 tbsp	60	17	0.0
strained or extracted	1 cup	1031	279	0.0
strained or extracted	1 tbsp	64	17	0.0
HONEY BUTTER *(Honey Butter)*	1 tbsp	50	11	1.0
HONEY MUSHROOM. See MUSHROOM, JAPANESE HONEY.				
HONEYDEW MELON. See MELON, HONEYDEW.				

Food Name	Serv. Size	Total Cal.	Carbs GMS	Fat GMS
HORSE				
raw	1 oz	38	0	1.3
roasted	3 oz	149	0	5.1
roasted, boneless, yield from 1 lb raw	11.9 oz	595	0	20.6
HORSE BEAN. See BEAN, FAVA.				
HORSERADISH				
Prepared				
	1 tbsp	7	2	0.1
	1 tsp	2	1	0.0
(Crowley)	1 oz	10	2	1.0
(Gold's) hot	1 tsp	4	1	1.0
(Gold's) red	1 tsp	4	1	0.0
(Gold's) white	1 tsp	4	1	1.0
(Kraft)	1 tbsp	10	1	0.0
(Kraft) cream style	1 tbsp	12	1	0.0
(Silver Spring) cream style	1 tsp	0	0	0.0
Raw	1 lb	288	65.3	1.0
HORSERADISH, JAPANESE. See WASABI ROOT.				
HORSERADISH SPREAD (Alouette) cheese and chive	1 oz	85	1	8.0
HORSERADISH TREE				
leafy tips, boiled, drained, chopped	1 cup	25	5	0.4
leafy tips, raw, chopped	1 cup	13	2	0.3
pods, boiled, drained, sliced	1 cup	42	10	0.2
pods, raw, sliced	1 cup	37	9	0.2
pods, raw, whole, approx 15 1/3 inch long	1 pod	4	1	0.0
HOT COCOA. See COCOA, HOT, MIX.				
HOT DOG. See FRANKFURTER.				
HOT DOG BUN. See BUN, FRANKFURTER.				
HUBBARD SQUASH. See SQUASH, HUBBARD.				
HUMMUS MIX				
(Fantastic Foods) mix only	2 tbsp	60	9	2.0
(Casbah) prepared	1 oz	160	14	8.0
HUMPBACK SALMON. See under SALMON.				
HUNGARIAN PEPPER. See PEPPER, HUNGARIAN.				
HUSHPUPPY				
(SeaPak) regular, frozen	4 oz	330	56	9.0
(Stilwell) jalapeño, frozen	3 pieces	70	4	5.0
(Stilwell) regular, frozen	3 pieces	140	19	6.0
HUSHPUPPY MIX				
(Golden Dipt)				
deluxe	1.25 oz	120	26	0.0
jalapeño	1.25 oz	120	27	0.0
w/onion	1.25 oz	120	27	0.0
HYACINTH BEAN. See BEAN, HYACINTH.				

I

Food Name	Serv. Size	Total Cal.	Carbs GMS	Fat GMS
ICE BAR/DESSERT. See also FRUIT BAR, FROZEN; SHERBET; SORBET.				
BAR				
(Cool Creations)				
fruit flavors, nonfat, 'Mickey & Minnie Surprise Pop'	1 pop	60	14	0.0
(Crystal Light) all flavors, nonfat	1 bar	14	2	0.0
(Eskimo Pie) vanilla, w/dark chocolate coating	1 bar	166	12	12.1
(Freezer Pleezer) assorted flavors, nonfat	1 bar	40	10	0.0

Food Name	Serv. Size	Total Cal.	Carbs GMS	Fat GMS
(Gold Bond) all flavors, nonfat, 'Twin Pop'	1 bar	60	14	0.0
(Good Humor)				
all flavors, nonfat, 'Ice Stripes'	1 bar	35	9	0.0
cherry, 'Calippo'	1 bar	138	35	0.1
cherry, Italian	6 oz	138	34	0.1
lemon, 'Calippo'	1 bar	112	28	0.1
orange, 'Calippo'	1 bar	111	27	0.2
(Jell-O)				
all flavors nonfat, 'Gelatin Pops'	1 bar	35	8	0.0
lemon, nonfat, 'Snowburst Bars'	1 bar	45	12	0.0
orange, nonfat, 'Snowburst Bars'	1 bar	45	12	0.0
(Klondike Bar) vanilla, w/chocolate coating	1 bar	489	36	35.7
(Kool-Aid)				
all flavors, 'Cream Pops'	1 bar	50	9	2.0
all flavors, 'Kool Pumps'	1 snack	80	16	1.0
all flavors, nonfat, 'Kool Pops'	1 bar	40	10	0.0
(Mama Tish's)				
Italian ice, cherry, made w/real fruit	4 oz	120	29	0.0
Italian ice, lemon, made w/real fruit	4 oz	90	24	0.0
Italian ice, strawberry, made w/real fruit	4 oz	80	21	0.0
Italian ice, tropical, made w/real fruit	4 oz	110	27	0.0
(Popsicle)				
all flavors, 'All Natural'	1 bar	60	14	0.0
all flavors, except cherry and wildberry, 'Water Ice'	1 bar	50	12	0.0
cherry, cola/cherry, 'Twister'	1 piece	45	10	0.0
cherry, 'Water Ice'	1 bar	70	17	0.0
wildberry, 'Water Ice'	1 bar	40	10	0.0
(Push-ups) assorted, orange, cherry, grape, 'Flintstones'	1 tube	100	20	2.0
(Tootsie Pop) assorted, cherry, grape, orange	1 bar	70	13	1.0
ITALIAN ICE				
(Luigi's)				
cherry	1 cup	120	28	0.0
chocolate fudge	1 cup	150	38	0.0
grape	1 cup	110	26	0.0
lemon	1 cup	110	25	0.0
strawberry	1 cup	110	26	0.0

ICE CREAM. See also ICE CREAM BAR/DESSERT; ICE CREAM CONE; ICE CREAM MIX; ICE CREAM SUBSTITUTE; ICE CREAM SUBSTITUTE BAR/DESSERT; ICE CREAM SUBSTITUTE MIX; ICE MILK.

Food Name	Serv. Size	Total Cal.	Carbs GMS	Fat GMS
(Borden)				
butter pecan, 'Lady Borden'	1/2 cup	180	16	12.0
chocolate swirl	1/2 cup	130	18	6.0
chocolate, Dutch, 'Olde Fashioned Recipe'	1/2 cup	130	16	6.0
strawberry	1/2 cup	130	18	6.0
strawberry cream, 'Olde Fashioned Recipe'	1/2 cup	130	19	5.0
vanilla, 'Olde Fashioned Recipe'	1/2 cup	130	15	7.0
(Breyers)				
butter almond	1/2 cup	170	15	10.0
butter pecan	1/2 cup	180	15	12.0
cherry vanilla	1/2 cup	150	17	7.0
chocolate	1/2 cup	160	20	8.0
chocolate chip	1/2 cup	170	18	10.0
coffee	1/2 cup	150	16	8.0
cookies and cream	1/2 cup	170	19	9.0
mint chocolate chip	1/2 cup	170	18	10.0
mocha almond fudge	1/2 cup	190	20	10.0
peach, natural	1/2 cup	130	18	6.0

Food Name	Serv. Size	Total Cal.	Carbs GMS	Fat GMS
strawberry	1/2 cup	130	16	6.0
vanilla	1/2 cup	150	15	8.0
vanilla fudge twirl	1/2 cup	160	19	8.0
vanilla-chocolate	1/2 cup	160	17	8.0
vanilla-chocolate-strawberry	1/2 cup	150	17	8.0
(Darigold)				
chocolate	1/2 cup	140	17	7.0
chocolate, 'Alpine'	1/2 cup	140	17	7.0
chocolate, 'Classic'	1/2 cup	180	16	13.0
vanilla	1/2 cup	130	15	7.0
vanilla, 'Alpine'	1/2 cup	130	15	7.0
vanilla, 'Classic'	1/2 cup	180	16	12.0
(Dreyer's/Edys)				
black cherry vanilla, fat-free	1/2 cup	100	22	0.0
black cherry vanilla, sugar-free	1/2 cup	90	12	3.0
butter pecan, light	1/2 cup	120	16	5.0
caramel cream, dreamy, light	1/2 cup	110	18	3.0
chocolate almond fudge, light	1/2 cup	120	16	5.0
chocolate chip	1/2 cup	150	16	9.0
chocolate fudge, fat-free	1/2 cup	110	25	0.0
chocolate fudge mousse, light	1/2 cup	110	17	3.0
cookie dough, light	1/2 cup	130	19	5.0
cookies and cream	1/2 cup	160	18	9.0
cookies and cream, light	1/2 cup	120	17	4.0
espresso fudge chip, light	1/2 cup	120	18	4.0
'French Silk' light	1/2 cup	120	19	4.0
fudge, marble	1/2 cup	150	18	8.0
marble fudge, fat-free	1/2 cup	110	24	0.0
marble fudge, sugar-free	1/2 cup	90	13	3.0
mint fudge, fat free	1/2 cup	110	24	0.0
mocha fudge, sugar-free	1/2 cup	90	13	3.0
peanut butter cup, light	1/2 cup	130	17	5.0
raspberry vanilla, fat free, sugar-free	1/2 cup	90	19	0.0
rocky road	1/2 cup	170	18	10.0
rocky road, light	1/2 cup	120	17	4.0
strawberry, sugar-free	1/2 cup	80	11	3.0
triple chocolate, sugar-free	1/2 cup	100	13	3.5
vanilla	1/2 cup	160	14	10.0
vanilla, fat-free	1/2 cup	100	22	0.0
vanilla, light	1/2 cup	100	15	3.0
vanilla, sugar-free	1/2 cup	80	11	3.0
vanilla and caramel, sugar-free	1/2 cup	90	13	3.0
vanilla-chocolate, fat free, sugar-free	1/2 cup	100	20	0.0
(Eagle Brand) vanilla, 'Homestyle'	1/2 cup	150	16	9.0
(Eskimo Pie) chocolate chip cone, 'Cookie Dough'	1 cone	280	33	14.0
(Frusen Gladje)				
butter pecan	1/2 cup	280	16	21.0
chocolate chocolate chip	1/2 cup	270	21	18.0
chocolate	1/2 cup	240	17	17.0
chocolate, Swiss candy almond	1/2 cup	270	18	19.0
strawberry	1/2 cup	230	20	15.0
vanilla	1/2 cup	230	16	17.0
vanilla Swiss almond	1/2 cup	270	18	19.0
vanilla toffee chunk	1/2 cup	270	22	17.0
(Good Humor)				
vanilla, 'Cup'	3 oz	98	12	5.1
vanilla-chocolate cup, 'Combo'	6 oz	201	26	9.2

Food Name	Serv. Size	Total Cal.	Carbs GMS	Fat GMS
(Häagen-Dazs)				
caramel nut sundae	1/2 cup	310	26	21.0
chocolate fudge, deep	1/2 cup	290	26	14.0
chocolate mint	1/2 cup	300	26	20.0
chocolate, deep	1/2 cup	290	26	14.0
chocolate, low-fat	1/2 cup	170	29	2.5
chocolate-peanut butter, deep	1/2 cup	330	25	19.0
coffee fudge, low-fat	1/2 cup	170	32	2.5
'Cookie Dough Dynamo'	4 oz	300	31	18.0
strawberry, low-fat	1/2 cup	150	28	2.0
vanilla, low-fat	1/2 cup	170	29	2.5
vanilla honey	1/2 cup	250	22	16.0
vanilla-peanut butter swirl	1/2 cup	280	19	21.0
(Healthy Choice)				
Black Forest, low-fat	1/2 cup	120	23	2.0
Bordeaux cherry, 'Dairy Dessert'	4 oz	120	23	2.0
Bordeaux cherry chocolate chip 'Dairy Dessert'	4 oz	120	23	2.0
butter pecan crunch, low-fat	1/2 cup	120	22	2.0
cappuccino chocolate chunk, low-fat	1/2 cup	120	22	2.0
cappuccino mocha fudge, low-fat	1/2 cup	120	23	2.0
chocolate, 'Dairy Dessert'	4 oz	130	24	2.0
chocolate chip, 'Dairy Dessert'	4 oz	130	24	2.0
coffee toffee, 'Dairy Dessert'	4 oz	130	25	2.0
cookies and cream, low-fat	1/2 cup	120	21	2.0
double fudge swirl, 'Dairy Dessert'	4 oz	130	24	2.0
fudge brownie, low-fat	1/2 cup	120	22	2.0
fudge brownie à la mode, low-fat	1/2 cup	120	22	2.0
mint chocolate chip, low-fat	1/2 cup	120	21	2.0
Neapolitan, 'Dairy Dessert'	4 oz	120	22	2.0
praline and caramel, low-fat	1/2 cup	130	25	2.0
praline caramel cluster, low-fat	1/2 cup	130	25	2.0
raspberry swirl, 'Dairy Dessert'	4 oz	120	23	2.0
rocky road, 'Dairy Dessert'	4 oz	160	32	2.0
strawberry, 'Dairy Dessert'	4 oz	120	23	2.0
turtle fudge cake, low-fat	1/2 cup	130	25	2.0
vanilla, 'Dairy Dessert'	4 oz	120	21	2.0
vanilla, old fashioned, 'Dairy Dessert'	4 oz	120	21	2.0
(Nutra/Balance) high-calorie and -protein	1 serving	232	25	12.0
(Sealtest)				
butter crunch	1/2 cup	150	18	7.0
butter pecan	1/2 cup	160	16	9.0
chocolate	1/2 cup	140	18	6.0
chocolate chip	1/2 cup	150	17	8.0
chocolate triple stripes	1/2 cup	140	17	7.0
chocolate-marshmallow sundae	1/2 cup	150	21	6.0
coffee	1/2 cup	140	16	7.0
fudge Royale	1/2 cup	140	19	7.0
heavenly hash	1/2 cup	150	19	7.0
maple walnut	1/2 cup	160	17	9.0
peanut fudge sundae	1/2 cup	140	17	7.0
strawberry	1/2 cup	130	18	5.0
vanilla	1/2 cup	140	16	7.0
vanilla, French	1/2 cup	140	16	7.0
vanilla-chocolate-strawberry 'Cubic Scoops'	1/2 cup	130	17	6.0
vanilla-chocolate-strawberry	1/2 cup	140	18	6.0
vanilla-orange sherbet, 'Cubic Scoops'	1/2 cup	130	22	4.0
vanilla-red raspberry sherbet, 'Cubic Scoops'	1/2 cup	130	22	4.0

Food Name	Serv. Size	Total Cal.	Carbs GMS	Fat GMS
(TCBY Treats)				
all flavors, hand-dipped	1/2 cup	140	17	7.0
all flavors, hand-dipped, low-fat, no added sugar	1/2 cup	100	19	2.5
all flavors, hand-dipped, nonfat	1/2 cup	100	23	0.0
(Weight Watchers)				
chocolate chip, 'ONE-ders'	4 oz	120	19	4.0
'Cookie Dough Craze'	1/2 cup	140	24	3.5
heavenly hash 'ONE-ders'	4 oz	130	22	3.0
'Oh! So Very Vanilla' light	1/2 cup	120	20	2.5
'Positively Praline Crunch' light	1/2 cup	140	25	3.0
pralines and creme, 'ONE-ders'	4 oz	120	19	4.0
'Reckless Rocky Road'	1/2 cup	140	23	3.0
'Triple Chocolate Tornado' light	1/2 cup	150	26	3.5

ICE CREAM BAR/DESSERT
BAR

Food Name	Serv. Size	Total Cal.	Carbs GMS	Fat GMS
(Baker's)				
chocolate fudge sundae 'Fudgetastic'	1 bar	220	23	15.0
chocolate fudge sundae, crunchy, 'Fudgetastic'	1 bar	230	24	14.0
(Eskimo Pie)				
vanilla, w/dark chocolate coating	1 bar	180	16	12.0
vanilla, w/milk chocolate coating	1 bar	190	18	12.0
vanilla, w/milk chocolate coating, almonds	1 bar	140	12	13.0
vanilla, w/milk chocolate coating, crisp rice	1 bar	150	12	11.0
(Freezer Pleezer) vanilla, w/chocolate flavored coating	1 bar	140	13	9.0
(Good Humor)				
'Fat Frog'	1 bar	154	16	9.2
'Halo Bar'	1 bar	230	23	13.7
'Whammy' assorted flavors	1 bar	95	7	7.2
chip candy crunch	1 bar	255	21	17.9
chocolate éclair	1 bar	188	23	9.9
chocolate fudge cake	1 bar	214	18	15.0
strawberry shortcake	1 bar	176	24	8.2
toasted almond	1 bar	212	24	11.8
vanilla, w/chocolate flavor coating	1 bar	198	17	13.7
(Haagen-Dazs)				
caramel almond, 'Crunch Bar'	1 bar	240	17	18.0
peanut butter, 'Crunch Bar'	1 bar	270	16	21.0
vanilla, 'Crunch Bar'	1 bar	220	16	16.0
vanilla, w/milk chocolate-brittle coating	1 bar	370	32	25.0
(Heath) 1 bar	1 bar	170	16	13.0
(Klondike)				
chocolate	1 bar	270	23	19.0
'Krispy'	1 bar	290	26	19.0
'Lite'	1 bar	140	10	10.0
w/chocolate flavored coating, 'Lite'	1 bar	110	14	6.0
(Natural Nectar)				
banana cream, 'Stick Novelties'	1 bar	170	22	8.0
cocoa fudge and cream, 'Stick Novelties'	1 bar	170	22	8.0
strawberries and cream, 'Stick Novelties'	1 bar	120	18	5.0
wildberry cream, 'Stick Novelties'	1 bar	120	22	3.0
(Nestlé)				
chocolate, w/milk chocolate coating, 'Quik'	1 bar	210	19	14.0
milk chocolate, w/almonds, milk chocolate coated	1 bar	350	28	23.0
vanilla, w/chocolate coating, crisp rice, 'Crunch'	1 bar	180	15	13.0
vanilla, w/chocolate coating, crisp rice, 'Crunch Lite'	1 bar	120	16	5.0
vanilla, w/white chocolate coating, 'Alpine Premium'	1 bar	350	25	25.0

Food Name	Serv. Size	Total Cal.	Carbs GMS	Fat GMS
(Oh Henry!)				
vanilla, w/caramel peanut, milk chocolate coating .... 1 bar		320	34	20.0
(Weight Watchers)				
chocolate, 'Treat Bars' .... 1 bar		100	18	1.0
chocolate fudge, double .... 1 bar		60	12	1.0
chocolate mousse, sugar-free .... 1 bar		35	9	1.0
CONE				
(Good Humor)				
'King Cone' .... 5.5 oz		290	41	12.0
boysenberry, 'King Cone' .... 5 oz		340	52	13.1
NOVELTY				
(Carnation)				
vanilla nuggets, w/dark chocolate coating, 'Bon Bons' .... 5 pieces		170	15	11.0
vanilla nuggets, w/milk chocolate coating, 'Bon Bons' .... 5 pieces		165	14	11.0
(Natural Nectar)				
mocha 'Round Novelties' .... 4 oz		300	40	14.0
nectar 'Round Novelties' .... 4 oz		300	38	15.0
SANDWICH				
(Eskimo Pie) vanilla, w/chocolate wafer .... 1 sandwich		170	26	6.0
(Good Humor)				
vanilla .... 1 sandwich		191	31	5.7
vanilla, w/chocolate chip cookie .... 1 sandwich		246	35	10.5
(Klondike)				
vanilla, 'Lite' .... 1 sandwich		100	18	2.0
vanilla .... 1 sandwich		230	33	9.0
(Weight Watchers)				
sandwich snack .... 1 sandwich		90	17	2.0
vanilla .... 1 sandwich		150	28	3.0
ICE CREAM CONE				
(Bozo)				
cake cup .... 1 cone		16	3	0.0
sugar .... 1 cone		53	11	1.0
(Comet)				
sugar .... 1 cone		50	11	0.0
waffle .... 1 cone		70	14	0.5
(Ener-G Foods) gluten free .... 1 cone		154	36	1.1
(Joy) .... 1 cone		16	3	1.0
(Keebler)				
cup, assorted colors .... 1 cone		15	4	1.0
cup, large, food service product .... 1 serving		15	4	0.0
plain .... 1 cone		15	4	1.0
sugar .... 1 cone		45	11	1.0
sugar, food service product .... 1 serving		47	10	0.2
waffle bowl, large, food service product .... 1 serving		60	12	1.5
waffle cone, large, food service product .... 1 serving		100	20	2.0
(Little Debbie) plain, 'Ice Cream Cup' .... 1 cone		15	3	0.1
(Nabisco)				
cup .... 1 cone		18	4	1.0
cup, 'Comet' .... 1 cone		18	4	1.0
sugar .... 1 cone		50	11	1.0
ICE CREAM MIX				
(Salada)				
Dutch chocolate, mix only .... 1 oz		110	26	0.0
Dutch chocolate, prepared .... 1 cup		310	31	19.0
peach, vanilla, mix only .... 1 oz		110	27	0.0
peach, vanilla, prepared .... 1 cup		310	32	18.0
peach, wild strawberry, mix only .... 1 oz		110	27	0.0
peach, wild strawberry, prepared .... 1 cup		310	32	18.0

Food Name	Serv. Size	Total Cal.	Carbs GMS	Fat GMS
ICE CREAM SANDWICH. See under ICE CREAM BAR/DESSERT.				
ICE CREAM SUBSTITUTE. See also YOGURT, FROZEN.				
(Freezees Nutcreem)				
butter pecan, nondairy, 100% natural	3 oz	131	17	7.0
cashew vanilla, nondairy, 100% natural	3 oz	131	17	7.0
lemon, nondairy, 100% natural	3 oz	131	17	7.0
orange, nondairy, 100% natural	3 oz	131	17	7.0
peanut, nondairy, 100% natural, 'Delight'	3 oz	131	17	7.0
strawberry, nondairy, 100% natural	3 oz	131	17	7.0
(Ice Bean)				
almond espresso, nondairy	4 oz	150	13	10.0
chocolate, nondairy, nonfat, 'Thunder'	1/2 cup	110	27	0.0
peanut butter carob chip, nondairy	4 oz	200	18	13.0
'Raspberry Patch' nondairy, nonfat	1/2 cup	110	27	0.0
'Vanilla Wavy' nondairy, nonfat	1/2 cup	110	27	0.0
(Living Rightly)				
almond pecan, nondairy	1/2 cup	140	21	5.0
carob peppermint, nondairy	1/2 cup	100	21	1.5
chocolate almond, nondairy	1/2 cup	140	21	5.0
vanilla, nondairy	1/2 cup	110	22	1.0
vanilla Swiss almond, nondairy	1/2 cup	140	21	5.0
(Low, Lite 'n Luscious)				
chocolate chip	1/2 cup	100	19	2.0
Jamoca Swiss almond	1/2 cup	90	19	2.0
pineapple coconut	1/2 cup	90	19	1.0
strawberry	1/2 cup	80	17	1.0
(Mocha Mix)				
strawberry swirl, nondairy, 100% milk-free	1/2 cup	140	20	6.0
vanilla, nondairy, 100% milk-free	1/2 cup	140	18	7.0
(Rice Dream)				
cappuccino flavor, nondairy	1/2 cup	130	17	5.0
carob almond, nondairy	1/2 cup	140	20	6.0
carob chip, nondairy	1/2 cup	130	20	6.0
carob, nondairy	1/2 cup	130	20	5.0
cocoa marble fudge, nondairy	1/2 cup	140	19	6.0
cookies and cream, nondairy	1/2 cup	130	21	5.0
lemon, nondairy	1/2 cup	130	17	5.0
mint carob chip, nondairy	1/2 cup	130	20	6.0
Neapolitan, nondairy	1/2 cup	130	21	5.0
peanut butter cup, nondairy	1/2 cup	130	21	6.0
peanut butter fudge, nondairy	1/2 cup	160	19	7.0
vanilla fudge, nondairy	1/2 cup	130	20	5.0
vanilla Swiss almond, nondairy	1/2 cup	130	20	6.0
vanilla, nondairy	1/2 cup	130	19	5.0
wildberry, nondairy	1/2 cup	130	17	5.0
(Sealtest)				
black cherry, nonfat, 'Free'	1/2 cup	100	25	0.0
chocolate, nonfat, 'Free'	1/2 cup	100	23	0.0
peach, nonfat, 'Free'	1/2 cup	100	23	0.0
strawberry, nonfat, 'Free'	1/2 cup	100	23	0.0
vanilla, nonfat, 'Free'	1/2 cup	100	24	0.0
vanilla-chocolate strawberry, nonfat, 'Free'	1/2 cup	100	23	0.0
vanilla-fudge royale, nonfat, 'Free'	1/2 cup	100	24	0.0
vanilla-strawberry royale, nonfat, 'Free'	1/2 cup	100	25	0.0
(Simple Pleasures)				
chocolate	1/2 cup	140	25	1.0
coffee	4 oz	120	22	1.0
peach	4 oz	135	24	1.0

Food Name	Serv. Size	Total Cal.	Carbs GMS	Fat GMS
rum raisin	4 oz	130	25	1.0
strawberry	4 oz	120	22	1.0
(Sweet Nothings)				
berry blackberry, nondairy, nonfat	1/2 cup	110	26	0.0
'Black Leopard' nondairy, nonfat	1/2 cup	100	23	0.0
chocolate Mandarin, nondairy, nonfat	1/2 cup	100	23	0.0
chocolate, nondairy, nonfat	1/2 cup	100	23	0.0
espresso fudge, nondairy, nonfat	1/2 cup	110	25	0.0
mango raspberry, nondairy, nonfat	1/2 cup	110	26	0.0
raspberry swirl, nondairy, nonfat	1/2 cup	110	26	0.0
'Tiger Stripes' nondairy, nonfat	1/2 cup	110	25	0.0
vanilla, nondairy, nonfat	1/2 cup	110	25	0.0
(Tofutti)				
all flavors, 'Lite Lite'	1/2 cup	90	20	1.0
all flavors, nondairy, 'Fruitti'	1/2 cup	100	20	0.0
butter pecan, nondairy	1 fl oz	55	6	3.3
chocolate cookie, nondairy, 'Supreme'	1 fl oz	53	7	2.8
chocolate fudge, nondairy, 'Better Than Yogurt'	1/2 cup	120	25	2.0
chocolate supreme, nondairy	1/2 cup	210	20	13.0
coffee marshmallow, nondairy, 'Better Than Yogurt'	1/2 cup	100	24	1.0
passion island fruit, nondairy, 'Better Than Yogurt'	1/2 cup	100	21	1.0
peach mango, nondairy, 'Better Than Yogurt'	1/2 cup	100	23	1.0
strawberry banana, nondairy, 'Better Than Yogurt'	1/2 cup	100	23	1.0
vanilla almond bark, nondairy	1 fl oz	53	5	3.3
vanilla fudge, nondairy, 'Better Than Yogurt'	1/2 cup	120	24	2.0
vanilla, nondairy	1 fl oz	48	5	2.8
'Wildberry Supreme' nondairy	1 fl oz	48	6	2.3
(Weight Watchers)				
'Arctic D'Lights'	1 serving	130	14	7.0
berries 'n creme mousse	1 serving	35	4	0.8
chocolate, nonfat	1/2 cup	80	19	0.0
chocolate swirl, nonfat	1/2 cup	90	22	0.0
chocolate treat	1 serving	100	21	1.0
Neapolitan, nonfat	1/2 cup	80	19	0.0
vanilla, nonfat	1/2 cup	80	20	0.0

ICE CREAM SUBSTITUTE BAR/DESSERT. See also YOGURT BAR, FROZEN BAR

(Crystal Light)				
Amaretto chocolate swirl, 'Cool N'Creamy'	1 bar	60	10	2.0
chocolate vanilla, 'Cool N'Creamy'	1 bar	50	7	2.0
double chocolate fudge, 'Cool N'Creamy'	1 bar	50	7	2.0
orange vanilla, 'Cool N'Creamy'	1 bar	30	5	1.0
(Freezer Pleezer)				
fudge flavored	1 bar	100	20	1.0
orange cream treats	1 bar	80	16	1.5
(Good Humor)				
chocolate fudge	1 bar	127	27	0.6
'Cool Shark'	1 bar	68	17	0.1
'Jumbo Jet Star'	1 bar	85	20	0.7
'Milky Pop'	1 bar	45	8	0.2
strawberry finger	1 bar	49	12	0.1
(Light n' Lively)				
chocolate mousse, nonfat	1 bar	50	12	0.0
double chocolate fudge, nonfat	1 bar	50	11	0.0
orange vanilla, nonfat	1 bar	40	10	0.0
strawberry, nonfat	1 bar	80	12	0.0
vanilla, chocolate dipped	1 bar	110	14	6.0

Food Name	Serv. Size	Total Cal.	Carbs GMS	Fat GMS
(Rice Dream)				
chocolate, nondairy	1 bar	270	33	16.0
chocolate, nutty, nondairy	1 bar	330	29	23.0
strawberry, nondairy	1 bar	260	31	14.8
vanilla, nondairy	1 bar	275	33	15.8
vanilla, nutty, nondairy	1 bar	330	29	23.0
(Sealtest)				
chocolate, w/fudge swirl, nonfat, 'Free'	1 bar	80	19	0.0
vanilla, w/fudge swirl, nonfat, 'Free'	1 bar	80	18	0.0
vanilla, w/strawberry swirl, nonfat, 'Free'	1 bar	70	17	0.0
(Trix)				
assorted flavors, nonfat	1 bar	40	10	0.0
'Fudge N' Fruity'	1 bar	80	17	1.0
(Weight Watchers)				
chocolate dip	1 bar	100	21	1.0
'Crispy Pralines & Creme'	1 bar	120	13	6.0
NOVELTY				
(Rice Dream)				
'Dream Pie' mint, nondairy	1 pie	380	47	19.0
'Dream Pie' vanilla, nondairy	1 pie	380	47	19.0
(Tofutti)				
'Love Drops' cappuccino flavored	1/2 cup	230	26	12.0
'Love Drops' chocolate	1/2 cup	230	26	13.0
'Love Drops' vanilla	1/2 cup	220	26	12.0
'O's' vanilla, chocolate dipped	1 piece	40	4	2.0
(Weight Watchers)				
'ONE-ders' brownies and creme	4 oz	130	20	4.0
parfait, double fudge brownie	1 serving	190	39	2.5
parfait, praline toffee crunch	1 serving	190	40	3.0
parfait, strawberry royale	1 serving	180	35	2.0
SUNDAE				
(Weight Watchers)				
chocolate chip cookie dough	1 serving	180	33	4.0
hot caramel fudge	4.5 oz	160	27	4.0
hot chocolate fudge	4.5 oz	160	26	4.0
hot mocha fudge	4.5 oz	160	24	5.0
ICE CREAM SUBSTITUTE MIX				
(Tofutti)				
soft serve	1 oz	48	5	1.0
soft serve, light	1 oz	23	5	0.3
ICE MILK				
(Borden)				
chocolate	1/2 cup	100	18	2.0
strawberry	1/2 cup	90	17	2.0
vanilla	1/2 cup	90	17	2.0
(Breyers)				
chocolate, 'Light'	1/2 cup	120	18	4.0
chocolate chocolate chip, 'Light'	1/2 cup	140	20	5.0
chocolate fudge twirl, 'Light'	1/2 cup	130	21	4.0
heavenly hash, 'Light'	1/2 cup	150	21	5.0
praline almond, 'Light'	1/2 cup	130	19	5.0
strawberry, 'Light'	1/2 cup	110	18	3.0
Swiss almond fudge twirl	1/2 cup	150	21	6.0
toffee fudge parfait, 'Light'	1/2 cup	140	22	5.0
vanilla, 'Light'	1/2 cup	120	18	4.0
vanilla-chocolate-strawberry, 'Light'	1/2 cup	120	18	4.0
vanilla-raspberry parfait, 'Light'	1/2 cup	130	23	3.0

Food Name	Serv. Size	Total Cal.	Carbs GMS	Fat GMS
(Darigold)				
chocolate, 'Lite'	1/2 cup	110	19	3.0
vanilla	1/2 cup	110	18	3.0
(Light n' Lively)				
caramel nut	1/2 cup	120	18	4.0
chocolate chip	1/2 cup	120	18	4.0
coffee	1/2 cup	100	16	3.0
cookies and cream	1/2 cup	110	18	3.0
heavenly hash	1/2 cup	120	20	4.0
vanilla	1/2 cup	100	16	3.0
vanilla, w/chocolate covered almonds	1/2 cup	120	17	4.0
vanilla-chocolate-strawberry	1/2 cup	100	17	3.0
vanilla-fudge twirl	1/2 cup	110	18	3.0
vanilla-raspberry swirl	1/2 cup	110	19	3.0
(Ponderosa)				
chocolate	3.5 oz	152	30	2.9
vanilla	3.5 oz	150	30	2.6
(Weight Watchers)				
chocolate, 'Grand Collection'	1/2 cup	110	18	3.0
chocolate chip, 'Grand Collection'	1/2 cup	120	19	4.0
chocolate swirl, 'Grand Collection'	1/2 cup	120	19	3.0
Neapolitan, 'Grand Collection'	1/2 cup	110	18	3.0
pecan pralines and creme, 'Grand Collection'	1/2 cup	120	20	4.0
vanilla, 'Grand Collection'	1/2 cup	100	16	3.0
ICE MILK BAR/DESSERT				
bar, 'Chocolate Almond Crunch' *(Weight Watchers)*	1 bar	120	12	7.0
cone, w/nuts 'Olde Nut Sundae' *(Gold Bond)*	3 oz	230	36	8.0

ICEBERG LETTUCE. See LETTUCE, ICEBERG.
ICED TEA. See TEA, ICED.
IMBU. See JOBO.
INDIAN DATE. See TAMARIND.
INDIAN FRY BREAD. See under BREAD.
INFANT FORMULA. See under BABY FOOD.
IRISH MOSS. See under SEA VEGETABLE.
ITALIAN BEAN. See BEAN, ITALIAN.
ITALIAN CHESTNUT. See CHESTNUT, EUROPEAN.
ITALIAN MUSHROOM. See MUSHROOM, CRIMINI.
ITALIAN SEASONING. See under SEASONING MIX.
ITALIAN STONE PINE NUT. See PINE NUT.

J

Food Name	Serv. Size	Total Cal.	Carbs GMS	Fat GMS
JACK BEAN. See BEAN, FAVA.				
JACK MACKEREL. See under MACKEREL.				
JACKFRUIT				
Fresh, raw, sliced	1 cup	155	40	0.5
Canned, in syrup, drained	1 cup	164	43	0.2
JALAPEÑO. See PEPPER, JALAPEÑO.				
JAM AND PRESERVES. See also FRUIT SPREAD.				
(Estee) all flavors	1 tsp	2	0	0.0
(Featherweight) all flavors	1 tsp	4	1	0.0
(Kraft) all flavors	1 tsp	17	4	0.0
(S&W) all flavors, 'Nutradiet'	1 tsp	4	1	0.0
APRICOT				
(Finast)	2 tsp	35	9	0.0

Food Name	Serv. Size	Total Cal.	Carbs GMS	Fat GMS
(Knott's Berry Farm) pure preserves	1 tsp	18	4	0.0
(Polaner)	2 tsp	35	9	0.0
(Smucker's) natural ingredients	1 tsp	18	4	0.0
APRICOT-PINEAPPLE				
(Knott's Berry Farm) pure preserves	1 tsp	18	4	0.0
(Knudsen)	2 tsp	35	8	1.0
(Smucker's) natural ingredients	1 tsp	18	4	0.0
BLACK CHERRY (Knudsen)	2 tsp	35	8	1.0
BLACKBERRY				
(Finast)	2 tsp	16	4	0.0
(Knott's Berry Farm) seedless, pure preserves	1 tsp	18	4	0.0
(Knudsen)				
	2 tsp	35	8	1.0
organic	2 tsp	25	7	1.0
(Polaner) seedless	2 tsp	35	9	0.0
(Smucker's) natural ingredients	1 tsp	18	4	0.0
(Stilwell) freezer jam	1 tbsp	36	8	0.0
BLUEBERRY				
(Finast)	2 tsp	16	4	0.0
(Knott's Berry Farm) pure preserves	1 tsp	18	4	0.0
(Knudsen)				
	2 tsp	35	8	1.0
organic	2 tsp	25	7	1.0
(Polaner)	2 tsp	35	9	0.0
(Smucker's) natural ingredients	1 tsp	18	4	0.0
BOYSENBERRY				
(Knott's Berry Farm) pure preserves	1 tsp	18	4	0.0
(Knudsen)	2 tsp	35	8	1.0
(Smucker's) natural ingredients	1 tsp	18	4	0.0
CHERRY				
(Finast)	2 tsp	25	9	0.0
(Knott's Berry Farm)				
Bing, pure preserves	1 tsp	18	4	0.0
red, pure preserves	1 tsp	18	4	0.0
(Smucker's) natural ingredients	1 tsp	18	4	0.0
FIG (Knott's Berry Farm) Kadota, pure preserves	1 tsp	18	4	0.0
GRAPE				
(Finast)				
	2 tsp	35	9	0.0
Concord	2 tsp	35	9	0.0
(Knudsen) Concord	2 tsp	35	8	1.0
(Polaner)	2 tsp	35	9	0.0
(Smucker's) Concord, natural ingredients	1 tsp	18	4	0.0
(Welch's)	2 tsp	35	9	0.0
ORANGE				
(Fifty 50) no sugar added	1 tsp	2	1	0.0
(Finast) marmalade	2 tsp	35	9	0.0
(Knott's Berry Farm) marmalade, w/NutraSweet, 'Light'	1 tsp	8	2	0.0
(Knudsen) marmalade	2 tsp	35	8	1.0
(Smucker's)				
marmalade	1 tsp	18	4	0.0
marmalade, low-sugar	1 tsp	8	2	0.0
marmalade, 'Simply Fruit'	1 tsp	16	4	0.0
marmalade, sweet, natural ingredients	1 tsp	18	4	0.0
(Polaner) marmalade	2 tsp	35	9	0.0
PEACH				
(Bama)	2 tsp	30	8	0.0
(Finast)	2 tsp	35	9	0.0

Food Name	Serv. Size	Total Cal.	Carbs GMS	Fat GMS
(Knudsen)	2 tsp	35	8	1.0
(Polaner)	2 tsp	35	9	0.0
(Smucker's) natural ingredients	1 tsp	18	4	0.0
PINEAPPLE				
(Finast)	2 tsp	35	9	0.0
(Polaner)	2 tsp	35	9	0.0
(Smucker's) natural ingredients	1 tsp	18	4	0.0
PLUM				
(Bama) red	2 tsp	30	8	0.0
(Smucker's) natural ingredients	1 tsp	18	4	0.0
RASPBERRY				
(Finast) red	2 tsp	35	9	0.0
(Knott's Berry Farm) seedless, pure preserves	1 tsp	18	4	0.0
(Knudsen)				
red	2 tsp	35	8	1.0
red, organic	2 tsp	25	7	1.0
(Polaner)				
red	2 tsp	35	9	0.0
red, seedless	2 tsp	35	9	0.0
(Smucker's)				
black, natural ingredients	1 tsp	18	4	0.0
red, seedless, natural ingredients	1 tsp	18	4	0.0
(Stilwell) freezer jam	1 tbsp	33	8	0.0
RASPBERRY-APPLE (Welch's)	2 tsp	35	9	0.0
STRAWBERRY				
(Bama)	2 tsp	30	8	0.0
(Finast)	2 tsp	35	9	0.0
(Knott's Berry Farm) seedless, pure preserves	1 tsp	18	4	0.0
(Knudsen)				
	2 tsp	35	8	1.0
organic	2 tsp	25	7	1.0
(Kraft) reduced calorie	1 tsp	6	2	0.0
(Piedmont)	2 tsp	35	9	0.0
(Polaner) strawberry	2 tsp	35	9	0.0
(Smucker's) seedless, natural ingredients	1 tsp	18	4	0.0
(Stilwell) freezer jam	1 tbsp	37	9	0.0
(Welch's)	2 tsp	35	9	0.0
TOMATO (Smucker's) natural ingredients	1 tsp	18	4	0.0
JAMAICAN BREADNUT. See BREADNUT TREE SEEDS.				
JAMBALAYA. See under SHRIMP DISH/ENTRÉE.				
JAMBERRY, fresh (Frieda's)	3.5 oz	25	4.2	0.5
JAMBOLAN. See JAVA PLUM.				
JAPANESE HONEY MUSHROOM. See MUSHROOM, JAPANESE HONEY.				
JAPANESE MEDLAR. See LOQUAT.				
JAPANESE WHITE RADISH. See DAIKON.				
JASMINE RICE. See under RICE.				
JAVA PLUM/jambolan				
cut up	1 cup	81	21	0.3
whole	3 med fruits	5	1	0.0
JELL-O. See under GELATIN DESSERT; GELATIN DESSERT MIX.				
JELLY. See also FRUIT SPREAD; JAM AND PRESERVES.				
(Estee) all flavors	1 tsp	2	0	0.0
(Featherweight) all flavors, except grape	1 tsp	4	1	0.0
(Kraft) all flavors	1 tsp	17	4	0.0
APPLE				
(Bama)	2 tsp	30	8	0.0
(Finast)	2 tsp	35	9	0.0
(Lucky Leaf)	1 oz	80	20	0.0

Food Name	Serv. Size	Total Cal.	Carbs GMS	Fat GMS
(Musselman's)	1 oz	80	20	0.0
(Polaner)	2 tsp	35	9	0.0
(Smucker's)				
cinnamon-flavored, natural ingredients	1 tsp	18	4	0.0
mint-flavored, natural ingredients	1 tsp	18	4	0.0
natural ingredients	1 tsp	18	4	0.0
APPLE BLACKBERRY *(Musselman's)*	1 oz	80	19	0.0
APPLE CHERRY *(Musselman's)*	1 oz	80	19	0.0
APPLE GRAPE				
(Musselman's)	1 oz	80	20	0.0
(Welch's)	2 tsp	35	9	0.0
APPLE RASPBERRY *(Musselman's)*	1 oz	80	19	0.0
APPLE STRAWBERRY *(Musselman's)*	1 oz	80	20	0.0
APRICOT-PINEAPPLE				
(Knott's Berry Farm) w/NutraSweet, 'Light'	1 tsp	8	2	0.0
BLACKBERRY				
(Bama)	2 tsp	30	8	0.0
(Knott's Berry Farm) w/NutraSweet, 'Light'	1 tsp	8	2	0.0
(Smucker's) natural ingredients	1 tsp	18	4	0.0
BOYSENBERRY				
(Knott's Berry Farm) w/NutraSweet, 'Light'	1 tsp	8	2	0.0
CHERRY *(Smucker's)* natural ingredients	1 tsp	18	4	0.0
CRABAPPLE *(Smucker's)* natural ingredients	1 tsp	18	4	0.0
CURRANT				
(Finast)	2 tsp	35	9	0.0
(Polaner)	2 tsp	35	9	0.0
(Smucker's) natural ingredients	1 tsp	18	4	0.0
ELDERBERRY *(Smucker's)* natural ingredients	1 tsp	18	4	0.0
GRAPE				
(Bama)	2 tsp	30	8	0.0
(Featherweight)	1 tsp	4	1	0.0
(Finast)	2 tsp	35	9	0.0
(Kraft) reduced calorie	1 tsp	6	2	0.0
(Musselman's)	1 oz	80	20	0.0
(Polaner)	2 tsp	35	9	0.0
(Smucker's) Concord, natural ingredients	1 tsp	18	4	0.0
(Welch's)	2 tsp	35	9	0.0
GREEN PEPPER *(Great Impressions)*	1 tbsp	50	13	0.0
GUAVA *(Smucker's)* natural ingredients	1 tsp	18	4	0.0
JALAPEÑO				
(Great Impressions)	1 tbsp	58	15	0.0
(Knott's Berry Farm) pure	1 tsp	18	4	0.0
MINT				
(Finast)	2 tsp	35	9	0.0
(Polaner)	2 tsp	35	9	0.0
MIXED FRUIT *(Smucker's)* natural ingredients	1 tsp	18	4	0.0
PLUM *(Smucker's)* natural ingredients	1 tsp	18	4	0.0
QUINCE *(Smucker's)* natural ingredients	1 tsp	18	4	0.0
RASPBERRY				
(Knott's Berry Farm) red, w/NutraSweet, 'Light'	1 tsp	8	2	0.0
(Polaner) raspberry	2 tsp	35	9	0.0
(Smucker's)				
black, natural ingredients	1 tsp	18	4	0.0
red, natural ingredients	1 tsp	18	4	0.0
RED PEPPER *(Great Impressions)*	1 tbsp	50	13	0.0
STRAWBERRY				
(Finast)	2 tsp	35	9	0.0
(Knott's Berry Farm) w/NutraSweet, 'Light'	1 tsp	8	2	0.0

Food Name	Serv. Size	Total Cal.	Carbs GMS	Fat GMS
(Polaner)	2 tsp	35	9	0.0
(Smucker's) natural ingredients	1 tsp	18	4	0.0
STRAWBERRY APPLE *(Polaner)*	2 tsp	35	9	0.0
JELLYBEAN. See under CANDY, JELLIED AND GUMMED.				
JERKY. See BEEF JERKY; BEEF SUBSTITUTE JERKY; TURKEY JERKY.				
JERUSALEM ARTICHOKE. See ARTICHOKE, JERUSALEM.				
JEW'S EAR. See CHINESE FUNGUS.				
JICAMA/Chinese yam/Mexican potato/sicama/yambean tuber				
raw, sliced	1 cup	46	11	0.1
raw, trimmed *(Frieda of California)*	1 oz	13	3	0.1
raw, whole	1 medium	250	58	0.6
JOBO/hog plum/imbu/yellow mombin				
seeded	1 oz	20	3.9	0.6
JUICE. See FRUIT JUICE BLEND; individual listings.				
JUJUBE, CHINESE				
dried	3.5 oz	287	73.6	1.1
dried	1 oz	81	20.1	0.3
raw	3.5 oz	79	20.2	0.1
raw	1 oz	22	5.7	0.1
JUNKET MIX				
CHOCOLATE				
mix only *(Junket)*	3/8 oz	40	10	0.0
prepared w/nonfat milk *(Junket)*	1/2 cup	90	15	0.0
prepared w/whole milk *(Junket)*	1/2 cup	120	15	4.0
RASPBERRY				
mix only *(Junket)*	3/8 oz	40	10	0.0
prepared w/nonfat milk *(Junket)*	1/2 cup	90	16	0.0
prepared w/whole milk *(Junket)*	1/2 cup	120	16	4.0
STRAWBERRY				
mix only *(Junket)*	3/8 oz	40	10	0.0
prepared w/nonfat milk *(Junket)*	1/2 cup	90	16	0.0
prepared w/whole milk *(Junket)*	1/2 cup	120	16	4.0
VANILLA				
mix only *(Junket)*	3/8 oz	40	10	0.0
prepared w/nonfat milk *(Junket)*	1/2 cup	90	16	0.0
prepared w/whole milk *(Junket)*	1/2 cup	120	16	4.0
JUTE POTHERB				
boiled, drained	1 cup	32	6	0.2
raw	1 cup	10	2	0.1

K

Food Name	Serv. Size	Total Cal.	Carbs GMS	Fat GMS
KAISER ROLL. See under ROLL.				
KALE/borecole/cole/colewort				
Canned, chopped *(Allens)*	1/2 cup	25	3	1.0
Fresh				
boiled, drained	4 oz	36	6.4	0.5
boiled, drained, chopped	1 cup	42	7.3	0.5
raw, chopped	1 cup	34	7	0.5
raw, chopped *(Dole)*	1/2 cup	17	3	0.5
boiled, drained, chopped	1 cup	36	7	0.5
Frozen				
boiled, drained, chopped	1 cup	39	7	0.6
boiled, drained, chopped or diced	1/2 cup	20	3	0.3
chopped *(Frosty Acres)*	3.3 oz	25	5	0.0

Food Name	Serv. Size	Total Cal.	Carbs GMS	Fat GMS
chopped (Seabrook)	3.3 oz	25	5	0.0
chopped (Southern)	3.5 oz	30	5	0.5
unprepared	10-oz pkg	80	14	1.3
KALE, SCOTCH				
boiled, drained, chopped	1 cup	36	7	0.5
raw, chopped	1 cup	28	6	0.4
KANPYO/dried gourd strips	1/2 cup	70	18	0.2
KANTEN				
raw	1 lb	116	30.6	0.1
raw	1 oz	7	1.9	tr
KASHA. See BUCKWHEAT GROATS, ROASTED.				
KATSUO. See under TUNA, SKIP JACK.				
KATURAY/sesbania flower				
flowers, raw, whole	1 cup	5	1	0.0
flowers, raw, whole	1 medium	1	0	0.0
flowers, steamed	1 cup	23	5	0.1
KEFIR				
black cherry flavored, cultured (Alta Dena)	1 cup	200	24	9.0
boysenberry flavored, cultured (Alta Dena)	1 cup	200	24	9.0
peach flavored, cultured (Alta Dena)	1 cup	200	24	9.0
plain, cultured, including acidophilus (Alta Dena)	1 oz	70	1	6.0
red raspberry flavored, cultured (Alta Dena)	1 cup	200	24	9.0
KELP. See under SEA VEGETABLE.				
KETA SALMON. See under SALMON.				
KETCHUP. See CATSUP.				
KIDNEY BEAN. See BEAN, KIDNEY.				
KIELBASA. See under SAUSAGE.				
KING CRAB. See under CRAB.				
KING MACKEREL. See under MACKEREL.				
KING SALMON. See under SALMON.				
KIWI FRUIT/Chinese gooseberry				
Fresh				
raw, cut up	1 cup	108	26	0.8
raw, peeled	1 large	56	14	0.4
raw, peeled	1 medium	46	11	0.3
KOHLRABI/cabbage turnip				
boiled, drained, sliced	1 cup	48	11	0.2
raw, sliced	1 cup	36	8	0.1
KOLBASSY. See under SAUSAGE.				
KOMBU. See under SEA VEGETABLE.				
KOOL-AID. See under FRUIT DRINK; FRUIT DRINK MIX.				
KOTTERIN MIRIN. See under SEASONING MIX.				
KUMQUAT				
raw, trimmed	1 med fruit	12	3	0.0
raw, w/seeds	1 lb	266	69.3	0.4

L

Food Name	Serv. Size	Total Cal.	Carbs GMS	Fat GMS
LAMB, AUSTRALIAN				
(NOTE: All USDA choice grade. TRIMMED = Lean; separable fat removed. UNTRIMMED = Separable fat not removed.)				
COMPOSITE CUTS				
Trimmed				
cooked	3 oz	171	0	8.2
raw	3 oz	121	0	5.3

Food Name	Serv. Size	Total Cal.	Carbs GMS	Fat GMS
raw	1 oz	40	0	1.8
Untrimmed				
cooked	3 oz	218	0	14.3
raw	3 oz	195	0	14.4
raw	1 oz	65	0	4.8
LEG/CENTER SLICE				
Trimmed				
center slice, raw	9.8 oz	403	0	17.1
center slice, w/bone, broiled	3 oz	156	0	6.5
center slice, w/bone, raw	1 oz	41	0	1.7
Untrimmed				
center slice, broiled	3 oz	183	0	10.0
center slice, raw	11 oz	616	0	39.7
center slice, w/bone, raw	1 oz	55	0	3.6
LEG/FORESHANK				
Trimmed				
braised	3 oz	140	0	4.4
raw	3 oz	105	0	3.2
raw	1 oz	35	0	1.1
Untrimmed				
braised	3 oz	201	0	12.3
raw	3 oz	100	0	10.8
raw	1 oz	55	0	3.6
LEG/SHANK				
Trimmed				
raw	3 oz	113	0	4.3
raw	1 oz	38	0	1.4
roasted	3 oz	155	0	6.2
Untrimmed				
raw	3 oz	171	0	11.5
raw	1 oz	57	0	3.8
roasted	3 oz	196	0	11.6
LEG/SIRLOIN				
Trimmed				
raw	3 oz	117	0	4.8
raw	1 oz	39	0	1.6
roasted	3 oz	183	0	9.1
Untrimmed				
raw	3 oz	216	0	17.0
raw	1 oz	72	0	5.7
roasted	3 oz	239	0	16.5
LEG/WHOLE				
Trimmed				
raw	3 oz	115	0	4.4
raw	1 oz	38	0	1.5
roasted	3 oz	162	0	6.9
Untrimmed				
raw	3 oz	183	0	12.9
raw	1 oz	61	0	4.3
roasted	3 oz	207	0	12.9
LOIN				
Trimmed				
broiled	3 oz	163	0	7.4
broiled, yield from 1 med chop	3.7 oz	111	0	5.1
raw	3 oz	124	0	5.3
raw	1 oz	41	0	1.8
Untrimmed				
broiled	3 oz	186	0	10.4

Food Name	Serv. Size	Total Cal.	Carbs GMS	Fat GMS
broiled, yield from 1 med chop	2.2 oz	136	0	7.6
raw	3 oz	173	0	11.4
raw	1 oz	58	0	3.8
RIB				
Trimmed				
raw	3 oz	136	0	7.0
raw	1 oz	45	0	2.3
roasted	3 oz	179	0	9.9
Untrimmed				
raw	3 oz	246	0	20.6
raw	1 oz	82	0	6.9
roasted	3 oz	235	0	17.2
SHOULDER/ARM				
Trimmed				
braised	3 oz	264	0	17.3
braised, yield from 1 med chop	6.5 oz	289	0	19.0
raw	3 oz	116	0	4.9
raw	1 oz	39	0	1.6
Untrimmed				
raw	1 oz	69	0	5.4
raw	3 oz	207	0	16.1
SHOULDER/BLADE				
Trimmed				
broiled	3 oz	196	0	12.2
raw	3 oz	139	0	7.7
raw	1 oz	46	0	2.6
Untrimmed				
broiled	3 oz	247	0	18.7
raw	3 oz	223	0	18.1
raw	1 oz	74	0	6.0
SHOULDER/WHOLE				
Trimmed				
cooked	3 oz	198	0	11.4
raw	3 oz	132	0	6.8
raw	1 oz	44	0	2.3
Untrimmed				
cooked	3 oz	252	0	18.4
raw	3 oz	218	0	17.4
raw	1 oz	73	0	5.8
SIRLOIN CHOP				
Trimmed				
broiled	3 oz	200	0	11.8
broiled, yield from 1 med chop	5.3 oz	247	0	14.5
raw	1 oz	59	0	4.1
Untrimmed				
broiled	3 oz	160	0	6.6
broiled, yield from 1 med chop	5.3 oz	179	0	7.4
raw	1 oz	37	0	1.4
LAMB, NEW ZEALAND				
COMPOSITE CUTS				
Trimmed				
cooked	4 oz	234	0.0	10.0
raw	1 oz	36	0.0	1.3
Untrimmed				
raw	1 oz	182	0.0	19.2
LEG/FORESHANK				
Trimmed				
braised	3 oz	158	0.0	5.1

Food Name	Serv. Size	Total Cal.	Carbs GMS	Fat GMS
braised, diced	1 cup	260	0.0	8.5
raw	1 lb	535	0.0	14.9
raw	1 oz	33	0.0	0.9
stewed	4 oz	211	0.0	6.8
stewed, diced	1 cup	260	0.0	8.5
Untrimmed				
braised	3 oz	219	0.0	13.5
braised, diced	1 cup	361	0.0	22.2
raw	1 lb	1012	0.0	73.3
raw	1 oz	62	0.0	4.5
stewed	4 oz	293	0.0	18.0
stewed, diced	1 cup	361	0.0	22.2
LEG/WHOLE				
Trimmed				
raw	1 lb	558	0.0	17.2
raw	1 oz	34	0.0	1.1
roasted	3 oz	154	0.0	6.0
roasted, diced	1 cup	253	0.0	9.8
Untrimmed				
raw	1 lb	980	0.0	69.4
raw	1 oz	60	0.0	4.3
roasted	3 oz	209	0.0	13.2
roasted, diced	1 cup	344	0.0	21.8
LOIN				
Trimmed				
broiled	4 oz	226	0.0	9.3
raw	1 oz	36	0.0	1.2
roasted	3 oz	169	0.0	7.0
Untrimmed				
broiled	3 oz	268	0.0	20.3
raw	1 oz	85	0.0	7.3
RIB				
Trimmed				
raw	1 lb	644	0.0	27.5
raw	1 oz	40	0.0	1.7
roasted	3 oz	167	0.0	8.6
Untrimmed				
raw	1 lb	1569	0.0	142.0
raw	1 oz	97	0.0	8.8
roasted	3 oz	289	0.0	24.4
SHOULDER/WHOLE				
Trimmed				
braised	3 oz	242	0.0	13.2
braised, diced	1 cup	399	0.0	21.7
raw	1 lb	612	0.0	24.6
raw	1 oz	38	0.0	1.5
stewed	6.5 oz	522	0.0	28.3
stewed, diced	1 cup	399	0.0	21.7
Untrimmed				
braised	3 oz	303	0.0	22.3
braised, diced	1 cup	491	0.0	35.5
raw	1 lb	1234	0.0	100.8
stewed	4 oz	398	0.0	28.8
stewed, diced	1 cup	491	0.0	35.5

LAMB, U.S.
(NOTE: All USDA choice grade. TRIMMED = Lean; separable fat removed. UNTRIMMED = Separable fat not removed.)

Food Name	Serv. Size	Total Cal.	Carbs GMS	Fat GMS
BRAIN				
braised	3 oz	123	0.0	8.6
braised, yield from 1 lb raw	12.25 oz	503	0.0	35.3
pan-fried	3 oz	232	0.0	18.9
raw	4 oz	138	0.0	9.7
COMPOSITE CUTS/LEG AND SHOULDER				
Trimmed				
braised, cubed	3 oz	190	0.0	7.5
broiled, cubed	3 oz	158	0.0	6.2
broiled, ground	3 oz	241	0.0	16.7
raw, cubed	1 lb	608	0.0	24.0
raw, cubed	1 oz	38	0.0	1.5
raw, ground	1 lb	1279	0.0	106.2
raw, ground	1 oz	79	0.0	6.6
stewed, cubed	4 oz	253	0.0	10.0
GROUND				
broiled	3 oz	241	0	16.7
raw	4 oz	319	0	26.5
raw	1 oz	80	0	6.6
HEART				
braised	3 oz	157	1.6	6.7
raw	4 oz	138	0.2	6.4
simmered	4 oz	210	2.2	9.0
KIDNEYS				
braised	3 oz	116	0.8	3.1
raw	4 oz	110	0.9	3.3
LEG/FORESHANK				
Trimmed				
braised	3 oz	159	0.0	5.1
braised	1 oz	53	0.0	1.7
braised, diced	1 cup	262	0.0	8.4
broiled, ground	1 cup	328	0.0	23.1
broiled, ground	4 oz	321	0.0	22.3
raw	1 lb	544	0.0	14.9
raw	1 oz	34	0.0	0.9
raw, ground	1 cup	637	0.0	52.9
stewed	4 oz	212	0.0	6.8
stewed	1 oz	53	0.0	1.7
stewed, diced	1 cup	262	0.0	8.4
Untrimmed				
braised	3 oz	207	0.0	11.4
braised	1 oz	69	0.0	3.8
braised, diced	1 cup	340	0.0	18.8
raw	1 lb	912	0.0	60.7
raw	1 oz	56	0.0	3.8
stewed	1 oz	69	0.0	3.8
stewed, diced	1 cup	340	0.0	18.8
LEG/SHANK				
Trimmed				
raw	1 lb	567	0.0	19.0
raw	1 oz	35	0.0	1.2
roasted	3 oz	153	0.0	5.7
roasted	1 oz	51	0.0	1.9
roasted, diced	1 cup	252	0.0	9.3
Untrimmed				
raw	1 lb	912	0.0	61.2
raw	1 oz	56	0.0	3.8

Food Name	Serv. Size	Total Cal.	Carbs GMS	Fat GMS
roasted	3 oz	191	0.0	10.6
roasted	1 oz	64	0.0	3.5
roasted, diced	1 cup	315	0.0	17.4
LEG/SIRLOIN				
Trimmed				
raw	1 lb	608	0.0	23.0
raw	1 oz	38	0.0	1.4
roasted	3 oz	173	0.0	7.8
roasted	1 oz	58	0.0	2.6
roasted, diced	1 cup	286	0.0	12.8
Untrimmed				
raw	1 lb	1234	0.0	100.3
raw	1 oz	76	0.0	6.2
roasted	3 oz	248	0.0	17.6
roasted	1 oz	83	0.0	5.9
roasted, diced	1 cup	409	0.0	28.9
LEG/WHOLE				
Trimmed				
raw	1 lb	581	0.0	20.5
raw	1 oz	36	0.0	1.3
roasted	3 oz	162	0 0	6.6
roasted	1 oz	54	0.0	2.2
roasted, diced	1 cup	267	0.0	10.8
Untrimmed				
raw	1 lb	1043	0.0	77.4
raw	1 oz	64	0.0	4.8
roasted	3 oz	219	0.0	14.0
roasted	1 oz	73	0.0	4.7
roasted, diced	1 cup	361	0.0	23.0
LIVER				
braised	3 oz	187	2.2	7.5
pan-fried	3 oz	202	3.2	10.8
raw	4 oz	158	2.0	5.7
LOIN				
Trimmed				
broiled	3 oz	184	0.0	8.3
raw	1 oz	40	0.0	1.7
roasted	3 oz	172	0.0	8.3
Untrimmed				
broiled	3 oz	269	0.0	19.6
roasted	3 oz	263	0.0	20.0
LUNGS				
braised	3 oz	96	0.0	2.6
raw	4 oz	108	0.0	3.0
PANCREAS				
braised	3 oz	199	0.0	12.8
raw	4 oz	172	0.0	11.1
RIB				
Trimmed				
broiled	3 oz	200	0.0	11.0
raw	1 lb	767	0.0	41.9
raw	1 oz	47	0.0	2.6
roasted	3 oz	197	0.0	11.3
Untrimmed				
broiled	3 oz	307	0.0	25.1
raw	1 lb	1687	0.0	156.0
raw	1 oz	104	0.0	9.6

Food Name	Serv. Size	Total Cal.	Carbs GMS	Fat GMS
roasted	3 oz	305	0.0	25.3
SHOULDER/ARM				
Trimmed				
braised	3 oz	237	0.0	12.0
broiled	3 oz	170	0.0	7.7
raw	1 oz	37	0.0	1.5
roasted	3 oz	163	0.0	7.9
Untrimmed				
braised	3 oz	294	0.0	20.4
broiled	3 oz	239	0.0	16.6
raw	1 oz	73	0.0	5.8
roasted	3 oz	237	0.0	17.2
SHOULDER/BLADE				
Trimmed				
braised	1 oz	81	0.0	4.7
broiled	3 oz	179	0.0	9.6
raw	3 oz	128	0.0	6.5
roasted	3 oz	178	0.0	9.8
Untrimmed				
braised	3 oz	293	0.0	21.0
broiled	3 oz	236	0.0	17.0
raw	1 lb	1175	0.0	94.6
raw	1 oz	73	0.0	5.8
roasted	3 oz	239	0.0	17.5
SHOULDER/WHOLE				
Trimmed				
braised	4 oz	321	0.0	10.0
braised, diced	1 cup	396	0.0	22.2
broiled	4 oz	238	0.0	11.9
roasted	4 oz	231	0.0	12.2
roasted, diced	1 cup	286	0.0	15.1
stewed	4 oz	321	0.0	10.0
stewed, diced	1 cup	396	0.0	22.2
Untrimmed				
braised, diced	1 cup	482	0.0	34.4
broiled	4 oz	315	0.0	21.8
broiled, diced	1 cup	389	0.0	27.0
roasted	4 oz	313	0.0	22.6
roasted, diced	1 cup	386	0.0	28.0
stewed	4 oz	390	0.0	27.8
stewed, diced	1 cup	482	0.0	34.4
SPLEEN				
braised	3 oz	133	0.0	4.1
raw	4 oz	115	0.0	3.5
TONGUE				
braised	3 oz	234	0.0	17.2
raw	4 oz	252	0.0	19.5
LAMB DINNER/ENTRÉE				
(Stouffer's) shepherd's pie, frozen, food service product	1 oz	36	3	1.8
LAMB'S QUARTERS				
Fresh				
boiled, drained	4 oz	36	5.7	0.8
boiled, drained, chopped	1 cup	58	9.0	1.3
raw	3.5 oz	43	7.3	0.8
raw, trimmed	1 lb	195	33.1	3.6
raw, trimmed	1 oz	12	2.1	0.2
LARD				
	1 cup	1849	0	205.0

Food Name	Serv. Size	Total Cal.	Carbs GMS	Fat GMS
.... 1 tbsp	115	0	12.8

LASAGNA/LASAGNA ENTRÉE
(Amy's Kitchen)
| tofu and vegetable .... 1 serving | 300 | 41 | 10.0 |
| vegetable, w/cheese .... 1 serving | 300 | 39 | 10.0 |

(Banquet)
| frozen, 'Extra Helping' .... 16.5 oz | 645 | 88 | 23.0 |
| w/meat sauce .... 1 entrée | 260 | 38 | 8.0 |

(Bernardi)
'Solito' .... 1 cup	380	33	18.0
'Supreme' .... 1 cup	310	32	13.0
supreme, portioned .... 1-1/4 cup	369	38	15.0
vegetable, 'Supreme' .... 1 cup	360	35	17.0

(Budget Gourmet)
sausage, Italian .... 1 entrée	430	40	21.0
three cheese .... 1 entrée	370	38	16.0
vegetable, 'Light' .... 1 entrée	290	36	9.0
w/cheese and meat sauce .... 1 entrée	326	35	12.0
w/Italian sausage .... 1 entrée	456	40	23.8
w/meat sauce, 'Light' .... 1 entrée	250	31	7.0

(Buitoni)
| in sauce, frozen, 'Family Style' .... 7.3 oz | 370 | 30 | 13.0 |
| meat, frozen, 'Single Serving' .... 9 oz | 580 | 57 | 19.0 |

(Celentano)
.... 10-oz tray	400	51	14.0
.... 1 cup	320	41	11.0
frozen, 14-oz tray .... 7 oz	280	33	10.0
low-fat, frozen, 'Great Choice' .... 10-oz tray	260	42	2.5
primavera, 'Great Choice' .... 10-oz tray	240	33	7.0
primavera, 'Selects' .... 10-oz tray	220	32	5.0

(Chef Boyardee)
.... 1 cup	270	41	8.0
hearty, microwave cup, 'Main Meals' .... 10.5 oz	290	41	8.0
in garden vegetable sauce, canned, microwave .... 7.5 oz	170	14	1.0
microwave .... 7.5 oz	230	31	9.0

(Contadina)
chicken, food service product, frozen .... 1 oz	44	3	2.6
classic, frozen, food service product .... 1 oz	39	4	1.6
precut, classic, frozen, food service product .... 1 oz	39	3	2.2

(Dining Lite)
| cheese, frozen .... 9 oz | 260 | 36 | 6.0 |
| w/meat sauce, frozen .... 9 oz | 240 | 36 | 5.0 |

(Dinty Moore)
w/meat sauce, packaged, 'American Classics' .... 10 oz	320	33	14.0
(Freezer Queen) w/meat sauce, 'Deluxe Family Suppers' .... 7 oz	200	28	6.0
(Green Giant) frozen, 'Entrées' .... 12 oz	490	44	20.0

(Healthy Choice)
Roma, w/meat sauce .... 1 entrée	400	59	7.0
w/meat sauce, frozen .... 10 oz	260	37	5.0
zucchini, frozen .... 11.5 oz	250	41	3.0
(Hormel) microwave cup .... 7.5 oz	250	25	13.0

(Le Menu)
| garden vegetable, 'Light Style' .... 10.5 oz | 260 | 35 | 8.0 |
| w/meat sauce, frozen, 'LightStyle' .... 10 oz | 290 | 36 | 8.0 |

(Lean Cuisine)
chicken, scaloppini, frozen, 'Café Classics' .... 1 pkg	290	34	8.0
classic .... 1 entrée	290	38	6.0
5-cheese, frozen, food service product .... 1 oz	27	3	0.7

Food Name	Serv. Size	Total Cal.	Carbs GMS	Fat GMS
'Hearty Portions'	1 entrée	440	64	9.0
tuna, w/spinach noodles, frozen	9.75 oz	240	29	7.0
vegetable	1 entrée	260	35	7.0
w/meat sauce	1 entrée	290	35	8.0
w/meat sauce, frozen	10.25 oz	280	36	6.0
(Legume)				
vegetable, w/tofu and sauce	12 oz	240	26	8.0
vegetarian, nondairy, classic, w/organic pasta and tofu	1 serving	340	37	13.0
vegetable, vegetarian, nondairy, w/organic pasta and tofu	1 serving	210	24	7.0
(Libby's) w/meat sauce, microwave cup, 'Diner'	7.75 oz	200	29	5.0
(Lunch Bucket) w/meat sauce, microwave lunch cup	7.5 oz	220	38	4.0
(Lunch Express)				
casserole, cheese	1 entrée	270	38	7.0
w/meat sauce	1 entrée	330	42	10.0
(Marie Callender's)				
extra cheese	1 cup	350	36	16.0
w/meat sauce	15 oz	370	34	18.0
w/meat sauce, frozen, family size	1 cup	350	32	16.0
(Mrs. Paul's) seafood, frozen, 'Light'	9.5 oz	290	39	8.0
(Nalley's) canned	7.5 oz	180	24	5.0
(Smart Ones)				
Alfredo	1 entrée	300	46	7.0
Florentine	1 entrée	200	34	2.0
w/meat sauce	1 entrée	240	43	2.0
(Stouffer's)				
fiesta, w/meat, frozen, food service product	1 oz	43	4	2.0
frozen, 96-oz pkg.	9 3/5 oz	400	37	14.0
frozen, 21-oz pkg.	10.5 oz	360	33	13.0
frozen, 10-oz pkg.	10 oz	340	40	12.0
vegetable	1 entrée	450	41	23.0
vegetable, frozen, 96-oz pkg.	9.6 oz	400	33	20.0
w/meat and sauce, frozen	1 pkg	768	73	29.8
w/meat and sauce	1 serving	277	26	10.8
w/meat and sauce, frozen, food service product	1 entrée	40	4	1.7
w/meat sauce	1 entrée	360	34	13.0
w/meat sauce, frozen, food service product	1 oz	39	3	1.6
(Swanson)				
w/meat sauce	1 entrée	340	37	12.0
w/meat sauce, frozen, 'Homestyle Recipe'	10.5 oz	400	39	15.0
(Top Shelf)				
Italian, packaged	10 oz	350	30	16.0
vegetable, packaged	10.6 oz	275	34	8.0
(Tyson) frozen 'Gourmet Selection'	11.5 oz	380	47	14.0
(Ultra Slim Fast)				
vegetable	12 oz	240	39	4.0
w/meat sauce	12 oz	330	38	9.0
(Weight Watchers)				
Bolognese	1 entrée	300	45	7.0
cheese, Italian	1 entrée	300	38	8.0
garden	1 entrée	270	36	7.0
w/cheese, meat, and tomato sauce	11-oz entrée	358	38	13.2
w/meat sauce	1 entrée	270	38	7.0

LASAGNA NOODLE. See under PASTA.
LAVER. See under SEA VEGETABLE.
LEEK
Fresh

boiled, drained, chopped	1/4 cup	8	2	0.1

Food Name	Serv. Size	Total Cal.	Carbs GMS	Fat GMS
boiled, drained, whole	1 medium	38	9	0.2
raw, chopped	1 cup	54	13	0.3
raw, whole	1 medium	54	13	0.3
Freeze-dried				
bulb/lower leaf portion	1/4 cup	3	1	0.0
bulb/lower leaf portion	1 tbsp	1	0	0.0
LEMON				
Fresh				
raw, sectioned, w/o peel	1 cup	61	20	0.6
raw, sliced, w/o peel, 1/8 of 2 1/8 inch diam lemon	1 wedge	2	1	0.0
raw, whole, w/o peel, 2 1/8 inch diam	1 lemon	17	5	0.2
raw, w/peel, w/o seeds, 2 3/8 inch diam	1 lemon	22	12	0.3
LEMON HERB SEASONING. See under SEASONING MIX.				
LEMON JUICE				
Canned or bottled				
	1 cup	51	16	0.7
	1 fl oz	6	2	0.1
	1 tbsp	3	1	0.0
unsweetened, single strength	1 cup	54	16	0.8
unsweetened, single strength	1 fl oz	7	2	0.1
(A&P) reconstituted, natural strength	1 fl oz	6	2	1.0
(Lucky Leaf)	6 fl oz	30	6	0.0
(ReaLemon)				
reconstituted, natural strength	1 fl oz	6	2	0.0
reconstituted, '100%'	1 fl oz	6	2	0.0
Fresh				
	1 cup	61	21	0.0
	1 fl oz	8	3	0.0
juice of 1/8 of 2 1/8 inch-diam lemon	0.2 oz	1	1	0.0
juice of 2 1/8 inch-diam lemon	1.6 oz	12	4	0.0
Frozen				
(Minute Maid) concentrate, prepared.	6 fl oz	8	2	0.0
(Sunkist)	1 fl oz	7	2	0.1
LEMON PEEL				
raw, grated	1 tbsp	3	1	0.0
raw, grated	1 tsp	1	0	0.0
raw, grated (Tone's)	1 tsp	0	0	0.0
LEMON PEPPER. See under SEASONING MIX.				
LEMONADE. See under FRUIT DRINK; FRUIT DRINK MIX.				
LEMONGRASS/citronella				
raw	1 cup	66	17	0.3
raw	1 tbsp	5	1	0.0
LEMON-LIME DRINK. See under FRUIT DRINK.				
LENTIL				
Canned, organic (Eden Foods)	1/2 cup	90	13	0.0
Dried				
boiled (A&P)	1 cup	210	39	1.0
green, raw (Arrowhead Mills)	2 oz	190	35	1.0
mature seeds, boiled	1 cup	230	40	0.8
mature seeds, boiled	1 tbsp	14	2	0.0
mature seeds, raw	1 cup	649	110	1.8
mature seeds, raw	1 tbsp	41	7	0.1
pink, raw	1 cup	664	114	4.2
red, raw (Arrowhead Mills)	2 oz	195	34	1.0
Sprouted, raw	1 cup	82	17	0.4
LENTIL DISH/ENTRÉE				
(Casbah) pilaf, prepared	3/4 cup	240	38	0.5

Food Name	Serv. Size	Total Cal.	Carbs GMS	Fat GMS
(Health Valley) canned, w/garden vegetables, nonfat, canned,				
'Fast Menu'	7.5 oz	160	18	4.0
(Natural Touch) lentil rice loaf	1 slice	166	15	8.6
LETTUCE				
BIBB, BOSTON, OR BUTTERHEAD				
leaf, large	1 leaf	2	0	0.0
leaf, medium	1 leaf	1	0	0.0
leaf, small	1 leaf	1	0	0.0
shredded	1 cup	7	1	0.1
whole *(Dole)*	1 med head	21	4	0.1
whole, approx 5-inch diam	1 head	21	4	0.4
COS				
inner leaf, whole	1 med leaf	1	0	0.0
shredded	1/2 cup	4	1	0.1
ICEBERG				
leaf, large	1 leaf	2	0	0.0
leaf, medium	1 leaf	1	0	0.0
leaf, small	1 leaf	1	0	0.0
shredded or chopped	1 cup	7	1	0.1
wedge, 1/6 of med head *(Dole)*	1 wedge	20	4	0.0
whole, approx 6-inch diam	1 head	65	11	1.0
LEAF, shredded *(Dole)*	1.5 cup	12	1	0.0
LOOSELEAF				
leaf, medium	1 leaf	2	0	0.0
shredded	1/2 cup	5	1	0.1
ROMAINE				
inner leaf, whole	1 leaf	1	0	0.0
shredded	1/2 cup	4	1	0.1
shredded *(Dole)*	1.5 cup	18	2	1.0
LICHI. See LITCHI.				
LIMA BEAN. See BEAN, LIMA; BEAN DISH/ENTRÉE.				
LIME				
fresh, raw, peeled and seeded	1 oz	9	3.0	0.1
fresh, raw, whole, approx 2-inch dia	1 lime	20	7	0.1
LIME DRINK. See under FRUIT DRINK.				
LIME JUICE				
Canned or bottled				
unsweetened	1 cup	52	16	0.6
unsweetened	1 fl oz	6	2	0.1
(ReaLime)				
original, unsweetened	1 tbsp	0	0	0.0
reconstituted, natural strength	1 fl oz	6	2	0.0
(Roses)	1 fl oz	48	12	0.0
(Santa Cruz Natural) organic, 'Cruz'	8 fl oz	120	27	1.0
Fresh				
	1 cup	66	22	0.2
	1 fl oz	8	3	0.0
juice of 2 1/8 inch-diam lime	1.3 oz	10	3	0.0
juice of 1/8 of 2 1/8 inch-diam lime	0.2 oz	1	0	0.0
LIMEADE. See under FRUIT DRINK.				
LING				
baked, broiled, grilled, or microwaved	3 oz	94	0	0.7
raw	3 oz	74	0	0.5
LINGCOD				
baked, broiled, grilled, or microwaved	3 oz	93	0	1.2
raw	3 oz	72	0	0.9
LINGUINE. See under PASTA.				

Food Name	Serv. Size	Total Cal.	Carbs GMS	Fat GMS
LINGUINE DISH/ENTRÉE. See under PASTA DISH/ENTRÉE.				
LIQUEUR				
COFFEE				
w/cream, 34 proof	1 fl oz	102	7	4.9
53 proof	1 fl oz	117	16	0.1
63 proof	1 fl oz	107	11	0.1
CRÈME DE MENTHE				
72 proof	1 fl oz	125	14	0.1
LIQUOR. See individual listings.				
LITCHI/lychee				
dried	3.5 oz	277	70.7	1.2
dried	1 oz	79	20.0	0.3
dried	1 medium	7	2	0.0
raw	1 cup	125	31	0.8
raw, shelled and seeded	1/2 cup	63	15.7	0.4
raw, shelled and seeded	1 oz	19	4.7	0.1
raw, trimmed, approx 0.6 oz	1 medium	6	2	0.0
raw, untrimmed	1 lb	179	45.0	1.2
LIVER. See under individual meat listings. Also see PÂTÉ, CANNED.				
LIVERWURST. See under LUNCHEON MEAT.				
LOBSTER				
NORTHERN				
boiled, poached, or steamed	1 cup	142	1.9	0.9
boiled, poached or steamed	4 oz	111	1.5	0.7
raw	1 lb	410	2.3	4.1
raw	3 oz	77	0.4	0.8
raw	1 oz	26	0.1	0.3
SPINY, MIXED SPECIES				
boiled, poached or steamed	3 oz	122	2.7	1.6
raw	1 lb	506	11.0	6.9
raw	3 oz	95	2.1	1.3
raw	1 oz	32	0.7	0.4
LOGANBERRY				
Fresh				
raw, trimmed	1 lb	281	67.6	2.7
raw, trimmed	1 cup	89	21.5	0.9
raw, untrimmed	1 lb	267	64.2	2.6
Frozen				
	1 cup	81	19.1	0.5
	4 oz	62	14.8	0.4
LONGAN/dragon's eye				
Dried	1 oz	81	21.0	0.1
Fresh				
raw, approx 0.2 oz	1 medium	2	0.5	tr
raw, shelled and seeded	1 oz	17	4.3	<.1
raw, untrimmed	1 lb	144	36.4	0.2
LONGBEAN				
Fresh				
boiled, drained	4 oz	53	10.4	0.1
boiled, drained, sliced	1/2 cup	25	4.8	0.1
boiled, drained, 13 1/4 inches long x 1/4 inch diam	1 pod	7	1.3	<.1
raw, sliced	1/2 cup	22	3.8	0.2
raw, 13 1/4 inches long x 1/4 inch diam	1 pod	6	1.0	0.1
raw, trimmed	1 oz	13	2.4	0.1
raw, untrimmed	1 lb	203	36.0	1.7
Dried				
boiled	1/2 cup	102	18.1	0.4

Food Name	Serv. Size	Total Cal.	Carbs GMS	Fat GMS
boiled	4 oz	134	23.9	0.5
raw	1/2 cup	292	52.0	1.1
raw	1 oz	98	17.6	0.4

LOOFAH GOURD. See GOURD, DISHCLOTH.

LOQUAT/Japanese medlar

raw, cubed	1 cup	70	18	0.3
raw, whole, large	1 fruit	9	2	0.0
raw, whole, medium	1 fruit	8	2	0.0
raw, whole, small	1 fruit	6	2	0.0

LOTTE. See MONKFISH.

LOTUS ROOT

boiled, drained, sliced	1/2 cup	40	10	0.0
raw, whole, 9.5-inch long	1 root	85	20	0.1

LOTUS SEED

dried	1 cup	106	21	0.6
dried, whole, approx 42 kernels	1 oz	94	18	0.6
raw	1 oz	25	5	0.1

LOX. See under SALMON, CHINOOK.

LUNCH COMBINATION, PACKAGED

(Eckrich)

ham and Swiss, crackers, 'Lunch Makers'	1 piece	40	2	2.0
turkey and cheddar, crackers, 'Lunch Makers'	1 piece	40	2	2.0

(Hillshire Farm)

bologna and American, cracker, Snickers, 6-oz drink	1 lunch	590	55	34.0
bologna and American, cracker, Snickers, w/o drink	1 lunch	490	31	34.0
chicken and Monterey Jack, cracker, Snickers	1 lunch	400	31	23.0
ham and cheddar, cracker, Snickers, w/o drink	1 lunch	400	32	23.0
ham and cheddar, cracker, Snickers, 6 oz drink	1 lunch	500	56	23.0
ham and Swiss, cracker, Oreo, 'Lunch'n Munch'	1 lunch	370	30	21.0
turkey and cheddar, cracker, brownie	1 lunch	400	34	22.0

(Louis Rich)

turkey breast and cheddar cheese, 'Lunch Breaks'	1 pkg	410	23	26.0
turkey ham and Swiss cheese, 'Lunch Breaks'	1 pkg	380	25	22.0
turkey salami and cheddar cheese, 'Lunch Breaks'	1 pkg	430	25	29.0
turkey, w/Monterey Jack cheese, 'Lunch Breaks'	1 pkg	400	27	25.0

(Oscar Mayer)

bologna and American lunch, 'Lunchables'	1 lunch	470	22	35.0
bologna and wild cherry lunch, 'Lunchables'	1 lunch	530	60	28.0
chicken and turkey lunch, 'Deluxe' 'Lunchables'	1 lunch	390	25	23.0
chicken w/Monterey Jack, cracker, pudding, 'Lunchables'	1 lunch	380	32	21.0
ham and cheddar lunch, 'Lunchables'	1 lunch	360	21	22.0
ham and Swiss lunch, 'Lunchables'	1 lunch	340	20	20.0
ham w/American cheese, cracker, pudding, 'Lunchables'	1 lunch	410	33	23.0
ham w/fruit punch, 'Lunchables'	1 lunch	440	54	20.0
ham w/Surfer Cooler, low-fat, 'Lunchables'	1 lunch	390	58	11.0
ham w/Swiss, cracker, cookie, 'Lunchables'	1 lunch	380	29	23.0
ham w/fruit punch, low-fat, 'Lunchables'	1 lunch	330	48	9.0
pepperoni pizza, 'Lunchables'	1 lunch	310	30	15.0
pepperoni pizza and orange, 'Lunchables'	1 lunch	460	62	16.0
pizza lunch, extra cheesy, 'Lunchables'	1 lunch	300	30	13.0
pizza lunch, extra cheesy, w/fruit punch, 'Lunchables'	1 lunch	450	63	15.0
smokie links sausage, 'Lunchables'	1 lunch	130	1	12.0
turkey, lowfat, w/Pacific Cooler, 'Lunchables'	1 lunch	360	56	9.0
turkey, w/Pacific Cooler, 'Lunchables'	1 lunch	450	54	20.0
turkey, w/Surfer Cooler, 'Lunchables'	1 lunch	430	61	15.0
turkey and cheddar, 'Lunchables'	1 lunch	350	22	20.0
turkey and ham, deluxe, 'Lunchables'	1 lunch	370	25	21.0

Food Name	Serv. Size	Total Cal.	Carbs GMS	Fat GMS
turkey w/cheddar, cracker, trail mix	1 lunch	460	41	26.0
turkey w/Monterey Jack, wheat cracker, 'Lunchables'	1 lunch	360	18	22.0
(Star-Kist) 'Charlie's Lunch Kit' w/1 mayo packet	4.6 oz	290	16	15.0
LUNCHEON MEAT				
BARBECUE LOAF *(Oscar Mayer)*	1 oz	46	2	2.3
BEEF				
(Boar's Head)				
roast, top round, oven-roasted	1 oz	40	1	1.0
roast, top round, oven-roasted, 'Deluxe'	1 oz	45	1	2.0
(Carl Budding)				
peppered, smoked, sliced, chopped, 'Lean'	1 oz	40	1	2.0
smoked, sliced	1 pkg	99	0	4.6
smoked, sliced	2 oz	79	0	3.7
smoked, sliced, chopped, 'Lean'	1 oz	40	1	2.0
(Eckrich) 'Slender Sliced'	1 oz	35	1	1.0
(Healthy Deli)				
roast	1 oz	30	0	0.4
roast, Italian	1 oz	31	0	0.6
(Hillshire Farm) roast, cured 'Deli Select'	1 oz	31	1	0.5
(Hormel)				
jellied, 'Perma-Fresh'	2 slices	90	0	4.0
smoked, cured	1 oz	50	0	2.0
smoked, cured, dried	1 oz	45	0	1.0
(Oscar Mayer)				
'Deli Thin'	4 slices	60	1	1.5
roast, 'Thin Sliced'	0.4 oz	14	0	0.4
smoked	0.5 oz	14	0	0.3
BOLOGNA				
(Bar-S) chicken, 'Tasty Bolony'	1 slice	70	3	5.0
(Boar's Head)				
beef	1 oz	74	1	7.0
ham	1 oz	40	1	2.0
pork and beef	1 oz	80	1	7.0
(Butterball)				
'Turkey Variety Pak'	3/4 oz	50	1	4.0
turkey 'Deli/Slice 'n Serve'	1 oz	70	2	6.0
turkey, 'Cold Cuts'	1 oz	70	2	6.0
(Eckrich)				
	1 oz	100	1	9.0
beef	1 oz	90	1	8.0
beef, 'Thick Sliced'	1.5 oz	130	2	12.0
garlic	1 oz	90	1	9.0
'German Brand'	1 oz	80	1	7.0
'Lean Supreme'	1 oz	70	1	6.0
'Sandwich'	1 oz	100	1	9.0
'Smorgas Pac'	1 oz	100	1	9.0
thick sliced, 1-lb pkg	1.8 oz	170	2	15.0
w/cheese	1 oz	90	1	9.0
(Empire Kosher)				
chicken, kosher	3 slices	200	2	7.0
turkey, kosher, sliced	3 slices	90	3	5.5
(Grillmaster) chicken	1 slice	70	1	6.0
(Health Valley) chicken	1 slice	85	1	8.0
(Healthy Choice)				
beef, low-fat, 'Cold Cuts'	1 slice	35	3	1.0
low-fat, 'Deli-Thin'	4 slices	60	5	1.5
turkey, pork and beef, low-fat, 'Cold Cuts'	1 slice	30	3	1.0

Food Name	Serv. Size	Total Cal.	Carbs GMS	Fat GMS
(Healthy Deli) beef and pork	1 oz	41	1	2.0
(Healthy Favorites) sliced	21 grams	20	1	0.3
(Hebrew National) beef, 'Original Deli Style'	1 oz	90	1	3.0
(Hillshire Farm)				
'Large'	1 oz	90	1	8.0
'Ring'	1 oz	89	1	8.0
(Hormel)				
beef, 'Coarse Ground, 1 lb.'	2 oz	160	1	14.0
beef, 'Perma-Fresh'	2 slices	170	1	16.0
'Fine Ground, 1-lb.'	2 oz	170	1	16.0
'Perma-Fresh'	2 slices	180	0	16.0
(JM)				
'German Brand'	1 oz	70	1	6.0
beef	1 oz	90	1	8.0
garlic	1 oz	90	1	8.0
(Kahn's)				
beef	1 slice	90	1	8.0
beef, 'Family Pack'	1 slice	70	1	6.0
beef, 'Giant'	1 slice	90	1	8.0
beef, 'Pounder'	1 slice	90	1	8.0
beef and cheddar	1 slice	90	1	8.0
'Deluxe Club Family Pack'	1 slice	70	1	6.0
'Deluxe Club'	1 slice	90	1	8.0
garlic	1 slice	90	1	8.0
'Giant Deluxe'	1 slice	90	1	8.0
'Giant Thick Deluxe'	1 slice	110	1	10.0
'Thick Deluxe'	1 slice	140	1	13.0
'Thin Sliced Deluxe'	1 slice	60	1	5.0
(Light and Lean)				
	2 slices	140	2	12.0
'Thin Sliced'	2 slices	70	1	6.0
(Longacre) turkey, sliced	1 oz	61	0	5.0
(Louis Rich)				
turkey, mild	1 oz	59	1	4.5
turkey	1 slice	52	1	3.7
(Mr. Turkey) turkey	1 slice	67	1	5.6
(Norbest) turkey, 'Blue Label' 2–2.5 lb.	1 oz	68	1	5.6
(OHSE)				
	1 slice	130	1	11.0
	1 oz	75	3	6.0
beef	1 oz	85	1	8.0
'15% Chicken'	1 oz	90	1	8.0
turkey	1 oz	70	2	6.0
(Oscar Mayer)				
	1 slice	90	1	8.0
beef	1 slice	89	1	8.2
beef, Lebanon	0.8 oz	46	0	2.9
beef, light	1 slice	55	2	4.0
chicken, pork, and beef	1 slice	89	1	8.2
fat-free	1 slice	22	2	0.2
garlic	1 slice	130	1	12.0
light	1 slice	60	2	4.0
pork, chicken, and beef, light	1 slice	56	2	4.1
Wisconsin made ring	1 slice	175	1	15.9
w/cheese	0.8 oz	74	1	6.8
(Pilgrim's Pride)	1 oz	59	1	4.4
(Smok-a-Roma) chicken, pork, and beef	1 slice	80	1	6.0

Food Name	Serv. Size	Total Cal.	Carbs GMS	Fat GMS
(Tyson) chicken	1 slice	44	4	0.5
CHICKEN BREAST				
(Carl Budding)				
smoked, sliced, chopped, 'Lean'	1 oz	50	1	3.0
smoked, w/dark meat, sliced	1 pkg	117	0	7.2
smoked, w/dark meat, sliced	2 oz	94	0	5.7
(Healthy Choice)				
roasted, 'Cold Cuts'	1 slice	25	2	0.0
roasted, 'Fresh Trak'	1 slice	35	2	1.0
smoked, 'Cold Cuts'	1 slice	30	2	1.0
(Healthy Favorites)				
oven-roasted, fat-free, thin sliced	4 slices	40	1	0.0
oven-roasted, thin sliced	1 slice	12	1	1.0
(Hillshire Farm) smoked, boneless, 'Deli Select'	1 slice	31	1	0.2
(Land O'Frost) smoked, thin sliced	2.5 oz	120	0	7.0
(Longacre) 'Premium'	1 slice	45	1	3.0
(Louis Rich)				
baked, 'Classic Baked Grill'	1 slice	44	2	0.2
baked, thin sliced, 'Classic Baked Grill'	1 slice	22	1	0.1
hickory smoked, boneless	1 slice	30	1	0.8
hickory smoked, boneless, 97% fat-free	1 slice	30	1	1.0
honey glazed, 'Carving Board'	1 slice	23	1	0.3
roasted, 'Cold Cuts'	1 slice	36	1	1.6
roasted, deluxe, 'Cold Cuts'	1 slice	28	1	0.6
roasted, thin sliced, 'Deli Thin'	1 slice	15	0	0.4
(Mr. Turkey)				
boneless	1 slice	32	1	1.1
smoked, 'Deli Cut'	3 slices	28	2	0.1
(Oscar Mayer)				
honey glazed, roasted	1 slice	57	2	0.7
honey glazed, roasted, thin sliced	1 slice	14	1	0.2
oven-roasted	1 slice	29	1	0.7
roasted, fat-free	1 slice	44	1	0.3
roasted, fat-free, thin sliced	1 slice	11	0	0.1
smoked	1 slice	25	0	0.4
'Thin Sliced'	1 slice	13	0	0.4
(Tyson)				
breast, hickory smoked	1 slice	25	1	1.0
honey flavored	1 slice	25	1	1.0
mesquite, oven-roasted	1 slice	25	1	1.0
oven-roasted	1 slice	25	1	0.5
CHICKEN ROLL				
(Longacre) sliced	1 slice	60	1	5.0
(Pilgrim's Pride)	1 slice	35	0	1.2
(Tyson)	1 slice	26	1	0.5
CORNED BEEF LOAF				
jellied	1 slice	43	0	1.7
(Carl Budding)				
chopped, pressed	1 pkg	101	1	4.8
chopped, pressed	2 oz	81	1	3.9
DUTCH LOAF				
(Eckrich)				
'Lean Supreme'	1 slice	60	2	4.0
'Smorgas Pac'	1 slice	70	2	6.0
(Kahn's)	1 slice	80	1	7.0
HAM				
(Boar's Head)				
boiled, 'Deluxe'	1 oz	28	1	1.0

Food Name	Serv. Size	Total Cal.	Carbs GMS	Fat GMS
'Lower Salt'	1 slice	28	1	1.0
(Butterball)				
turkey, 'Cold Cuts'	1 oz	35	1	1.0
turkey, honey cured, chopped 'Cold Cuts'	1 oz	35	2	1.0
turkey, honey cured, 'Cold Cuts'	1 oz	35	1	1.0
turkey, honey cured, 'Slice 'n Serve'	1 oz	40	1	2.0
turkey, 'Slice 'n Serve'	1 oz	35	1	2.0
turkey, sliced, 'Deli Thin'	1 oz	35	1	1.0
(Carl Budding)				
honey, smoked, sliced, chopped, 'Lean'	1 slice	50	1	3.0
smoked, sliced	1 pkg	116	1	6.6
smoked, sliced	2 oz	92	1	5.3
smoked, sliced, chopped, 'Lean'	1 slice	50	1	3.0
(Danola)				
Danish, premium, 97% fat-free	1 slice	30	1	1.0
Danish, premium, 97% fat-free, thin sliced	2 slices	45	0	1.0
(Decker) chopped	1 slice	100	2	8.0
(Eckrich)				
chopped	1 slice	45	1	2.0
chopped, 'Lean Supreme'	1 slice	35	1	2.0
smoked, 'Slender Sliced'	1 slice	40	1	2.0
(Healthy Choice)				
baked, water added, 'Cold Cuts'	1 slice	30	1	1.0
cooked, water added, 'Fresh Trak'	1 slice	30	1	1.0
honey, water added, 'Cold Cuts'	1 slice	30	1	1.0
honey, water added, 'Fresh Trak'	1 slice	30	1	1.0
smoked, water added, 'Cold Cuts'	1 slice	30	1	1.0
(Healthy Deli)				
baked, Virginia	1 slice	34	2	0.9
baked, Virginia, less salt	1 slice	32	1	0.9
Black Forest	1 slice	32	0	0.6
cooked, fresh	1 slice	33	0	0.8
'Deluxe'	1 slice	31	1	0.9
honey, 'Honey Valley'	1 slice	31	1	0.8
jalapeño	1 slice	25	1	0.6
'Lessalt'	1 slice	32	1	0.9
'Taverne'	1 slice	31	0	0.8
(Healthy Favorites)				
baked, 98% fat-free	4 slices	50	1	1.0
boiled, thin sliced	1 slice	12	1	1.0
chicken, smoked, w/natural juices, thin sliced	1 slice	13	0	0.4
honey, thin sliced	1 slice	14	1	1.0
honey, water added, 'Breakfast'	1 slice	30	1	0.9
honey baked, 98% fat-free, thin sliced	4 slices	50	2	1.5
smoked, cooked, thin sliced	1 slice	14	1	1.0
(Hormel)				
'Cure 81'	1 slice	89	0	3.0
deli, cooked	1 slice	29	1	1.0
chopped, 'Black Label'	1 slice	70	1	6.0
chopped, 'Perma-Fresh'	2 slices	88	0	5.0
(Jennie-O)				
turkey, cooked, natural smoked flavoring, cured	2 oz	80	1	4.5
turkey, cooked, smoke flavoring, lean, 20% water added	2 oz	70	0	3.5
(JM)				
chopped	1 slice	80	1	7.0
cooked	1 slice	30	1	1.0
'Slice 'n Eat 93% Fat-Free'	2 oz	70	1	3.0

Food Name	Serv. Size	Total Cal.	Carbs GMS	Fat GMS
'Slice 'n Eat 95% Fat-Free Presliced'	2 slices	60	1	2.0
smoked, golden	2 slices	80	1	5.0
smoked, golden, water added	2 slices	70	4	2.0
(Jones Dairy Farm)				
'Farm'	1 slice	50	0	1.1
'Farm Family Ham'	1 slice	35	0	1.2
hickory smoked, 97% fat-free, 'Lean Choice'	2 slices	50	0	1.5
(Kahn's)				
low-salt	1 slice	30	1	1.0
chopped	1 slice	50	1	3.0
cooked, sliced	1 slice	30	1	1.0
(Light and Lean)				
barbecue	2 slices	50	0	2.0
black peppered	2 slices	50	0	2.0
chopped	2 slices	70	0	4.0
cooked, sliced	2 slices	50	0	2.0
glazed	2 slices	50	0	2.0
red peppered	2 slices	50	0	2.0
smoked, cooked	2 slices	50	0	2.0
(Longacre)				
turkey, chunk	1 oz	37	0	2.0
turkey, lean, lite, 'Deli'	1 oz	37	0	2.0
turkey, sliced	1 oz	33	0	1.0
(Louis Rich)				
baked, dinner slices	1 slice	80	1	1.5
turkey, chopped	1 oz	46	0	2.8
turkey, cured	1 oz	25	1	0.7
turkey, 'Deli Thin'	1 slice	15	0	0.4
turkey, 15% water added, 'Cold Cuts'	1 slice	45	1	2.5
turkey, honey cured, 'Cold Cuts' 15% water added	1 slice	30	1	1.0
turkey, 96% fat-free, 'Deli-Thin'	1 slice	15	1	1.0
turkey, 96% fat-free, square	1 slice	25	1	1.0
turkey, 'Round'	1 oz	34	0	1.2
turkey, 'Square'	1 slice	24	0	0.7
turkey, 10% water added, 'Cold Cuts'	1 slice	35	0	1.0
turkey, 10% water added, 'Square'	1 serving	32	0	1.1
turkey, thin sliced	1 slice	12	0	0.4
turkey, water added	1 oz	33	0	1.4
turkey, water added, 94% fat-free	1 oz	35	1	2.0
turkey, water added, 95% fat-free, round	1 slice	30	1	1.0
(Mr. Turkey)				
turkey	1 slice	33	0	1.4
turkey, chopped	1 oz	37	0	1.6
turkey, smoked	1 slice	33	0	1.4
turkey, smoked, breakfast	1 oz	33	0	1.3
turkey, smoked, buffet style	1 oz	32	0	1.3
turkey, smoked, 'Chub'	1 oz	32	0	1.3
(Norbest)				
turkey, dark meat, hickory smoked	1 oz	39	0	2.2
turkey, thigh meat, cured, Canadian style	1 oz	35	0	1.4
turkey, thigh meat, cured, 'Gold Label'	1 oz	27	0	0.7
turkey, thigh meat, cured, half, 'Tavern'	1 oz	29	1	0.8
turkey, thigh meat cured, whole, 'Tavern'	1 oz	27	0	0.8
(OHSE)				
chopped	1 slice	65	1	5.0
cooked	1 slice	30	1	1.0
pit	1 slice	40	1	2.0

Food Name	Serv. Size	Total Cal.	Carbs GMS	Fat GMS
smoked, 95% fat-free	1 slice	30	1	1.0
turkey	1 oz	30	2	1.0
(Oscar Mayer)				
baked	1 slice	21	0	0.5
baked, water added, 96% fat free	1 slice	65	1	2.3
baked, water added, 96% fat free, thin sliced	1 slice	22	0	0.8
black peppered, cracked	1 slice	22	0	0.8
boiled	1 slice	23	0	0.7
boiled, thin sliced	1 slice	13	0	0.4
boiled, water added, thin sliced	4 slices	50	0	2.0
chopped	1 slice	50	1	3.0
chopped, w/natural juice	1 slice	52	1	3.4
honey, thin sliced	1 slice	13	0	0.4
'Jubilee'	1 slice	43	0	2.4
peppered, chopped	1 slice	55	1	3.7
smoked, 40% ham/water product	1 slice	34	1	0.3
smoked, 40% ham/water product, thin sliced	1 slice	12	0	0.1
water added, boiled	1 slice	22	0	0.8
water added, smoked, cooked	1 slice	21	0	0.8
(Pilgrim's Pride) chicken	1 slice	35	1	1.8
(Smok-a-Roma) cooked, 95% fat-free	1 slice	35	0	1.5
(Swift)				
'Premium Hostess'	1 slice	30	0	1.0
'Premium Sugar Plum'	1 slice	30	1	1.0
(Tyson) turkey	1 slice	23	1	0.2
HEAD CHEESE *(Oscar Mayer)*	1 slice	52	0	3.8
HAM LOAF *(Eckrich)*	1 slice	50	1	4.0
HAM AND CHEESE LOAF				
(Eckrich)	1 oz slice	50	1	4.0
(Hormel)				
canned, 8-lb	3 oz	260	1	22.0
'Perma-Fresh'	2 slices	110	0	7.0
(Kahn's)	1 slice	70	1	6.0
(Light and Lean)	2 slices	90	0	6.0
(OHSE)	1 oz	65	2	5.0
(Oscar Mayer)	1 slice	66	1	5.0
HONEY LOAF				
(Eckrich) 'Smorgas Pac'	1 oz slice	35	2	1.0
(Hormel) 'Perma-Fresh'	2 slices	90	0	5.0
(Kahn's)	1 slice	40	1	2.0
(Oscar Mayer)	1 slice	34	1	1.0
IOWA BRAND LOAF *(Hormel)* 'Perma-Fresh'	2 slices	90	0	6.0
JALAPEÑO LOAF *(Kahn's)*	1 slice	70	2	6.0
LIVER CHEESE				
(JM)	1 oz slice	70	1	6.0
(Oscar Mayer) pork fat wrapped	1 slice	114	1	9.9
LIVER LOAF				
(Hormel) 'Perma-Fresh'	2 slices	160	1	13.0
(Kahn's)	1 slice	170	3	15.0
LIVERWURST				
(Hickory Farms)	1 oz	97	1	9.0
(Hormel) canned	0.5 oz	35	0	3.0
(Jones Dairy Farm)				
'Farm Club'	1 oz	80	0	6.3
'Farm Slices'	1 slice	75	0	6.6
(Oscar Mayer)				
Braunschweiger, sliced	1 slice	94	1	8.5

Food Name	Serv. Size	Total Cal.	Carbs GMS	Fat GMS
Braunschweiger, tube	1 serving	191	1	17.1
(Underwood) canned	2 1/8 oz	180	4	15.0
LOAF				
(Armour)				
canned, 'Treet'	2 oz	200	3	17.0
low-salt, canned, 'Treet'	2 oz	190	3	16.0
(Hormel)				
pork w/chicken, light, 'Spam'	2 oz	108	1	7.8
pork w/ham, 'Spam'	2 oz	172	1	15.6
pork w/ham, less salt, 'Spam'	2 oz	176	1	15.0
pork w/ham, light, 'Spam'	2 oz	140	1	12.0
pork w/ham, smoke-flavored, 'Spam'	2 oz	170	0	15.0
pork w/ham, w/cheese chunks, 'Spam'	2 oz	170	0	16.0
(JM) 'P&B'	1 slice	70	2	5.0
(Kahn's) 'P&B'	1 slice	40	1	2.0
(OHSE)				
	1 slice	100	2	8.0
	1 oz	75	1	6.0
(Oscar Mayer) spiced	1 slice	70	2	5.0
(Smok-a-Roma)				
	2 slices	90	0	8.0
spiced	1 slice	90	2	7.0
MACARONI AND CHEESE LOAF				
(Eckrich)	1 slice	75	3	6.0
(OHSE)	1 slice	60	4	3.0
OLD FASHIONED LOAF *(Oscar Mayer)*	1 slice	65	2	4.6
OLIVE LOAF				
(Eckrich)	1 slice	80	2	6.0
(Hormel) 'Perma-Fresh'	2 slices	110	5	7.0
(Oscar Mayer) chicken, pork, turkey	1 slice	74	2	6.1
PASTRAMI				
(Boar's Head) 'Round'	1 slice	40	1	1.5
(Butterball)				
turkey, 'Cold Cuts'	1 oz	30	0	1.0
turkey, 'Slice 'n Serve'	1 oz	35	1	1.0
(Carl Budding)				
beef, smoked, chopped, pressed	1 pkg	100	1	4.6
beef, smoked, chopped, pressed	2 oz	80	1	3.7
smoked, sliced, chopped, 'Lean'	1 slice	40	1	2.0
(Empire Kosher) turkey, kosher, sliced	3 slices	60	0	2.0
(Healthy Deli) 'Deli Round'	1 slice	34	1	1.1
(Longacre) turkey, sliced	1 oz	32	0	1.0
(Louis Rich)				
turkey	1 slice	30	0	1.0
turkey, 96% fat-free, 'Deli-Thin'	1 slice	10	1	1.0
turkey, 96% fat-free, square	1 oz slice	25	1	1.0
turkey, 'Round'	1 oz	32	0	1.1
turkey, 'Square'	1 oz	24	0	0.7
turkey, thin sliced	1 oz	11	0	0.4
(Mr. Turkey)				
turkey	1 slice	31	1	1.0
turkey, sliced, 'Deli Cut'	3 slices	36	1	1.4
(Norbest) turkey, 3 lb	1 oz	29	0	0.8
(Oscar Mayer) thin sliced	1 slice	16	0	0.3
PEPPERED LOAF				
(Eckrich)	1 slice	35	2	1.0
(Kahn's)	1 slice	40	1	2.0

Food Name	Serv. Size	Total Cal.	Carbs GMS	Fat GMS
(Oscar Mayer)	1 slice	39	1	1.5
PICKLE AND PIMIENTO LOAF				
(Oscar Mayer)				
	1 slice	80	3	6.0
w/chicken	1 serving	75	3	6.0
PICKLE LOAF				
(Eckrich) 'Smorgas Pac'	1 slice	80	2	6.0
(Hormel) 'Perma-Fresh'	2 slices	102	3	7.0
(Kahn's)				
	1 slice	80	2	7.0
beef 'Family Pack'	1 slice	60	1	5.0
'Family Pack'	1 slice	70	2	6.0
(Light and Lean)	2 slices	100	3	6.0
(OHSE)	1 oz	60	2	4.0
(Smok-a-Roma) w/turkey and pork	1 slice	90	4	6.0
PORK *(Eckrich)* 'Slender Sliced'	1 oz	45	1	2.0
SALAMI				
(Boar's Head) beef	1 oz	60	1	4.0
(Eckrich)				
beer	1 slice	70	1	6.0
cotto	1 slice	70	1	6.0
cotto, beef	1.3 oz	100	2	8.0
(Gallo Salame)				
dry, Italian, light, w/turkey, pork, and beef	7 slices	70	1	5.0
(Hebrew National) beef, 'Original Deli Style'	1 oz	80	1	7.0
(Hickory Farms)				
dry or hard	1 oz	120	0	10.0
Genoa	1 oz	110	0	10.0
(Hormel)				
beef, 'Perma-Fresh'	2 slices	50	0	5.0
cotto, 'Club'	1 oz	100	0	5.0
cotto, 'Perma-Fresh'	2 slices	105	1	7.0
dry or hard	1 oz	110	0	10.0
dry or hard, 'Homeland'	1 oz	117	2	10.0
dry or hard, 'National Brand'	1 oz	120	0	11.0
dry or hard, 'Perma-Fresh'	2 slices	80	0	7.0
dry or hard, 'Sliced'	1 oz	110	0	10.0
Genoa	1 oz	110	0	10.0
Genoa, 'DiLusso'	1 oz	100	0	8.0
Genoa, 'Gran Valore'	1 oz	110	0	10.0
Genoa, 'San Remo Brand'	1 oz	118	0	10.0
'Party'	1 oz	90	0	8.0
piccolo, 'Stick'	1 oz	120	0	11.0
(JM)				
cotto	1 oz slice	80	2	6.0
dry or hard	1 oz slice	110	1	9.0
Genoa	1 oz slice	100	1	8.0
(Kahn's)				
beef	1 slice	70	1	6.0
beef, 'Family Pack'	1 slice	60	1	5.0
cooked	1 slice	60	1	4.0
cotto, 'Family Pack'	1 slice	45	1	3.0
(Light and Lean) cotto	2 slices	80	0	6.0
(Mr. Turkey) cotto, turkey	1 slice	49	1	3.3
(OHSE) cooked	1 oz	65	1	5.0
(Oscar Mayer)				
beef, 'Machiaeh Brand'	1 slice	60	0	5.0

Food Name	Serv. Size	Total Cal.	Carbs GMS	Fat GMS
beer	1 slice	52	0	4.2
cotto	1 slice	70	1	5.0
cotto, beef	1 slice	47	0	3.6
cotto, beef, pork, and chicken	1 slice	56	1	4.7
Genoa	1 slice	35	0	3.0
hard	1 slice	36	0	2.8
SPICE LOAF				
(Hormel)				
canned	3 oz	280	2	26.0
'Perma-Fresh'	2 slices	118	1	9.0
(JM)	1 slice	70	1	6.0
(Kahn's)				
beef, 'Family Pack'	1 slice	60	1	5.0
'Family Pack'	1 slice	70	1	6.0
'Luncheon Loaf'	1 slice	80	1	7.0
(Oscar Mayer)	1 serving	66	2	4.7
TURKEY BREAST				
(Boar's Head)				
golden	1 oz	35	1	1.0
golden, skinless	1 oz	30	1	1.0
(Butterball)				
barbecue seasoned, 'Slice 'n Serve'	1 oz	40	1	2.0
'Cold Cuts'	1 oz	30	1	1.0
hickory smoked, 'Slice 'n Serve'	1 oz	35	1	1.0
no salt added, 'Deli'	1 oz	45	0	2.0
'Slice 'n Serve'	1 oz	35	1	1.0
smoked, 'Cold Cuts'	1 oz	35	0	1.0
smoked, 'Turkey Variety Pak'	3/4 oz	25	1	1.0
(Carl Budding)				
and dark meat, smoked, sliced	1 pkg	114	1	6.5
and dark meat, smoked, sliced	2 oz	91	1	5.2
smoked, sliced, chopped, 'Lean'	1 oz	50	1	3.0
(Carving Board)				
hickory-smoked	1 slice	40	0	0.5
traditional	1 slice	40	0	0.5
(Empire Kosher)				
oven prepared, kosher, sliced	3 slices	50	1	0.5
smoked, kosher, sliced	3 slices	40	0	0.0
(Healthy Choice)				
and white meat, honey roasted and smoked, 'Cold Cuts'	1 slice	35	2	1.0
honey roasted and smoked	1 slice	35	1	1.0
honey roasted and smoked, 'Fresh Trak'	1 slice	35	2	1.0
roasted, 'Cold Cuts'	1 slice	30	1	1.0
roasted, 'Fresh Trak'	1 slice	30	1	1.0
roasted, 97% fat-free	1 slice	30	1	1.0
smoked, 'Cold Cuts'	1 slice	30	2	1.0
(Healthy Deli)				
'Gourmet'	1 oz	28	1	0.6
honey	1 oz	28	1	0.5
'Lessalt'	1 oz	25	0	0.5
oven cooked	1 oz	26	0	0.2
smoked 'Gourmet'	1 oz	31	0	0.5
smoked, 3-lb	1 oz	29	1	0.5
(Healthy Favorites)				
oven-roasted	1 slice	12	1	1.0
oven-roasted, fat-free	4 slices	40	2	0.0

Food Name	Serv. Size	Total Cal.	Carbs GMS	Fat GMS
smoked . . . . 1 slice		12	1	1.0
(Hormel)				
'Perma-Fresh' . . . . 2 slices		60	0	2.0
smoked, 'Perma-Fresh' . . . . 2 slices		60	0	2.0
(Land O'Frost) smoked, thin sliced . . . . 2.5 oz		110	0	7.0
(Light and Lean) breast . . . . 2 slices		60	0	2.0
(Longacre)				
and white meat, browned and roasted . . . . 1 oz		40	1	2.0
and white meat, 'Deli Chef' . . . . 1 oz		35	1	1.0
and white meat, skinless 'Deli Chef' . . . . 1 oz		40	1	2.0
browned, glazed, 'Gourmet' . . . . 1 oz		35	1	1.0
browned, glazed, 'Premium' . . . . 1 oz		30	1	1.0
browned, roasted, 'Gourmet' . . . . 1 oz		35	1	1.0
browned, roasted, 'Premium' . . . . 1 oz		30	1	1.0
'Catering' . . . . 1 oz		35	1	1.0
'Gourmet' . . . . 1 oz		35	1	1.0
lean, lite, 'Deli' . . . . 1 oz		35	0	1.0
lean, lite, skinless, 'Deli' . . . . 1 oz		35	0	1.0
lean, lite, smoked, 'Deli' . . . . 1 oz		35	0	1.0
low-salt, 'Gourmet' . . . . 1 oz		30	1	1.0
'Premium' . . . . 1 oz		30	1	1.0
'Salt Watchers' . . . . 1 oz		32	0	1.0
skinless, 'Catering' . . . . 1 oz		35	1	1.0
skinless, 'Gourmet' . . . . 1 oz		30	1	1.0
skinless, 'Premium' . . . . 1 oz		30	1	1.0
sliced . . . . 1 oz		30	1	1.0
smoked . . . . 1 oz		35	0	1.0
smoked, sliced . . . . 1 oz		26	1	1.0
(Louis Rich)				
and white meat, roasted . . . . 1 serving		27	1	0.5
and white meat, smoked . . . . 1 serving		28	1	0.6
'Carving Board' . . . . 22 grams		21	0	0.3
cooked, barbecued, no skin . . . . 1 oz		30	1	1.0
hickory smoked . . . . 1 slice		60	2	0.0
hickory smoked, nonfat, 'Cold Cuts' . . . . 1 slice		25	1	0.0
honey roasted, 95% fat-free . . . . 1 slice		35	1	1.0
nonfat, 'Deli-Thin' . . . . 4 slices		40	2	0.0
oven-roasted . . . . 1 oz		31	1	0.8
oven-roasted, 97% fat-free, 'Deli-Thin' . . . . 1 slice		10	1	1.0
roasted . . . . 1 slice		50	1	0.0
roasted, fat-free . . . . 1 slice		24	1	0.2
roasted, nonfat, 'Cold Cuts' . . . . 1 slice		25	1	0.0
roasted, thin sliced . . . . 1 slice		12	0	0.3
smoked . . . . 1 slice		21	0	0.3
smoked, 'Carving Board' . . . . 1 slice		21	0	0.2
smoked, 98% fat-free . . . . 1 slice		20	1	1.0
smoked, 97% fat-free, 'Deli-Thin' . . . . 1 slice		10	1	1.0
smoked, 96% fat-free' . . . . 1 oz		35	1	1.0
smoked, thin sliced . . . . 0.4 oz slice		11	0	0.1
white, smoked, 'Cold Cuts' . . . . 1 slice		30	0	1.0
(Mr. Turkey)				
. . . . 1 oz		31	0	0.7
smoked . . . . 1 oz		31	0	0.7
honey roasted, 'Deli Cut' . . . . 3 slices		30	2	0.5
roasted . . . . 1 slice		33	2	0.8
roasted, quartered . . . . 3.5 oz		94	3	2.2

Food Name	Serv. Size	Total Cal.	Carbs GMS	Fat GMS
smoked, 'Deli Cut'	3 slices	24	2	0.2
smoked, quartered	3.5 oz	89	4	0.5
(Norbest)				
and thigh,'Blue Label'	1 oz	31	0	0.9
skinless, 'Blue Label'	1 oz	24	1	0.3
skinless, 'Orange Label'	1 oz	26	1	0.2
skinless, 'Tan Label'	1 oz	24	1	0.5
skinless, 'Yellow Label'	1 oz	24	0	0.5
skinless, salt-free, 'Blue Label'	1 oz	33	0	0.3
smoked, 'Gold Label'	1 oz	29	0	0.6
w/skin, 'Blue Label'	1 oz	28	0	0.7
w/skin, 'Orange Label'	1 oz	26	0	0.3
w/skin, 'Yellow Label'	1 oz	25	0	0.5
w/skin, prebrowned, 'Orange Label'	1 oz	29	0	0.8
w/skin, salt-free, 'Blue Label'	1 oz	35	0	0.5
w/skin, smoked, 'Orange Label'	1 oz	30	1	0.5
(OHSE)				
oven cooked	1 oz	30	1	1.0
smoked	1 oz	30	1	1.0
(Oscar Mayer)				
cooked, oven-roasted, thin sliced	1 slice	12	0	0.2
smoked	1 slice	20	0	0.2
roasted	4 slices	50	2	1.0
roasted, nonfat	4 slices	40	2	0.0
smoked, fat-free	1 slice	10	0	0.1
smoked, honey roasted	4 slices	60	2	1.0
smoked, nonfat	4 slices	40	2	0.0
white, roasted	1 slice	30	1	1.0
(Tyson) breast	1 slice	20	0	0.4
TURKEY HAM. See under LUNCHEON MEAT, HAM.				
TURKEY LOAF				
(Louis Rich) 89% fat-free	1 oz	45	0	2.8
(Mr. Turkey) spiced	1 oz	51	1	3.6
TURKEY ROLL				
(Norbest)				
	1 oz	31	1	1.1
white and dark meat, 'Orange Label'	1 oz	36	0	2.0
white meat, diced	1 oz	31	1	0.9
white meat, 'Orange Label'	1 oz	29	1	0.9
LUNCHEON MEAT SPREAD				
(Hormel)				
deviled, 'Spam'	1 oz	78	2	7.0
deviled, 'Spam'	1 tbsp	35	0	3.0
LUNCHEON MEAT SUBSTITUTE				
(White Wave)				
chicken style, sandwich sliced *(White Wave)*	1 slice	80	8	0.0
pastrami style, vegetarian, sandwich sliced	1 slice	90	8	0.0
(Worthington)				
bologna style, vegetarian, 'Bolono'	3 slices	79	2	3.3
salami style, vegetarian, 'Meatless Salami'	3 slices	130	2	8.0
smoked turkey style slices, vegetarian*(Worthington)*	3 slices	142	3	9.9
vegetarian, 'Numete'	3/8-inch slice	130	5	10.0
vegetarian, 'Protose'	3/8-inch slice	131	5	6.7
LUPIN				
mature seeds, boiled	1 cup	198	16	4.8
mature seeds, raw	1 cup	668	73	17.5

M

Food Name	Serv. Size	Total Cal.	Carbs GMS	Fat GMS
MACADAMIA NUT				
dried, whole, 10-12 kernels	1 oz	204	4	21.5
dried, whole or halves	1 cup	962	19	101.5
dry-roasted, salted, whole, 10-12 kernels	1 oz	203	4	21.6
dry-roasted, salted, whole or halves	1 cup	959	17	101.9
dry-roasted, unsalted, whole, 10-12 kernels	1 oz	204	4	21.6
dry-roasted, unsalted, whole or halves	1 cup	962	18	101.9
salted *(Maunu Loa)*	1 oz	210	4	21.0
shelled, salted *(Maunu Loa)*	1 oz	210	4	21.0
unsalted, natural *(Flanigan Farms)*	1/4 cup	200	4	21.0
MACADAMIA NUT BUTTER				
roasted *(Maranatha Natural)*	2 tbsp	200	6	19.0
roasted, organic *(Maranatha Natural)*	2 tbsp	230	5	24.0
MACARONI. See under PASTA.				
MACARONI DISH/ENTRÉE. See under PASTA DISH ENTRÉE.				
MACE				
ground	1 tbsp	25	3	1.7
ground	1 tsp	8	1	0.6
ground *(Durkee)*	1 tsp	10	0	0.0
ground *(Laurel Leaf)*	1 tsp	10	0	0.0
ground *(McCormick/Schilling)*	1 tsp	8	1	0.4
ground *(Spice Islands)*	1 tsp	10	1	0.7
ground *(Tone's)*	1 tsp	8	1	0.6
MACKEREL				
ATLANTIC				
baked, broiled, grilled, or microwaved	4 oz	297	0.0	20.2
baked, broiled, grilled, or microwaved	3 oz	223	0.0	15.1
raw	1 lb	929	0.0	63.0
raw	3 oz	174	0.0	11.8
JACK, mixed species				
Canned				
drained	1 cup	296	0.0	12.0
drained	4 oz	177	0.0	7.1
Fresh				
baked, broiled, grilled, or microwaved	3 oz	171	0.0	8.6
raw	1 lb	712	0.0	35.8
raw	3 oz	134	0.0	6.7
KING				
baked, broiled, grilled, or microwaved	3 oz	114	0.0	2.2
raw	1 lb	475	0.0	9.1
raw	3 oz	89	0.0	1.7
PACIFIC, mixed species				
baked, broiled, grilled, or microwaved	3 oz	171	0.0	8.6
raw	1 lb	712	0.0	35.8
raw	3 oz	134	0.0	6.7
SPANISH				
baked, broiled, grilled, or microwaved	5.1-oz fillet	231	0.0	9.2
baked, broiled, grilled, or microwaved	4 oz	179	0.0	7.2
baked, broiled, grilled, or microwaved	3 oz	134	0.0	5.4
raw	1 lb	631	0.0	28.6
raw	3 oz	118	0.0	5.3
MAHI MAHI/dolphin fish				
Fresh				
baked, broiled, grilled, or microwaved	3 oz	93	0	0.8

Food Name	Serv. Size	Total Cal.	Carbs GMS	Fat GMS
raw	3 oz	72	0	0.6
Frozen *(Peter Pan Seafoods)* fillets, boneless, skinless	3.5 oz	85	0	0.7
MAI TAI. See under COCKTAIL; COCKTAIL MIX.				
MALABAR SPINACH. See SPINACH, MALABAR.				
MALACCA APPLE, w/o seeds	1 oz	9	2.3	<.1
MALT, dry	1 oz	103	21.7	0.5
MALT EXTRACT, dried	1 oz	103	25.0	0.0
MALT SYRUP. See under SYRUP.				
MALTED MILK FLAVOR DRINK MIX				
CHOCOLATE FLAVOR				
w/added nutrients, powder, mix only	1 cup	279	66	2.7
w/added nutrients, powder, prepared w/milk	8 fl oz	225	29	8.7
w/o added nutrients, powder, mix only	1 envelope	79	18	0.8
w/o added nutrients, powder, prepared w/milk	8 fl oz *(1 cup)*	228	30	9.0
(Kraft) powder, 'Instant' mix only	3 tsp	90	18	1.0
NATURAL FLAVOR				
w/added nutrients, powder, prepared	8 fl oz *(1 cup)*	231	28	8.7
w/oadded nutrients, powder, prepared	8 fl oz *(1 cup)*	236	27	9.8
(Kraft) powder, 'Instant'	3 tsp	90	16	2.0
MAMMY APPLE				
peeled, w/o seeds	1 oz	14	3.5	0.1
raw	3-1/2 oz	51	12.5	0.5
raw, trimmed, whole, approx 3.1 lb	1 medium	431	105.8	4.2
raw, untrimmed	1 lb	139	34.0	1.4
MANDARIN ORANGE. See also TANGERINE.				
Canned				
in juice	1 cup	92	24	0.1
in light syrup	1 cup	154	41	0.3
MANGO				
Canned or jarred, sliced, chilled *(Sun Fresh)*	3.5 oz	89	21.0	0.3
Fresh				
raw, peeled, w/o seed	1 oz	18	4.8	0.1
raw, sliced	1 cup	107	28.1	0.5
raw, trimmed, whole, medium, approx 10.6 oz	1 mango	135	35.2	0.6
raw, untrimmed	1 lb	204	53.2	0.9
MANGOSTEEN				
Canned				
in syrup	1 cup	158	39	1.3
in syrup, drained	1 cup	143	35	1.1
MANICOTTI/MANICOTTI ENTRÉE				
(Bernardi)				
cheese	2 pieces	300	27	14.0
cheese, large	1 piece	170	16	8.0
(Budget Gourmet)				
cheese, w/meat sauce	1 entrée	420	38	22.0
frozen, w/meat sauce, frozen	1 entrée	440	34	26.0
(Buitoni) frozen 'Single Serving' one package	9 oz	470	45	14.0
(Celentano)				
	10-oz tray	450	41	21.0
Florentine, 'Great Choice'	10-oz tray	210	29	6.0
Florentine, 'Selects'	10-oz tray	230	29	7.0
mini	4.8 oz	280	32	12.0
w/sauce	8 oz	320	28	15.0
w/o sauce	7 oz	410	40	19.0
(Contadina) cheese, frozen	1 oz	31	3	1.4
(Healthy Choice)				

Food Name	Serv. Size	Total Cal.	Carbs GMS	Fat GMS
cheese, frozen	9.25 oz	220	34	3.0
w/three cheeses	1 entrée	300	40	9.0
(Le Menu) three cheese, frozen	11.75 oz	390	44	15.0
(Lean Cuisine) cheese and spinach, 'Hearty Portions'	1 entrée	340	52	7.0
(Legume)				
cheese, w/spinach, tofu, and sauce, frozen	11 oz	260	30	7.0
classic, vegetarian, nondairy, w/organic pasta and tofu	1 serving	360	40	13.0
Florentine, nondairy, w/organic pasta and tofu	1 serving	300	39	8.0
(Stouffer's) cheese	1 entrée	340	32	16.0
(Weight Watchers)				
cheese	1 entrée	260	31	7.0
cheese, frozen	9.25 oz	260	31	8.0

MANICOTTI NOODLE. See under PASTA.
MANIOC. See CASSAVA.
MAPLE SYRUP. See under SYRUP.
MARGARINE

Food Name	Serv. Size	Total Cal.	Carbs GMS	Fat GMS
coconut, hydrogenated and regular, w/safflower and hydrogenated palm	1 stick	815	1	91.3
coconut, hydrogenated and regular, w/safflower and hydrogenated palm	1 tsp	34	0	3.8
corn, hydrogenated	1 stick	815	1	91.3
corn, hydrogenated	1 tsp	34	0	3.8
corn, hydrogenated and regular	1 stick	815	1	91.3
corn, hydrogenated and regular	1 tsp	34	0	3.8
corn, hydrogenated and regular, soft	1 cup	1626	1	182.5
corn, hydrogenated and regular, soft	1 tsp	34	0	3.8
corn, w/hydrogenated soybean and cottonseed	1 stick	815	1	91.3
corn, w/hydrogenated soybean and cottonseed	1 tsp	34	0	3.8
corn, w/hydrogenated soybean and cottonseed, unsalted	1 stick	810	1	91.1
corn, w/hydrogenated soybean and cottonseed, unsalted	1 tsp	34	0	3.8
lard, hydrogenated	1 stick	831	1	91.3
lard, hydrogenated	1 tsp	34	0	3.8
safflower, hydrogenated and regular	1 cup	1626	1	182.5
safflower, hydrogenated and regular	1 tsp	34	0	3.8
safflower, w/hydrogenated cottonseed and peanut, soft	1 cup	1626	1	182.5
safflower, w/hydrogenated cottonseed and peanut, soft	1 tsp	34	0	3.8
safflower, w/hydrogenated soybean	1 stick	815	1	91.3
safflower, w/hydrogenated soybean	1 tsp	34	0	3.8
safflower, w/hydrogenated soybean and cottonseed	1 stick	815	1	91.3
safflower, w/hydrogenated soybean and cottonseed	1 tsp	34	0	3.8
soybean, hydrogenated	1 stick	812	1	91.0
soybean, hydrogenated	1 tsp	34	0	3.8
soybean, hydrogenated and regular	1 stick	815	1	91.3
soybean, hydrogenated and regular	1 tsp	34	0	3.8
soybean, hydrogenated and regular, soft, salted	1 cup	1626	1	182.5
soybean, hydrogenated and regular, soft, salted	1 tsp	34	0	3.8
soybean, hydrogenated and regular, soft, unsalted	1 cup	1626	2	182.3
soybean, hydrogenated and regular, soft, unsalted	1 tsp	34	0	3.8
soybean, hydrogenated, w/corn and hydrogenated cottonseed	1 stick	815	1	91.3
soybean, hydrogenated, w/corn and hydrogenated cottonseed	1 tsp	34	0	3.8
soybean, hydrogenated, w/cottonseed	1 stick	815	1	91.3
soybean, hydrogenated, w/cottonseed	1 tsp	34	0	3.8
soybean, hydrogenated, w/cottonseed, soft	1 cup	1626	1	182.5
soybean, hydrogenated, w/cottonseed, soft	1 tsp	34	0	3.8
soybean, hydrogenated, w/hydrogenated and regular palm	1 stick	815	1	91.3
soybean, hydrogenated, w/hydrogenated and regular palm	1 tsp	34	0	3.8

Food Name	Serv. Size	Total Cal.	Carbs GMS	Fat GMS
soybean, hydrogenated, w/hydrogenated and regular palm, soft ...	1 cup	1626	1	182.5
soybean, hydrogenated, w/hydrogenated and regular palm, soft ...	1 tsp	34	0	3.8
soybean, hydrogenated, w/safflower, soft	1 cup	1626	1	182.5
soybean, hydrogenated, w/safflower, soft	1 tsp	34	0	3.8
soybean and cottonseed, hydrogenated	1 stick	815	1	91.3
soybean and cottonseed, hydrogenated	1 tsp	34	0	3.8
soybean and cottonseed, hydrogenated, soft	1 cup	1626	1	182.5
soybean and cottonseed, hydrogenated, soft	1 tsp	34	0	3.8
soybean and cottonseed, hydrogenated, soft, salted	1 cup	1626	1	182.5
soybean and cottonseed, hydrogenated, soft, salted	1 tsp	34	0	3.8
soybean and cottonseed, hydrogenated, soft, unsalted	1 cup	1626	2	182.3
soybean and cottonseed, hydrogenated, soft, unsalted	1 tsp	34	0	3.8
soybean and cottonseed, hydrogenated and regular, liquid	1 cup	1637	0	183.0
soybean and cottonseed, hydrogenated and regular, liquid	1 tsp	34	0	3.8
soybean and palm, hydrogenated	1 stick	815	1	91.3
soybean and palm, hydrogenated	1 tsp	34	0	3.8
sunflower, w/hydrogenated cottonseed and peanut, soft	1 cup	1626	1	182.5
sunflower, w/hydrogenated cottonseed and peanut, soft	1 tsp	34	0	3.8
sunflower, w/hydrogenated soybean and cottonseed	1 stick	815	1	91.3
sunflower, w/hydrogenated soybean and cottonseed	1 tsp	34	0	3.8
(A&P)				
premium	1 tbsp	100	1	11.0
quarters, corn oil.......................................	1 tbsp	100	1	11.0
soft, bowl	1 tbsp	100	1	11.0
(Blue Bonnet)				
soft	1 tbsp	100	0	11.0
stick	1 tbsp	100	0	11.0
whipped, stick	1 tbsp	70	0	7.0
(Cannola) soft	1 tbsp	100	0	11.0
(Canoleo) 100% Canola oil, all natural, dairy-free	1 tbsp	100	0	11.0
(Chiffon)				
soft, cup	1 tbsp	90	0	10.0
soft, stick	1 tbsp	100	0	11.0
soft, unsalted	1 tbsp	90	0	10.0
whipped	1 tbsp	70	0	8.0
(Country Morning)				
light, stick	1 tsp	20	0	2.0
light, tub	1 tsp	20	0	2.0
regular, stick	1 tsp	35	0	4.0
regular, tub	1 tsp	30	0	3.0
unsalted, stick	1 tsp	35	0	4.0
unsalted, tub	1 tsp	30	0	3.0
(Fleischmann's)				
diet, lower calorie	1 tbsp	50	0	6.0
40% corn oil, less fat, stick	1 tbsp	52	1	5.6
regular, soft...	1 tbsp	100	0	11.0
regular, stick	1 tbsp	100	0	11.0
sweet, unsalted, soft	1 tbsp	100	0	11.0
sweet, unsalted, stick	1 tbsp	100	0	11.0
sweet, unsalted, stick	1 tbsp	100	0	11.0
whipped, lightly salted	1 tbsp	70	0	7.0
whipped, unsalted......................................	1 tbsp	70	0	7.0
(Hain)				
safflower..	1 tbsp	100	0	11.0
safflower, soft	1 tbsp	100	0	11.0
safflower, unsalted	1 tbsp	100	0	11.0

Food Name	Serv. Size	Total Cal.	Carbs GMS	Fat GMS
(Hollywood)				
safflower	1 tbsp	100	0	11.0
safflower, unsalted	1 tbsp	100	0	11.0
(I Can't Believe It's Not Butter)	1 tbsp	90	0	10.0
(Imperial)				
lower calorie, 'Diet'	1 tbsp	50	0	6.0
soft	1 tbsp	100	0	11.0
(Land O'Lakes)				
corn oil, premium, stick	1 tbsp	35	0	4.0
regular, stick	1 tsp	35	0	4.0
soy oil, regular, stick	1 tbsp	35	0	4.0
soy oil, soft	1 tbsp	35	0	4.0
tub	1 tsp	35	0	4.0
(Mazola)				
	1 tbsp	100	0	11.0
lower calorie	1 tbsp	50	0	5.5
unsalted	1 tbsp	100	0	11.0
(Miracle Brand)				
whipped, cup	1 tbsp	60	0	7.0
whipped, stick	1 tbsp	70	0	7.0
(Fleischmann's) 'Move Over Butter'	1 tbsp	60	0	6.0
(Nucoa)				
	1 tbsp	100	0	11.0
'Heart Beat'	1 tbsp	25	0	3.0
soft	1 tbsp	90	0	10.0
unsalted, 'Heart Beat'	1 tbsp	24	0	3.0
(P&Q) quarters, 60% vegetable oil	1 tbsp	80	1	8.0
(Parkay)				
	1 tbsp	100	0	11.0
diet, soft	1 tbsp	50	0	6.0
regular, soft	1 tbsp	100	0	11.0
squeezable	1 tbsp	90	0	10.0
whipped, cup	1 tbsp	70	0	7.0
whipped, stick	1 tbsp	70	0	7.0
(Saffola) soft	1 tbsp	100	0	11.0
(Smart Beat)				
super light	1 tbsp	20	0	2.0
trans fat-free, lactose-free	1 tbsp	20	0	2.0
(Weight Watchers)				
light	1 tbsp	45	2	4.0
stick	1 tbsp	60	0	7.0
tub	1 tbsp	50	0	6.0
unsalted	1 tbsp	50	0	6.0
MARGARINE SPREAD				
margarine-butter blend, 60% corn oil margarine, 40% butter	1 stick	811	1	91.2
margarine-butter blend, 60% corn oil margarine, 40% butter	1 tsp	36	0	4.0
(Blue Bonnet)				
48% vegetable oil	1 tbsp	60	1	6.0
75% vegetable oil	1 tbsp	90	0	11.0
soft, 'Better Blend'	1 tbsp	90	0	11.0
stick, 'Better Blend'	1 tbsp	90	0	11.0
unsalted, 'Better Blend'	1 tbsp	90	0	11.0
whipped, 60% vegetable oil	1 tbsp	80	0	8.0
(Brummel & Brown)				
58% vegetable oil, 10% yogurt	1 tbsp	70	0	8.0
35% vegetable oil, 25% yogurt	1 tbsp	50	0	5.0
(Country Crock)				
48% vegetable oil	1 tbsp	60	0	7.0

Food Name	Serv. Size	Total Cal.	Carbs GMS	Fat GMS
48% vegetable oil, churn style	1 tbsp	60	0	7.0
52% vegetable oil	1 tbsp	60	0	7.0
52% vegetable oil, churn style, stick	1 tbsp	80	0	9.0
64% vegetable oil, stick	1 tbsp	80	0	9.0
squeezable	1 tbsp	80	0	9.0
(Fleischmann's)				
'Move Over Butter'	1 tbsp	90	0	10.0
72% vegetable oil w/cream buttermilk, tub, whipped,				
'Move Over Butter'	1 tbsp	60	0	7.0
72% vegetable. oil w/sweet cream buttermilk, stick,				
'Move Over Butter'	1 tbsp	90	0	10.0
(Hollywood) soft	1 tbsp	90	1	10.0
(I Can't Believe It's Not Butter)				
	1 tbsp	90	0	10.0
40% vegetable oil w/cream buttermilk, tub	1 tbsp	50	0	6.0
52% vegetable oil w/cream buttermilk, quarters	1 tbsp	60	0	7.0
single portion	1 tbsp	90	0	10.0
68% vegetable oil w/buttermilk, squeezable	1 tbsp	90	0	10.0
70% vegetable oil w/cream buttermilk, stick	1 tbsp	90	0	10.0
70% vegetable oil w/cream buttermilk, tub	1 tbsp	90	0	10.0
light	1 tbsp	60	0	7.0
(Imperial) 45% vegetable oil, 'Light'	1 tbsp	60	0	6.0
(Kraft)				
bowl, 'Touch of Butter'	1 tbsp	50	0	6.0
stick, 'Touch of Butter'	1 tbsp	90	0	10.0
(Land O'Lakes)				
w/sweet cream, stick	1 tsp	30	0	4.0
w/sweet cream, tub	1 tsp	25	0	3.0
w/sweet cream, unsalted	1 tsp	30	0	4.0
lightly salted, soft, 'Country Morning Blend'	1 tbsp	30	0	3.0
lightly salted, soft, 'Country Morning Light'	1 tbsp	20	0	3.0
lightly salted, soft, 64% soy oil	1 tbsp	25	0	3.0
lightly salted, soft, w/sweet cream	1 tbsp	25	0	3.0
lightly salted, stick, 'Country Morning Blend'	1 tbsp	35	0	4.0
lightly salted, stick, 'Country Morning Light'	1 tbsp	20	0	3.0
lightly salted, stick, w/sweet cream	1 tbsp	30	0	4.0
unsalted, soft, 'Country Morning Blend'	1 tbsp	30	0	3.0
unsalted, stick, 'Country Morning Blend'	1 tbsp	35	0	4.0
unsalted, stick, w/sweet cream	1 tbsp	30	0	4.0
(Parkay) 50% vegetable oil	1 tbsp	60	0	7.0
(Promise)				
24% vegetable oil, 'Ultra'	1 tbsp	30	0	3.5
40% vegetable oil, soft	1 tbsp	50	0	6.0
40% vegetable oil, stick	1 tbsp	50	0	6.0
68% vegetable oil	1 tbsp	90	0	10.0
extra light	1 tbsp	50	0	6.0
lower calorie	1 tbsp	70	0	7.0
w/Canola oil, 'Ultra'	1 tbsp	35	0	4.0
whipped	1 tbsp	60	0	7.0
(Shedd's Spread) 52% vegetable oil	1 tbsp	60	0	7.0
(Touch of Butter) 47% vegetable oil and dairy spread	1 tbsp	60	0	7.0
(Weight Watchers)				
extra light, sweet, no salt, 'Country Cottage'	1 tbsp	50	0	6.0
extra light, tub 'Country Cottage Farms'	1 tbsp	45	2	4.0
light, 'Country Cottage Farms'	1 tbsp	50	0	6.0
light, stick	1 tbsp	60	0	7.0
MARGARINE SUBSTITUTE				
corn, hydrogenated and regular, 40% fat	1 cup	801	1	90.0

Food Name	Serv. Size	Total Cal.	Carbs GMS	Fat GMS
corn, hydrogenated and regular, 40% fat	1 tsp	17	0	1.9
soybean, hydrogenated, 40% fat	1 cup	801	1	90.0
soybean, hydrogenated, 40% fat	1 tsp	17	0	1.9
soybean, hydrogenated, w/cottonseed, 40% fat	1 cup	801	1	90.0
soybean, hydrogenated, w/cottonseed, 40% fat	1 tsp	17	0	1.9
soybean, hydrogenated, w/hydrogenated and regular palm, 40% fat	1 cup	801	1	90.0
soybean, hydrogenated, w/hydrogenated and regular palm, 40% fat	1 tsp	17	0	1.9
soybean, hydrogenated, w/hydrogenated and regular palm, 60% fat, tub	1 cup	1236	0	139.2
soybean, hydrogenated, w/hydrogenated and regular palm, 60% fat, tub	1 tsp	26	0	2.9
soybean and cottonseed, hydrogenated, 40% fat	1 cup	801	1	90.0
soybean and cottonseed, hydrogenated, 40% fat	1 tsp	17	0	1.9
soybean and cottonseed, hydrogenated, 60% fat, tub	1 cup	1236	0	139.2
soybean and cottonseed, hydrogenated, 60% fat, tub	1 tsp	26	0	2.9
soybean and palm, hydrogenated, 60% fat, stick	1 cup	1236	0	139.2
soybean and palm, hydrogenated, 60% fat, stick	1 tsp	26	0	2.9
(Promise Ultra) nonfat	1 tbsp	5	1	0.0
MARGARITA. See under COCKTAIL MIX.				
MARINADE				
(DiGiorno) refrigerated	5 oz	110	12	6.0
CALCUTTA MASALA *(TAJ Cuisine of India)*	4 oz	100	13	5.0
FAJITA				
(Old El Paso)	1/8 jar	14	3	0.0
(Tone's)	1 tsp	9	2	0.1
FOR MEAT *(Crown Colony)*	1/2 tsp	5	1	0.0
FRENCH *(Litehouse)* country herb, refrigerated	1 tbsp	54	2	5.0
KASHMIR TANDOOKI *(TAJ Cuisine of India)*	2 oz	50	5	3.0
Lemon Herb *(Golden Dipt)*	1 oz	130	2	14.0
LEMON PEPPER *(Lawry's)*	1 oz	20	2	1.1
MESQUITE *(S&W)*	1 tbsp	10	3	0.0
OYSTER AND SHRIMP *(Caribbean Clipper)*	1 tsp	10	2	0.0
SEAFOOD *(Golden Dipt)* honey soy, nonfat	1 tbsp	30	5	0.0
STIR-FRY *(La Choy)* food service product	1 tbsp	25	5	0.1
TERIYAKI				
(Golden Dipt) ginger	1 oz	120	12	7.0
(Kikkoman)				
	1 tbsp	15	2	0.0
light	1 tbsp	15	3	0.0
(LaChoy)	1 oz	30	5	0.0
(Lawry's)				
	2 tbsp	72	11	0.4
barbecue	1/4 cup	164	27	2.3
barbecue	1/8 cup	82	14	1.1
(S&W)				
	1 tbsp	25	5	0.0
light	1 tbsp	25	5	0.0
WHITE WINE DIJON *(Golden Dipt)*	1 tbsp	10	1	0.0
WINE AND GARLIC *(Charcoal Companion)* glaze, spray	2 tbsp	40	4	0.0
MARINADE MIX				
BARBECUE *(Adolph's)* 'Marinade in Minutes'	1/2 tsp	5	1	0.0
BEEF				
(Durkee)	1/2 tsp	0	1	0.0
(Lawry's)	1 pkg	49	11	0.2
(Marinade Magic)	1/2 tsp	10	2	0.0

Food Name	Serv. Size	Total Cal.	Carbs GMS	Fat GMS
CAJUN				
(Adolph's) 'Marinade in Minutes'	1/2 tsp	5	1	0.0
(Luzianne)	1/4 tsp	0	0	0.0
(Tone's)	1 tsp	9	2	0.2
CHICKEN				
(Adolph's)				
	3/4 tsp	5	1	0.0
salt-free	3/4 tsp	5	2	0.0
(McCormick/Schilling) mesquite, 'Sauce Blends'	1 pkg	132	24	3.0
(Schilling) mesquite	1/6 pkg	20	4	0.0
CITRUS *(Lawry's)* grill	2 tbsp	34	3	0.4
FAJITA				
(Marinade Magic)	1/2 tsp	5	1	0.0
(McCormick/Schilling)	2 tsp	15	3	0.0
FOR MEAT				
(Adolph's)				
	1/2 tsp	5	1	0.0
no salt	1/2 tsp	5	2	0.0
(French's)	1/8 pkg	10	2	0.0
(Kikkoman)	1 tsp	10	2	0.0
(McCormick/Schilling)	1 tsp	15	2	0.0
GARLIC				
(Adolph's)				
Dijon, 'Marinade in Minutes'	3/4 tsp	10	1	0.0
'Marinade in Minutes'	1/2 tsp	0	1	0.0
HERB				
(Adolph's)				
Italian, 'Marinade in Minutes'	1/4 tsp	0	1	0.0
lemon, 'Marinade in Minutes'	1/2 tsp	10	2	0.0
Parmesan, 'Marinade in Minutes'	3/4 tsp	10	1	0.0
(Lawry's) herb and garlic, w/lemon	2 tbsp	36	4	1.0
(Marinade Magic) lemon	1/2 tsp	5	1	0.0
HICKORY *(Adolph's)* grill, 'Marinade in Minutes'	1 tbsp	20	4	0.5
HOT AND SPICY *(Adolph's)* 'Marinade in Minutes'	3/4 tsp	5	1	0.0
LEMON GARLIC *(Adolph's)* 'Marinade in Minutes'	1 tbsp	30	2	2.5
LEMON PEPPER *(Adolph's)* 'Marinade in Minutes'	1/2 tsp	10	2	0.0
MESQUITE				
(Adolph's)				
'Marinade in Minutes' dry	3/4 tsp	10	2	0.0
'Marinade in Minutes' liquid	1 tbsp	45	5	2.5
(Lawry's)	2 tbsp	24	3	0.4
SCAMPI *(Adolph's)* 'Marinade in Minutes'	1/2 tsp	10	2	0.0
STEAK *(Adolph's)* 'Marinade in Minutes'	1/4 tsp	0	1	0.0
TERIYAKI				
(Adolph's)				
'Marinade in Minutes' dry	1 1/2 tsp	15	3	0.0
'Marinade in Minutes' liquid	1 tbsp	20	5	0.0
MARIONBERRY TOPPING *(Flav-R-Pac)*	2 tbsp	40	10	0.0
MARJORAM				
dried	1 tbsp	5	1	0.1
dried	1 tsp	2	0	0.0
dried *(Durkee)*	1 tbsp	7	0	0.0
dried *(Durkee)*	1 tsp	2	0	0.0
dried *(Laurel Leaf)*	1 tbsp	7	0	0.0
dried *(McCormick/Schilling)*	1 tsp	4	1	0.0
dried *(Laurel Leaf)*	1 tsp	2	0	0.0
dried *(Spice Islands)*	1 tsp	4	1	0.1

Food Name	Serv. Size	Total Cal.	Carbs GMS	Fat GMS
dried *(Tone's)*	1 tsp	2	0	0.1
MARMALADE. See under JAM AND PRESERVES.				
MARMALADE PLUM. See SAPOTE.				
MARROW BEAN. See BEAN, MARROW.				
MARROW SQUASH. See SQUASH, MARROW.				
MARSHMALLOW. See under CANDY.				
MARSHMALLOW TOPPING				
(Finast) creme	1 oz	95	23	0.0
(Kraft) creme	1 oz	90	23	0.0
(Marshmallow Fluff)	1 tsp	59	15	0.0
(Smucker's)	2 tbsp	120	29	0.0
MATAI. See under WATER CHESTNUT.				
MATZO. See under CRACKER.				
MATZO MEAL. See under CRACKER MEAL.				
MAYONNAISE				
(Bama)	1 tbsp	100	0	11.0
(Bennett's) 'Real'	1 tbsp	110	1	12.0
(Best Foods)				
cholesterol-free	1 tbsp	50	1	5.0
light	1 tbsp	50	1	5.0
low-fat	1 tbsp	25	4	1.0
'Real'	1 tbsp	100	0	11.0
(Blue Plate)				
less fat, cholesterol-free	1 tbsp	50	1	5.0
100% natural, no additives	1 tbsp	100	0	11.0
(Cains)	1 tbsp	100	0	11.0
(Estee)				
lower calorie	1 tbsp	50	1	5.0
lower calorie	1 packet	15	2	1.0
(Featherweight)				
lower calorie	1 tbsp	30	3	2.0
soy, 'Soyamaise'	1 tbsp	100	0	11.0
(Finast)				
....	1 tbsp	100	0	11.0
lower calorie, 'Lite'	1 tbsp	40	1	4.0
(Hain)				
Canola	1 tbsp	100	1	11.0
cold processed	1 tbsp	110	0	12.0
less fat, no salt added, 'Real'	1 tbsp	110	0	12.0
lower calorie, low sodium, 'Light'	1 tbsp	60	2	6.0
low-sodium, all natural	1 tbsp	110	0	12.0
no salt added, 'Real'	1 tbsp	110	0	12.0
safflower	1 tbsp	110	0	12.0
(Hellmann's)				
cholesterol-free	1 tbsp	50	1	5.0
lower calorie, 'Light'	1 tbsp	50	1	5.0
low-fat	1 tbsp	25	4	1.0
'Real'	1 tbsp	100	0	11.0
(Hollywood)				
....	1 tbsp	110	0	12.0
Canola	1 tbsp	100	1	11.0
safflower	1 tbsp	100	0	12.0
(Janet Lee) lower calorie, 'Light'	1 tbsp	50	1	5.0
(JFG)				
'Creamy Velvet'	1 tbsp	100	0	11.0
less fat, cholesterol free	1 tbsp	50	0	5.0

Food Name	Serv. Size	Total Cal.	Carbs GMS	Fat GMS
(Kraft)				
light	1 tbsp	50	2	5.0
lower calorie, 'Light'	1 tbsp	50	1	5.0
nonfat	1 tbsp	10	2	0.0
'Real'	1 tbsp	100	0	11.0
w/lime juice, 'Mayonesa'	1 tbsp	64	0	12.0
(Pathmark)				
	1 tbsp	100	0	11.0
lower calorie	1 tbsp	40	1	4.0
low-sodium	1 tbsp	100	0	11.0
'No Frills'	1 tbsp	100	0	11.0
(Rokeach)	1 tbsp	100	0	11.0
(Smart Beat) lower calorie, 'Golden Corn Light'	1 tbsp	40	1	4.0
(Spectrum) Canola, eggless, lite	1 tbsp	35	1	3.0
(Weight Watchers)				
light	1 tbsp	25	1	2.0
lower calorie	1 tbsp	50	1	5.0
lower calorie, low-sodium	1 tbsp	50	1	5.0
(Westbrae)				
	1 tbsp	100	0	11.0
Canola	1 tbsp	100	0	11.0

MAYONNAISE SUBSTITUTE

Food Name	Serv. Size	Total Cal.	Carbs GMS	Fat GMS
(Best Foods) vegetarian	1 tbsp	50	2	5.0
(Hain)				
Canola, lower calorie	1 tbsp	60	2	5.0
eggless, no salt added	1 tbsp	110	0	12.0
(Hellmann's)				
cholesterol-free	1 tbsp	50	1	5.0
vegetarian	1 tbsp	50	2	5.0
(Kraft) vegetarian	1 tbsp	50	3	5.0
(Life) sunflower, all natural	1 tbsp	71	1	8.0
(Nasoya) 'Nayonaise'	1 tbsp	35	1	3.3
(Nayonnaise) vegetable dressing and dip	1 tbsp	35	1	3.0
(Nucoa) 'Heart Beat'	1 tbsp	40	1	4.0
(Weight Watchers) cholesterol-free	1 tbsp	50	1	5.0

MEAT LOAF DINNER/ENTRÉE

Food Name	Serv. Size	Total Cal.	Carbs GMS	Fat GMS
(Banquet) w/tomato sauce, potatoes, carrots in sauce, frozen, 'Extra Helping'	1 pkg	612	34	40.0
(Healthy Choice) traditional, w/potato, vegetable, apple praline	1 pkg	316	52	5.0
(Lean Magic) flame broiled	1 piece	148	4	7.2
(Lean Magic 30) flame broiled	1 piece	110	4	3.6
(Stouffer's) w/gravy, frozen, food service product	1 oz	40	2	2.4

MEAT LOAF SEASONING. See under SEASONING MIX.

MEAT STICKS, SMOKED

Food Name	Serv. Size	Total Cal.	Carbs GMS	Fat GMS
	1 oz	156	2	14.1
	1 stick	109	1	9.8

MEAT SUBSTITUTE. See also individual meat substitute listings.

Food Name	Serv. Size	Total Cal.	Carbs GMS	Fat GMS
(Heartline) vegetarian, unflavored, lite	0.5 oz	22	1	0.0
(Worthington)				
multigrain cutlets, vegetarian	1 slice	99	5	1.8
vegetarian, 'Choplets'	1 slice	94	3	1.6
vegetarian, cutlets	1 slice	66	3	1.1
vegetarian, 'Diced Chik'	1/4 cup	57	1	3.5
vegetarian, 'Numete'	1 slice	132	5	9.6
vegetarian, patties, 'Crispychik'	1 serving	175	15	9.4

Food Name	Serv. Size	Total Cal.	Carbs GMS	Fat GMS
MEAT TENDERIZER				
(Adolph's)				
seasoned, '100% Natural'	1/4 tsp	0	0	0.0
sodium-free, '100% Natural'	1/4 tsp	0	1	0.0
spiced, sodium-free, '100% Natural'	1/4 tsp	0	1	0.0
unseasoned, '100% Natural'	1/4 tsp	0	0	0.0
(Tone's)				
seasoned	1 tsp	7	1	0.2
unseasoned	1 tsp	7	1	0.2
MEATBALL DINNER/ENTRÉE				
(Armour)				
Swedish, 'Classics'	11.25 oz	330	23	18.0
Swedish, beef, 'Classics'	11.25 oz	360	32	17.0
(Banquet) Swedish, beef, frozen	11 oz	440	27	27.0
(Bernardi) meatballs	6 meatballs	270	5	22.0
(Budget Gourmet)				
Swedish, beef, frozen	11.2 oz	450	40	22.0
Swedish, w/cream sauce and noodles, frozen	1 entrée	550	40	34.0
(Chef Boyardee) stew, canned	8 oz	350	24	24.0
(Dinty Moore)				
stew	8 oz	240	14	16.0
stew, microwave cup	7.5 oz	240	14	16.0
(Freezer Queen) Swedish, beef, frozen	10 oz	350	26	19.0
(Healthy Choice)				
Italian style, 'Hearty Handfuls'	1 entrée	320	51	5.0
Swedish, frozen	1 entrée	280	35	6.0
(Lean Cuisine)				
Swedish	1 entrée	280	33	7.0
Swedish, w/pasta, frozen	1 entrée	290	32	8.0
Swedish, w/pasta, frozen	1 pkg	276	31	7.2
(Lunch Express) Swedish, w/pasta, frozen	1 entrée	530	41	32.0
(Marie Callender's) Swedish, frozen	12.5 oz	520	44	26.0
(Morton) Swedish, beef, frozen	10 oz	310	26	17.0
(Smart Ones) Swedish	1 entrée	300	33	10.0
(Stouffer's)				
Swedish, frozen	1 entrée	440	36	23.0
Swedish, w/gravy, food service product	1 oz	48	2	3.3
(Swanson) Swedish, beef, frozen	10 oz	350	37	11.0
(Weight Watchers) Swedish, frozen	1 entrée	280	34	8.0
MEATBALL SEASONING. See under SEASONING MIX.				
MEDICAL NUTRITIONALS				
CARBOHYDRATE SUPPLEMENT				
(Mead Johnson Nutritionals)				
'Moducal, 100% maltodextrin, powder	1/2 cup	240	64	0.0
(Ross)				
'Polycose' for oral or tube feeding (not parenteral use), kosher, gluten- and lactose-free, low-residue, liquid	100 ml	200	50	0.0
'Polycose' for oral or tube feeding (not parenteral use), kosher, gluten- and lactose-free, low-residue, powder	100 gm	380	94	0.0
CRITICAL CARE SUPPORT				
(Nestlé Clinical Nutrition)				
'Crucial' for tube feeding, lactose- and gluten-free, low-residue, ready to use	1000 ml	1500	135	68.0
'Crucial' for tube feeding, lactose- and gluten-free, low-residue, ready to use	250 ml	375	34	16.9
(Novartis [Sandoz])				
'Impact' ready to use	1000 ml	1000	130	28.0

Food Name	Serv. Size	Total Cal.	Carbs GMS	Fat GMS
'Impact' ready to use, 1 can,	250 ml	250	33	6.9
'Impact 1.5' for fluid restriction or high caloric needs, ready to use,	1000 ml	1500	140	69.0
'Impact 1.5' for fluid restriction or high caloric needs, ready to use, 1 can	250 ml	375	35	17.2
'Impact with Fiber' ready to use	1000 ml	1000	140	28.0
'Impact with Fiber' ready to use, 1 can,	250 ml	250	34	6.9
(Ross)				
'Perative' for tube feeding (not parenteral use), kosher, gluten- and lactose-free, low-residue, ready to use,	1 liter	1300	177	37.4
'Perative' for tube feeding (not parenteral use), kosher, gluten- and lactose-free, low-residue, ready to use	8 fl oz	308	42	8.8
DIABETES/GLUCOSE INTOLERANCE SUPPORT				
(Mead Johnson Nutritionals)				
'Choice DM' for oral or tube feeding, ready to use	1000 ml	1060	106	51.0
'Choice DM' for oral or tube feeding, ready to use	8 fl oz	250	25	12.0
(Nestlé Clinical Nutrition)				
'Glytrol with Fiber' for oral or tube feeding, kosher, sucrose-, lactose-, and gluten-free, ready to use	1000 ml	1000	100	47.5
'Glytrol with Fiber' for oral or tube feeding, kosher, sucrose-, lactose-, and gluten-free, ready to use	250 ml	250	25	11.9
(Novartis [Sandoz])				
'Diabetisource with Fiber' ready to use	1000 ml	1000	90	49.0
'Diabetisource with Fiber' ready to use, 1 can	250 ml	250	23	12.2
'Resource Diabetic with Fiber' for oral or tube feeding, ready to use	1000 ml	1060	99	47.0
'Resource Diabetic with Fiber' for oral or tube feeding, ready to use	237 ml	250	23	11.1
(Ross)				
'Glucerna with Fiber' for oral or tube feeding (not parenteral use), kosher, gluten- and lactose-free, low-residue, ready to use	1 liter	1000	96	54.4
'Glucerna with Fiber' for oral or tube feeding (not parenteral use), kosher, gluten- and lactose-free, low-residue, ready to use	8 fl oz	237	23	12.9
ELEMENTAL DIET				
(B. Braun/McGaw)				
'Immun-Aid' for oral or tube feeding, high-nitrogen, powder, prepared, daily dose	2000 ml	2000	240	44.0
'Immun-Aid' for oral or tube feeding, high-nitrogen, powder, prepared, 1 serving	500 ml	500	60	11.0
(Mead Johnson Nutritionals)				
'Criticare HN' high-nitrogen, ready to use	1000 ml	1060	220	5.3
'Criticare HN' high-nitrogen, ready to use	8 fl oz	250	51	1.3
(Nestlé Clinical Nutrition)				
'Peptamen' for tube feeding, isotonic, lactose- and gluten-free, low-residue, ready to use	1000 ml	1000	127	39.0
'Peptamen' for tube feeding, isotonic, lactose- and gluten-free, low-residue, ready to use	250 ml	250	32	9.8
'Peptamen Oral' oral, lactose- and gluten-free, low-residue, ready to use	1000 ml	1000	127	39.0
'Peptamen Oral' oral, lactose- and gluten-free, low-residue, ready to use	250 ml	250	32	9.8
'Peptamen VHP' for tube feeding, very high protein, isotonic, lactose- and gluten-free, low-residue, ready to use	1000 ml	1000	105	39.0
'Peptamen VHP' for tube feeding, very high protein, isotonic, lactose- and gluten-free, low-residue, ready to use	250 ml	250	26	9.8

Food Name	Serv. Size	Total Cal.	Carbs GMS	Fat GMS
'Peptamen VHP' oral, very high protein, lactose- and gluten-free, low-residue, ready to use .... 1000 ml	1000	105	39.0
'Peptamen VHP' oral, very high protein, lactose- and gluten-free, low-residue, ready to use .... 250 ml	250	26	9.8
'Reabilan' for tube feeding, lactose and gluten-free, low-residue, ready to use .... 1000 ml	1000	132	40.5
'Reabilan' for tube feeding, lactose and gluten-free, low-residue, ready to use .... 375 ml	375	49	15.2
'Reabilan HN' for tube feeding, high-nitrogen, lactose- and gluten-free, low-residue, ready to use .... 1000 ml	1333	158	54.0
'Reabilan HN' for tube feeding, high-nitrogen, lactose- and gluten-free, low-residue, ready to use .... 375 ml	500	59	20.2
(Novartis [Sandoz])			
'Tolerex' powder, prepared .... 1000 ml	1000	230	1.5
'Tolerex' powder, prepared, 1 packet .... 300 ml	300	68	0.4
'Vivonex Plus' high-nitrogen, powder, prepared .... 1000 ml	1000	190	6.7
'Vivonex Plus' high-nitrogen, powder, prepared .... 300 ml	300	57	2.0
'Vivonex T.E.N' for gastrointestinal impairment, powder, prepared .... 1000 ml	1000	210	2.8
'Vivonex T.E.N' for gastrointestinal impairment, powder, prepared, 1 packet .... 300 ml	300	62	0.8
FAT MALABSORPTION SUPPORT			
(Mead Johnson Nutritionals)			
'Lipisorb' lactose-free, low-residue, powder, prepared .... 8 fl oz	480	56	23.0
'Lipisorb' lactose-free, low-residue, ready to use .... 1000 ml	1350	161	57.0
'Lipisorb' lactose-free, low-residue, ready to use .... 8 fl oz	320	38	13.4
GASTROINTESTINAL SUPPORT			
(Nestlé Clinical Nutrition)			
'Elementra' for oral or tube feeding, elemental protein, powder, 2 scoops .... 6.6 gm	25	0	0.3
(Novartis [Sandoz])			
'Sandosource Peptide' semi-elemental, low-fat, ready to use ... 1000 ml	1000	160	17.0
'Sandosource Peptide' semi-elemental, low-fat, ready to use .... 250 ml	250	41	4.4
(Ross)			
'Alitraq' for oral or tube feeding (not parenteral use), kosher, gluten-free, low-residue, powder, prepared .... 1 liter	1000	165	15.5
'Alitraq' for oral or tube feeding (not parenteral use), kosher, gluten-free, low-residue, powder, prepared .... 300 ml	300	50	4.7
'Vital High Nitrogen' for oral or tube feeding (not parenteral use), kosher, gluten- and lactose-free, low-residue, powder, prepared .... 1 liter	1000	185	10.8
'Vital High Nitrogen' for oral or tube feeding (not parenteral use), kosher, gluten- and lactose-free, low-residue, powder, prepared .... 300 ml	300	55	3.3
GENERAL PURPOSE			
(Mead Johnson Nutritionals)			
'Boost' oral, milk-based, cholesterol- and lactose-free .... 8 fl oz	240	41	4.2
'Sustacal' oral, milk-based, lactose-free cholesterol-free, powder, prepared .... 8 fl oz	200	36	0.7
'Sustacal' oral, milk-based, moderate protein, fiber-free, lactose-free, low-residue, ready to use .... 8 fl oz	240	33	5.5
'Sustacal Pudding' lactose-free, fiber-free .... 8 fl oz	240	32	9.5
'Sustacal with Fiber' oral, milk-based, w/fiber, lactose-free, ready to use .... 8 fl oz	250	33	8.3
(Novartis [Sandoz])			
'Resource' fruit beverage, low-electrolyte, fat-free .... 1000 ml	760	150	0.0
'Resource' fruit beverage, low-electrolyte, fat-free, 1 Brik Pak .... 237 ml	180	36	0.0

Food Name	Serv. Size	Total Cal.	Carbs GMS	Fat GMS
(Ross)				
'Ensure' for oral or tube feeding (not parenteral use), kosher, gluten- and lactose-free, low-residue, powder, prepared .... 1 liter		1060	145	37.2
'Ensure' for oral or tube feeding (not parenteral use), kosher, gluten- and lactose-free, low-residue, powder, prepared .... 8 fl oz		250	34	8.8
'Ensure' for oral or tube feeding (not parenteral use), kosher, gluten- and lactose-free, low-residue, ready to use ..... 1 liter		1060	169	25.8
'Ensure' for oral or tube feeding (not parenteral use), kosher, gluten- and lactose-free, low-residue, ready to use ..... 8 fl oz		250	40	6.1
'Ensure Pudding' oral, patients w/swallowing impairments, kosher, gluten-free, 9.2 g lactose/serving .... 5-oz can		250	34	9.7
'Ensure with Fiber' for oral or tube feeding (not parenteral use), fiber-fortified, kosher, gluten- and lactose-free, low-residue, ready to use .... 1 liter		1100	162	37.2
'Ensure with Fiber' for oral or tube feeding (not parenteral use), fiber-fortified, kosher, gluten- and lactose-free, low-residue, ready to use .... 8 fl oz		260	38	8.8
GERIATRIC				
(Nestlé Clinical Nutrition)				
'Probalance with Fiber' for oral or tube feeding, high-fiber, kosher, lactose- and gluten-free, ready to use .... 1000 ml		1200	156	40.6
'Probalance with Fiber' for oral or tube feeding, high-fiber, kosher, lactose- and gluten-free, ready to use .... 250 ml		300	39	10.2
HEALING SUPPORT				
(Mead Johnson Nutritionals)				
'Protain XL' for tube feeding, high-protein, w/fiber, ready to use ... 1000 ml		1000	129	30.0
'Protain XL' for tube feeding, high-protein, w/fiber, ready to use ... 8 fl oz		237	31	7.1
'Traumacal' for oral or tube feeding, high-calorie, high-nitrogen ... 1000 ml		1500	142	68.0
'Traumacal' for oral or tube feeding, high-calorie, high-nitrogen ... 8 fl oz		355	34	16.2
(Nestlé Clinical Nutrition)				
'Replete' isotonic, kosher, lactose- and gluten-free, low-residue, ready to use .... 1000 ml		1000	113	34.0
'Replete' isotonic, kosher, lactose- and gluten-free, low-residue, ready to use .... 250 ml		250	28	8.5
'Replete with Fiber' for oral or tube feeding, isotonic, high-fiber, kosher, lactose- and gluten-free, ready to use ..... 1000 ml		1000	113	34.0
'Replete with Fiber' for oral or tube feeding, isotonic, high-fiber, kosher, lactose- and gluten-free, ready to use ...... 250 ml		250	28	8.5
(Ross)				
'Ensure' oral, coffee flavored, canned .... 8 fl oz		250	34	8.8
'Promote' for oral or tube feeding, high-protein, kosher, gluten- and lactose-free, low-residue, ready to use .... 1 liter		1000	130	26.0
'Promote' for oral or tube feeding, high-protein, kosher, gluten- and lactose-free, low-residue, ready to use .... 8 fl oz		237	31	6.2
'Promote with Fiber' for oral or tube feeding, high-protein, kosher, gluten- and lactose-free, low-residue, ready to use ..... 1 liter		1000	139	28.2
'Promote with Fiber' for oral or tube feeding, high-protein, kosher, gluten- and lactose-free, low-residue, ready to use ..... 8 fl oz		237	33	6.7
HEPATIC SUPPORT				
(B. Braun/McGaw)				
'Hepatic-Aid II' for oral or tube feeding, amino acid and calories, powder, prepared .... 340 ml		400	57	12.3
(Nestlé Clinical Nutrition)				
'Nutrihep' for oral or tube feeding, kosher, lactose- and gluten-free, ready to use .... 1000 ml		1500	290	21.2
'Nutrihep' for oral or tube feeding, kosher, lactose- and gluten-free, ready to use .... 250 ml		375	73	5.3

Food Name	Serv. Size	Total Cal.	Carbs GMS	Fat GMS
HIV/AIDS SUPPORT				
(Ross)				
'Advera with Fiber' for oral or tube feeding (not parenteral use), kosher, gluten- and lactose-free, ready to use	1 liter	1280	216	22.8
'Advera with Fiber' for oral or tube feeding (not parenteral use), kosher, gluten- and lactose-free, ready to use	8 fl oz	303	51	5.4
HYDRATION SUPPORT				
(Ross)				
'Equalyte' enteral rehydration solution	8 fl oz	24	7	0.0
'Equalyte' rehydration solution, for oral or tube feeding (not parenteral use), kosher, gluten- and lactose-free, ready to use	1 liter	100	25	na
'Introlite' rehydration solution, for tube feeding (not parenteral use), low calorie, kosher, gluten- and lactose-free, low-residue, ready to use	1 liter	530	71	18.4
'Pedialyte' for children	8 fl oz	24	6	0.0
HYPEROSMOLAR SENSITIVITY SUPPORT				
(Ross)				
for oral or tube feeding (not parenteral use), kosher, gluten- and lactose-free, low-residue, ready to use	1 liter	1060	152	34.7
for oral or tube feeding (not parenteral use), kosher, gluten- and lactose-free, low-residue, ready to use	8 fl oz	250	36	8.2
INTACT PROTEIN DIET				
(Mead Johnson Nutritionals)				
'Comply' for tube feeding, high-calorie, lactose-free, ready to use	1000 ml	1500	180	61.0
'Comply' for tube feeding, high-calorie, lactose-free, ready to use	8 fl oz	355	43	14.5
'Deliver 2.0' for oral or tube feeding, high-calorie, high-nitrogen, lactose-free	1000 ml	2000	200	102.0
'Deliver 2.0' for oral or tube feeding, high-calorie, high-nitrogen, lactose-free	8 fl oz	470	47	24.0
'Isocal' for tube feeding, lactose-free, low-residue, ready to use	1000 ml	1060	135	44.0
'Isocal' for tube feeding, lactose-free, low-residue, ready to use	8 fl oz	250	32	10.5
'Isocal HN' for tube feeding, high-nitrogen, isotonic, low-residue, ready to use	1000 ml	1060	123	145.0
'Isocal HN' for tube feeding, high-nitrogen, isotonic, low-residue, ready to use	8 fl oz	250	29	10.7
'Ultracal with Fiber' for tube feeding, high-nitrogen, w/fiber, ready to use	1000 ml	1060	123	45.0
'Ultracal with Fiber' for tube feeding, high-nitrogen, w/fiber, ready to use	8 fl oz	250	29	10.7
(Nestlé Clinical Nutrition)				
'Nubasics' oral, low-sodium, kosher, lactose-, gluten-, and cholesterol-free, low-residue, ready to use	250 ml	250	33	9.2
'Nubasics Complete Nutrition Bar' oral, low-sodium, kosher, lactose- and gluten-free	1 bar	125	17	4.6
'Nubasics Complete Nutrition Soup' oral, low-cholesterol, lactose- and gluten-free, low-residue, 1 envelope	56 g	250	33	9.2
Nubasics Decaffeinated Coffee Beverage' oral, kosher, lactose-, gluten-, and cholesterol-free, powder	2 scoops level	125	19	2.8
'Nubasics Juice Drink' oral, kosher, lactose-, gluten-, and cholesterol-free; low-residue	163 ml	163	34	0.1
'Nubasics Plus' oral, high-calorie, low-sodium, kosher, lactose-, gluten-, and cholesterol-free, low-residue, ready to use	250 ml	375	44	16.2

Food Name	Serv. Size	Total Cal.	Carbs GMS	Fat GMS
'Nubasics 2.0' oral, very high calorie; kosher, lactose- and gluten-free, low-residue, ready to use	250 ml	500	49	26.5
'Nubasics VHP' oral, high-protein, low-sodium, kosher, lactose-, gluten-, and cholesterol-free, ready to use	250 ml	250	28	8.3
'Nubasics with Fiber' oral, high-protein with fiber, low-sodium, kosher, lactose-, gluten-, and cholesterol-free, low-residue, ready to use	250 ml	250	33	9.2
'Nutren 1.0' for oral or tube feeding, kosher, lactose- and gluten-free, low-residue, ready to use	250 ml	250	32	9.5
'Nutren 1.0' for oral or tube feeding, kosher, lactose- and gluten-free, low-residue, ready to use	1000 ml	1000	127	38.0
'Nutren 1.0 with Fiber' for oral or tube feeding, high-fiber, kosher, lactose- and gluten-free, ready to use	1000 ml	1000	127	38.0
'Nutren 1.0 with Fiber' for oral or tube feeding, high-fiber, kosher, lactose- and gluten-free, ready to use	250 ml	250	32	9.5
'Nutren 1.5' for oral or tube feeding, high-calorie, kosher, lactose- and gluten-free, low-residue, ready to use	1000 ml	1500	169	67.6
'Nutren 1.5' for oral or tube feeding, high-calorie, kosher, lactose- and gluten-free, low-residue, ready to use	250 ml	375	42	16.9
'Nutren 2.0' for oral or tube feeding, very high calorie, kosher, lactose- and gluten-free, low-residue, ready to use . . .	1000 ml	2000	196	106.0
'Nutren 2.0' for oral or tube feeding, very high calorie, kosher, lactose- and gluten-free, low-residue, ready to use	250 ml	500	49	26.5
(Novartis [Sandoz])				
'Citrotein' fruit-flavored, lactose-free, low-residue, powder, prepared, 1 serving	254 ml	170	31	0.4
'Citrotein' fruit-flavored, lactose-free, low-residue, powder, prepared	100 ml	670	120	1.6
'Compleat' for tube feeding, blenderized, ready to use	1000 ml	1070	130	43.0
'Compleat' for tube feeding, blenderized, ready to use, 1 can	250 ml	265	32	10.7
'Compleat Modified with Fiber' for tube feeding, blenderized, lactose-free, isotonic, ready to use	1000 ml	1070	140	37.0
'Compleat Modified with Fiber' for tube feeding, blenderized, lactose-free, isotonic, ready to use, 1 can	250 ml	265	35	9.2
'Fibersource HN' for oral or tube feeding, high-fiber, high-nitrogen, lactose- and gluten-free, ready to use	1000 ml	1200	160	41.0
'Fibersource HN' for oral or tube feeding, high-fiber, high-nitrogen, lactose- and gluten-free, ready to use, 1 can	250 ml	300	40	10.4
'Fibersource' for oral or tube feeding, high-fiber, lactose- and gluten-free, ready to use	1000 ml	1200	170	41.0
'Fibersource' for oral or tube feeding, high-fiber, lactose- and gluten-free, ready to use, 1 can	250 ml	300	42	10.4
'Isosource HN' for oral or tube feeding, protein maintenance, lactose-, gluten-, and fiber-free, ready to use . . .	1000 ml	1200	160	41.0
'Isosource HN' for oral or tube feeding, protein maintenance, lactose-, gluten-, and fiber-free, ready to use	250 ml	300	39	10.4
'Isosource 1.5 with Fiber' high-calorie, high-nitrogen, ready to use	1000 ml	1500	68	65.0
'Isosource 1.5 with Fiber' high-calorie, high-nitrogen, ready to use, 1 can	250 ml	375	17	16.2
'Isosource Standard' for oral or tube feeding, protein maintenance, lactose-, gluten-, and fiber-free, ready to use . . .	1000 ml	1200	170	41.0
'Isosource Standard' for oral or tube feeding, protein maintenance, lactose-, gluten-, and fiber-free, ready to use	250	300	42	10.4
'Isosource VHN with Fiber' for oral or tube feeding, w/fiber, ready to use	1000 ml	1000	130	29.0
'Isosource VHN with Fiber' for oral or tube feeding, w/fiber, ready to use	250 ml	250	32	7.2

Food Name	Serv. Size	Total Cal.	Carbs GMS	Fat GMS
'Resource Plus' for oral or tube feeding, high-calorie, lactose- and gluten-free, ready to use .... 1000 ml		1500	200	53.0
'Resource Plus' for oral or tube feeding, high-calorie, lactose- and gluten-free, ready to use, 1 Brik Pak .... 237 ml		355	47	12.6
'Resource Standard' maintenance protein and calorie, lactose- and gluten-free, ready to use .... 1000 ml		1100	140	37.0
'Resource Standard' maintenance protein and calorie, lactose- and gluten-free, ready to use, 1 Brik Pak .... 237 ml		250	34	8.8
(Ross)				
'Ensure High Protein' oral (not parenteral use), kosher, gluten- and lactose-free, low-residue, ready to use .... 8 fl oz		225	31	6.0
'Ensure Plus' for oral or tube feeding (not parenteral use), high-calorie, kosher, gluten- and lactose-free, low-residue, ready to use .... 1 liter		1500	200	53.3
'Ensure Plus' for oral or tube feeding (not parenteral use), high-calorie, kosher, gluten- and lactose-free, low-residue, ready to use .... 8 fl oz		355	47	12.6
'Ensure Plus HN' for oral or tube feeding (not parenteral use), high calorie, kosher, gluten- and lactose-free, low-residue, ready to use .... 1 liter		1500	200	50.0
'Ensure Plus HN' for oral or tube feeding (not parenteral use), high-calorie, kosher, gluten- and lactose-free, low-residue, ready to use .... 8 fl oz		355	47	11.8
'Jevity with Fiber' for tube feeding (not parenteral use), fiber-fortified, isotonic, kosher, gluten-and lactose-free, low-residue, ready to use .... 1 liter		1060	154	34.7
'Jevity with Fiber' for tube feeding (not parenteral use), fiber-fortified, isotonic, kosher, gluten-and lactose-free, low-residue, ready to use .... 8 fl oz		250	36	8.2
'Jevity Plus with Fiber' for tube feeding (not parenteral use), high-nitrogen, kosher, gluten- and lactose-free, ready to use .... 1 liter		1200	175	39.3
'Jevity Plus with Fiber' for tube feeding (not parenteral use), high-nitrogen, kosher, gluten- and lactose-free, ready to use ... 8 fl oz		285	42	9.3
'Osmolite' for oral or tube feeding (not parenteral use), high-nitrogen, isotonic, kosher, gluten- and lactose-free, low-residue, ready to use .... 1 liter		1060	144	34.7
'Osmolite' for oral or tube feeding (not parenteral use), high-nitrogen, isotonic, kosher, gluten- and lactose-free, low-residue, ready to use .... 8 fl oz		250	34	8.2
'Osmolite HN Plus' for tube feeding (not parenteral use), high-calorie, high-nitrogen, kosher, gluten- and lactose-free, low-residue, ready to use .... 1 liter		1200	158	39.3
'Osmolite HN Plus' for tube feeding (not parenteral use), high-calorie, high-nitrogen, kosher, gluten- and lactose-free, low-residue, ready to use .... 8 fl oz		285	38	9.3
'Twocal HN' for oral or tube feeding (not parenteral use), high-calorie, high-protein, kosher, gluten- and lactose-free, low-residue, ready to use .... 1 liter		2000	217	90.9
'Twocal HN' for oral or tube feeding (not parenteral use), high-calorie, high-protein, kosher, gluten- and lactose-free, low-residue, ready to use .... 8 fl oz		475	51	21.5
PARENTERAL SUPPORT (NUTRIENT INJECTIONS)				
(B. Braun/McGaw)				
'Freamine HBC' 6.9% amino acids, sterile, nonpyrogenic, hypertonic solution .... 100 ml		na	na	na
'Freamine III' 8.5% amino acids, nonpyrogenic, hypertonic solution .... 100 ml		na	na	na

Food Name	Serv. Size	Total Cal.	Carbs GMS	Fat GMS
'Freamine III' 10% amino acids, sterile, nonpyrogenic, hypertonic solution, w/electrolytes	100 ml	na	na	na
'Freamine III with Electrolytes' 8.5% amino acids, sterile, nonpyrogenic, hypertonic solution, w/electrolytes	100 ml	na	na	na
'Freamine II' 3% amino acids, sterile, nonpyrogenic, slightly hypertonic solution, w/electrolytes	100 ml	na	na	na
'Hepatamine' 8% amino acids, for patients w/cirrosis or hepatitis, sterile, nonpyrogenic, hypertonic solution	500 ml	na	na	na
'Hepatamine' 8% amino acids, for patients w/hepatic encephalopathy, injection	100 ml	na	na	na
'Procalamine' 3% amino acids, 3% glycerine, sterile, nonpyrogenic, moderately hypertonic injection, w/electrolytes	100 ml	na	na	na
'Trophanine' 10% amino acids, sterile, nonpyrogenic, hypertonic solution, w/electrolytes	100 ml	na	na	na
'Trophanine' 6% amino acids, sterile, nonpyrogenic, hypertonic solution, w/electrolytes	100 ml	na	na	na

PEDIATRIC

(Mead Johnson Nutritionals)

Food Name	Serv. Size	Total Cal.	Carbs GMS	Fat GMS
'Kindercal with Fiber' for oral or tube feeding, lactose-free, isotonic, ready to use	1000 ml	1060	135	44.0
'Kindercal with Fiber' for oral or tube fooding, lactose-free, isotonic, ready to use	8 fl oz	250	32	10.5
'Portagen' for GI disorders, children under 2 years, powder, prepared	5 fl oz	100	12	4.8

(Nestlé Clinical Nutrition)

Food Name	Serv. Size	Total Cal.	Carbs GMS	Fat GMS
'Nutren Junior' for oral or tube feeding, children 1–10 years, kosher, lactose- and gluten-free, low-residue, ready to use	1000 ml	1000	128	42.0
'Nutren Junior' for oral or tube feeding, children 1–10 years, kosher, lactose- and gluten-free, low-residue, ready to use	250 ml	250	32	10.5
'Nutren Junior with Fiber' for oral or tube feeding, children 1-10 years, kosher, lactose- and gluten-free, low-residue, ready to use	1000 ml	1000	128	42.0
'Nutren Junior with Fiber' for oral or tube feeding, children 1–10 years, kosher, lactose- and gluten-free, low-residue, ready to use	250 ml	250	32	10.5
'Peptamen Junior' for tube feeding, GI patients, children 1-10 years, lactose- and gluten-free, low-residue, ready to use	1000 ml	1000	138	38.5
'Peptamen Junior' for tube feeding, GI patients, children 1-10 years, lactose- and gluten-free, low-residue, ready to use	250 ml	250	34	9.6
'Peptamen Junior Oral' oral, for children 1-10 years, lactose- and gluten-free, low-residue, ready to use	1000 ml	1000	138	38.5
'Peptamen Junior Oral' oral, for children 1-10 years, lactose- and gluten-free, low-residue, ready to use	250 ml	250	34	9.6

(Novartis [Sandoz])

Food Name	Serv. Size	Total Cal.	Carbs GMS	Fat GMS
'Vivonex Pediatric' for oral or tube feeding, children 1–10 years, powder, prepared	1000 ml	800	130	24.0
'Vivonex Pediatric' for oral or tube feeding, children 1–10 years, powder, prepared	250 ml	200	32	5.9

(Ross)

Food Name	Serv. Size	Total Cal.	Carbs GMS	Fat GMS
'Pediasure with Fiber' for oral or tube feeding (not parenteral use), kosher, gluten- and lactose-free, ready to use, not for children with galactosemia	1 liter	1000	114	49.7

Food Name	Serv. Size	Total Cal.	Carbs GMS	Fat GMS
'Pediasure with Fiber' for oral or tube feeding (not parenteral use), kosher, gluten- and lactose-free, ready to use, not for children with galactosemia . . . . 8 fl oz		237	27	11.8
'Pediasure' for oral or tube feeding (not parenteral use) kosher, gluten- and lactose-free, low-residue, not for children with galactosemia . . . . 1 liter		1000	110	49.7
'Pediasure' for oral or tube feeding (not parenteral use) kosher, gluten- and lactose-free, low-residue, not for children with galactosemia. . . . . 8 fl oz		237	26	11.8
PROTEIN SUPPLEMENT				
(Mead Johnson Nutritionals)				
'Casec' . . . . 100 gm		380	0	2.0
(Novartis [Sandoz])				
'Meritene' oral, powder, prepared . . . . 1000 ml		1100	120	34.0
'Meritene' oral, powder, prepared, 1 serving . . . . 275 ml		275	31	8.8
(Ross)				
for oral or tube feeding (not parenteral use), powder, gluten-free, low-residue, kosher, 2 scoops . . . . 6.6 gm		28	1	0.6
PULMONARY SUPPORT				
(Mead Johnson Nutritionals)				
'Respalor' for oral or tube feeding, high-nitrogen, high-calorie, ready to use . . . . 1000 ml		1520	148	71.0
'Respalor' for oral or tube feeding, high-nitrogen, high-calorie, ready to use . . . . 8 fl oz		360	35	16.8
(Nestlé Clinical Nutrition)				
'Nutrivent' for tube feeding, kosher, lactose- and gluten-free, low-residue, ready to use . . . . 1000 ml		1500	100	94.0
'Nutrivent' for tube feeding, kosher, lactose- and gluten-free, low-residue, ready to use . . . . 250 ml		375	25	23.7
(Ross)				
'Pulmocare' for oral or tube feeding (not parenteral use), kosher, gluten- and lactose-free, low-residue, ready to use . . . . . 1 liter		1500	106	93.3
'Pulmocare' for oral or tube feeding (not parenteral use), kosher, gluten- and lactose-free, low-residue, ready to use . . . . . 8 fl oz		355	25	22.1
RENAL SUPPORT				
(Mead Johnson Nutritionals)				
'Magnacal' for oral or tube feeding, high-calorie, ready to use . . . 1000 ml		2000	200	101.0
'Magnacal' for oral or tube feeding, high-calorie, ready to use . . . . 8 fl oz		470	47	24.0
(Nestlé Clinical Nutrition)				
'Renalcal Diet' for oral or tube feeding, patients w/renal failure, high-calorie, kosher, lactose- and gluten-free, low-residue, ready to use . . . . 1000 ml		2000	290	82.4
'Renalcal Diet' for oral or tube feeding, patients w/renal failure, high-calorie, kosher, lactose- and gluten-free, low-residue, ready to use . . . . 250 ml		500	73	20.6
(Ross)				
'Nepro' for oral or tube feeding (not parenteral use), dialyzed patients, kosher, gluten- and lactose-free, low-residue, ready to use . . . . 1 liter		2000	222	95.6
'Nepro' for oral or tube feeding (not parenteral use), dialyzed patients, kosher, gluten- and lactose-free, low-residue, ready to use . . . . 8 fl oz		475	52	22.7
'Suplena' for oral or tube feeding (not parenteral use), predialyzed patients, kosher, gluten- and lactose-free, low-residue, ready to use . . . . 1 liter		2000	255	95.6
'Suplena' for oral or tube feeding (not parenteral use), predialyzed patients, kosher, gluten- and lactose-free, low-residue, ready to use . . . . 8 fl oz		475	61	22.7

Food Name	Serv. Size	Total Cal.	Carbs GMS	Fat GMS
MEDLAR, JAPANESE. See LOQUAT.				
MELBA TOAST. See under CRACKER.				
MELON, CANTALOUPE/muskmelon				
Fresh				
balls	1 cup	62	15	0.5
balls	10 balls	48	12	0.4
cubed	1 cup	56	13	0.4
diced	1 cup	55	13	0.4
wedges, 1/8 of large melon	1 wedge	36	9	0.3
wedges, 1/8 of medium melon	1 wedge	24	6	0.2
wedges, 1/8 of small melon	1 wedge	19	5	0.2
whole, large, approx 6 1/2 inch diam	1 melon	285	68	2.3
whole, medium, approx 5-inch diam	1 melon	193	46	1.5
whole, small, approx 4 1/4 inch diam	1 melon	154	37	1.2
Frozen, balls *(Flav-R-Pac)*	3/4 cup	40	10	0.0
MELON, CASABA				
cubed	1 cup	44	11	0.2
sliced, medium	1/10 melon	43	10	0.2
whole, medium	1 melon	426	102	1.6
MELON, HONEYDEW				
Fresh				
balls	1 cup	62	16	0.2
diocd	1 cup	60	16	0.2
wedges, 1/8 of 5.25-inch diam melon	1 wedge	44	11	0.1
wedges, 1/8 of 6- to 7-inch diam melon	1 wedge	56	15	0.2
whole, approx 5.25-inch diam	1 melon	350	92	1.0
whole, 6- to 7-inch diam	1 melon	448	118	1.3
Frozen				
balls, *(Flav-R-Pac)*	3/4 cup	45	11	0.0
balls, unthawed	1 cup	57	14	0.4
MENHADEN OIL. See under FISH OIL.				
MENUDO MIX. See under SEASONING MIX.				
MESQUITE SEASONING. See under MARINADE MIX; SEASONING MIX.				
MEXICAN OREGANO. See OREGANO, MEXICAN.				
MEXICAN POTATO. See JICAMA.				
MEXICAN SEASONING. See under SEASONING MIX.				
MEXICAN STYLE DINNER/ENTRÉE. See also individual listings.				
(Amy's Kitchen) tamale pie	1 serving	220	41	3.0
(Banquet)				
combination, frozen	12 oz	520	72	17.0
frozen	12 oz	490	62	18.0
(Morton) Mexican style, frozen	10 oz	300	44	10.0
(Patio)				
'Fiesta' frozen	12.25 oz	470	55	20.0
frozen	13.25 oz	540	64	25.0
w/tamale, beef enchilada, beans, rice, rice	1 pkg	508	68	19.9
(Stouffer's) 'Mexi-Mac' frozen, food service product	1 oz	26	4	0.9
(Swanson) 'Hungry Man'	1 entrée	690	87	27.0
(Van de Kamp's) frozen	1/2 pkg	220	25	10.0
MILK				
COW				
Canned				
Low-fat				
(Carnation)	1/2 cup	110	12	3.0
Nonfat/skim				
(Carnation)	1/2 cup	100	14	0.3
(Diehl)	1/2 cup	100	14	1.0

Food Name	Serv. Size	Total Cal.	Carbs GMS	Fat GMS
(Finast)	1/2 cup	100	14	1.0
(Pathmark)	1/2 cup	100	14	0.0
(Pet)	1/2 cup	100	14	1.0
Whole				
(Carnation)	1/2 cup	110	12	3.0
Condensed				
sweetened, canned	1 cup	982	166	26.6
sweetened, canned	1 fl oz	123	21	3.3
sweetened, canned *(Borden)*	1/3 cup	320	54	8.0
sweetened, canned *(Carnation)*	1/3 cup	320	56	8.0
sweetened, canned *(Eagle)*	1/2 cup	320	52	9.0
sweetened, canned, 'Jerzee' *(Diehl)*	1/3 cup	320	52	9.0
sweetened, freeze-dried *(Crystalac)*	1 oz	139	22	3.4
Evaporated				
Low-fat				
(Carnation)	1/2 cup	110	12	3.0
canned *(Pathmark)*	1/2 cup	100	14	0.0
Nonfat/skim				
	1 cup	199	29	0.5
	1/2 cup	100	15	0.3
	1 fl oz	25	4	0.1
(Carnation)	1/2 cup	100	14	1.0
(Pet)	1/2 cup	100	14	1.0
Whole				
	1 cup	339	25	19.1
	1/2 cup	169	13	9.5
	1 fl oz	42	3	2.4
(Finast)	1/2 cup	170	12	10.0
(IGA)	1/2 cup	170	12	10.0
(Pathmark)	1/2 cup	170	12	10.9
(Pet)	1/2 cup	170	12	10.0
canned *(Carnation)*	1/2 cup	170	12	10.0
canned *(Diehl)*	1/2 cup	170	12	10.0
filled *(Pet)*	1/2 cup	150	12	8.0
imitation, filled *(Diehl)*	1/2 cup	150	12	8.0
vitamin A, canned	1/2 cup	169	13	9.5
vitamin A, canned	1 fl oz	42	3	2.4
Dry				
Nonfat/skim				
calcium reduced	1 oz	100	15	0.1
calcium reduced	1/4 lb	400	59	0.2
extra grade, instant *(Saco Foods)*	5 tbsp	80	12	1.0
instant	1 cup	244	35	0.5
instant	1/3 cup	82	12	0.2
instant *(Carnation)*	5 tbsp	80	12	0.2
instant, 'Dairy Creamer' *(Weight Watchers)*	1 pkt	10	1	0.0
instant, 'Dairy Fresh' *(Sanalac)*	0.8 oz	80	12	0.1
instant, prepared *(Alba)*	8 fl oz	80	12	0.0
low lactose *(Nutra/Balance)*	1/4 cup	20	3	0.1
regular	1 cup	435	62	0.9
regular	1/4 cup	109	16	0.2
vitamin A	1 cup	435	62	0.9
vitamin A	1/4 cup	109	16	0.2
Whole				
	1 cup	635	49	34.2
	1/4 cup	159	12	8.5

Food Name	Serv. Size	Total Cal.	Carbs GMS	Fat GMS
Fresh				
Low-fat, 1% fat				
(Crowley)	1 cup	100	11	2.0
protein fortified (A&P)	1 cup	100	12	3.0
protein fortified (Borden)	1 cup	100	11	2.0
protein fortified (Crowley)	1 cup	100	11	2.0
protein fortified (Darigold)	1 cup	100	13	2.0
protein fortified 'Nice n' Light' (Knudsen)	1 cup	130	15	3.0
protein fortified, calcium added (Darigold)	1 cup	100	11	2.0
protein fortified, lactose added, 'Lactaid' (Crowley)	1 cup	100	11	2.0
vitamin A	1 quart	409	47	10.3
vitamin A	1 cup	102	12	2.6
vitamin A, protein fortified	1 quart	477	54	11.5
vitamin A, protein fortified	1 cup	119	14	2.9
vitamin A, school milk carton	1/2 pint	102	12	2.6
vitamin A, w/added nonfat milk solids	1 quart	418	49	9.5
vitamin A, w/added nonfat milk solids	1 cup	104	12	2.4
vitamin A and D enriched (Lucerne)	1 cup	110	13	2.5
Low-fat, 2% fat				
(Lucerne) vitamin A and D enriched	1 cup	130	13	5.0
protein fortified (A&P)	1 cup	120	12	5.0
protein fortified (Crowley)	1 cup	120	11	5.0
protein fortified (Darigold)	1 cup	120	11	5.0
protein fortified (Finast)	1 cup	130	12	5.0
protein fortified (Knudsen)	1 cup	140	13	5.0
protein fortified (Viva)	1 cup	120	11	5.0
protein fortified, 'Hi-Protein' (Borden)	1 cup	140	13	5.0
protein fortified, 'Nutrish Acidophilus' (Darigold)	1 cup	120	11	5.0
protein fortified, 'Sweet Acidophilus' (Knudsen)	1 cup	140	13	5.0
protein fortified, 'Tone Acidophilus' (Crowley)	1 cup	120	11	5.0
vitamin A	1 quart	485	47	18.7
vitamin A	1 cup	121	12	4.7
vitamin A, protein fortified	1 quart	546	54	19.5
vitamin A, protein fortified	1 cup	137	14	4.9
vitamin A, school milk carton	1/2 pint	121	12	4.7
vitamin A, w/added nonfat milk solids	1 quart	500	49	18.8
vitamin A, w/added nonfat milk solids	1 cup	125	12	4.7
w/added nonfat milk solids	1 quart	544	54	19.4
w/added nonfat milk solids	1 cup	136	13	4.9
Nonfat/skim				
	1 quart	343	48	1.8
	1 cup	86	12	0.4
protein fortified (A&P)	1 cup	90	12	1.0
protein fortified (Crowley)	1 cup	90	12	1.0
protein fortified (Knudsen)	1 cup	80	12	0.0
protein fortified (Weight Watchers)	1 cup	90	13	1.0
protein fortified, 'Skim-Line' (Borden)	1 cup	100	13	1.0
protein fortified, 'Trim' (Darigold)	1 cup	80	11	1.0
vitamin A, nonfat	1 quart	342	48	1.8
vitamin A, nonfat	1 cup	86	12	0.4
vitamin A, protein fortified, nonfat	1 quart	400	55	2.5
vitamin A, protein fortified, nonfat	1 cup	100	14	0.6
vitamin A, w/added nonfat milk solids	1 quart	361	49	2.5
vitamin A, w/added nonfat milk solids	1 cup	90	12	0.6
vitamin A and D enriched (Lucerne)	1 cup	90	13	0.0
Whole				
(Carnation)	1 cup	150	12	8.0

Food Name	Serv. Size	Total Cal.	Carbs GMS	Fat GMS
low-salt	1 quart	594	44	33.8
low-salt	1 cup	149	11	8.4
low-sodium *(A&P)*	1 cup	150	11	8.0
low-sodium *(Borden)*	1 cup	150	11	8.0
low-sodium *(Crowley)*	1 cup	150	11	8.0
low-sodium *(Darigold)*	1 cup	150	11	8.0
low-sodium *(Knudsen)*	1 cup	160	12	8.0
low-sodium, 'Hi-Calcium' *(Borden)*	1 cup	150	11	8.0
3.7% fat	1 quart	626	45	35.7
3.7% fat	1 cup	157	11	8.9
3.25% fat	1 quart	600	45	32.6
3.25% fat	1 cup	150	11	8.2
3.25% fat	1 tbsp	9	1	0.5
3.25% fat, school milk carton	1/2 pint	150	11	8.2
vitamin A and D enriched *(Lucerne)*	1 cup	150	12	8.0
vitamin D, homogenized *(Borden)*	1 cup	150	11	8.0
vitamin D, homogenized *(Trader Joe's)*	1 cup	150	11	8.0
GOAT				
Evaporated, canned, undiluted *(Meyenberg)*	4 fl oz	143	10	7.9
Fresh				
	1 quart	672	43	40.4
	1 cup	168	11	10.1
	1 fl oz	21	1	1.3
INDIAN BUFFALO				
	1 quart	943	51	67.2
	1 cup	236	13	16.8
HUMAN				
	1 cup	171	17	10.8
	1 fl oz	21	2	1.3
SHEEP				
	1 quart	1057	53	68.6
	1 cup	264	13	17.1
MILK SUBSTITUTE. See also RICE BEVERAGE; SOYMILK.				
w/lauric acid oil, fluid	1 quart	600	60	33.3
w/lauric acid oil, fluid	1 cup	150	15	8.3
w/hydrogenated vegetable oils, fluid	1 quart	600	60	33.3
w/hydrogenated vegetable oils, fluid	1 cup	150	15	8.3
w/hydrogenated vegetable oils, fluid	1 fl oz	19	2	1.0
(Ener-G Foods) lactose-free	3 tbsp	85	7	1.6
(First Alternative) 1%, lactose-free	1 cup	80	6	2.0
MILKFISH. See AWA.				
MILKSHAKE				
(Killer Shake)				
banana, 'Bodacious Bananaberry'	1 carton	420	62	14.0
chocolate, 'Totally Chocolate'	1 carton	470	65	17.0
(MicroMagic)				
chocolate, frozen	11.5 fl oz	340	55	8.0
strawberry, frozen	11.5 fl oz	340	54	9.0
vanilla, frozen	11.5 fl oz	380	60	13.0
MILKSHAKE MIX, CHOCOLATE				
chocolate fudge *(Weight Watchers)*	1 pkt	70	11	1.0
orange sherbet *(Weight Watchers)*	1 pkt	70	11	0.0
MILLET				
pearl, cooked	1/2 cup	143	28.4	1.2
pearl, cooked	4 oz	135	26.8	1.1
pearl, raw	1/2 cup	378	72.9	4.2
pearl, raw	1 oz	107	20.7	1.2

Food Name	Serv. Size	Total Cal.	Carbs GMS	Fat GMS
pearl, raw, hulled *(Arrowhead Mills)*	1 oz	90	21.0	1.0
Proso/hog millet, whole grain	3 1/2 oz	327	72.9	2.9
MINCEMEAT. See under PIE FILLING.				
MISO				
	1 cup	567	77	16.7
barley, mugi, organic *(Eden Foods)*	1 tbsp	25	3	1.0
barley, pasteurized *(Westbrae)*	1 tsp	12	2	0.0
brown rice, genmai, organic *(Eden Foods)*	1 tbsp	25	3	1.0
brown rice, pasteurized *(Westbrae)*	1 tsp	10	2	0.0
hacho *(Westbrae)*	1 tsp	14	1	0.0
hacho, organic *(Eden Foods)*	1 tbsp	35	2	1.5
red, instant *(Westbrae)*	.35 oz	35	3	1.0
red, pasteurized *(Westbrae)*	1 tsp	10	1	0.0
rice, kome, organic *(Eden Foods)*	1 tbsp	25	3	1.0
rice, sweet white shiro, organic *(Eden Foods)*	1 tbsp	35	5	1.0
soy and rice, red, kome, organic *(Eden Foods)*	1 tbsp	25	3	1.0
soy, hacho, organic *(Eden Foods)*	1 tbsp	35	2	2.0
soy, pasteurized *(Westbrae)*	1 tsp	12	1	0.0
white, instant *(Westbrae)*	.35 oz	35	4	1.0
MOLASSES				
	1 cup	872	226	0.3
	1 tbsp	53	14	0.0
bead *(LaChoy)*	1/2 tsp	7	2	1.0
blackstrap	1 cup	771	199	0.0
blackstrap	1 tbsp	47	12	0.0
dark *(Br'er Rabbit)*	1 oz	110	28	0.0
gold *(Grandma's)*	1 tbsp	70	17	0.0
gold, mild flavor *(Grandma's)*	1 tbsp	70	17	0.0
green, robust flavor *(Grandma's)*	1 tbsp	70	16	0.0
light *(Br'er Rabbit)*	1 oz	110	29	0.0
MOMBIN, YELLOW. See JOBO.				
MONKFISH/angler fish/bellyfish/frogfish/goosefish/lotte/sea devil				
baked, broiled, grilled, or microwaved	3 oz	82	0	1.7
raw	3 oz	65	0	1.3
MONOSODIUM GLUTAMATE				
flavor enhancer, 'MSG' *(Accent)*	0.13 tsp	0	0	0.0
flavor enhancer, 'MSG' *(Tone's)*	1 tsp	0	0	0.0
MOOSE				
raw	1 oz	29	0	0.2
roasted	3 oz	114	0	0.8
roasted, boneless, yield from 1 lb raw	11.9 oz	456	0	3.3
MOSTACCIOLI. See under PASTA.				
MOSTACCIOLI DISH/ENTRÉE. See under PASTA DISH/ENTRÉE.				
MOTH BEAN. See BEAN, MOTH.				
MOUNTAIN YAM. See under YAM.				
MOUSSE				
(Estee) orange chocolate	1/2 cup	70	9	3.0
(Weight Watchers)				
chocolate	1 serving	190	31	5.0
pecan praline	1 serving	170	31	3.5
triple chocolate caramel	1 serving	200	34	4.0
MOUSSE BAR chocolate *(Weight Watchers)*	1 bar	35	9	0.5
MOUSSE MIX				
(Alsa) dark chocolate	2.5 tbsp	105	13	5.1
(Jell-O)				
chocolate, 'Rich & Luscious' mix only	1 pkg	110	18	3.0
chocolate, 'Rich & Luscious' prepared w/whole milk	1/2 cup	150	21	6.0

Food Name	Serv. Size	Total Cal.	Carbs GMS	Fat GMS
chocolate fudge, 'Rich & Luscious' prepared w/whole milk	1/2 cup	140	20	6.0
chocolate fudge 'Rich & Luscious' mix only	1 pkg	110	18	4.0
(Sans Sucre de Paris)				
cheesecake, w/NutraSweet, mix only	1/2 cup	60	7	1.5
cheesecake, w/NutraSweet, prepared w/skim milk	1/2 cup	73	10	1.5
chocolate, w/NutraSweet, mix only	1/2 cup	55	6	3.0
chocolate, w/NutraSweet, prepared w/skim milk	1/2 cup	75	8	3.0
chocolate cheesecake, w/NutraSweet, prepared w/skim milk ...	1/2 cup	75	10	1.5
chocolate cheesecake, w/NutraSweet, mix only	1/2 cup	60	7	1.5
key lime, w/NutraSweet, mix only	4 oz	60	6	4.0
key lime w/NutraSweet, prepared w/skim milk	4 oz	75	6	4.0
lemon, w/NutraSweet, mix only	1/2 cup	50	7	2.0
lemon, w/NutraSweet, prepared w/skim milk	1/2 cup	70	9	2.0
strawberry, w/NutraSweet, mix	1/2 cup	50	7	2.0
strawberry, w/NutraSweet, prepared w/skim milk	1/2 cup	70	9	2.0
(Weight Watchers)				
chocolate, prepared w/nonfat milk	1/2 cup	60	9	3.0
chocolate cheesecake, prepared w/nonfat milk	1/2 cup	60	12	2.0
chocolate raspberry, prepared w/nonfat milk	1/2 cup	60	12	3.0
white chocolate, almond, prepared w/nonfat milk	1/2 cup	60	6	3.0

MUFFIN. See also ENGLISH MUFFIN; MUFFIN MIX.
APPLE
(Awrey's)

1.5 oz	1 muffin	130	17	6.0
streusel, 4.2 oz, 'Grande'	1 muffin	340	50	13.0
2.5 oz	1 muffin	220	30	10.0
(Muffin-A-Day) bran, 'Total Health Muffin'	1 muffin	120	31	0.0

APPLE BANANA NUT

(Awrey's) 4.2 oz, 'Grande'	1 muffin	260	27	16.0
(Hostess) w/walnuts, mini	5 muffins	160	17	9.0

APPLE SPICE

(Health Valley) nonfat	1 muffin	130	30	0.0
(Healthy Choice) frozen, 2.5 oz	1 muffin	190	40	4.0
(Sara Lee) frozen, 2.5 oz	1 muffin	220	36	8.0
(Weight Watchers) 'Microwave' 2.5 oz	1 muffin	160	29	5.0

BANANA

(Health Valley) nonfat	1 muffin	130	29	0.0
(Hostess) bran, low-fat	1 serving	240	47	3.0

BANANA NUT

(Break Cake) 5 oz	1 muffin	60	7	3.0
(Healthy Choice) frozen, 2.5 oz	1 muffin	180	32	6.0
(Weight Watchers)	1 muffin	180	34	4.0

BLUEBERRY
(Awrey's)

4.2 oz, 'Grande'	1 muffin	360	52	14.0
1.5 oz	1 muffin	130	18	5.0
(Break Cake) 5 oz	1 muffin	60	8	3.0
(Ener-G Foods) gluten-free	1 muffin	51	8	1.9
(Entenmann's)				
....	1 muffin	200	29	8.0
nonfat, no cholesterol	1 muffin	120	26	0.0
(Healthy Choice) frozen, 2.5 oz	1 muffin	190	39	4.0
(Hostess)				
low-fat	1 serving	230	47	2.5
mini, 'Breakfast Bake Shop'	5 muffins	240	29	13.0
(Muffin-A-Day) bran, 'Total Health Muffin'	1 muffin	120	31	0.0
(Natural Ovens) low-fat	1 muffin	160	32	1.0

Food Name	Serv. Size	Total Cal.	Carbs GMS	Fat GMS
(Pepperidge Farm) frozen, 'Old Fashioned'	1 muffin	170	27	7.0
(Sara Lee)				
frozen, 'Free & Light'	1 muffin	120	28	0.0
frozen, 2.5 oz	1 muffin	200	34	8.0
(Weight Watchers)	1 muffin	180	33	4.0
BLUEBERRY APPLE *(Health Valley)* twin pack	1 muffin	140	32	0.0
BRAN				
(Awrey's)				
w/raisins, 1.5 oz	1 muffin	110	18	4.0
w/raisins, 2.5 oz	1 muffin	190	30	7.0
w/raisins, 4.2 oz, 'Grande'	1 muffin	320	50	12.0
(Pepperidge Farm) w/raisins, cholesterol-free, frozen, 'Old Fashioned	1 muffin	170	30	6.0
(Sara Lee) w/raisins, 2.5 oz, frozen	1 muffin	220	37	7.0
(Weight Watchers) 'Harvest Honey'	1 muffin	220	42	4.5
BUTTERMILK *(Ener-G Foods)* gluten-free	1 muffin	195	30	6.9
CARROT				
(Health Valley) nonfat, twin pack	1 muffin	130	30	0.0
(Muffin-A-Day) 'Total Health Muffin'	1 muffin	120	31	0.0
(Natural Ovens) low-fat	1 muffin	150	30	2.0
CHEESE *(Sara Lee)* streusel, 2.1 oz	1 muffin	220	27	11.0
CHOCOLATE CHIP				
(Sara Lee) chocolate chunk, frozen, 2.1 oz	1 muffin	220	33	8.0
(Weight Watchers)	1 muffin	200	39	4.0
CINNAMON *(Pepperidge Farm)* swirl, frozen, 'Old Fashioned'	1 muffin	190	30	6.0
CORN				
(Awrey's) 1.5 oz	1 muffin	130	20	5.0
(Pepperidge Farm) frozen, 'Old Fashioned'	1 muffin	180	27	7.0
(Sara Lee) golden, frozen, 2.5 oz	1 muffin	250	31	13.0
CRANBERRY				
(Awrey's) 1.5 oz	1 muffin	120	20	4.0
(Natural Ovens) low-fat	1 muffin	140	26	2.0
OAT BRAN				
(Awrey's)				
2.75 oz	1 muffin	180	27	7.0
w/pineapple and raisins, 2.75 oz	1 muffin	180	26	6.0
(Health Valley)				
w/almonds and dates	1 muffin	180	31	4.0
w/blueberries	1 muffin	180	32	4.0
w/raisins	1 muffin	180	31	5.0
(Hostess)				
'Breakfast Bake Shop'	1 muffin	160	21	7.0
'Snack Cake'	1 serving	160	21	8.0
w/banana and nuts, 'Breakfast Bake Shop'	1 muffin	140	20	5.0
(Pepperidge Farm) w/apple, cholesterol-free, frozen, 'Old Fashioned'	1 muffin	190	29	7.0
(Sara Lee)				
2.5 oz	1 muffin	210	35	8.0
w/apple, 2.5 oz	1 muffin	210	35	8.0
RAISIN				
(Awrey's)				
bran, 1.5 oz	1 muffin	110	18	4.0
bran, 4.2 oz, 'Grande'	1 muffin	320	50	12.0
(Health Valley) spice	1 muffin	140	32	0.0
(Pepperidge Farm) bran, cholesterol-free, frozen, 'Old Fashioned'	1 muffin	170	30	6.0
(Sara Lee) bran, 2.5 oz	1 muffin	220	37	7.0

Food Name	Serv. Size	Total Cal.	Carbs GMS	Fat GMS
(Wonder) 'Raisin Rounds'	1 muffin	140	27	2.0
RASPBERRY *(Health Valley)* nonfat, twin pack	1 muffin	130	30	0.0
RICE BRAN				
(Ener-G Foods) gluten-free	1 serving	257	32	11.8
(Health Valley) w/raisins	1 muffin	215	35	7.0
SOURDOUGH *(Wonder)*	1 muffin	130	27	1.0
MUFFIN MIX				
(Gluten-Free Pantry) gluten-free	1 serving	100	24	0.0
ALMOND				
(Krusteaz) w/poppyseeds, prepared	1 muffin	167	30	4.0
APPLE				
(Betty Crocker)				
cinnamon, prepared w/egg, 2% milk	1/12 pkg	120	18	4.0
cinnamon, prepared w/egg white, nonfat milk	1/12 pkg	110	18	3.0
streusel, Dutch, prepared w/egg, whole milk	1/12 pkg	200	32	7.0
(General Mills)				
and cinnamon, prepared	1 muffin	100	17	3.0
and cinnamon, prepared w/egg white, nonfat milk	1 muffin	110	18	3.0
and cinnamon, prepared w/2% milk, 1 egg	1 muffin	120	18	4.0
(Krusteaz) and cinnamon, prepared	1 muffin	180	36	3.0
(Martha White) and cinnamon, prepared w/2% milk	1 muffin	140	25	3.0
APPLESAUCE				
(Gold Medal) prepared w/egg, whole milk	1/6 pkg	160	26	5.0
(Robin Hood) prepared w/egg, whole milk	1/6 pkg	160	26	5.0
BANANA				
(Gold Medal) prepared w/egg, whole milk	1/12 pkg	150	24	5.0
(Robin Hood) prepared w/egg, whole milk	1/12 pkg	150	24	5.0
BANANA NUT				
(Betty Crocker)				
prepared w/egg, 2% milk	1/12 pkg	120	17	5.0
prepared w/egg white, nonfat milk	1/12 pkg	110	17	4.0
(General Mills)				
prepared	1 muffin	110	17	4.0
prepared w/egg white, nonfat milk	1 muffin	120	18	4.0
prepared w/2% milk, 1 egg	1 muffin	120	18	4.0
(Martha White) prepared w/2% milk	1 muffin	180	23	8.0
BERRY				
(General Mills)				
wild, prepared	1 muffin	100	18	3.0
wild, 'Light' prepared	1 muffin	90	20	1.0
wild, 'Light' prepared w/1 egg	1 muffin	90	20	1.0
wild, prepared w/2% milk, 1 egg	1 muffin	120	19	4.0
wild, prepared w/egg white, skim milk	1 muffin	110	19	3.0
BLACKBERRY *(Martha White)* prepared	1 muffin	140	25	3.0
BLUEBERRY				
(Betty Crocker)				
streusel 'Bake Shop' prepared	1/12 pkg	210	31	8.0
wild, mix only	1 serving	128	26	1.8
wild, prepared w/egg, 2% milk	1/12 pkg	120	18	4.0
wild, prepared w/egg white, skim milk	1/12 pkg	110	18	3.0
(Duncan Hines)				
bakery style, mix only	1 muffin	180	32	5.0
bakery style, prepared	1 muffin	190	32	6.0
regular style, mix only	1 muffin	110	21	2.0
regular style, prepared	1 muffin	120	21	3.0
(General Mills)				
prepared w/egg white, nonfat milk	1 muffin	110	18	3.0

Food Name	Serv. Size	Total Cal.	Carbs GMS	Fat GMS
prepared w/2% milk, 1 egg	1 muffin	120	18	4.0
'Twice the Blueberries' prepared	1 muffin	100	17	3.0
'Twice the Blueberries' prepared, cholesterol-free recipe	1 muffin	110	18	3.0
'Twice the Blueberries' prepared w/2% milk, 1 egg	1 muffin	120	18	4.0
(Gold Medal) imitation, mix only	1 serving	127	24	2.7
(Krusteaz) prepared	1 muffin	150	27	4.0
(Lovin' Lites)				
prepared w/water, 1 egg	1/12 pkg	100	21	1.0
prepared w/water, 2 egg whites	1/12 pkg	100	21	1.0
(Martha White)				
artificial flavor	1 serving	162	30	3.5
prepared	1/6 pkg	140	25	3.0
prepared w/2% milk	1 muffin	140	25	3.0
(Robin Hood) 'Pouch Mix' prepared w/egg, whole milk	1/6 pkg	170	26	6.0
BRAN				
(Duncan Hines) and honey, bakery style, prepared	1 muffin	200	32	7.0
(Gold Medal) w/honey, prepared w/egg, whole milk	1/6 pkg	170	25	6.0
(Hodgson Mill) stone ground, whole grain	1/4 cup	130	27	1.0
(Krusteaz) w/honey, prepared	1 muffin	140	23	4.0
(Martha White) prepared w/2% milk	1 muffin	150	24	5.0
(Robin Hood) w/honey, prepared w/egg, whole milk	1/6 pkg	170	25	6.0
CARAMEL				
(Gold Medal) 'Pouch Mix' prepared w/egg, whole milk	1/6 pkg	150	23	5.0
(Robin Hood) 'Pouch Mix', prepared w/egg, whole milk	1/6 pkg	150	23	5.0
CARROT NUT				
(Betty Crocker)				
prepared w/egg, 2% milk	1/12 pkg	150	22	5.0
prepared w/egg white, nonfat milk	1/12 pkg	150	22	5.0
CHOCOLATE CHIP				
(Betty Crocker)				
prepared	1/12 pkg	140	22	5.0
prepared w/egg, 2% milk	1/12 pkg	150	22	6.0
(Krusteaz)				
chocolate, prepared	1 muffin	200	36	5.0
chocolate, prepared	1 muffin	200	35	5.0
CINNAMON				
(Betty Crocker) streusel, prepared w/egg, 2% milk	1/12 pkg	200	27	9.0
(Duncan Hines)				
swirl, bakery style, mix only	1 muffin	190	32	6.0
swirl, bakery style, prepared	1 muffin	200	32	7.0
(General Mills)				
'Streusel' prepared	1 muffin	190	27	8.0
'Streusel' prepared w/2% milk, 1 egg	1 muffin	200	27	9.0
CORN				
(Arrowhead Mills) blue, prepared	1 muffin	110	15	4.0
(Dromedary)				
mix only	3 1/2 tbsp	110	20	3.0
prepared	1 muffin	120	20	4.0
(Flako)				
mix only	1/3 cup	160	29	4.0
prepared	1 muffin	116	20	3.3
(Gold Medal) prepared w/egg, whole milk	1/6 pkg	130	24	2.0
(Krusteaz) prepared, 1.48 oz	1 muffin	220	36	7.0
(Martha White) yellow, prepared w/water	1 muffin	160	30	3.0
(Robin Hood) prepared w/egg, whole milk	1/6 pkg	130	24	2.0
CRANBERRY ORANGE NUT				
(Duncan Hines) bakery style, prepared	1 muffin	200	30	8.0

Food Name	Serv. Size	Total Cal.	Carbs GMS	Fat GMS
LEMON				
(Martha White) and poppy seed, prepared w/2% milk	1 muffin	200	30	9.0
OAT				
(Gold Medal) prepared w/egg & 2% milk	1/6 pkg	150	23	5.0
(Robin Hood) prepared w/egg & 2% milk	1/6 pkg	150	23	5.0
OAT BRAN				
(Arrowhead Mills)				
w/apple and spice, prepared	1 muffin	120	15	4.0
wheat-free, prepared	1 muffin	100	11	5.0
(Betty Crocker)				
prepared w/egg, 2% milk	1/8 pkg	190	25	8.0
prepared w/egg white, nonfat milk	1/8 pkg	180	25	7.0
w/oatmeal and raisins, prepared w/egg, 2% milk	1/12 pkg	140	22	4.0
(General Mills) prepared	1 muffin	170	26	6.0
prepared w/nonfat milk, egg white	1 muffin	170	26	6.0
prepared w/2% milk, 1 egg	1 muffin	180	26	7.0
(Hain)				
w/apple and cinnamon, prepared	1 muffin	140	28	3.0
w/banana and nuts, prepared	1 muffin	140	26	4.0
w/raspberry and spice, prepared	1 muffin	140	27	3.0
(Krusteaz) prepared	1 muffin	190	33	5.0
OATMEAL				
(Betty Crocker)				
and raisin, prepared w/egg white, nonfat milk	1/12 pkg	130	22	3.0
ORANGE				
(Martha White) and berry, prepared w/2% milk	1 muffin	140	25	3.0
PECAN				
(Duncan Hines) crunch, bakery style, prepared	1 muffin	220	27	11.0
RASPBERRY				
(Martha White) raspberry, prepared w/2% milk	1 muffin	140	25	3.0
STRAWBERRY				
(Arrowhead Mills) wheat bran, prepared	2 muffins	270	43	7.0
(Betty Crocker)				
crown, prepared w/egg, 2% milk	1/10 pkg	150	24	5.0
crown, prepared w/egg white, nonfat milk	1/10 pkg	140	24	4.0
(Martha White)				
prepared	1/6 pkg	140	25	3.0
prepared w/2% milk	1 muffin	140	25	3.0
WHOLE WHEAT				
(Hodgson Mill) stone ground, whole grain	1/4 cup	130	27	1.0
MULBERRY				
fresh, raw	1 cup	60	14	0.5
fresh, raw	10 medium	6	1	0.1
MULLET, STRIPED				
baked, broiled, grilled, or microwaved	4 oz	170	0.0	5.5
raw	1 lb	530	0.0	17.2
raw	3 oz	99	0.0	3.2
MUNG BEAN. See BEAN, MUNG.				
MUNGO BEAN. See BEAN, MUNGO.				
MUSHROOM, BUTTON. See MUSHROOM, WHITE.				
MUSHROOM, CRIMINI, brown, Italian, fresh, raw	1 piece	3	1	0.0
MUSHROOM, ENOKI				
Fresh				
raw, whole	1 large	2	0	0.0
raw, whole	1 medium	1	0	0.0
MUSHROOM, JAPANESE HONEY/hon shimeji				
Fresh				
(Frieda of California) trimmed	1 oz	9	1	0.1

Food Name	Serv. Size	Total Cal.	Carbs GMS	Fat GMS
MUSHROOM, OYSTER/abalone/hiritake/shimeji/tree mushroom				
Fresh				
raw *(Frieda of California)*	1 oz	7	1	0.1
raw, whole	1 large	55	9	0.8
raw, whole	1 small	6	1	0.1
MUSHROOM, SHIITAKE				
Dried				
whole	4 medium	44	11	0.1
whole	1 medium	11	3	0.0
Fresh				
cooked, pieces	1 cup	80	21	0.3
cooked, whole	4 medium	40	10	0.2
MUSHROOM, STRAW				
Canned				
in salt water, imported *(Orchids)*	11 med pieces	16	2	0.0
Oriental *(Green Giant)*	2 oz	12	2	0.0
pieces, drained	1 cup	58	8	1.2
pieces, drained	1 med piece	2	0	0.0
whole *(Green Giant)*	1/4 cup	12	2	0.0
MUSHROOM, TREE. See MUSHROOM, OYSTER.				
MUSHROOM, WHITE				
Canned				
(B in B)	1/4 cup	12	2	0.0
caps, drained	8 caps	11	2	0.1
pieces, drained	1 cup	37	8	0.5
pieces, drained	1/2 cup	19	4	0.2
pieces and stems *(Allens)*	1/2 cup	20	3	1.0
pieces and stems, broiled in butter, 'BinB' *(Green Giant)*	1/2 cup	30	4	0.0
sliced *(Green Giant)*	1/2 cup	30	4	0.0
sliced, broiled in butter, 'BinB' *(Green Giant)*	1/2 cup	30	4	0.0
slices, drained	10 slices	10	2	0.1
stems and pieces *(Brandywine)*	1/2 cup	20	3	0.0
w/garlic *(B in B)*	1/4 cup	12	2	0.0
whole, broiled in butter, 'BinB' *(Green Giant)*	1 can	30	4	0.0
whole, drained, medium	1 mushroom	3	1	0.0
whole, pieces, and stems *(Green Giant)*	1/4 cup	12	2	0.0
Fresh				
boiled, drained, chopped	1 tbsp	3	1	0.0
boiled drained, sliced	1 cup	42	8	0.7
boiled, drained, sliced	1/2 cup	21	4	0.4
boiled, drained, whole, medium	1 mushroom	3	1	0.1
raw, pieces or slices	1 cup	18	3	0.2
raw, sliced	1/2 cup	9	1	0.1
raw, whole	1 cup	24	4	0.3
raw, whole, medium	1 mushroom	5	1	0.1
Frozen				
(Freshlike)	3.5 oz	30	4	0.0
(Veg-All)	3.5 oz	30	4	0.0
whole, 'Deluxe' *(Birds Eye)*	2.6 oz	20	4	0.0
MUSHROOM DISH/ENTRÉE				
(Empire Kosher) breaded, frozen	7 mushrooms	90	16	1.0
(Gardenburger) patty, savory, vegetarian, 'Gourmet'	2.5 oz	120	18	3.0
(Green Giant) creamy, 'Right for Lunch'.	9.5 oz	220	29	11.0
(Stilwell)				
battered, 'Quick Krisp'	5 pieces	90	13	2.5
breaded	6 pieces	90	17	0.0
MUSKMELON. See MELON, CANTALOUPE.				

Food Name	Serv. Size	Total Cal.	Carbs GMS	Fat GMS
MUSKRAT				
raw	1 oz	46	0	2.3
roasted	3 oz	199	0	10.0
roasted, boneless, yield from 1 lb raw	11 oz	732	0	36.7
MUSSEL, BLUE				
boiled, poached, or steamed	3 oz	146	6	3.8
raw	1 cup	129	6	3.4
raw	3 oz	73	3	1.9
raw, large	1 mussel	17	1	0.4
raw, medium	1 mussel	14	1	0.4
raw, small	1 mussel	9	0	0.2
raw, w/o shell	1 oz	24	1	0.6
MUSTARD, DRY				
(Spice Islands)	1 tsp	9	0	0.6
ground *(Durkee)*	1 tsp	19	0	0.1
ground *(Eden Foods)*	1 tsp	0	1	0.0
ground *(Laurel Leaf)*	1 tsp	19	0	0.1
MUSTARD, PREPARED				
yellow	1 cup	165	19	7.8
yellow	1 tsp	3	0	0.2
(Dietsource) lower calorie, low sodium	1 serving	15	1	1.0
(Featherweight)	1 tsp	5	0	0.0
(French's)				
'Bold'n Spicy'	1 tsp	5	0	0.0
Dijon	1 tsp	10	0	0.5
horseradish	1 tsp	0	0	0.0
Medford	1 tbsp	16	1	1.0
w/onion	1 tsp	8	2	0.0
yellow	1 tsp	0	0	0.0
(Great Impressions) jalapeño	2 tsp	7	1	0.3
(Grey Poupon)				
Dijon	1 tsp	6	1	0.4
Dijon, country	1 tsp	6	0	0.0
Parisian	1 tsp	6	0	0.0
(Gulden's)				
hot, 'Diablo'	.25 oz	8	0	0.0
mild, yellow, creamy	.25 oz	6	0	0.0
spicy, brown	.25 oz	8	0	0.0
(Hain)				
stone ground	1 tbsp	14	1	1.0
stone ground, no salt added	1 tbsp	14	1	1.0
(Heinz)				
mild, yellow	1 tbsp	8	1	1.0
spicy, brown	1 tbsp	14	1	1.0
yellow	1 tsp	3	0	0.2
(Kraft)				
horseradish	1 tbsp	14	1	1.0
'Pure'	1 tbsp	11	1	1.0
(Westbrae)				
Dijon	1 tbsp	16	1	1.0
'Mt. Fuji'	1 tbsp	16	1	1.0
stone ground, no salt	1 tbsp	16	1	1.0
yellow	1 tbsp	16	1	1.0
MUSTARD BLEND				
(Best Foods/Hellmann's) blend, 'Creamy Dijonniase'	1 tsp	10	1	1.0
(Luzianne) 'Creole' yellow and brown	1 tbsp	10	2	0.0
MUSTARD FLOUR. See under FLOUR.				

Food Name	Serv. Size	Total Cal.	Carbs GMS	Fat GMS
MUSTARD GREENS				
Fresh				
boiled, drained, chopped	1 cup	21	3	0.3
raw, chopped	1 cup	15	3	0.1
Canned, chopped *(Allens)*	1/2 cup	20	2	1.0
Frozen				
(Frosty Acres)	3.3 oz	20	3	0.0
chopped *(Flav-R-Pac)*	1/3 cup	25	2	0.0
chopped *(Seabrook)*	3.3 oz	20	3	0.0
chopped *(Southern)*	3.5 oz	25	4	0.3
chopped, unprepared	1 cup	29	5	0.4
unprepared	10-oz pkg	57	10	0.8
w/o salt, chopped, drained	1 cup	29	5	0.4
w/o salt, drained	10-oz pkg	40	7	0.5
w/salt, chopped or diced, drained	1/2 cup	14	2	0.2
w/salt, drained	10-oz pkg	40	7	0.5
MUSTARD OIL				
	1 cup	1927	0	218.0
	1 tbsp	124	0	14.0
MUSTARD SEED				
(McCormick/Schilling)	1 tsp	17	1	0.8
yellow	1 tbsp	53	4	3.2
yellow	1 tsp	15	1	0.9
MUSTARD SPINACH/tendergreen				
boiled, drained, chopped	1 cup	29	5	0.4
raw, chopped	1 cup	33	6	0.5
MUTTON TALLOW				
	1 cup	1849	0	205.0
	1 tbsp	115	0	12.8

MUTTONFISH. See OCEAN POUT.

N

Food Name	Serv. Size	Total Cal.	Carbs GMS	Fat GMS
NACHO CHIPS. See under CORN CHIPS AND SNACKS.				
NACHO SEASONING. See under SEASONING MIX.				
NAPA. See BOK CHOY.				
NAPOLES				
cooked	1 med pad	4	1	0.0
cooked, sliced	1 cup	22	5	0.1
raw, sliced	1 cup	14	3	0.1
NATAL PLUM. See CARISSA.				
NATTO. See SOYBEAN, FERMENTED.				
NAVY BEAN. See BEAN, NAVY.				
NECTAR. See under FRUIT DRINK.				
NECTARINE				
Fresh				
raw, pitted	1 oz	14	3.3	0.1
raw, sliced	1 cup	68	16.3	0.6
raw, trimmed, whole, approx 2.5 inch diam	1 nectarine	67	16.0	0.6
raw, untrimmed *(Dole)*	1 medium	70	16.0	1.0
raw, whole	1 lb	204	48.6	1.9

NEW ZEALAND SPINACH. See SPINACH, NEW ZEALAND.
NONDAIRY DESSERT, FROZEN. See ICE CREAM SUBSTITUTE; ICE CREAM SUBSTITUTE BAR/DESSERT.

Food Name	Serv. Size	Total Cal.	Carbs GMS	Fat GMS
NONDAIRY DESSERT MIX. See ICE CREAM SUBSTITUTE MIX.				
NOODLE. See also PASTA.				
CELLOPHANE. See under NOODLE, CHINESE.				
CHINESE				
cellophane/long rice, mung bean, dry	1 cup	491	121	0.1
chow mein	1 cup	237	26	13.8
chow mein	1.5 oz	227	25	13.2
rice, cooked	1 cup	192	44	0.4
(China Boy) chow mein	1/2 cup	130	16	5.0
(Chun King)				
chow mein, w/almonds	1/3 cup	140	15	7.0
chow mein, w/sesame bits	1/3 cup	140	16	7.0
(La Choy)				
chow mein, food service product	1/2 cup	140	17	6.1
chow mein, wide, crispy	1 cup	296	32	16.5
rice, canned	1 cup	242	43	6.1
rice, food service product	1/2 cup	122	22	3.1
CHOW MEIN. See under NOODLE, CHINESE.				
EGG				
enriched, cooked	1 cup	213	40	2.4
enriched, dry	1 cup	145	27	1.6
enriched, dry	2 oz	217	41	2.4
spinach, enriched, cooked	1 cup	211	39	2.5
spinach, enriched, dry	1 cup	145	27	1.7
spinach, enriched, dry	2 oz	218	40	2.6
unenriched, dry	1 cup	145	27	1.6
(American Beauty)				
extra wide, enriched, dry	2 oz	220	42	3.0
fine, enriched, dry	2 oz	220	42	3.0
medium, enriched, dry	2 oz	220	42	3.0
wide, enriched, dry	2 oz	220	42	3.0
(Borden) kluski, enriched, dry	1 cup	220	40	3.0
(Creamette)				
plain, enriched, dry	2 oz	221	40	2.5
w/pasteurized eggs, wide, 'Fancy' dry	2 oz	220	40	3.0
(De Boles)				
Jerusalem artichoke, dry	2 oz	210	41	1.0
Jerusalem artichoke, garlic and parsley, dry	2 oz	210	41	1.0
(De Cecco) spinach, dry	2 oz	210	41	1.0
(Eden Foods)				
bifun, rice	2 oz	200	44	0.5
fine, dry, 'Herb's'	2 oz	220	42	2.0
kluski, medium, dry, 'Herb's'	2 oz	220	42	2.0
kluski, wide, dry, 'Herb's'	2 oz	220	42	2.0
medium, dry, 'Herb's'	2 oz	220	42	2.0
(Gioia) plain, dry	2 oz	220	40	3.0
(Golden Grain) plain, dry	2 oz	210	39	2.2
(Goodman's) plain, 'Country Style' dry	2 oz	220	40	3.0
(Hodgson Mill)				
spinach, whole wheat, dry	2 oz	190	32	2.0
vegetable, dry	2 oz	200	37	2.0
whole wheat, wide, dry	2 oz	190	34	2.0
(Hospitality) wide, enriched, 'Valu Pack' dry	1 1/4 cup	235	43	2.5
(Mrs. Grass) plain, dry	2 oz	220	40	3.0
(Mueller's)				
kluski, dry	2 oz	220	38	3.0
plain, dry	2 oz	220	40	3.0

Food Name	Serv. Size	Total Cal.	Carbs GMS	Fat GMS
(No Yolks) no egg yolks, broad, dry	2 oz	200	40	1.0
(P&R) plain, dry	2 oz	220	42	3.0
(Prince) plain, dry	2 oz	210	40	2.0
(Reames) homestyle, frozen	1/2 cup	170	32	2.0
(Ronzoni)				
very low-sodium, dry, 'Egg Pastina'	2 oz	220	42	3.0
wide, enriched, 'Country Kitchen Style' dry	2 oz	220	42	3.0
(San Giorgio) plain, dry	2 oz	220	42	3.0
JAPANESE				
soba, cooked	1 cup	113	24	0.1
soba, dry	2 oz	192	43	0.4
somen, cooked	1 cup	231	48	0.3
somen, dry	2 oz	203	42	0.5
(Eden Foods)				
harusame, mung bean, dry	2 oz	190	47	0.0
jinenjo soba, wild yam, dry	2 oz	190	37	0.5
kuzu and sweet potato, dry	2 oz	190	47	0.0
soba, 40% buckwheat	2 oz	190	37	1.0
soba, buckwheat, 100% buckwheat, dry	2 oz	200	41	1.5
soba, lotus root	2 oz	190	37	1.0
soba, mugwort	2 oz	190	37	0.5
soba, traditional	2 oz	190	37	1.0
soba, wild yam	2 oz	190	37	0.5
udon, brown rice	2 oz	190	38	1.0
(Westbrae)				
buckwheat, dry	2 oz	190	40	2.0
genmai, dry	2 oz	200	41	1.0
somen, whole wheat, dry	2 oz	200	41	1.0
traditional, dry	2 oz	190	41	2.0
udon, whole wheat, organic, dry	2 oz	200	41	1.0
SOBA. See under NOODLE, JAPANESE.				
UDON. See under NOODLE, JAPANESE.				
NOODLE DISH/ENTRÉE See also PASTA DISH/ENTRÉE.				
(Banquet)				
and julienne beef, w/sauce, frozen, 'Family Entrées'	7 oz	170	22	3.0
w/beef gravy, frozen, 'Family Entrées'	8 oz	200	22	7.0
w/chicken, frozen	10 oz	350	42	15.0
w/chicken, frozen, 'Family Favorites'	10 oz	340	42	15.0
(Dinty Moore)				
and chicken, packaged, 'American Classics'	10 oz	230	24	7.0
tuna noodle casserole, packaged, 'American Classics'	10 oz	240	28	7.0
(Heinz)				
and chicken, canned	7.5 oz	160	19	7.0
w/beef, in sauce, canned	7.5 oz	170	17	8.0
w/tuna, canned	7.5 oz	170	20	5.0
(Hormel) w/chicken, 'Micro-Cup'	7.5 oz	180	18	8.0
(Kid's Kitchen) rings and chicken, microwave cup	7.5 oz	150	17	4.0
(La Choy)				
and vegetables	1 cup	131	27	1.3
chow mein, canned	1 cup	300	32	16.0
w/beef, bi-pack	1 cup	148	24	1.2
w/beef, vegetables	1 cup	156	27	3.5
w/chicken, bi-pack	1 cup	161	23	3.8
w/chicken, vegetables	1 cup	163	24	3.3
(Marie Callender's) w/chicken, escalloped	1 cup	420	44	21.0
(Nalley's)				
and chicken, canned	7 3/8 oz	150	17	5.0

Food Name	Serv. Size	Total Cal.	Carbs GMS	Fat GMS
and chicken, w/vegetables, canned	7 3/8 oz	160	18	5.0
(Stouffer's)				
Romanoff	1 entrée	490	48	25.0
Romanoff, frozen, food service product	1 oz	41	4	2.2
(Swanson) w/chicken, frozen	10.5 oz	280	45	8.0
(Van Camp's) w/franks, canned, 'Noodle Weenee'	1 cup	245	33	8.5
(Weight Watchers) kung pao	1 entrée	260	35	10.0

NOODLE DISH/ENTRÉE MIX. See also PASTA DISH/ENTRÉE MIX.

(Kraft)

cheese, 'Dinner'	3/4 cup	340	37	17.0
chicken flavor, 'Dinner'	3/4 cup	240	32	9.0

(Lipton)

egg noodles Alfredo, mix only	1 cup	389	58	11.0
egg noodles Alfredo, mix only	1 pkg	518	77	14.6
egg noodles Alfredo, prepared	1 serving	259	39	7.3
(Mountain House) w/chicken, freeze-dried, prepared	1 cup	270	34	10.0
(Ultra Slim Fast) w/Alfredo sauce, prepared	8 oz	240	47	4.0

NORI. See under SEA VEGETABLE.

NORTHERN PIKE. See under PIKE.

NORWAY HADDOCK. See OCEAN PERCH, ATLANTIC.

NUT SNACK

(Fisher)

crisp, golden, 'Nut 'N Crunchies'	1/4 cup	140	15	7.0
fiesta, 'Nut 'N Crunchies'	1/4 cup	140	16	7.0
honey crunch, 'Nut 'N Crunchies'	1/4 cup	140	17	6.0

NUT TOPPING

(Fisher)

fancy	1 oz	170	7	15.0
oil roasted, w/peanuts	1 oz	160	7	14.0
(Planters)	1 oz	180	6	16.0

(Smucker's)

pecan, in syrup	2 tbsp	130	28	1.0
walnut, in syrup	2 tbsp	130	27	1.0

NUTMEG

ground	1 tbsp	37	3	2.5
ground	1 tsp	12	1	0.8
ground *(Durkee)*	1 tsp	12	0	0.0
ground *(Laurel Leaf)*	1 tsp	12	0	0.0
ground *(McCormick/Schilling)*	1 tsp	11	1	0.8
ground *(Spice Islands)*	1 tsp	11	1	0.7

NUTMEG BUTTER OIL

	1 cup	1927	0	218.0
	1 tbsp	120	0	13.6

NUTS, MIXED

(Eagle)

	1/4 cup	200	6	17.0
lightly salted	1/4 cup	200	6	17.0
w/o peanuts, deluxe	1/4 cup	200	8	14.0

(Fisher)

cashews, honey-glazed 'Favorites'	1/4 cup	170	9	13.0
cashews, praline-glazed, 'Favorites'	1/4 cup	170	11	12.0
cashews, toffee-glazed, 'Favorites'	1/4 cup	170	11	11.0
cashews, tropical fruit, 'Favorites'	1/4 cup	140	14	8.0
lightly salted	1/4 cup	180	5	16.0
salted	1/4 cup	180	5	16.0
(Flanigan Farms) natural, unsalted	1 oz	180	5	17.0
(Guy's) w/peanuts	1 oz	170	3	14.0

Food Name	Serv. Size	Total Cal.	Carbs GMS	Fat GMS
(Planters)				
cashews, almonds, and peanuts, 'Select Mix'	1 oz	170	7	14.0
cashews, almonds, and pecans, 'Select Mix'	1 oz	180	6	16.0
cashews, pecans, and peanuts, 'Select Mix'	1 oz	180	6	16.0
Dry-roasted				
(Eden Foods) sunflower, peanuts, cashews, almonds	1 oz	170	9	11.0
(Finast)				
lightly salted	1 oz	170	7	15.0
salted	1 oz	170	7	15.0
salted, w/peanuts, 'No Frills'	1 oz	180	7	14.0
w/peanuts, salted, 'No Frills'	1 oz	180	7	14.0
(Pathmark) w/peanuts, salted, 'No Frills'	1 oz	180	7	14.0
(Planters)				
	1 oz	160	7	14.0
sesame nut mix	1 oz	160	8	12.0
unsalted	1 oz	170	7	15.0
Honey-roasted				
(Eagle) cashews and peanuts	1/4 cup	180	8	14.0
(Fisher) cashews and peanuts	1/4 cup	170	8	13.0
(Planters)				
	1 oz	170	9	13.0
cashews and peanuts	1 oz	170	9	12.0
Oil-roasted				
(Flavor House)	1 oz	180	6	18.0
(Planters)				
	1 oz	180	6	16.0
'Deluxe'	1 oz	180	6	17.0
lightly salted	1 oz	180	6	16.0
sesame nut mix	1 oz	160	8	13.0
unsalted	1 oz	180	6	16.0
(Pathmark)				
w/peanuts, salted, 'No Frills'	1 oz	180	5	15.0
w/o peanuts, salted, fancy, 'No Frills'	1 oz	180	7	15.0

O

Food Name	Serv. Size	Total Cal.	Carbs GMS	Fat GMS
OAT. See also under CEREAL, HOT.				
	1 cup	607	103	10.8
steel cut *(Arrowhead Mills)*	2 oz	220	37	4.0
OAT BRAN				
cooked	1 cup	88	25	1.9
raw	1 cup	231	62	6.6
OAT FLOUR. See under FLOUR.				
OAT MIX, gluten free *(Ener-G Foods)*	1 cup	376	7	7.7
OAT VEGETABLE OIL				
	1 cup	1927	0	218.0
	1 tbsp	120	0	13.6
OCEAN CATFISH. See WOLF FISH.				
OCEAN PERCH, ATLANTIC/Norway haddock/red perch/rose perch				
Fresh				
baked, broiled, or grilled	3 oz	103	0	1.8
raw	3 oz	80	0	1.4
raw, boneless	1 oz	27	0	0.5
Frozen				
(Booth)	4 oz	100	0	1.0

Food Name	Serv. Size	Total Cal.	Carbs GMS	Fat GMS
fillet, light *(Van de Kamp's)*	1 piece	280	21	14.0
'Fishmarket Fresh' *(Gorton's)*	5 oz	140	2	3.0
natural *(Van de Kamp's)*	4 oz	130	0	5.0
OCEAN POUT/muttonfish				
baked, broiled, or grilled	3 oz	87	0	1.0
raw	3 oz	67	0	0.8
OCEANIC BONITO. See under TUNA., SKIPJACK				
OCTOPUS				
common, boiled, poached, or steamed	3 oz	139	4	1.8
common, raw	3 oz	70	2	0.9
OHELOBERRY, RAW				
fresh, raw	1 cup	39	10	0.3
fresh, raw	10 medium	3	1	0.0
OKRA				
Fresh				
boiled, drained, sliced	1/2 cup	26	6	0.1
boiled, drained, whole, approx 3-inch long	8 med pods	27	6	0.1
raw, sliced	1 cup	33	8	0.1
raw, whole, approx 3-inch long	8 med pods	31	7	0.1
Frozen				
cut *(Flav-R-Pac)*	3/4 cup	25	4	0.0
cut *(Freshlike)*	3.3 oz	25	6	0.0
cut *(Pictsweet)*	3/4 cup	25	5	0.0
cut *(Seabrook)*	3.3 oz	25	6	0.0
cut *(Southern)*	3.5 oz	31	7	0.2
cut *(Veg-All)*	3.3 oz	25	6	0.0
drained	10-oz pkg	71	15	0.8
sliced, drained	1/2 cup	26	5	0.3
unprepared	10-oz pkg	85	19	0.7
unprepared	3-lb pkg	408	90	3.4
whole *(Flav-R-Pac)*	9 pieces	35	6	0.5
whole *(Freshlike)*	3.3 oz	30	7	0.0
whole *(Seabrook)*	3.3 oz	30	7	0.0
whole *(Southern)*	3.5 oz	35	7	0.2
whole *(Veg-All)*	3.3 oz	30	7	0.0
whole, baby *(Frosty Acres)*	3.3 oz	30	7	0.0
OLD-FASHIONED. See under COCKTAIL MIX.				
OLIVE				
all varieties, all sizes, pickled *(S&W)*	1 oz	46	0	5.1
mixed sizes, chopped	1 tbsp	10	1	0.9
mixed varieties, pickled, chopped *(Lindsay)*	1 oz	29	2	2.7
mixed varieties, pickled, pitted *(Vlasic)*	1 oz	37	1	3.9
mixed varieties, pickled, sliced *(Lindsay)*	1 oz	29	2	2.7
salad, pickled *(Progresso)*	1/2 cup	120	1	15.0
whole, large	1 olive	5	0	0.5
whole, small	1 olive	4	0	0.3
ASCOLANO				
all sizes, pickled, pitted *(Lindsay)*	1 oz	23	2	1.9
colossal, pickled, pitted *(Lindsay)*	10 olives	90	6	7.7
jumbo, pickled, pitted *(Lindsay)*	10 olives	66	5	5.7
super colossal, pickled, pitted *(Lindsay)*	10 olives	122	9	10.4
BLACK				
colossal, w/pits *(S&W)*	1 piece	15	1	1.5
extra large, pitted *(S&W)*	3 pieces	25	1	2.5
extra large, pitted, 'Black Pearls' *(Musco)*	3 olives	25	1	2.0
jumbo, pitted *(S&W)*	3 pieces	25	1	2.0
medium, pitted, 'Black Pearls' *(Musco)*	5 olives	25	1	2.0

Food Name	Serv. Size	Total Cal.	Carbs GMS	Fat GMS
GREEK				
all sizes, salt-cured, oil-coated, pickled, pitted	1 oz	96	2.5	10.2
extra large, salt-cured, oil-coated, pickled, w/pits	10 olives	89	2.3	9.5
extra large, salt-cured, pickled, w/pits	10 olives	89	2.3	9.5
medium, salt-cured, oil-coated, pickled, w/pits	10 olives	65	1.7	6.9
medium, salt-cured, pickled, w/pits	10 olives	65	1.7	6.9
GREEN				
chopped (Early California)	14 grams	18	1	2.0
extra large, pitted (Vlasic)	14 grams	18	1	2.0
jumbo	1 olive	7	0	0.6
large, pitted (Vlasic)	15 grams	25	1	2.5
martini, pimento stuffed (Santa Barbara Olive Co.)	0.5 oz	25	0	2.0
medium, pitted (Vlasic)	14 grams	18	1	2.0
pimento stuffed (Golden Gate)	15 grams	15	1	1.0
pitted, pitted (Vlasic)	14 grams	18	1	2.0
queen (S&W)	2 olives	20	1	2.0
small, pitted (Vlasic)	14 grams	18	1	2.0
Spanish, pimento stuffed (Star)	15 grams	15	1	1.0
super colossal	1 olive	12	1	1.0
w/jalapeño (Santa Barbara Olive Co.)	0.5 oz	25	0	2.0
MANZANILLA				
all sizes, pickled, pitted (Lindsay)	1 oz	32	2	3.0
extra large, pickled, pitted (Lindsay)	10 olives	63	4	5.9
large, pickled, pitted (Lindsay)	10 olives	50	3	4.8
medium, pickled, pitted (Lindsay)	10 olives	44	2	4.1
small, pickled, pitted (Lindsay)	10 olives	37	2	3.5
stuffed (S&W)	3 olives	25	1	2.0
w/pimento (S&W)	3 olives	25	1	2.0
MISSION				
all sizes, pickled, pitted (Lindsay)	1 oz	32	2	3.0
extra large, pickled, pitted (Lindsay)	10 olives	63	4	5.9
large, pickled, pitted (Lindsay)	10 olives	50	3	4.8
medium, pickled, pitted (Lindsay)	10 olives	44	2	4.1
small, pickled, pitted (Lindsay)	10 olives	37	2	3.5
SEVILLANO				
all sizes, pickled, pitted (Lindsay)	1 oz	23	2	1.9
colossal, pickled, pitted (Lindsay)	10 olives	90	6	7.7
jumbo, pickled, pitted (Lindsay)	10 olives	66	5	5.7
super colossal, pickled, pitted (Lindsay)	10 olives	122	9	10.4
OLIVE APPETIZER				
(Progresso)				
	1/2 cup	180	6	21.0
'Condite'	1/2 cup	130	5	14.0
OLIVE SALAD (Progresso) drained	2 tbsp	25	1	2.5
OLIVE OIL				
salad or cooking	1 cup	1909	0	216.0
salad or cooking	1 tbsp	119	0	13.5
(Amore)				
'Pure'	1 tbsp	130	0	14.0
extra virgin	1 tbsp	130	0	14.0
(Bertolli)	1 tbsp	120	0	14.0
(Filippo Berio)	1 tbsp	120	0	14.0
(Hain)	1 tbsp	120	0	14.0
(Pope) Italian, cold press, no salt	1 tbsp	120	0	14.0
(Progresso)				
'Riviera Blend'	1 tbsp	120	0	14.0
extra mild	1 tbsp	120	0	14.0

Food Name	Serv. Size	Total Cal.	Carbs GMS	Fat GMS
extra virgin	1 tbsp	120	0	14.0
oil cured	6 olives	80	3	6.0
(Spectrum) extra virgin, pure pressed, organic	1 tbsp	120	0	14.0
(Wesson)	1 tbsp	122	0	13.6

ONION
COCKTAIL

large *(S&W)*	8 onions	5	1	0.0
lightly spiced *(Vlasic)*	1 oz	4	1	0.0
small *(S&W)*	12 onions	5	1	0.0

GREEN. See SCALLION.
RED, WHITE, OR YELLOW
Canned

chopped or diced, w/liquid	1/2 cup	21	4	0.1
sweet *(Heinz)*	1 oz	40	9	0.0
whole, small *(Green Giant)*	1/2 cup	35	8	0.0
whole, small *(Pathmark)*	1/2 cup	35	7	0.0
whole, w/liquid	1 medium	12	3	0.1

Dried

(Basic American)	1 oz	99	22	0.3
minced, w/green onion *(Lawry's)*	1 tsp	7	2	0.2

Fresh

boiled, drained, chopped	1 cup	92	21	0.4
boiled, drained, chopped	1 tbsp	7	2	0.0
boiled, drained, chopped or diced	1/2 cup	29	7	0.1
boiled, drained, chopped or diced	1 tbsp	4	1	0.0
boiled, drained, whole, medium, approx 2.5-inch diam	1 onion	41	10	0.2
boiled, drained, sliced, medium, 1/8 inch thick	1 slice	5	1	0.0
raw, chopped	1 cup	61	14	0.3
raw, chopped	1 tbsp	4	1	0.0
raw, sliced	1 cup	44	10	0.2
raw, sliced, medium, 1/8-inch thick	1 slice	5	1	0.0
raw, whole, medium, approx 2.5-inch diam	1 onion	42	9	0.2

Frozen

chopped *(Ore-Ida)*	2 oz	20	4	1.0
chopped *(Seabrook)*	1 oz	8	2	0.0
diced *(Flav-R-Pac)*	2/3 cup	30	6	0.0
diced *(Freshlike)*	3.3 oz	8	2	0.0
diced *(Veg-All)*	3.3 oz	8	2	0.0
unprepared	10-oz pkg	82	19	0.3
whole *(Freshlike)*	3.3 oz	35	8	0.0
whole *(Veg-All)*	3.3 oz	35	8	0.0
whole, small *(Birds Eye)*	4 oz	40	10	0.0
whole, small *(Flav-R-Pac)*	1/2 cup	25	7	0.0
whole, small *(Seabrook)*	3.3 oz	35	8	0.0

WELSH

trimmed	1 lb	160	28.8	1.6
trimmed	1 oz	10	1.8	0.1

ONION DISH MIX *(Vidalia Sweet)* rings,

all purpose	1/4 cup	100	21	na

ONION FLAKES

dehydrated	1 tbsp	17	4	0.0
dehydrated	1/4 cup	49	12	0.1
minced *(Lawry's)*	1 tsp	7	2	0.2

ONION POWDER

	1 tbsp	23	5	0.1
	1 tsp	7	2	0.0
ground *(Durkee)*	1 tsp	8	0	0.0

Food Name	Serv. Size	Total Cal.	Carbs GMS	Fat GMS
ground *(Laurel Leaf)*	1 tsp	8	0	0.0
ground *(McCormick/Schilling)*	1 tsp	10	2	0.0
ground *(Spice Islands)*	1 tsp	8	2	0.1
ground *(Tone's)*	1 tsp	5	2	0.1
ONION SALT				
(Schilling) 'California blend'	1/4 tsp	0	0	0.0
(Tone's)	1 tsp	1	0	0.0
ONION SNACK *(Wise)* rings	1 oz	130	21	5.0
OPOSSUM				
roasted	3 oz	188	0	8.7
roasted, boneless, yield from 1 lb raw	14 oz	882	0	40.7
roasted, diced	1 cup	309	0.0	14.3
ORANGE				
ALL VARIETIES				
raw, peeled, sections	1 cup	85	21	0.2
raw, peeled, whole, large, approx 3 1/16 inch diam.	1 orange	86	22	0.2
raw, peeled, whole, medium, approx 2 5/8 inch diam	1 orange	62	15	0.2
raw, peeled, whole, small, approx 2 3/8 inch diam	1 orange	45	11	0.1
raw, w/peel	1 cup	68	26	0.5
raw, medium, w/peel, w/o seeds	1 orange	64	25	0.5
CALIFORNIA				
Navel				
peeled, raw, sections, w/o membranes	1 cup	76	19	0.1
peeled, raw, whole, medium, approx 2 7/8 inch diam	1 orange	64	16	0.1
Valencia				
peeled, raw, sections, w/o membranes	1 cup	88	21	0.5
peeled, raw, whole, medium, approx 2 5/8 inch diam	1 orange	59	14	0.4
FLORIDA				
raw, whole, peeled, medium, approx 2 11/16 inch diam	1 orange	69	17	0.3
raw, whole, peeled, medium, approx 2 5/8 inch diam	1 orange	65	16	0.3
raw, sections, peeled, w/o membranes	1 cup	85	21	0.4
ORANGE DRINK. See under FRUIT DRINK; FRUIT JUICE DRINK.				
ORANGE JUICE				
canned or boxed	1 cup	105	25	0.3
fresh squeezed	1 cup	112	26	0.5
fresh squeezed	1 fl oz	14	3	0.1
fresh squeezed, juice from 1 med fruit	3 oz	39	9	0.2
(A&P) frozen concentrate, prepared	6 fl oz	80	19	1.0
(Citrus Hill)				
'Plus Calcium'	6 fl oz	90	20	1.0
'Select'	6 fl oz	90	20	1.0
(Crowley)	8 fl oz	110	26	0.0
(Del Monte) canned or boxed, 'Unsweetened'	6 fl oz	80	19	0.0
(Donald Duck)				
100% orange juice, from concentrate	8 fl oz	120	29	0.0
100% pure, from concentrate	6 fl oz	90	22	0.0
(Flav-R-Pac)	1 cup	120	29	0.0
(Florida's Natural)				
homestyle, Florida fruit, not from concentrate	8 fl oz	120	29	0.0
(Knudsen)				
	8 fl oz	100	23	0.0
float	8 fl oz	120	27	0.0
(Kraft) chilled, 'Pure 100% Unsweetened'	6 fl oz	80	19	0.0
(Minute Maid)				
calcium-fortified	6 fl oz	80	20	0.0
calcium-fortified, frozen concentrate, prepared	6 fl oz	80	20	0.0
country style	6 fl oz	80	20	0.0

Food Name	Serv. Size	Total Cal.	Carbs GMS	Fat GMS
country style, frozen concentrate, prepared .... 6 fl oz		80	20	0.0
premium choice .... 6 fl oz		90	21	0.0
pulp-free .... 6 fl oz		80	20	0.0
pulp-free, frozen concentrate, prepared .... 6 fl oz		80	20	0.0
reduced acid, frozen concentrate, prepared .... 6 fl oz		80	20	0.0
regular .... 6 fl oz		80	20	0.0
regular, frozen concentrate, prepared .... 6 fl oz		80	20	0.0
(Ocean Spray) .... 6 fl oz		80	19	0.0
(S&W) .... 6 fl oz		90	22	0.0
(Sippin' Pak) .... 8.45 fl oz		110	26	0.0
(Stokely) canned or boxed, 'Unsweetened' .... 6 fl oz		89	21	1.0
(Sunkist)				
.... 6 fl oz		84	20	0.1
8–16 servings per pkg, frozen concentrate, prepared .... 6 fl oz		112	27	0.1
'Fresh Squeezed' .... 6 fl oz		77	18	0.3
(Tree Top) 100% .... 8 fl oz		120	28	0.0
(TreeSweet)				
.... 6 fl oz		78	18	0.0
frozen concentrate, prepared .... 6 fl oz		84	20	0.0
(Tropicana)				
from concentrate .... 60 ml		110	27	0.0
homestyle, 'Season's Best' .... 8 fl oz		110	27	0.0
plus calcium, 'Pure Premium' .... 8 fl oz		110	26	0.0
plus calcium, 'Season's Best' .... 8 fl oz		110	27	0.0
plus fiber, 'Pure Premium' .... 8 fl oz		120	30	0.0
plus vitamins, 'Pure Premium' .... 8 fl oz		110	26	0.0
plus vitamins, 'Season's Best' .... 8 fl oz		110	27	0.0
'Pure Premium' .... 8 fl oz		110	26	0.0
reconstituted, 100% pure .... 6 fl oz		80	16	1.0
(Veryfine)				
blend, '100%' .... 8 fl oz		120	30	0.0
'100%' .... 8 fl oz		121	24	0.0
ORANGE JUICE BLEND. See under FRUIT JUICE BLEND.				
ORANGE PEEL				
grated, raw .... 1 tbsp		6	2	0.0
grated, raw .... 1 tsp		2	1	0.0
ORANGE ROUGHY/slimehead				
baked, broiled, or grilled .... 3 oz		76	0	0.8
raw .... 3 oz		59	0	0.6
ORANGEADE. See under FRUIT DRINK.				
OREGANO				
(McCormick/Schilling) .... 1 tsp		6	1	0.0
dried *(Golden Dipt)* .... 2 grams		6	1	0.0
dried *(Spice Islands)* .... 1 tsp		6	1	0.1
dried *(Tone's)* .... 1 tsp		5	1	0.2
ground .... 1 tbsp		14	3	0.5
ground .... 1 tsp		5	1	0.2
ground *(Durkee)* .... 1 tsp		5	0	0.0
ground *(Laurel Leaf)* .... 1 tsp		5	0	0.0
OREGANO, MEXICAN *(McCormick/Schilling)* .... 1 tsp		4	1	0.0
ORIENTAL STYLE DINNER/ENTRÉE. See also individual listings.				
(Le Menu) Empress, w/seasoned rice, frozen, ... 8.25 oz		210	26	5.0
(Pasta Roni) stir-fry .... 1 serving		131	17	5.4
(Rice A Roni) stir-fry, 'Fast Cook' .... 2.5 oz		164	24	5.6
ORIENTAL RADISH. See DAIKON.				
ORIENTAL SEASONING MIX. See under SEASONING MIX.				

Food Name	Serv. Size	Total Cal.	Carbs GMS	Fat GMS
OYSTER				
ALL SPECIES				
Canned				
(Bumble Bee) . . . . 1 cup		218	15	5.3
(S&W) . . . . 2 oz		70	2	3.0
'Fancy' *(S&W)* . . . . 2 oz		95	4	3.0
cherrywood smoked, petite, in cottonseed oil, w/salt *(Reese)* . . . . . . 2 oz		110	6	6.0
salt and water added, whole *(Crown Prince)* . . . . 3 pieces		70	4	3.0
smoked *(S&W)* . . . . ,. 2 oz		100	6	6.0
smoked, whole, in cottonseed oil *(Crown Prince)* . . . . 1 can		170	8	9.0
EASTERN				
Canned				
. . . . 3 oz		59	3	2.1
. . . . 1 medium		6	0	0.2
drained . . . . 1 oz		16	1	0.6
drained . . . . 1 cup		112	6	4.0
w/liquid . . . . 12 oz		188	11	6.7
w/liquid . . . . 1 cup		171	10	6.1
Fresh				
breaded and fried . . . . 3 oz		167	10	10.7
breaded and fried . . . . ,. . . . 6 medium		173	10	11.1
farmed, cooked . . . . 3 oz		67	6	1.8
farmed, cooked . . . . 6 medium		47	4	1.3
farmed, raw . . . . 3 oz		50	5	1.3
farmed, raw . . . . 6 medium		50	5	1.3
wild, cooked, dry heat . . . . 3 oz		61	4	1.6
wild, cooked, dry heat . . . . 6 medium		42	3	1.1
wild, cooked, moist heat . . . . 3 oz		116	7	4.2
wild, cooked, moist heat . . . . 6 medium		58	3	2.1
wild, raw . . . . 1 cup		169	10	6.1
wild, raw . . . . 6 medium		57	3	2.1
PACIFIC				
cooked . . . . 3 oz		139	8	3.9
cooked . . . . 1 medium		41	2	1.1
raw . . . . 3 oz		69	4	2.0
raw . . . . 1 medium		41	2	1.1
OYSTER DISH/ENTRÉE				
(Campbell's) stew, canned, condensed, prepared . . . . 8 oz		70	5	5.0
OYSTER MUSHROOM. See MUSHROOM, OYSTER.				
OYSTER PLANT. See SALSIFY.				

P

Food Name	Serv. Size	Total Cal.	Carbs GMS	Fat GMS
PACIFIC COD. See COD, PACIFIC.				
PACIFIC MACKEREL. See MACKEREL, PACIFIC.				
PACIFIC ROCKFISH. See ROCKFISH, PACIFIC.				
PAD THAI SEASONING. See under SEASONING MIX.				
PAK-CHOI. See BOK CHOY.				
PALM, HEARTS OF				
Canned				
. . . . 1 cup		41	7	0.9
. . . . 1 med piece		9	2	0.2
Brazilian *(Reese)* . . . . 1/3 cup		15	1	1.0

Food Name	Serv. Size	Total Cal.	Carbs GMS	Fat GMS
PALM KERNEL OIL/babassu oil				
.... 1 cup		1879	0	218.0
.... 1 tbsp		117	0	13.6
.... 2 tbsp		234	0	27.2
PALM OIL				
.... 1 cup		1909	0	216.0
.... 1 tbsp		120	0	13.6
PANCAKE				
(Aunt Jemima)				
homestyle, frozen	3 pancakes	210	40	3.5
low-fat, frozen	3 pancakes	150	30	1.5
original, frozen, microwave	3 pancakes	211	40	3.6
(Downyflake) frozen	3 pancakes	280	45	9.0
(Krusteaz) mini, frozen, microwave	6 pancakes	120	21	2.0
(Pillsbury) original, frozen, microwave	3 pancakes	240	47	4.0
BLUEBERRY				
(Aunt Jemima) frozen	3 pancakes	210	40	3.5
(Downyflake) frozen	3 pancakes	290	48	9.0
(Krusteaz) frozen, 4.5-oz serving	3 pancakes	280	49	5.0
(Pillsbury) frozen, microwave	3 pancakes	250	49	4.0
BUTTERMILK				
(Aunt Jemima)				
frozen, microwave	3 pancakes	210	40	3.5
frozen, microwave, 'Lite'	3 pancakes	140	28	3.0
(Downyflake) frozen	3 pancakes	280	45	9.0
(Krusteaz)				
frozen, 4.75-oz serving	3 pancakes	290	53	5.0
mini, frozen, microwave	1 serving	116	22	1.6
(Pillsbury)				
frozen, microwave	3 pancakes	260	51	4.0
mini, frozen, microwave	11 pancakes	230	44	4.0
(Weight Watchers) frozen, microwave, 2.5-oz serving	1/2 pkg	140	22	3.0
WHOLE WHEAT				
(Krusteaz) whole, and honey, frozen, 4.75-oz serving	3 pancakes	250	45	4.0
(Pillsbury) harvest, frozen, microwave	3 pancakes	240	48	4.0
PANCAKE BATTER				
(Aunt Jemima)				
blueberry, frozen	3.6 oz	204	39	4.0
buttermilk, frozen	3.6 oz	180	36	2.3
plain, frozen	3.6 oz	183	37	2.4
PANCAKE DISH/MEAL				
(Aunt Jemima)				
and sausages, frozen, 'Homestyle'	6 oz	420	57	16.0
breakfast, lite, w/lite syrup, frozen, 'Homestyle'	6 oz	260	53	3.0
w/lite links, lite, frozen, 'Homestyle'	6 oz	310	43	10.0
(Downyflake) and sausages, frozen	5.5 oz	430	47	23.0
(Great Starts)				
silver dollar sized, w/sausage	1 meal	340	36	18.0
w/bacon	1 meal	400	42	20.0
w/sausage	1 meal	490	52	25.0
(Swanson) whole wheat, w/lite links, 'Great Starts'	5.5 oz	350	39	16.0
PANCAKE MIX. See also PANCAKE/WAFFLE MIX.				
(Betty Crocker) complete, mix only	1/3 cup	200	39	3.0
(Gluten Free Pantry) gluten-free, mix only	1 serving	130	28	1.0
(Sweet 'n Low) low-salt and -cholesterol, w/Sweet 'n Low, prepared, 3-inch diam	5 pancakes	160	32	2.0

Food Name	Serv. Size	Total Cal.	Carbs GMS	Fat GMS
BUCKWHEAT				
(Hodgson Mill) whole grain, stone ground, mix only	1/3 cup	190	40	1.0
BUTTERMILK				
(Aunt Jemima) lower calorie, complete, mix only	1/3 cup	131	28	1.4
(Betty Crocker) complete, mix only	1/3 cup	200	39	2.5
(Hungry Jack)				
complete, mix only	1/3 cup	160	32	1.5
mix only	1/3 cup	160	33	1.5
(MET-RX Caffe) mix only	1/2 cup	200	33	3.0
(Robin Hood) mix only	1/3 cup	180	31	3.0
WHOLE WHEAT *(Hodgson Mill)* w/buttermilk, mix only	1/3 cup	120	28	1.0
PANCAKE SYRUP. See under SYRUP.				
PANCAKE/WAFFLE MIX				
(Arrowhead Mills)				
'Griddle Lite' mix only	1/2 cup	260	50	3.0
original style, mix only	1/4 cup	130	24	2.0
(Aunt Jemima)				
'Original' prepared, 4-inch diam	3 pancakes	116	25	0.8
complete, mix only	1/3 cup	165	34	1.7
(Bisquick) 'Shake 'n Pour' prepared, 4-inch diam	3 pancakes	260	48	5.0
(Downyflake) plain, prepared, 'Crisp & Healthy'	1 waffle	80	16	1.0
(Estee) prepared, 3-inch diam	3 pancakes	100	21	0.0
(Featherweight) prepared, 4-inch diam	3 pancakes	140	24	2.0
(Gold Medal) 'Pouch Mix' prepared w/egg	1/8 pouch	100	17	2.0
(Hungry Jack)				
'Panshakes' prepared, 4-inch diam	3 pancakes	250	43	6.0
light, complete, 'Extra Lights' mix only	1/17 pkg	180	38	3.0
light, complete, 'Extra Lights' prepared w/water, 4-inch diam	3 pancakes	180	38	3.0
light, complete, 'Extra Lights' prepared, 4-inch diam	3 pancakes	190	37	2.0
light, prepared w/3/4 cup skim milk, 2 tbsp oil, 2 egg whites, 4-inch diam	3 pancakes	170	28	4.0
light, regular, 'Extra Lights' mix only	1/17 pkg	180	38	3.0
light, regular, 'Extra Lights' prepared w/3/4 cup 2% milk, 2 tbsp oil, 1 egg, 4-inch diam	3 pancakes	190	28	6.0
light, regular, 'Extra Lights' prepared w/nonfat milk, 2 egg whites, 4-inch diam	3 pancakes	170	28	4.0
light, regular, 'Extra Lights' prepared w/water, 4-inch diam	3 pancakes	180	38	3.0
light, regular, 'Extra Lights' prepared, 4-inch diam	3 pancakes	210	30	7.0
pre-measured, mix only	1/2 pkt	200	38	3.5
pre-measured, prepared w/water, 4-inch diam	3 pancakes	180	33	3.0
regular, mix only	1/3 cup	150	32	1.5
(Martha White)				
'FlapStax' prepared w/water	1 pancake	80	17	1.0
'Light Crust' mix only	2 oz	120	20	3.0
(Robin Hood) 'Pouch Mix' prepared w/egg	1/8 pouch	100	17	2.0
APPLE CINNAMON				
(Bisquick) 'Shake 'n Pour' 4', prepared	3 pancakes	270	49	5.0
(Downyflake) 'Crisp & Healthy'	1 waffle	80	16	1.0
CORN *Arrowhead Mills)* blue corn, mix only	1/3 cup	150	28	2.0
BLUEBERRY				
(Hungry Jack)				
microwave, mix only	3/4 pkg	230	47	4.0
prepared, 4-inch diam	3 pancakes	320	41	15.0
wild, mix only	1/5 pkg	170	38	1.0
wild, prepared w/ 1-1/4 cup milk, 1/4 cup oil, 1 egg, 4-inch diam	3 pancakes	320	41	14.0

Food Name	Serv. Size	Total Cal.	Carbs GMS	Fat GMS
(Krusteaz) imitation, prepared, 4 inch diam	3 pancakes	205	39	4.0
BUCKWHEAT				
(Arrowhead Mills) mix only	1/2 cup	270	53	2.0
(Aunt Jemima) mix only	1/4 cup	105	24	0.9
(Don's Chuck Wagon) buckwheat, compete, mix only	1/3 cup	160	33	1.0
(Krusteaz) buckwheat, prepared, 4-inch diam	3 pancakes	215	40	3.0
BUTTERMILK				
(Aunt Jemima)				
complete, 'Lite' prepared, 4-inch diam	3 pancakes	130	25	2.0
complete, mix only	1/3 cup	162	32	1.7
original, prepared, 4-inch diam	3 pancakes	122	26	0.7
(Betty Crocker)				
complete, prepared, 4-inch diam	3 pancakes	210	41	3.0
original, mix only	1/2 cup	170	36	1.0
original, prepared, 4-inch diam	3 pancakes	210	41	3.0
original, prepared w/2/3 cup milk, 1 tbsp oil, egg, 4-inch diam	3 pancakes	280	39	10.0
(Bob's Red Mill) mix only	1/2 cup	190	11	1.0
(Downyflake) 'Jumbo'	2 waffles	170	30	4.0
(Health Valley) 'Biscuit & Pancake' mix only	1 oz	100	20	1.0
(Hungry Jack) complete, mix only	1/17 pkg	180	38	1.0
complete, packets, prepared, 4-inch diam	3 pancakes	180	35	3.0
complete, prepared, 4-inch diam	3 pancakes	180	39	1.0
complete, prepared w/water, 4-inch diam	3 pancakes	180	38	1.0
microwave, mix ony	3/4 pkg	260	51	4.0
original, mix only	1/25 pkg	120	26	0.0
original, prepared, 4-inch diam	3 pancakes	240	29	11.0
original, prepared w/2/3 cup 2% milk, 2 tbsp oil, 1 egg, 4-inch diam	3 pancakes	210	28	9.0
original, prepared w/2/3 cup nonfat milk, 2 tbsp oil, 2 egg whites, 4-inch diam	3 pancakes	200	28	7.0
(Krusteaz) prepared, 4-inch diam	3 pancakes	200	39	3.0
MULTIGRAIN *(Arrowhead Mills)* mix only	1/2 cup	350	70	2.0
OAT BRAN				
(Arrowhead Mills) oat bran, mix only	1/2 cup	200	64	2.0
(Bisquick) 'Shake 'n Pour' prepared, 4-inch diam	3 pancakes	240	45	4.0
(Hungry Jack) microwave, mix onlry	3/4 pkg	230	45	4.0
(Krusteaz) 'Lite' prepared, 4-inch diam	3 pancakes	130	36	1.0
WHOLE WHEAT				
(Aunt Jemima)				
mix only	1/4 cup	120	26	0.5
prepared, 4-inch diam	3 pancakes	161	35	1.0
(Hungry Jack) harvest, microwave, mix only	3/4 pkg	230	46	4.0
(Krusteaz) w/honey, prepared, 4-inch diam	3 pancakes	215	42	1.0
(Stone-Buhr) mix only	1/4 cup	120	28	1.0
PAPAYA				
raw, cubed	1 cup	55	14	0.2
raw, mashed	1 cup	90	23	0.3
raw, whole, large, 5.75 inch long, 3.25 inch diam.	1 papaya	148	37	0.5
raw, whole, medium, 5 1/8 inch long, 3 inch diam	1 papaya	119	30	0.4
raw, whole, small, 4.5 inch long, 2.75 inch diam.	1 papaya	59	15	0.2
PAPAYA DRINK. See under FRUIT DRINK; FRUIT JUICE DRINK.				
PAPAYA JUICE *(Knudsen)* creamed	8 fl oz	160	40	0.0
PAPRIKA				
ground	1 tbsp	20	4	0.9
ground	1 tsp	6	1	0.3

Food Name	Serv. Size	Total Cal.	Carbs GMS	Fat GMS
ground *(Durkee)*	1 tsp	8	0	0.0
ground *(Laurel Leaf)*	1 tsp	8	0	0.0
ground *(McCormick/Schilling)*	1 tsp	9	1	0.4
ground *(Spice Islands)*	1 tsp	7	1	0.2
PARANUT. See BRAZIL NUT.				
PARROTFISH/pollyfish				
raw	1 lb	390	0.0	1.8
raw	1 oz	24	0.0	0.1
PARSLEY				
dried	1 tbsp	4	1	0.1
dried	1 tsp	1	0	0.0
dried *(McCormick/Schilling)*	1 tsp	2	0	0.0
freeze-dried	1/4 cup	4	1	0.1
freeze-dried	1 tbsp	1	0	0.0
fresh, raw	1 cup	22	4	0.5
fresh, raw	10 sprigs	4	1	0.1
fresh, raw	1 tbsp	1	0	0.0
PARSLEY FLAKES				
(Spice Islands)	1 tsp	4	1	0.1
ground *(Durkee)*	1 tsp	1	0	0.0
ground *(Laurel Leaf)*	1 tsp	1	0	0.0
PARSLEY ROOT/Hamburg parsley/turnip-rooted parsley				
fresh	1 lb	50	10.4	2.7
fresh	1 oz	3	0.7	0.2
PARSLEY SEASONING. See under SEASONING MIX.				
PARSNIP				
boiled, drained, sliced	1/2 cup	63	15	0.2
boiled, drained, whole, approx 9 inch long	1 parsnip	130	31	0.5
raw, sliced	1 cup	100	24	0.4
PARTY MIX				
(Michael Season's)				
spicy, low-fat, original	1 oz	110	23	1.5
traditional, low-fat	1 oz	120	23	1.5
PASSIONFRUIT/granadilla				
purple, raw, sliced	1 cup	229	55	1.7
purple, raw, whole, trimmed	1 fruit	17	4	0.1
PASSIONFRUIT JUICE				
purple	1 cup	126	34	0.1
purple	1 fl oz	16	4	0.0
yellow	1 cup	148	36	0.4
yellow	1 fl oz	19	4	0.1
PASTA. See also NOODLE.				
(NOTE: 2 ounces uncooked pasta = approximately 1 cup cooked.)				
(Al Dente) wild mushroom, dry	2 oz	220	40	2.0
(Creamette)				
dry	2 oz	210	42	1.0
rainbow, dry	2 oz	210	42	1.0
vegetable, dry	2 oz	210	42	1.0
w/egg, dry	2 oz	221	40	2.5
(De Boles)				
rainbow, dry, 'Primavera'	2 oz	200	41	1.0
vegetable, dry, 'Primavera' dry	2 oz	200	41	1.0
(Golden Grain) dry	2 oz	203	41	0.7
(Misura) whole wheat, w/bran, dry	2 oz	197	40	1.0
(Mueller's) 'Super Shapes' dry	2 oz	210	42	1.0
(Pastamania!)				
beet, spinach, and tomato	2 oz	200	40	1.0

Food Name	Serv. Size	Total Cal.	Carbs GMS	Fat GMS
oat bran, natural, gourmet, dry	2 oz	209	41	1.0
(Ronzoni) dry	2 oz	210	41	1.0
ACINI PEPE *(Ronzoni)* enriched, dry	2 oz	210	42	1.0
AGNOLOTTI *(Contadina)* refrigerated, 'Fresh'	3 oz	270	38	7.0
ANGEL HAIR				
(American Beauty) 100% durum wheat semolina, dry	2 oz	210	42	1.0
(Contadina)	1 1/4 cup	240	43	3.0
(Creamette) enriched, dry	2 oz	210	42	1.0
(De Boles)				
Jerusalem artichoke, dry	2 oz	210	41	1.0
Jerusalem artichoke, garlic and parsley, dry	2 oz	210	41	1.0
Jerusalem artichoke, tomato and basil, dry	2 oz	210	41	1.0
Jerusalem artichoke, tomato and lemon pepper, dry	2 oz	200	40	1.0
Jerusalem artichoke, whole wheat, dry	2 oz	210	40	2.0
(DiGiorno) refrigerated, uncooked	3 oz	250	47	3.0
(Hodgson Mill) 100% durum whole wheat flour, dry	2 oz	190	34	1.0
(Westbrae) corn, dry	2 oz	210	46	2.0
BOW TIE				
(De Cecco) farfelle, enriched, dry	2 oz	210	41	1.0
(Garden Time) four-color, dry	2 oz	203	41	1.0
(Hodgson Mill) whole wheat, dry	2 oz	190	34	1.0
(Mueller's) dry	2 oz	220	38	3.0
(Pasta Perfect) dry	1 cup	140	26	2.0
(Ronzoni) enriched, dry	2 oz	210	42	1.0
(Westbrae) vegetable, dry	2 oz	190	39	2.0
CAPELLINI				
(American Beauty) 100% durum wheat semolina, dry	2 oz	210	42	1.0
CORN *(Westbrae)* corn, dry	2 oz	210	46	2.0
CURLS *(Ancient Harvest)* quinoa, wheat-free, dry	2 oz	180	35	2.0
FARFALLE. See BOW TIE.				
FETTUCCINE				
(Al Dente)				
basil, dry	2 oz	220	40	2.0
curry, dry	2 oz	220	40	2.0
dill, dry	2 oz	220	40	2.0
spinach, dry	2 oz	220	40	2.0
tarragon, dry	2 oz	220	40	2.0
whole wheat, dry	2 oz	210	42	1.0
(American Beauty)				
spinach and egg, enriched, dry, 'Florentine'	2 oz	220	42	3.0
(Antoine's) egg, enriched, dry	2 oz	210	41	1.0
(Contadina)				
....	1 1/4 cup	250	45	3.5
cholesterol-free	1 cup	240	46	3.0
(De Boles)				
cholesterol-free, low-sodium, low-fat	2 oz	210	41	1.0
Jerusalem artichoke, dry	2 oz	210	41	1.0
Jerusalem artichoke, spinach, dry	2 oz	210	41	1.0
Jerusalem artichoke, tomato and lemon pepper, dry	2 oz	200	40	1.0
Jerusalem artichoke, tomato and pesto, dry	2 oz	210	41	1.0
(De Cecco) egg, dry, 'Home-Style'	2 oz	210	40	3.0
(DiGiorno)				
dry, approx 1 1/3 cups cooked	3 oz	250	47	3.0
spinach, dry, approx 1 1/3 cups cooked	3 oz	250	46	3.0
(Eden Foods)				
bell pepper basil, dry, 'Herb's'	2 oz	220	42	2.0
parsley garlic, dry, 'Herb's'	2 oz	220	42	2.0

Food Name	Serv. Size	Total Cal.	Carbs GMS	Fat GMS
spinach, dry, 'Herb's'	2 oz	220	42	2.0
(Hodgson Mill) whole wheat, dry	2 oz	190	34	1.0
(Pastamania!)				
durum wheat, dry	2 oz	200	38	2.0
garlic and parsley, dry	2 oz	200	38	2.0
garlic, parsley, and basil, dry	2 oz	200	38	2.0
spinach and durum wheat, dry	2 oz	200	38	2.0
w/lemon and pepper, dry	2 oz	220	40	3.0
w/mushrooms, dry	2 oz	210	41	2.0
w/Jerusalem artichoke	2 oz	210	41	2.0
(Ronzoni) egg, extra long, enriched, dry	2 oz	220	42	3.0
(Rummo) nested, dry	2 oz	210	41	1.0
FUSILLI				
(Antoine's)				
rainbow, dry	2 oz	210	41	1.0
tricolor, dry	2 oz	210	41	1.0
tricolor, vegetable, enriched, dry	2 oz	210	41	1.0
vegetable, dry	2 oz	210	41	1.0
(De Cecco)				
enriched, dry	2 oz	210	41	1.0
spinach, enriched, dry	2 oz	210	41	1.0
(Pastamania!) tomato and spinach, tre colore, dry	2 oz	200	40	1.0
GEMELLI				
(Antoine's) macaroni, enriched, dry	2 oz	210	41	1.0
LASAGNA				
(American Beauty) 100% durum wheat semolina, dry	2 oz	210	42	1.0
(Bernardi)				
sheets	1 piece	250	47	3.0
sheets, wavy	1 piece	310	60	2.5
(Creamette) 100% semolina, enriched, dry	2 oz	210	42	1.0
(De Boles)				
Jerusalem artichoke, dry	2 oz	210	41	1.0
whole wheat, dry	2 oz	210	40	2.0
(De Cecco) 100% semolina, dry	2 oz	210	41	1.0
(Ener-G Foods) gluten-free, dry	2 oz	214	42	0.1
(Health Valley)				
whole wheat, dry	2 oz	170	40	1.0
whole wheat, spinach, dry	2 oz	170	40	1.0
(Hodgson Mill) whole wheat, dry	2 oz	190	34	1.0
(Mueller's) dry	2 oz	210	42	1.0
(Ronzoni) curly edge, enriched, dry	2 oz	210	42	1.0
(Westbrae)				
spinach, whole wheat, no egg, dry	2 oz	210	40	2.0
whole wheat, no egg, dry	2 oz	210	40	2.0
LINGUINE				
(Ancient Harvest) quinoa, wheat-free, dry	2 oz	180	35	2.0
(Creamette) enriched, dry	2 oz	210	42	1.0
(De Boles) Jerusalem artichoke, dry	2 oz	210	41	1.0
(De Cecco) enriched, dry	2 oz	210	41	1.0
(DiGiorno)				
dry, approx 1-1/3 cups cooked	3 oz	250	46	3.0
refrigerated, uncooked	3 oz	250	47	3.0
(Pastamania!) durum wheat, dry	2 oz	200	38	2.0
(Quinoa) quinoa, wheat-free, dry	2 oz	180	35	2.0
(Ronzoni) enriched, dry	2 oz	210	42	1.0
MACARONI				
	2 oz	211	43	0.9
elbows, enriched, cooked	1 cup	197	40	0.9

Food Name	Serv. Size	Total Cal.	Carbs GMS	Fat GMS
elbows, enriched, dry	1 cup	390	78	1.7
elbows, unenriched, cooked	1 cup	197	40	0.9
elbows, unenriched, dry	1 cup	390	78	1.7
elbows, whole wheat, cooked	1 cup elbows	174	37	0.8
elbows, whole wheat, dry	1 cup elbows	198	43	0.8
small shells, dry	1 cup	345	69	1.5
spirals, enriched, cooked	1 cup	189	38	0.9
spirals, enriched, dry	1 cup	312	63	1.3
spirals, vegetable, enriched, dry	1 cup spirals	209	43	0.6
spirals, whole wheat, dry	1 cup spirals	365	79	1.5
vegetable, enriched, cooked	1 cup	172	36	0.1
vegetable, enriched, dry	1 cup	308	63	0.9
(American Beauty)				
elbows, 100% durum wheat semolina, dry	2 oz	210	42	1.0
100% durum wheat semolina, dry, 'Curly-Roni'	2 oz	210	42	1.0
(Ancient Harvest)				
elbows, quinoa, wheat-free, dry	2 oz	180	36	2.0
elbows, wheat-free, gluten-free	2 oz	180	35	2.0
(Creamette) elbows, enriched, dry	2 oz	210	42	1.0
(De Boles)				
elbows, corn, wheat-free, dry	2 oz	210	45	1.0
elbows, dry, 'Primavera'	2 oz	210	41	1.0
elbows, Jerusalem artichoke, dry	2 oz	210	41	1.0
elbows, whole wheat and Jerusalem artichoke, dry	2 oz	210	40	2.0
(Delmonico) dry	2 oz	210	42	1.0
(Eden Foods)				
elbows, whole wheat, vegetable	2 oz	210	42	1.0
elbows, whole-grain, organic, dry	2 oz	210	39	1.5
(Eden Foods) elbows, whole-grain, organic, dry	2 oz	210	39	1.5
(Ener-G Foods)				
brown rice, gluten-free, dry	2 oz	212	44	0.1
rice, gluten-free, dry	2 oz	214	42	0.1
shells, rice, gluten free, dry	2 oz	214	42	0.1
(Gioia) dry	2 oz	210	41	1.0
(Hodgson Mill) elbows, whole wheat, dry	2 oz	190	34	1.0
(Hospitality) elbows, enriched, dry, 'Valu Pack'	1/2 cup	240	48	0.5
(P&R) dry	2 oz	210	42	1.0
(Prince) dry	2 oz	210	43	1.0
(Quinoa) elbows, quinoa, wheat-free, dry	2 oz	180	36	2.0
(Ronzoni) dry	2 oz	210	41	1.0
(San Giorgio) dry, 'Italian/American Style'	2 oz	210	42	1.0
(Westbrae) elbows, corn, dry	2 oz	210	46	2.0
MANICOTTI *(Ronzoni)* extra fancy, enriched, dry	2 oz	210	42	1.0
MOSTACCIOLI				
(American Beauty)				
100% durum wheat semolina, dry	2 oz	210	42	1.0
tricolor, 'Italiano' dry	2 oz	210	42	1.0
(Creamette) enriched, dry	2 oz	210	42	1.0
(Ronzoni) enriched, dry	2 oz	210	40	1.0
ORZO *(Ronzoni)* enriched, dry	2 oz	210	42	3.0
PAGODAS				
(Ancient Harvest)				
garden	2 oz	180	35	2.0
garden, gluten-free	2 oz	180	35	2.0
PENNE *(Hodgson Mill)* whole wheat, dry	2 oz	190	34	1.0
PENNE RIGATI				
(Antoine's) uncooked	2 oz	210	41	1.0
(De Cecco) macaroni, enriched, dry	2 oz	210	41	1.0

Food Name	Serv. Size	Total Cal.	Carbs GMS	Fat GMS
PENNONI *(De Cecco)* macaroni, enriched, dry	2 oz	210	41	1.0
RADIATORE				
(Antoine's) macaroni, enriched, dry	2 oz	210	41	1.0
(Hodgson Mill)				
four colors	2 oz	200	41	1.0
whole wheat, dry	2 oz	190	34	1.0
(Ronzoni) tomato and spinach, tri-color, macaroni, dry	2 oz	210	42	1.0
RIBBON				
(Creamette)				
spinach, enriched, dry	2 oz	210	42	1.0
yolk-free, dry, 'Dutch'	2 oz	210	42	1.0
(De Boles) whole wheat and Jerusalem artichoke, dry	2 oz	210	40	2.0
(Eden Foods)				
extra fine, organic, dry	2 oz	220	44	1.0
mixed vegetable, dry, 'Herb's'	2 oz	220	42	2.0
paella, organic, dry	2 oz	220	44	1.0
paella, wheat, w/saffron, organic, dry	2 oz	228	44	1.0
parsley garlic, organic, dry	2 oz	220	44	1.0
pesto, organic, dry	2 oz	220	44	1.0
wheat, parsley garlic, organic, dry	2 oz	228	44	1.0
whole grain, dry, 'Herb's' dry	2 oz	200	40	1.5
whole grain, spinach, organic, dry	2 oz	200	40	1.5
(Hodgson Mill) whole wheat, dry	2 oz	190	34	1.0
RIGATONI				
(Creamette) enriched, dry	2 oz	210	42	1.0
(De Boles)				
Jerusalem artichoke, dry	2 oz	210	41	1.0
Jerusalem artichoke, dry, 'Primavera'	2 oz	210	41	1.0
(De Cecco) enriched, dry	2 oz	210	41	1.0
(Ronzoni) enriched, dry	2 oz	210	42	1.0
ROTELLE				
(American Beauty) 100% durum wheat semolina, dry	2 oz	210	42	1.0
(Ancient Harvest) quinoa, wheat-free, dry	2 oz	180	35	2.0
(Creamette) enriched, dry	2 oz	210	42	1.0
(De Cecco) enriched, dry	2 oz	210	41	1.0
(Pastamania!) beet, spinach, and tomato, dry	2 oz	200	40	1.0
(Quinoa)				
quinoa, dry	2 oz	210	40	1.0
quinoa, wheat-free, dry	2 oz	180	35	2.0
(Ronzoni) enriched, dry	2 oz	210	40	1.0
ROTINI				
(American Beauty)				
100% durum wheat semolina, dry	2 oz	210	42	1.0
quinoa, dry	2 oz	210	40	1.0
tricolor, 'Italiano' dry	2 oz	210	42	1.0
wheat and quinoa, organic, low-salt, no cholesterol	2 oz	210	42	1.0
(Bernardi) vegetable	1 1/4 cup	220	44	1.0
(Creamette) enriched, dry	2 oz	210	42	1.0
(De Boles)				
Jerusalem artichoke, dry	2 oz	210	41	1.0
Jerusalem artichoke, garlic and parsley, dry	2 oz	210	41	1.0
Jerusalem artichoke, tomato and basil, dry	2 oz	210	41	1.0
vegetable, dry, 'Primavera'	2 oz	210	41	1.0
(Eden Foods) mixed vegetable	2 oz	210	42	1.0
(Hodgson Mill) vegetable, four flavors, dry	2 oz	200	na	1.0
(Pasta Perfect)				
	1 cup	140	28	0.0
spinach	1 cup	140	27	0.0

Food Name	Serv. Size	Total Cal.	Carbs GMS	Fat GMS
RUFFLE				
(Mueller's) trio, dry	2 oz	210	42	1.0
SHELLS				
(American Beauty)				
100% durum wheat semolina, dry	2 oz	210	40	1.0
100% durum wheat semolina, macaroni, dry	2 oz	210	42	1.0
large, durum wheat semolina, dry	2 oz	210	42	1.0
medium, durum wheat semolina, dry	2 oz	210	42	1.0
tricolor, 'Italiano' dry	2 oz	210	42	1.0
(Ancient Harvest) quinoa, wheat-free, dry	2 oz	180	35	2.0
(Creamette) medium, enriched, dry	2 oz	210	42	1.0
(De Boles)				
	2 oz	210	41	1.0
corn, wheat-free, dry	2 oz	210	45	1.0
dry, 'Primavera'	2 oz	210	41	1.0
whole wheat and Jerusalem artichoke, dry	2 oz	210	40	2.0
(Eden Foods)				
vegetable, organic, dry	2 oz	210	42	1.0
w/mixed vegetable, dry, 'Herb's'	2 oz	210	42	1.0
wheat, vegetable, no eggs, organic, dry	2 oz	228	44	1.0
(Hodgson Mill) whole wheat, medium	2 oz	190	34	1.0
(Mueller's)				
dry	2 oz	210	42	1.0
jumbo, dry	2 oz	210	42	1.0
(Pasta Perfect)	1 cup	140	28	0.0
(Pastamania!) tomato and spinach, dry	2 oz	200	40	1.0
(Quinoa) quinoa 'Supergrain Wheat-free' dry	2 oz	180	35	2.0
(Ronzoni)				
enriched, dry	2 oz	210	42	1.0
extra fancy, enriched, dry	2 oz	210	42	1.0
jumbo, enriched, dry	2 oz	210	42	1.0
(Westbrae) corn, dry	2 oz	210	46	2.0
SPAGHETTI				
enriched, cooked	1 cup	197	40	0.9
protein-fortified, cooked	1 cup	230	44	0.3
unenriched, cooked	1 cup	197	40	0.9
(Al Dente) pepper, 'Three Pepper Pasta' dry	2 oz	220	40	2.0
(American Beauty) 100% durum wheat semolina, dry	2 oz	210	42	1.0
(Ancient Harvest) quinoa, wheat-free, dry	2 oz	180	35	2.0
(Creamette)				
dry	2 oz	210	42	1.0
enriched, thin, dry	2 oz	210	42	1.0
spinach, w/egg, uncooked	2 oz	220	40	3.0
(De Boles)				
corn, wheat-free, dry	2 oz	210	45	1.0
Jerusalem artichoke, dry	2 oz	210	41	1.0
Jerusalem artichoke, spinach	2 oz	200	41	1.0
whole wheat and Jerusalem artichoke, dry	2 oz	210	40	2.0
(DiGiorno) uncooked, approx 1 1/3 cups cooked	3 oz	250	47	3.0
(Eden Foods)				
durum wheat, organic, dry	2 oz	210	42	1.0
kamut, whole grain, organic, dry	2 oz	210	38	1.5
parsley garlic, organic, dry	2 oz	210	42	1.0
whole grain, organic, dry	2 oz	210	39	1.5
(Ener-G Foods)				
brown rice, gluten-free, dry	2 oz	212	44	0.1
rice, gluten-free, dry	2 oz	214	42	0.1

Food Name	Serv. Size	Total Cal.	Carbs GMS	Fat GMS
(Health Valley)				
amaranth, dry	2 oz	170	40	1.0
oat bran, dry	2 oz	120	23	1.0
whole wheat, dry	2 oz	170	40	1.0
whole wheat, spinach, dry	2 oz	170	40	1.0
(Hodgson Mill)				
durum whole wheat, thin, dry	2 oz	190	34	1.0
whole wheat, spinach, dry	2 oz	190	35	2.0
(Hospitality) enriched, 100% semolina, dry	2 oz	210	42	0.5
(Quinoa) quinoa, 'Supergrain'	2 oz	210	40	1.0
(Ronzoni)				
enriched, dry	2 oz	210	42	1.0
enriched, thin, dry	2 oz	210	42	1.0
(Rummo) dry	2 oz	210	41	1.0
(Westbrae)				
corn, dry	2 oz	210	46	2.0
whole wheat, no egg, dry	2 oz	210	40	2.0
whole wheat, spinach, no egg, dry	2 oz	210	40	2.0
SPAGHETTINI *(De Cecco)* enriched, dry	2 oz	210	41	1.0
SPIRAL				
(American Beauty)				
rainbow, 100% durum wheat semolina, dry	2 oz	210	42	1.0
(Antoine's) spicy, uncooked	2 oz	210	41	1.0
(Eden Foods)				
kamut, whole grain, organic, dry	2 oz	210	38	1.5
sesame rice, whole grain, organic, dry	2 oz	200	37	2.0
vegetable, whole grain, organic, dry	2 oz	210	39	1.5
wheat, sesame rice, organic, dry	2 oz	212	40	1.0
wheat, vegetable, no eggs, organic, dry	2 oz	228	44	1.0
(Hodgson Mill) whole wheat, whole grain, dry	2 oz	190	34	1.0
(Mueller's) 'Twist Trio' dry	2 oz	210	42	1.0
TAGLIATELLE				
(Contadina) spinach	1 1/4 cup	270	46	4.0
(Ener-G Foods)				
brown rice, gluten-free, dry	2 oz	212	44	0.1
rice, gluten-free, dry	2 oz	214	42	0.1
TAGLIERINI *(Pastamania!)* tomato and spinach, dry	2 oz	210	40	2.0
TRICOLOR				
(Creamette) dry	2 oz	210	42	1.0
TRICOLOR PASTA, PRIMAVERA				
(De Boles) tricolor, 'Primavera' dry	2 oz	200	41	1.0
WAGON WHEEL *(Hodgson Mill)* four flavors, dry	2 oz	200	41	1.0
VERMICELLI				
(American Beauty) 100% durum wheat semolina, dry	2 oz	210	42	1.0
(Creamette) enriched, extra thin, dry	2 oz	210	42	1.0
(Ener-G Foods) rice, gluten-free, dry	2 oz	214	42	0.1
(Ronzoni) enriched, dry	2 oz	210	42	1.0
WHEAT				
(De Boles) whole wheat 'Natural Gourmet' dry	2 oz	200	40	1.0
ZITI				
(De Boles)				
....	2 oz	210	41	1.0
Jerusalem artichoke, dry	2 oz	210	41	1.0
(Ronzoni) enriched, dry	2 oz	210	42	1.0
PASTA CHIPS				
(Bachman) pasta snack chip 'Pastapazazz'	1 oz	150	15	9.0

Food Name	Serv. Size	Total Cal.	Carbs GMS	Fat GMS
PASTA DISH/ENTRÉE. See also LASAGNA/LASAGNA ENTRÉE; MANICOTTI/MANICOTTI ENTRÉE; RAVIOLI DISH/ENTRÉE; TORTELLINI DISH/ENTRÉE.				
(Budget Gourmet)				
w/chicken, in wine and mushroom sauce w/chicken .... 1 entrée		280	40	7.0
(Celentano) and cheese, baked, frozen .... 6 oz		290	29	13.0
(Chef Boyardee)				
rings and franks, microwave .... 7.5 oz		190	31	5.0
rings and meatballs, microwave .... 7.5 oz		220	33	8.0
(Contadina) chicken, herb, w/tomato sauce, frozen .... 1 oz		27	4	0.6
(Green Giant)				
Dijon, frozen, 'Microwave Garden Gourmet' .... 1 pkg		300	24	20.0
Parmesan, w/sweet peas, frozen, 'One Serving' .... 5.5 oz		160	21	5.0
(Healthy Choice)				
primavera, microwave .... 11 oz		280	51	3.0
vegetable, Italiano .... 1 entrée		250	48	3.0
w/chicken, teriyaki, frozen, 'Classics' .... 12.6 oz		350	58	3.0
w/shrimp, frozen, 'Classics' .... 12.5 oz		270	44	4.0
(Lean Cuisine)				
cheddar bake .... 1 entrée		220	29	6.0
w/chicken and herb tomato sauce, frozen .... 9.5 oz		270	38	6.0
w/turkey, Dijon sauce, frozen, 'Lunch Express' .... 9 7/8 oz		290	39	7.0
(Lunch Bucket)				
chicken, Italian, lunch cup, 'Light'n Healthy' .... 7.5 oz		130	23	1.0
(Lunch Express)				
and tuna, casserole .... 1 entrée		280	39	6.0
and turkey, Dijon .... 1 entrée		270	37	6.0
(Marie Callender's)				
frozen, 'Callender's Deluxe' .... 1 cup		350	4	23.0
primavera, w/chicken, frozen .... 1 cup		310	22	19.0
w/beef and broccoli .... 15 oz		570	73	15.0
(MET-RX) cafe pasta meal .... 1 cup		190	27	1.0
(Smart Ones)				
and spinach, Romano .... 1 entrée		260	35	8.0
Portafino, in wine sauce, frozen .... 9.5 oz		160	30	1.0
(Tyson) trio, frozen, 'Gourmet Selection' .... 11 oz		450	53	17.0
(Weight Watchers)				
and spinach, Romano .... 1 entrée		240	32	8.0
Italiano, frozen, 'Ultimate 200' .... 8 oz		190	19	4.0
w/tomato basil sauce .... 1 entrée		260	33	9.0
ANGEL HAIR				
(Budget Gourmet) .... 1 entrée		230	38	5.0
(Lean Cuisine) frozen .... 1 entrée		220	41	3.0
(Marie Callender's) w/sausage and breadstick, frozen .... 1 entrée		370	43	15.0
(Smart Ones) .... 1 entrée		170	29	2.0
BOW TIES				
(Marie Callender's)				
Alfredo .... 13 oz		620	40	42.0
and meat sauce .... 13 oz		480	44	22.0
marinara .... 13 oz		430	46	19.0
(Lean Cuisine) and chicken, 'Café Classics' .... 1 entrée		270	34	6.0
(Pasta Perfect) w/vegetables .... 1/2 cup		110	19	1.0
(Weight Watchers) Marsala .... 1 entrée		280	36	9.0
CANNELLONI				
(Bernardi) w/beef .... 1 piece		200	19	10.0
(Celentano) Florentine, frozen .... 12 oz		350	48	8.0
(Dining Lite) cheese, frozen .... 9 oz		310	38	9.0

Food Name	Serv. Size	Total Cal.	Carbs GMS	Fat GMS
(Lean Cuisine)				
beef, w/tomato sauce, frozen	9 5/8 oz	200	28	3.0
cheese	1 entrée	240	29	5.0
cheese, w/tomato sauce, frozen	9 1/8 oz	270	27	8.0
CAVATELLI *(Celentano)*	2/3 cup	400	79	1.5
FETTUCCINE				
(Armour) chicken, frozen, 'Classics'	11 oz	260	28	9.0
(Banquet)				
Alfredo	1 entrée	350	40	16.0
Alfredo, four cheeses, frozen	1 entrée	480	48	24.0
chicken, frozen, 'Healthy Balance'	11.25 oz	320	47	7.0
w/meat sauce, frozen	10 oz	290	34	10.0
(Budget Gourmet) primavera, w/chicken	1 entrée	280	38	8.0
(Contadina) grilled chicken, frozen, food service product	1 oz	42	3	2.7
(Dining Lite) w/broccoli, frozen	9 oz	290	33	12.0
(Green Giant)				
primavera, frozen	1 pkg	230	26	8.0
primavera, 'Microwave Garden Gourmet'	1 pkg	260	25	13.0
(Hain) Alfredo, 'Pasta & Sauce'	1/4 pkg	180	27	4.0
(Healthy Choice)				
Alfredo	1 entrée	250	39	5.0
chicken, Alfredo	1 entrée	280	35	7.0
chicken, frozen	8.5 oz	240	29	4.0
(Kraft) Alfredo, 'Pasta & Cheese' prepared	1/2 cup	180	19	9.0
(Lean Cuisine)				
Alfredo, frozen	9 oz	280	41	7.0
chicken	1 entrée	270	33	6.0
chicken, Alfredo sauce, frozen 'Lunch Express'	10.25 oz	240	31	6.0
chicken, frozen	9 oz	280	33	6.0
primavera, frozen	10 oz	260	32	8.0
(Lunch Express) primavera	1 entrée	420	33	25.0
(Marie Callender's)				
Alfredo, frozen	1 cup	190	29	21.0
Alfredo, supreme	1 cup	450	35	27.0
Alfredo, w/bread	14 oz	800	71	47.0
primavera, w/tortellini	1 cup	430	35	27.0
w/broccoli and chicken	13 oz	410	32	24.0
(Michelinas) w/creamy pesto sauce 'Lean 'n Tasty'	1 entrée	250	38	6.0
(Right Course) chicken, Italiano, w/vegetables, frozen	9 5/8 oz	280	29	8.0
(Stouffer's)				
Alfredo	1 entrée	580	42	39.0
chicken, 'Homestyle'	1 entrée	390	32	15.0
chicken, homestyle, w/vegetable medley, frozen	9.5 oz	350	27	17.0
(Ultra Slim-Fast)	12 oz	390	38	12.0
(Weight Watchers)				
Alfredo, w/broccoli	1 entrée	230	34	6.0
chicken	1 entrée	290	39	7.0
LINGUINE				
(Banquet) w/meat sauce, frozen, 'Healthy Balance'	11.5 oz	290	49	6.0
(Budget Gourmet)				
w/shrimp, frozen	10 oz	330	33	15.0
w/shrimp and clams, 'Light'	1 entrée	280	38	8.0
w/tomato sauce, sausage, 'Special Selections'	1 entrée	360	43	14.0
(Healthy Choice) w/shrimp, frozen	9.5 oz	230	40	2.0
(Lean Cuisine)				
w/clam sauce, frozen	9 5/8 oz	280	36	8.0
w/meatballs, frozen, food service product	1 oz	25	3	0.8

Food Name	Serv. Size	Total Cal.	Carbs GMS	Fat GMS
(Marie Callender's) and Italian sausage	15 oz	710	70	36.0
(Top Shelf) w/clam sauce, packaged	1 serving	330	30	18.0
MACARONI				
(Amy's Kitchen)				
and cheese	1 serving	390	50	14.0
and soy cheese	1 serving	360	42	14.0
(Banquet)				
and beef, shells, frozen	10 oz	340	34	14.0
and cheese	1 entrée	320	44	11.0
and cheese, frozen	10 oz	420	46	20.0
and cheese, frozen, 'Family Entrées'	8 oz	290	32	13.0
(Budget Gourmet)				
and cheese	1 entrée	270	45	6.0
and cheese, frozen, 'Side Dish'	5.3 oz	210	23	8.0
and cheese, frozen, 'Special Selections'	1 entrée	400	38	20.0
(Chef Boyardee)				
and cheese, canned	7.5 oz	170	33	2.0
and cheese, w/shells, canned	7.5 oz	150	31	1.0
and chicken, canned	7.5 oz	180	30	2.0
canned, 'Roller Coasters'	7.5 oz	230	28	10.0
dinosaurs, in tomato and cheese sauce	1 cup	210	45	0.0
dinosaurs, w/mini meatballs, in tomato sauce	1 cup	270	38	9.0
elbows w/beef, in sauce, microwave	7.5 oz	210	29	7.0
in cheese sauce, canned, 'ABC's & 123's'	8.6 oz	200	42	1.0
in cheese sauce, canned, 'Sharks'	7.5 oz	170	34	1.0
in cheese sauce, canned, 'Smurfs'	7.5 oz	150	29	1.0
in cheese sauce, canned, 'Tic Tac Toes'	8.6 oz	190	41	1.0
in cheese sauce, canned, 'Tic Tac Toes'	7.5 oz	160	31	1.0
in cheese sauce, microwave, 'ABC's & 123's'	7.5 oz	180	37	1.0
in cheese sauce, microwave, 'Dinosaurs'	7.5 oz	180	36	1.0
in cheese sauce, microwave, 'Tic Tac Toes'	7.5 oz	170	36	1.0
in chicken sauce, canned, 'Pac Man'	7.5 oz	170	22	7.0
in sauce, canned 'ABC's & 123's'	7.5 oz	160	31	1.0
in sauce, canned 'Turtles'	7.5 oz	150	31	1.0
in sauce, microwave, 'Turtles'	7.5 oz	160	33	1.0
in tomato and cheese sauce, 'Street Sharks'	1 cup	210	47	0.0
in tomato sauce, canned, 'Pac Man'	7.5 oz	150	30	1.0
mini bites, canned	7.5 oz	260	30	12.0
shells, in meat sauce, canned	7.5 oz	190	31	6.0
shells, in meat sauce, microwave	7.5 oz	210	32	6.0
shells, in mushroom sauce, microwave	7.5 oz	170	35	1.0
'Teenage Mutant Ninja Turtles'	1 pkg	227	34	6.8
w/beef, canned, 'Beefaroni'	1 cup	260	37	7.0
w/beef, microwave, 'Beefaroni'	7.5 oz	220	31	7.0
w/meatballs, canned, 'ABC's & 123's'	8.6 oz	280	35	11.0
w/meatballs, canned, 'Dinosaurs'	8.6 oz	280	36	11.0
w/meatballs, canned, 'Pac Man'	7.5 oz	230	32	9.0
w/meatballs, canned, 'Smurfs'	7.5 oz	240	31	9.0
w/meatballs, canned, 'Tic Tac Toes'	7.5 oz	240	31	9.0
w/meatballs, canned, 'Tic Tac Toes'	8.6 oz	290	39	11.0
w/meatballs, canned, 'Turtles'	7.5 oz	220	30	8.0
w/meatballs, in sauce, canned, 'Zooroni'	7.5 oz	240	33	8.0
w/meatballs, 'Street Sharks' *(Chef Boyardee)*	1 cup	250	37	8.0
(Franco-American) and cheese	1 cup	210	29	7.0
(Green Giant)				
and cheese, frozen, 'One Serving'	5.7 oz	230	28	9.0

Food Name	Serv. Size	Total Cal.	Carbs GMS	Fat GMS
(Healthy Choice)				
and cheese	1 entrée	290	50	7.0
and cheese, meatless	1 entrée	320	50	7.0
(Heinz)				
and cheese, canned	7.5 oz	190	26	8.0
w/beef, in tomato sauce, canned	7.5 oz	200	23	8.0
(Hormel) and cheese, micro cup	7.5 oz	189	26	6.0
(Kid Cuisine)				
and cheese, frozen, 'Mega Meal'	12.45 oz	470	75	13.0
and cheese, w/apples, corn, fudge brownie, frozen	1 meal	310	54	7.0
and cheese, w/mini franks, frozen	9 oz	380	55	14.0
(Kid's Kitchen)				
beefy, microwave cup	7.5 oz	200	25	6.0
and cheese, microwave cup	7.5 oz	260	28	11.0
(Lean Cuisine)				
and beef	1 entrée	280	40	8.0
and beef, frozen, food service product	1 oz	27	3	0.9
and beef, in tomato sauce, frozen	1 pkg	249	37	5.4
and cheese	1 entrée	290	43	7.0
and cheese, frozen, food service product	1 oz	33	4	1.1
(Libby's) and cheese, microwave cup, 'Diner'	7.5 oz	360	27	22.0
(Lipton) and cheese, w/shells, 'Hearty Ones'	11 oz	367	60	7.4
(Lunch Bucket) and cheese, microwave lunch cup	7.5 oz	210	24	9.0
(Lunch Express) and cheese, w/broccoli	1 entrée	240	35	6.0
(Marie Callender's)				
and beef, w/tomatoes and soft breadstick, frozen	1 entrée	310	40	11.0
and cheese	13.5 oz	510	65	18.0
and cheese, frozen, 'Marie's Special'	1 cup	420	47	17.0
(Michelina's)				
and beef, 'Lean 'n Tasty'	1 entrée	230	34	6.0
and cheese, 'Lean 'n Tasty'	1 entrée	270	41	6.0
(Morton) and cheese casserole, frozen	6.5 oz	290	30	14.0
(Myers) and cheese, frozen	3.5 oz	168	16	9.0
(Nalley's) w/beef	7.5 oz	180	29	3.0
(Nestlé)				
and cheese, canned, 'Chef Mate'	1 pkg	3397	425	131.9
and cheese, canned, 'Chef Mate'	1 cup	283	35	11.0
(Pathmark) w/beef, in tomato sauce, canned, 'No Frills'	7.5 oz	200	22	8.0
(Smart Ones) and cheese	1 entrée	220	42	2.0
(Stouffer's)				
and beef	1 entrée	420	40	20.0
and beef, w/tomato	10 oz	270	43	4.0
and cheese	6 oz	330	31	17.0
and cheese, frozen, food service product	1 oz	39	4	1.6
(Swanson)				
and beef, frozen	12 oz	370	48	15.0
and cheese, frozen	12.25 oz	370	43	15.0
and cheese, frozen	7 oz	200	24	8.0
and cheese, frozen, 'Homestyle Recipe'	10 oz	390	37	19.0
(Tyson)				
and cheese, frozen, 'Tweety'	8 oz	340	49	10.0
frozen, 'Bugs Bunny/Tazmanian Devil'	8 oz	290	41	8.0
frozen, 'Daffy Duck & Elmer Fudd'	8 oz	270	40	7.0
frozen, 'Foghorn Leghorn/Henry Hawk'	8 oz	230	39	4.0
frozen, 'Looney Tunes Sylvester & Tweety'	8 oz	250	41	4.0
(Weight Watchers)				
and beef	1 entrée	220	32	4.5

Food Name	Serv. Size	Total Cal.	Carbs GMS	Fat GMS
in tomato sauce, frozen .... 1 pkg		282	45	4.6
and cheese .... 1 entrée		280	42	7.0
MOSTACCIOLI				
(Banquet) w/meat sauce, frozen, 'Family Entrées' .... 7 oz		170	28	3.0
(Contadina) w/meat sauce, frozen, food service product .... 1 oz		35	5	1.2
PENNE				
(Budget Gourmet)				
w/tomato sauce, Italian sausage, frozen .... 10 oz		320	53	9.0
w/tomato andsausage, 'Special Selections' .... 1 entrée		330	49	8.0
(Healthy Choice) w/roasted tomato sauce .... 1 entrée		230	36	5.0
(Marie Callender's) and pepperoni .... 15 oz		800	74	43.0
(Michelina's) w/mushrooms, 'Lean 'n Tasty' .... 1 entrée		250	38	6.0
(Weight Watchers)				
and ricotta, spicy .... 1 entrée		280	45	6.0
pollo .... 1 entrée		290	40	5.0
w/sun dried tomatoes .... 1 entrée		290	40	9.0
RIGATONI				
(Chef Boyardee)				
canned, 'Special Recipe' 'Ragatoni' .... 7.5 oz		210	33	6.0
microwave 'Ragatoni' .... 7.5 oz		210	31	6.0
(Budget Gourmet)				
tomato sauce, frozen, 'Special Selections' .... 1 entrée		420	41	22.0
w/broccoli and chicken, in cream sauce, frozen .... 10.8 oz		290	44	7.0
w/broccoli, white chicken, in cream sauce .... 1 entrée		250	37	7.0
(Healthy Choice)				
in meat sauce, frozen .... 9.5 oz		260	34	6.0
w/chicken, frozen, 'Classics' .... 12.5 oz		360	50	4.0
(Lean Cuisine)				
.... 1 entrée		180	25	4.0
jumbo, w/meatballs, 'Hearty Portions' .... 1 entrée		440	62	9.0
(Marie Callender's)				
Parmigiana, family size, frozen .... 1 cup		320	32	14.0
Parmigiana, w/breadstick, frozen .... 1 cup + bread		300	32	14.0
(Stouffer's) w/meat sauce, homestyle, frozen .... 12 oz		400	49	13.0
ROTINI				
(Green Giant)				
cheddar cheese, 'Microwave Garden Gourmet' .... 1 pkg		230	32	10.0
(Mrs. Paul's) seafood, frozen, 'Light' .... 9 oz		240	34	6.0
(Norpac)				
w/spinach rotini and vegetables, 'Pasta Perfect' .... 1/2 cup		100	19	0.0
w/vegetables, vegetarian, 'Pasta Perfect' .... 1/2 cup		110	20	1.0
(Weight Watchers) three cheese, w/vegetables, frozen .... 9 oz		270	34	8.0
SHELLS				
(Bernardi)				
cheese stuffed .... 2 pieces		240	25	11.0
cheese stuffed, large .... 1 piece		160	13	9.0
Florentine .... 1 piece		190	17	8.0
(Buitoni) shells, stuffed, frozen, 'Single Serving' .... 9 oz		460	46	13.0
(Celentano)				
broccoli stuffed, frozen, 'Great Choice' .... 10 oz		190	31	4.0
stuffed, frozen .... 8 oz		330	41	11.0
stuffed, lowfat, frozen 'Great Choice' .... 10 oz		250	41	2.0
stuffed, w/sauce, frozen .... 10 oz		410	51	14.0
stuffed, w/sauce, frozen .... 6.25 oz		340	31	16.0
(Healthy Choice)				
stuffed, in tomato sauce, frozen, 'Classics' .... 12 oz		330	53	3.0
(Le Menu) stuffed, 3-cheese, frozen 'LightStyle' .... 10 oz		280	34	8.0

Food Name	Serv. Size	Total Cal.	Carbs GMS	Fat GMS
(Lean Cuisine) cheese stuffed, frozen .... 1 oz		25	3	0.8
(Norpac)				
seashells w/vegetables, vegetarian, 'Pasta Perfect' .... 1/2 cup		130	25	1.0
(Stouffer's) cheese, w/tomato sauce, frozen .... 9.25 oz		300	28	13.0
SPAGHETTI				
(Banquet)				
w/meat sauce, frozen, 'Casserole' .... 8 oz		270	35	8.0
w/meatballs, frozen .... 10 oz		290	44	10.0
(Budget Gourmet)				
marinara .... 1 entrée		290	50	6.0
w/tomato and meat sauce, 'Special Selections' .... 1 entrée		320	49	7.0
(Buitoni) and meatballs, in sauce, canned .... 7.5 oz		190	21	8.0
(Chef Boyardee)				
and beef, in tomato sauce, canned .... 7.5 oz		240	30	9.0
and meatballs .... 1 cup		250	32	10.0
and meatballs, in tomato sauce, canned .... 1 pkg		442	60	15.3
and meatballs, in tomato sauce, canned .... 1 serving		250	34	8.6
and meatballs, canned, 'Microwave' .... 7.5 oz		230	29	10.0
w/beef, 'Beefagetti' .... 1 cup		250	37	7.0
(Dining Lite) w/beef, frozen .... 9 oz		220	25	8.0
(Estee) meatballs, canned .... 7.5 oz		240	19	14.0
(Featherweight) and meatballs, canned .... 7.5 oz		160	23	3.0
(Finast) rings, in tomato sauce, canned .... 7.5 oz		150	31	1.0
(Franco-American)				
in tomato and cheese sauce .... 1 cup		210	41	2.0
in tomato and cheese sauce, 'Spaghettio's' .... 1 cup		190	36	2.0
in tomato sauce .... 1 cup		270	35	10.0
w/meatballs, 'Spaghettio's' .... 1 cup		260	31	11.0
w/sliced frankfurters, 'Spaghettio's' .... 1 cup		250	32	11.0
(Freezer Queen) w/meat sauce, frozen 'Single Serve' .... 10 oz		350	47	12.0
(Healthy Choice) Bolognese, frozen .... 1 serving		255	43	2.9
(Kid Cuisine) w/meat sauce, frozen .... 9.25 oz		310	43	12.0
(Le Menu)				
w/beef, sauce, and mushrooms, frozen, 'LightStyle' .... 9 oz		280	45	6.0
(Lean Cuisine)				
.... 1 entrée		290	50	5.0
w/meat sauce .... 1 entrée		290	45	6.0
w/meat sauce, frozen .... 1 entrée		313	51	5.9
w/meatballs .... 1 entrée		290	40	7.0
w/neatballs and sauce, frozen .... 1 entrée		299	40	7.5
(Legume)				
and neatballs, vegetarian .... 1 serving		330	46	4.0
w/organic pasta and tofu, vegetarian .... 1 serving		240	23	11.0
w/veggie protein cutlet, vegetarian .... 1 serving		380	47	10.0
(Lunch Express) w/meat sauce .... 1 entrée		320	43	10.0
(Marie Callender's)				
and meat sauce, w/garlic bread .... 1 cup		380	51	13.0
marinara, w/cheese garlic bread .... 1 cup		410	61	13.0
(Michelina's)				
and meatballs, w/Pomodoro sauce, low-fat, frozen .... 1 pkg		312	49	7.1
and meatballs, w/Pomodoro sauce, low-fat, frozen .... 1 serving		312	49	7.1
(Morton) w/meatballs, frozen .... 10 oz		200	39	3.0
(Nalley's) and meatballs, canned .... 7.5 oz		190	29	4.0
(Pathmark)				
w/meatballs, in tomato sauce, canned 'No Frills' .... 7.5 oz		200	22	8.0
(Stouffer's)				
and meatballs .... 1 entrée		420	51	15.0

Food Name	Serv. Size	Total Cal.	Carbs GMS	Fat GMS
Parmesan, w/Italian-style green beans, frozen .... 10.25 oz		240	30	9.0
w/meat sauce, frozen .... 12 7/8 oz		320	38	12.0
(Swanson)				
w/Italian meatballs, frozen, 'Homestyle Recipe' .... 13 oz		490	60	18.0
w/meatballs, frozen.................................... 12.5 oz		390	46	17.0
(Top Shelf)				
spaghettini, packaged .... 1 serving		240	35	5.0
w/meat sauce .... 10 oz		260	37	6.0
(Tyson) w/meatballs, frozen, 'Daffy Duck' .... 8.65 oz		340	49	10.0
(Ultra Slim-Fast) w/beef and mushroom sauce .... 12 oz		370	49	10.0
(Van Camp's) w/franks, canned, 'Spaghettee Weenee' .... 1 cup		243	35	7.4
(Weight Watchers)				
marinara .... 1 entrée		280	46	7.0
w/meat sauce .... 1 entrée		290	45	6.0
SPIRALS *(Chef Boyardee)* canned, spirals, in pizza sauce .... 7.5 oz		180	35	3.0
ZITI				
(Budget Gourmet) Parmesano .... 1 entrée		260	39	7.0
(Healthy Choice)				
w/zesty tomato sauce, frozen, 'Classics' .... 12 oz		350	59	5.0
(Weight Watchers) w/mozzarella .... 1 entrée		280	45	6.0
PASTA DISH/ENTRÉE MIX. See also NOODLE DISH/ENTRÉE MIX.				
(Fantastic Foods)				
salad, Italian herb, prepared .... 1 cup		170	34	1.5
salad, Oriental, spicy, prepared .... 1 cup		200	37	3.0
(Kraft) salad, Italian, 97% fat free, prepared .... 3/4 cup		190	35	2.0
(Lunch Bucket)				
'Pasta 'n Chicken' microwave lunch cup .... 7.5 oz		180	22	6.0
w/beef, in wine sauce, micro cup, 'Light'n Healthy' .... 7.5 oz		130	21	3.0
(Pasta Roni) Parmesano pasta, 'Tenderthin' prepared .... 1 serving		226	28	9.6
(Suddenly Salad)				
salad, classic, mix only .... 3/4 cup		190	38	1.5
salad, classic, prepared .... 3/4 cup		250	38	8.0
(Ultra Slim-Fast)				
w/beef flavored sauce, prepared .... 8 oz		230	45	3.0
w/chicken flavored sauce, prep .... 8 oz		220	45	3.0
w/tomato herb sauce, prep .... 8 oz		220	46	3.0
w/zesty cheese sauce, prepared .... 8 oz		230	44	4.0
ANGEL HAIR				
(Golden Saute)				
w/chicken and broccoli, mix only .... 1/3 pkg		220	44	1.0
w/chicken and broccoli, prepared .... 1 cup		270	44	7.0
w/Parmesan, mix only .... 1/4 pkg		130	21	3.0
w/Parmesan, prepared .... 1/2 cup		160	21	6.0
(Pasta Roni)				
w/Parmesan cheese, prepared .... 1 serving		145	18	6.5
w/herb sauce, prepared .... 1 serving		145	19	6.3
CORKSCREW				
(Pasta Roni)				
w/creamy garlic sauce, prepared .... 1 serving		190	18	11.1
w/four cheese sauce, prepared .... 1 serving		231	28	10.2
FETTUCINE				
(Pasta Roni)				
broccoli au gratin, prepared .... 1 serving		164	22	5.6
cheddar, prepared .... 1 serving		169	23	5.9
chicken, prepared .... 1 serving		181	23	7.6
Romanoff, prepared .... 1 serving		231	27	10.7
Stroganoff, prepared .... 1 serving		209	27	7.9

Food Name	Serv. Size	Total Cal.	Carbs GMS	Fat GMS
w/Alfredo sauce, prepared .... 1 serving		265	27	14.1
LINGUINE				
(Pasta Roni)				
linguine w/chicken and broccoli sauce, prepared .... 1 serving		209	28	9.0
w/creamy chicken, Parmesan sauce, prepared .... 1 serving		231	26	10.4
MACARONI				
(De Boles)				
and cheddar, w/artichoke pasta shells, mix only .... 2 oz		210	40	2.0
and cheddar, w/artichoke pasta shells, prepared .... 3/4 cup		220	31	7.0
and cheese, w/artichoke pasta elbows, 'Mac & Cheese' mix only ... 2 oz		210	40	2.0
and cheese, w/artichoke pasta elbows, 'Mac & Cheese' prepared .... 3/4 cup		200	27	8.0
and cheese, w/artichoke pasta elbows, mix only .... 1/2 cup		200	33	3.5
and cheese, w/artichoke pasta elbows, prepared .... 3/4 cup		250	33	8.5
and cheese, w/artichoke pasta shells, mix only .... 1/2 cup		200	33	3.5
and cheese, w/artichoke pasta shells, prepared .... 3/4 cup		250	33	8.5
and cheese, w/wheat pasta elbows, mix only .... 1/2 cup		200	32	4.0
and cheese, w/wheat pasta elbows, prepared .... 3/4 cup		250	32	9.0
elbows, w/cheese sauce, mix only .... 2 oz		210	40	2.0
(Fantastic Foods)				
shells, w/curry, 'Tofu Classics' mix only .... 1/2 cup		200	40	1.5
(Hodgson Mill)				
and cheese, w/whole wheat pasta, mix only .... 1 pkg		774	143	9.7
and cheese, w/whole wheat pasta, mix only .... 2.5 oz		263	48	3.3
(Hormel) and cheese, micro cup .... 7.5 oz		189	26	6.0
(Kraft)				
and cheese, 'Deluxe Dinner' prepared .... 3/4 cup		260	36	8.0
and cheese, 'Dinner' prepared .... 3/4 cup		290	34	13.0
and cheese, 'Dinomac Dinner' prepared .... 3/4 cup		310	36	14.0
and cheese, 'Family Size Dinner' prepared .... 3/4 cup		290	34	13.0
and cheese, original flavor, mix only .... 1 serving		259	48	2.6
and cheese, 'Original' prepared .... 1 cup		410	49	18.0
and cheese, 'Teddy Bears Dinner' prepared .... 3/4 cup		310	36	14.0
and cheese, 'Wild Wheels Dinner' prepared .... 3/4 cup		310	36	14.0
and cheese, w/spirals, 'Dinner' prepared .... 3/4 cup		340	36	18.0
shells w/Velveeta, 'Original' .... 1 cup		360	44	13.0
(Libby's) and cheese, microwave cup, 'Diner' .... 7.5 oz		360	27	22.0
(Lipton) and cheese, w/shells, 'Hearty Ones' .... 11 oz		367	60	7.4
(Lunch Bucket)				
and cheese, microwave lunch cup .... 7.5 oz		210	24	9.0
and vegetables, micro cup, 'Light'n Healthy' .... 7.5 oz		150	30	1.0
elbows, in tomato sauce, microwave lunch cup .... 7.5 oz		190	38	2.0
(Nestlé) shells, w/sausage, canned, 'Chef-Mate' .... 1 cup		382	19	27.6
(Pasta Roni) shells w/white cheddar, prepared .... 1 serving		220	27	9.0
(Ultra Slim-Fast) and cheese, prepared .... 1 cup		230	46	3.0
PENNE				
(Golden Saute)				
stir-fry, w/chicken, mix only .... 1/2 cup		220	45	2.0
stir-fry, w/chicken, prepared .... 1 cup		270	45	8.0
(Pasta Roni) w/herb and butter sauce .... 1 serving		194	19	11.1
RIGATONI				
(Pasta Roni)				
w/tomato basil sauce, prepared .... 1 serving		81	12	3.0
w/white cheddar and broccoli sauce, prepared .... 1 serving		181	22	8.6
ROTINI				
(Golden Saute)				
w/chicken, herbs, and Parmesan, mix only .... 1 cup		280	45	9.0

Food Name	Serv. Size	Total Cal.	Carbs GMS	Fat GMS
SPAGHETTI				
(Chef Boyardee)				
w/condensed meat sauce, 'Dinner' prepared	3.25 oz	250	37	6.0
w/meat sauce, 'Dinner' prepared	7.9 oz	240	42	3.0
w/mushroom sauce, 'Dinner' prepared	7.9 oz	210	41	1.0
(Fantastic Foods) w/whole wheat noodles, low-fat, 'All-O-Round'				
prepared	10 oz	211	45	2.0
(Hormel) w/meatballs, micro cup	7.5 oz	210	27	7.0
(Kid's Kitchen)				
rings, microwave cup, mix only	7.5 oz	180	35	1.0
rings and franks, w/tomato sauce, micro cup, mix only	7.5 oz	290	33	12.0
w/meatballs, microwave cup	7.5 oz	220	26	8.0
(Kraft)				
mild, 'American Style Dinner' prepared	1 cup	300	50	7.0
tangy, 'Italian Style Dinner' prepared	1 cup	310	49	8.0
w/meat sauce, 'Dinner' prepared	1 cup	360	47	14.0
(Libby's) w/meatballs, in sauce, 'Diner' micro cup	7.75 oz	190	31	3.0
(Lunch Bucket) and meat sauce' microwave lunch cup	7.5 oz	240	39	5.0
(Mountain House)				
w/meat and sauce, freeze-dried, prepared	1 cup	260	41	5.0
VERMICELLI				
(Pasta Roni) w/garlic and olive oil sauce, prepared	1 serving	203	27	8.8
PASTA SAUCE. See under SAUCE.				
PASTA SEASONING. See under SEASONING MIX.				
PASTRY. See also CAKE, SNACK; PASTRY, TOASTER.				
(Tio Pepe's) churro, original	1 serving	140	14	9.0
(Entenmann's) Danish ring	1.5 oz	180	18	10.0
APPLE				
(Aunt Fanny's)				
cinnamon roll, old-fashioned, individual	2 oz	180	34	1.0
strudel, individual	3 oz	330	38	18.0
(Awrey's)				
filled Danish, 2.75 oz, 'Round'	1 piece	270	34	14.0
filled Danish, 4.5 oz, 'Round'	1 piece	390	50	20.0
filled Danish, 3 oz, 'Square'	1 piece	220	34	8.0
filled Danish, 1.7 oz, miniature	1 piece	160	21	8.0
(Break Cake)				
roll, sweet, 1.4 oz, multi-pak	1 roll	120	24	2.0
roll, sweet, 4.5 oz	2 rolls	380	75	5.0
(Entenmann's)				
'Apple Puffs'	1 puff	280	39	13.0
strudel, old-fashioned	1.5 oz	120	17	5.0
(Hormel) 'Apple Dulcita'	4 oz	290	44	10.0
(Hostess) filled Danish, fried, 'Breakfast Bake Shop'	1 piece	400	46	22.0
(Pepperidge Farm)				
crisp, 'Berkshire'	1 ramekin	250	43	8.0
Danish, 2 1/4 oz	1 piece	220	35	8.0
fruit square	1 piece	220	27	12.0
turnover, frozen	1 piece	300	34	17.0
turnover, ready to bake	1 serving	284	31	16.0
(Pillsbury)				
cinnamon roll, w/icing, ready to bake	1 roll	140	21	5.0
pocket	1 piece	240	25	13.0
turnover, refrigerated	1 piece	170	23	8.0
(Sara Lee)				
Danish twist	1/8 pkg	190	22	10.0
Danish, 'Free & Light'	1/8 pkg	130	30	0.0
Danish, 'Individual' 1.3 oz	1 piece	120	15	6.0

Food Name	Serv. Size	Total Cal.	Carbs GMS	Fat GMS
(Tastykake) pocket	3 oz	323	38	17.6
(Tio Pepe's) churro, apple filled, regular size	1 serving	160	22	7.0
(Weight Watchers)				
crisp, 'Sweet Celebrations'	1/2 pkg	190	40	5.0
roll, sweet 'Microwave'	1/2 pkg	160	27	4.0
APRICOT				
(Entenmann's) Danish twist, fat-free, cholesterol-free	1 slice	150	34	0.0
(Tio Pepe's) filled churro, regular size	1 serving	170	25	7.0
BAVARIAN CREAM				
(Entenmann's)	1.3 oz	80	20	0.0
(Rich's) cream puff	1 piece	150	17	8.0
(Tio Pepe's) filled churro, regular size	1 serving	160	22	7.0
BLACK FOREST *(Entenmann's)* fat-free, cholesterol-free	1 slice	130	32	0.0
BLUEBERRY, turnover *(Pepperidge Farm)*	1 piece	310	32	19.0
CARAMEL *(Pillsbury)* w/nuts	1 piece	160	19	8.0
CHEESE				
(Awrey's)				
filled Danish, 4.5 oz, 'Round'	1 piece	420	52	22.0
filled Danish, 2.75 oz, 'Round'	1 piece	280	34	15.0
filled Danish, 2.5 oz, 'Square'	1 piece	210	25	11.0
filled Danish, miniature 1.7 oz	1 piece	170	21	9.0
(Pepperidge Farm) Danish, 2 1/4 oz	1 piece	240	25	14.0
(Sara Lee)				
Danish, 'Individual' 1.3 oz	1 piece	130	13	8.0
Danish twist	1/8 pkg	200	21	12.0
(Tastykake) pocket	3 oz	325	41	16.7
CHERRY				
(Aunt Fanny's) strudel, individual	3 oz	320	39	16.0
(Hormel) 'Cherry Dulcita'	4 oz	300	48	9.0
(Pepperidge Farm) turnover	1 piece	310	32	19.0
(Pillsbury) turnover	1 piece	170	23	8.0
CHOCOLATE				
Fresh				
churro, creme filled, regular size *(Tio Pepe's)*	1 serving	180	28	7.0
fudge tart, frosted *(Toastettes)*	1 serving	190	34	5.0
Frozen or refrigerated				
éclair *(Weight Watchers)*	1 serving	150	25	4.0
éclair, 'Sweet Celebrations' *(Weight Watchers)*	2.1 oz	150	26	4.0
éclair, triple chocolate *(Weight Watchers)*	1 serving	160	25	5.0
éclair, 2 oz *(Rich's)*	1 piece	210	27	10.0
CINNAMON				
(Awrey's) cinnamon-walnut Danish, 'Round' 2.75 oz	1 piece	300	31	18.0
(Entenmann's) filbert ring	1.5 oz	190	19	12.0
(Tio Pepe's) churro	1 churro	110	14	5.0
CINNAMON-RAISIN				
(Awrey's)				
filled Danish, 3 oz, 'Square'	1 piece	290	41	12.0
filled Danish, miniature 1.5 oz	1 piece	160	21	8.0
(Entenmann's) bun, nonfat, no cholesterol	1 serving	160	36	0.0
(Pepperidge Farm) Danish, 2 1/4 oz	1 piece	250	35	11.0
(Pillsbury) Danish, w/icing	1 piece	150	20	7.0
(Sara Lee) Danish, individual, 1.3 oz	1 piece	150	17	8.0
DATE NUT *(Awrey's)* 1 piece	1.6 oz	230	35	10.0
ÉCLAIR *(Tasty-Klair)* custard-filled, prepared	1 pie	296	27	17.7
LEMON				
(Entenmann's)				
lemon Danish twist	1.2 oz	140	17	7.0
twist, fat-free, cholesterol-free	1 slice	130	31	0.0

Food Name	Serv. Size	Total Cal.	Carbs GMS	Fat GMS
NUT				
(Flanigan Farms)				
and fruit, almond, raisin, date, sunflower seed, no salt .... 1/4 cup		130	12	8.0
peanut, raisin, and sunflower seed, no salt .... 1/4 cup		130	11	10.0
ORANGE *(Pillsbury)* Danish, w/icing .... 1 piece		150	19	7.0
PEACH *(Pepperidge Farm)* turnover .... 1 piece		310	34	18.0
PECAN *(Entenmann's)* Danish ring .... 1.5 oz		190	19	12.0
PINEAPPLE *(Awrey's)* filled Danish, miniature, 1.7 oz .... 1 piece		157	21	8.0
RASPBERRY				
(Awrey's) filled Danish, 3 oz, 'Square' .... 1 piece		260	45	8.0
(Entenmann's)				
cheese, fat-free, cholesterol-free .... 1 slice		140	32	0.0
Danish twist .... 1.2 oz		140	18	7.0
(Hostess) raspberry-filled Danish, fried .... 1 piece		390	49	20.0
(Pepperidge Farm)				
raspberry Danish, 2 1/4 oz .... 1 piece		220	31	9.0
turnover .... 1 piece		310	36	17.0
(Sara Lee) raspberry Danish twist, 1/8 pkg .... 1/8 pkg		200	25	9.0
(Tio Pepe's) churro, regular size .... 1 serving		160	23	7.0
STRAWBERRY				
(Awrey's)				
filled Danish, 4.5 oz, 'Round' .... 1 piece		400	53	20.0
filled Danish, 2.75 oz, 'Round' .... 1 piece		270	34	14.0
filled Danish, miniature, 1.7 oz .... 1 piece		160	21	8.0
WALNUT *(Entenmann's)* Danish ring .... 1.5 oz		190	19	12.0
PASTRY, TOASTER				
APPLE				
(Auburn Farms)				
cinnamon, nonfat .... 1 pastry		157	36	0.5
cinnamon, 'Toast 'n Jammers' .... 1 pastry		180	42	0.0
(Kellogg's)				
cinnamon, frosted, low-fat, 'Pop Tarts' .... 1 pastry		191	40	2.9
cinnamon, 'Pop Tarts' .... 1 pastry		205	37	5.3
cinnamon Danish, 'Pastry Swirls' 'Pop Tarts' .... 1 pastry		256	37	11.0
(Pastry Poppers) fruit juice sweetened, low-sodium .... 2 oz		212	38	5.4
(Pepperidge Farm)				
cinnamon, 'Croissant Toaster Tarts' .... 1 pastry		170	25	7.0
(Pillsbury)				
'Danish' 'Toaster Strudel' .... 1 pastry		197	25	9.8
spice, 'Muffins' 'Toaster Strudel' .... 1 pastry		130	21	5.0
'Toaster Strudel' .... 1 pastry		180	9	7.0
(Toastettes)				
'Frosted Tarts' .... 1 pastry		190	35	5.0
'Tarts' .... 1 pastry		190	36	5.0
BANANA NUT				
(Pillsbury)				
'Muffins' 'Toaster Strudel' .... 1 pastry		130	19	6.0
'Strudel Breakfast Pastries' 'Toaster Strudel' .... 1 pastry		190	28	8.0
BERRY *(Kellogg's)* wild, frosted, 'Pop Tarts' .... 1 pastry		210	39	5.0
BLUEBERRY				
(Auburn Farms) nonfat .... 1 pastry		165	38	0.5
(Howard Johnson's) frozen, ready to eat, 'Toasties' .... 1 serving		235	32	9.7
(Kellogg's)				
frosted, 'Pop Tarts' .... 1 pastry		203	37	5.2
low-fat, 'Pop Tarts' .... 1 pastry		192	40	2.9
plain, 'Pop Tarts' .... 1 pastry		212	36	6.9
(Pastry Poppers) fruit juice sweetened, low-sodium .... 2 oz		212	38	4.5

Food Name	Serv. Size	Total Cal.	Carbs GMS	Fat GMS
(Pillsbury)				
....	1 pastry	180	9	7.0
'Strudel Breakfast Pastries' 'Toaster Strudel'	1 pastry	190	28	8.0
'Toaster Strudel'	1 pastry	190	26	9.0
wild, Maine, 'Toaster Strudel'	1 pastry	120	23	3.0
(Toastettes)				
'Frosted Tarts'	1 pastry	190	35	5.0
'Tarts'	1 pastry	190	35	5.0
BRAN *(Thomas')* 'Toast-r-Cakes'	1 pastry	103	18	2.9
BROWN SUGAR CINNAMON				
(Kellogg's)				
frosted, 'Pop Tarts'	1 pastry	211	34	7.4
frosted w/cinnamon, low-fat, 'Pop Tarts'	1 pastry	188	39	2.8
plain, 'Pop Tarts'	1 pastry	219	32	9.2
CHEESE				
(Kellogg's) Danish, 'Pastry Swirls' 'Pop Tarts'	1 pastry	252	37	11.0
(Pepperidge Farm) 'Croissant Toaster Tarts'	1 pastry	190	22	10.0
(Pillsbury)				
cream cheese	1 pastry	190	9	10.0
cream cheese, w/blueberry	1 pastry	190	9	9.0
cream cheese, w/strawberry	1 pastry	190	9	9.0
CHERRY				
(Kellogg's)				
low-fat, 'Pop Tarts'	1 pastry	192	40	2.9
plain, 'Pop Tarts'	1 pastry	204	37	5.4
(Pastry Poppers) fruit juice sweetened, low-sodium	2 oz	212	38	4.5
(Pillsbury)				
....	1 pastry	180	9	7.0
'Strudel Breakfast Pastries' 'Toaster Strudel'	1 pastry	190	26	9.0
'Toaster Strudel'	1 pastry	190	26	8.0
(Toastettes)				
'Frosted Tarts'	1 pastry	190	35	5.0
'Tarts'	1 pastry	190	35	5.0
CHOCOLATE FUDGE				
(Kellogg's)				
fudge, frosted, 'Pop Tarts'	1 pastry	201	37	4.8
fudge, frosted, low-fat, 'Pop Tarts'	1 pastry	190	40	3.0
milk chocolate, 'Pop Tarts' *(Kellogg's)*	1 pastry	205	36	5.8
vanilla creme, frosted, 'Pop Tarts'	1 pastry	203	37	5.3
CINNAMON				
(Pillsbury)				
....	1 pastry	190	9	8.0
'Danish' 'Toaster Strudel'	1 pastry	214	24	11.9
'Strudel Breakfast Pastries' 'Toaster Strudel'	1 pastry	190	26	8.0
'Toaster Strudel'	1/6 pkg	200	23	10.0
(Toastettes) frosted, brown sugar cinnamon	1 pastry	190	35	5.0
CORN				
(Pillsbury) old-fashioned, 'Muffins' 'Toaster Strudel'	1 pastry	120	17	5.0
(Oroweat) toaster biscuit	1 biscuit	200	39	3.0
FRENCH TOAST *(Pillsbury)*	1 pastry	190	9	7.0
FRUIT PUNCH *(Toastettes)* 'Frosted Tarts'	1 pastry	190	35	5.0
GRAPE *(Kellogg's)* frosted, 'Pop Tarts'	1 pastry	203	38	5.1
LEMON *(Pillsbury)* 'Danish' 'Toaster Strudel'	1 pastry	197	25	9.8
OAT BRAN *(Awrey's)* w/raisins, 'Toastums'	1 pastry	130	17	5.0
PEACH-APRICOT				
(Pastry Poppers) fruit juice sweetened, low-salt	2 oz	212	38	4.5

Food Name	Serv. Size	Total Cal.	Carbs GMS	Fat GMS
RAISIN				
RAISIN BRAN				
(Pillsbury)				
bran, 'Muffins' 'Toaster Strudel'	1 pastry	120	16	5.0
'Danish' 'Toaster Strudel'	1 pastry	197	25	9.8
RASPBERRY				
(Auburn Farms)				
nonfat	1 pastry	180	42	0.0
'Toast 'n Jammers' *(Auburn Farms)*	1 pastry	180	42	0.0
(Kellogg's) frosted, 'Pop Tarts'	1 pastry	205	37	5.5
(Pastry Poppers) fruit juice sweetened, low-sodium	2 oz	212	38	4.5
(Pillsbury)				
. . . .	1 pastry	180	9	7.0
'Danish' 'Toaster Strudel'	1 pastry	197	25	9.8
'Strudel Breakfast Pastries' 'Toaster Strudel'	1 pastry	190	27	8.0
'Toaster Strudel'	1 pastry	180	26	7.0
S'MORES *(Kellogg's)* 'Pop Tarts'	1 pastry	204	36	5.5
STRAWBERRY				
(Auburn Farms) nonfat	1 pastry	180	42	0.0
(Kellogg's)				
frosted, 'Pop Tarts'	1 pastry	203	38	5.0
frosted, low-fat, 'Pop Tarts'	1 pastry	191	40	3.0
low-fat, 'Pop Tarts'	1 pastry	192	40	2.9
'Pastry Swirls' 'Pop Tarts'	1 pastry	254	37	11.0
'Pop Tarts'	1 pastry	210	37	6.0
(Pastry Poppers) fruit juice sweetened, low-sodium	2 oz	212	38	4.5
(Pepperidge Farm) 'Croissant Toaster Tarts'	1 pastry	190	28	7.0
(Pillsbury)	1 pastry	180	9	7.0
'Danish' 'Toaster Strudel'	1 pastry	197	25	9.8
'Strudel Breakfast Pastries' 'Toaster Strudel'	1 pastry	190	27	8.0
'Toaster Strudel'	1 pastry	180	26	7.0
(Toast N' Jammers) 100% juice sweetened, whole wheat	1 pastry	165	38	0.5
(Toastettes) frosted	1 pastry	190	35	5.0
PÂTÉ, CANNED				
chicken liver	1 oz	57	2	3.7
chicken liver	1 tbsp	26	1	1.7
goose liver, de foie gras, smoked	1 oz	131	1	12.4
goose liver, de foie gras, smoked	1 tbsp	60	1	5.7
liver *(Sells)*	2.25 oz	190	3	16.0
PATTYPAN SQUASH. See SQUASH, SCALLOP.				
PEACH				
Canned				
extra light, halves or slices, w/liquid	1 cup	104	27	0.2
halves *(Hunt's)*	1/2 cup	100	24	0.0
in extra heavy syrup, halves or slices, w/liquid	1 cup	252	68	0.1
in heavy syrup, halves, w/liquid	1/2 med fruit	73	20	0.1
in heavy syrup, slices, w/liquid	1 cup	194	52	0.3
in juice, halves, w/liquid	1/2 fruit	43	11	0.0
in juice, halves or slices, w/liquid	1 cup	109	29	0.1
in light syrup, halves, w/liquid	1/2 fruit	53	14	0.0
in light syrup, halves or slices, w/liquid	1 cup	136	37	0.1
in water, halves, w/liquid	1/2 fruit	24	6	0.1
in water, halves or slices, w/liquid	1 cup	59	15	0.1
sliced *(Hunt's)*	1/2 cup	100	24	0.0
spiced, in heavy syrup, whole, w/liquid	1 cup	182	49	0.2

Food Name	Serv. Size	Total Cal.	Carbs GMS	Fat GMS
Dried				
sulfured, stewed	1 cup	322	83	1.0
sulfured, uncooked	1 cup	377	96	1.2
sulfured, uncooked, halves	1 cup	382	98	1.2
sulfured, uncooked, halves	1/2 medium	31	8	0.1
sulfured, w/added sugar	1 cup	278	72	0.6
sulfured, w/o added sugar	1 cup	199	51	0.6
Fresh				
raw, sliced	1 cup	73	19	0.2
raw, whole, large, 2.75 inch diam, 2.5 per lb	1 peach	68	17	0.1
raw, whole, medium, 2.5 inch diam, 4 per lb	1 peach	42	11	0.1
raw, whole, small, 2 inch diam, 5 per lb	1 peach	34	9	0.1
Frozen				
in syrup, sliced (Flav-R-Pac)	2/3 cup	100	25	0.0
sliced (Flav-R-Pac)	2/3 cup	50	13	0.0
sliced, thawed	1 cup	235	60	0.3
sweetened, sliced	10-oz pkg	267	68	0.4
sweetened, sliced	10 med slices	146	37	0.2
PEACH BUTTER, nonfat (Smucker's)	1 tsp	15	4	0.0
PEACH DRINK. See under FRUIT DRINK; FRUIT JUICE BLEND; FRUIT JUICE DRINK; PEACH JUICE.				
PEACH JUICE				
(Dole) orchard blend, 'Pure & Light'	6 fl oz	90	24	0.0
(Mountain Sun) 'Mountain Peach' organic	8 fl oz	112	27	0.0
(Smucker's) 'Naturally 100%'	8 fl oz	120	30	0.0
PEANUT				
ALL TYPES				
lightly salted, shelled (Eagle)	1 oz	180	5	15.0
salted (Frito-Lay's)	1 oz	170	6	15.0
salted in shell, shelled (Fisher)	1/4 cup	170	6	14.0
salted, shelled (Little Debbie)	1.25 oz	230	5	18.0
shelled (Beer Nuts)	1 oz	180	7	14.0
shelled (Weight Watchers)	1 pouch	100	4	7.0
shelled, 'Ballpark' (Eagle)	1 oz	180	5	15.0
shelled, 'Sweet & Crunchy' (Pathmark)	1 oz	140	15	8.0
shelled, 'Sweet-N-Crunchy' (Planters)	1 oz	140	15	8.0
spicy, hot, shelled, 'Heat' (Planters)	1 oz	170	5	14.0
spicy, mild, shelled, 'Heat' (Planters)	1 oz	170	5	14.0
unsalted, shelled (Little Debbie)	1.25 oz	230	5	18.0
Dry roasted				
lightly salted (Finast)	1 oz	160	6	14.0
lightly salted (Fisher)	1 oz	160	6	14.0
lightly salted (Planters)	1 oz	170	5	15.0
salted (Fisher)	1 oz	160	6	14.0
salted (Flavor House)	1 oz	180	5	14.0
salted (Frito-Lay's)	1 1/8 oz	190	7	16.0
salted (Guy's)	1 oz	170	3	14.0
salted (Pathmark)	1 oz	170	5	14.0
salted (Planters)	1 oz	160	6	14.0
unsalted (Finast)	1 oz	160	5	14.0
unsalted (Flavor House)	1 oz	180	5	14.0
unsalted (Pathmark)	1 oz	170	5	14.0
unsalted (Planters)	1 oz	170	5	15.0
unsalted, natural (Flanigan Farms)	1 oz	170	6	14.0
unsalted, 'No Frills' (Pathmark)	1 oz	180	5	14.0

Food Name	Serv. Size	Total Cal.	Carbs GMS	Fat GMS
Golden roasted				
(Fisher)	1/4 cup	160	10	12.0
barbecue, crunchy (Fisher)	1/4 cup	160	10	11.0
Honey roasted				
(Fisher)	1/4 cup	170	7	13.0
(Flavor House)	1 oz	160	9	11.0
(Little Debbie)	1.13 oz	190	9	13.0
(Pathmark)	1 oz	170	8	13.0
(Planters)	1 oz	170	8	13.0
(Weight Watchers)	1 pouch	100	4	7.0
'Honey Roast' (Eagle)	1 oz	170	7	13.0
unsalted (Fisher)	1 oz	150	4	13.0
Oil roasted				
(Fisher)	1/4 cup	170	5	15.0
(Planters)	1 oz	170	5	14.0
lightly salted (Planters)	1 oz	170	5	14.0
lightly salted	1 oz	160	6	14.0
redskin (Planters)	1 oz	170	5	15.0
salted (Flavor House)	1 oz	170	5	15.0
salted (Pathmark)	1 oz	180	5	14.0
salted (Planters)	1 oz	170	5	15.0
salted, cocktail (Planters)	1 oz	170	5	15.0
unsalted (Planters)	1 oz	170	5	14.0
unsalted, cocktail (Planters)	1 oz	170	5	15.0
Raw				
	1 cup	828	24	71.9
	1 oz	161	5	14.0
Roasted				
salted, in shell (Planters)	1.5 oz	170	5	14.0
unsalted, in shell (Planters)	1.5 oz	170	5	14.0
Yogurt coated (Harmony)	17 pieces	210	21	13.0
SPANISH				
shelled, salted (Guy's)	1 oz	170	3	14.0
Dry roasted (Planters)	1 oz	160	6	14.0
Oil roasted				
(Flavor House)	1 oz	170	5	15.0
(Planters)	1 oz	170	5	15.0
Raw				
	1 cup	832	23	72.4
	1 oz	162	4	14.1
(Planters)	1 oz	160	5	14.0
salted (Fisher)	1 oz	160	5	14.0
Roasted				
salted (Eagle)	1 oz	180	5	15.0
salted (Fisher)	1/4 cup	180	6	16.0
VALENCIA				
Oil roasted				
unsalted	1 cup	848	23	73.8
unsalted	1 oz	167	5	14.5
Raw				
unsalted	1 cup	832	31	69.5
unsalted	1 oz	162	6	13.5
VIRGINIA				
Oil roasted				
unsalted	1 cup	827	28	69.5
unsalted	1 oz	164	6	13.8

Food Name	Serv. Size	Total Cal.	Carbs GMS	Fat GMS
Raw				
unsalted	1 cup	822	24	71.2
unsalted	1 oz	160	5	13.8
PEANUT BUTTER				
chunky	1 cup	1520	56	128.8
chunky	2 tbsp	188	7	16.0
chunky, no salt added	1 cup	1520	56	128.8
chunky, no salt added	2 tbsp	188	7	16.0
smooth	1 cup	1530	50	131.7
smooth	2 tbsp	190	6	16.3
smooth, no salt added	1 cup	1530	50	131.7
smooth, no salt added	2 tbsp	190	6	16.3
(Arrowhead Mills)				
chunky	2 tbsp	190	6	16.0
creamy	2 tbsp	190	6	16.0
(Bama)				
chunky	2 tbsp	200	6	17.0
creamy	2 tbsp	200	6	17.0
crunchy	2 tbsp	200	6	17.0
smooth	2 tbsp	200	6	17.0
(Estee)				
chunky	2 tbsp	200	6	18.0
creamy	2 tbsp	200	6	18.0
(Featherweight)				
chunky	1 tbsp	90	2	7.0
smooth	1 tbsp	90	2	7.0
(Finast)				
chunky, 'Crunchy'	2 tbsp	195	6	17.0
smooth	2 tbsp	195	6	17.0
(Health Valley)				
chunky, no salt added	2 tbsp	180	6	14.0
creamy, no salt added	2 tbsp	180	6	14.0
(Hollywood)				
chunky	1 tbsp	35	1	3.0
creamy	1 tbsp	35	1	3.0
no salt added	1 tbsp	35	1	3.0
(JFG)				
creamy	2 tbsp	200	8	16.0
creamy, 50% less salt	2 tbsp	200	8	16.0
crunchy	2 tbsp	200	8	16.0
(Jif)				
creamy	2 tbsp	190	7	16.0
creamy, 'Simply Jif'	2 tbsp	190	6	16.0
crunchy, 'Simply Jif'	2 tbsp	190	7	16.0
extra crunchy	2 tbsp	190	7	16.0
smooth	2 tbsp	190	6	16.0
(Maranatha Natural) crunchy	2 tbsp	190	7	15.0
(Pathmark)				
chunky, 'Super Chunky'	2 tbsp	200	6	17.0
'Natural'	2 tbsp	200	5	17.0
smooth, 'Creamy'	2 tbsp	200	6	17.0
smooth, 'No Frills'	2 tbsp	200	6	17.0
(Peter Pan)				
creamy	2 tbsp	189	7	16.0
creamy, low salt	2 tbsp	197	6	17.5
creamy, whipped	2 tbsp	148	5	12.6
crunchy	2 tbsp	188	6	15.9

Food Name	Serv. Size	Total Cal.	Carbs GMS	Fat GMS
crunchy, low salt	2 tbsp	197	6	17.3
crunchy, salt-free	2 tbsp	190	5	17.0
crunchy, whipped	2 tbsp	148	5	12.5
smooth, no salt added	2 tbsp	195	5	17.1
(Real Brand)				
creamy	2 tbsp	189	5	16.4
crunchy	2 tbsp	189	5	16.3
(Reese) creamy	2 tbsp	204	6	16.1
(Roaster Fresh) gourmet	1 oz	166	5	14.0
(S&W) 'Nutradiet'	1 tbsp	93	2	8.0
(Skippy)				
chunky, roasted honey nut	2 tbsp	190	6	17.0
chunky, 'Super Chunk'	2 tbsp	190	5	17.0
creamy	2 tbsp	190	5	17.0
creamy, roasted honey nut	2 tbsp	190	6	17.0
(Smucker's)				
chunky, 'Chunky Natural'	2 tbsp	200	6	16.0
honey sweetened	2 tbsp	200	7	16.0
no salt added, 'Natural'	2 tbsp	200	6	16.0
smooth, 'Natural'	2 tbsp	200	6	16.0
smooth, no salt added, 'Natural'	2 tbsp	200	6	17.0
(Westbrae)				
crunchy, no salt added, 'Natural'	2 tbsp	190	7	16.0
crunchy, w/salt, 'Natural'	2 tbsp	190	7	16.0
smooth, no salt added, 'Natural'	2 tbsp	190	7	16.0
(Woodstock) smooth, unsalted, 'Old Fashioned'	2 tbsp	200	6	16.0
PEANUT BUTTER CHIPS				
for baking, 'Reese's' *(Hershey's)*	1.5 oz	230	19	13.0
PEANUT BUTTER SPREAD				
(Bama) w/jelly	2 tbsp	150	20	7.0
(Bama) w/jelly	2 tbsp	150	20	7.0
(Jif) creamy, less fat	2 tbsp	190	15	12.0
(Peter Pan) creamy, less fat	2 tbsp	180	15	11.0
(Peter Pan) crunchy, less fat	2 tbsp	195	15	11.7
(Skippy) chunky, less fat	2 tbsp	180	13	12.4
(Skippy) creamy, less fat	2 tbsp	190	13	12.5
(Smucker's) w/grape jelly, 'Goober Grape'	2 tbsp	180	18	10.0
(Smucker's) w/strawberry jelly, 'Goober Strawberry'	2 tbsp	180	18	10.0
PEANUT BUTTER TOPPING, w/caramel				
(Smucker's)	2 tbsp	150	29	2.0
PEANUT OIL				
	1 cup	1909	0	216.0
	1 tbsp	119	0	13.5
(Hain)	1 tbsp	120	0	14.0
(Wesson)	1 tbsp	122	0	13.6
100% pure *(Hollywood)*	1 tbsp	120	0	14.0
100% pure *(Planters)*	1 tbsp	120	0	14.0
pure pressed, organic *(Spectrum)*	1 tbsp	120	0	14.0
PEAR				
Canned				
in extra heavy syrup, halves, w/liquid	1 cup	258	67	0.3
in extra heavy syrup, halves, w/1.75 tbsp liquid	1 med half	77	20	0.1
in extra light syrup, halves, w/liquid	1 cup	116	30	0.2
in extra light syrup, halves, w/liquid	1 med half	36	9	0.1
in heavy syrup, w/liquid	1 cup	197	51	0.3
in heavy syrup, w/liquid	1 med half	56	15	0.1
in juice, halves, w/liquid	1 cup	124	32	0.2

Food Name	Serv. Size	Total Cal.	Carbs GMS	Fat GMS
in juice, halves, w/liquid	1 med half	38	10	0.1
in light syrup, halves, w/liquid	1 cup	143	38	0.1
in light syrup, halves, w/liquid	1/2 fruit	43	12	0.0
in water, halves, w/liquid	1 cup	71	19	0.1
in water, halves, w/liquid	1 med half	22	6	0.0
Dried				
sulfured, stewed, halves	1 cup	324	86	0.8
sulfured, uncooked, halves	1 cup	472	125	1.1
sulfured, uncooked, halves	1 med half	47	13	0.1
Fresh				
sliced	1 cup	97	25	0.7
whole, large, 2 per lb	1 pear	123	32	0.8
whole, medium, 2.5 per lb	1 pear	98	25	0.7
whole, small, 3 per lb	1 pear	82	21	0.6
PEAR JUICE				
(Knudsen)	8 fl oz	110	28	0.0
(Mountain Sun) organic, 'Mountain pear'	8 fl oz	102	25	0.0
(Santa Cruz Natural) organic, 'Cruz'	8 fl oz	135	32	1.0
PEAR NECTAR. See under FRUIT JUICE DRINK.				
PEAS, BLACK-EYED. See BLACK-EYED PEAS.				
PEAS, CROWDER. See under BLACK-EYED PEAS.				
PEAS, FIELD				
Canned				
'Fresh' (Allens)	1/2 cup	100	18	1.0
tiny, w/snaps 'Fresh' (Allens)	1/2 cup	70	13	1.0
w/snaps (Bush's Best)	1/2 cup	80	16	0.0
w/snaps, 'Fresh' (Allens)	1/2 cup	100	20	1.0
w/snaps, seasoned w/pork (Luck's)	1/2 cup	130	19	3.0
PEAS, GREEN				
Canned				
dry, early June (Allens)	1/2 cup	80	15	1.0
early (A&P)	1/2 cup	70	15	1.0
early (Stokely)	1/2 cup	60	12	0.0
early, 'LeSueur' (Green Giant)	1/2 cup	60	12	0.0
early, 50% less sodium, 'LeSueur' (Green Giant)	1/2 cup	60	11	0.0
early June (Green Giant)	1/2 cup	50	12	0.0
early June, 'Petit Pois' (S&W)	1/2 cup	70	12	0.0
early June (Veg-All)	1/2 cup	50	10	0.0
early June, medium (TenderSweet)	1/2 cup	70	11	0.5
early June, medium, no salt added (TenderSweet)	1/2 cup	50	10	0.0
early June, 'Sun-Vista' (S&W)	1/2 cup	80	18	0.0
early June, tiny, party (Stokely)	1/2 cup	60	10	0.0
early, very young, small (Green Giant)	1/2 cup	50	12	0.0
mixed, no salt or sugar added (IGA)	1/2 cup	50	10	0.0
mixed sizes (A&P)	1/2 cup	60	12	1.0
no salt added, w/liquid (Del Monte)	1/2 cup	60	11	0.0
no salt or sugar added (Stokely)	1/2 cup	50	9	0.0
seasoned, w/liquid (Del Monte)	1/2 cup	60	11	0.0
small, w/liquid (Del Monte)	1/2 cup	50	9	0.0
sweet (Featherweight)	1/2 cup	70	12	0.0
sweet (Finast)	1/2 cup	70	13	1.0
sweet (Green Giant)	1/2 cup	60	11	0.0
sweet (Stokely)	1/2 cup	70	11	0.5
sweet (Veg-All)	1/2 cup	50	10	0.0
sweet, 50% less sodium (Green Giant)	1/2 cup	60	11	0.0
sweet, 50% less sodium, 'LeSueur' (Green Giant)	1/2 cup	60	11	0.0
sweet, garden (Freshlike)	1/2 cup	50	10	0.0

Food Name	Serv. Size	Total Cal.	Carbs GMS	Fat GMS
sweet, garden, no salt added *(Freshlike)*	1/2 cup	50	10	0.0
sweet, garden, fancy *(Pathmark)*	1/2 cup	70	12	1.0
sweet, large, tender *(Pathmark)*	1/2 cup	70	12	1.0
sweet, 'LeSueur' *(Green Giant)*	1/2 cup	60	12	0.0
sweet, 'Little Gem' *(Pathmark)*	1/2 cup	70	12	1.0
sweet, mini, in brine *(Green Giant)*	1/2 cup	60	12	1.0
sweet, mixed sizes *(Veg-All)*	1/2 cup	50	10	0.0
sweet, mixed sizes, no salt added *(Pathmark)*	1/2 cup	50	10	0.0
sweet, no salt added *(Finast)*	1/2 cup	60	12	0.0
sweet, 'No Frills' *(Pathmark)*	1 cup	120	25	1.0
sweet, 'Nutradiet' *(S&W)*	1/2 cup	40	8	0.0
sweet, 'Perfection' *(S&W)*	1/2 cup	70	12	0.0
sweet, small *(Freshlike)*	1/2 cup	50	10	0.0
sweet, small *(Pathmark)*	1/2 cup	70	12	1.0
sweet, small *(Veg-All)*	1/2 cup	50	10	0.0
sweet, tiny, early June *(IGA)*	1/2 cup	70	12	0.0
sweet, very young, small *(Green Giant)*	1/2 cup	50	12	0.0
sweet, very young, tender *(Green Giant)*	1/2 cup	50	11	0.0
sweet, water packed, no sugar or salt added *(Freshlike)*	1/2 cup	50	10	0.0
very young, sweet, 'LeSueur' *(Green Giant)*	1/2 cup	50	12	0.0
w/liquid *(Del Monte)*	1/2 cup	60	10	0.0
Freeze-dried, prepared *(Mountain House)*	1/2 cup	70	12	1.0
Fresh				
boiled, drained	1 cup	134	25	0.4
boiled, drained	1/2 cup	62	11	0.2
raw	1 cup	117	21	0.6
Frozen				
(Birds Eye)	3.3 oz	80	13	0.0
(Flav-R-Pac)	2/3 cup	70	12	0.5
(Freshlike)	3.3 oz	80	13	0.0
(Frosty Acres)	3.3 oz	80	13	0.0
(Health Valley)	1/2 cup	65	11	0.0
(Seabrook)	3.3 oz	80	13	0.0
(Southern)	3.5 oz	79	14	0.5
(Veg-All)	3.3 oz	80	13	0.0
boiled, drained	10-oz pkg	197	36	0.7
early, baby, 'LeSueur Select' *(Green Giant)*	1/2 cup	60	13	0.0
early, very young, small, 50% less sodium, 'LeSueur' *(Green Giant)*	1/2 cup	60	11	0.0
early June, 'Harvest Fresh' *(Green Giant)*	1/2 cup	60	12	1.0
LeSueur style, 'Valley Combinations' *(Green Giant)*	1/2 cup	70	12	2.0
no salt added *(Flav-R-Pac)*	2/3 cup	70	12	0.5
petite *(C&W)*	2/3 cup	70	12	0.5
petite *(Flav-R-Pac)*	2/3 cup	70	12	0.5
petite *(Southern)*	3.5 oz	64	11	0.4
petite, no salt added *(C&W)*	2/3 cup	70	12	0.5
'Portion Pack' *(Birds Eye)*	3 oz	70	12	0.0
'Singles' *(Stokely)*	3 oz	65	12	1.0
sweet *(Finast)*	3.3 oz	80	13	0.0
sweet *(Green Giant)*	1/2 cup	50	11	0.0
sweet, baby, 'LeSueur Select' *(Green Giant)*	2/3 cup	60	11	0.0
sweet, 'Harvest Fresh' *(Green Giant)*	1/2 cup	50	12	0.0
sweet, no salt added *(Del Monte)*	1/2 cup	60	11	0.0
sweet 'Plain Polybag' *(Green Giant)*	2/3 cup	70	13	0.0
tender, tiny, 'Deluxe' *(Birds Eye)*	3.3 oz	60	11	0.0
tiny *(Freshlike)*	3.3 oz	60	11	0.0
tiny *(Frosty Acres)*	3.3 oz	60	11	0.0
tiny *(Seabrook)*	3.3 oz	60	11	0.0

Food Name	Serv. Size	Total Cal.	Carbs GMS	Fat GMS
tiny *(Veg-All)*	3.3 oz	60	11	0.0
Sprouted, mature seeds, raw	1 cup	154	34	0.8
PEAS, GREEN, DISH/ENTRÉE				
(A&P)				
and carrots, frozen	3.3 oz	60	11	1.0
early June, and carrots, canned, no salt added	1/2 cup	60	12	1.0
mixed sizes, and carrots, canned	1/2 cup	60	12	1.0
sweet, and carrots, frozen	1/2 cup	80	13	1.0
(Allens) creamed, 'Fresh'	1/2 cup	90	14	1.0
(Birds Eye)				
and pearl onions, frozen, 'Combination Vegetables'	3.3 oz	70	13	0.0
(Budget Gourmet)				
w/water chestnuts, Oriental, 'Side Dish'	5 oz	120	15	3.0
(Del Monte) and carrots, canned, w/liquid	1/2 cup	50	10	0.0
(Finast) and carrots, canned	1/2 cup	55	9	0.0
(Flav-R-Pac)				
and carrots, frozen	2/3 cup	50	9	0.0
and pearl onions, frozen	2/3 cup	70	12	0.5
(Freshlike)				
and carrots, frozen	3.3 oz	60	11	0.0
and onions, frozen	3.3 oz	70	13	0.0
sweet, and diced carrots, canned, in water, no salt added	1/2 cup	50	12	0.0
sweet, and diced carrots, canned, in water, no sugar added	1/2 cup	50	12	0.0
sweet, and sliced carrots, canned	1/2 cup	50	12	0.0
sweet, and tiny onions, canned	1/2 cup	60	12	0.0
(Frosty Acres)				
and carrots, frozen	3.3 oz	60	11	0.0
and pearl onions, frozen	3.3 oz	70	13	0.0
(Green Giant) and pearl onions, canned, w/liquid	1/2 cup	50	11	0.0
(Kohl's) and carrots, canned	1/2 cup	50	20	1.0
(Pathmark) and carrots, canned	1/2 cup	60	18	1.0
(S&W) and carrots, canned, 'Nutradiet'	1/2 cup	35	7	0.0
(Seabrook)				
and carrots, frozen	3.3 oz	60	11	0.0
and onions, frozen	3.3 oz	70	13	0.0
(Southern) and carrots, frozen	3.5 oz	64	12	0.0
(Stokely)				
and carrots, canned	1/2 cup	50	9	0.0
and diced carrots, no salt or sugar added	1/2 cup	45	8	0.0
and sliced carrots, no salt or sugar added	1/2 cup	45	8	0.0
(Veg-All)				
and carrots, frozen	3.3 oz	60	11	0.0
and onions, frozen	3.3 oz	70	13	0.0
sweet, and diced carrots, canned	1/2 cup	50	12	0.0
sweet, and sliced carrots, canned	1/2 cup	50	12	0.0
PEAS, PIGEON				
immature seeds, boiled, drained	1 cup	170	30	2.1
immature seeds, raw	1 cup	209	37	2.5
immature seeds, raw	10 seeds	5	1	0.1
red gram, mature seeds, boiled	1 cup	203	39	0.6
red gram, mature seeds, raw	1 cup	703	129	3.1
PEAS, PURPLE HULLED				
canned, 'Fresh' *(Allens)*	1/2 cup	100	16	1.0
frozen *(Frosty Acres)*	3.3 oz	130	23	0.0
PEAS, SNAP				
sugar snap *(Green Giant)*	1/2 cup	30	8	0.0
sugar snap, 'Deluxe' *(Birds Eye)*	2.6 oz	45	9	0.0
sugar snap, frozen *(Flav-R-Pac)*	3/4 cup	30	7	0.0

Food Name	Serv. Size	Total Cal.	Carbs GMS	Fat GMS
sugar snap, 'Harvest Fresh' *(Green Giant)*	1/2 cup	30	8	0.0
sugar snap, 'Select' *(Green Giant)*	1/2 cup	30	8	0.0
PEAS, SNOW/Chinese pea pods				
Fresh				
edible-podded, boiled, drained	1 cup	67	11	0.4
edible-podded, raw, whole	10 pods	14	3	0.1
edible-podded, raw, chopped	1 cup	41	7	0.2
edible-podded, raw, whole	1 cup	26	5	0.1
Frozen				
(Chun King)	1.5 oz	20	3	0.0
(Flav-R-Pac)	1 cup	50	6	0.0
(Seabrook)	2 oz	20	4	0.0
baby, pods *(C&W)*	2/3 cup	40	7	0.0
'Deluxe' *(Birds Eye)*	3 oz	35	6	0.0
edible-podded, drained	1 cup	83	14	0.6
edible-podded, drained	1/2 cup	42	7	0.3
edible-podded, drained	10 oz pkg	132	23	1.0
edible-podded, unprepared	10-oz pkg	119	20	0.9
edible-podded, unprepared	1/2 cup	30	5	0.2
pods, food service product *(La Choy)*	1 cup	41	9	0.0
PEAS, SPLIT				
boiled *(A&P)*	1 cup	220	40	1.0
green, raw *(Arrowhead Mills)*	2 oz	200	35	1.0
mature seeds, boiled	1 cup	231	41	0.8
mature seeds, boiled	1 tbsp	14	3	0.0
mature seeds, raw	1 cup	672	119	2.3
PEAS AND CARROTS. See under PEAS, GREEN, DISH/ENTRÉE.				
PECAN				
Dried				
chopped	1 cup	822	16	85.6
halves	1 cup	746	15	77.7
halves, approx 20 pieces	1 oz	196	4	20.4
Dry roasted				
unsalted	1 oz	201	4	21.1
salted	1 oz	201	4	21.1
Honey roasted *(Planters)*	1 oz	200	8	18.0
Oil roasted				
salted	1 cup	787	14	82.8
salted, halves, approx 15 pieces	1 oz	203	4	21.3
unsalted	1 cup	787	14	82.8
unsalted, halves, approx 15 pieces	1 oz	203	4	21.3
Raw				
(Fisher)	1 oz	190	5	19.0
chips *(Planters)*	1 oz	190	5	20.0
halves *(Planters)*	1 oz	190	5	20.0
pieces *(Planters)*	1 oz	190	5	20.0
Roasted				
chipped pieces, shelled *(Azar)*	2 oz	370	10	38.0
chopped, shelled *(Fisher)*	1 oz	190	5	19.0
ground, shelled *(Fisher)*	1 oz	190	5	19.0
halves, pieces, or chips, shelled *(Planters)*	1 oz	190	5	20.0
halves and pieces, shelled, *(Azar)*	2 oz	370	10	38.0
pieces, shelled *(Azar)*	2 oz	370	10	38.0
pieces, shelled, natural, unsalted *(Flanigan Farms)*	1 oz	190	4	20.0
shelled, natural, unsalted *(Flanigan Farms)*	1/4 cup	190	5	19.0
PECAN BUTTER roasted, organic				
(Maranatha Natural)	2 tbsp	220	7	21.0

Food Name	Serv. Size	Total Cal.	Carbs GMS	Fat GMS
PECTIN MIX, unsweetened .... 1.75 oz		163	45	0.1
PENNE. See under PASTA.				
PENNE DISH/ENTRÉE. See under PASTA DISH/ENTRÉE.				
PEPITAS				
dried, in shell .... 1 lb		1817	59.8	153.9
dried, shelled .... 1 cup		747	24.6	63.3
dried, shelled, approx 142 kernels .... 1 oz		154	5.1	13.0
natural, unsalted *(Flanigan Farms)* .... 1/4 cup		150	5	13.0
roasted, shelled .... 1 cup		1184	30.5	95.6
roasted, shelled .... 1 oz		148	3.8	12.0
roasted, whole, in shell .... 1 cup		285	34.4	12.4
roasted, whole, in shell, approx 85 seeds .... 1 oz		127	15.3	5.5
shelled, salted .... 1 cup		285	34.4	12.4
shelled, salted.. 1 lb		2021	243.8	88.0
shelled, salted .... 1 oz		127	15.3	5.5
PEPEAO. See CHINESE FUNGUS.				
PEPPER, ANCHO, dried, whole .... 1 medium		48	9	1.4
PEPPER, BANANA				
Canned or jarred, hot *(Vlasic)* .... 1 oz		5	1	0.0
Fresh				
raw, chopped .... 1 cup		33	7	0.6
raw, whole, small, approx 4-inch long .... 1 pepper		9	2	0.1
raw, whole, medium, approx 4.5-inch long .... 1 pepper		12	2	0.2
raw, whole, large, approx 5-inch long .... 1 pepper		20	4	0.3
PEPPER, BELL/green pepper/red pepper/sweet pepper/yellow pepper				
Canned or jarred				
California roasted *(Mezzetta)* .... 1 oz		8	0	0.0
fried *(Progresso)*....................................... 1/2 jar		37	4	3.0
green, halves, w/liquid .... 1 cup		25	5	0.4
red, halves, w/liquid .... 1 cup		25	5	0.4
red, halves, w/liquid .... 1/2 cup		13	3	0.2
roasted *(Progresso)* .... 1/2 cup		20	5	1.0
'Sweet Pepper Mementos' *(Heinz)* .... 1 oz		6	1	0.0
Freeze-Dried				
.... 1/4 cup		5	1	0.0
.... 1 tbsp		1	0	0.0
red .... 1/4 cup		5	1	0.0
red .... 1 tbsp		1	0	0.0
Fresh				
(Dole) .... 1 medium		25	5	1.0
green, boiled, drained, chopped .... 1/2 cup		19	5	0.1
green, boiled, drained, minced .... 1 tbsp		3	1	0.0
green, boiled, drained, strips .... 1 cup		38	9	0.3
green, raw, chopped .... 1 cup		40	10	0.3
green, raw, minced .... 1 tbsp		3	1	0.0
green, raw, rings, 3-inch diam, 1/4-inch thick .... 1 ring		3	1	0.0
green, raw, sliced....................................... 1 cup		25	6	0.2
green, raw, strips .... 10 strips		7	2	0.1
green, raw, whole, approx 2.75-inch long, 2.5-inch diam. ...... 1 pepper		32	8	0.2
green, raw, whole, approx 3.75-inch long, 3-inch diam .... 1 pepper		44	11	0.3
red, boiled, drained, chopped .... 1/2 cup		19	5	0.1
red, boiled, drained, minced .... 1 tbsp		3	1	0.0
red, boiled, drained, strips .... 1 cup		38	9	0.3
red, raw .... 1 small		20	5	0.1
red, raw, chopped .... 1 cup		40	10	0.3
red, raw, minced .... 1 tbsp		3	1	0.0
red, raw, rings, 3-inch diam, 1/4-inch thick .... 1 ring		3	1	0.0

Food Name	Serv. Size	Total Cal.	Carbs GMS	Fat GMS
red, raw, sliced	1 cup	25	6	0.2
red, raw, whole, approx 2.75-inch long, 2.5-inch diam.	1 medium	32	8	0.2
red, raw, whole, approx 3.75-inch long, 3-inch diam	1 large	44	11	0.3
yellow, raw, strips	10 strips	14	3	0.1
yellow, whole, approx 3.75-inch long, 30inch diam	1 pepper	50	12	0.4
Frozen				
green *(Seabrook)*	1 oz	6	1	0.0
green, chopped, unprepared	10-oz pkg	57	13	0.6
green, diced *(Flav-R-Pac)*	3/4 cup	20	4	0.0
red *(Seabrook)*	1 oz	8	1	0.0
red, chopped, unprepared	10-oz pkg	57	13	0.6
red, chopped, unprepared	1 oz	6	1	0.1
red, diced *(Flav-R-Pac)*	3/4 cup	20	4	0.0
red, strips *(Flav-R-Pac)*	3/4 cup	20	4	0.0
strips *(Flav-R-Pac)*	3/4 cup	20	4	0.0
PEPPER, BELL, DISH/ENTRÉE				
(Celentano) red, sweet, stuffed, frozen	13 oz	350	28	20.0
(Lean Cuisine) red, stuffed, frozen, 'Salsa'lito'	1 oz	26	4	0.6
(Stouffer's)				
stuffed, frozen	1 entrée	200	24	8.0
stuffed, w/beef, in tomato sauce	1 pkg	378	42	16.2
stuffed, w/beef, in tomato sauce	1 serving	189	21	8.1
stuffed, w/sauce, frozen, food service product	1 oz	25	3	1.1
stuffed, w/o sauce, food service product	1 oz	31	3	1.4
PEPPER, CHERRY				
Canned or jarred				
diced, drained *(Progresso)*	2 tbsp	30	2	2.0
diced, fried *(Progresso)*	2 tbsp	60	3	5.0
hot *(Progresso)*	1/2 cup	190	3	20.0
hot *(Vlasic)*	1 oz	10	2	0.0
hot, pickled *(Progresso)*	1/2 cup	130	3	12.0
hot, whole *(Progresso)*	1 med pepper	15	3	0.0
hot or mild, rings *(Vlasic)*	1 oz	5	1	0.0
mild *(Vlasic)*	1 oz	10	2	0.0
PEPPER, CHILI/chile				
Canned or jarred				
green *(Santiago)*	2 oz	13	3	0.1
green, chopped *(Old El Paso)*	2 tbsp	8	2	1.0
green, chopped, no seeds, w/liquid	1/2 cup	14	3	0.1
green, diced *(Pancho Villa)*	2 tbsp	5	1	0.0
green, diced *(Rosarita)*	2 tbsp	6	1	0.1
green, diced, food service product *(Rosarita)*	2 tbsp	6	1	0.1
green, diced, w/liquid *(Del Monte)*	1/2 cup	20	5	0.0
green, strips, food service product *(Rosarita)*	1/4 cup	4	1	0.1
green, whole *(Old El Paso)*	1 med pepper	8	1	1.0
green, whole *(Rosarita)*	2 tbsp	4	1	0.1
green, whole, diced, sliced, or strips *(Ortega)*	1 oz	10	3	0.0
green, whole, food service product *(Rosarita)*	2 tbsp	4	1	0.1
green, whole, no seeds, w/liquid	1 med pepper	15	4	0.1
green, whole, w/liquid *(Del Monte)*	1/2 cup	20	5	0.0
hot, diced *(Ortega)*	1 oz	8	2	0.0
hot, whole *(Ortega)*	1 oz	8	2	0.0
hot, tiny, Mexican *(Vlasic)*	1 oz	6	2	0.0
red, chopped, no seeds, w/liquid	1/2 cup	14	3	0.1
red, whole, no seeds, w/liquid	1 med pepper	15	4	0.1
Fresh				
green, chopped or diced	1/2 cup	30	7	0.1

Food Name	Serv. Size	Total Cal.	Carbs GMS	Fat GMS
green, raw, whole	1 med pepper	18	4	0.1
red, chopped or diced	1/2 cup	30	7	0.1
red, raw, whole	1 med pepper	18	4	0.1
Frozen				
green *(Santiago)*	2 oz	15	3	0.2
green, chopped *(Old El Paso)*	2 tbsp	5	1	0.0
hot, roasted, peeled, chopped *(Baca's)*	2 tbsp	5	1	0.0
Sun-dried				
hot, chopped	1 cup	120	26	2.1
hot, whole	1 med pepper	2	0	0.0
PEPPER, GREEN. See PEPPER, BELL.				
PEPPER, GROUND				
BLACK				
	1 tbsp	16	4	0.2
	1 dash	0	0	0.0
(Durkee)	1 tsp	8	0	0.0
(Laurel Leaf)	1 tsp	8	0	0.0
(McCormick/Schilling)	1 tsp	7	1	0.0
(Spice Islands)	1 tsp	9	2	0.2
coarse grind, 'Mr. Pepper' *(Tone's)*	1 tsp	8	2	0.1
fine grind, 'Mr. Pepper' *(Tone's)*	1 tsp	8	2	0.1
CAYENNE *(Spice Islands)*	1 tsp	9	1	0.3
CHILI				
(Spice Islands)	1 tsp	9	1	0.3
fresh ground *(Durkee)*	1 tsp	11	0	0.0
fresh ground *(Laurel Leaf)*	1 tsp	11	0	0.0
red *(McCormick/Schilling)*	1 tsp	10	1	0.4
RED				
(Spice Islands)	1 tsp	9	1	0.3
(Spice Islands)	1 tsp	9	1	0.3
fresh-ground *(Durkee)*	1 tsp	8	0	0.0
fresh-ground *(Laurel Leaf)*	1 tsp	8	0	0.0
WHITE				
	1 tbsp	21	5	0.2
	1 tsp	7	2	0.1
(Durkee)	1 tsp	9	0	0.0
(Laurel Leaf)	1 tsp	9	0	0.0
(McCormick/Schilling)	1 tsp	8	2	0.0
(Spice Islands)	1 tsp	9	2	0.2
PEPPER, HUNGARIAN, raw	1 med pepper	8	2	0.1
PEPPER, JALAPEÑO				
Canned or jarred				
(Old El Paso)	2 tbsp	16	4	0.0
chopped, w/liquid	1 cup	37	6	1.3
diced *(Ortega)*	1 oz	10	3	0.0
diced *(Rosarita)*	2 tbsp	5	1	0.2
for nachos *(La Victoria)*	14 pieces	5	1	0.0
for nachos *(La Victoria)*	1 tbsp	2	1	1.0
hot *(Vlasic)*	1/4 cup	10	2	0.0
marinated *(La Victoria)*	1 tbsp	4	1	1.0
marinated *(La Victoria)*	1.5 pieces	10	2	0.0
nacho sliced *(Rosarita)*	2 tbsp	4	1	0.1
nacho sliced, food service product *(Rosarita)*	2 tbsp	4	1	0.1
pickled *(Old El Paso)*	2 peppers	5	1	0.0
sliced, w/liquid *(Del Monte)*	1/2 cup	30	6	1.0
sliced, w/liquid	1 cup	28	5	1.0
slices, pickled *(Old El Paso)*	2 tbsp	15	3	0.0

Food Name	Serv. Size	Total Cal.	Carbs GMS	Fat GMS
whole *(Old El Paso)*	2 peppers	14	1	1.0
whole *(Ortega)*	1 oz	10	3	0.0
whole *(Rosarita)*	2 tbsp	8	1	0.1
whole, food service product *(Rosarita)*	2 peppers	6	1	0.1
whole, w/escabeche *(Rosarita)*	1.16 oz	8	1	0.2
whole, w/liquid	1 med pepper	6	1	0.2
whole, w/liquid *(Del Monte)*	1/2 cup	30	6	1.0
Fresh				
raw, whole	1 pepper	4	1	0.1
raw, sliced	1 cup	27	5	0.6
PEPPER, PEPPERONCINI				
(Progresso) Tuscan	1/2 cup	20	7	0.0
(Vlasic)	1 oz	5	1	0.0
PEPPER, PERSIL, dried	1 medium	24	4	1.1
PEPPER, RED. See PEPPER, BELL.				
PEPPER, SERRANO				
Fresh				
raw, chopped	1 cup	34	7	0.5
raw, whole	1 medium	2	0	0.0
PEPPER, SWEET. See PEPPER, BELL.				
PEPPER, TUSCAN, canned or jarred, drained				
(Progresso)	3 medium	10	1	0.0
PEPPER, YELLOW. See PEPPER, BANANA, PEPPER, BELL.				
PEPPER DISH/ENTRÉE. See PEPPER, BELL, DISH/ENTRÉE.				
PEPPER DILL SEASONING. See under SEASONING MIX.				
PEPPERMINT				
fresh, raw, whole	2 leaves	0	0	0.0
fresh, raw, chopped	2 tbsp	2	0	0.0
PEPPERONCINI. See PEPPER, PEPPERONCINI.				
PEPPERONI. See under SAUSAGE.				
PERCH				
Fresh				
mixed species, baked, broiled, grilled, or microwaved	3 oz	99	0	1.0
mixed species, raw	3 oz	77	0	0.8
Frozen				
(Booth)	4 oz	100	0	1.0
(SeaPak)	4 oz	100	0	2.0
fillet, battered *(Van de Kamp's)*	2 pieces	310	18	21.0
PERSIL PEPPER. See PEPPER, PERSIL.				
PERSIMMON				
dried, organic *(Flanigan Farms)*	1 pkg	90	20	0.0
dried, whole, trimmed, medium, approx 2.5 inch diam	1 fruit	93	25	0.2
raw, Japanese, whole, medium, approx 2.5 inch diam	1 fruit	118	31	0.3
raw, native, trimmed, medium, approx 2.5 inch diam	1 fruit	32	8	0.1
PESTO. See under SAUCE.				
PE-TSAI. See BOK CHOY.				
PHEASANT				
breast, meat only, raw	6.4 oz	242	0	5.9
leg, meat only, raw, 1 medium	3.5 oz	133	0	4.3
leg, meat only, raw, 1 medium, boneless/skinless	3.3 oz	143	0	4.6
PHYLLO DOUGH				
	1 oz	85	15	1.7
frozen, ready-to-use *(Apollo)*	1 oz	80	18	0.4
PICCALILLI. See under RELISH.				
PICKLE				
BREAD AND BUTTER				
(Claussen)				
chips	4 slices	20	4	0.0

Food Name	Serv. Size	Total Cal.	Carbs GMS	Fat GMS
sandwich slices	2 slices	25	5	0.0
(Heinz) slices 'Cucumber Slices'	1 oz	25	6	0.0
(Mrs. Fanning's) slices	2 slices	16	3	0.0
(Vlasic)				
chunks, 'Old-Fashion'	1 oz	25	6	0.0
'Deli'	1 oz	25	6	0.0
'Sandwich Stackers'	1 oz	25	6	0.0
sweet, 'Sweet Butter Chips'	1 oz	30	7	0.0
sweet, 'Sweet Butter Stix'	1 oz	18	5	0.0
DILL				
(Claussen)				
halves, kosher	1 oz	5	1	0.0
miniature, kosher	1 piece	5	1	0.0
no garlic	1 piece	17	3	0.3
sandwich slices, kosher	2 slices	5	1	0.0
whole, kosher	1 oz	5	1	0.0
(Featherweight) whole	1 piece	4	1	0.0
(Heinz)				
baby	1 oz	4	1	0.0
chips	1 oz	4	1	0.0
halves, 'Deli Style'	1 oz	4	1	0.0
hamburger slices	1 oz	2	0	0.0
spears, kosher	1 oz	4	1	0.0
spears, Polish style	1 oz	4	1	0.0
whole, 'Genuine'	1 oz	2	0	0.0
whole, kosher	1 oz	4	1	0.0
whole, kosher, 'Old Fashioned'	1 oz	4	1	0.0
whole, Polish style	1 oz	4	1	0.0
whole, processed	1 oz	2	0	0.0
(Steinfeld)				
baby, kosher	1 oz	5	1	0.0
hamburger chips	1 oz	5	1	0.0
(Vlasic)				
baby, whole, kosher	1 oz	5	1	0.0
chunks, Polish, snack	1 oz	4	1	0.0
chunks, zesty, snacks	1 oz	4	1	0.0
crunchy	1 oz	4	1	0.0
crunchy, half salt	1 oz	4	1	0.0
crunchy, zesty	1 oz	4	1	0.0
gherkins	1 oz	4	1	0.0
hamburger chips, half salt	1 oz	2	1	0.0
original	1 oz	5	1	0.0
'Sandwich Stackers' kosher	1 oz	5	1	0.0
'Sandwich Stackers' Polish	1 oz	5	1	0.0
'Sandwich Stackers' zesty	1 oz	5	1	0.0
spears, deli style	1 oz	5	1	0.0
spears, half salt	1 oz	4	1	0.0
spears, kosher	1 oz	4	1	0.0
spears, no garlic	1 oz	4	1	0.0
spears, Polish	1 oz	5	1	0.0
spears, zesty	1 oz	4	1	0.0
HOT AND SPICY (Vlasic) garden, mixed	1 oz	4	1	0.0
KOSHER. See also DILL.				
(Heinz)				
chips, 'Old Fashioned'	1 oz	4	1	0.0
halves, 'Old Fashioned Deli Halves'	1 oz	4	1	0.0
(Vlasic) chunks, snack	2 pieces	5	1	0.0
SOUR (Claussen) halves, deli style	1 oz	5	1	0.0

Food Name	Serv. Size	Total Cal.	Carbs GMS	Fat GMS
SWEET				
(Featherweight) sliced	3.5 pieces	24	6	0.0
(Heinz)				
cubes, salad,	1 oz	30	7	0.0
'Cucumber Stix'	1 oz	25	6	0.0
gherkins	1 oz	35	8	0.0
mixed, low-sodium	1 oz	40	9	0.0
sliced	1 oz	35	8	0.0
sliced, 'Cucumber Slices'	1 oz	20	5	0.0
(Steinfeld) chips	1 oz	30	8	0.0
(Vlasic)	1 oz	35	9	0.0
PICKLING SPICE. See under SEASONING MIX.				
PIE				
APPLE				
(Amy's Kitchen) single serving	1 pie	220	35	8.0
(Banquet)				
'Family Size'	1/6 pie	250	37	11.0
frozen, ready to bake	1 serving	292	41	13.2
(Entenmann's)				
beehive, nonfat, cholesterol free	1 piece	270	65	0.0
homestyle	2.1 oz	140	21	7.0
(McMillin's)	4 oz	430	51	23.0
(Mrs. Smith's)				
'Pie In Minutes'	1/8 pie	210	29	9.0
less fat, frozen	1 slice	250	43	8.0
(Pet-Ritz)	1/16 pie	330	53	12.0
(Sara Lee)				
'Homestyle'	1/10 pie	280	42	12.0
'Homestyle High'	1/10 pie	400	46	23.0
streusel, frozen, 'Free & Light'	1/8 pie	170	36	2.0
BANANA CREAM				
(Banquet)	1/6 pie	180	21	10.0
(Mrs. Smith's)	1 slice	280	37	14.0
(Pet-Ritz)	1/6 pie	170	22	9.0
BERRY *(McMillin's)*	4 oz	430	52	23.0
BLACKBERRY *(Banquet)* frozen, 'Family Size'	1/6 pie	270	40	11.0
BLUEBERRY				
(Banquet) 'Family Size'	1/6 pie	270	40	11.0
(Mrs. Smith's) 'Pie In Minutes'	1/8 pie	220	32	9.0
(Pet-Ritz)	1/6 pie	370	50	12.0
(Sara Lee) 'Homestyle'	1/10 pie	300	45	12.0
CHERRY				
(Banquet) frozen, 'Family Size'	1/6 pie	250	36	11.0
(Entenmann's) beehive, nonfat, cholesterol free	1 piece	270	64	0.0
(Mrs. Smith's)				
frozen, 'Pie In Minutes'	1/8 pie	220	32	9.0
less fat, frozen	1 slice	250	44	8.0
(Pet-Ritz) frozen	1/6 pie	300	48	12.0
(Sara Lee)				
frozen, 'Homestyle'	1/10 pie	270	37	13.0
streusel, frozen, 'Free & Light'	1/10 pie	160	34	2.0
CHOCOLATE				
(Banquet) cream, frozen	1/6 pie	190	24	10.0
(McMillin's) pudding	4 oz	420	54	21.0
(Pet-Ritz) cream, frozen	1/6 pie	190	27	8.0
(Weight Watchers)				
Mississippi mud	1 serving	160	24	5.0

Food Name	Serv. Size	Total Cal.	Carbs GMS	Fat GMS
mocha	1 serving	170	31	4.0
COCONUT				
(Banquet) cream, frozen	1/6 pie	190	22	11.0
(Entenmann's) custard	1.8 oz	140	16	8.0
(McMillin's) pudding	4 oz	450	50	26.0
(Pet-Ritz) cream, frozen	1/6 pie	190	27	8.0
EGG CUSTARD (Pet-Ritz) frozen	1/6 pie	200	28	8.0
KEY LIME (Mrs. Smith's)	1 slice	380	58	14.0
LEMON				
(Banquet) cream, frozen	1/6 pie	170	23	9.0
(McMillin's)	4 oz	450	52	25.0
(Mrs. Smith's) meringue, frozen	1/8 pie	210	38	5.0
(Pet-Ritz) cream, frozen	1/6 pie	190	26	9.0
MINCEMEAT				
(Banquet) frozen, 'Family Size'	1/6 pie	260	38	11.0
(Mrs. Smith's) frozen	1 slice	300	48	11.0
(Pet-Ritz) frozen	1/6 pie	280	48	9.0
(Sara Lee) frozen, 'Homestyle'	1/10 pie	300	43	13.0
NEAPOLITAN (Pet-Ritz) cream, frozen	1/6 pie	180	17	10.0
PEACH				
(Banquet) frozen, 'Family Size'	1/6 pie	245	35	11.0
(McMillin's)	4 oz	430	52	24.0
(Pet-Ritz) frozen	1/6 pie	320	51	12.0
(Sara Lee) frozen, 9-inch, 'Homestyle'	1/10 pie	280	41	12.0
PECAN				
(Mrs. Smith's) frozen	1 slice	520	73	23.0
(Sara Lee) frozen, 'Homestyle'	1/10 pie	400	56	18.0
PUMPKIN				
(Banquet) frozen, 'Family Size'	1/6 pie	200	29	8.0
(Mrs. Smith's) frozen	1 slice	270	44	8.0
(Pet-Ritz) custard, frozen	1/6 pie	250	39	9.0
(Sara Lee) frozen, 'Homestyle'	1/10 pie	240	34	10.0
RASPBERRY (Sara Lee) frozen, 'Homestyle'	1/10 pie	280	39	13.0
STRAWBERRY				
(Banquet) cream, frozen	1/6 pie	170	22	9.0
(McMillin's)	4 oz	400	50	20.0
(Mrs. Smith's) frozen	1 slice	280	45	11.0
(Pet-Ritz) cream, frozen	1/6 pie	170	20	9.0
STRAWBERRY RHUBARB (Mrs. Smith's) frozen	1 slice	280	44	11.0
SWEET POTATO PIE				
(Mrs. Smith's) frozen	1 slice	280	43	11.0
(Pet-Ritz) frozen	1/6 pie	150	21	7.0
PIE, SNACK				
(Tastykake) 'Klair'	1 piece	402	51	20.1
APPLE				
(Break Cake) 'Fried Pie' 4.5 oz	2 pies	430	63	18.0
(Drake's)	1 piece	210	29	10.0
(Hostess)				
French	1 piece	430	60	20.0
'Snack Cake'	1 serving	480	67	22.0
(Little Debbie)				
Dutch apple, 2.5 oz	1 piece	270	48	8.0
Dutch apple, 2.17 oz	1 piece	230	42	8.0
(Tastykake)				
	1 piece	296	46	12.3
French, 4.2 oz	1 piece	353	63	10.7
(Weight Watchers)	1/2 pkg	200	39	5.0

Food Name	Serv. Size	Total Cal.	Carbs GMS	Fat GMS
BANANA CREAM *(Tastykake)* 4.2 oz	1 piece	382	54	16.1
BLACKBERRY *(Hostess)*	1 piece	420	59	18.0
BLUEBERRY				
(Drake's) w/apple	1 piece	210	30	10.0
(Hostess) 'Snack Cake'	1 serving	480	70	21.0
(Tastykake)	1 piece	308	55	9.4
CHERRY				
(Break Cake) 'Fried Pie'	2 pies	410	64	16.0
(Drake's) w/apple	1 piece	220	30	10.0
(Hostess) 'Snack Cake'	1 serving	470	65	22.0
(McMillin's)	4 oz	430	51	24.0
(Tastykake)	1 piece	298	49	9.7
CHOCOLATE				
(Hostess) pudding	1 piece	490	76	19.0
(Pepperidge Farm) Mississippi mud, 'American Collection'	1 ramekin	310	23	23.0
(Tastykake) pudding	1 piece	443	68	16.2
COCONUT *(Tastykake)* creme	1 piece	377	46	20.2
LEMON				
(Break Cake) 'Fried Pie'	2 pies	490	66	23.0
(Drake's)	1 piece	210	27	11.0
(Hostess) 'Snack Cake'	1 serving	500	66	24.0
(Tastykake)	1 piece	319	48	13.2
LEMON-LIME *(Tastykake)*	1 piece	310	54	8.8
OATMEAL				
(Little Debbie)				
cream, 2.75 oz	1 piece	350	51	14.0
cream, 1.33 oz	1 piece	160	25	6.0
PEACH				
(Hostess) 'Snack Cake'	1 serving	480	68	21.0
(Tastykake)	1 piece	310	54	8.8
PECAN				
(Little Debbie)				
3 oz	1 piece	280	60	3.0
1.83 oz	1 piece	170	37	2.0
PINEAPPLE CHEESE *(Tastykake)*	1 piece	343	54	13.2
PUMPKIN *(Tastykake)*	1 piece	324	47	14.2
STRAWBERRY				
(Hostess)	1 piece	410	56	19.0
(Tastykake)	1 piece	342	57	11.4
PIE CRUST				
(Keebler)				
shell, chocolate, food service product, 'Ready Crust'	1 slice	100	13	4.5
tart shell, graham, food service product, 'Ready Crust'	1 serving	120	15	6.0
(Mrs. Smith's)				
shell, 8-inch	1/8 shell	80	8	5.0
shell, 9-inch	1/8 shell	90	10	5.0
shell, 9-5/8 inch	1/8 shell	120	12	7.0
shell, less fat, frozen, 9-inch	1 slice	100	13	5.0
(Nabisco)				
chocolate cookie crumb, 'Oreo'	1 slice	140	18	7.0
vanilla wafer crumb, 'Nilla'	1 slice	144	18	7.6
(Oronoque)				
deep dish, 9-inch	1/8 crust	100	8	7.0
deep dish, 9-inch, frozen	1/6 shell	130	11	9.0
deep dish, 10-inch	1/8 crust	130	10	8.0
regular, 9-inch	1/8 crust	90	7	6.0
regular, 9-inch, frozen	1/6 shell	120	9	8.0

Food Name	Serv. Size	Total Cal.	Carbs GMS	Fat GMS
regular, 6-inch	1/4 crust	110	9	7.0
tart shell, 3-inch	1 tart	140	11	9.0
(Pet-Ritz)				
	1/6 shell	110	11	7.0
all vegetable shortening	1/6 shell	110	10	8.0
deep dish	1/6 shell	130	12	8.0
deep dish, whole grain	1/6 shell	130	14	8.0
deep dish, w/vegetable shortening	1/6 shell	140	12	9.0
graham cracker	1/6 shell	110	8	6.0
9 5/8-inch	1/6 shell	170	15	11.0
tart shell, 3-inch	1 shell	150	12	10.0
(Pillsbury)	1 slice	110	12	7.0

PIE CRUST MIX
(Betty Crocker)

Food Name	Serv. Size	Total Cal.	Carbs GMS	Fat GMS
	1 serving	110	9	8.0
stick	1/8 stick	120	10	8.0
(Flako)				
mix only	1/4 cup	130	13	8.0
prepared	1 serving	247	24	15.0
(General Mills) mix only	1/16 pkg	120	10	8.0
(Krusteaz) prepared	1/8 shell	90	10	5.0
(Nabisco)				
chocolate cookie crumbs, 'Oreo' mix only	2 tbsp	80	13	3.0
graham cracker crumbs 'Honey Maid' mix only	2 1/2 tbsp	70	13	2.0
vanilla wafer crumbs, 'Nilla' mix only	2 tbsp	70	12	2.0
(Pillsbury)				
mix only	2 tbsp	100	10	6.0
prepared w/water	1/8 pkg	200	20	13.0

PIE FILLING. See also PUDDING/PIE FILLING MIX.
APPLE PIE FILLING
(Comstock)

Food Name	Serv. Size	Total Cal.	Carbs GMS	Fat GMS
canned	3.5 oz	120	30	0.0
canned, 'Lite'	3.5 oz	80	20	0.0
(Lucky Leaf)				
canned	4 oz	120	30	0.0
canned, 'Deluxe'	4 oz	120	35	0.0
canned, 'Plus'	4 oz	121	30	0.0
turnover, diced, canned	4 oz	120	30	0.0
(Musselman's)				
canned	4 oz	120	30	0.0
canned, 'Deluxe'	4 oz	120	35	0.0
canned, 'Plus'	4 oz	121	30	0.0
turnover, diced, canned	4 oz	120	30	0.0
(Pathmark) canned 'No Frills'	4 oz	130	33	0.0
(White House) canned	3.5 oz	121	29	1.0

APRICOT

Food Name	Serv. Size	Total Cal.	Carbs GMS	Fat GMS
(Comstock) canned	3.5 oz	110	29	0.0
(Lucky Leaf) canned	4 oz	150	39	0.0
(Musselman's) canned	4 oz	150	39	0.0
BANANA *(Comstock)* canned	3.5 oz	110	22	2.0

BLACKBERRY
(Lucky Leaf)

Food Name	Serv. Size	Total Cal.	Carbs GMS	Fat GMS
canned	4 oz	120	31	0.0
canned, 'Plus'	4 oz	121	30	0.0
(Musselman's)				
canned	4 oz	120	31	0.0
canned 'Plus'	4 oz	121	30	0.0

Food Name	Serv. Size	Total Cal.	Carbs GMS	Fat GMS
BLUEBERRY				
(Comstock)				
canned	3.5 oz	110	28	0.0
canned, 'Lite'	3.5 oz	75	17	0.0
(Lucky Leaf)				
canned, cultivated	4 oz	120	31	0.0
canned, 'Plus'	4 oz	145	35	0.0
(Musselman's)				
canned, cultivated	4 oz	120	31	0.0
canned 'Plus'	4 oz	145	35	0.0
(White House) canned	3.5 oz	118	28	1.0
BOYSENBERRY				
(Lucky Leaf) canned	4 oz	120	31	0.0
(Musselman's) canned	4 oz	120	31	0.0
CHERRY				
(Comstock)				
canned	3.5 oz	110	28	0.0
canned, 'Lite'	3.5 oz	75	19	0.0
(Lucky Leaf) canned	4 oz	120	29	0.0
(Musselman's)				
canned	4 oz	120	29	0.0
canned, 'Plus'	4 oz	108	26	0.2
(Pathmark) canned 'No Frills'	4 oz	130	33	0.0
(White House) canned	3.5 oz	141	33	1.0
CHOCOLATE				
(Comstock) canned	3.5 oz	130	26	3.0
(Royal) mousse, 'No-Bake'	1/8 pie	130	21	4.0
COCONUT *(Comstock)* canned	3.5 oz	120	22	3.0
GOOSEBERRY				
(Lucky Leaf) canned	4 oz	180	45	0.0
(Musselman's) canned	4 oz	180	45	0.0
LEMON				
(Comstock) canned	3.5 oz	140	34	1.0
(Lucky Leaf) canned	4 oz	200	48	2.0
(Lucky Leaf) canned, 'French'	4 oz	180	42	1.0
(Musselman's) canned	4 oz	200	48	2.0
(Musselman's) canned, 'French'	4 oz	180	42	1.0
MINCEMEAT				
(Comstock) canned	3.5 oz	150	39	1.0
(Lucky Leaf) canned	4 oz	190	48	1.0
(Musselman's) canned	4 oz	190	48	1.0
(None Such)				
canned	1/3 cup	200	48	1.0
canned, condensed	1/4 pkg	220	50	2.0
w/brandy and rum, canned	1/3 cup	220	48	2.0
(S&W)	1/4 cup	180	43	2.5
PEACH				
(Comstock) canned	3.5 oz	110	26	0.0
(Lucky Leaf)				
canned	4 oz	150	37	0.0
canned, 'Plus'	4 oz	113	27	0.0
(Musselman's)				
canned	4 oz	150	37	0.0
canned 'Plus'	4 oz	113	27	0.0
(White House) canned	3.5 oz	117	28	1.0
PINEAPPLE				
(Comstock) canned	3.5 oz	100	28	0.0

Food Name	Serv. Size	Total Cal.	Carbs GMS	Fat GMS
(Lucky Leaf) canned	4 oz	110	30	0.0
(Musselman's) canned	4 oz	110	30	0.0
PUMPKIN				
(Comstock) canned	3.5 oz	100	24	0.0
(Libby's)				
canned	1 cup	260	64	0.3
canned	1/2 cup	100	25	0.0
(Lucky Leaf) canned	4 oz	170	33	4.0
(Musselman's) canned	4 oz	170	33	4.0
(Stokely) canned	1/2 cup	170	44	0.0
RAISIN				
(Comstock) canned	3.5 oz	120	32	0.0
(Lucky Leaf) canned	4 oz	130	34	1.0
(Musselman's) canned	4 oz	130	34	1.0
RASPBERRY				
(Lucky Leaf) black, canned	4 oz	190	43	0.0
(Lucky Leaf) red, canned	4 oz	190	46	0.0
(Musselman's) black, canned	4 oz	190	43	0.0
(Musselman's) red, canned	4 oz	190	46	0.0
STRAWBERRY				
(Comstock) canned	3.5 oz	100	25	0.0
(Lucky Leaf)				
canned	4 oz	120	30	0.0
canned, 'Plus'	4 oz	138	34	0.0
(Musselman's)				
canned	4 oz	120	30	0.0
canned, 'Plus'	4 oz	138	34	0.0
STRAWBERRY-RHUBARB				
(Lucky Leaf) canned	4 oz	120	31	0.0
(Musselman's) canned	4 oz	120	31	0.0
VANILLA CREME				
(Lucky Leaf)	4 oz	150	32	3.0
(Musselman's)	4 oz	150	32	3.0
PIE MIX				
BANANA CREAM				
(Jell-O)				
'No Bake' prepared	1/8 pie	240	27	14.0
'No Bake' mix only	1 pkg	140	25	5.0
'No Bake' prepared w/whole milk	1/8 pie	240	27	14.0
CHOCOLATE PIE MIX, MOUSSE				
(Jell-O)				
mousse, 'No Bake' mix only	1 pkg	160	22	7.0
mousse, 'No Bake' prepared	1/8 pie	260	25	17.0
mousse, 'No Bake' prepared w/whole milk	1/8 pie	260	25	17.0
(Royal)				
mint, 'No-Bake' prepared	1/8 pie	260	25	15.0
mousse, 'No Bake' prepared	1/8 pie	230	27	12.0
COCONUT CREAM				
(Jell-O)				
'No Bake' mix only	1 pkg	160	25	7.0
'No Bake' prepared	1/8 pie	260	27	16.0
'No Bake' prepared w/whole milk	1/8 pie	260	27	16.0
LEMON MERINGUE				
(Royal) 'No Bake' prepared	1/8 pie	310	50	11.0
PUMPKIN				
(Jell-O)				
'No Bake' mix only	1 pkg	140	28	3.0

Food Name	Serv. Size	Total Cal.	Carbs GMS	Fat GMS
'No Bake' prepared	1/8 pie	250	31	13.0
'No Bake' prepared w/whole milk	1/8 pie	250	31	13.0
(Libby's) prepared	1/6 pie	390	53	17.0
PIEROGI				
(Mrs. T's)				
potato and American cheese filled	3 pierogies	220	32	6.0
potato and onion filled	3 pierogies	180	34	2.0
sauerkraut filled	3 pierogies	160	32	1.5
PIGEON. See SQUAB.				
PIGEON PEA. See PEAS, PIGEON.				
PIGNOLI NUT. See PINE NUT.				
PIG'S EAR. See under PORK.				
PIG'S FEET. See under PORK.				
PIG'S HEART. See under PORK.				
PIG'S JOWL. See under PORK.				
PIG'S KNUCKLES. See under PORK.				
PIG'S TAIL. See under PORK.				
PIG'S TONGUE. See under PORK.				
PIKE				
NORTHERN				
baked, broiled, grilled, or microwaved	3 oz	96	0	0.7
raw	3 oz	75	0	0.6
WALLEYE				
baked, broiled, grilled, or microwaved	3 oz	101	0	1.3
raw	3 oz	79	0	1.0
PILAF ENTRÉE				
(Health Valley)				
oat bran, w/garden vegetables 'Fast Menu'	7.5 oz	210	31	7.0
(Weight Watchers) Florentine	1 entrée	290	47	7.0
PILI NUT/Canary Tree				
dried	1 cup	863	5	95.5
dried, approx 15 kernels	1 oz	204	1	22.6
PIMIENTO				
Canned or jarred				
	1 cup	44	10	0.6
all varieties, drained (Dromedary)	1 oz	10	2	0.0
chopped	1 tbsp	3	1	0.0
sliced	1 slice	<1	0	0.0
whole	1 whole pimiento	15	3	0.2
PIMIENTO SPREAD (Price's)	1 oz	80	2	6.0
PIÑA COLADA. See under COCKTAIL; COCKTAIL MIX.				
PINE NUT/Colorado pinyon/Italian stone pine nut/pignoli/pinnochio/piñon				
(Progresso)	1 oz jar	170	2	13.0
dried	1 cup	770	19	69.0
dried	1 oz	160	4	14.4
dried	1 tbsp	49	1	4.4
dried	10 med nuts	10	0	0.9
natural, unsalted (Flanigan Farms)	1/4 cup	150	4	14.0
PINEAPPLE				
Canned				
chunks, in extra heavy syrup, w/liquids	1 cup	216	56	0.3
chunks, in heavy syrup, w/liquid	1 cup	198	51	0.3
chunks, in juice, w/liquid	1 cup	149	39	0.2
chunks, in light syrup, w/liquid	1 cup	131	34	0.3
chunks, in water, w/liquid	1 cup	79	20	0.2
crushed, in extra heavy syrup, w/liquids	1 cup	216	56	0.3
crushed, in heavy syrup, w/liquid	1 cup	198	51	0.3

Food Name	Serv. Size	Total Cal.	Carbs GMS	Fat GMS
crushed, in juice, w/liquid	1 cup	149	39	0.2
crushed, in light syrup, w/liquid	1 cup	131	34	0.3
crushed, in water, w/liquid	1 cup	79	20	0.2
rings, in heavy syrup, 3-inch diam, w/liquid	1 ring	38	10	0.1
rings, in juice, 3-inch diam, w/liquid	1 ring w/liquid	28	7	0.0
rings, in light syrup, 3-inch diam, w/liquid	1 ring w/liquid	25	6	0.1
rings, in water, 3-inch diam, w/liquid	1 ring w/liquid	15	4	0.0
sliced (S&W)	1 slice	90	23	0.0
sliced, in extra heavy syrup, w/liquids	1 cup	216	56	0.3
sliced, in heavy syrup, w/liquid	1 cup	198	51	0.3
sliced, in juice, w/liquid	1 cup	149	39	0.2
sliced, in light syrup, w/liquid	1 cup	131	34	0.3
sliced, in water, w/liquid	1 cup	79	20	0.2
Fresh				
raw, diced	1 cup	76	19	0.7
raw, sliced, 3.5 inch diam, 1/2 inch thick	1 slice	27	7	0.2
raw, sliced, 3.5 inch diam, 3/4 inch thick	1 slice	41	10	0.4
raw, whole, trimmed	1 med fruit	231	58	2.0
Frozen				
chunks (Flav-R-Pac)	2/3 cup	75	19	0.0
chunks, sweetened	1 cup	208	54	0.2

PINEAPPLE DRINK. See under FRUIT DRINK; FRUIT JUICE DRINK.
PINEAPPLE JUICE. See also under FRUIT JUICE BLEND; FRUIT JUICE DRINK.
Can, bottle, box, or carton

Food Name	Serv. Size	Total Cal.	Carbs GMS	Fat GMS
unsweetened, w/added ascorbic acid	1 cup	140	34	0.2
unsweetened, w/o added ascorbic acid	1 cup	140	34	0.2
(Del Monte)				
	8 fl oz	110	29	0.0
unsweetened	6 fl oz	100	25	0.0
(Dole)	6 fl oz	103	25	0.2
(IGA) unsweetened	6 fl oz	100	25	0.0
(J. Hungerford)				
100% juice	9.03 fl oz	124	31	0.0
regular	9.03 fl oz	114	29	0.0
(Knudsen)	8 fl oz	110	25	0.0
(Minute Maid)	6 fl oz	90	23	0.0
(Mott's)	9.5 fl oz	169	42	0.0
(Pathmark)				
'Hawaiian'	6 fl oz	100	25	0.0
unsweetened, 'No Frills'	6 fl oz	100	25	0.0
(S&W)				
	8 fl oz	110	29	0.0
unsweetened	6 fl oz	90	23	0.0
(Veryfine) '100%'	8 fl oz	125	31	0.0
Frozen or chilled				
concentrate, prepared	1 cup	130	32	0.1
concentrate, unprepared	6 fl oz	387	96	0.2
(Minute Maid)	6 fl oz	90	23	0.0
PINEAPPLE TOPPING				
(Kraft)	1 tbsp	50	13	0.0
(Smucker's)	2 tbsp	130	32	0.0

PINK BEAN. See BEAN, PINK.
PINK GRAPEFRUIT JUICE. See under GRAPEFRUIT JUICE.
PINK SALMON. See under SALMON.
PINNOCHIO. See PINE NUT.
PIÑON. See PINE NUT.
PINTO BEAN. See BEAN, PINTO.

Food Name	Serv. Size	Total Cal.	Carbs GMS	Fat GMS
PISTACHIO				
in shell *(Dole)*	1 oz	90	3	7.0
natural *(Blue Diamond)*	1 oz	140	4	12.0
natural, in shell *(Fisher)*	1 oz	170	7	14.0
natural, unsalted *(Flanigan Farms)*	1/4 cup	180	8	14.0
red *(Blue Diamond)*	1 oz	140	3	12.0
red *(Fisher)*	1/4 cup	111	4	9.8
Dried				
raw	1 cup	705	37	55.3
raw	30 nuts	99	5	7.8
raw, approx 47 kernels	1 oz	156	8	12.2
Dry roasted				
(Dole)	1 oz	163	7	14.0
natural or red *(Planters)*	1 oz	170	6	14.0
salted	1 cup	726	35	58.5
salted, approx 47 kernels	1 oz	161	8	13.0
unsalted	1 cup	730	36	58.5
unsalted, approx 47 kernels	1 oz	162	8	13.0
Roasted, *(David's)* salted	1 pkg	270	11	21.0
PISTACHIO BUTTER, roasted *(Maranatha Natural)*	2 tbsp	170	7	13.0
PITA. See under BREAD.				
PITANGA/Surinam cherry				
raw	1 cup	57	13.0	0.7
raw, trimmed	1/2 cup	29	6.5	0.3
raw, trimmed	1 oz	9	2.1	0.1
raw, trimmed, approx .3 oz	1 medium	2	0.5	0.0
raw, untrimmed	1 lb	132	29.9	1.6
PIZZA				
(Banquet)				
cheese, on French bread, frozen, 'Zap'	4.5 oz	310	41	10.0
deluxe, on French bread, frozen, 'Zap'	4.8 oz	330	39	13.0
pepperoni, 'Pizza Pie'	1 pizza	470	45	27.0
pepperoni, on French bread, 'Zap'	4.5 oz	350	36	16.0
sausage, 'Pizza Pie'	6 oz	500	48	29.0
sausage and pepperoni, 'Pizza Pie'	6 oz	470	43	27.0
(Celentano)				
cheese, 5.5 oz	2 1/4 slices	340	46	11.0
thick crust, 6.5 oz	1/2 pizza	390	62	12.0
(Celeste)				
cheese, individual	1 pizza	420	42	20.0
cheese, large	1 slice	320	32	16.0
four cheese, individual, 'Original'	1 pizza	480	41	26.0
four cheese, zesty, individual	1 pizza	470	44	24.0
individual, 'Deluxe'	1 pizza	470	46	25.0
large, 'Deluxe'	1 slice	350	35	18.0
pepperoni, individual	1 pizza	470	41	27.0
pepperoni, large	1 slice	350	33	20.0
sausage	1/4 pizza	375	30	22.0
sausage, individual sized	1 pizza	530	52	27.0
sausage, w/green and red peppers, mushrooms, frozen, 'Deluxe'	1 pkg	1538	133	82.6
sausage, w/green and red peppers, mushrooms, frozen, 'Deluxe'	1 serving	386	33	20.7
suprema, individual	1 pizza	500	49	27.0
suprema, large	1 slice	290	27	16.0
vegetable, individual sized	1 pizza	420	46	21.0

Food Name	Serv. Size	Total Cal.	Carbs GMS	Fat GMS
(Crisp 'N Tasty)				
combination	1/2 serving	280	27	15.0
pepperoni	1/2 serving	280	28	15.0
sausage	1/2 serving	280	27	15.0
(Empire Kosher)				
kosher	1 piece	150	15	5.0
kosher, on English muffin	1 muffin	130	15	5.0
kosher, 3 pack.	1 pizza	210	23	9.0
kosher, 10 oz.	1/2 pizza	340	38	13.0
(Graindance Pizza)				
cheese, whole wheat crust, all natural	1 slice	200	23	8.0
(Healthy Choice)				
cheese, on French bread	1 entrée	340	51	5.0
deluxe, on French bread, frozen	6.25 oz	330	41	8.0
pepperoni, on French bread	1 entrée	340	49	5.0
sausage, on French bread	1 entrée	320	48	5.0
supreme, on French bread	1 entrée	330	51	5.0
vegetable, on French bread	1 entrée	280	45	4.0
(Jack's)				
pepperoni, frozen, 'Jack's Original'	1 pkg	1288	118	64.2
pepperoni, frozen, 'Jack's Original'	1 serving	323	30	16.1
sausage and pepperoni, 'Great Combinations'	1 pkg	1389	120	70.0
sausage and pepperoni, 'Great Combinations'	1 serving	348	30	17.5
(Jeno's)				
cheese, microwave, individual	1 serving	240	25	11.0
combination, microwave, individual	1 serving	310	25	18.0
pepperoni, 'Pizza Pocket'	1 serving	370	35	20.0
pepperoni, frozen, 'Crisp 'n Tasty'	1 pkg	516	46	28.8
pepperoni, individual, microwave	1 serving	280	25	16.0
sausage, individual	1 serving	280	25	16.0
sausage, 'Pizza Pocket'	1 serving	360	35	19.0
sausage and pepperoni, 'Crisp 'n Tasty'	1 pkg	491	52	24.2
sausage and pepperoni, 'Pizza Pocket'	1 serving	360	35	20.0
supreme, 'Pizza Pocket'	1 serving	370	36	19.0
(Kashi) spicy Southwest, vegetarian, frozen	1 slice	210	28	7.0
(Kid Cuisine)				
cheese	6.85 oz	380	57	12.0
hamburger	6.85 oz	330	50	10.0
(Lean Cuisine)				
cheese, on French bread	1 entrée	350	48	8.0
deluxe, on French bread	1 entrée	330	45	6.0
pepperoni, on French bread	1 entrée	330	46	7.0
sausage, on French bread, frozen	6 oz	350	42	10.0
(Mrs. Paterson's)				
supreme, hand held, frozen, 'Aussie Pie'	5.5 oz	470	44	27.0
(Nature's Hilights)				
Italian cheese	1/2 pizza	360	46	12.0
soy cheese	1/2 pizza	290	52	1.5
(Oven Lovin')				
cheese, microwave	1/2 pizza	250	24	12.0
cheese, on French bread, frozen, microwave	1 serving	350	40	14.0
combination, microwave	1/2 pizza	310	26	18.0
combination, on French bread, frozen, microwave	1 serving	420	41	21.0
pepperoni, microwave	1/2 pizza	300	25	17.0
pepperoni, on French bread, frozen, microwave	1 serving	410	40	21.0
sausage, microwave	1/2 pizza	290	26	16.0
sausage, on French bread, frozen, microwave	1 serving	400	41	20.0

Food Name	Serv. Size	Total Cal.	Carbs GMS	Fat GMS
supreme, microwave	1/2 pizza	310	27	18.0
(Pappalo's)				
cheese, on French bread, frozen	1 piece	360	40	15.0
combination, on French bread, frozen	1 piece	430	41	21.0
pepperoni, deep dish	1 slice	340	37	14.0
pepperoni, deep dish, individual, frozen, 'For One'	1 pizza	525	65	19.5
pepperoni, on French bread, frozen	1 piece	410	41	20.0
pepperoni, pan pizza	1/5 pizza	350	40	11.0
pepperoni, pizzeria style, 12 inch	1 slice	380	38	17.0
pepperoni, traditional crust, 9 inch	1/2 pizza	390	47	14.0
sausage, deep dish	1 slice	330	36	13.0
sausage, on French bread, frozen	1 piece	410	41	18.0
sausage, pan pizza	1/5 pizza	350	39	11.0
sausage, pizzeria style crust, 12 inch	1 slice	370	38	16.0
sausage, traditional crust, 9 inch	1/2 pizza	380	47	13.0
sausage and pepperoni, deep dish	1 slice	330	36	14.0
sausage and pepperoni, pan pizza	1/5 pizza	360	40	12.0
sausage and pepperoni, pizzeria style, 12 inch	1 slice	380	39	17.0
sausage and pepperoni, traditional crust, 9 inch	1/2 pizza	390	45	15.0
supreme, pan pizza	1/5 pizza	340	37	12.0
supreme, traditional crust, 12 inch	1/4 pizza	350	38	12.0
supreme, traditional crust, 9 inch	1/2 pizza	400	46	16.0
three cheese, pan	1/5 pizza	310	39	8.0
three cheese, traditional crust, 12 inch	1/4 pizza	310	41	7.0
three cheese, traditional crust, 9 inch	1/2 pizza	350	47	11.0
(Pepperidge Farm)				
cheese, on croissant pastry	1 pizza	430	41	23.0
deluxe, on croissant pastry	1 pizza	440	43	23.0
pepperoni, on croissant pastry	1 pizza	420	43	22.0
(Pillsbury)				
cheese, on French bread, frozen, 'Microwave'	1 piece	370	41	15.0
pepperoni, on French bread, frozen, 'Microwave'	1 piece	430	45	19.0
sausage, on French bread, frozen, 'Microwave'	1 piece	410	48	16.0
sausage combo, w/pepperoni, on French bread, frozen, 'Microwave'	1 piece	450	47	21.0
(Pizsoy)				
cheese, w/tofu mozzarella, whole wheat crust, original	1 slice	165	28	5.0
(Red Baron)				
cheese	1/5 pizza	350	33	17.0
cheese, 'Deep Dish Singles'	1 pizza	460	41	23.0
cheese, sausage, mushrooms, pepperoni, and vegetable	1/5 pizza	340	31	18.0
pepperoni, 'Deep Dish Singles'	1 pizza	530	47	31.0
pepperoni, frozen, 'Premium Deep Dish Singles'	1 pkg	961	96	50.1
pepperoni, frozen, 'Premium Deep Dish Singles'	1 serving	480	48	25.0
pepperoni, frozen	1 pkg	1788	146	101.5
pepperoni, frozen	1 serving	442	36	25.1
sausage	1/5 pizza	340	32	18.0
sausage, ham, and pepperoni, 'Deep Dish Singles'	1 pizza	490	41	26.0
sausage, pepperoni, mushroom, pepper, and onion	1/5 pizza	360	33	19.0
supreme, w/sausage, mushrooms, pepperoni, frozen	1 pkg	1736	161	91.2
supreme, w/sausage, mushrooms, pepperoni, frozen	1 serving	344	32	18.1
two cheese, w/sausage, pepperoni, onions, 'Deluxe'	1 pkg	1746	166	92.3
two cheese, w/sausage, pepperoni, onions, 'Deluxe'	1 serving	337	32	17.8
(Smart Ones) combo, deluxe, pizza	1 entrée	380	47	11.0
(Soypreme)				
cheese, w/tofu mozzarella, whole wheat crust	1 slice	209	22	7.0
cheese, w/tofu mozzarella, whole wheat crust, 'Garden Patch'	1 slice	211	24	7.0

Food Name	Serv. Size	Total Cal.	Carbs GMS	Fat GMS
(Stouffer's)				
bacon cheddar, on French bread	1 entrée	440	44	22.0
Canadian bacon, on French bread.	5.5 oz	370	40	15.0
cheese, on French bread	1/2 pizza	350	42	14.0
cheeseburger, on French bread	1/2 pizza	440	31	26.0
deluxe, w/sausage, pepperoni, mushroom, on French bread, frozen	1 pkg	858	89	41.3
deluxe, w/sausage, pepperoni, mushroom, on French bread, frozen	1 serving	429	44	20.6
double cheese, on French bread	1/2 pizza	420	44	19.0
hamburger, on French bread, frozen	1 pkg	410	39	18.0
on French bread, 'Deluxe'	1/2 pizza	440	42	22.0
pepperoni, on French bread	1/2 pizza	420	42	20.0
pepperoni, w/mushrooms, on French bread	1/2 pizza	430	43	21.0
sausage, on French bread	1/2 pizza	420	41	20.0
sausage and pepperoni, on French bread	1/2 pizza	490	45	25.0
vegetable, deluxe, on French bread	1/2 pizza	400	43	17.0
w/sausage and pepperoni, on French bread, frozen	1 pkg	896	87	45.0
w/sausage and pepperoni, on French bread, frozen	1 serving	448	44	22.5
(Tombstone)				
bacon, Canadian style, 12 inch, 'Original'	3.6 oz	230	23	10.0
bacon cheeseburger, 12 inch, 'Special Order'	4.7 oz	330	29	16.0
cheese, microwave, 7 inch	7.7 oz	500	45	24.0
cheese, original, 12 inch	3.4 oz	230	23	10.0
cheese, original, 9 inch	5.6 oz	380	40	17.0
cheese, sausage, and mushroom, original, 12 inch	3.8 oz	240	23	11.0
cheese, w/hamburger, original, 12 inch	3.7 oz	250	23	12.0
cheese, w/pepperoni, 'Italian Thincrust'	3 oz	230	15	14.0
cheese, w/sausage, 12' 'Original'	3.7 oz	240	23	11.0
cheese and hamburger, original, 9 inch	6.3 oz	440	41	21.0
cheese and pepperoni, microwave, 7 inch	7.5 oz	550	38	32.0
cheese and pepperoni, original, 9 inch	6.3 oz	480	40	26.0
cheese and sausage 'Italian Thincrust'	3.2 oz	220	15	13.0
cheese and sausage, original, 9 inch	6.3 oz	420	41	19.0
chicken, deluxe, light,	1/2 pizza	180	23	4.0
chicken, light, 8 inch	4.5 oz	240	28	8.0
deluxe, original, 12 inch	1 slice	310	29	14.0
double cheese, w/pepperoni, double top, 12 inch	4.8 oz	360	24	20.0
four cheese, 'Special Order'	4.3 oz	300	28	14.0
four meat, 'Special Order'	4.6 oz	320	28	15.0
four meat, 9 inch, 'Special Order'	3.9 oz	280	24	14.0
Italian sausage, 'Special Order'	4.5 oz	300	28	13.0
Italian sausage, microwave, 7 inch	8.0 oz	550	38	32.0
pepperoni and sausage, original, 9 inch	6.6 oz	490	40	26.0
pepperoni and sausage, original, frozen	1 pkg	952	82	51.7
pepperoni and sausage, original, frozen	1 serving	317	27	17.2
pepperoni, 'Special Order'	4.4 oz	320	28	16.0
pepperoni, 8 inch, 'Light'	4.0 oz	250	27	10.0
pepperoni, 9 inch, 'Special Order'	3.7 oz	280	24	14.0
pepperoni, original, 12 inch	1 slice	400	35	21.0
pepperoni, original, frozen, 12 inch	1 pkg	938	85	47.3
pepperoni, original, frozen, 12 inch	1 serving	312	28	15.7
pepperoni, original, frozen, 9 inch	1 pkg	1659	155	83.6
pepperoni, original, frozen, 9 inch	1 serving	413	39	20.8
pepperoni, thin crust	1 slice	400	25	25.0
ranchero, deluxe, 'Mexican Style Thincrust'	3.4 oz	230	16	13.0
sausage, double top, w/double cheese, 12 inch	4.8 oz	330	24	16.0

Food Name	Serv. Size	Total Cal.	Carbs GMS	Fat GMS
sausage and mushroom, original	1 pkg	1496	152	67.1
sausage and mushroom, original	1 serving	306	31	13.7
sausage and pepperoni, double top, 12 inch	4.8 oz	340	24	18.0
sausage and pepperoni, microwave, 7 inch	8 oz	570	39	32.0
sausage and pepperoni, original	1 pkg	1635	153	81.7
sausage and pepperoni, original	1 serving	328	31	16.4
sausage and pepperoni, original, 12 inch	3.7 oz	260	23	13.0
supreme, 'Italian Style Thincrust'	3.38 oz	230	16	14.0
supreme, 'Special Order'	4.4 oz	320	29	15.0
supreme, 9 inch, 'Special Order'	4.0 oz	280	24	14.0
supreme, light	1 slice	270	30	9.0
supreme, microwave, 7 inch	8.5 oz	550	40	31.0
supreme, original, 12 inch	3.8 oz	270	24	14.0
supreme, thin crust	1 slice	380	26	22.0
taco, microwave, 7 inch	8.4 oz	590	41	34.0
three sausage, 9 inch, 'Special Order'	3.8 oz	260	24	12.0
vegetable, light	1 slice	240	31	7.0
(Tony's)				
pepperoni, w/Italian style pastry crust, frozen	1 pkg	1232	110	67.9
pepperoni, w/Italian style pastry crust, frozen	1 serving	406	36	22.4
sausage, deep dish, frozen, 'D'Primo'	1 pkg	1576	164	80.2
sausage, deep dish, frozen, 'D'Primo'	1 serving	391	41	19.9
sausage and pepperoni, w/Italian style pastry crust	1 pkg	1319	126	70.2
sausage and pepperoni, w/Italian style pastry crust	1 serving	434	41	23.1
supreme, w/sausage, pepperoni, mushroom, peppers, onion, Italian crust	1 pkg	1213	118	60.6
supreme, w/sausage, pepperoni, mushroom, peppers, onion, Italian crust	1 serving	400	39	20.0
taco style, w/sausage, sauce, corn style crust	1 pkg	1326	130	70.5
taco style, w/sausage, sauce, corn style crust	1 serving	437	43	23.3
(Totino's)				
baconburger, on French bread, 'Party'	1/2 pizza	370	33	20.0
Canadian bacon, 'Party'	1/2 pizza	320	33	15.0
cheese, 'Pan Pizza'	1/6 pizza	290	35	10.0
cheese, family size, 'Party Pizza'	1/3 pizza	320	43	11.0
cheese, microwaveable, individual	1 pizza	240	25	11.0
cheese, on French bread, 'Party'	1/2 pizza	320	33	14.0
combination, 'Party'	1/2 pizza	390	34	21.0
combination, family size, 'Party Pizza'	1/3 pizza	400	47	18.0
combination, microwaveable, individual	1 pizza	310	25	18.0
hamburger, 'Party'	1/2 pizza	350	33	18.0
Mexican, zesty, 'Party'	1/2 pizza	370	34	19.0
pepperoni, 'Pan Pizza'	1/6 pizza	330	35	15.0
pepperoni, 'Party Pizza Family Size'	1/3 pizza	410	44	20.0
pepperoni, crisp crust, frozen	1 pkg	728	69	38.9
pepperoni, crisp crust, frozen	1 serving	364	35	19.4
pepperoni, microwaveable, individual	1 pizza	280	25	16.0
pepperoni, zesty	1/2 pizza	380	33	21.0
sausage, 'Pan Pizza'	1/6 pizza	320	35	13.0
sausage, 'Party'	1/2 pizza	380	34	20.0
sausage, family size, 'Party Pizza'	1/3 pizza	410	48	18.0
sausage, individual, microwaveable	1 pizza	280	25	16.0
sausage and pepperoni, 'Pan Pizza'	1/6 pizza	330	35	15.0
sausage and pepperoni, crisp crust	1 pkg	769	72	40.7
sausage and pepperoni, crisp crust	1 serving	385	36	20.4
(Tyson)				
hamburger, 'Looney Tunes Wile E. Coyote'	6 oz	310	40	11.0

Food Name	Serv. Size	Total Cal.	Carbs GMS	Fat GMS
pepperoni, 'Looney Tunes Foghorn Leghorn'	6.35 oz	400	57	13.0
(Weight Watchers)				
cheese	6.03 oz	300	36	7.0
combination, 'Deluxe'	1 serving	380	47	11.0
extra cheese	1 serving	390	49	12.0
pepperoni	1 serving	390	46	12.0
(Wolfgang Puck's)				
chicken, spicy, 'Pizza California'	1/2 pizza	360	36	16.0
mushroom and spinach, 'Pizza California'	1/2 pizza	270	36	8.0
PIZZA CRUST				
(Boboli) cheese, 6 inch	1/2 crust	150	25	3.5
(Ener-G Foods) gluten-free, 10 inch	1 slice	134	20	5.7
(Pillsbury) 'All Ready'	1/8 crust	90	16	1.0
PIZZA CRUST DOUGH *(Rhodes)* frozen	1 slice	130	23	2.0
PIZZA CRUST MIX				
(Chef Boyardee) 'Quick & Easy' mix only	1/6 pkg	150	26	2.0
(French Meadow) spelt, organic, yeast-free, prepared	1/6 crust	90	10	2.0
(Gold Medal)				
just add water, prepared	1/4 crust	160	32	2.0
'Pouch Mix' mix only	1/6 pkg	110	22	1.0
(Martha White)				
deep dish, prepared w/water	1 slice	110	23	1.0
regular, prepared w/water	1 slice	100	19	2.0
(Robin Hood) 'Pouch Mix' mix only	1/6 pkg	110	22	1.0
PIZZA DINNER/ENTRÉE				
(Kid Cuisine)				
cheese, 'Mega Meal'	9.7 oz	430	75	7.0
w/hamburger, apples, corn, chocolate pudding	1 meal	330	50	9.0
PIZZA KIT				
(Chef Boyardee)				
cheese, 'Complete'	1/4 pkg	230	36	6.0
cheese, '2 Complete'	1/8 pkg	210	31	5.0
pepperoni, 'Complete'	1/4 pkg	250	31	9.0
pepperoni, '2 Complete'	1/8 pkg	210	31	7.0
plain	1/4 pkg	180	32	3.0
sausage	1/4 pkg	270	34	10.0
(Contadina)				
cheese	4.94 oz	320	41	10.0
pepperoni	4.94 oz	370	38	16.0
PIZZA SNACK				
(Jenny's Cuisine) puffs, cheese, w/vegetables, thick crust	1 puff	252	34	8.5
(Totino's)				
roll, hamburger, frozen	1 pkg	577	66	24.4
roll, hamburger, frozen	1 serving	231	26	9.8
roll, pepperoni, frozen	1 pkg	579	59	28.4
roll, pepperoni, frozen	1 serving	385	39	18.9
roll, sausage, frozen	1 pkg	528	60	22.5
roll, sausage, frozen	1 serving	351	40	14.9
PLANTAIN				
cooked, mashed	1 cup	232	62	0.4
cooked, sliced	1 cup	179	48	0.3
raw, sliced	1 cup	181	47	0.5
raw, whole	1 medium	218	57	0.7
PLUM				
Canned				
purple, in heavy syrup, w/liquid	1 medium	41	11	0.0
purple, in juice, w/liquid	1 medium	27	7	0.0

Food Name	Serv. Size	Total Cal.	Carbs GMS	Fat GMS
purple, in light syrup, w/liquid	1 medium	29	7	0.0
purple, in water, w/liquid	1 medium	19	5	0.0
purple, pitted, in extra heavy syrup, w/liquid	1 cup	264	69	0.3
purple, pitted, in heavy syrup, w/liquid	1 cup	230	60	0.3
purple, pitted, in juice, w/liquid	1 cup	146	38	0.1
purple, pitted, in light syrup, w/liquid	1 cup	159	41	0.3
purple, pitted, in water, w/liquid	1 cup	102	27	0.0
Fresh				
raw, sliced	1 cup	91	21	1.0
raw, whole, approx 2 1/8 inch diam	1 plum	36	9	0.4
PLUM, JAPANESE. See UMEBOSHI.				
POI				
	1 cup	269	65	0.3
crumbles *(Ener-G Foods)*	1 cup	376	75	8.0
POKEBERRY SHOOT				
boiled, drained	1 cup	33	5	0.7
boiled, drained	1 tbsp	2	0	0.0
raw	1 cup	37	6	0.6
POLENTA MIX *(Fantastic Foods)* 'Polenta'				
prepared	1/2 cup	106	18	2.0
POLISH SAUSAGE. See under SAUSAGE.				
POLLACK				
ALASKAN				
baked, broiled, grilled, or microwaved	4 oz	128	0.0	1.3
raw	1 lb	365	0.0	3.6
raw	1 oz	23	0.0	0.2
ATLANTIC				
baked, broiled, grilled, or microwaved	3 oz	100	0	1.1
raw	3 oz	78	0	0.8
WALLEYE				
baked, broiled, grilled, or microwaved	3 oz	96	0	1.0
raw	3 oz	69	0	0.7
POLLYFISH. See PARROTFISH.				
POMEGRANATE/Chinese apple				
raw, trimmed	1 oz	19	4.9	0.1
raw, untrimmed	1 lb	172	43.6	0.8
raw, whole, medium, approx 3 3/8 inch diam	1 pomegranate	105	26.4	0.5
POMEGRANATE JUICE				
(Knudsen)	8 fl oz	85	21	0.0
(Knudsen) fruit juice sweetened	8 fl oz	150	37	0.0
POMELO/pummelo				
raw, sections	1/2 cup	36	9.1	<.1
raw, trimmed	1 oz	11	2.7	<.1
raw, untrimmed	1 lb	95	24.4	0.1
raw, whole, medium, approx 5 1/2 inches diam, 2.4 lbs	1 pomelo	228	58.6	0.2
POMFRET				
raw	1 lb	663	0.0	36.4
raw	1 oz	41	0.0	2.3
POMPANO, FLORIDA				
baked, broiled, grilled, or microwaved	3 oz	179	0	10.3
raw	3 oz	139	0	8.1
raw, boneless	1 oz	46	0	2.7
POP. See SOFT DRINKS AND MIXERS.				
POPCORN				
(NOTE: All popcorn is popped unless otherwise noted.)				
(Act II)				
artificial butter flavor, 'Butter Lovers' unpopped	3 tbsp	170	19	11.0

Food Name	Serv. Size	Total Cal.	Carbs GMS	Fat GMS
butter flavor, microwave, unpopped	3 tbsp	170	19	11.0
natural, microwave, unpopped	3 tbsp	180	19	12.0
(Auburn Farms) caramel, nonfat	2/3 cup	120	28	0.0
(Bachman)				
	0.5 oz	80	7	6.0
cheese flavor	0.5 oz	90	7	6.0
'Lite'	0.5 oz	50	10	1.0
white cheddar cheese flavor	0.5 oz	70	7	4.0
(Bearitos)				
buttery	1 cup	60	4	4.0
cheese flavor, 'Organic'	1 oz	137	13	8.0
herb, lite, organic	3.5 cups	140	20	6.0
no salt, no oil	1 cup	30	6	0.5
no salt, organic	1 oz	108	22	0.8
'Organic Lite'	1 oz	132	15	6.9
'Organic Traditional'	1 oz	140	12	9.2
(Betty Crocker)				
butter flavor, microwave, 'Pop Secret'	3 cups	100	11	6.0
butter flavor, microwave, 'Pop Secret By Request'	3 cups	60	12	1.0
butter flavor, microwave, 'Pop Secret Light'	3 cups	70	12	3.0
butter flavor, no salt, 'Pop Secret'	3 cups	100	11	6.0
butter flavor, original, microwave, 'Pop Secret'	1 cup	35	4	2.5
butter flavor, 'Pop Secret'	1/4 bag	120	13	8.0
butter flavor, 'Pop Secret Light'	1/4 bag	90	13	4.0
butter flavor, 'Pop Secret Pop Qwiz'	1 bag	110	11	7.0
butter flavor, 'Pop Secret Pop Qwiz'	2 3/4 cups	80	9	5.0
butter flavor, salt-free, 'Pop Secret'	1/4 bag	120	13	7.0
butter flavor, singles 'Pop Secret Light'	1 bag	180	28	8.0
butter flavor, singles, 'Pop Secret Light'	6 cups	140	23	6.0
butter flavor, singles, 'Pop Secret'	1 bag	250	27	16.0
butter flavor, singles, 'Pop Secret'	6 cups	200	23	12.0
buttery burst, microwave, 'Pop Secret'	1 cup	35	4	2.5
buttery burst, light, microwave, 'Pop Secret'	1 cup	25	4	1.0
cheese flavor, microwave, 'Pop Secret' 1/3 pkg.	3 cups	170	15	11.0
natural, 'Pop Secret'	1/4 bag	120	13	8.0
natural, 'Pop Secret Light'	1/4 bag	90	13	4.0
natural, 'Pop Secret Pop Qwiz'	2 3/4 cups	80	9	5.0
natural, 'Pop Secret Pop Qwiz'	1 bag	110	11	7.0
natural, microwave, 'Pop Secret'	3 cups	100	11	6.0
natural, microwave, 'Pop Secret By Request'	3 cups	60	12	1.0
natural, microwave, 'Pop Secret Light'	3 cups	70	12	3.0
natural, singles, 'Pop Secret Light'	1 bag	170	26	7.0
natural, singles 'Pop Secret Light'	6 cups	150	23	6.0
(Bonnie Lee)				
air popped, salted	1 qt	109	20	1.0
oil popped, salted	1 qt	172	20	8.0
(Cape Cod)				
all natural	3.5 cups	160	18	9.0
butter, old fashioned	3 cups	170	16	10.0
white cheddar cheese flavor	0.5 oz	80	6	5.0
(Clover Club) white cheddar cheese flavor	0.5 oz	70	6	5.0
(Country Grown) no added fat or salt, microwave	3 cups	85	17	1.0
(Cracker Jack)				
butter toffee, w/almonds, pecans, 'Nutty Delux'	1 oz	130	19	6.0
caramel, w/peanuts	1/2 cup	120	23	2.0
(Estee) caramel coated, bag	1 oz	140	25	3.0
(Featherweight)				
butter flavor, low-salt, microwave	3 cups	100	14	3.0

Food Name	Serv. Size	Total Cal.	Carbs GMS	Fat GMS
natural, low-salt, microwave	3 cups	80	14	1.0
(Frito-Lay's)				
	0.5 oz	70	9	3.0
cheese flavor	0.5 oz	80	7	5.0
(Good Health) butterscotch, 100% natural	30-g pkg	110	24	0.0
(Healthy Choice) natural flavor	1 cup	15	4	0.0
(Jiffy Pop)				
butter flavor 'Pan Popcorn'	4 cups	130	16	6.0
butter flavor, microwave	4 cups	140	17	7.0
microwave	4 cups	140	17	7.0
'Pan Popcorn'	4 cups	130	16	6.0
(Jolly Time)				
butter flavored, light, microwave	3 cups	60	12	2.0
butter flavored, microwave	3 cups	90	13	5.0
cheddar flavor, microwave	3 cups	155	17	10.0
natural flavor, light, microwave	3 cups	70	13	2.0
natural flavor, microwave	3 cups	120	15	7.0
white, air-popped	3 cups	60	15	1.0
white, unsalted	4 cups	75	20	1.0
yellow, air-popped	3 cups	60	14	1.0
yellow, unsalted	4 cups	75	19	1.0
(Keebler)				
honey caramel, 'Pop Deluxe'	1 oz	120	22	3.0
white cheddar cheese flavor	1 oz	140	13	10.0
(Kettle Poppins)				
brewer's yeast	0.5 oz	70	8	2.5
lightly salted	0.5 oz	70	9	2.5
white cheddar	0.5 oz	70	9	2.5
(Lapidus Popcorn Company)				
herb, organic	2 cups	170	15	11.0
white cheddar, organic	2 cups	180	13	13.0
(Laura Scudder's)				
'Tender Baby White Corn'	0.5 oz	80	6	6.0
white cheddar cheese flavor	0.5 oz	70	6	5.0
(Louise's)				
nonfat	1 oz	100	24	0.0
toffee caramel, buttery, nonfat	1 oz	100	24	0.0
(Nature's Choice)				
caramel, original	1 oz	108	25	1.0
caramel, w/peanuts	1 oz	114	23	1.0
(Orville Redenbacher)				
butter flavored, light, microwave, 'Gourmet'	3 cups	80	14	4.0
butter flavored, light, microwave, snack size	3 cups	70	11	3.0
butter flavored, microwave, 'Gourmet'	3 cups	110	12	8.0
butter flavored, microwave, 'Smart Pop'	3 cups	50	11	1.0
butter flavored, microwave, snack size	3 cups	100	11	6.0
butter flavored, salt-free, microwave, 'Gourmet'	3 cups	110	12	8.0
butter toffee, microwave, 'Gourmet'	2 1/2 cups	210	26	12.0
caramel, 'Ready-to-Eat'	1 oz	112	22	3.5
caramel, microwave, 'Gourmet'	2 1/2 cups	240	29	14.0
cheddar cheese, microwave, 'Gourmet'	3 cups	130	14	8.0
cheddar cheese, microwave, 'Gourmet'	3 cups	150	13	10.0
hot air, 'Gourmet'	3 cups	40	10	1.0
hot air, unpopped	2 tbsp	92	24	0.8
natural, light, microwave, 'Gourmet'	3 cups	80	14	4.0
natural, microwave, 'Gourmet'	3 cups	110	12	8.0
natural, salt-free, microwave 'Gourmet'	3 cups	110	12	8.0

Food Name	Serv. Size	Total Cal.	Carbs GMS	Fat GMS
original, 'Gourmet'.	3 cups	80	10	4.0
regular	1 oz	138	17	8.7
sour cream and onion, microwave, 'Gourmet'	3 cups	180	16	13.0
white cheddar cheese, 'Ready-to-Eat'	1.06 oz	139	17	8.6
white, 'Gourmet'	3 cups	80	10	4.0
(Painted Desert) microwave	1 cup	27	6	1.0
(Pillsbury)				
butter flavor, frozen, microwave	3 cups	210	20	13.0
original, frozen, microwave	3 cups	210	20	13.0
salt-free, frozen, microwave	3 cups	170	23	7.0
(Planters)				
butter flavor, microwave	3 cups	140	13	10.0
natural, microwave	3 cups	140	14	9.0
(Pop Weaver's)				
butter flavor, microwave	4 cups	140	20	8.0
natural, microwave	3 cups	140	20	8.0
(Pops-Rite)				
butter flavor, microwave	3 cups	90	13	5.0
microwave, 'Natural'	3 cups	90	13	5.0
white, air popped, no salt	1 oz	100	20	2.0
white, oil popped, unsalted	1 oz	220	20	15.0
yellow, air popped, no salt	1 oz	100	21	2.0
yellow, oil popped, unsalted	1 oz	220	21	15.0
(Smartfood) white cheddar cheese flavor	0.5 oz	80	7	5.0
(Tone's)	1 cup	30	6	0.4
(Ultra Slim-Fast) butter flavor, 'Lite 'N Tasty'	0.5 oz	60	10	2.0
(Vic's)				
caramel, lite, 'Gourmet'	1/2 cup	60	10	2.0
white cheddar cheese, lite, 'Gourmet'	2/3 cup	40	4	2.0
white, lite, 'Gourmet'	1 cup	35	6	2.0
yellow cheddar cheese, lite, 'Gourmet'	2/3 cup	40	4	2.0
(Weight Watchers)				
butter	0.66 oz	90	13	3.0
caramel	1 serving	100	22	1.0
'Lightly Salted'	0.66 oz	80	12	4.0
microwave	1 oz pkg	100	22	1.0
white cheddar cheese flavor	0.66 oz pkg	100	10	6.0
(Wise)				
butter flavor	1 cup	80	7	5.0
'Tender Baby White Corn'	0.5 oz	80	6	6.0
'Tender Eating Baby Popcorn'	0.5 oz	70	4	6.0
white cheddar cheese flavor	0.5 oz	70	6	5.0
POPCORN OIL				
(Orville Redenbacher) and topping oil	1 tbsp	120	0	13.5
(Planters)	1 tbsp	120	0	14.0
(Wesson)				
buttery flavor	1 tbsp	120	0	13.5
popping and topping oil, food service product	1 tbsp	122	0	13.5
POPCORN SEASONING. See under SEASONING MIX.				
POPPY SEED				
	1 tbsp	47	2	3.9
	1 tsp	15	1	1.3
(McCormick/Schilling)	1 tsp	17	1	1.2
(Spice Islands)	1 tsp	13	1	0.9
whole (Durkee)	1 tsp	15	0	0.0
whole (Laurel Leaf)	1 tsp	15	0	0.0
POPPY SEED FILLING (Solo) 'Sokal'	2 tbsp	119	21	3.2

Food Name	Serv. Size	Total Cal.	Carbs GMS	Fat GMS
POPPY SEED OIL				
..../......................	1 cup	1927	0	218.0
....	1 tbsp	120	0	13.6
PORK. See also HAM.				
(NOTE: TRIMMED = Lean; separable fat removed. UNTRIMMED = Separable fat not removed.)				
BACKFAT				
Fresh				
wholesale cuts, raw	1 lb	3683	0.0	402.3
wholesale cuts, raw	1 oz	230	0.0	25.1
BACKRIB				
Fresh				
Untrimmed				
raw	1 lb	1279	0.0	107.0
raw	1 oz	80	0.0	6.7
raw 'Gourmet' *(JM)*	5.5 oz	220	0.0	18.0
roasted	3 oz	315	0.0	25.1
BELLY				
Fresh				
wholesale cuts, raw	1 lb	2350	0.0	240.5
wholesale cuts, raw	1 oz	147	0.0	15.0
BRAIN				
Fresh				
braised	3 oz	117	0.0	8.1
in milk gravy *(Armour)*	2.75 oz	110	1.0	8.0
raw	1 oz	36	0.0	2.6
CENTER LOIN				
Fresh				
Trimmed				
chop, bone in, braised	3 oz	172	0.0	7.1
chop, bone in, broiled	3 oz	172	0.0	6.9
chop, bone in, pan fried	3 oz	197	0.0	8.9
roast, bone in, roasted	3 oz	169	0.0	7.7
Untrimmed				
chop, bone in, braised	3 oz	210	0.0	12.0
chop, bone in, broiled	3 oz	204	0.0	11.1
chop, bone in, pan fried	3 oz	235	0.0	14.1
roast, bone in, roasted	3 oz	199	0.0	11.4
CENTER RIB				
Fresh				
Trimmed				
chop, bone in, braised	3 oz	179	0.0	8.6
chop, bone in, broiled	3 oz	186	0.0	8.3
chop, bone in, pan-fried	3 oz	185	0.0	9.2
roast, bone in, roasted	3 oz	182	0.0	8.6
Untrimmed				
chop, bone in, braised	3 oz	217	0.0	13.4
chop, bone in, broiled	3 oz	224	0.0	13.2
chop, bone in, pan-fried	3 oz	225	0.0	14.4
roast, bone in, roasted	3 oz	217	0.0	13.0
CHITTERLINGS				
Fresh				
raw	1 oz	71	0.1	6.5
simmered	3 oz	258	0.0	24.4
CHOP				
Refrigerated or frozen				
boneless, 'America's Cut' *(JM)*	6 oz	330	0.0	20.0
center cut, 'Always Tender' *(Hormel)*	4 oz	187	1.0	10.8
center cut, 'Always Tender' *(Hormel)*	1 oz	47	0.0	2.7

Food Name	Serv. Size	Total Cal.	Carbs GMS	Fat GMS
COMPOSITE CUTS				
Canned				
(Hormel)	3 oz	240	2.0	21.0
chopped (Hormel)	3 oz	200	2.0	16.0
Fresh				
Trimmed				
leg, loin, and shoulder, cooked	3 oz	180	0.0	8.2
leg, loin, and shoulder, raw	1 oz	41	0.0	1.7
loin and shoulder, cooked	3 oz	179	0.0	8.0
loin and shoulder, raw	1 oz	41	0.0	1.7
retail cuts, cooked	3 oz	232	0.0	14.6
retail cuts, raw	1 lb	980	0.0	67.8
retail cuts, raw	1 oz	61	0.0	4.2
roasted	3 oz	180	0.0	8.2
Untrimmed				
leg, loin, shoulder, spareribs, cooked	3 oz	232	0.0	14.6
leg, loin, shoulder, spareribs, raw	1 oz	64	0.0	4.7
loin and shoulder, cooked	3 oz	214	0.0	12.6
loin and shoulder, raw	1 lb	907	0.0	58.5
loin and shoulder, raw	1 oz	57	0.0	3.7
raw	1 lb	1030	0.0	74.8
raw	1 oz	64	0.0	4.7
EAR				
Fresh				
raw	1 oz	66	0	4.3
simmered	1 medium	184	0	12.0
FEET				
Fresh				
raw	1 oz	75	0	5.3
simmered	3 oz	165	0	10.5
Pickled				
approx 6 oz (Penrose)	1 piece	220	2	15.0
cured	1 oz	58	0	4.6
GROUND				
Fresh				
cooked	3 oz	252	0.0	17.6
raw	4 oz	297	0	23.9
Refrigerated or frozen (JM)	3 oz	190	0.0	14.0
HEART				
Fresh				
braised	1 cup	215	1	7.3
braised	1 medium	191	1	6.5
raw	1 medium	267	3	9.9
raw	1 oz	33	0	1.2
HOCKS, refrigerated, hickory smoked (Cook's)	3 oz	270	5	20.0
JOWL				
Fresh				
raw	4 oz	740	0	78.7
raw	1 oz	186	0	19.7
KIDNEYS				
Fresh				
braised	1 cup	211	0.0	6.6
braised	3 oz	128	0.0	4.0
raw	1 oz	28	0.0	0.9
KNUCKLES, jarred, pickled, approx 6 oz (Penrose)	1 piece	290	1	21.0
LEG, RUMP HALF				
Fresh				
Trimmed				
raw	1 lb	621	0.0	23.5

Food Name	Serv. Size	Total Cal.	Carbs GMS	Fat GMS
raw	1 oz	39	0.0	1.5
roasted	3 oz	175	0.0	6.9
roasted, diced	1 cup	278	0.0	11.0
Untrimmed				
raw	1 lb	1007	0.0	71.2
raw	1 oz	63	0.0	4.4
roasted	3 oz	214	0.0	12.1
roasted	1.5 oz	117	0.0	7.6
roasted, diced	1 cup	340	0.0	19.3
LEG, SHANK HALF				
Fresh				
Trimmed				
raw	1 lb	631	0.0	25.5
raw	1 oz	39	0.0	1.6
roasted	3 oz	183	0.0	8.9
roasted, diced	1 cup	290	0.0	14.2
Untrimmed				
raw	1 lb	1193	0.0	95.4
raw	1 oz	75	0.0	6.0
roasted	3 oz	246	0.0	17.0
roasted	1.5 oz	129	0.0	9.4
roasted, diced	1 cup	390	0.0	27.1
LEG, WHOLE				
Fresh				
Trimmed				
raw	1 lb	617	0.0	24.5
raw	1 oz	39	0.0	1.5
roasted	3 oz	179	0.0	8.0
roasted	1.5 oz	94	0.0	4.7
roasted	1 cup	285	0.0	12.7
Untrimmed				
raw	1 lb	1111	0.0	85.6
raw	1 oz	69	0.0	5.3
roasted	3 oz	232	0.0	15.0
roasted	1.5 oz	125	0.0	8.8
roasted, diced	1 cup	369	0.0	23.8
LIVER				
Fresh				
braised	3 oz	140	3.2	3.7
fried	3 oz	205	2.1	9.8
raw	1 oz	38	0.7	1.0
LOIN				
Fresh				
Trimmed				
blade, braised	3 oz	191	0.0	11.1
blade, broiled	3 oz	199	0.0	11.8
blade, pan-fried	3 oz	205	0.0	12.8
blade, pan-fried in vegetable oil	4 oz	321	0.0	22.5
blade, roasted	3 oz	210	0.0	12.6
ribs, country-style, braised	3 oz	199	0.0	11.6
ribs, country-style, raw	1 oz	45	0.0	2.3
ribs, country-style, roasted	3 oz	210	0.0	12.6
whole, braised	3 oz	173	0.0	7.8
whole, broiled	3 oz	178	0.0	8.3
whole, chopped, braised	1 cup	382	0.0	20.4
whole, chopped, broiled	1 cup	360	0.0	21.4
whole, chopped, roasted	1 cup	336	0.0	19.5

Food Name	Serv. Size	Total Cal.	Carbs GMS	Fat GMS
whole, raw	1 oz	44	0.0	2.1
whole, roasted	3 oz	178	0.0	8.2
Untrimmed				
blade, braised	3 oz	275	0.0	21.6
blade, broiled	3 oz	272	0.0	21.1
blade, pan-fried	3 oz	291	0.0	23.6
blade, pan-fried in vegetable oil	4 oz	469	0.0	41.9
blade, roasted	3 oz	275	0.0	20.9
ribs, country-style, braised	3 oz	252	0.0	18.3
ribs, country-style, raw	1 oz	68	0.0	5.3
ribs, country-style, roasted	3 oz	279	0.0	21.5
whole, braised	3 oz	203	0.0	11.6
whole, broiled	3 oz	206	0.0	11.8
whole, roasted	3 oz	211	0.0	12.4
Refrigerated or frozen				
boneless, 'Always Tender' *(Hormel)*	1 oz	41	0.0	2.0
boneless, 'Always Tender' *(Hormel)*	4 oz	163	1.0	8.0
whole or half, center cut, boneless *(JM)*	3 oz	190	0.0	13.0
LUNGS				
Fresh				
braised	3 oz	84	0.0	2.6
raw	1 oz	24	0.0	0.8
PANCREAS				
Fresh				
braised	3 oz	186	0.0	9.2
raw	4 oz	225	0.0	15.0
SHOULDER				
Fresh				
Trimmed				
arm picnic, braised	3 oz	211	0.0	10.4
arm picnic, raw	1 oz	40	0.0	1.8
arm picnic, roasted	3 oz	194	0.0	10.7
Boston blade, braised	3 oz	232	0.0	13.2
Boston blade, broiled	3 oz	193	0.0	10.7
Boston blade, raw	1 oz	47	0.0	2.6
Boston blade, roasted	3 oz	197	0.0	12.2
whole, chopped, roasted	1 cup	341	0.0	21.0
whole, raw	1 lb	671	0.0	32.4
whole, raw	1 oz	42	0.0	2.0
whole, roasted	3 oz	195	0.0	11.5
whole, roasted, diced	1 cup	310	0.0	18.3
Untrimmed				
arm picnic, braised	3 oz	280	0.0	19.7
arm picnic, braised, diced	1 cup	444	0.0	31.3
arm picnic, raw	1 oz	72	0.0	5.7
arm picnic, roasted	3 oz	269	0.0	20.4
arm picnic, roasted, diced	1 cup	428	0.0	32.4
Boston blade, braised	3 oz	271	0.0	18.5
Boston blade, broiled	3 oz	220	0.0	14.1
Boston blade, raw	1 lb	989	0.0	71.8
Boston blade, roasted	3 oz	229	0.0	16.0
whole, raw	1 oz	67	0.0	5.1
whole, roasted	3 oz	248	0.0	18.2
whole, roasted, diced	1 cup	394	0.0	28.9
SIRLOIN				
Fresh				
Trimmed				
chop, bone in, braised	3 oz	167	0.0	7.7

Food Name	Serv. Size	Total Cal.	Carbs GMS	Fat GMS
chop, bone in, broiled	3 oz	181	0.0	8.6
chop, boneless, braised	3 oz	149	0.0	5.6
chop, boneless, broiled	3 oz	164	0.0	5.7
chop, boneless, raw	1 lb	581	0.0	19.1
chop or roast, raw	1 oz	43	0.0	1.9
roast, bone in, roasted	3 oz	184	0.0	8.8
roast, boneless, roasted	3 oz	168	0.0	7.0
Untrimmed				
chop, bone in, braised	3 oz	208	0.0	12.8
chop, bone in, broiled	3 oz	220	0.0	13.7
chop, boneless, braised	3 oz	161	0.0	7.1
chop, boneless, broiled	3 oz	177	0.0	7.3
chop or roast, raw	1 oz	78	0.0	6.3
roast, bone in, roasted	3 oz	222	0.0	13.6
roast, boneless, roasted	3 oz	176	0.0	8.0
SPARERIBS				
Fresh				
Untrimmed				
braised	3 oz	337	0.0	25.8
raw	1 oz	81	0.0	6.7
Refrigerated or frozen, raw, 'Gourmet' *(JM)*	4.5 oz	250	0.0	22.0
SPLEEN				
Fresh				
braised	3 oz	127	0.0	2.7
raw	1 oz	28	0.0	0.7
STOMACH				
Fresh				
raw	4 oz	177	0.0	10.8
raw	1 oz	45	0.0	2.7
TAIL				
Fresh				
raw	4 oz	427	0	37.9
raw	1 oz	107	0	9.5
simmered	3 oz	337	0	30.4
TENDERLOIN				
Fresh				
Trimmed				
broiled	3 oz	159	0.0	5.4
raw	1 lb	544	0.0	15.5
raw	1 oz	34	0.0	1.0
roasted	3 oz	139	0.0	4.1
roasted, chopped or diced	1 cup	232	0.0	6.7
Untrimmed				
broiled	3 oz	171	0.0	6.9
raw	1 oz	39	0.0	1.5
roasted	3 oz	147	0.0	5.1
Refrigerated, boneless *(JM)*	3 oz	120	0.0	5.0
TONGUE				
Canned, cured, '8-lb. can' *(Hormel)*	3 oz	190	0	13.0
Fresh				
braised	3 oz	230	0	15.8
raw	4 oz	254	0	19.4
raw	1 oz	64	0	4.9
TOP LOIN				
Fresh				
Trimmed				
chop or roast, raw	1 oz	46	0.0	2.1
chop, boneless, braised	3 oz	172	0.0	7.3

Food Name	Serv. Size	Total Cal.	Carbs GMS	Fat GMS
chop, boneless, broiled	3 oz	173	0.0	6.6
chop, boneless, pan-fried in vegetable oil	4 oz	291	0.0	17.4
chop, boneless, pan-fried	3 oz	191	0.0	8.9
roast, boneless, raw	1 oz	40	0.0	1.5
roast, boneless, roasted	3 oz	165	0.0	6.1
roast, boneless, roasted, chopped	1 cup	343	0.0	19.3
Untrimmed				
chop, boneless, braised	3 oz	198	0.0	10.8
chop, boneless, broiled	3 oz	195	0.0	9.6
chop, boneless, pan-fried in vegetable oil	3 oz	337	0.0	28.6
chop, boneless, pan-fried	3 oz	218	0.0	12.6
chop or roast, boneless, raw	1 oz	54	0.0	3.3
roast, boneless, roasted	3 oz	192	0.0	9.7
roast, boneless, roasted, chopped	1 cup	462	0.0	35.2
PORK, SALT				
cured *(Hormel)*	2 oz	320	0.0	33.0
cured, raw	8 oz	1698	0.0	182.7
cured, raw	1 oz	212	0.0	22.8
PORK AND BEANS. See under BAKED BEANS, CANNED.				
PORK DINNER/ENTRÉE				
(Armour) brain, in milk gravy	2.75 oz	110	1.0	8.0
(Banquet) cutlet	1 entrée	420	38	25.0
(Bryan Foods) puréed	1/3 cup	140	0	11.0
(Chun King) sweet and sour, frozen	13 oz	400	78	5.0
(Cook's) picnic, smoked, whole, super trim, water added	3 oz	160	1	13.0
(Healthy Choice) patty, grilled, glazed	1 entrée	300	44	6.0
(Hormel)				
loin fillet, lemon garlic, 'Always Tender'	1 oz	33	1	1.2
loin fillet, lemon garlic, 'Always Tender'	4 oz	132	2	4.7
steak, breaded, frozen	3 oz	220	11	15.0
tenderlion, peppercorn, 'Always Tender'	4 oz	123	2	4.3
tenderloin, teriyaki, 'Always Tender'	4 oz	134	5	3.4
(John Morrell)				
back rib, barbecued, frozen 'Classics'	4.75 oz	240	8	17.0
chop, center cut, barbecued, frozen	4.5 oz	230	7	9.0
loin, thin sliced, barbecued, frozen	5 slices	150	5	6.0
tenderloin, barbecued, frozen, 'Pork Classics'	3 oz	130	3	5.0
(La Choy)				
chow mein, bi-pack	1 cup	78	9	2.2
sweet and sour, frozen, food service product	1 cup	241	43	6.2
(Lloyds)				
baby back rib, w/barbecue sauce, fully cooked	3 ribs	350	17	23.0
sparerib, w/barbecue sauce, fully cooked	3 ribs	380	13	27.0
(Marie Callender's) chop, country fried	15 oz	550	50	27.0
(Pierre)				
nuggets, breaded, frozen, product 1921	1 piece	42	2	2.8
patty, country fried, frozen, product 1920	1 piece	279	14	18.7
patty, country fried, frozen, product 3701	1 piece	241	13	15.0
patty, country fried, frozen, product 3801	1 piece	242	13	15.0
steak, country fried, frozen, product 3700	1 piece	293	15	18.7
steak, country fried, frozen, product 3800	1 piece	370	17	25.0
(Swanson) loin, frozen	10.75 oz	280	27	12.0
(Tyson)				
patty, deluxe, frozen, 'Looney Tunes Porky Pig'	6.5 oz	370	48	14.0
(Wonderbites)				
and turkey, barbecue, flame broiled, product 9119, 'Lean Magic 30'	1 piece	132	8	4.1

Food Name	Serv. Size	Total Cal.	Carbs GMS	Fat GMS
barbecue, flame broiled, product 1830	1 piece	207	3	16.2
barbecue, flame broiled, product 3734	1 piece	153	3	8.6
barbecue, flame broiled, product 3735	1 piece	36	1	2.0
barbecue, flame broiled, product 3834	1 piece	152	3	9.0
barbecue, flame broiled, product 3835, 'Dippers'	1 piece	41	1	2.9
barbecue, flame broiled, product 9800	1 piece	184	3	11.8
barbecue, flame broiled, product 9966, 'Dippers'	1 piece	44	1	2.9
barbecue, flame broiled, w/100 serving trays, product 9968	1 piece	50	1	3.6
barbecue, less fat, flame broiled, product 3730	1 piece	35	1	1.8
barbecue, less fat, flame broiled, product 3731	1 piece	140	3	7.4
barbecue, ready to cook, product 1190	1 piece	224	4	18.7
barbecue, ready to cook, product 1330	1 piece	267	5	22.7
Oriental crunch, flame-broiled, frozen,'Dippers'	1 piece	90	5	6.2
Oriental crunch, product 3702	1 piece	87	5	5.9
rib, barbecue, flame broiled, frozen, product 3736	1 piece	40	2	1.8
rib, barbecue, flame broiled, product 1805, 'Lean Magic'	1 piece	160	8	6.7
rib, barbecue, flame broiled, product 1809, 'Lean Magic'	1 piece	47	2	2.6
rib, flame broiled, frozen, product 3831, 'Lean Magic'	1 piece	132	3	6.3
(Rib-B-Q) rib, barbecue, flame broiled, product 3830, 'Lean Magic'	1 piece	39	1	2.5
teriyaki, flame broiled, product 3759	1 piece	45	2	2.3
PORK FAT				
leaf, raw	1 oz	243	0.0	26.7
leaf, fresh	4 oz	968	0.0	106.4
separable fat from fully cooked ham, roasted	1 oz	167	0.0	17.5
separable fat from fully cooked ham, unheated	1 oz	164	<.1	17.4
separable fat from ham and arm picnic, roasted	3 oz	502	0.0	52.6
separable fat from ham and arm picnic, roasted	1 oz	168	0.0	17.5
separable fat from ham and arm picnic, unheated	1 oz	164	0.0	17.4
PORK SEASONING. See under SEASONING MIX.				
PORK SEASONING AND COATING MIX. See under SEASONING AND COATING MIX.				
PORK SKINS				
barbecue	1 oz	153	0	9.0
barbecue	1/2 oz	76	0	4.5
plain	1 oz	155	0	8.9
plain	1/2 oz	77	0	4.4
PORK SUBSTITUTE				
(Worthington) vegetarian, 'Choplets'	2 slices	90	3	1.5
POT ROAST SEASONING. See under SEASONING MIX.				
POTATO				
Canned				
(Stokely)	1/2 cup	50	11	0.0
(Veg-All)	1/2 cup	60	13	0.0
diced (Bush's Best)	1/2 cup	40	8	0.0
diced (Taylor's Brand)	1 cup	90	25	0.0
new, extra small, whole (IGA)	1/2 cup	45	9	0.0
new, small, whole (IGA)	1/2 cup	45	9	0.0
new, whole, drained (Hunt's)	4 oz	70	15	1.0
sliced (Bush's Best)	1/2 cup	40	8	0.0
sliced (Taylor's Brand)	1 cup	90	25	0.0
sliced, w/liquid (Del Monte)	1/2 cup	45	10	0.0
white, diced (Allens)	1/2 cup	45	10	1.0
white, double diced (Allens)	1/2 cup	45	10	1.0
white, sliced (A&P)	1/2 cup	45	11	1.0
white, sliced (Allens)	1/2 cup	45	10	1.0
white, sliced, no salt added (Pathmark)	1 cup	100	20	0.0

Food Name	Serv. Size	Total Cal.	Carbs GMS	Fat GMS
white, small, sliced *(Finast)*	1/2 cup	55	13	0.0
white, small, whole *(Finast)*	1/2 cup	55	13	0.0
white, whole *(A&P)*	1/2 cup	45	11	1.0
white, whole, no salt added *(Pathmark)*	1 cup	100	20	0.0
whole *(Bush's Best)*	1/2 cup	40	8	0.0
whole *(Stokely)*	2/3 cup	70	14	0.0
whole, w/liquid *(Del Monte)*	1/2 cup	45	10	0.0
Dried, slices and dices, rehydrated *(Basic American)*	1/2 cup	72	16	0.1
Fresh				
baked, flesh and skin, 2 1/3 x 4 3/4 inch	1 potato	220	51	0.2
baked, flesh only	1/2 cup	57	13	0.1
baked, flesh only, 2 1/3 x 4 3/4 inch	1 potato	145	34	0.2
boiled, cooked in skin, flesh only	1/2 cup	68	16	0.1
boiled, cooked in skin, flesh only, 2.5 inch diam	1 potato	118	27	0.1
boiled, cooked w/o skin, flesh only	1/2 cup	67	16	0.1
boiled, cooked w/o skin, flesh only, 2.5 inch diam	1 potato	116	27	0.1
Finnish yellow, raw *(Frieda's)*	3.5 oz	100	22.0	na
microwaved, cooked in skin, flesh and skin, 2.5 inch diam	1 potato	212	49	0.2
microwaved, cooked in skin, flesh and skin	1/2 cup	78	18	0.1
microwaved, cooked in skin, flesh/skin, 2-1/3 x 4.75 inch	1 potato	156	36	0.2
raw, diced, flesh and skin	1/2 cup	59	13	0.1
raw, sliced	1 cup	142	32	0.3
raw, whole, large, 3–4.25 inch diam, flesh and skin	1 potato	145	33	0.2
raw, whole, long, 2 1/3 x 4 3/4 inch, flesh and skin	1 potato	160	36	0.2
raw, whole, medium, 2.25–3 inch diam, flesh and skin	1 potato	96	22	0.1
raw, whole, small, 1.75–2.25 inch diam, flesh and skin	1 potato	73	17	0.1
skin, baked	1 skin	115	27	0.1
skin, boiled	1 skin	27	6	0.0
skin, microwaved	1 skin	77	17	0.1
skin, raw	1 skin	22	5	0.0
Frozen				
red, whole, 2 to 3 potatoes *(C&W)*	85 grams	60	15	0.0
redskin, diced, frozen *(Flav-R-Pac)*	3/4 cup	60	16	0.0
redskin, tri-cut, frozen *(Flav-R-Pac)*	2/3 cup	60	15	0.0
redskin, wedges, frozen *(Flav-R-Pac)*	3/4 cup	60	15	0.0
skin, baked *(Tato Skins)*	1 oz	150	17	8.0
white, whole *(Southern)*	3.5 oz	69	15	0.1
white, whole, boiled *(Seabrook)*	3.2 oz	60	13	0.0
whole, small *(Ore-Ida)*	3 oz	70	16	1.0

POTATO CHIPS AND SNACKS
CHIPS

(Auburn Farms)

Food Name	Serv. Size	Total Cal.	Carbs GMS	Fat GMS
barbecue, nonfat	1 oz	100	23	0.0
Cajun, nonfat	1 oz	99	23	0.0
cheddar cheese, 96% fat free, Spudbakes'	1 oz	100	22	1.0
cheddar, nonfat	1 oz	99	22	0.0
mesquite barbecue, 98% fat free, Spudbakes'	1 oz	110	25	0.5
original, nonfat	1 oz	99	23	0.0
sour cream and onion, 98% fat free, Spudbakes'	1 oz	100	21	0.5
sour cream and onion, nonfat	1 oz	99	22	0.0

(Bachman)

Food Name	Serv. Size	Total Cal.	Carbs GMS	Fat GMS
barbecue flavor	1 oz	150	14	9.0
barbecue flavor, hot	1 oz	150	14	9.0
'Kettle Cooked'	1 oz	140	16	8.0
plain	1 oz	160	14	10.0
'Ridge'	1 oz	160	14	10.0
'Ruffled'	1 oz	160	14	10.0

Food Name	Serv. Size	Total Cal.	Carbs GMS	Fat GMS
Saratoga style, 'Kettle Cooked'	1 oz	140	16	8.0
sour cream and onion flavor	1 oz	150	14	9.0
unsalted	1 oz	160	14	10.0
vinegar flavor	1 oz	150	15	9.0
(Barbara's Bakery)				
herb and garlic, 'True Blues'	1 oz	140	15	9.0
no salt added	1 1/4 cup	150	15	10.0
plain	1 1/4 cup	150	15	10.0
rippled	1 1/4 cup	150	15	10.0
yogurt and green onion	1 1/4 cup	150	15	9.0
yogurt and green onion, no salt added	1 1/4 cup	150	15	9.0
(Barrel O'Fun) plain	1 oz	150	14	10.0
(Cape Cod)				
dill and sour cream flavor	1 oz	150	16	8.0
dill and sour cream flavor, no salt added	1 oz	150	16	8.0
no salt added	1 oz	150	16	8.0
plain	1 oz	150	16	8.0
plain, 'Selects'	1 oz *(19 chips)*	130	18	6.0
sea salt and vinegar, approx 18 chips	1 oz	150	17	8.0
sour cream and chives, approx 18 chips	1 oz	150	15	9.0
'Waves'	1 oz	150	16	8.0
(Cottage Fries) no salt added	1 oz	160	14	11.0
(Eagle)				
barbecue flavor, 'Extra Crunchy'	1 oz	150	16	8.0
barbecue flavor, 'Extra Crunchy Louisiana'	1 oz	150	16	8.0
barbecue flavor, 'Thins'	1 oz	150	15	10.0
cheddar and sour cream, rippled, crispy	1 oz	160	14	11.0
'Eagle Thins'	1 oz	150	15	10.0
'Extra Crunchy'	1 oz	150	16	8.0
extra crunchy, 'Hawaiian Kettle'	1 oz	150	17	8.0
Idaho russet	1 oz	150	16	8.0
Idaho russet, dark and crunchy	1 oz	140	17	7.0
mesquite BBQ, rippled	1 oz	160	15	10.0
'Ridged Thins'	1 oz	150	15	10.0
ripple chips	1 oz	150	14	10.0
sour cream and onion flavor, 'Ridged'	1 oz	150	15	10.0
sour cream and onion flavor, thins	1 oz	160	14	10.0
spicy, fiesta thins	1 oz	160	15	9.0
thins, no salt added	1 oz	150	14	10.0
(Featherweight) low salt	1 oz	160	14	11.0
(Great Snackers)				
barbecue flavor	1 serving	60	8	3.0
cheddar cheese flavor	1 serving	60	8	3.0
sour cream and onion	0.5 oz	70	10	3.0
toasted onion flavor	1 serving	60	8	3.0
(Guiltless Gourmet)				
baked, less salt	1 oz	110	22	1.5
baked, seasoned salt	1 oz	110	22	1.5
barbecue, baked	1 oz	110	22	1.5
sour cream and onion	1 oz	110	22	1.5
(Health Valley)				
'Country Dip'	1 oz	160	15	10.0
'Country Ripple'	1 oz	160	15	10.0
'Country'	1 oz	160	15	10.0
'Natural'	1 oz	160	15	10.0
no salt added, 'Country Dip'	1 oz	160	15	10.0
no salt added, 'Country Natural'	1 oz	160	15	10.0

Food Name	Serv. Size	Total Cal.	Carbs GMS	Fat GMS
no salt added, 'Country Ripple'	1 oz	160	15	10.0
no salt added, 'Country'	1 oz	160	15	10.0
(Keebler)				
lightly seasoned	1 oz	140	18	7.0
sour cream and onion	1 oz	140	17	7.0
(Kettle Chips)				
jalapeño Jack	1 oz	150	15	9.0
lightly salted	1 oz	150	15	9.0
New York cheddar	1 oz	150	15	9.0
no salt added	1 oz	150	15	9.0
organically grown, w/sea salt	1 oz	150	15	9.0
salsa w/mesquite	1 oz	150	15	9.0
sea salt and vinegar	1 oz	150	15	9.0
yogurt and green onion	1 oz	150	15	9.0
(King Kold)				
'Rip-L'	1 oz	150	16	9.0
au gratin flavor	1 oz	150	15	8.0
barbecue flavor 'BBQ'	1 oz	140	16	8.0
dill flavor	1 oz	150	16	8.0
onion-garlic flavor	1 oz	150	15	9.0
plain	1 oz	150	16	9.0
sour cream and onion flavor	1 oz	150	15	10.0
(Lay's)				
au gratin, wavy	1 oz	150	14	10.0
baked, low-fat	1 oz	110	23	1.5
barbecue flavor, approx. 15-20 chips	1 oz	150	15	9.0
barbecue flavor, baked, low-fat, 'KC Masterpiece'	1 oz	120	22	3.0
barbecue flavor, 'KC Masterpiece'	1 oz	160	15	10.0
Cajun flavor, 'Crunch Tators Amazin Cajun'	1 oz	150	17	8.0
cheddar cheese flavor, 15–20 chips	1 oz	150	14	10.0
cheddar, deli style	1 oz	150	16	10.0
chili, deli style	1 oz	150	16	10.0
deli style	1 oz	150	16	10.0
'Flamin' Hot' 15–20 chips	1 oz	150	15	9.0
jalapeño flavor, 'Crunch Tators Hoppin' Jalapeño'	1 oz	140	18	7.0
mesquite barbecue flavor 'Crunch Tators Mighty Mesquite'	1 oz	150	17	8.0
original	1 oz	150	15	10.0
original, 'Crunch Tators' approx 16 chips	1 oz	150	17	8.0
ranch flavor, wavy	1 oz	160	14	11.0
salt and vinegar flavor	1 oz	150	15	10.0
sour cream and onion	1 oz	150	15	9.0
sour cream and onion, baked, lowfat	1 oz	120	21	3.0
tangy ranch flavor, approx 15–20 chips	1 oz	160	15	10.0
unsalted	1 oz	150	15	10.0
wavy	1 oz	160	15	10.0
(Louise's)				
barbecue, nonfat	1 oz	110	23	0.0
Maui onion, nonfat	1 oz	110	24	0.0
mesquite barbecue flavor	1 oz	100	23	1.0
nonfat, no salt added	1 oz	110	24	0.0
original	1 oz	100	23	1.0
original, nonfat	1 oz	110	23	0.0
vinegar and salt flavor	1 oz	100	23	1.0
vinegar and salt, nonfat	1 oz	110	23	0.0
(Michael Season's)				
baked, less salt	1 oz	110	21	1.5
French onion flavor, baked	1 serving	110	21	1.5

Food Name	Serv. Size	Total Cal.	Carbs GMS	Fat GMS
hickory barbecue, baked	1 oz	110	21	1.5
honey barbecue	1 oz	140	20	6.0
honey barbecue, 40% less fat	1 oz	140	20	6.0
less fat, rippled	1 oz	140	17	6.7
lightly salted, 40% less fat	1 oz	130	17	6.0
no salt added, 40% less fat	1 oz	130	17	6.0
yogurt and green onion, 40% lower fat	1 oz	130	17	6.0
(Mr. Phipps)				
barbecue, tater crisps	0.5 oz	60	10	2.0
sour cream 'n onion, tater crisps	0.5 oz	60	10	2.0
(Munchos) plain, approx 16 chips	1 oz	160	15	10.0
(Nabisco)				
baked, baked, snack chips, 'Zings'	0.5 oz	70	10	3.0
cheese, cheddar, baked, cracker chips, 'Zings'	0.5 oz	70	9	3.0
cheese, cheddar, cracker chips, 'Zings'	15 pieces	70	9	3.0
ranch, baked, cracker chips, 'Zings'	0.5 oz	70	9	3.0
(O'Boisies)				
plain	1 oz	150	16	9.0
sour cream and onion flavor	1 oz	150	15	9.0
(Pacific Grain)				
'Rancho-O's'	1 oz	130	22	1.0
baked, 100% natural	1 oz	120	23	1.0
BBQ, baked, 100% natural	1 oz	120	23	2.0
(Poore Brothers)				
barbecue	1 oz	150	15	10.0
Cajun	1 oz	140	16	8.0
dill pickle	1 oz	140	16	8.0
grilled steak and onion	1 oz	140	15	8.0
jalapeño	1 oz	140	16	9.0
Parmesan and garlic	1 oz	140	16	9.0
regular	1 oz	140	17	8.0
salt and vinegar	1 oz	140	15	9.0
unsalted	1 oz	140	17	8.0
(Pringle's)				
barbecue flavor, 'Light'	1 oz	150	17	8.0
barbecue flavor, 'Right Crisp'	1 oz	140	18	7.0
cheddar and sour cream, 'Ridges'	1 oz	150	15	10.0
'Cheez Ums'	1 oz	150	14	10.0
French onion flavor, 'Idaho Rippled'	1 oz	170	13	12.0
'Idaho Rippled'	1 oz	170	13	12.0
'Light'	1 oz	150	17	8.0
mesquite barbecue, 'Ridges'	1 oz	150	15	10.0
mesquite barbecue, ridged	1 oz	150	15	10.0
original flavor, 1/3 less fat	16 chips	140	19	7.0
ranch flavor, 'Light'	1 oz	150	17	8.0
ranch	1 oz	150	15	10.0
ranch, 'Right Crisp'	1 oz	140	18	7.0
'Right Crisp'	1 oz	140	19	7.0
sour cream and onion	1 oz	160	15	10.0
sour cream and onion, 'Right Crisp'	1 oz	140	18	7.0
taco and cheddar flavor, 'Idaho Rippled'	1 oz	170	13	12.0
(Ruffles)				
barbecue flavor	1 oz	150	16	9.0
barbecue, mesequite, 'KC Masterpiece'	1 oz	150	15	9.0
Cajun flavor, 'Cajun Spice'	1 oz	150	15	10.0
cheddar and sour cream	1 oz	160	14	10.0
40% less fat 'Choice' approx 16 chips	1 oz	130	18	6.0

Food Name	Serv. Size	Total Cal.	Carbs GMS	Fat GMS
French onion flavor	1 oz	150	15	10.0
low-fat	1 oz	130	18	6.7
mesquite barbecue flavor, 'Mesquite Grille'	1 oz	160	14	10.0
1/3 less fat, 'Light Choice'	1 oz	130	19	6.0
original	1 serving	150	14	10.0
ranch flavor	1 oz	150	15	9.0
sour cream and onion flavor	1 oz	150	15	9.0
(Snacktime)				
jalapeño flavor, 'Krunchers!'	1 oz	150	16	9.0
'Krunchers!'	1 oz	150	16	9.0
mesquite barbecue flavor, 'Krunchers!'	1 oz	150	16	9.0
(Spicer's)				
barbecue wheat, for weight control	1 oz	100	12	5.0
dietetic, natural, for weight control	1 oz	100	11	4.0
sour cream and onion, for weight control	1 oz	100	12	4.0
(Tato Skins)				
cheese and bacon flavor, potato skins	1 oz	150	17	8.0
sour cream n' chives flavor, potato skins	1 oz	150	17	8.0
(Westbrae)				
potato chips, no salt added	1 oz	150	16	8.0
'Ripple'	1 oz	150	16	8.0
salted	1 oz	160	15	10.0
(Wise)				
barbecue flavor	1 oz	150	14	10.0
barbecue flavor, 'Ridgies'	1 oz	150	14	10.0
hot	1 oz	160	14	11.0
'New York Deli'	1 oz	160	14	11.0
onion-garlic flavor	1 oz	150	14	10.0
'Plain'	1 oz	150	14	10.0
'Ridgies Super Crispy'	1 oz	150	14	10.0
'Ridgies'	1 oz	150	14	10.0
'Rippled'	1 oz	150	14	10.0
sour cream and onion flavor 'Ridgies'	1 oz	160	14	11.0
(Zapp's)				
Cajun flavor, 'Lite Kettle'	1 oz	150	16	8.0
Cajun flavor, 'Original Kettle'	1 oz	150	16	8.0
jalapeño flavor, 'Original Kettle'	1 oz	150	16	8.0
'Lite Kettle'	1 oz	150	16	8.0
mesquite barbecue flavor, 'Lite Kettle'	1 oz	150	16	8.0
mesquite barbecue flavor, 'Original Kettle'	1 oz	150	16	8.0
no salt added, 'Lite Kettle'	1 oz	150	16	8.0
no salt added, 'Original Kettle'	1 oz	150	16	8.0
'Original Kettle'	1 oz	150	16	8.0
sour cream and onion flavor 'Lite'	1 oz	150	16	8.0
STICKS				
(Allens)				
shoestring, canned	1 oz	140	16	8.0
shoestring, no salt added, canned	1 oz	140	16	8.0
(Flavor Tree) sour cream and onion	1/4 cup	127	13	8.3
(Planters)				
	1 oz	160	15	10.0
barbecue flavor	1 oz	160	15	10.0
(S&W)				
fabulous fries, 'Pik-Nik'	2/3 cup	150	16	9.0
ketchup and fries, 'Pik-Nik'	2/3 cup	160	17	10.0
shoestring, 'Pik-Nik'	2/3 cup	280	26	18.0
shoestring, 50% less salt, 'Pik-Nik'	3/4 cup	165	16	12.0

Food Name	Serv. Size	Total Cal.	Carbs GMS	Fat GMS
shoestring, Sante Fe BBQ, 'Pik-Nik'	2/3 cup	180	18	12.0
shoestring, sour cream and cheddar, 'Pik-Nik'	2/3 cup	180	17	13.0
POTATO DISH/ENTRÉE				
(A&P)				
fried, crinkle cut	3.5 oz	140	25.0	4.0
fried, regular	3.5 oz	140	25.0	4.0
fried, shoestring	3.5 oz	170	24.0	6.0
fried, steak fries	3.5 oz	140	24.0	4.0
hash brown	3.5 oz	80	17.0	0.0
morsels	3.5 oz	140	23.0	4.0
(Basic American)				
au gratin, 'Classic Casseroles'	3 oz	81	13	2.6
hash brown, 'Golden Grill'	1/2 cup	118	13	6.8
hash brown, 'ReddiShred'	1/2 cup	134	16	6.8
scalloped, 'Classic Casseroles'	3 oz	81	13	2.3
(Bernardi) gnocchi, uncooked	2/3 cup	281	56	2.0
(Budget Gourmet)				
w/broccoli, cheese sauce, frozen, 'Light and Healthy'	10.5 oz	300	40	10.0
(Crispy Crowns) puffs, frozen, prepared	10 puffs	133	18	6.4
(Empire Kosher)				
potato pancake, triangle, latkes w/onions, frozen	2 oz	77	13.0	2.4
(Healthy Choice)				
casserole, frozen, 'Garden Style'	1 meal	200	30	4.0
cheddar broccoli, w/cheese Sauce, frozen	1 pkg	328	53	7.0
garden casserole	1 serving	220	30	6.0
w/broccoli and cheddar cheese	1 entrée	330	53	7.0
(Heinz)				
fried, crinkle cut 'Deep Fries'	3 oz	150	22.0	6.0
fried 'Deep Fries'	3 oz	160	23.0	6.0
fried, shoestring 'Deep Fries'	3 oz	200	25.0	10.0
hash brown, w/butter and onions 'Deep Fries'	3 oz	110	14.0	7.0
(Hormel) scalloped, w/ham, microwaveable	1 cup	240	20	14.0
(Joan of Arc)				
salad, German style, canned	1/2 cup	120	23.0	3.0
salad, homestyle, canned	1/2 cup	340	32.0	22.0
(Lean Cuisine)				
baked, w/broccoli and cheddar, frozen	10 3/8 oz	290	37	9.0
baked, w/sour cream, frozen	10 3/8 oz	230	38	5.0
cheddar, 'Deluxe'	1 entrée	230	32	6.0
roasted, w/broccoli, cheddar cheese sauce	1 entrée	260	39	6.0
scalloped	1 entrée	250	38	6.0
(Lunch Bucket) scalloped, microwave cup	7.5 oz	160	20	7.0
(MicroMagic)				
fried	3 oz	290	40.0	13.0
fried, skinny	3 oz	350	49.0	15.0
sticks, 'Tater Sticks'	4 oz	390	43.0	22.0
(Mountain House) hash brown, freeze-dried, prepared	1 cup	150	36.0	0.0
(Ore-Ida)				
fried, cottage cut	3 oz	120	19.0	5.0
fried, 'Country Style Dinner Fries'	3 oz	110	19.0	3.0
fried, crinkle cut, 'Golden Crinkles'	3 oz	120	19.0	4.0
fried, crinkle cut, 'Lites'	3 oz	90	16.0	2.0
fried, crinkle cut, microwave	3.5 oz	180	26.0	8.0
fried, crinkle cut, 'Pixie Crinkles'	3 oz	140	21.0	6.0
fried, 'Crisp Crowns'	3 oz	160	20.0	9.0
fried, 'Crispers!'	3 oz	230	25.0	15.0
fried, French, extra crispy 'Nacho Crispers'	3 oz	180	21.0	10.0

Food Name	Serv. Size	Total Cal.	Carbs GMS	Fat GMS
fried, French, 'Fast Fries'	3 oz	150	23.0	7.0
fried, 'Golden Fries'	3 oz	120	19.0	4.0
fried, 'Lites'	3 oz	90	16.0	2.0
fried, shoestring	3 oz	140	21.0	6.0
fried, shoestring, 'Lites'	3 oz	90	15.0	4.0
fried, wedges, 'Home Style Potato Wedges'	3 oz	100	17.0	3.0
fried, w/onions, 'Crispy Crowns'	3 oz	170	20.0	9.0
hash brown, 'Golden Patties'	2.5 oz	140	15.0	8.0
hash brown, microwave	2 oz	130	12.0	8.0
hash brown, shredded	3 oz	70	15.0	<1.0
hash brown, 'Southern Style'	3 oz	70	16.0	<1.0
hashbrown, w/cheddar, 'Cheddar Browns'	3 oz	90	13.0	2.0
puffs, bacon flavored 'Tater Tots'	3 oz	140	19.0	6.0
puffs 'Tater Tots'	3 oz	140	19.0	7.0
puffs, microwave, 'Tater Tots'	4 oz	200	29.0	9.0
puffs, w/onion, 'Tater Tots'	3 oz	140	19.0	6.0
(Pik-Nik) shoestring	1 oz	160	15	10.3
(Quick 'n Crispy)				
fried, crinkle cut	4 oz	370	44.0	19.0
fried, shoestring	4 oz	390	48.0	20.0
fried, thin cuts	4 oz	370	44.0	19.0
wedges	4 oz	280	36.0	13.0
(Read)				
salad, German style, canned	1/2 cup	120	23.0	3.0
salad, homestyle, canned	1/2 cup	340	32.0	22.0
(Seabrook)				
fried	3 oz	120	20.0	4.0
fried, cottage cut	2.8 oz	110	17.0	4.0
fried, crinkle cut	3 oz	120	20.0	4.0
fried, shoestring	3 oz	140	20.0	6.0
(Stouffer's)				
au gratin	1/2 cup	130	15	6.0
au gratin, frozen, food service product	1 oz	32	4	1.3
scalloped	1/2 cup	140	17	6.0
scalloped, frozen, food service product	1 oz	31	4	1.3
(Weight Watchers)				
baked, vegetable primavera, frozen	11.15 oz	320	49	9.0
baked, w/broccoli and ham, frozen	11.5 oz	240	30	5.0
baked, w/turkey, homestyle, frozen	11.25 oz	230	27	7.0
w/broccoli and cheese	1 serving	250	35	7.0
POTATO DISH/ENTRÉE MIX				
(Arrowhead Mills) Western, flakes	2 oz	140	44.0	0.0
(Barbara's Bakery)				
mashed, mix only	1/3 cup	70	17	0.0
Western, mix only	4 oz	389	89.0	1.0
(Betty Crocker)				
au gratin, prepared w/margarine and skim milk	1/2 cup	150	21.0	5.0
hash brown, mix only	1/2 cup	120	30	0.0
hash brown, w/onions, prepared w/margarine	1/2 cup	160	24.0	6.0
hash brown, w/onions, prepared	1/6 pkg	110	24.0	1.0
mashed, cheddar cheese, 'Potato Buds' mix only	1/12 pkg	110	20.0	2.0
mashed, cheddar cheese, 'Potato Buds' prepared	1/2 cup	180	21.0	9.0
mashed, cheddar cheese, 'Potato Buds' reduced fat recipe, mix only	1/12 pkg	140	21.0	5.0
mashed, 'Potato Buds' mix only	1/3 cup	80	18	0.0
mashed, 'Potato Buds' prepared w/o added salt	1/2 cup	130	17.0	6.0
mashed, 'Potato Buds' prepared	1/2 cup	130	17.0	6.0

Food Name	Serv. Size	Total Cal.	Carbs GMS	Fat GMS
scalloped, cheesy, mix only	1/6 pkg	90	19.0	1.0
scalloped, cheesy, prepared	1/2 cup	140	20.0	5.0
scalloped, mix only	1/6 pkg	90	19.0	1.0
scalloped, prepared	1/2 cup	140	20.0	5.0
scalloped, sour cream and chives, mix only	1/6 pkg	100	19.0	2.0
scalloped, sour cream and chives, prepared	1/2 cup	140	21.0	5.0
scalloped, w/ham, mix only	1/5 pkg	100	20.0	1.0
scalloped, w/ham, prepared	1/2 cup	160	22.0	6.0
stuffed, butter, herbed, 'Twice Baked' prepared	1/2 cup	220	20.0	13.0
stuffed, butter, herbed, 'Twice Baked' mix only	1/6 pkg	100	18.0	2.0
stuffed, cheddar, mild, w/onion, 'Twice Baked' mix only	1/6 pkg	100	18.0	2.0
stuffed, cheddar, mild, w/onion, 'Twice Baked' prepared	1/2 cup	190	19.0	11.0
stuffed, sour cream and chives, 'Twice Baked' mix only	1/6 pkg	90	17.0	2.0
stuffed, sour cream and chives, 'Twice Baked' prepared	1/2 cup	200	19.0	11.0
stuffed, w/bacon and cheddar, 'Twice Baked' mix only	1/6 pkg	110	19.0	2.0
stuffed, w/bacon and cheddar, 'Twice Baked' prepared	1/2 cup	210	21.0	11.0
(Country Store) mashed, prepared	1/3 cup	70	16.0	0.0
(Ener-G Foods) mix, gluten-free	1 cup	878	226	0.0
(Fantastic Foods)				
au gratin, prepared w/whole milk	1/2 cup	156	25.0	4.0
au gratin, prepared w/whole milk and salted butter	1/2 cup	196	25.0	8.0
country style, prepared	1/2 cup	85	19.0	0.3
country style, prepared w/salted butter	1/2 cup	118	19.0	4.0
(French's)				
au gratin, tangy, prepared	1/2 cup	130	20.0	5.0
casserole, cheddar and bacon, prepared	1/2 cup	130	18.0	5.0
scalloped, creamy Italian, prepared	1/2 cup	120	19.0	3.0
scalloped, crispy top, w/savory onion, prepared	1/2 cup	140	20.0	5.0
scalloped, real cheese, prepared	1/2 cup	140	19.0	5.0
scalloped, sour cream and chives, prepared	1/2 cup	150	19.0	7.0
Western, creamy, prepared	1/2 cup	130	20.0	4.0
(General Mills)				
au gratin, mix only	1/6 pkg	100	20.0	1.0
au gratin, prepared w/margarine and 2% milk	1/2 cup	150	21.0	6.0
au gratin, w/broccoli, homestyle, mix only	1/6 pkg	90	18.0	1.0
au gratin, w/broccoli, homestyle, prepared w/margarine and 2% milk	1/2 cup	140	19.0	6.0
hash brown	1/6 pkg	110	24.0	<1.0
hash brown, prepared w/margarine	1/2 cup	160	24.0	6.0
julienne, mix only	1/6 pkg	90	17.0	1.0
julienne, prepared w/margarine and 2% milk	1/2 cup	130	19.0	5.0
mashed, American cheese, homestyle, mix only	1/6 pkg	100	20.0	1.0
mashed, American cheese, homestyle, prepared w/margarine and 2% milk	1/2 cup	150	21.0	6.0
mashed, cheddar and bacon, mix only	1/6 pkg	100	20.0	1.0
mashed, cheddar and bacon, prepared w/margarine and 2% milk	1/2 cup	150	21.0	6.0
mashed, cheddar cheese, homestyle, mix only	1/6 pkg	90	19.0	1.0
mashed, cheddar cheese, homestyle, prepared w/margarine and 2% milk	1/2 cup	150	21.0	6.0
scalloped, mix only	1/6 pkg	90	19.0	1.0
scalloped, prepared w/margarine and 2% milk	1/2 cup	140	20.0	5.0
scalloped, smoky cheddar, mix only	1/6 pkg	100	20.0	1.0
scalloped, smoky cheddar, prepared w/margarine and 2% milk	1/2 cup	140	21.0	5.0
scalloped, sour cream and chive	1/6 pkg	100	19.0	2.0

Food Name	Serv. Size	Total Cal.	Carbs GMS	Fat GMS
scalloped, sour cream and chives, prepared				
w/margarine and 2% milk	1/2 cup	150	20.0	6.0
scalloped, w/ham, mix only	1/5 pkg	100	20.0	1.0
scalloped, w/ham, prepared w/margarine and 2% milk	1/2 cup	170	22.0	7.0
Western, cheesy, homestyle, mix only	1/6 pkg	100	19.0	2.0
Western, cheesy, homestyle, prepared w/margarine				
and 2% milk	1/2 cup	150	20.0	6.0
Western, potato buds, mix only	1/8 pkg	70	16.0	0.0
Western, potato buds, prepared w/o salt	1/2 cup	130	17.0	6.0
Western, potato buds, prepared	1/2 cup	130	17.0	6.0
(Hungry Jack)				
mashed, 'Flakes' prepared	1/2 cup	140	17.0	7.0
Western, flakes	13.3 oz	70	16.0	0.0
Western, flakes, prepared w/margarine, 2% milk, salt, water	1/2 cup	130	17.0	6.0
Western, flakes, prepared w/margarine, 2% milk, water	1/2 cup	130	17.0	6.0
(Idaho) potato pancake, prepared, 3 inch diam	3 pancakes	90	16	2.0
(Idaho Spuds)				
potato pancake, prepared, 3 inch diam	3 cakes	90	16.0	2.0
Western, flakes	13.3 oz	70	15.0	0.0
Western, granules	13.3 oz	60	14.0	0.0
Western, granules, prepared	1/2 cup	130	16.0	6.0
Western, granules, prepared w/margarine, 2% milk, water	1/2 cup	120	16.0	5.0
Western, granules, prepared w/margarine, 2% milk,				
salt, water	1/2 cup	120	16.0	5.0
(Idaho Spuds)				
Western, flakes, prepared	1/2 cup	140	17.0	7.0
Western, flakes, prepared w/margarine, 2% milk, water	1/2 cup	130	16.0	6.0
Western, flakes, prepared w/margarine, 2% milk, salt, water	1/2 cup	130	16.0	6.0
(Idahoan)				
au gratin, prepared	1/2 cup	130	18.0	5.0
hash brown, herb and butter, mix only	1/6 pkg	90	16.0	2.0
hash brown, prepared w/unsalted butter	1/2 cup	140	18.0	7.0
hash brown, 'Quick One-Pan' prepared	1/2 cup	140	18.0	7.0
mashed, cheddar, spicy, mix only	1/6 pkg	90	17.0	1.0
mashed, cheddar, spicy, prepared	1/2 cup	140	21.0	5.0
scalloped, prepared	1/2 cup	140	20.0	5.0
scalloped, prepared w/o added salt, w/unsalted butter	1/2 cup	140	16.0	7.0
scalloped, sour cream and chives, mix only	1/6 pkg	90	15.0	2.0
scalloped, sour cream and chives, prepared	1/2 cup	130	18.0	5.0
Western, 'Complete' mix only	1/3 cup	100	19.0	2.0
Western, mix only	1/3 cup	80	18.0	0.0
(Ore-Ida)				
mashed, natural butter flavor, prepared w/2% milk	1/2 cup	170	23.0	5.0
mashed, natural butter flavor, unprepared	2.25 oz	100	14.0	3.0
(Pillsbury)				
au gratin, tangy, 'Specially' mix only	1/6 pkg	90	19.0	1.0
au gratin, tangy, prepared w/butter and whole milk	1/2 cup	140	20.0	6.0
mashed, cheddar and bacon, 'Specialty' mix only	1/6 pkg	90	18.0	1.0
mashed, cheddar and bacon, 'Specialty' prepared w/butter				
and whole milk	1/2 cup	140	19.0	6.0
potato pancake, 'Specialty'	1/8 pkg	70	16.0	0.0
potato pancake, 'Specialty' prepared w/water and egg,				
3 inch diam each	3 cakes	90	16.0	2.0
scalloped, sour cream and chives, 'Specialty,' mix only	1/6 pkg	100	18.0	2.0
scalloped, sour cream and chives, 'Specialty,' prepared				
w/butter and whole milk	1/2 cup	150	20.0	6.0
Western, cheesy, 'Specialty' mix only	1/6 pkg	100	19.0	2.0

Food Name	Serv. Size	Total Cal.	Carbs GMS	Fat GMS
Western, cheesy, 'Specialty,' prepared w/butter, whole milk . . . . . 1/2 cup		150	20.0	6.0
Western, creamy white sauce, 'Specialty,' mix only . . . . 1/6 pkg		100	19.0	2.0
POTATO JUICE, bottled *(Biotta)* . . . . 6 fl oz		144	31	0.1
POTATO SALAD. See under POTATO DISH/ENTRÉE.				
POTATO SALAD DRESSING. See under SALAD DRESSING.				
POTATO SALAD SEASONING. See under SEASONING MIX.				
POTATO SEASONING. See under SEASONING MIX.				
POTATO STARCH *(Featherweight)* . . . . 1 cup		620	154	1.0
POTATO STICKS. See under POTATO CHIPS AND SNACKS.				
POTTED MEAT SPREAD				
(Armour) . . . . 1.83 oz		100	1	7.0
(Hormel) . . . . 1 oz		53	2	4.0
(Libby's) . . . . 1/4 cup		110	0	7.0
POULTRY SEASONING. See under SEASONING MIX.				
POWER BAR. See under SPORTS AND DIET/NUTRITION BAR.				
PRESERVES. See JAM AND PRESERVES.				
PRETZEL				
(A & Eagle) . . . . 1 oz		110	22	2.0
(Bachman)				
hard . . . . 1 oz		110	23	1.0
hard, unsalted . . . . 1 oz		110	23	1.0
logs . . . . 1 oz		110	21	2.0
'Nutzels' . . . . 1 oz		110	21	2.0
'Petite' . . . . 1 oz		110	21	2.0
rings . . . . 1 oz		110	21	2.0
rod . . . . 1 oz		110	21	2.0
sodium-free, 'Petite' . . . . 1 oz		110	21	2.0
thin . . . . 1 oz		110	21	2.0
thin, 'Thin'n Light' . . . . 1 oz		110	21	2.0
treats . . . . 1 oz		110	21	2.0
twist . . . . 1 oz		110	21	2.0
(Barbara's Bakery)				
Bavarian . . . . 2 pretzels		100	20	1.5
Bavarian, no salt added . . . . 2 pretzels		100	20	1.5
mini, no salt added . . . . 18 pretzels		100	21	1.5
mini, no salt added, 17 pretzels . . . . 1 oz		110	21	1.0
none-grain . . . . 2 pretzels		100	20	1.5
(Bearitos) stick, thin, organic . . . . 30 grams		110	24	0.5
(Benzel's Bretzles) tiny, thin . . . . 1 oz		104	23	0.0
(Cape Cod) multigrain, no fat . . . . 30 pretzels		110	25	0.0
(Delicious)				
party . . . . 1 oz		110	23	1.0
stick . . . . 1 oz		110	23	1.0
twist . . . . 1 oz		110	23	1.0
(Eagle)				
Bavarian, sourdough, no fat . . . . 1 oz		110	24	0.0
Bavarian, sourdough, no fat, no salt added . . . . 1 oz		110	24	0.0
mini bites, low-fat . . . . 1 oz		110	22	10.0
stick, low-fat . . . . 1 oz		110	24	1.0
twist, thin, low-fat . . . . 1 oz		110	22	10.0
twist, thin, no fat . . . . 1 oz		100	22	0.0
(Estee)				
Dutch style, unsalted . . . . 2 pretzels		110	23	1.0
unsalted . . . . 15 pretzels		75	16	1.0
unsalted . . . . 5 pretzels		25	5	1.0
(Featherweight) low-salt . . . . 20 pieces		110	23	1.0
(Harmony) yogurt coated . . . . 1/3 cup		140	21	5.0

Food Name	Serv. Size	Total Cal.	Carbs GMS	Fat GMS
(J&J Snack Foods)				
Bavarian, soft	1 pretzel	180	34	2.5
Bavarian, twist, soft	1 pretzel	210	41	3.0
cheese-filled, soft, 'Superpretzel'	1 pretzel	380	61	7.0
cinnamon-raisin, soft, king size, 'Superpretzel'	1 pretzel	390	76	4.0
cinnamon-raisin, soft, regular size, 'Superpretzel'	1 pretzel	190	38	2.0
cinnamon-raisin, w/icing, soft, king size, 'Superpretzel'	1 pretzel	420	85	4.0
cinnamon-raisin, w/icing, soft, regular size, 'Superpretzel'	1 pretzel	210	43	2.0
jalapeño, soft, 'Superpretzel'	1 pretzel	360	78	0.0
rod, sweet dough, soft	1 pretzel	300	60	3.0
soft, all natural, regular size	1 pretzel	190	41	0.0
soft, king size, 'Superpretzel'	1 pretzel	390	83	0.0
soft, no salt, frozen, 'Superpretzel'	1 pretzel	170	37	0.0
stick, cheese-filled, nacho, 'Superpretzel'	2 softstix	140	24	2.5
stick, cheese-filled, pizza, 'Superpretzel'	2 softstix	140	24	2.5
stick, sweet dough, soft	1 pretzel	170	34	1.5
(Keebler)				
braids, 'Butter Pretzels'	1 oz	110	21	1.0
knots, 'Butter Pretzels'	1 oz	110	21	1.0
(Louise's) sourdough, nonfat	1 oz	90	19	0.0
(M&M Mars) w/cheddar, 'Combos'	10 combos	130	20	5.1
(Michael Season's) mini	18 pretzels	120	21	1.0
(Mister Salty)				
Dutch style	2 pretzels	120	25	1.0
'Juniors'	1 oz	110	22	2.0
rings	1 oz	110	21	2.0
rings, butter flavor	1 oz	110	21	2.0
stick	1 oz	110	23	1.0
stick, butter flavor	1 oz	110	22	1.0
stick, nonfat	47 stick	110	23	0.0
stick, very thin, approx 92 pieces	1 oz	110	22	3.0
twist, nonfat	9 pieces	110	23	0.0
(Mr. Phipps)				
less salt	16 pretzels	120	21	2.5
original, nonfat	16 pretzels	100	22	0.0
(Mr. Salty)				
30% less sodium	88 stick	110	25	0.0
nonfat	16 pretzels	100	22	0.0
(Nabisco) chips, sesame	8 pieces	60	10	2.0
(Pepperidge Farm) 'Snack Stick'	8 pieces	120	23	3.0
(Quinlan)				
beer	1 oz	110	22	1.4
logs	1 oz	103	22	0.8
oat bran	1 oz	115	22	1.5
rice bran, no salt	1 oz	101	20	2.3
stick	1 oz	105	22	0.6
thin	1 oz	104	22	0.6
thin, 'Ultra Thin'	1 oz	106	23	0.6
tiny, thin	1 oz	109	21	1.5
tiny, thin, no salt	1 oz	115	22	1.6
(Rokeach)				
Dutch style	1 oz	110	24	0.0
Dutch style, unsalted	1 oz	110	20	0.0
'Party'	1 oz	110	23	1.0
unsalted, 'Baldies'	1 oz	110	20	0.0
(Rold Gold)				
baked, 33% less sodium	10 pretzels	110	23	0.0

Food Name	Serv. Size	Total Cal.	Carbs GMS	Fat GMS
Bavarian, 3 pretzels	1 oz	120	22	2.0
rod	1 oz	110	22	1.0
stick	1 oz	110	23	1.0
stick, nonfat	1 oz	110	23	0.0
thin twist	1 oz	110	23	1.0
thin, baked, 33% less sodium, fat-free'	1 oz	110	23	0.0
tiny, twist, nonfat	1 oz	100	23	0.0
'Tiny Tim'	1 oz	110	23	1.0
twist, thin, 10 twists	1 oz	110	23	1.0
(Seyfert's) rod, butter flavor	1 oz	110	21	1.0
(Snyder's) pieces, buttermilk ranch, sourdough	1 oz	130	19	5.0
(Ultra Slim Fast) twist	1 oz	100	21	1.0

PRICKLY PEAR

raw, sliced	1 cup	61	14	0.8
raw, whole, trimmed	1 medium	42	10	0.5

PROTEIN BAR. See under SPORTS AND DIET/NUTRITION BAR.

PRUNE

Canned

in heavy syrup, w/liquid	1 cup	246	65	0.5
in heavy syrup, w/liquid	5 medium	90	24	0.2

Dried

low-moisture, stewed	1 cup	316	83	0.7
low-moisture, uncooked	1 cup	447	118	1.0
pitted, stewed	1 cup	265	70	0.6
pitted, uncooked	1 cup	406	107	0.9
uncooked	1 medium	20	5	0.0

PRUNE JUICE

Canned or bottled

	1 cup	182	45	0.1
	1 fl oz	23	6	0.0
(Del Monte) unsweetened	6 fl oz	120	33	0.0
(J. Hungerford) 100% juice	9.03 fl oz	178	44	0.0
(Knudsen) organic	8 fl oz	170	42	0.0
(Lucky Leaf)	6 fl oz	150	36	0.0
(Mott's)				
	6 fl oz	130	32	0.0
country style	6 fl oz	130	32	0.0
(Pathmark)				
'All Natural'	6 fl oz	120	30	0.0
w/prune pulp, 'Homestyle'	6 fl oz	130	32	0.0
(S&W) unsweetened	6 fl oz	120	31	0.0
(SunSweet)	6 fl oz	130	33	0.0

PSYLLIUM FIBER, smooth texture (Metamucil) .... 1 heaping tsp | 20 | 5 | 0.0

PUDDING. See also PUDDING MIX; PUDDING/PIE FILLING MIX.

ALMOND

(Imagine Foods) nondairy, low-fat, 'Dream Pudding'	4 oz	150	31	2.0

BANANA

(Del Monte) 'Pudding Cup'	5 oz	180	30	5.0
(Hunt's) 'Snack Pack'	1/2 cup	158	25	5.8
(Imagine Foods) nondairy, 'Dream Pudding'	4 oz	120	30	0.0
(Lucky Leaf)	4 oz	150	24	5.0
(Musselman's)	4 oz	150	24	5.0

BUTTERSCOTCH

(Crowley)	4.5 oz	150	27	3.0
(Del Monte) 'Pudding Cup'	5 oz	180	31	5.0
(Featherweight)	1/2 cup	100	21	1.0

Food Name	Serv. Size	Total Cal.	Carbs GMS	Fat GMS
(Hunt's) 'Snack Pack'	4 oz	153	24	5.7
(Imagine Foods) nondairy	1 cup	150	31	3.0
(Lucky Leaf)	4 oz	170	26	7.0
(Musselman's)	4 oz	170	26	7.0
(Rich's) frozen	3 oz	130	18	6.0
(Ultra Slim Fast) 'Lite 'N Tasty'	4 oz	100	21	1.0
(White House)	3.5 oz	113	20	3.0
BUTTERSCOTCH-CHOCOLATE-VANILLA				
(Jell-O) swirl	4 oz	180	28	5.0
CARAMEL (Hershey's) caramello	4 oz	180	28	6.0
CAROB				
(Imagine Foods) nondairy, nonfat, 'Dream Pudding'	4 oz	130	31	0.0
CHOCOLATE				
(Crowley)	4.5 oz	190	29	3.0
(Del Monte)				
'Pudding Cup'	5 oz	190	31	6.0
'Pudding Snack Light'	4.25 oz	100	19	1.0
fudge, 'Pudding Cup'	5 oz	190	31	6.0
(Estee)	1/2 cup	70	12	1.0
(Featherweight)	1/2 cup	100	21	1.0
(Hershey's)				
	4 oz	180	29	5.0
fudge, 'Snack Pack'	4 oz	158	24	5.9
'Hershey's Special Dark'	4 oz	180	30	5.0
'Light' 'Snack Pack'	4 oz	100	20	2.0
milk chocolate variety, 'Snack Pack'	4 oz	166	26	5.9
nonfat, 'Snack Pack'	4 oz	96	21	0.4
'Snack Pack'	4 oz	161	25	5.9
(Imagine Foods) nondairy	1 cup	170	36	3.0
(Jell-O)				
	4 oz	170	28	6.0
fat free	1 serving	102	23	0.5
fudge	4 oz	170	28	6.0
fudge, 'Light Pudding Snacks'	4 oz	100	22	1.0
fudge, 'Pudding Snacks'	4 oz	170	28	6.0
fudge-milk chocolate swirl	4 oz	170	28	6.0
'Light Pudding Snacks'	4 oz	100	21	2.0
milk chocolate 'Pudding Snacks'	4 oz	170	29	6.0
nonfat	1 serving	100	23	0.0
nonfat, 'Free'	4 oz	100	24	0.0
(Lucky Leaf)				
	4 oz	180	27	7.0
fudge	4 oz	180	25	8.0
(Musselman's)				
	4 oz	180	27	7.0
fudge	4 oz	180	25	8.0
(Pathmark) 'No Frills'	5 oz	200	30	8.0
(Rich's) frozen	3 oz	140	18	7.0
(Swiss Miss)				
fudge	4 oz	175	28	5.6
fudge, 'Light'	4 oz	100	20	1.0
fudge, nonfat	1/2 cup	103	23	0.3
milk chocolate variety	4 oz	166	26	2.9
nonfat	1/2 cup	100	22	0.4
sundae	4 oz	220	36	7.0
(Ultra Slim Fast) chocolate	4 oz	100	21	1.0
(White House) chocolate	3.5 oz	120	22	4.0

Food Name	Serv. Size	Total Cal.	Carbs GMS	Fat GMS
CHOCOLATE ALMOND (Hershey's)	4 oz	180	29	6.0
CHOCOLATE AND VANILLA				
(Hershey's)				
'Kisses'	4 oz	180	29	6.0
'Kisses-Free'	4 oz	100	22	0.0
(Jell-O)				
'Light Pudding Snacks'	4 oz	100	21	2.0
nonfat	1 serving	100	23	0.0
swirl	4 oz	170	28	6.0
swirl, 'Free'	4 oz	100	24	0.0
swirl, 'Pudding Snacks'	4 oz	180	28	6.0
swirl, variety pack	1 snack	100	23	0.0
(Swiss Miss)				
parfait, 'Light'	4 oz	100	20	1.0
nonfat	1/2 cup	104	23	0.3
chocolate-vanilla-chocolate swirl	4 oz	172	27	6.0
variety	4 oz	171	27	6.0
CHOCOLATE-CARAMEL				
(Hunt's) swirl, 'Snack Pack'	4 oz	165	25	5.9
(Jell-O) swirl, 'Pudding Snacks'	4 oz	170	28	6.0
CHOCOLATE MARSHMALLOW				
(Hunt's)				
'Snack Pack'	4 oz	155	23	5.9
s'mores, 'Snack Pack'	4 oz	154	25	5.6
CHOCOLATE MINT				
(Hershey's) 'York Peppermint Pattie'	4 oz	180	29	6.0
(Jell-O) swirl, 'Free'	4 oz	100	24	0.0
CHOCOLATE PEANUT BUTTER				
(Hunt's) chocolate peanut butter swirl, 'Snack Pack'	4 oz	169	26	6.3
CHOCOLATE RASPBERRY (Healthy Choice)	1 cup	110	22	2.0
COCONUT				
(Imagine Foods) nondairy, low-fat, 'Dream Pudding'	4 oz	150	32	2.0
LEMON				
(Imagine Foods) nondairy	1 cup	150	33	3.0
(Hunt's) 'Snack Pack'	4 oz	138	28	2.8
(White House)	3.5 oz	152	37	1.0
RICE				
(Crowley)	4.5 oz	125	22	2.0
(Lucky Leaf)	4 oz	120	20	3.0
(Musselman's)	4 oz	120	20	3.0
(White House)	3.5 oz	111	20	3.0
TAPIOCA				
(Crowley)	4.5 oz	135	27	1.0
(Del Monte) 'Pudding Cup'	5 oz	180	30	4.0
(Healthy Choice) French creme	1 cup	110	21	2.0
(Hunt's)				
nonfat, 'Snack Pack'	1/2 cup	95	21	0.3
'Snack Pack'	4 oz	151	23	5.7
'Snack Pack Light'	4 oz	100	18	2.0
(Jell-O)	4 oz	170	27	4.0
(Lucky Leaf)	4 oz	140	20	6.0
(Musselman's)	4 oz	140	20	6.0
(Swiss Miss)				
'Light'	4 oz	100	18	2.0
nonfat	1/2 cup	99	22	0.3
(White House)	3.5 oz	131	19	6.0

Food Name	Serv. Size	Total Cal.	Carbs GMS	Fat GMS
VANILLA				
(Crowley)	4.5 oz	140	26	3.0
(Del Monte)				
'Pudding Cup'	5 oz	180	32	5.0
'Pudding Snack Light'	4.25 oz	100	19	1.0
(Estee)	1/2 cup	70	12	1.0
(Featherweight)	1/2 cup	100	20	2.0
(Healthy Choice) French	1 cup	110	20	2.0
(Hunt's)				
'Snack Pack'	4 oz	158	25	5.7
'Snack Pack Light'	4 oz	93	21	0.4
(Jell-O)				
	4 oz	180	28	7.0
fat free	1 serving	104	23	0.2
'Free'	4 oz	100	23	0.0
'Light Pudding Snacks'	4 oz	100	20	2.0
pudding snack	1 serving	100	23	0.0
(Lucky Leaf)	4 oz	170	25	7.0
(Musselman's)	4 oz	170	25	7.0
(Pathmark) 'No Frills'	5 oz	200	28	8.0
(Rich's) frozen	3 oz	130	18	6.0
(Swiss Miss)				
'Light'	4 oz	100	18	2.0
nonfat	1/2 cup	99	22	0.4
sundae	4 oz	175	27	6.8
(Ultra Slim-Fast) 'Lite 'N Tasty'	4 oz	100	21	1.0
(White House)	3.5 oz	111	20	3.0
PUDDING BAR, FROZEN				
(Jell-O)				
chocolate fudge, 'Pudding Pops'	1 bar	80	13	2.0
chocolate-peanut butter swirl 'Pudding Pops'	1 bar	80	12	3.0
chocolate-vanilla swirl, 'Pudding Pops'	1 bar	80	13	2.0
double chocolate swirl, 'Pudding Pops'	1 bar	80	13	2.0
milk chocolate, 'Pudding Pops'	1 bar	80	13	2.0
PUDDING MIX. See also PUDDING/PIE FILLING MIX.				
BANANA				
(Jell-O)				
cream, instant, prepared w/whole milk	1/2 cup	160	28	4.0
cream, microwave, prepared w/whole milk	1/2 cup	150	25	4.0
instant, sugar-free, prepared w/2% milk	1/2 cup	80	11	2.0
(Royal)				
cream, instant, prepared w/whole milk	1/2 cup	180	29	5.0
cream, prepared w/whole milk	1/2 cup	160	27	4.0
BUTTER ALMOND				
(Royal) toasted, instant, prepared w/whole milk	1/2 cup	170	30	4.0
BUTTER PECAN (Jell-O) instant, prepared w/whole milk	1/2 cup	170	28	5.0
BUTTERSCOTCH				
(D-Zerta) low-calorie, prepared w/nonfat milk	1/2 cup	70	12	0.0
(Featherweight)				
instant, prepared w/whole milk	1/2 cup	100	19	0.0
prepared as directed	1/2 cup	12	3	0.0
(Jell-O)				
cook and serve	1 serving	80	20	0.0
instant, prepared w/whole milk	1/2 cup	160	28	4.0
instant, sugar-free, prepared w/2% milk	1/2 cup	90	12	2.0
microwave, prepared w/whole milk	1/2 cup	170	28	4.0
prepared, w/whole milk	1/2 cup	170	30	4.0

Food Name	Serv. Size	Total Cal.	Carbs GMS	Fat GMS
(Royal)				
instant, prepared w/whole milk	1/2 cup	180	29	5.0
instant, sugar-free, prepared w/2% milk	1/2 cup	100	16	2.0
prepared, w/whole milk	1/2 cup	160	27	4.0
CHOCOLATE				
(D-Zerta) lower calorie	1 serving	20	5	0.0
(Featherweight)				
instant, prepared	1/2 cup	110	22	0.0
prepared	1/2 cup	12	3	0.0
(Jell-O)				
cook and serve, sugar-free, mix only	1/2 cup	30	7	0.0
cook and serve, sugar-free, prepared w/nonfat milk	1/2 cup	70	13	3.0
cook and serve, sugar-free, prepared w/2% milk	1/2 cup	90	13	3.0
fudge, instant, sugar-free, prepared w/2% milk	1/2 cup	100	14	3.0
fudge, instant, sugar-free, prepared w/whole milk	1/2 cup	180	31	5.0
fudge, prepared w/whole milk	1/2 cup	160	28	4.0
instant, prepared w/whole milk	1/2 cup	180	31	4.0
instant, sugar-free, prepared w/2% milk	1/2 cup	90	13	3.0
microwave, prepared w/whole milk	1/2 cup	170	28	5.0
milk chocolate, instant, prepared w/whole milk	1/2 cup	180	31	5.0
milk chocolate, microwave, prepared w/whole milk	1/2 cup	160	27	5.0
milk chocolate, prepared w/whole milk	1/2 cup	160	28	4.0
prepared w/whole milk	1/2 cup	160	28	4.0
(Royal)				
chocolate chip, prepared w/whole milk	1/2 cup	190	35	4.0
dark and sweet, prepared w/whole milk	1/2 cup	190	35	4.0
instant, prepared w/whole milk	1/2 cup	190	35	4.0
instant, sugar-free, prepared w/2% milk	1/2 cup	110	17	3.0
prepared w/whole milk	1/2 cup	180	33	4.0
(Weight Watchers) instant, prepared w/nonfat milk	1/2 cup	90	18	1.0
CHOCOLATE MINT				
(Royal) instant, prepared w/whole milk	1/2 cup	190	35	4.0
COCONUT				
(Jell-O) cream, instant, prepared w/whole milk	1/2 cup	180	27	6.0
(Royal) toasted, instant, prepared w/whole milk	1/2 cup	170	30	4.0
CUSTARD				
(Jell-O)				
egg, golden, 'Americana' prepared w/whole milk	1/2 cup	160	23	5.0
(Royal) prepared w/whole milk	1/2 cup	150	22	5.0
FLAN				
(Jell-O) prepared w/whole milk	1/2 cup	150	26	4.0
(Royal) w/caramel sauce, prepared w/whole milk	1/2 cup	150	22	5.0
KEY LIME *(Royal)* prepared w/whole milk	1/2 cup	160	30	3.0
LEMON				
(Featherweight) custard, prepared w/whole milk	1/2 cup	40	8	0.0
(French's) prepared	1/2 cup	110	22	1.0
(Jell-O) instant, prepared w/whole milk	1/2 cup	170	29	4.0
(Royal)				
instant, prepared w/whole milk	1/2 cup	180	29	5.0
lemon, prepared w/whole milk	1/2 cup	160	30	3.0
PISTACHIO				
(Jell-O)				
instant, prepared w/whole milk	1/2 cup	170	28	5.0
instant, sugar-free, prepared w/2% milk	1/2 cup	90	12	3.0
(Royal) instant, prepared w/whole milk	1/2 cup	170	30	4.0
RASPBERRY				
(Salada) and pie glaze, prepared w/whole milk	1/2 cup	130	32	0.0

Food Name	Serv. Size	Total Cal.	Carbs GMS	Fat GMS
RICE *(Jell-O)* rice 'Americana' prepared w/whole milk .... 1/2 cup		170	30	4.0
STRAWBERRY				
(Salada) and pie glaze, prepared w/whole milk .... 1/2 cup		130	32	0.0
TAPIOCA				
(Jell-O) vanilla, 'Americana' prepared w/whole milk .... 1/2 cup		160	27	4.0
(Minute) mix only .... 1 1/2 tsp		20	5	0.0
(Royal) vanilla, prepared w/whole milk .... 1/2 cup		160	27	4.0
VANILLA				
(D-Zerta) low-calorie, prepared w/nonfat milk .... 1/2 cup		70	12	0.0
(Featherweight)				
instant, prepared .... 1/2 cup		100	19	0.0
custard, prepared w/whole milk .... 1/2 cup		40	8	0.0
(Jell-O)				
cook and serve, sugar-free, prepared w/skim milk .... 1/2 cup		60	11	2.0
cook and serve, sugar-free, prepared w/2% milk .... 1/2 cup		80	11	2.0
cook and serve, sugar-free, mix only .... 1/2 cup		20	5	0.0
French, instant, prepared w/whole milk .... 1/2 cup		160	28	4.0
instant, prepared w/whole milk .... 1/2 cup		170	29	4.0
instant, sugar-free, prepared w/2% milk .... 1/2 cup		90	12	2.0
microwave, prepared w/whole milk .... 1/2 cup		160	26	4.0
prepared w/whole milk .... 1/2 oup		160	26	4.0
(Royal)				
instant, prepared w/whole milk .... 1/2 cup		180	29	5.0
instant, sugar-free, prepared w/2% milk .... 1/2 cup		100	16	2.0
prepared w/whole milk .... 1/2 cup		160	27	4.0
PUDDING/PIE FILLING MIX. See also PUDDING MIX.				
BANANA				
(Jell-O)				
cream, instant, prepared w/whole milk .... 1/2 cup		160	28	4.0
cream, mix only .... 1 pkg		50	14	0.0
cream, prepared w/whole milk .... 1/6 pkg		100	17	3.0
instant, sugar-free, mix only .... 1 pkg		25	6	0.0
instant, sugar-free, prepared w/2% milk .... 1/2 cup		80	11	2.0
microwave, cream, mix only .... 1 pkg		80	19	0.0
microwave, cream, prepared w/whole milk .... 1/2 cup		150	25	4.0
(Royal)				
cream, instant, mix only .... 1 serving		90	22	0.0
cream, mix only .... 1 serving		80	20	0.0
BUTTER PECAN *(Jell-O)* instant, prepared w/whole milk .... 1/2 cup		170	28	5.0
BUTTERSCOTCH				
(D-Zerta)				
lower calorie, mix only .... 1 pkg		25	6	0.0
lower calorie, prepared .... 1/2 cup		70	12	0.0
(Jell-O)				
instant, sugar-free, mix only .... 1 pkg		25	6	0.0
instant, sugar-free, prepared w/2% milk .... 1/2 cup		90	12	2.0
instant, prepared w/whole milk .... 1/2 cup		160	28	4.0
microwave, mix only .... 1 pkg		90	23	0.0
microwave, prepared w/whole milk .... 1/2 cup		170	28	4.0
regular, mix only .... 1 pkg		90	24	0.0
regular, prepared w/whole milk .... 1/2 cup		170	30	4.0
(My-T-Fine) prepared .... 1/2 cup		90	22	0.0
(Royal)				
instant, mix only .... 1 serving		90	22	0.0
prepared .... 1/2 cup		90	23	0.0
CHERRY VANILLA *(Royal)* instant, mix only .... 1 serving		90	23	0.0

Food Name	Serv. Size	Total Cal.	Carbs GMS	Fat GMS
CHOCOLATE				
(D-Zerta)				
lower calorie, mix only	1 pkg	20	5	0.0
lower calorie, prepared	1/2 cup	60	11	0.0
(Jell-O)				
cook and serve, nonfat, lower calorie	1 serving	90	23	0.3
cook and serve, sugar-free, prepared	1 serving	31	7	0.3
fat-free, sugar-free, prepared	1 serving	34	8	0.3
fudge, instant, mix only	1 pkg	100	25	1.0
fudge, instant, prepared w/whole milk	1/2 cup	180	31	5.0
fudge, instant, sugar-free, mix only	1 pkg	35	8	1.0
fudge, mix only	1 pkg	90	22	0.0
instant, mix only	1 pkg	100	25	0.0
instant, mix only	1 serving	99	25	0.3
instant, prepared w/whole milk	1/2 cup	180	31	4.0
instant, sugar-free, mix only	1 pkg	30	7	0.0
instant, sugar-free, prepared w/2% milk	1/2 cup	100	14	3.0
instant, sugar-free, prepared w/2% milk	1/2 cup	90	13	3.0
microwave, mix only	1 pkg	90	22	1.0
microwave, prepared w/whole milk	1/2 cup	170	28	5.0
milk chocolate, instant, mix only	1 pkg	100	25	1.0
milk chocolate, instant, prepared w/whole milk	1/2 cup	180	31	5.0
milk chocolate, microwave, mix only	1 pkg	90	21	1.0
milk chocolate, microwave, prepared w/whole milk	1/2 cup	160	27	5.0
milk chocolate, mix only	1 pkg	90	22	0.0
milk chocolate, prepared w/whole milk	1/2 cup	160	28	4.0
sugar-free, mix only,	1 pkg	30	7	0.0
prepared w/whole milk	1/2 cup	160	28	4.0
sugar-free, prepared w/2% milk	1/2 cup	90	13	3.0
(My-T-Fine)				
fudge, prepared	1/2 cup	100	24	0.0
prepared	1/2 cup	100	23	0.0
(Royal)				
chocolate chip, instant, mix only	1 serving	110	26	1.0
dark and sweet, prepared	1/2 cup	90	22	0.0
instant, mix only	1 serving	110	27	0.0
instant, sugar-free, prepared	1/2 cup	50	11	0.0
prepared	1/2 cup	90	22	0.0
CHOCOLATE ALMOND				
(My-T-Fine) prepared	1/2 cup	100	23	1.0
(Royal) instant, prepared	1/2 cup	120	26	1.0
CHOCOLATE PEANUT BUTTER CHIP				
(Royal) instant, mix only	1 serving	110	26	1.0
COCONUT				
(Jell-O)				
cream, mix only	1 pkg	60	12	2.0
cream, prepared w/whole milk	1/6 pkg	110	16	4.0
cream, instant, prepared w/whole milk	1/2 cup	180	27	6.0
(Royal) toasted, instant	1/2 cup	100	20	2.0
CUSTARD *(Royal)*	1/2 cup	60	16	0.0
FLAN				
(Jell-O)				
flan, mix only	1 pkg	80	20	0.0
flan, prepared w/whole milk	1/2 cup	150	26	4.0
(Royal) caramel, prepared	1/2 cup	60	15	0.0
KEY LIME *(Royal)* mix only	1 serving	50	13	0.0

Food Name	Serv. Size	Total Cal.	Carbs GMS	Fat GMS
LEMON				
(Jell-O)				
instant, mix only	1 pkg	90	23	0.0
instant, prepared w/whole milk	1/2 cup	170	29	4.0
mix only	1 pkg	50	13	0.0
prepared	1/6 pkg	170	38	2.0
(My-T-Fine) mix only	1 serving	90	22	0.0
(Royal)				
instant, mix only	1 serving	90	23	0.0
meringue, 'No-Bake'	1/8 pie	210	38	5.0
mix only	1 serving	50	13	0.0
PISTACHIO				
(Jell-O)				
instant, mix only	1 pkg	100	22	1.0
instant, prepared w/whole milk	1/2 cup	170	28	5.0
instant, sugar-free, mix only	1 pkg	30	6	1.0
instant, sugar-free, prepared w/2% milk	1/2 cup	90	12	3.0
(Royal) instant, mix only	1 serving	90	22	1.0
STRAWBERRY *(Royal)* instant, mix only	1 serving	100	24	0.0
TAPIOCA *(My-T-Fine)* mix only	1 serving	80	19	0.0
VANILLA				
(D-Zerta)				
lower calorie, mix only	1 pkg	25	6	0.0
lower calorie, prepared	1/2 cup	70	12	0.0
(Jell-O)				
cook and serve, nonfat, lower calorie	1 serving	86	22	0.0
cook and serve, sugar-free, prepared	1 serving	21	5	0.0
fat-free, sugar-free, prepared	1 serving	26	6	0.1
French, instant, mix only	1 pkg	90	23	0.0
French, instant, prepared w/whole milk	1/2 cup	160	28	4.0
French, mix only	1 pkg	90	24	0.0
French, prepared w/whole milk	1/2 cup	170	30	4.0
instant, mix only	1 pkg	94	23	0.2
instant, prepared w/whole milk	1/2 cup	170	29	4.0
instant, sugar-free, mix only	1 pkg	25	6	0.0
instant, sugar-free, prepared w/2% milk	1/2 cup	90	12	2.0
microwave, mix only	1 pkg	80	21	0.0
microwave, prepared w/whole milk	1/2 cup	160	26	4.0
mix only	1 pkg	80	21	0.0
prepared w/whole milk	1/2 cup	160	26	4.0
sugar-free, mix only	1 pkg	20	5	0.0
sugar-free, prepared w/2% milk	1/2 cup	80	11	2.0
(My-T-Fine)				
mix only	1 serving	80	20	0.0
prepared	1/2 cup	90	22	0.0
(Nutra/Balance) low-lactose	1 serving	242	36	7.5
(Royal)				
chocolate chip, instant, mix only	1 serving	90	22	1.0
(Royal) instant, mix only	1 serving	90	23	0.0
PUERTO RICAN CHERRY. See ACEROLA.				
PUFF PASTRY				
ready-to-bake, frozen, baked	1 oz	158	13	10.9
ready-to-bake, frozen, unprepared	1 oz	156	13	10.8
(Pepperidge Farm)				
sheet, frozen	1/4 sheet	260	22	17.0
shell, mini, frozen	1 shell	50	4	4.0
shell, patty, frozen	1 shell	210	16	15.0

Food Name	Serv. Size	Total Cal.	Carbs GMS	Fat GMS
PUMMELO, RAW. See POMELO.				
PUMPKIN				
Fresh				
boiled, drained, mashed	1 cup	49	12	0.2
raw, cubed, 1-inch cubes	1 cup	30	8	0.1
Canned				
	1 cup	83	20	0.7
(Del Monte)	1/2 cup	35	9	0.0
solid pack (Libby's)	1/2 cup	40	9	0.5
(Stokely)	1/2 cup	40	10	0.0
PUMPKIN FLOWER				
boiled, drained	1 cup	20	4	0.1
raw	1 cup	5	1	0.0
raw, whole	1 medium	<1	0	0.0
PUMPKIN LEAF				
boiled, drained	1 cup	15	2	0.2
raw	1 cup	7	1	0.2
PUMPKIN PIE SPICE. See under SEASONING MIX.				
PUMPKIN SEED				
dried, kernels	1 cup	747	25	63.3
dried, kernels, hulled, approx 142 seeds	1 oz	153	5	13.0
dry roasted, w/tamari, garlic, and cayenne (Eden Foods)	1 oz	170	5	11.0
roasted, kernels	1 cup	1185	30	95.6
roasted, kernels	1 oz	148	4	11.9
roasted, salted (David's)	1 pkg	320	6	25.0
roasted, whole	1 cup	285	34	12.4
roasted, whole, approx 85 seeds	1 oz	126	15	5.5
PUMPKINFISH. See SUNFISH.				
PUNCH. See under FRUIT DRINK; FRUIT DRINK MIX; FRUIT JUICE DRINK.				
PURPLE HULLED PEAS. See PEAS, PURPLE HULLED.				
PURSLANE/pussley				
boiled, drained	1 cup	21	4	0.2
boiled, drained	1/2 cup	10	2.1	0.1
raw	1 cup	7	1.5	0.0
raw	1/2 cup	4	0.7	<.1
PUSSLEY. See PURSLANE.				

Q

Food Name	Serv. Size	Total Cal.	Carbs GMS	Fat GMS
QUAIL/bobwhite				
breast, meat only, raw	1 oz	35	0.0	0.8
giblets, raw	3.5 oz	176	6.7	6.2
meat and skin, raw	1 oz	54	0.0	3.4
meat only, raw	1 oz	34	0.0	0.9
QUEEN CRAB. See under CRAB.				
QUICHE				
(Nancy's)				
broccoli-cheddar, frozen, microwave, 'French Baked'	1 quiche	490	33	33.0
Monterey Jack, w/Swiss and bacon, 'Classic French'	1 quiche	520	30	37.0
(Stilwell)				
bacon and onion	1/6 carton	210	4	16.0
broccoli and cheese	1/6 carton	180	4	14.0
ham	1/6 carton	190	4	15.0
spinach and onion	1/6 carton	190	7	13.0

Food Name	Serv. Size	Total Cal.	Carbs GMS	Fat GMS
three cheese	1/6 carton	200	4	16.0
QUINCE				
raw, trimmed	1 medium	52	14.1	0.1
raw, trimmed	1 oz	16	4.3	<.1
raw, untrimmed	1 lb	158	42.3	0.3
QUINOA				
flakes, steam-rolled, uncooked *(Ancient Harvest)*	1/3 cup	105	23	1.0
flakes, steam-rolled, uncooked *(Quinoa)*	1/3 cup	105	23	1.0
organic, uncooked *(Arrowhead Mills)*	1/4 cup	140	25	2.0
uncooked *(Eden Foods)*	2 oz	200	38	4.0
uncooked	1 cup	636	117	9.9
whole grain, uncooked *(Ancient Harvest)*	1/4 cup	159	28	2.0
whole grain, uncooked *(Quinoa)*	1/4 cup	159	28	2.0
QUINOA FLOUR. See under FLOUR.				
QUINOA SEED				
(Arrowhead Mills)	2 oz	200	35	3.0
wild, uncooked *(Eden Foods)*	1/4 cup	170	31	2.5

R

Food Name	Serv. Size	Total Cal.	Carbs GMS	Fat GMS
RABBIT				
domesticated, composite cuts, raw	1 oz	39	0	1.6
domesticated, composite cuts, roasted	3 oz	167	0	6.8
domesticated, composite cuts, stewed	3 oz	175	0	7.1
wild, raw	1 oz	32	0	0.7
wild, stewed	3 oz	147	0	3.0
RACCOON, roasted	3 oz	217	0	12.3
RADICCHIO				
fresh, raw, leaf	1 med leaf	2	0	0.0
fresh, raw, shredded	1 cup	9	2	0.1
RADISH				
fresh, raw, sliced	1 cup	23	4	0.6
fresh, raw, sliced	1/2 cup	12	2	0.3
fresh, raw, whole *(Dole)*	7 med radishes	20	3	0.0
fresh, raw, whole, large, 1–1.25-inch diam	1 radish	2	0	0.0
fresh, raw, whole, medium, 3/4–1-inch diam	1 radish	1	0	0.0
fresh, raw, whole, small, under 3/4-inch diam	1 radish	<1	0	0.0
BLACK/winter radish				
raw, trimmed	1 lb	77	16.3	0.5
raw, trimmed	1 oz	5	1.0	<.1
ORIENTAL. See DAIKON.				
RED				
fresh, raw, sliced	1 cup	23	4	0.6
fresh, raw, sliced	1/2 cup	12	2	0.3
fresh, raw, whole *(Dole)*	7 med radishes	20	3	0.0
fresh, raw, whole, large, 1–1.25-inch diam	1 radish	2	0	0.0
fresh, raw, whole, medium, 3/4–1-inch diam	1 radish	1	0	0.0
fresh, raw, whole, small, under 3/4-inch diam	1 radish	<1	0	0.0
WHITE ICICLE				
raw, sliced	1/2 cup	7	1.3	0.1
raw, trimmed	1 oz	4	0.7	<.1
raw, untrimmed	1 lb	41	7.7	0.3
raw, whole, approx 7-inch long	1 medium	2	0.5	0.0
RADISH JUICE, bottled *(Biotta)*	6 fl oz	39	8	0.1

Food Name	Serv. Size	Total Cal.	Carbs GMS	Fat GMS
RADISH LEAVES, trimmed	1 oz	15	2.8	0.1
RADISH SEED				
sprouted	1 lb	186	13.9	11.5
sprouted	1 oz	12	0.9	0.7
sprouted, raw	1 cup	16	1	1.0
sprouted, raw	1/2 cup	8	0.7	0.5
RAG GOURD. See GOURD, DISHCLOTH.				
RAINBOW SMELT. See SMELT, RAINBOW.				
RAISIN				
Golden				
seedless	1 cup packed	498	131	0.8
seedless	1 cup	438	115	0.7
seedless *(S&W)*	1/4 cup	130	31	0.0
seedless *(Sun-Maid)*	1/4 cup	130	31	0.0
Dark				
seeded	1 cup packed	488	129	0.9
seeded	1 cup	429	114	0.8
seedless	1 cup packed	495	131	0.8
seedless	1 cup	435	115	0.7
seedless	50 medium	78	21	0.1
seedless *(S&W)*	1/4 cup	130	31	0.0
seedless, for baking *(Sun-Maid)*	1/4 cup	124	30	0.0
seedless, mini-box	0.5 oz	42	11	0.1
seedless, natural *(Sun-Maid)*	1/4 cup	130	31	0.0
RAMBUTAN				
canned, in syrup	1 cup	175	45	0.4
canned, in syrup	1 medium	7	2	0.0
canned, in syrup, drained	1 cup	123	31	0.3
RASPBERRY/bramble				
Canned, in heavy syrup, w/liquid	1 cup	233	60	0.3
Fresh				
raw	1 pint	153	36	1.7
raw	1 cup	60	14	0.7
raw	10 medium	9	2	0.1
Frozen				
(Flav-R-Pac)	1 cup	50	11	0.0
in syrup *(Flav-R-Pac)*	2/3 cup	230	57	0.0
red, sweetened	10-oz pkg	293	74	0.5
red, sweetened, unthawed	1 cup	258	65	0.4
RASPBERRY JUICE *(Smucker's)* red, 'Naturally 100%'	8 fl oz	120	30	0.0
RASPBERRY SYRUP. See under SYRUP.				
RASPBERRY TOPPING				
(Flav-R-Pac)	2 tbsp	45	11	0.0
(Knudsen) pourable	1 oz	75	18	1.0
(Smucker's) nonfat, 'Light'	2 tbsp	55	14	0.0
RAVIOLI DISH/ENTRÉE				
(Amy's Kitchen)				
cheese, in sauce, organic, frozen	8-oz entrée	340	44	12.0
cheese, organic, frozen	1 cup	215	26	5.0
(Bernardi)				
beef, breaded	1 cup	270	43	6.0
beef, jumbo, round	1 cup	450	48	19.0
beef, square	1 cup	280	37	9.0
beef ravioletti, square	1 cup	330	47	10.0
cheese, jumbo	1 cup	380	47	9.0
cheese, round, jumbo	1 cup	410	48	15.0

Food Name	Serv. Size	Total Cal.	Carbs GMS	Fat GMS
cheese, square.	1 cup	260	36	7.0
cheese ravioletti.	1 cup	280	40	8.0
chicken, jumbo, round	1 cup	450	52	17.0
Espanol, breaded	1 cup	290	43	6.0
Florentine, round, jumbo	1 cup	370	53	10.0
pesto, round, jumbo	1 cup	480	57	19.0
seafood, round, jumbo	1 cup	440	57	15.0
vegetable, jumbo, round	1 cup	430	59	15.0
(Buitoni)				
cheese, frozen.	4 oz	360	31	8.0
cheese, in sauce, canned	7.5 oz	190	27	6.0
meat, in sauce, canned	7.5 oz	180	28	4.0
(Celentano)				
cheese, mini	12 ravioli	270	42	6.0
cheese, round	6 raviolis	400	61	9.0
frozen	6.5 oz	380	50	11.0
frozen, 'Great Choice'	6 ravioli	360	69	4.0
mini, frozen	4 oz	250	39	5.0
(Chef Boyardee)				
beef, canned, microwave	7.5 oz	190	31	4.0
beef, canned 'Sir Chomps'	7.5 oz	170	32	3.0
beef, in tomato and meat sauce, canned	1 pkg	400	64	9.4
beef, in tomato and meat sauce, canned	1 cup	230	37	5.0
beef, microwave cup, 'Main Meals'	10.5 oz	290	52	4.0
beef, mini, in tomato and meat sauce	1 pkg	404	69	8.0
beef, mini, in tomato and beef sauce	1 cup	240	37	6.0
beef, w/meat sauce, canned, 'Smurfs'	7.5 oz	230	38	5.0
beef and cheese, in tomato sauce	1 cup	220	38	3.0
cheese, canned 'Sir Chomps'	7.5 oz	170	38	1.0
cheese, in meat sauce, canned, microwave	7.5 oz	200	37	3.0
cheese, in tomato sauce	1 cup	210	44	0.0
chicken, canned	7.5 oz	180	29	4.0
chicken, mini, canned	7.5 oz	220	29	8.0
(Contadina)				
beef, refrigerated, 'Fresh'	3 oz	270	30	11.0
beef and garlic	1 1/4 cup	350	39	14.0
cheese	1 cup	280	31	12.0
cheese, light	1 cup	240	35	5.0
chicken, refrigerated, 'Fresh'	3 oz	260	32	10.0
chicken and rosemary	1 1/4 cup	330	43	12.0
garden vegetable, light	1 1/4 cup	290	43	6.0
(DiGiorno)				
cheese, w/herb, Italian, refrigerated, cooked	1 cup	280	35	10.0
sausage, Italian, refrigerated, cooked	1 cup	270	34	9.0
(Estee) beef, canned	7.5 oz	230	25	11.0
(Finast) beef, in sauce, canned	7.5 oz	250	33	10.0
(Franco-American) beef, in meat sauce	1 cup	280	38	9.0
(Healthy Choice) cheese, Parmigiana	1 entrée	260	44	5.0
(Hormel) beef, in tomato sauce, micro cup	7.5 oz	247	28	11.0
(Kid Cuisine)				
cheese, mini, frozen	8.75 oz	250	52	2.0
cheese, mini, w/applesauce, corn, and brownie, frozen	1 meal	310	61	4.0
(Kid's Kitchen)				
mini, microwave cup	7.5 oz	230	34	6.0
(Lean Cuisine) cheese	1 entrée	270	40	7.0
(Libby's) beef, in sauce, microwave cup, 'Diner'	7.75 oz	240	35	5.0

Food Name	Serv. Size	Total Cal.	Carbs GMS	Fat GMS
(Lucca)				
beef	1 cup	190	28	5.0
chicken, w/savory herbs	1 cup	180	26	4.0
Italian sausage, w/herbs and seasonings	1 cup	200	29	6.0
(Lunch Express) cheese	1 entrée	360	43	14.0
(Marie Callender's)				
w/marinara sauce and 1 oz				
garlic bread, frozen	1 serving	370	47	14.0
(Nalley's) beef, canned	7.5 oz	180	30	3.0
(Pathmark)				
beef, bite size, in tomato sauce, 'No Frills'	7.5 oz	180	28	4.0
cheese in tomato sauce, canned, 'No Frills'	7.5 oz	185	27	6.0
(Progresso)				
beef, frozen	1 cup	260	45	5.0
cheese, frozen	1 cup	220	43	2.0
(Smart Ones) Florentine	1 entrée	220	43	2.0
(Weight Watchers) cheese, baked, frozen	9 oz	240	27	6.0
RED BEAN. See BEAN, RED.				
RED CABBAGE. See CABBAGE, RED.				
RED CURRANT. See under CURRANT.				
RED CURRY BASE. See under SEASONING MIX, CURRY.				
RED PEPPER. See PEPPER, BELL. See also under PEPPER, CHILI; PEPPER, GROUND.				
RED PERCH. See OCEAN PERCH, ATLANTIC.				
RED SALMON. See under SALMON.				
REFRIED BEANS. See under BEAN DISH/ENTRÉE.				
RELISH				
CORN, canned *(Green Giant)*	1 tbsp	20	5	0.0
CRANBERRY-ORANGE, for chicken, canned *(Ocean Spray)*	1/4 cup	120	29	0.0
DILL, nonfat *(Vlasic)*	1 oz	2	1	0.0
HAMBURGER *(Heinz)*	1 oz	40	9	0.0
HOT DOG *(Vlasic)*	1 oz	40	8	1.0
INDIA *(Heinz)*	1 oz	35	9	0.0
PICCALILLI				
(Heinz)	1 oz	30	7	0.0
(Progresso)	1/2 cup	190	4	20.0
not *(Vlasic)*	1 oz	35	8	0.0
PICKLE				
dill *(Vlasic)*	1 tbsp	5	1	0.0
hot dog *(Heinz)*	1 tbsp	15	4	0.0
India *(Vlasic)*	1 tbsp	15	4	0.0
sweet *(Claussen)*	1 tbsp	15	3	0.0
sweet *(Heinz)*	1 tbsp	15	4	0.0
sweet *(Vlasic)*	1 tbsp	15	4	0.0
RENNIN, enzyme tablet, unsweetened	0.35 oz	8	2	0.0
RHUBARB				
Fresh				
raw, whole	1 med stalk	11	2	0.1
raw, diced	1 cup	26	6	0.2
Frozen				
(Flav-R-Pac)	1 cup	30	5	0.5
w/sugar, cooked	1 cup	278	75	0.1
uncooked, diced	1 cup	29	7	0.2
RICE				
ARBORIO				
(Colavita) dry	1 oz	100	22	0.0
(Fantastic Foods) dry, 'Elegant Grains'	1/4 cup	210	45	0.0

Food Name	Serv. Size	Total Cal.	Carbs GMS	Fat GMS
BASMATI				
(Arrowhead Mills)				
brown, long-grain, dry	2 oz	200	44	1.0
white, long grain, dry	1/4 cup	150	33	1.0
(Fantastic Foods)				
brown, cooked, w/1 tbsp salted butter	1/2 cup	115	22	2.0
brown, dry, 'Elegant Grains'	1/4 cup	170	36	1.5
white, cooked, prep w/1 tbsp salted butter	1/2 cup	116	23	1.0
white, dry, 'Elegant Grains'	1/4 cup	180	38	0.0
(Texmati) white, long-grain, cooked w/o salt or butter	1/2 cup	82	31	0.0
BROWN				
long grain, cooked	1 cup	216	45	1.8
long grain, raw	1 cup	685	143	5.4
medium grain, cooked	1 cup	218	46	1.6
medium grain, raw	1 cup	688	145	5.1
(Arrowhead Mills)				
long grain, raw	2 oz	200	44	1.0
medium grain, raw	2 oz	200	44	1.0
short grain, raw	2 oz	200	44	1.0
Spanish, quick, dry	1/3 cup	150	30	1.0
vegetable, quick, dry	1/3 cup	150	30	1.0
wild, dry	1/3 cup	140	28	1.0
(Carolina) long grain, cooked, no salt or butter	1/2 cup	110	23	0.0
(Eden Foods)				
traditional	1/2 cup	200	38	2.0
udon, organic, traditional, dry	1/2 cup	200	38	2.0
(Fantastic Foods)				
cooked	1 cup	240	55	2.0
w/miso, dry	1/2 cup	250	55	3.0
(Lundberg Family)				
golden rose, organic	1/4 cup	160	34	2.0
long grain, cooked	1 cup	232	50	1.2
(Mahatma) long grain, cooked, no salt or butter	1/2 cup	110	23	0.0
(Minute) instant	1/2 cup	120	25	1.0
(River) long grain, cooked, no salt or butter	1/2 cup	110	23	0.0
(S&W)				
long grain, cooked, no salt or butter	3.5 oz	110	25	0.0
long grain, dry	1/4 cup	150	32	1.0
(Uncle Ben's)				
instant, original, dry	1/4 cup	170	37	1.5
long grain, cooked, no salt or butter	2/3 cup	130	27	1.0
precooked, prepared, no salt or butter	1/2 cup	90	21	1.0
GLUTINOUS				
white, cooked	1 cup	169	37	0.3
white, raw	1 cup	685	151	1.0
JASMINE *(Fantastic Foods)* uncooked, 'Elegant Grains'	1/4 cup	170	38	0.0
WHITE				
long grain, cooked	1 cup	205	45	0.4
long grain, dry	1 cup	675	148	1.2
long grain, parboiled, cooked	1 cup	200	43	0.5
long grain, parboiled, dry	1 cup	686	151	1.0
long grain, precooked or instant, enriched, dry	1 cup	360	79	0.3
long grain, precooked or instant, enriched, prepared	1 cup	162	35	0.3
medium grain, cooked	1 cup	242	53	0.4
medium grain, dry	1 cup	702	155	1.1
short grain, cooked	1 cup	242	53	0.4
short grain, dry	1 cup	716	158	1.0

Food Name	Serv. Size	Total Cal.	Carbs GMS	Fat GMS
(Botan) long grain, Calrose	1/4 cup	150	33	0.0
(Carolina)				
long grain, cooked, w/o salt, butter	1/2 cup	100	22	0.0
long grain, instant, cooked, w/o salt, butter	1/2 cup	110	23	0.0
(Dynasty) long grain, enriched	1 oz	118	26	0.0
(Finast) long grain, cooked, w/o salt, butter	1/2 cup	115	26	0.0
(Mahatma) long grain, cooked, w/o salt, butter	1/2 cup	110	23	0.0
(Minute)				
long grain, cooked, w/o salt, butter	2/3 cup	120	27	0.0
long grain, cooked, w/o salt, butter	1/2 cup	90	20	0.0
long grain, 'Premium' cooked, w/o salt, butter	2/3 cup	120	27	0.0
'Original'	2/3 cup	120	27	0.0
(River) long grain, cooked, w/o salt, butter	1/2 cup	100	22	0.0
(S&W) long grain, cooked, w/o salt, butter	3.5 oz	106	23	0.0
(Success) long grain, enriched, cooked, w/o salt, butter	1/2 cup	100	21	0.0
(Uncle Ben's)				
long grain, cooked, w/o salt and butter	2/3 cup	130	28	1.0
long grain, cooked, w/o salt, butter	1/2 cup	90	20	1.0
long grain, instant, cooked, w/salt and butter	2/3 cup	130	27	2.0
long grain, instant, cooked, w/o salt, butter	2/3 cup	120	27	1.0
long grain, 'Natural' cooked, w/salt, butter	2/3 cup	150	28	3.0
long grain, parboiled, cooked, w/salt, butter	2/3 cup	140	28	2.0
long grain, parboiled, cooked, w/o salt, butter	2/3 cup	120	28	1.0
(Water Maid) long grain, cooked, w/o salt, butter	1/2 cup	100	22	0.0
RICE, WILD				
cooked *(Fantastic Foods)*	1/2 cup	83	18	0.0
cooked	1 cup	166	35	0.6
extra fancy, prepared *(Gourmet House)*	1 oz	107	22	0.3
giant, prepared *(Gourmet House)*	1 oz	106	22	0.3
raw	1 cup	571	120	1.7
select, prepared *(Gourmet House)*	1 oz	106	22	0.3
RICE AND BEANS. See under RICE DISH/ENTRÉE.				
RICE BEVERAGE				
(Amazake Light) nondairy, original flavor	1 cup	90	20	0.0
(Don Jose)				
original flavor, 'Horchata'	8 fl oz	70	6	4.0
strawberry flavor, 'Horchata'	8 fl oz	70	7	3.5
(Eden Foods) original flavor, organic, w/soy	8 fl oz	120	16	3.0
(Grainaissance)				
almond flavor, sweet brown rice, 'Amazake'	8 fl oz	198	37	4.0
apricot flavor, sweet brown rice, 'Amazake'	8 fl oz	158	36	0.0
cocoa-almond flavor, brown rice, 'Amazake'	8 fl oz	198	36	4.0
mocha java flavor, sweet brown rice, 'Amazake'	8 fl oz	178	37	2.0
original flavor, brown rice, 'Amazake'	8 fl oz	148	34	0.0
sesame flavor, sweet brown rice, 'Amazake'	8 fl oz	198	37	1.0
vanilla pecan flavor, brown rice, 'Amazake'	8 fl oz	198	37	4.0
(Imagine Foods)				
carob flavor, brown rice, nondairy, 'Rice Dream Lite'	8 fl oz	150	32	3.0
carob flavor, nondairy, 'Rice Dream'	8 fl oz	150	32	2.5
chocolate flavor, brown rice, nondairy, 'Rice Dream'	8 fl oz	190	44	3.0
chocolate flavor, enriched, nondairy, 'Rice Dream'	8 fl oz	170	36	3.0
chocolate flavor, nondairy, 'Rice Dream'	8 fl oz	160	35	2.5
nondairy, 'Rice Dream'	8 fl oz	130	28	2.0
original flavor, enriched, nondairy, 'Rice Dream'	8 fl oz	120	25	2.0
vanilla flavor, brown rice, nondairy, 'Rice Dream Lite'	8 fl oz	120	28	2.0
vanilla flavor, enriched, nondairy, 'Rice Dream'	8 fl oz	130	28	2.0
(Sovex) original vanilla flavor, 'Better Than Milk'	2 tbsp	72	17	0.0

Food Name	Serv. Size	Total Cal.	Carbs GMS	Fat GMS
(Westbrae Naturals)				
plain	8 fl oz	100	18	3.0
vanilla flavor	8 fl oz	120	22	3.0
RICE BEVERAGE MIX				
Devan Sweet) made from organic brown rice	1 1/2 tsp	25	2	0.0
RICE BRAN, crude	1 cup	373	59	24.6
RICE BRAN OIL				
	1 cup	1927	0	218.0
	1 tbsp	120	0	13.6
(Hain)	1 tbsp	120	0	14.0
RICE CAKE				
(Lundberg Family)				
all flavors, sodium-free	1 cake	60	14	0.5
all flavors, very low sodium	1 cake	60	14	0.5
APPLE CINNAMON				
(Hain)	1 serving	50	11	0.0
(Quaker) nonfat	1 cake	40	9	0.0
BROWN RICE				
	1 cake	35	7	0.3
buckwheat	1 cake	34	7	0.3
buckwheat, unsalted	1 cake	34	7	0.3
corn	1 cake	35	7	0.3
multigrain	1 cake	35	7	0.3
multigrain, unsalted	1 cake	35	7	0.3
unsalted	1 cake	35	7	0.3
rye	1 cake	35	7	0.3
w/sesame seed	1 cake	35	7	0.3
w/sesame seed, unsalted	1 cake	35	7	0.3
(Lundberg) unsalted	1 cake	70	16	0.0
BARBECUE *(Hain)* mini	0.5 oz	70	10	3.0
CARAWAY RYE *(Lundberg)*	1 cake	60	14	0.0
CAROB COATED				
(Carafection)				
'Mint Rice Crisps'	1 oz	139	17	7.0
'Rice Crisps'	1 oz	139	17	7.0
CHEESE				
(Hain)				
mini	0.5 oz	60	10	2.0
nacho, mini	0.5 oz	70	10	2.0
(Lundberg Family)				
mini	5 cakes	57	13	1.0
mini	5 cakes	57	13	1.0
CINNAMON				
(Quaker) crunch	1 serving	50	11	0.0
(Chico-San) sugar, mini	5 cakes	50	12	0.0
CORN *(Quaker)*	1 cake	35	7	0.2
DILL *(Lundberg Family)* creamy, mini	5 cakes	60	13	1.0
HONEY NUT *(Chico-San)* unglazed, mini	4 cakes	60	2	1.0
HONEY NUT *(Hain)*	1 serving	50	11	0.0
MUGWORT *(Grainaissance)* bake and serve, 'Mochi'	2 oz	140	29	1.3
MULTIGRAIN				
(Chico-San) very low sodium	1 cake	35	8	0.0
(Hain) five grain	1 cake	40	8	1.0
(Pritikin)				
sodium-free *(Pritikin)*	1 cake	35	7	0.0
very low sodium	1 cake	35	7	0.0
(Quaker)	0.32 oz	34	7	0.4

Food Name	Serv. Size	Total Cal.	Carbs GMS	Fat GMS
PLAIN				
(Chico-San) nonfat, original	1 cake	35	8	0.0
(Grainaissance) organic, bake and serve, 'Mochi'	2 oz	140	29	1.3
(Hain)				
	1 cake	40	8	1.0
mini	0.5 oz	60	12	1.0
mini, unsalted	0.5 oz	60	12	1.0
unsalted	1 cake	40	8	1.0
unsalted, mini	0.5 oz	60	12	1.0
(Konriko) unsalted, original	1 cake	30	7	0.0
(Koyo)				
organic, lightly salted	1 cake	40	8	0.0
organic, no added salt	1 cake	40	8	0.0
(Lundberg Family) organic, lightly salted	1 cake	60	14	0.5
(Pritikin)				
sodium-free	1 cake	35	7	0.0
very low sodium	1 cake	35	7	0.0
(Quaker)				
	0.32 oz	35	7	0.3
lightly salted	1 cake	35	7	0.0
unsalted	1 cake	35	7	0.3
RAISIN				
(Grainaissance) cinnamon, bake and serve, 'Mochi'	2 oz	143	30	1.2
RYE *(Quaker)*	1 cake	34	7	0.4
SESAME				
(Chico-San) original	1 cake	35	8	0.0
(Grainaissance) garlic, bake and serve, 'Mochi'	2 oz	143	28	1.9
(Hain)				
unsalted	1 cake	40	8	1.0
	1 cake	40	8	1.0
(Pritikin)				
nonfat, sodium-free	1 cake	35	7	0.0
nonfat, very low sodium	1 cake	35	7	0.0
(Quaker)	0.32 oz	35	7	0.3
(Westbrae)				
double sesame	0.28 oz	30	6	1.0
garlic	0.28 oz	30	6	1.0
TERIYAKI				
(Hain) mini	0.5 oz	50	12	1.0
(Westbrae)	0.28 oz	30	6	1.0
WHEAT *(Quaker)*	1 cake	34	7	0.3
WHOLE GRAIN, herb and garlic *(American Grains)*	0.5 oz	60	11	1.7
RICE CHIPS, brown rice *(Eden Foods)*	1-oz bag	130	19	5.0
RICE DISH/ENTRÉE				
(Bearitos)				
rice and beans, Cajun style	1 cup	140	26	1.0
rice and beans, Cuban style	1 cup	150	27	1.0
rice and beans, Mexican style	1 cup	160	30	1.0
(Lean Cuisine)				
Mexican style, w/chicken, frozen, 'Lunch Express'	9 1/8 oz	270	43	5.0
(Lunch Express) stir-fry, w/chicken	1 entrée	280	39	9.0
(Marie Callender's) w/chicken and broccoli, cheesy	12 oz	390	44	13.0
(Smart Ones) Santa Fe style rice and beans	1 entrée	290	43	8.0
(Suzi Wan) sweet and sour	1 cup	268	46	6.9
(Weight Watchers)				
and vegetables, Hunan style	1 entrée	250	39	7.0
and vegetables, Peking style	1 entrée	270	48	6.0

Food Name	Serv. Size	Total Cal.	Carbs GMS	Fat GMS
paella	1 entrée	280	48	7.0
rice and beans, Santa Fe style, 'Smart Ones'	1 entrée	290	41	9.0
risotto, w/cheese and mushrooms	1 entrée	290	44	8.0
RICE DISH/ENTRÉE MIX				
(Casbah)				
pilaf, nutted, prepared	3/4 cup	190	35	2.0
pilaf, prepared	3/4 cup	210	38	0.5
Spanish pilaf *(Casbah)* prepared	3/4 cup	200	40	0.5
tabbouleh rice, mix only	1 oz	90	20	1.0
(Ener-G Foods)				
brown rice pilaf, 'Old World' prepared	1 cup	364	76	3.0
gluten-free, low-sodium, mixonly	1 cup	507	111	2.0
gluten-free, mix only	1 cup	528	97	1.8
(Fantastic Foods)				
rice and beans, Caribbean, mix only	1 serving	230	44	1.5
rice and beans, northern Italian, mix only	1 serving	240	49	1.5
rice and beans, Szechuan, mix only	1 serving	210	41	2.0
rice and pinto beans, Tex-Mex, mix only	2.3 oz	240	48	2.5
rice and red beans, Cajun, mix only	2.3 oz	230	46	3.0
(La Choy) fried, prepared	1 cup	236	53	1.1
(Lundberg Family)				
blend, brown and white, mix only	1/4 cup	150	35	1.5
brown rice picante, prepared, 'Spanish Fiesta' 'Quick'	1 cup	260	53	2.5
brown rice, exotic wild rice, and mushrooms, prepared, 'Quick'	1 cup	260	53	3.0
(Minute)				
long grain and wild, mix only	1/2 cup	120	25	0.0
long grain and wild, prepared w/salted butter	1/2 cup	150	25	4.0
(Rice A Roni)				
beef flavored, 1/3 less sodium, prepared	2.5 oz	158	30	2.8
beef flavored, prepared	2.5 oz	169	27	4.5
chicken flavored, 'Fast Cook' prepared	2.5 oz	141	23	3.7
chicken flavored, 1/3 less sodium, prepared	2.5 oz	158	30	2.8
chicken flavored, prepared	2.5 oz	181	29	5.4
fried, 1/3 less sodium, prepared	2.5 oz	147	29	2.0
fried, prepared	2.5 oz	181	29	6.2
herb and butter, prepared	2.5 oz	175	30	5.1
long grain and wild, original, prepared	2.5 oz	164	28	4.8
long grain and wild, w/chicken, almond, prepared	2.5 oz	164	28	4.8
pilaf, long grain and wild, prepared	2.5 oz	135	24	3.1
pilaf, prepared	2.5 oz	175	30	5.1
Spanish, 'Fast Cook' prepared	2.5 oz	141	25	3.1
Spanish, prepared	2 oz	122	21	3.6
Stroganoff, prepared	2.5 oz	203	28	8.2
w/chicken, broccoli, prepared	2.5 oz	164	29	4.2
white cheddar and herb, prepared	2.5 oz	192	28	7.9
RICE FLOUR. See under FLOUR.				
RICE SEASONING. See under SEASONING MIX.				
RICE STICK, wild rice *(Golden Flavor)* wild	1 oz	150	17	7.0
RICE SYRUP. See under SYRUP.				
RISOTTO. See under RICE DISH/ENTRÉE.				
ROAST BEEF HASH. See under HASH.				
ROCKFISH, PACIFIC				
baked, broiled, grilled, or microwaved	3 oz	103	0	1.7
raw	3 oz	80	0	1.3
ROE				
mixed species, cooked	3 oz	173	2	7.0
mixed species, cooked	1 oz	58	1	2.3

Food Name	Serv. Size	Total Cal.	Carbs GMS	Fat GMS
mixed species, raw	3 oz	119	1	5.5
mixed species, raw	1 oz	40	0	1.8
ROLL. See also BREAD; BUN; CROISSANT; ENGLISH MUFFIN; ROLL, SWEET.				
(Brownberry) assorted, 'Hearth'	1 roll	124	24	2.3
(Country Oven) enriched, brown and serve	1 roll	80	13	2.0
(King's Hawaiian Bread) ready-to-eat	1 roll	90	15	2.0
(Pepperidge Farm) brown and serve, 'Hearth'	1 roll	50	10	1.0
(Wonder)				
gem style, brown and serve	1 roll	80	13	2.0
plain pan	1 roll	80	14	1.0
CLUB *(Pepperidge Farm)* brown and serve, 'Deli Classic'	1 roll	100	19	1.0
CRESCENT *(Pepperidge Farm)* butter, 'Deli Classic'	1 roll	110	13	6.0
DINNER				
(Arnold) '24 Dinner Party'	1 roll	51	9	1.2
(Awrey's)				
'Black Forest'	1 roll	50	10	1.0
cracked wheat	1 roll	50	10	1.0
crusty	1 roll	70	12	1.0
plain	1 roll	60	11	1.0
w/poppy seed	1 roll	59	11	1.0
w/sesame seed	1 roll	60	11	1.0
(Ener-G Foods) tapioca, gluten-free	1 serving	151	24	5.7
(Home Pride)				
wheat	1 roll	70	12	1.0
white	1 roll	80	14	2.0
(Pepperidge Farm)				
country style, 'Classic'	1 roll	50	9	1.0
'Old Fashioned'	1 roll	50	7	2.0
'Party'	1 roll	30	5	1.0
(Pillsbury)				
butterflake	1 serving	130	19	5.0
hot	1 serving	130	21	3.0
(Roman Meal)	1 roll	69	13	1.2
(Wonder)				
	1 roll	80	14	1.0
brown and serve	1 serving	80	13	2.0
EGG *(Levy's)* 'Old Country Deli'	1 roll	146	28	2.8
FINGER w/poppy seeds	1 roll	50	8	2.0
FRENCH				
(Du Jour) petite, brown and serve	1 roll	230	45	2.0
(Francisco) 'International'	1 roll	108	21	1.5
(Pepperidge Farm)				
brown and serve, 'Deli Classic'	1/2 roll	120	24	1.0
'Deli Classic' 4 per pkg.	1/2 piece	120	22	2.0
'Deli Classic' 9 per pkg.	1 roll	100	20	1.0
sourdough	1 piece	100	19	1.0
HARD, including Kaiser	1 oz	83	15	1.2
HOAGIE				
(Wonder)	1 roll	400	73	7.0
(Pepperidge Farm) soft, 'Deli Classic'	1 roll	210	34	5.0
ITALIAN *(Du Jour)* crusty, brown and serve	1 roll	80	16	1.0
KAISER				
(Arnold) 'Francisco'	1 roll	184	35	2.9
(Brownberry) 'Hearth'	1 roll	152	29	2.8
(Holsum) 'Big'	1 bun	200	38	3.0
LUIGI 'Twin Pack' *(Colombo Brand)*	2 oz piece	146	25	1.6

Food Name	Serv. Size	Total Cal.	Carbs GMS	Fat GMS
ONION				
(Holsum) 'Big'	1 bun	190	32	4.0
(Levy's) 'Old Country Deli'	1 roll	153	31	1.9
(Pepperidge Farm) w/poppy seeds, sandwich	1 roll	150	26	3.0
PARKER HOUSE				
(Bridgford)	1 roll	85	16	1.3
(Pepperidge Farm)	1 roll	60	9	1.0
POTATO				
(Mrs. Wright's) Dutch style, long	1 roll	150	27	2.5
(Pepperidge Farm)				
	1 roll	160	28	4.0
'Hearty Classic'	1 roll	90	14	3.0
SANDWICH				
(Arnold) w/egg, 'Dutch'	1 roll	123	22	3.3
(Awrey's) oat bran	1 roll	120	22	2.0
(Pepperidge Farm)				
'Deli Classic'	1 roll	110	16	4.0
w/sesame seeds	1 roll	140	23	3.0
SOFT (Pepperidge Farm) 'Family'	1 roll	100	18	2.0
SOUR (Colombo Brand) 'Sour '49er'	1.2-oz roll	90	16	0.6
SWEET (Colombo Brand) 'Sweet '49er'	1.2-oz roll	96	15	1.8
STEAK				
(Colombo Brand)				
sour	2.6-oz roll	200	35	2.2
sweet	2.6-oz roll	206	34	3.3
TWIST (Pepperidge Farm) golden, 'Heat 'n Serve'	1 piece	110	14	5.0
WHEAT				
(Country Oven) w/honey, brown and serve	1 roll	70	13	2.0
(King's Hawaiian Bread) w/honey, ready-to-eat	1 roll	90	15	2.0
ROLL, SWEET. See also BUN, SWEET; PASTRY.				
CARAMEL NUT (Aunt Fanny's) individual	2 oz	190	33	6.0
CHEESE (Weight Watchers) frozen, microwave	1/2 pkg	180	32	4.0
CHERRY				
(Break Cake)				
4.5 oz	2 rolls	400	79	3.0
multi-pak, 1.4 oz	1 roll	130	25	2.0
CINNAMON				
(Aunt Fanny's)				
11-oz size, rectangular	2 oz	181	34	3.0
individual	1.9 oz	180	32	5.0
(Awrey's)				
homestyle	1 piece	240	40	7.0
swirl, 'Grande'	1 piece	340	46	16.0
(Break Cake)				
4.5 oz	2 rolls	420	73	10.0
multi pak, 1.3 oz	1 roll	120	22	3.0
nut, 3 oz	2 rolls	330	52	11.0
(Hostess Snack Cake)	1 serving	210	34	7.0
(Hungry Jack) iced, refrigerated	2 pieces	290	37	14.0
(Pillsbury)				
iced, refrigerated	1 piece	110	17	5.0
raisin, w/icing	1 serving	180	26	7.0
w/icing	1 serving	140	21	5.0
(Sara Lee) all butter	2 oz piece	230	31	11.0
(Weight Watchers) glazed	1 serving	200	33	5.0
FRUIT (Aunt Fanny's) Dixie, individual	2 oz	180	34	4.0
ORANGE (Hostess) swirl, 'Breakfast Bake Shop'	1 piece	230	26	12.0

Food Name	Serv. Size	Total Cal.	Carbs GMS	Fat GMS
PECAN				
(Aunt Fanny's) 11-oz size, rectangular .... 2 oz		184	32	4.0
(Break Cake) multi pak, 1.3 oz .... 1 roll		120	22	3.0
(Hostess) caramel swirl, 'Breakfast Bake Shop' .... 1 piece		240	23	15.0
(Hostess) spinner, 'Breakfast Bake Shop' .... 1 piece		220	30	10.0
RAISIN *(Break Cake)* cinnamon, multi pak, 1.25 oz .... 1 roll		120	21	3.0
STRAWBERRY				
(Aunt Fanny's) 11-oz size, rectangular .... 2 oz		190	35	4.0
(Weight Watchers) frozen, microwave .... 1/2 pkg		170	29	5.0
ROLL, SWEET, DOUGH				
(Pillsbury)				
apple cinnamon, w/icing, refrigerated, prepared .... 1 roll		140	21	5.0
cinnamon raisin, w/icing, refrigerated, prepared .... 1 roll		180	26	7.0
cinnamon, w/icing, refrigerated, prepared .... 1 roll		150	24	5.0
ROLL DOUGH				
(Mrs. Wright's) crescent, refrigerated .... 1 roll		80	13	3.0
(Pillsbury)				
butterflake, refrigerated .... 1 roll		140	20	5.0
crescent, cheese, refrigerated .... 2 rolls		210	21	12.0
(Rhodes)				
cinnamon, frozen .... 1 roll		236	35	9.6
nonfat, no preservatives, 'Lite' .... 1 roll		89	18	0.4
Parker House style, frozen .... 1 oz		90	14	2.0
wheat, flaked, frozen .... 1 roll		140	24	3.0
white, frozen .... 1 roll		98	17	2.1
white, Texas style, frozen .... 1 roll		156	28	3.3
whole wheat, Texas style, frozen .... 1 roll		140	24	3.0
ROLL MIX				
(Dromedary)				
hot, mix only .... 1/8 pkg		209	41	2.0
hot, prepared .... 2 pieces		239	41	5.0
(Krusteaz) hot, prepared .... 1 roll		150	28	3.0
(Pillsbury)				
hot .... 1/4 cup		110	21	1.0
'Hot Roll Mix' prepared .... 1/16 pkg		120	21	2.0
ROMAN BEAN. See BEAN, CRANBERRY.				
ROOT BEER. See under SOFT DRINKS AND MIXERS.				
ROSE COCO BEAN. See BEAN, CRANBERRY.				
ROSE PERCH. See OCEAN PERCH, ATLANTIC.				
ROSELLE				
raw, trimmed .... 1 cup		28	6.4	0.4
trimmed .... 1 oz		14	3.2	0.2
untrimmed .... 1 lb		136	31.3	1.8
ROSEMARY				
Dried				
.... 1 tbsp		11	2	0.5
.... 1 tsp		4	1	0.2
(McCormick/Schilling) .... 1 tsp		6	1	0.0
(Spice Islands) .... 1 tsp		5	1	0.2
Fresh				
.... 1 tbsp		2	0	0.1
.... 1 tsp		1	0	0.0
Ground				
(Durkee) .... 1 tsp		5	0	0.0
(Laurel Leaf) .... 1 tsp		5	0	0.0
ROTINI. See under PASTA.				
ROTINI DISH/ENTRÉE. See under PASTA DISH/ENTRÉE.				

Food Name	Serv. Size	Total Cal.	Carbs GMS	Fat GMS
ROTINI DISH/ENTRÉE MIX. See under PASTA DISH/ENTRÉE MIX.				
RUCOLA. See ARUGULA.				
RUGULA. See ARUGULA.				
RUM				
80 proof	1 fl oz	64	0	0.0
86 proof	1 fl oz	70	0	0.0
90 proof	1 fl oz	73	0	0.0
94 proof	1 fl oz	76	0	0.0
100 proof	1 fl oz	82	0	0.0
RUM RUNNER. See under COCKTAIL MIX.				
RUTABAGA				
Fresh				
boiled, drained, cubed	1 cup	66	15	0.4
boiled, drained, mashed	1 cup	94	21	0.5
raw, cubed	1 cup	50	11	0.3
raw, whole	1 medium	139	31	0.8
Canned, diced *(Allens)*	1/2 cup	20	4	1.0
RYE				
	1 cup	566	118	4.2
flakes, rolled *(Arrowhead Mills)*	1/3 cup	110	24	0.5
whole-grain *(Arrowhead Mills)*	2 oz	190	42	1.0
RYE CAKE *(Quaker)* 'Grain Cakes'	.32 oz piece	35	7	0.3
RYE FLOUR. See under FLOUR.				
RYE WHISKEY. See WHISKEY.				

S

Food Name	Serv. Size	Total Cal.	Carbs GMS	Fat GMS
SABLEFISH. See COD, ALASKAN.				
SACCHARIN. See under SUGAR SUBSTITUTE.				
SAFFLOWER OIL				
expeller pressed *(Hollywood)*	1 tbsp	120	0	14.0
'Hi-Oleic' *(Hain)*	1 tbsp	120	0	14.0
100% pure pressed *(Loriva')*	1 tbsp	120	0	12.0
over 70% oleic	1 cup	1927	0	218.0
over 70% oleic	1 tbsp	124	0	14.0
pure pressed, organic *(Spectrum)*	1 tbsp	120	0	14.0
salad or cooking, over 70% linoleic	1 cup	1927	0	218.0
salad or cooking, over 70% linoleic	1 tbsp	120	0	13.6
salad or cooking, over 70% oleic	1 cup	1927	0	218.0
salad or cooking, over 70% oleic	1 tbsp	120	0	13.6
SAFFLOWER SEED, kernels, dried	1 oz	147	10	10.9
SAFFLOWER SEED MEAL, partially defatted	1 oz	97	14	0.7
SAFFRON				
dried	1 tbsp	7	1	0.1
dried	1 tsp	2	0	0.0
SAGE				
ground	1 tbsp	6	1	0.3
ground	1 tsp	2	0	0.1
ground *(Durkee)*	1 tbsp	9	0	0.0
ground *(Durkee)*	1 tsp	3	0	0.0
ground *(Laurel Leaf)*	1 tbsp	9	0	0.0
ground *(Laurel Leaf)*	1 tsp	3	0	0.0
ground *(McCormick/Schilling)*	1 tsp	4	0	0.0
ground *(Spice Islands)*	1 tsp	4	1	0.1

Food Name	Serv. Size	Total Cal.	Carbs GMS	Fat GMS
SALAD DRESSING				
(Estee) regular	1 tbsp	4	1	0.0
(Johnny's) lite	2 tbsp	70	14	2.0
(Ott's) lower calorie, 'Famous'	1 tbsp	26	4	1.3
BACON				
(Estee) and tomato	1 tbsp	8	1	1.0
(Kraft)				
and tomato	2 tbsp	140	2	14.0
and tomato, reduced calorie	1 tbsp	30	2	2.0
creamy, lower calorie	1 tbsp	30	2	2.0
(T. Marzetti) buttermilk, refrigerated	1 tbsp	93	0	10.0
BLUE CHEESE				
(Estee)	1 tbsp	8	1	1.0
(Featherweight) 'Neu Bleu'	1 tbsp	4	1	0.0
(Hidden Valley Ranch)				
	2 tbsp	20	4	0.0
low-fat'	1 tbsp	10	3	0.0
(Kraft)				
	2 tbsp	45	11	0.0
chunky	1 tbsp	60	2	6.0
chunky, lower calorie	1 tbsp	30	2	2.0
(La Martinique) vinaigrette	2 tbsp	160	0	17.0
(Lawry's) 'Classic' 1 oz	1 tbsp	186	2	2.0
(Litehouse)				
and dip, refrigerated, 'Lite'	1 tbsp	33	1	3.0
and dip, refrigerated, 'Original'	1 tbsp	77	0	8.0
country, and dip, refrigerated	1 tbsp	76	0	8.0
(Roka)				
	1 tbsp	60	1	6.0
lower calorie	1 tbsp	16	1	1.0
(S&W) 'Nutradiet'	1 tbsp	25	2	2.0
(T. Marzetti)				
	1 tbsp	90	1	9.0
buttermilk, refrigerated	1 tbsp	90	1	10.0
chunky, refrigerated	1 tbsp	78	1	8.0
'Light'	1 tbsp	90	1	9.0
refrigerated, 'Lite'	1 tbsp	45	0	5.0
(Walden Farms) calorie-free	2 tbsp	0	0	0.0
(Wish-Bone)				
chunky	1 tbsp	75	1	7.9
chunky, light	2 tbsp	80	2	8.0
BUTTERMILK				
(Hain) buttermilk, 'Old Fashioned'	1 tbsp	70	0	7.0
(Hollywood) 'Old Fashioned'	1 tbsp	75	1	8.0
(Kraft)				
creamy	1 tbsp	80	1	8.0
creamy, lower calorie	1 tbsp	30	1	3.0
(Seven Seas) 'Buttermilk Recipe'	1 tbsp	80	1	8.0
(T. Marzetti) and herbs	1 tbsp	95	0	10.0
CAESAR				
(Cardini's)	2 tbsp	80	1	8.0
(Cook's Classics)	1 tbsp	50	1	5.0
(Estee)	2 tbsp	8	1	1.0
(Hain)				
creamy	1 tbsp	60	1	6.0
creamy, low-salt	1 tbsp	60	1	6.0
(Hollywood)	1 tbsp	70	2	7.0

Food Name	Serv. Size	Total Cal.	Carbs GMS	Fat GMS
(Johnny's) 'Great Caesar'	2 tbsp	170	1	18.0
(Kraft) golden	1 tbsp	70	1	7.0
(Lawry's) 'Classic'	1 tbsp	130	1	13.5
(Litehouse) and dip, refrigerated	1 tbsp	57	0	6.0
(T. Marzetti)				
	1 tbsp	80	1	8.0
light, 50% less fat	2 tbsp	80	1	7.0
refrigerated	1 tbsp	75	0	8.0
house	1 tbsp	75	1	8.0
(Walden Farms) calorie-free	2 tbsp	0	0	0.0
(Weight Watchers)				
nonfat	1 tbsp	5	1	0.0
(Weight Watchers) nonfat, 'Single Serve'	1 tbsp	6	1	0.0
(Wish-Bone)				
	1 tbsp	77	1	8.0
w/olive oil	2 tbsp	100	2	10.0
w/olive oil, 'Lite'	2 tbsp	60	3	5.0
CATALINA *(Kraft)* Catalina, nonfat	2 tbsp	35	8	0.0
CELERY SEED				
(T. Marzetti)				
and onion	1 tbsp	75	9	6.0
refrigerated	1 tbsp	72	5	5.0
CHEESE				
(Bernstein's) 'Cheese Fantastico Parmesan'	2 tbsp	30	5	1.0
(Featherweight)	1 tbsp	20	1	2.0
(Hollywood)	1 tbsp	80	2	8.0
(Lawry's) creamy, w/Parmesan, 'Classic'	1 oz	156	5	15.1
(Wish-Bone)	1 tbsp	89	1	9.2
CILANTRO *(Paula's)* and tomato, 'Herb Garden'	0.5 oz	54	1	6.0
CITRUS *(Hain)* tangy, 'Canola'	1 tbsp	50	1	5.0
COLESLAW				
(Best Foods) 'One Step'	2 tbsp	160	4	16.0
(Hellmann's) 'One Step'	2 tbsp	160	4	16.0
(Hidden Valley Ranch) nonfat	2 tbsp	35	9	0.0
(Blue Plate)	2 tbsp	140	5	13.0
(JFG)	2 tbsp	140	5	13.0
(Kraft)	1 tbsp	70	4	6.0
(Litehouse) refrigerated	1 tbsp	80	2	8.0
(T. Marzetti)				
light	1 tbsp	50	6	3.0
original	1 tbsp	79	3	7.0
'South Recipe'	1 tbsp	66	6	5.0
CREAMY				
(Estee) nonfat	1 tbsp	4	1	0.0
(Hain)				
	1 tbsp	80	0	8.0
no salt added	1 tbsp	80	1	8.0
(Hollywood) creamy	1 tbsp	90	2	9.0
(Kraft)				
house,	1 tbsp	60	1	6.0
house, lower calorie	1 tbsp	30	1	2.0
lower calorie	1 tbsp	25	1	2.0
nonfat, no oil, lower calorie	1 tbsp	4	1	0.0
w/real sour cream	1 tbsp	50	1	5.0
zesty	1 tbsp	50	1	5.0
zesty, lower calorie	1 tbsp	20	1	2.0
(Life) creamy, egg-free, 'All Natural'	1 tbsp	39	2	4.0

Food Name	Serv. Size	Total Cal.	Carbs GMS	Fat GMS
(Pathmark)				
....	1 tbsp	70	1	7.0
zesty	1 tbsp	70	1	8.0
zesty, nonfat, lower calorie	1 tbsp	6	1	0.0
(Rancher's Choice)				
....	1 tbsp	90	1	10.0
lower calorie	1 tbsp	30	1	3.0
(S&W)				
nonfat, no oil	1 tbsp	2	0	0.0
'Nutradiet'	1 tbsp	10	1	1.0
(Seven Seas) creamy	1 tbsp	70	1	7.0
(Weight Watchers) creamy, nonfat, 'Single Serve'.	1 tbsp	9	2	0.0
(Wish-Bone)				
....	1 tbsp	56	2	5.5
herbal, 'Classics'	1 tbsp	70	1	7.3
'Lite'	1 tbsp	26	2	2.0
CUCUMBER				
(Featherweight) creamy, nonfat	1 tbsp	4	1	0.0
(Hain) dill, creamy	1 tbsp	80	0	8.0
(Herb Magic) creamy, no oil	2 tbsp	15	4	0.0
(Kraft)				
creamy	1 tbsp	70	1	8.0
creamy, less fat, lower calorie	1 tbsp	25	1	2.0
DIJON				
(Cook's Classics) oil-free	1 tbsp	8	2	0.0
(Estee) creamy	1 tbsp	8	1	1.0
(Featherweight) creamy	1 tbsp	20	1	2.0
(Great Impressions) mustard	1 tbsp	57	0	6.1
(Pritikin) w/balsamic vinegar, nonfat	2 tbsp	30	6	0.0
DILL				
(Nasoya) creamy	2 tbsp	63	3	5.4
(Hain) cucumber, creamy	1 tbsp	80	0	8.0
(Paula's) and garlic, 'Herb Garden'	0.5 oz	54	1	6.0
FRENCH				
(Catalina)				
....	1 tbsp	60	4	5.0
reduced calorie	1 tbsp	18	3	1.0
(Cook's Classics) 'Country French'	1 tbsp	10	3	0.0
(Estee)				
....	1 tbsp	4	1	0.0
creamy	2 tbsp	10	2	0.0
(Featherweight)	1 tbsp	14	3	0.0
(Great Impressions) w/green pepper, low-calorie	1 tbsp	64	4	5.2
(Hain)				
creamy	1 tbsp	60	1	6.0
spicy mustard, 'Canola'	1 tbsp	50	1	5.0
(Hollywood) creamy	1 tbsp	70	2	7.0
(Kraft)				
....	1 tbsp	60	2	6.0
'Miracle'	1 tbsp	70	3	6.0
reduced calorie	1 tbsp	20	3	1.0
(Litehouse) country herb, and marinade, refrigerated	1 tbsp	54	2	5.0
(Pathmark)				
creamy	1 tbsp	60	2	5.0
reduced calorie	1 tbsp	20	3	1.0
(Pritikin)	2 tbsp	35	8	0.0

Food Name	Serv. Size	Total Cal.	Carbs GMS	Fat GMS
sodium-free	1 tbsp	10	3	0.0
(S&W) 'Nutradiet'	1 tbsp	18	3	0.0
(Seven Seas)				
creamy	1 tbsp	60	2	6.0
'French! Light'	1 tbsp	35	2	3.0
(T. Marzetti)				
California French	1 tbsp	90	5	6.0
California, 'Light'	1 tbsp	40	3	3.0
country	1 tbsp	72	4	6.0
fat-free, 'California French'	1 tbsp	16	4	0.0
'Frenchette'	1 tbsp	10	3	0.0
honey, blue, refrigerated	1 tbsp	70	5	6.0
honey, refrigerated	1 tbsp	74	5	6.0
honey, refrigerated, 'Lite'	1 tbsp	48	5	3.0
'Light'	1 tbsp	16	3	1.0
(Ultra Slim-Fast) cholesterol-free	1 tbsp	20	4	1.0
(Weight Watchers) low-calorie	1 tbsp	10	2	0.0
(Wish-Bone)				
'Deluxe Food Service'	1 tbsp	61	2	5.6
'Deluxe'	1 tbsp	60	2	5.4
garlic, creamy	1 tbsp	55	2	5.3
'Lite'	1 tbsp	31	2	2.5
'Lite Sweet 'n Spicy'	1 tbsp	18	3	0.5
low-calorie, 'Lite'	1 tbsp	30	2	2.5
red, low-calorie, 'Lite'	1 tbsp	17	3	0.4
'Sweet'n Spicy'	1 tbsp	63	3	5.7
FRUIT SALAD				
(Knott's Berry Farm)	1 tbsp	50	3	5.0
(Great Impressions) orange marmalade	1 tbsp	87	5	7.1
GARLIC				
(Cook's Classics) 'Garlic Lover's'	1 tbsp	50	1	5.0
(Estee) creamy, nonfat	1 tbsp	2	0	0.0
(Hain) and sour cream	1 tbsp	70	0	7.0
(Kraft)				
creamy	2 tbsp	110	2	11.0
creamy	1 tbsp	50	1	5.0
(Life) w/tofu, and dip, 'All Natural'	1 tbsp	70	1	7.1
(Pritikin) herb, nonfat, sodium-free	1 tbsp	6	2	0.0
(Wish-Bone) creamy	1 tbsp	74	1	8.0
HERB				
(Featherweight)				
	1 tbsp	25	2	2.0
nonfat	1 tbsp	6	1	0.0
(Hain) savory, 'No Salt Added'	1 tbsp	90	0	10.0
(Nasoya)				
garden	2 tbsp	62	3	5.4
garlic, 'Vegi-Dressing'	1 tbsp	40	1	3.0
(Pritikin) garlic and, nonfat, sodium-free	1 tbsp	6	2	0.0
(Seven Seas)				
and spice, 'Viva'	1 tbsp	60	1	6.0
'Viva Herbs and Spices! Light'	1 tbsp	30	1	3.0
HOMESTYLE				
(Dorothy Lynch)				
	1 tbsp	55	5	3.8
lower calorie	1 tbsp	30	7	1.0
HONEY (Hain) and sesame	1 tbsp	60	2	5.0

Food Name	Serv. Size	Total Cal.	Carbs GMS	Fat GMS
HONEY MUSTARD				
(Cook's Classics) apple	1 tbsp	50	2	6.0
(Knott's Berry Farm) 'Peggy Jane's'	1 tbsp	60	2	6.0
(Kraft) Dijon, nonfat	2 tbsp	45	10	0.0
(Litehouse) and dip, refrigerated	1 tbsp	67	2	7.0
(Marzetti) Dijon, peppercorn	2 tbsp	150	7	13.0
(Pritikin) Dijon	2 tbsp	45	11	0.0
(T. Marzetti)				
Dijon	1 tbsp	67	3	6.0
Dijon, light	1 tbsp	24	6	0.0
Dijon, refrigerated	1 tbsp	68	3	6.0
Dijon ranch	1 tbsp	89	1	9.0
(Weight Watchers) Dijon, nonfat	1 tbsp	23	6	0.0
(Wish-Bone) Dijon, 'Healthy Sensation!'	1 tbsp	25	5	0.0
ITALIAN				
(Bernstein's) herb and garlic, creamy	1 tbsp	60	1	6.0
(Best Foods) creamy, homestyle	2 tsp	60	0	7.0
(Cardini's)	2 tbsp	130	1	14.0
(Cook's Classics) garlic gusto, oil free	1 tbsp	6	1	0.0
(Estee)				
creamy	2 tbsp	14	2	1.0
nonfat	2 tbsp	4	1	0.0
(Featherweight) nonfat	1 tbsp	4	1	0.0
(Hain)				
'Canola'	1 tbsp	50	1	5.0
no oil	1 tbsp	2	1	0.0
no salt added, 'Traditional'	1 tbsp	60	1	6.0
Thousand Island, no oil	1 tbsp	12	3	0.0
'Traditional'	1 tbsp	80	0	8.0
(Herb Magic) no oil	2 tbsp	10	2	0.0
(Hidden Valley Ranch) parmesan, lowfat	1 tbsp	16	3	1.0
(Hollywood)	1 tbsp	90	1	9.0
(Kraft)				
creamy, 'Deliciously Light'	1 tbsp	25	1	2.0
creamy, 'Reduce-Calorie'	1 tbsp	25	1	2.0
creamy, w/real sour cream	1 tbsp	50	1	5.0
'Deliciously Light'	1 tbsp	35	1	3.0
house	1 tbsp	60	1	6.0
house, reduced calorie	1 tbsp	30	1	2.0
nonfat	2 tbsp	20	4	0.0
nonfat, 'Free'	2 tbsp	20	4	0.3
nonfat, 'Healthy Sensation'	2 tbsp	15	2	0.0
nonfat, oil-free 'Reduce-Calorie'	1 tbsp	4	1	0.0
'Presto'	1 tbsp	70	1	7.0
zesty	2 tbsp	109	2	11.1
zesty	1 tbsp	50	1	5.0
zesty, reduced calorie	1 tbsp	20	1	2.0
(Litehouse) creamy, and dip, refrigerated	1 tbsp	60	0	6.0
(Nasoya)				
creamy	2 tbsp	61	3	5.2
'Vegi-Dressing'	1 tbsp	40	1	3.0
(Ott's)	1 tbsp	80	0	9.1
(Pritikin)				
sodium-free, nonfat	1 tbsp	8	2	0.0
zesty, nonfat	2 tbsp	20	5	0.0
(Seven Seas)				
creamy	2 tbsp	120	1	12.0

Food Name	Serv. Size	Total Cal.	Carbs GMS	Fat GMS
nonfat	2 tbsp	50	12	0.0
nonfat, 'Free Viva'	1 tbsp	4	1	0.0
'Viva'	1 tbsp	50	1	5.0
'Viva Creamy Italian! Light'	1 tbsp	45	1	4.0
'Viva Italian! Light'	1 tbsp	30	1	3.0
(T. Marzetti)				
creamy	1 tbsp	80	1	8.0
garlic, refrigerated	1 tbsp	81	1	9.0
gusto	1 tbsp	58	0	8.0
'Light'	1 tbsp	35	1	3.0
nonfat, 'Fat-Free'	1 tbsp	5	1	0.0
nonfat, 'Frenchette'	1 tbsp	6	2	0.0
'Olde Venice'	2 tbsp	130	2	13.0
Romano cheese, refrigerated	1 tbsp	77	1	8.0
Romano	1 tbsp	80	0	8.0
w/olive oil	1 tbsp	60	1	7.0
(Ultra Slim-Fast) cholesterol-free	1 tbsp	6	1	1.0
(Walden Farms)				
calorie-free	2 tbsp	0	0	0.0
country, calorie-free	2 tbsp	0	0	0.0
w/sun-dried tomatoes, calorie-free	2 tbsp	0	0	0.0
(Weight Watchers)				
	1 tbsp	2	0	0.0
creamy	1 tbsp	3	1	0.0
creamy, nonfat	1 tbsp	12	3	0.0
creamy, whipped	1 tbsp	50	2	5.0
nonfat	1 tbsp	6	1	0.0
nonfat, 'Single Serve'	0.75 oz	8	2	0.0
(Wish-Bone)				
	1 tbsp	46	2	4.5
'Lite'	1 tbsp	7	1	0.3
nonfat, 'Healthy Sensation!'	1 tbsp	6	1	0.0
olive oil, 'Classic'	1 tbsp	34	2	3.0
'Robusto'	1 tbsp	47	2	4.5
MAYONNAISE TYPE				
(A&P)	1 tbsp	70	2	7.0
(Bama)	1 tbsp	50	3	4.0
(Blue Plate)	1 tbsp	70	2	7.0
(Finast)	1 tbsp	70	2	7.0
(Hain) eggless, no salt added	1 tbsp	110	0	12.0
(JFG)	1 tbsp	50	2	5.0
(Kraft)				
light	1 tbsp	50	1	4.9
'Miracle Whip'	1 tbsp	70	2	7.0
'Miracle Whip Light'	1 tbsp	45	2	4.0
nonfat	1 tbsp	11	2	0.4
nonfat, 'Miracle Whip-Free'	1 tbsp	20	5	0.0
(Ott's) 'Famous'	1 tbsp	40	4	2.7
(P&Q)	1 tbsp	50	3	5.0
(Pathmark) 'No Frills'	1 tbsp	50	3	5.0
(Spin Blend)				
	1 tbsp	60	3	5.0
cholesterol-free	1 tbsp	40	2	4.0
(Weight Watchers)				
whipped	1 tbsp	45	3	4.0
whipped, low-sodium	1 tbsp	50	1	5.0
whipped, nonfat	1 tbsp	12	4	0.0

Food Name	Serv. Size	Total Cal.	Carbs GMS	Fat GMS
ONION				
(Kraft) and chives, creamy	1 tbsp	70	1	7.0
(Paula's) toasted, nonfat	2 tbsp	10	3	0.0
(Wish-Bone) and chives, 'Lite'	1 tbsp	37	2	3.3
ORIENTAL STYLE *(Featherweight)*	1 tbsp	20	1	2.0
PARMESAN *(T. Marzetti)* peppercorn, refrigerated	1 tbsp	81	1	9.0
PEANUT *(A Taste of Thai)* spicy	1 tbsp	40	6	1.5
PEPPERCORN				
(Litehouse) and dip, refrigerated	1 tbsp	67	0	7.0
(T. Marzetti) cracked, refrigerated	1 tbsp	62	0	7.0
(Weight Watchers) creamy, nonfat	1 tbsp	8	2	0.0
PESTO *(Cardini's)* pasta, w/basil	2 tbsp	140	0	14.0
POPPYSEED				
(Great Impressions)	2 tbsp	131	8	11.0
(Hain) Natural Classics	2 tbsp	140	3	14.0
(Knott's Berry Farm)				
	2 tbsp	120	10	9.0
Peggy Jane's'	1 tbsp	60	4	5.0
(La Martinique)	2 tbsp	170	8	15.0
(Litehouse) and dip, refrigerated	1 tbsp	65	3	6.0
(T. Marzetti) refrigerated	1 tbsp	72	5	6.0
POTATO SALAD				
(Best Foods) One Step	2 tbsp	160	2	17.0
(Blue Plate)	2 tbsp	130	1	14.0
(Hellmann's) One Step	2 tbsp	160	2	17.0
(JFG)	2 tbsp	130	1	14.0
(T. Marzetti)	1 tbsp	80	3	7.0
RANCH				
(Bernstein's) Parmesan garlic	2 tbsp	45	7	1.0
(Best Foods)				
homestyle	2 tsp	70	1	7.0
homestyle, light,	1 1/3 tbsp	70	2	7.0
(Hellmann's)				
homestyle	2 tsp	70	1	7.0
light, homestyle	1 1/3 tbsp	70	2	7.0
(Herb Magic) no oil	2 tbsp	15	4	0.0
(Hidden Valley Ranch)				
94% fat-free	2 tbsp	40	5	2.0
honey Dijon	2 tbsp	35	7	0.0
honey Dijon, low-fat	1 tbsp	20	3	1.0
original, 'Light'	1 tbsp	40	2	4.0
(Kraft)				
	2 tbsp	148	1	15.6
buttermilk	2 tbsp	150	1	16.0
cucumber	2 tbsp	140	2	15.0
light, 'Light Done Right!'	2 tbsp	77	3	6.8
nonfat	2 tbsp	48	11	0.3
nonfat, 'Healthy Sensation'	2 tbsp	40	9	0.0
peppercorn, nonfat	2 tbsp	45	11	0.0
w/salsa	2 tbsp	130	1	13.0
(Litehouse)				
and dip, refrigerated	1 tbsp	59	1	6.0
and dip, refrigerated, 'Lite'	1 tbsp	35	1	3.0
country, and dip, refrigerated	1 tbsp	61	1	7.0
jalapeño, and dip, refrigerated	1 tbsp	60	1	6.0
(Pritikin) sodium-free, nonfat	1 tbsp	16	4	0.0

Food Name	Serv. Size	Total Cal.	Carbs GMS	Fat GMS
(Seven Seas)				
'Buttermilk Recipe Ranch! Light'	1 tbsp	50	1	5.0
nonfat	2 tbsp	45	11	0.0
'Viva Ranch! Light'	1 tbsp	50	2	5.0
'Viva'	1 tbsp	80	1	8.0
(T. Marzetti)				
(T. Marzetti)	1 tbsp	90	0	2.0
buttermilk, refrigerated	1 tbsp	93	0	10.0
buttermilk, refrigerated, 'Lite'	1 tbsp	45	1	5.0
Caesar	1 tbsp	95	1	10.0
fat-free	1 tbsp	12	3	0.0
garden	1 tbsp	100	1	10.0
honey Dijon	1 tbsp	89	1	9.0
'Light'	1 tbsp	40	2	4.0
Parmesan, refrigerated	1 tbsp	86	1	9.0
peppercorn	1 tbsp	85	1	9.0
peppercorn, fat-free	1 tbsp	14	3	0.0
(Walden Farms) calorie-free	2 tbsp	0	0	0.0
(Weight Watchers)				
creamy, nonfat	1 tbsp	25	6	0.0
creamy, nonfat, 'Single Serve'	1 pkt	35	8	0.0
(Wish-Bone)				
	1 tbsp	78	1	8.3
and salsa, 'Santa Fe'	2 tbsp	150	3	15.0
lite	2 tbsp	100	5	9.0
nonfat, 'Healthy Sensation!'	1 tbsp	16	3	0.0
RASPBERRY				
(Walden Farms) diet	2 tbsp	<1	0	0.0
(Pritikin) vinaigrette, w/olive oil	2 tbsp	45	11	0.0
RUSSIAN				
(Kraft)				
	1 tbsp	60	4	5.0
creamy	1 tbsp	60	2	5.0
reduced calorie	1 tbsp	30	4	1.0
w/pure honey, low-calorie	1 tbsp	60	4	5.0
(Featherweight) nonfat	1 tbsp	6	1	0.0
(S&W) Russian, 'Nutradiet'	1 tbsp	25	4	1.0
(Weight Watchers) whipped	1 tbsp	50	2	5.0
(Wish-Bone)				
	1 tbsp	46	6	2.5
'Food Service'	1 tbsp	47	6	2.5
'Lite'	1 tbsp	22	4	0.6
SAN FRANCISCO *(Lawry's)* w/Romano cheese, 'Classic'	1 oz	136	2	14.0
SESAME				
(Hain) honey and	1 tbsp	60	2	5.0
(Nasoya) garlic	2 tbsp	63	3	5.4
SOUR CREAM				
(Crowley) nondairy	1 oz	40	1	4.0
(Friendship) 'Sour Treat'	1 oz	36	2	3.0
SPINACH SALAD *(T. Marzetti)* refrigerated	1 tbsp	35	2	10.0
SWEET AND SOUR				
(Herb Magic) no oil	2 tbsp	35	9	0.0
(Old Dutch) oil-, fat-, and cholesterol-free	2 tbsp	50	13	0.0
(T. Marzetti)				
'Fat-Free'	1 tbsp	20	5	0.0
'Light'	1 tbsp	45	5	3.0
refrigerated	1 tbsp	72	5	6.0

Food Name	Serv. Size	Total Cal.	Carbs GMS	Fat GMS
THOUSAND ISLAND				
(Best Foods) homestyle	1 1/3 tbsp	80	3	8.0
(Estee)	1 tbsp	8	2	0.0
(Featherweight)	1 tbsp	18	3	0.0
(Hain)	1 tbsp	50	0	5.0
(Hollywood)	1 tbsp	60	3	6.0
(Kraft)				
	1 tbsp	60	2	5.0
'Free'	1 tbsp	20	5	0.0
reduced calorie	1 tbsp	20	3	1.0
w/bacon	1 tbsp	60	2	6.0
(Litehouse) and dip, refrigerated	1 tbsp	65	1	7.0
(S&W) 'Nutradiet'	1 tbsp	25	2	2.0
(Seven Seas)				
creamy	1 tbsp	50	2	5.0
'Thousand Island! Light'	1 tbsp	30	3	2.0
(T. Marzetti)				
	1 tbsp	74	2	7.0
fat-free	1 tbsp	17	4	0.0
'Frenchette'	1 tbsp	20	3	0.0
light	1 tbsp	35	3	3.0
refrigerated	1 tbsp	82	6	5.0
(Ultra Slim-Fast) cholesterol-free	1 tbsp	18	4	1.0
(Walden Farms)	2 tbsp	0	0	0.0
(Weight Watchers) whipped	1 tbsp	50	2	5.0
(Wish-Bone)				
	1 tbsp	63	3	5.6
'Lite'	1 tbsp	36	2	3.0
TOMATO				
(Cook's Classics) basil	1 tbsp	12	1	1.0
(Featherweight) zesty, nonfat	1 tbsp	2	0	0.0
TUNA SALAD				
(Best Foods) 'One Step'	2 tbsp	140	4	14.0
(Blue Plate)	2 tbsp	130	1	13.0
(Hellmann's) 'One Step'	2 tbsp	140	4	14.0
(JFG)	2 tbsp	130	1	13.0
VINAIGRETTE				
(Great Impressions) balsamic vinegar and oil	1 tbsp	67	2	6.5
(Hain)				
cheese	1 tbsp	55	0	6.0
Dijon	1 tbsp	50	0	5.0
Dijon, creamy, 'Natural Classics'	2 tbsp	130	3	13.0
Swiss cheese	1 tbsp	60	0	7.0
tomato, garden, 'Canola'	1 tbsp	60	1	6.0
(Herb Magic) no oil	2 tbsp	10	3	0.0
(Hollywood) Dijon	1 tbsp	60	2	6.0
(Knott's Berry Farm) w/sun dried tomato	1 tbsp	45	1	4.0
(Kraft) oil and vinegar	1 tbsp	70	1	8.0
(La Martinique) French	2 tbsp	170	0	19.0
(Lawry's)				
Chinese vinegar, w/sesame and ginger, 'Classic'	1 tbsp	145	2	15.0
(Litehouse) sour cream and chives, refrigerated	1 tbsp	63	1	7.0
(Marie's)				
herb, 'Lite and Zesty'	1 tbsp	16	4	0.0
Italian, 'Lite and Zesty'	1 tbsp	16	4	0.0
(Newman's Own) olive oil and vinegar	2 tbsp	150	1	16.0

Food Name	Serv. Size	Total Cal.	Carbs GMS	Fat GMS
(Pritikin)				
herb, sodium-free	1 tbsp	8	2	0.0
olive oil, raspberry	2 tbsp	45	11	0.0
(S&W)				
balsamic wine, 'Vintage Lites'	2 tbsp	35	8	0.0
mango key lime, 'Vintage Lites'	2 tbsp	30	7	0.0
Oriental rice wine, 'Vintage Lites'	2 tbsp	30	8	0.0
raspberry blush, 'Vintage Lites'	2 tbsp	40	10	0.0
red wine w/herb, 'Vintage Lites'	2 tbsp	40	11	0.0
white wine w/herb, 'Vintage Lites'	2 tbsp	40	10	0.0
(Seven Seas) red wine vinegar	2 tbsp	15	3	0.0
(Simply Delicious)				
ginger plum, 'Un-Dressing'	1 tbsp	36	1	4.0
herb garlic, 'Un-Dressing'	1 tbsp	43	1	4.0
honey mustard, 'Un-Dressing'	1 tbsp	41	2	4.0
lemon tahini, 'Un-Dressing'	1 tbsp	43	1	4.0
lime cilantro, 'Un-Dressing'	1 tbsp	41	1	4.0
pink peppercorn, 'Un-Dressing'	1 tbsp	40	1	4.0
(Walden Farms)				
balsamic, diet	2 tbsp	0	0	0.0
honey Dijon	2 tbsp	0	0	0.0
(Weight Watchers) tomato	1 tbsp	8	2	0.0
(Wish-Bone)				
Dijon, 'Classic'	1 tbsp	60	1	6.1
Dijon, lite	2 tbsp	60	3	5.0
olive oil	1 tbsp	28	2	2.3
olive oil, 'Lite'	1 tbsp	16	2	0.9
red wine	1 tbsp	51	4	3.8
VEGETABLE *(T. Marzetti)* and dip, refrigerated	1 tbsp	88	1	10.0
WINE VINEGAR				
(Estee) red wine, nonfat	1 tbsp	2	0	0.0
(Featherweight) red wine, nonfat	1 tbsp	6	1	0.0
(Great Impressions)				
red wine, and oil	1 tbsp	64	3	6.1
white wine, and oil	1 tbsp	63	1	6.6
(Kraft)				
red wine, and oil	1 tbsp	60	4	4.0
red wine, nonfat	2 tbsp	15	3	0.0
(Lawry's)				
red wine, w/Cabernet, 'Classics'	1 tbsp	138	5	13.7
vintage, w/sherry wine, 'Classics'	1 tbsp	110	3	10.5
white wine, w/Chardonnay, 'Classic'	1 tbsp	153	3	15.7
(Marie's) white wine, nonfat, 'Lite and Zesty'	1 tbsp	20	5	0.0
(Pathmark) red wine, and oil	1 tbsp	70	2	7.0
(Seven Seas)				
red wine, and oil, 'Viva Red Wine!'	1 tbsp	45	1	4.0
red wine, and oil, 'Viva'	1 tbsp	70	1	7.0
SALAD DRESSING MIX				
BACON *(Lawry's)* mix only	1 pkg	65	9	0.8
BLUE CHEESE				
(Best Foods) blue cheese, homestyle, mix only	2 tsp	45	1	4.5
(Good Seasons)				
and herbs, mix only	1 pkg	4	1	0.0
and herbs, prepared	1 tbsp	70	1	8.0
(Hain) 'No Oil' prepared	1 tbsp	14	1	1.0
(Hidden Valley Ranch)				
mix only	1.1 oz	112	19	2.0

Food Name	Serv. Size	Total Cal.	Carbs GMS	Fat GMS
prepared	1 tbsp	58	1	6.0
(Tone's) blue cheese, mix only	1 tsp	13	2	0.2
(Weight Watchers) mix only	1 tbsp	8	1	0.0
BUTTERMILK				
(Good Seasons)				
'Farm Style' prepared	1 tbsp	60	1	6.0
nonfat, 'Farm Style' mix only	1 pkg	4	1	0.0
(Hain) 'No Oil' prepared	1 tbsp	11	1	1.0
(Hidden Valley Ranch) original recipe, prepared	1 tbsp	58	1	3.0
(Tone's) mix only	1 tsp	10	2	0.2
CAESAR				
(Good Seasons) gourmet, prepared	2 tbsp	150	3	16.0
(Hain) 'No Oil' prepared	1 tbsp	6	1	1.0
(Lawry's) mix only	1 pkg	75	9	3.1
CHEESE				
(Good Seasons)				
garlic, mix only	1 serving	40	8	0.0
garlic, prepared	2 tbsp	140	1	16.0
Italian, mix only	1 pkg	4	1	0.0
CHICKEN SALAD *(Kikkoman)* Chinese, mix only	1 tbsp	30	6	0.0
DILL				
(Good Seasons)				
'Classic' mix only	1 tbsp	2	0	0.0
'Classic' prepared	1 tbsp	70	1	8.0
(Knorr) and dip, mix only	1 tbsp	2	1	1.0
FRENCH				
(Hain) 'No Oil' prepared	1 tbsp	12	3	0.0
(Weight Watchers) mix only	1 tbsp	3	1	0.0
GARLIC				
(Good Seasons)				
and herb, mix only	1 serving	40	8	0.0
and herb, prepared	1 tbsp	70	1	8.0
(Hain) and cheese, 'No Oil' prepared	1 tbsp	6	1	1.0
HERB				
(Good Seasons)				
'Classic' mix only	1 pkg	2	0	0.0
'Classic' prepared	1 tbsp	70	1	8.0
zesty, lowfat recipe, prepared	1 tbsp	12	1	1.0
zesty, mix only	1 tbsp	6	1	0.0
zesty, nonfat recipe, prepared	1 tbsp	6	1	0.0
(Hain) 'No Oil' prepared	1 tbsp	2	1	0.0
(Hidden Valley Ranch)				
creamy, mix only	0.9 oz	76	16	0.0
creamy, prepared	1 tbsp	58	1	6.0
HONEY MUSTARD				
(Good Seasons)				
low-fat recipe, prepared	1 tbsp	18	2	1.0
nonfat recipe, mix only	1 serving	160	40	0.0
nonfat recipe, prepared	1 tbsp	10	2	0.0
prepared	1 tbsp	80	2	8.0
ITALIAN				
(Good Seasons)				
cheese, 'Lite' mix only	1 tbsp	25	1	3.0
cheese, mix only	1 pkg	4	1	0.0
cheese, prepared	1 tbsp	70	1	8.0
creamy, fat-free recipe, prepared	1 tbsp	8	2	0.0
creamy, low-fat recipe, prepared	1 tbsp	16	2	1.0

Food Name	Serv. Size	Total Cal.	Carbs GMS	Fat GMS
creamy, nonfat, mix only	1 serving	80	24	0.0
lemon and herbs, mix only	1 tbsp	70	1	8.0
lemon and herbs, prepared	1 tbsp	70	1	8.0
'Lite' mix only	1 tbsp	25	1	3.0
mild, mix only	1 serving	80	16	0.0
mild, prepared	1 tbsp	70	1	8.0
mix only	1 serving	40	8	0.0
mix only	1 tbsp	6	1	0.0
'No Oil' mix only	1 tbsp	6	2	0.0
nonfat, mix only	1 serving	80	24	0.0
nonfat, prepared	2 tbsp	10	3	0.0
prepared w/o oil	1 tbsp	6	2	0.0
prepared	1 tbsp	70	1	8.0
prepared	2 tbsp	140	1	15.0
zesty, 'Lite' mix only	1 tbsp	25	1	3.0
zesty, 'Lite' prepared	1 tbsp	25	1	3.0
zesty, mix only	1 pkg	2	1	0.0
zesty, mix only	1 serving	40	8	0.0
zesty, prepared	1 tbsp	70	1	8.0
(Lawry's)				
mix only	1 pkg	45	9	0.2
w/chococ, mix only	1 pkg	74	12	2.1
(Tone's)				
creamy, mix only	1 tsp	13	3	0.1
mix only	1 tsp	12	3	0.1
LEMON				
(Good Seasons)				
and herbs, Italian, prepared	1 tbsp	70	1	8.0
and herbs, Italian, mix only	1 pkg	2	1	0.0
RANCH				
(Good Seasons)				
'Lite' prepared	1 tbsp	30	2	2.0
Italian, 'Lite' prepared	1 tbsp	30	2	2.0
Italian, prepared	1 tbsp	60	1	6.0
lower calorie, mix only	1 serving	160	32	0.0
mix only	1 serving	80	16	0.0
prepared	1 tbsp	60	1	6.0
(Hidden Valley Ranch)				
lower calorie, mix only	1.1 oz	98	17	2.0
lower calorie, prepared	1 tbsp	35	2	3.0
original, mix only	1 oz	93	18	1.0
original, prepared	1 tbsp	58	1	6.0
w/bacon, mix only	1.2 oz	118	1	2.0
w/bacon, prepared	1 tbsp	58	1	6.0
RUSSIAN *(Weight Watchers)* mix only	1 tbsp	4	1	0.0
SESAME, Oriental *(Good Seasons)* mix only	1/8 envelope	15	3	0.0
SOY SESAME *(Kikkoman)* mix only	2 tsp	15	3	1.0
THOUSAND ISLAND				
(Best Foods) homestyle, mix only	2 tsp	40	1	4.0
(Weight Watchers) nonfat, mix only	1 tbsp	4	1	0.0
VINAIGRETTE Oriental *(Kikkoman)* mix only	2 tsp	20	3	0.0
SALAD MIX				
(Suddenly Salad)				
Caesar, mix only	2/3 cup	150	30	1.0
Caesar, prepared	3/4 cup	220	30	9.0
ranch, and bacon, prepared	3/4 cup	330	30	20.0
ranch, and bacon, low-fat, prepared	3/4 cup	180	30	2.0

Food Name	Serv. Size	Total Cal.	Carbs GMS	Fat GMS
SALAD SEASONING. See under SEASONING MIX.				
SALAD TOPPING				
(Produce Partners) seasoned	1 tbsp	30	3	1.0
(Salad Crispins)				
bacon and onion, 'American Style'	1 tbsp	35	4	1.0
cheddar and onion	1 tbsp	35	4	1.0
Italian style, w/Parmesan cheese	1 tbsp	35	4	1.0
ranch	1 tbsp	35	4	1.0
(Salad Nibbler)				
buttermilk ranch, crouton topping	1 oz	128	13	5.0
cheddar, seasoned, crouton topping	1 oz	129	13	6.0
(Schilling) seasoned	1 tbsp	35	2	1.5
(Special Edition)				
garlic and cheese, sesame, nuggets	1 tbsp	40	3	2.5
sesame, nuggets	1 tbsp	35	3	2.5
(Tone's) 'American'	1 tsp	7	1	0.3
SALISBURY STEAK. See under BEEF DINNER/ENTRÉE.				
SALMON				
ATLANTIC				
Fresh				
farmed, baked, broiled, grilled, or microwaved	3 oz	175	0	10.5
farmed, raw	3 oz	156	0	9.2
wild, baked, broiled, grilled, or microwaved	3 oz	155	0	6.9
wild, raw	3 oz	121	0	5.4
BLUEBACK. See under SOCKEYE.				
CHINOOK/king				
Fresh				
baked, broiled, grilled, or microwaved	3 oz	196	0	11.4
raw	3 oz	153	0	8.9
Smoked				
	3 oz	99	0	3.7
boneless	1 oz	33	0	1.2
flaked	1 cup	159	0	5.9
lox	3 oz	99	0	3.7
lox	1 oz	33	0	1.2
CHUM/keta				
Canned				
(Bumble Bee)	1 cup	306	0	11.4
(Libby's)	3.7 oz	130	0	6.0
drained, w/bone	3 oz	120	0	4.7
drained, w/bone, no salt added	3 oz	120	0	4.7
w/liquid *(Bumble Bee)*	3.5 oz	160	0	8.0
Fresh				
baked, broiled, grilled, or microwaved	3 oz	131	0	4.1
raw	3 oz	102	0	3.2
Frozen				
(Peter Pan Seafoods) fillet portion, raw	3.5 oz	120	0	3.8
(Peter Pan Seafoods) side, pinbone in, raw	3.5 oz	120	0	3.8
(Peter Pan Seafoods) steak, raw	3.5 oz	120	0	3.8
COHO/silver				
Canned				
meat only *(Deming's)*	1/2 cup	140	0	5.0
Fresh				
farmed, baked, broiled, grilled, or microwaved	3 oz	151	0	7.0
farmed, raw	3 oz	136	0	6.5
wild, baked, broiled, grilled, or microwaved	3 oz	118	0	3.7
wild, boiled or poached	3 oz	156	0	6.4

Food Name	Serv. Size	Total Cal.	Carbs GMS	Fat GMS
wild, raw	3 oz	124	0	5.0
HUMPBACK. See PINK.				
KETA. See COHO.				
KING. See CHINOOK.				
MIXED SPECIES				
Canned, boneless, skinless *(Libby's)*	3.25 oz	110	1	4.0
Frozen, steak, w/o seasoning mix *(SeaPak)*	8-oz pkg	270	0	9.0
Smoked, Nova, sliced *(Lascco)*	3 oz	120	0	6.0
PINK/humpback				
Canned				
(Captain's Choice)	3 oz	110	0	5.0
Alaska, w/liquid *(Deming's)*	1/2 cup	140	0	6.0
Alaskan, fancy *(Crown Prince)*	3.5 oz	140	0	6.0
Alaskan, fresh packed *(Libby's)*	3.7 oz	130	0	6.0
boneless, skinless *(Chicken of the Sea)*	2 oz	60	0	2.0
boneless, skinless, w/liquid *(Bumble Bee)*	3.5 oz	120	0	5.0
chunk, boneless, skinless, w/liquid *(Deming's)*	3.25 oz	120	0	5.0
drained, w/bones	3 oz	118	0	5.1
w/bones and liquid	3 oz	118	0	5.1
w/liquid *(Bumble Bee)*	1 cup	310	0	13.0
w/liquid *(Bumble Bee)*	3.5 oz	160	0	8.0
w/liquid *(Del Monte)*	1/2 cup	160	0	7.0
w/liquid *(Featherweight)*	2 oz	70	0	3.0
w/liquid *(Libby's)*	7.75 oz	310	0	13.0
Fresh				
baked, broiled, grilled, or microwaved	3 oz	127	0	3.8
raw	3 oz	99	0	2.9
RED. See SOCKEYE.				
SILVER. See COHO.				
SOCKEYE/red				
Canned				
(Bumble Bee)	1 cup	376	0	20.5
(Libby's)	7.75 oz	380	0	21.0
(S&W)	3 oz	152	0	8.8
Alaska *(Deming's)*	1/2 cup	170	0	9.0
Alaska, medium *(Deming's)*	1/2 cup	150	0	7.0
blueback *(Rubinstein's)*	1/2 cup	170	0	9.0
blueback, 'Fancy' *(S&W)*	1/2 cup	190	0	10.0
boneless, skinless, w/liquid *(Bumble Bee)*	3.5 oz	130	0	6.0
drained, w/bone	3 oz	130	0	6.2
drained, w/bone, no salt added	3 oz	130	0	6.2
'Nutradiet' *(S&W)*	1/2 cup	188	0	11.0
w/liquid *(Bumble Bee)*	3.5 oz	180	0	10.0
w/liquid *(Del Monte)*	1/2 cup	180	0	9.0
Fresh				
baked, broiled, grilled, or microwaved	3 oz	184	0	9.3
raw	3 oz	143	0	7.3
SALMON OIL. See under FISH OIL.				
SALMON SUBSTITUTE *(Mox Lox)* smoked	1.5 oz	25	3	1.0
SALSA. See also under SAUCE, BARBECUE.				
(Arizona Cactus Ranch)				
cactus fruit or prickly pear, organic	2 tbsp	15	4	0.0
(Chi-Chi's)				
hot	1 oz	8	2	2.0
medium	1 oz	7	2	2.0
mild	1 oz	7	2	2.0

Food Name	Serv. Size	Total Cal.	Carbs GMS	Fat GMS
(Del Monte)				
burrito, can or jar	1/4 cup	20	4	0.0
green chili, mild	1/4 cup	20	3	0.0
roja, mild	1/4 cup	20	4	0.0
(Eagle)				
medium	2 tbsp	10	2	0.0
mild	2 tbsp	10	2	0.0
w/cheese, medium	2 tbsp	40	3	3.0
(Enrico's)				
hot, chunky style	2 tbsp	8	2	0.0
hot, chunky style, no salt added	2 tbsp	8	2	0.0
mild, chunky style	2 tbsp	8	2	0.0
mild, chunky style, no salt added	2 tbsp	8	2	0.0
(Garden of Eden)				
nonfat, organic, 'Great Garlic/Hot Habenero'	2 tbsp	10	2	0.0
(Guiltless Gourmet)				
medium	2 tbsp	10	2	0.0
red pepper, roasted	2 tbsp	10	2	0.0
Southwestern grill	2 tbsp	10	2	0.0
tomatillo	2 tbsp	10	2	0.0
(Hain)				
green chili, hot	1/4 cup	22	4	0.0
mild	1/2 cup	20	4	0.0
(Heluva Good)				
hot	2 tbsp	10	2	0.0
mild	2 tbsp	10	2	0.0
(Hot Cha Cha) 'Texas'	1 oz	6	3	0.0
(Kaukauna)				
Mexican, medium	2 tbsp	15	3	0.0
Mexican, mild	2 tbsp	15	3	0.0
(La Victoria)				
'Brava'	1 tbsp	6	1	1.0
'Casera'	1 tbsp	4	1	1.0
chili dip, chunky	2 tbsp	9	2	0.0
green chili	2 tbsp	10	2	0.0
green chili, mild	2 tbsp	8	1	0.1
green jalapeño	1 tbsp	4	1	1.0
green jalapeño	2 tbsp	10	1	0.3
hot	1 tbsp	2	0	0.1
hot	2 tbsp	9	2	0.1
hot, 'Victoria'	2 tbsp	7	1	0.1
hot, thick and chunky	2 tbsp	9	1	0.1
jalapeña	2 tbsp	12	2	0.2
medium	2 tbsp	8	1	0.1
medium, 'Suprema'	2 tbsp	8	1	0.1
medium, thick and chunky	2 tbsp	8	1	0.1
mild	2 tbsp	8	1	0.1
mild, 'Suprema'	2 tbsp	8	2	0.1
mild, thick and chunky	2 tbsp	8	1	0.1
omelet	1 tbsp	6	1	1.0
'Ranchera'	1 tbsp	6	1	1.0
red jalapeño	1 tbsp	6	1	1.0
'Suprema'	2 tbsp	10	2	0.0
'Victoria'	1 tbsp	4	1	1.0
(Litehouse) medium, 'Zesty'	1 tbsp	4	1	0.0
(Mi Ranchito)				
hot, restaurant style	2 tbsp	10	2	0.0

Food Name	Serv. Size	Total Cal.	Carbs GMS	Fat GMS
mild, fat-free, restaurant style	2 tbsp	10	2	0.0
(Millina's Finest) hot, mild or garlic, fat-free, organic	2 tbsp	10	2	0.0
(Mission)				
hot	2 tbsp	5	2	0.0
mild	2 tbsp	5	2	0.0
'Poco Picante'	2 tbsp	5	2	0.0
(Nabisco)				
green chili, hot	1 tbsp	6	2	0.0
green chili, medium	1 tbsp	6	1	0.0
green chili, mild	1 tbsp	8	2	0.0
taco, hot, can or jar, 'Thick & Smooth'	1 tbsp	8	2	0.0
taco, medium, can or jar, 'Thick & Smooth'	1 tbsp	8	2	0.0
taco, mild, can or jar, 'Thick & Smooth'	1 tbsp	8	2	0.0
(Old El Paso)				
green chili, medium	2 tbsp	10	2	0.0
green chili, 'Thick 'n Chunky'	2 tbsp	3	1	0.0
homestyle, medium	2 tbsp	5	1	0.0
homestyle, mild	2 tbsp	5	1	0.0
hot, 'Pico de Gallo'	2 tbsp	5	2	0.0
hot, 'Thick n' Chunky'	2 tbsp	10	2	0.0
medium, 'Pico de Gallo'	2 tbsp	5	2	0.0
medium, 'Salsa Verde'	2 tbsp	10	2	0.0
medium, 'Thick n'Chunky'	2 tbsp	10	2	0.0
mild or medium, chunky	2 tbsp	15	3	0.0
mild, 'Thick n' Chunky'	2 tbsp	10	2	0.0
taco, hot	1 tbsp	5	1	0.0
taco, medium	1 tbsp	5	1	0.0
taco, mild	1 tbsp	5	1	0.0
taco, mild, extra chunky	1 tbsp	5	1	0.0
verde, 'Thick 'n Chunky'	2 tbsp	10	2	1.0
(Ortega)				
green chili, hot	1 oz	10	2	0.0
green chili, medium	1 oz	8	2	0.0
green chili, mild	1 oz	8	2	0.0
medium, thick and chunky	1 tbsp	4	1	0.0
ranchera	1 oz	12	3	0.0
taco, hot, can or jar	1 oz	10	2	0.0
taco, mild, can or jar	1 oz	10	2	0.0
(Pablo's)				
hot, 'Deli Style'	1 oz	10	2	0.0
mild, 'Deli Style'	1 oz	10	2	0.0
(Pace)				
medium, thick and chunky	2 tbsp	4	1	1.0
mild, thick and chunky	2 tbsp	4	1	1.0
salsa dip, medium, 'Chunky'	2 tbsp	4	1	1.0
salsa dip, mild, 'Chunky'	2 tbsp	4	1	1.0
(Parrot Brand)				
black bean, medium, organic, nonfat	2 tbsp	10	2	0.0
hot, fat-free, organic	2 tbsp	10	2	0.0
pinto bean, medium, fat-free, organic	2 tbsp	9	2	0.0
tomatillo, spicy, all natural, 'Green Verde'	2 tbsp	17	2	0.0
(Pritikin) very low-sodium	1/4 cup	25	5	0.0
(Progresso)				
Italian, hot	2 tbsp	10	2	0.0
Italian, medium	2 tbsp	10	2	0.0
Italian, mild	2 tbsp	10	2	0.0

Food Name	Serv. Size	Total Cal.	Carbs GMS	Fat GMS
(Rosarita)				
green chile, mild, food service product	2 tbsp	7	2	0.1
green chili, extra chunky, 'de Mexico Style'	2 tbsp	30	7	1.0
green chili, mild	1.09 oz	7	2	0.1
green tomatillo, 'de Mexico Style'	2 tbsp	20	4	1.0
green tomatillo, medium	2 tbsp	8	2	0.2
hot, chunky	3 tbsp	25	6	1.0
jalapeño picante, hot	2 tbsp	8	2	0.1
jalapeño picante, medium	2 tbsp	8	2	0.1
jalapeño picante, mild	2 tbsp	8	2	0.1
medium, chunky	3 tbsp	25	6	1.0
medium, extra chunky	2 tbsp	7	1	0.2
mild, 'Casa Mamita'	1.13 oz	7	1	0.1
mild, chunky	3 tbsp	25	6	1.0
picante, food service product	2 tbsp	26	6	0.1
roasted, mild	2 tbsp	10	2	0.3
taco, medium, chunky	3 tbsp	25	6	1.0
taco, mild	2 oz	27	6	0.1
taco, mild, chunky	3 tbsp	25	6	1.0
traditional, 'de Mexico Style'	2 tbsp	12	3	0.0
traditional, medium	2 tbsp	7	2	0.1
traditional, mild	2 tbsp	7	1	0.1
(S&W)				
hot, 'Sun-Vista'	2 tbsp	5	2	0.0
medium, 'Ready Cut'	1/4 cup	20	4	0.0
mild, 'Ready Cut'	1/4 cup	20	4	0.0
w/chipotle, 'Ready Cut'	1/4 cup	20	4	0.0
w/cilantro, 'Ready Cut'	1/4 cup	20	4	0.0
(Santiago) chunky	1 fl oz	10	2	0.1
(Sun Vista) hot	2 tbsp	5	2	0.0
(Territorial House) green chili	0.5 oz	4	1	1.0
(Timpone's) tomato, fresh roasted, 'Salsa Muy Rica'	2 tbsp	10	2	0.0
(Tostitos)				
con queso	4 tbsp	80	10	5.0
con queso, low-fat	4 tbsp	80	8	3.0
medium or hot	4 tbsp	30	6	0.0
mild	4 tbsp	30	6	0.0
'Ultimate Garden'	4 tbsp	30	6	0.0
SALSIFY/oyster plant/vegetable oyster				
boiled, drained, sliced	1 cup	92	21	0.2
boiled, drained, sliced	1/2 cup	46	10.5	0.1
raw, sliced	1 cup	109	25	0.3
raw, sliced	1/2 cup	55	12.5	0.1
SALSIFY, BLACK/scorzonera				
raw	1 lb	372	84.4	0.1
raw	1 oz	23	5.3	tr
SALT				
iodized *(Morton)*	1 tsp	0	0	0.0
kosher *(Morton)*	1 tsp	0	0	0.0
'Nature's Seasons' *(Morton)*	1 tsp	3	1	0.1
non-iodized *(Morton)*	1 tsp	0	0	0.0
sea *(Hain)*	1 tsp	0	0	0.0
sea *(Tone's)*	1 tsp	0	0	0.0
table	1 cup	0	0	0.0
table	1 dash	0	0	0.0
table	1 tbsp	0	0	0.0
table	1 tsp	0	0	0.0

Food Name	Serv. Size	Total Cal.	Carbs GMS	Fat GMS

SALT PORK. See PORK, SALT.
SALT SEASONING. See under SEASONING MIX.
SALT SUBSTITUTE

(Featherweight)	1/4 tsp	0	0	0.0
(Morton)	1 tsp	1	0	0.0
'Chef Shaker' (Diamond Crystal)	1/2 tsp	0	0	0.0
extra spicy (Mrs. Dash)	0.13 tsp	2	0	0.0
'Lite' (Lawry's)	1 tsp	8	2	0.1
lite, 1/2 the salt of regular salt (Morton)	1/4 tsp	0	0	0.0
'Lite Salt' (Morton)	1 tsp	1	0	0.0
'Salt-Free' (Lawry's)	1 tsp	10	2	0.2
'Salt-It' (Estee)	1/8 tsp	0	0	0.0
seasoned (Adolph's)	1/4 tsp	0	0	0.0
seasoned (Featherweight)	1/4 tsp	0	0	0.0
seasoned (Morton)	1 tsp	2	1	0.1
seasoned (Mrs. Dash)	0.13 tsp	2	0	0.0
seasoned, 'Instead of Salt' (Health Valley)	1 tsp	11	2	0.5
seasoned, 'Salt-Free' (Lawry's)	1 tsp	3	1	0.1

SAND PEAR. See ASIAN PEAR.
SANDWICH
BEEF

(Healthy Choice) Philly beef steak, 'Hearty Handfuls'	1 entree	290	47	5.0
(Hot Pockets)				
beef and cheddar stuffed sandwich, frozen	1 pkg	403	39	20.2
pocket, w/cheddar, frozen	5 oz	370	36	17.0
pocket, w/cheese, no gravy, 'Beef & Cheddar'	1 pocket	524	36	34.8
(Igor's Piroshki) pocket, w/cheddar	1 sandwich	370	31	20.0
(Kid Cuisine)				
double patty w/cheese, frozen, 'Mega Meal'	9.1 oz	480	55	20.0
patty w/cheese, frozen	6.25 oz	400	47	19.0
(Lean Pockets) pocket, w/broccoli, frozen	1 pkg	250	30	8.0
(Manwich)				
'Chili Fixin's'	1 cup	290	20	14.0
extra thick and chunky, prepared	1 sandwich	330	36	13.0
Mexican, prepared	1 sandwich	310	30	13.0
'sloppy Joe', prepared	1 sandwich	310	31	13.0
(MicroMagic)				
burger, w/cheese, frozen	4.75 oz	450	29	25.0
hamburger, frozen	4 oz	350	26	18.0
(Mrs. Paterson's)				
steak, w/mushroom, pocket, hand held, 'Aussie Pie'	5.5 oz	410	43	20.0
(Pierre)				
submarine, flame-broiled	1 piece	152	2	8.9
submarine, flame-broiled, 'Hot Diggity Sub'	1 piece	158	2	9.5
(Tyson) barbecue, no bone, frozen, microwave	1 sandwich	200	29	2.7
CALZONE				
(Amy's Kitchen) cheese, pocket, organic, frozen	1 sandwich	290	38	9.0
CANADIAN BACON				
(Quick Meal)				
Canadian bacon, w/egg and cheese, on muffin	4.5 oz	250	29	8.0
CHICKEN				
(Banquet) breast patty, bun, microwave.	4 oz	310	31	14.0
(BestFresh)				
breast, teriyaki, charbroiled	1 sandwich	490	45	20.0
w/cucumber yogurt dressing	1 sandwich	390	38	15.0
(Hot Pockets)				
w/broccoli, cheese, stuffed, 'Croissant Pockets'	1 pkg	602	78	22.0

Food Name	Serv. Size	Total Cal.	Carbs GMS	Fat GMS
chicken, w/cheddar, pocket, frozen	5 oz	310	38	11.0
(Kid Cuisine) chicken, dinner	8.2 oz	470	61	17.0
(Lean Pockets)				
fajita, pocket, frozen	1 pocket	250	36	6.0
Oriental, pocket, frozen	1 pkg	250	35	6.0
supreme, glazed, frozen	1 pkg	464	68	12.5
supreme, glazed, frozen	1 serving	233	34	6.3
w/Parmesan, pocket, frozen	1 pkg	270	35	6.0
(MicroMagic) frozen	4.5 oz	390	42	16.0
(Quick Meal)				
	4.3 oz	320	40	11.0
biscuit	4.2 oz	310	36	13.0
grilled	4.7 oz	300	35	9.0
(Tyson)				
barbecue, frozen, microwave	4 oz	230	27	6.0
breast, frozen, microwave	3.5 oz	275	27	12.0
breast, grilled, boneless	3.5 oz	150	2	8.0
breast, grilled, microwave	1 entree	210	25	6.0
grilled, boneless	3.5 oz	200	25	5.0
mini, frozen, microwave	3.5 oz	230	39	5.0
(Weight Watchers)				
grilled, 'Ultimate 200'	4 oz	200	22	5.0
w/broccoli, cheese, pocket sandwich, 'On-The-Go'	1 pkg	266	40	6.1
EGG *(Great Starts)* w/bacon and cheese, muffin	1 sandwich	290	25	15.0
ENGLISH MUFFIN *(Weight Watchers)*	1 sandwich	210	28	5.0
FISH				
(Fisher Boy) burger, crunchy	1 burger	180	18	6.0
(Quick Meal)	5.2 oz	430	56	16.0
HAM				
(Hot Pockets)				
and cheese, pocket, frozen	5 oz	360	36	16.0
and cheese, stuffed	1 pkg	681	77	28.4
and cheese, stuffed	1 serving	340	38	14.2
w/cheese, no gravy, pocket, 'Ham 'n Cheese'	1 pocket	524	36	34.8
(Igor's Piroshki) and cheese, pocket	1 sandwich	370	46	15.0
(Owens) and cheese, refrigerated, 'Border Breakfasts'	2 oz	150	14	6.0
(Red Baron)				
and cheese, 'Premium Pockets'	1 pkg	721	73	34.2
and cheese, 'Premium Pockets'	1 serving	356	36	16.9
(Swanson)				
and cheese, on bagel, refrigerated, 'Great Starts'	3 oz	240	28	8.0
(Weight Watchers)				
and cheese, on bagel	3 oz	210	28	6.0
and cheese, pocket, frozen, 'Ultimate 200'	4 oz	200	24	6.0
HOT DOG				
(Kid Cuisine) w/bun	6.7 oz	450	27	19.0
(Kid Cuisine) w/bun, 'Mega Meal'	8.25 oz	500	52	25.0
PIZZA				
(Hot Pockets)				
pepperoni, pocket, frozen	5 oz	380	40	17.0
pepperoni, stuffed, frozen	1 pkg	735	77	35.3
pepperoni, stuffed, frozen	1 serving	367	39	17.7
sausage, pocket, frozen	5 oz	360	40	16.0
(Igor's Piroshki) pepperoni and sausage, pocket	1 sandwich	400	39	19.0
(Lean Pockets)				
pocket, frozen, 'Deluxe'	1 pkg	280	34	9.0
sausage and pepperoni, pocket, frozen, 'Deluxe'	1 pocket	300	37	11.0

Food Name	Serv. Size	Total Cal.	Carbs GMS	Fat GMS
(Weight Watchers) pocket, 'Deluxe' 'Ultimate 200'	4 oz	200	25	5.0
PORK				
(Quick Meal) barbecue	4.3 oz	350	40	14.0
(Swanson) rib, hot, smothered	10.25 oz	340	50	10.0
SUBMARINE *(BestFresh)* 'Deluxe'	1 sandwich	790	59	44.0
TURKEY				
(BestFresh) smoked	1 sandwich	580	49	26.0
(Healthy Deli)				
w/corned beef, 'Doubledecker'	1 oz	30	1	0.7
w/ham, 'Doubledecker'	1 oz	30	1	0.9
(Hot Pockets) w/ham and cheese, frozen	5 oz	320	37	11.0
(Igor's Piroshki) and Swiss, w/broccoli, frozen	1 sandwich	320	41	11.0
(Lean Pockets) w/broccoli and cheese, frozen	1 pocket	260	32	9.0
VEGGIE				
(Ken & Robert's)				
barbecue style, 'Truly Amazing'	5 oz	320	50	10.0
broccoli cheddar, 'Truly Amazing'	5 oz	275	37	9.0
Greek style, 'Truly Amazing'	5 oz	270	35	10.0
Indian style, 'Truly Amazing'	5 oz	300	41	12.0
Oriental style, 'Truly Amazing'	5 oz	295	41	12.0
pizza style, 'Truly Amazing'	5 oz	315	42	12.0
Tex Mex style, 'Truly Amazing'	5 oz	310	43	11.0
(Morningstar Farms)				
burger and cheese style, 'Stuffed Sandwiches'	1 sandwich	290	10	8.0
ham and cheese style, 'Stuffed Sandwiches'	1 sandwich	300	45	7.0
pepperoni pizza style, 'Stuffed Sandwiches'	1 sandwich	280	42	7.0
SANDWICH FILLING MIX				
(French's) sloppy Joe, mix only	1/8 pkg	16	4	0.0
(Hunt's)				
sloppy Joe, barbecue, 'Manwich' mix only	1/4 cup	57	14	0.2
sloppy Joe, bold, 'Manwich' mix only	1/4 cup	63	13	1.1
sloppy Joe, Mexican, 'Manwich' mix only	1/4 cup	27	5	0.2
sloppy Joe, original, 'Manwich' mix only	1/4 cup	32	6	0.4
sloppy Joe, thick and chunky, 'Manwich'	1/4 cup	44	9	0.5
(McCormick/Schilling) sloppy Joe, mix only	1 tsp	15	3	0.0
(Schilling) sloppy Joe, mix only	1/4 pkg	26	6	0.5
(Tone's) sloppy Joe, mix only	1 tsp	14	3	0.1
SANDWICH SPREAD. See also LUCHEON MEAT SPREAD; POTTED MEAT SPREAD.				
(Best Foods)	1 tbsp	50	3	5.0
(Blue Plate)	1 tbsp	75	3	7.0
(Hellmann's)	1 tbsp	50	3	5.0
(JFG)	1 tbsp	60	3	5.0
(Oscar Mayer)				
	2 oz	130	8	10.0
pork, chicken, and beef	1 serving	71	5	5.0
SAPODILLA				
fresh, raw, pulp	1 cup	200	48	2.7
fresh, raw, whole	1 medium	141	34	1.9
SAPOTE/marmalade plum				
fresh, raw, trimmed	1 oz	38	9.6	0.2
fresh, raw, trimmed, whole, approx 11.2 oz	1 medium	302	76	1.4
fresh, raw, untrimmed	1 lb	431	108.7	1.9
SARDINE				
ATLANTIC				
Canned				
in oil, drained, w/bone	1 oz	59	0	3.2
in oil, drained, w/bone	2 medium	50	0	2.7

Food Name	Serv. Size	Total Cal.	Carbs GMS	Fat GMS
in oil, drained, w/bone	1 cup	310	0	17.1
BRISLING/Norwegian				
Canned				
(S&W)	3 oz	257	0	20.9
in mild sardine oil, drained (Empress)	3.75 oz	260	1	20.0
in mustard sauce (Crown Prince)	3.75 oz	240	2	18.0
smoked, in oil (Crown Prince)	3.75 oz	260	1	42.0
w/liquid (Underwood)	3.75 oz	260	1	20.0
MAINE				
Canned				
in mustard, drained (Beach Cliff)	3 oz	227	4	18.0
in soybean oil, drained (Beach Cliff)	3 oz	240	0	20.0
in tomato sauce, drained (Beach Cliff)	3 oz	210	0	17.0
in water, drained (Beach Cliff)	3 oz	230	1	18.0
MIXED SPECIES				
Canned				
boneless, skinless (S&W)	3 oz	177	0	10.6
in mustard sauce (Underwood)	3.75 oz	220	2	16.0
in oil (Featherweight)	1 1/8 oz	130	1	10.0
in olive oil, boneless, skinless (Crown Prince)	1 pkg	230	0	15.0
in soya oil, drained (Underwood)	3.75 oz	230	1	18.0
in Tabasco sauce, drained (Underwood)	3 oz	220	1	16.0
in tomato sauce (Del Monte)	1/2 cup	360	45	12.0
in tomato sauce (Underwood)	3.75 oz	220	2	16.0
in tomato sauce, drained, w/bone	1 cup	158	0	10.7
in tomato sauce, drained, w/bone	1 medium	68	0	4.6
in water (Featherweight)	1 1/8 oz	95	1	7.0
kippered, 'Kippered Snacks' (Brunswick)	3.5 oz	185	1	14.0
NORWEGIAN. See BRISLING.				
SARDINE OIL. See under FISH OIL.				
SAUCE				
ALFREDO SAUCE				
(Bernardi)	1/2 cup	180	10	13.0
(Contadina)				
	1/2 cup	400	8	38.0
frozen, food service product	1 oz	67	3	5.7
light	1/2 cup	190	10	13.0
pouch, food service product	1 oz	70	2	6.1
refrigerated 'Fresh'	6 oz	540	10	53.0
(DiGiorno)				
light	1/4 cup	140	9	9.0
reduced-fat, 'Lighter Varieties'	1/4 cup	180	15	11.0
refrigerated	2 oz	200	2	20.0
(Five Brothers)				
	1/4 cup	120	2	11.0
w/mushrooms	1/4 cup	80	3	7.0
(Progresso) canned, 'Authentic Pasta Sauces'	1/2 cup	340	6	30.0
APPLE-APRICOT				
(Lucky Leaf) 'Fruit n' Sauce'	4 oz	90	22	0.0
(Musselman's) 'Fruit n' Sauce'	4 oz	90	22	0.0
APPLE-CHERRY				
(Lucky Leaf) 'Fruit n' Sauce'	4 oz	100	24	0.0
(Musselman's) 'Fruit n' Sauce'	4 oz	100	24	0.0
APPLE-CRANBERRY (Lucky Leaf)	4 oz	80	19	0.0
APPLE-PEACH				
(Lucky Leaf) 'Fruit n' Sauce'	4 oz	90	22	0.0
(Musselman's) 'Fruit n' Sauce'	4 oz	90	22	0.0

Food Name	Serv. Size	Total Cal.	Carbs GMS	Fat GMS
APPLE-PINEAPPLE				
(Lucky Leaf) 'Fruit n' Sauce'	4 oz	110	26	0.0
(Musselman's) 'Fruit n' Sauce'	4 oz	110	26	0.0
APPLE-STRAWBERRY				
(Lucky Leaf) 'Fruit n' Sauce'	4 oz	100	24	0.0
(Musselman's) 'Fruit n' Sauce'	4 oz	100	24	0.0
BARBECUE				
(Bull's Eye)				
regular	0.5 oz	22	5	0.0
Ridge's	2 tbsp	63	15	0.1
(Cattleman's)				
classic	2 tbsp	70	15	0.0
mild	1 tbsp	25	5	0.0
smoky	1 tbsp	25	5	0.0
(Enrico's)				
'Original'	1 tbsp	18	3	1.0
mesquite	1 tbsp	18	3	1.0
(Estee) regular	1 tbsp	18	3	1.0
(Golden Dipt) Cajun style	1 oz	90	5	8.0
(Hain) honey	1 tbsp	14	1	1.0
(Healthy Choice)				
hickory	1.13 oz	26	6	0.2
hot and spicy	1.13 oz	25	6	0.2
original	1.13 oz	25	6	0.2
(Heinz)				
Cajun style	1 tbsp	15	3	0.1
chunky, 'Thick & Rich'	1 tbsp	24	5	0.0
Hawaiian style	1 tbsp	19	4	0.1
Hawaiian style, 'Thick & Rich'	1 oz	40	10	0.0
hickory smoke	1 tbsp	19	4	0.1
hickory smoke, 'Thick & Rich'	1 tbsp	20	5	0.0
hickory, 'Select'	1 oz	35	8	0.0
hot, 'Thick & Rich'	1 tbsp	20	5	0.0
mesquite smoke, 'Thick & Rich'	1 oz	30	7	0.0
mushroom	1 tbsp	14	3	0.1
mushroom, 'Thick & Rich'	1 tbsp	20	5	0.0
'Old Fashioned'	1 tbsp	18	4	0.1
old fashioned, 'Thick & Rich'	1 oz	35	8	0.0
onion	1 tbsp	15	3	0.1
onion, 'Thick & Rich'	1 tbsp	20	5	0.0
original, 'Thick & Rich'	1 tbsp	20	5	0.0
'Select'	1 tbsp	18	4	0.1
Texas style, hot, 'Thick & Rich'	1 tbsp	15	3	0.2
(Hunt's)				
'Chicken Sensations'	1 tbsp	35	3	2.7
country style	1.2 oz	39	9	0.3
hickory	1 tbsp	20	5	1.0
hickory, 'Light'	1.13 oz	27	6	0.2
homestyle	1.23 oz	41	10	0.1
Kansas City style	1.23 oz	43	10	0.2
New Orleans style	1.23 oz	41	9	0.2
original recipe	2 tbsp	40	9	0.0
Southern style	1.2 oz	40	9	0.4
Texas style	1.23 oz	42	10	0.1
western style	1.23 oz	41	10	0.2
(Kraft)				
chunky, 'Thick 'n Spicy'	2 tbsp	60	13	1.0

Food Name	Serv. Size	Total Cal.	Carbs GMS	Fat GMS
hickory smoke	2 tbsp	39	9	0.1
hickory smoke, 'Thick 'N Spicy'	2 tbsp	50	12	0.0
hickory smoke, w/onion bits	2 tbsp	50	11	1.0
honey, 'Thick 'N Spicy'	2 tbsp	60	13	0.0
hot	2 tbsp	40	9	0.0
Kansas City style	2 tbsp	50	11	0.0
Kansas City style, 'Thick 'N Spicy'	2 tbsp	60	14	0.0
mesquite smoke	2 tbsp	40	9	0.0
mesquite smoke, 'Thick 'N Spicy'	2 tbsp	50	12	0.0
original	2 tbsp	39	9	0.1
original, 'Thick 'N Spicy'	2 tbsp	50	12	0.0
roasted garlic	2 tbsp	50	12	0.0
salsa style	2 tbsp	45	9	0.0
w/Italian seasonings	2 tbsp	50	10	1.0
w/onion bits	2 tbsp	45	11	0.0
(LaChoy) Oriental	1 tbsp	16	4	0.1
(Lawry's)				
Dijon and honey	1/2 cup	203	27	1.2
orange juice, 'California Grill'	1/4 cup	34	3	0.7
(Libby's) w/beef, 'Sloppy Joe'	1/3 cup	110	7	7.0
(Luzianne) mustard base, 'Cajun'	2 tbsp	110	19	4.0
(Marzetti) original, 'Texas Best'	2 tbsp	42	4	2.7
(Maull's) smoky	1 tbsp	20	4	1.0
(Open Pit)				
hickory	2 tbsp	50	11	0.5
original	2 tbsp	50	11	0.5
(Open Range)				
hickory	1.2 oz	37	9	0.2
hickory, food service product	2 tbsp	37	9	0.2
original	1.2 oz	38	9	0.2
original, food service product	2 tbsp	38	9	0.2
(Ott's)				
regular	1 tbsp	14	3	0.1
smoky	1 tbsp	14	3	0.1
(Woodys) sweet and sour	2 tbsp	70	17	0.0
BASIL-HERB				
(Golden Dipt) 'Nature Bay'	2 grams	8	1	0.0
(Nature Bay)	2 grams	8	1	0.0
BEARNAISE (Great Impressions)	2 tbsp	192	0	21.0
BEEF				
(Ragu)				
barbecue, 'Beef Tonight'	4 oz	70	15	1.0
skillet lasagna, 'Beef Tonight'	4 oz	60	9	1.0
stroganoff, 'Beef Tonight'	4 oz	130	6	12.0
(Simmer Chef) Stroganoff, family style	1/2 cup	110	8	7.0
BOLOGNESE				
(Contadina)				
	5 oz	130	0	7.0
refrigerated, 'Fresh'	7.5 oz	230	12	11.0
(Progresso) canned, 'Authentic Pasta Sauces'	1/2 cup	150	12	8.0
BROCCOLI (Simmer Chef) creamy	1/2 cup	110	9	8.0
BROWNING (Gravymaster)	1 tsp	12	2	0.0
CACCIATORE				
(Recipe Sauces)	3.9 oz	40	9	1.0
(Simmer Chef) old country	1/2 cup	110	15	4.0
CARBONARA (DiGiorno) refrigerated	2 oz	200	3	19.0
CHARDONNAY (Golden Dipt)	1 oz	60	1	6.0

Food Name	Serv. Size	Total Cal.	Carbs GMS	Fat GMS
CHEESE				
(Contadina)				
four cheese, refrigerated 'Fresh'	6 oz	470	8	45.0
four cheese, w/white wine & shallots	1/2 cup	320	8	28.0
(DiGiorno) four cheese	1/4 cup	160	3	15.0
(J. Hungerford)				
cheddar, 'Stadium'	2 oz	80	6	5.0
nacho	2.01 oz	120	7	9.0
nacho, 'Stadium'	2.01 oz	80	6	5.0
(Kaukauna)				
nacho	1 oz	80	4	6.0
nacho, medium, microwaveable	2 tbsp	90	4	7.0
nacho, mild, microwaveable	2 tbsp	90	4	7.0
(Kraft)				
jalapeño pepper, pasteurized process, 'Cheez Whiz'	2 tbsp	90	3	7.0
pasteurized process, 'Cheez Whiz'	2 tbsp	90	3	7.0
salsa, mild, pasteurized process, 'Cheez Whiz'	2 tbsp	100	3	7.0
(La Victoria)				
cheddar	1/4 cup	105	6	8.5
nacho, w/jalapeño peppers	1/4 cup	122	7	9.7
(Lucky Leaf)				
cheddar	4 oz	220	12	18.0
cheddar, aged	4 oz	240	11	20.0
cheddar, mild, aged	4 oz	200	9	18.0
cheddar, sharp, aged	4 oz	230	6	17.0
nacho	4 oz	220	11	18.0
(Musselman's)				
cheddar	4 oz	220	12	18.0
cheddar, aged	4 oz	240	11	20.0
cheddar, mild, aged	4 oz	200	9	18.0
cheddar, sharp, aged	4 oz	230	6	17.0
nacho	4 oz	220	11	18.0
(Nestlé)				
cheddar, 'Chef Mate'	1 cup	327	32	18.8
cheddar, 'Chef Mate'	1/4 cup	82	8	4.7
cheddar, sharp, 'Chef Mate'	1 cup	532	7	46.0
cheddar, sharp, 'Chef Mate'	1/4 cup	133	2	11.5
con queso, 'Que Bueno'	1 cup	335	14	24.1
con queso, 'Que Bueno'	1/4 cup	84	4	6.0
golden, 'Chef-Mate'	1 cup	554	9	45.5
golden, 'Chef-Mate'	1/4 cup	139	2	11.4
jalapeño, 'Que Bueno'	1 pkg	3876	370	224.2
jalapeño, 'Que Bueno	1/4 cup	81	8	4.7
nacho, mild, 'Que Bueno'	1 cup	476	10	40.5
nacho, mild, 'Que Bueno'	1/4 cup	119	3	10.1
nacho, 'Que Bueno'	1 cup	512	16	40.4
nacho, 'Que Bueno'	1/4 cup	128	4	10.1
(Pablo's)				
jalapeño, 'Deli Style'	1 oz	59	4	4.0
nacho, 'Deli Style'	1 oz	59	4	4.0
(Snow's) Welsh rarebit	1/2 cup	170	10	11.0
(Weight Watchers) cheddar, sharp	2 tbsp	70	7	3.0
(White House)				
cheddar, aged	3.5 oz	213	10	18.0
jalapeño	3.5 oz	193	10	16.0
nacho	3.5 oz	193	10	16.0

Food Name	Serv. Size	Total Cal.	Carbs GMS	Fat GMS
CHICKEN				
(Hunt's) Southwestern, 'Chicken Sensations'	1 tbsp	27	1	2.6
(Ragu)				
cacciatore, 'Chicken Tonight'	4 oz	70	12	2.0
French, country, 'Chicken Tonight'	4 oz	140	6	12.0
herbed, w/wine, 'Chicken Tonight'	4 oz	100	13	4.0
honey mustard, light, 'Chicken Tonight'	4 oz	50	12	1.0
Italian, primavera, 'Light'	4 oz	50	9	1.0
primavera, creamy, 'Chicken Tonight'	4 oz	90	9	6.0
sweet and sour, 'Chicken Tonight'	4 oz	80	19	0.0
sweet and spicy, light, 'Chicken Tonight'	4 oz	50	10	1.0
w/mushrooms, creamy, 'Chicken Tonight'	4 oz	110	5	10.0
CHILI				
(Chef Boyardee) hot dog, w/beef	1 oz	30	4	1.0
(Del Monte)	1 tbsp	20	5	0.0
(El Molino) green, mild	2 tbsp	10	2	0.0
(Featherweight)	1 tbsp	8	2	0.0
(Gebhardt) hot dog	2 tbsp	20	2	1.0
(Heinz)	1 oz	30	7	0.0
(Just Rite) hot dog sauce	2.19 oz	50	5	2.9
(Las Palmas) red	1/2 cup	25	3	1.0
(Manwich) 'Chili Fixin's'	5.3 oz	110	20	1.0
(Open Range) hot dog	2.22 oz	61	6	3.5
(S&W)				
'Chili Makin's'	1/2 cup	100	20	1.0
steakhouse	1 tbsp	15	4	0.0
(Wolf Brand) hot dog	1.25 oz	44	4	2.3
CHOCOLATE *(Chocolate Mountain)*	2 tbsp	120	20	4.0
CLAM				
(Buitoni) red, canned	5 oz	190	28	6.0
(Contadina)				
red, refrigerated, 'Fresh'	7.5 oz	120	15	4.0
white, refrigerated, 'Fresh'	6 oz	290	13	23.0
(Ferrara)				
red, canned	4 oz	70	8	2.0
white, canned	4 oz	80	4	5.0
(Progresso)				
red, canned	1/2 cup	70	7	3.0
white, canned	1/2 cup	110	1	8.0
COCKTAIL				
(Del Monte)	1/4 cup	100	24	0.0
(Estee)	1 tbsp	10	2	1.0
(Golden Dipt)				
extra hot	1 tbsp	20	5	0.0
regular	1 tbsp	20	5	0.0
(Great Impressions)				
	1 tbsp	21	5	0.1
'Brandy Glow'	1 tbsp	68	2	6.7
low-salt	1 tbsp	21	5	0.1
(Heinz)	1/4 cup	60	14	0.0
(S&W)	1 tsp	20	5	0.0
(Sauceworks)	1 tbsp	14	3	0.0
(Stokely)	1 tbsp	18	5	0.0
CRANBERRY-ORANGE				
(Ocean Spray) crushed, for chicken, 'CranFruit'	2 oz	90	23	0.0
CRANBERRY-RASPBERRY				
(Ocean Spray) crushed, for chicken, 'CranFruit'	2 oz	90	23	0.0

Food Name	Serv. Size	Total Cal.	Carbs GMS	Fat GMS
CRANBERRY-STRAWBERRY				
(Ocean Spray) crushed, for chicken, 'CranFruit'	2 oz	90	22	0.0
CREOLE				
(Enrico's) Cajun, 'Light'	4 oz	76	9	2.8
(Golden Dipt) cooking sauce	1 oz	20	2	1.0
(Nestlé)				
'Chef Mate'	1 cup	99	15	2.8
'Chef Mate'	1/4 cup	25	4	0.7
CURRY				
(Flavor of the Rain Forest) ginger, stir-fry	1 tbsp	15	2	1.0
(TAJ Cuisine of India) Bombay	4 oz	90	10	5.0
DIABLE (Escoffier) nonat	1 tbsp	20	4	0.0
DIJONAISSE (Golden Dipt)	1 oz	52	2	4.0
ENCHILADA				
(Del Monte)				
hot	1/2 cup	45	11	0.0
mild	1/2 cup	45	11	0.0
(El Molino) hot	2 tbsp	16	2	1.0
(Gebhardt)	1/4 cup	35	4	2.0
(La Victoria)				
	1 cup	80	10	5.0
	1/4 cup	20	3	0.9
(Las Palmas) hot	1/2 cup	25	3	1.0
(Nestlé)				
'Que Bueno'	1 pkg	1928	259	76.3
'Que Bueno'	2 tbsp	15	2	0.6
(Old El Paso)				
green	2 tbsp	11	3	0.0
green chili	1/4 cup	30	3	1.5
hot	1/4 cup	30	4	1.0
mild	1/4 cup	25	4	1.0
(Ortega)				
hot	1 oz	12	3	0.0
mild	1 oz	12	3	0.0
(Rosarita)				
	1/4 cup	23	3	1.1
food service product	1/4 cup	23	3	1.1
mild	2.5 oz	25	3	1.0
(Santiago)	1 fl oz	11	2	0.1
FAJITA				
(S&W) Southwestern	1 tbsp	10	2	0.0
(Tio Sancho) 'Skillet Sauce'	1 oz	14	2	0.5
FORESTIERA (Contadina) refrigerated, 'Fresh'	7.5 oz	270	15	9.0
GARLIC				
(A Taste of Thai) chili pepper	1 tbsp	10	2	0.0
(Golden Dipt) herb, nonfat, 'Nature Bay'	2 grams	8	1	0.0
(Hunt's) Italian, 'Chicken Sensations'	1 tbsp	30	1	2.7
GINGER				
(Flavor of the Rain Forest) curry, stir-fry	1 tbsp	15	2	1.0
(Mr. Spice) stir fry, fat-free, salt-free	1 tbsp	11	3	0.0
HERB (Lawry's) and garlic, w/lemon juice	1/4 cup	36	4	0.4
HOISIN (Dynasty)	2 tbsp	80	15	1.5
HOLLANDAISE (Great Impressions)	2 tbsp	192	0	21.0
HONEY MUSTARD				
(Ragu) light, Chicken Tonight'	4 oz	50	12	0.5
(Simmer Chef)	1/2 cup	150	30	2.0

Food Name	Serv. Size	Total Cal.	Carbs GMS	Fat GMS
HORSERADISH				
(Great Impressions)	1 tbsp	74	1	7.6
(Heinz)	1 tbsp	74	2	7.4
(Life) strong, 'All Natural'	1/2 tbsp	7	1	1.0
(Sauceworks)	1 tbsp	50	2	5.0
HOT DOG				
(Chili Bowl) chili, w/beef	1/4 cup	100	6	7.0
(Gebhardt)				
chili, food service product	1/4 cup	61	6	3.5
chili, w/beef	1/4 cup	57	6	3.2
(Hunt's) chili, w/beef	1/4 cup	61	6	3.5
(Just Rite)	1/4 cup	50	5	2.9
(Nestlé)				
chili, w/beef, 'Chef-Mate'	1 pkg	3368	449	115.7
chili, w/beef, 'Chef-Mate'	1/4 cup	69	9	2.4
Coney Island, 'Chef-Mate'	1 cup	303	23	19.7
Coney Island, 'Chef-Mate'	1/4 cup	76	6	4.9
HOT SAUCE				
(Gebhardt) pepper, 'Louisiana Style'	1/2 tsp	0	0	0.0
(Tabasco) pepper	1 tsp	1	0	0.0
(Tabasco) pepper	1/4 tsp	1	0	0.0
(Gebhardt)	1 tsp	1	0	0.0
HUNTER *(McCormick/Schilling)*	1 tbsp	25	4	0.0
ITALIAN				
(Nestlé) 'Chef-Mate'	1 cup	125	24	2.4
(Nestlé) 'Chef-Mate'	1/4 cup	61	11	1.2
JALAPEÑO *(Tabasco)*	1 tsp	0	0	0.0
KUNG PAO *(Dynasty)* spicy hot	2 tbsp	50	6	2.5
LEMON				
(Nestlé) 'Chef-Mate'	1 pkg	2849	679	12.5
(Nestlé) 'Chef-Mate'	2 tbsp	43	10	0.2
LEMON BUTTER DILL *(Golden Dipt)*	1 oz	100	4	9.0
LEMON DILL *(Golden Dipt)* 'Nature Bay'	1 oz	110	3	11.0
LEMON HERB *(Hunt's)* 'Chicken Sensations'	1 tbsp	31	2	2.7
LOBSTER SAUCE *(Progresso)* rock	1/2 cup	120	11	8.0
MARINARA. See also SAUCE, PASTA.				
(Angela Mia) food service product	1/2 cup	47	9	0.3
(Bernardi)	1/2 cup	120	20	4.0
(Buitoni)	1/2 cup	70	11	3.0
(Contadina)				
	1 cup	145	17	7.0
	1/2 cup	73	9	3.5
frozen, food service product	1 oz	18	2	0.9
(Five Brothers) w/burgundy wine	1/2 cup	80	9	4.0
(Hunt's) chunky	1/2 cup	60	12	1.6
(Millina's Finest)				
organic	4 oz	48	9	0.5
Zinfandel, organic	4 oz	44	9	0.5
(Pathmark)				
'All Natural'	1/2 cup	80	12	2.0
'No Frills'	1/2 cup	80	12	3.0
(Prego)	1/2 cup	110	12	6.0
(Progresso)				
	1/2 cup	90	9	5.0
'Authentic Pasta Sauces'	1/2 cup	110	10	6.0
(Ragu) 'Old World Style'	1/2 cup	90	9	5.0
(Rokeach)	3 oz	60	9	2.0

Food Name	Serv. Size	Total Cal.	Carbs GMS	Fat GMS
(Westbrae)				
....	4 oz	40	7	1.0
w/mushrooms	4 oz	50	7	1.0
MESQUITE				
(Lawry's) w/lime juice	1/4 cup	24	3	0.4
(S&W) and marinade	1 tbsp	10	3	0.0
MEXICAN *(S&W)* mild, 'Tomato Garden'	1/4 cup	20	4	0.0
MOLE POBLANO *(La Victoria)*	2 oz	240	28	10.3
MUSHROOM *(Simmer Chef)* and herb, creamy	1/2 cup	110	7	9.0
NEWBURG *(Snow's)* canned, w/sherry	1/3 cup	120	10	8.0
ONION *(Simmer Chef)* and mushroom, hearty	1/2 cup	50	9	1.0
ORANGE DIJON *(Golden Dipt)* 'Nature Bay'	1 oz	110	6	9.0
ORANGE *(LaChoy)* Mandarin	1 tbsp	24	6	0.0
OREGANO HERB *(Golden Dipt)* 'Nature Bay'	2 grams	6	1	0.0
PARMIGIANA *(Betty Crocker)* 'Recipe Sauces'	3.9 oz	50	9	1.0
PASTA/spaghetti. See also SAUCE, MARINARA; SAUCE, TOMATO.				
(Angela Mia)	1/2 cup	49	11	0.5
(Campbell's)				
extra garlic and onion	4 oz	50	12	1.0
'Homestyle'	4 oz	40	10	0.0
Italian style............	4 oz	50	12	0.0
mushroom	4 oz	50	11	1.0
traditional, 'Healthy Request'	4 oz	50	12	0.0
w/fresh mushrooms, 'Healthy Request'	4 oz	50	11	1.0
(Chef Boyardee)				
meat flavor	3.75 oz	80	11	3.0
meat flavor, 'Original'	3.75 oz	120	13	6.0
meatless, 'Jars'	4 oz	60	11	1.0
mushroom flavor	3.75 oz	60	11	1.0
mushroom flavor, 'Jars'	4 oz	70	11	2.0
mushroom flavor, 'Original'	3.75 oz	80	13	3.0
w/ground beef, 'Jars'	4 oz	90	14	3.0
(Classico) sun-dried tomato, 'Di Capri'	1/2 cup	80	8	4.5
(Contadina)				
meat flavored, 'Original Recipe'	1/2 cup	100	17	3.2
mushroom, 'Original Recipe'	1/2 cup	90	18	2.3
traditional, 'Original Recipe'	1/2 cup	90	17	2.3
(Del Monte) flavored w/meat	1/2 cup	70	9	2.0
traditional	1/2 cup	70	11	2.0
w/garlic and onion	1/2 cup	70	10	2.0
w/mushrooms	1/2 cup	70	11	2.0
(DiGiorno) plum tomato and mushroom, refrigerated	5 oz	100	20	1.0
(Eden Foods)				
and pizza sauce, organic............	4 oz	80	10	3.0
organic, no salt added	4 oz	80	14	2.0
(Enrico's)				
all natural, no salt added	4 oz	60	9	1.0
garlic and sun-dried tomatoes, all natural	3.5 oz	62	9	2.0
Italian style, all natural	3.5 oz	53	11	1.0
mushroom and green pepper, all natural	4 oz	60	9	1.0
mushroom and green pepper, no salt added	4 oz	60	9	1.0
mushroom flavor	4 oz	60	9	1.0
organic tomatoes, 'Hot & Spicy Arabiati'	3.5 oz	60	9	1.8
original, all natural	4 oz	60	9	1.0
peppers and mushrooms, all natural	4 oz	60	9	1.0
w/fresh mushrooms	4 oz	60	9	1.0
(Featherweight) mushroom flavor	4 oz	60	11	1.0

Food Name	Serv. Size	Total Cal.	Carbs GMS	Fat GMS
(Five Brothers)				
garden vegetable primavera	1/2 cup	70	9	3.0
tomato basil	1/2 cup	60	8	2.0
w/sautéed mushrooms	1/2 cup	90	10	4.0
(Healthy Choice)				
garlic and herb	4 oz	40	9	1.0
garlic and herb, original	1/2 cup	50	10	0.0
garlic and onion	1/2 cup	40	9	0.0
garlic and onion, chunky	4 oz	40	10	0.0
Italian vegetable, chunky	4.41 oz	50	11	0.6
mushroom and green pepper, super chunky	1/2 cup	45	9	0.0
mushroom, chunky	4 oz	45	10	0.0
mushroom, super chunky	1/2 cup	40	9	0.0
traditional	4 oz	40	9	1.0
vegetable primavera, super chunky	1/2 cup	45	9	0.0
w/chunky mushrooms, nonfat	4 oz	45	10	0.0
w/mushrooms	4 oz	40	9	1.0
w/vegetables, Italian style, chunky	4 oz	40	9	0.0
(Hunt's)				
'Homestyle'	4 oz	60	10	2.0
'Traditional'	4 oz	70	12	2.0
100% natural, 'Old Country'	4 oz	60	8	2.0
garlic and herb, 'Classic'	4.41 oz	58	10	2.1
garlic and herb, 'Light'	4.41 oz	39	7	0.8
garlic and herb, 'Old Country'	1/2 cup	63	9	2.7
garlic and onion, 'Classic Italian'	1/2 cup	58	10	2.1
Italian sausage	1/2 cup	77	12	2.7
Italian style vegetable, chunky	1/2 cup	63	13	1.0
Italian vegetable, 'Old Country'	1/2 cup	64	9	2.6
light meat	4.41 oz	45	8	1.2
meat flavor	4 oz	70	12	2.0
meat flavored, 'Home Style'	1/2 cup	57	7	2.6
meat flavored, 'Old Country'	1/2 cup	56	7	2.6
meat flavored, 'Original'	1/2 cup	65	11	2.3
meat	4.44 oz	65	11	2.3
meat, 'Homestyle'	4.41 oz	56	7	2.6
mushroom flavor	4 oz	70	12	2.0
mushroom	4.44 oz	65	11	2.3
mushroom, 'Home Style'	1/2 cup	57	7	2.6
mushroom, light	4.41 oz	39	7	0.8
mushroom, 'Old Country'	1/2 cup	53	7	2.7
mushroom, 'Original'	1/2 cup	65	11	2.3
Parmesan, 'Classic Italian'	1/2 cup	50	8	2.1
spaghetti, cheese and garlic, Italian style	1/2 cup	65	9	2.4
spaghetti, chunky	4 oz	50	12	1.0
spaghetti, tomato basil, 'Classic'	4.41 oz	48	8	2.1
spaghetti, tomato, garlic, and onion, chunky.	1/2 cup	61	13	1.0
spaghetti, w/tomato chunks, 'Chunky Style'	4 oz	50	12	1.0
tomato and basil, 'Classic Italian'	1/2 cup	48	8	2.1
traditional, 'Light'	4 oz	40	9	0.0
traditional, 'Home Style'	1/2 cup	57	7	2.6
traditional, 'Old Country'	1/2 cup	53	7	2.7
traditional, 'Original'	1/2 cup	65	11	2.3
w/meat	4 oz	70	12	2.0
w/mushrooms	4 oz	70	12	2.0
w/mushrooms, 'Light'	4 oz	40	9	0.0
(McCormick/Schilling) herb and garlic	1 tbsp	20	2	0.0

Food Name	Serv. Size	Total Cal.	Carbs GMS	Fat GMS
(Millina's Finest)				
sweet pepper and onion, nonfat organic	4 oz	41	7	0.5
tomato and mushroom, nonfat, organic	4 oz	45	9	0.0
tomato basil, nonfat, organic	4 oz	46	9	0.5
(Nestlé)	1/2 cup	70	12	1.6
(P&Q)				
meat flavor	1/2 cup	70	11	2.0
meatless	1/2 cup	70	14	1.0
mushroom flavor	1/2 cup	70	14	1.0
(Pastorelli) 'Italian Chef'	4 oz	81	11	3.0
(Pathmark)				
meat flavor, 'All Natural'	1/2 cup	80	11	3.0
meat flavor, 'No Frills'	1/2 cup	90	11	5.0
meatless, 'All Natural'	1/2 cup	70	11	2.0
meatless, 'No Frills'	1/2 cup	80	11	3.0
mushroom flavor, 'All Natural'	1/2 cup	70	11	2.0
(Prego)				
	1/2 cup	110	19	3.0
garden combination	4 oz	80	14	2.0
garden combination, chunky	1/2 cup	100	19	2.0
garlic and cheese, extra chunky	1/2 cup	130	22	3.5
low-salt	1/2 cup	110	11	6.0
meat flavored	1/2 cup	140	21	6.0
mushroom	1/2 cup	150	23	5.0
mushroom, extra chunky, extra spicy	1/2 cup	120	19	4.0
mushroom, w/onion, extra chunky	1/2 cup	110	18	3.0
mushroom, w/tomato, chunky	1/2 cup	110	19	3.0
mushroom and green pepper, chunky	1/2 cup	120	18	4.5
mushroom flavor	4 oz	130	20	5.0
onion, tomato-based, 'Extra Chunky'	4 oz	110	14	5.0
onion, w/garlic	1/2 cup	110	19	3.0
sausage, w/peppers, extra chunky	1/2 cup	180	22	9.0
spaghetti, traditional, '100% Natural'	2 tbsp	136	21	5.0
three cheese	1/2 cup	100	18	2.0
tomato and onion, w/garlic, extra chunky	1/2 cup	110	19	3.5
traditional	1/2 cup	140	23	4.5
(Pritikin)				
garden style, chunky	1/2 cup	50	11	0.0
original	1/2 cup	60	14	1.0
(Progresso)				
meat flavor	1/2 cup	110	13	5.0
mushroom flavor	1/2 cup	110	13	5.0
primavera, creamy, 'Authentic Pasta Sauces'	1/2 cup	190	8	17.0
Sicilian, 'Authentic Pasta Sauces'	1/2 cup	30	2	2.5
spaghetti	1/2 cup	110	13	5.0
(Ragu)				
beef flavored, 'Hearty'	1/2 cup	130	19	4.5
'Fresh Italian'	4 oz	90	13	3.0
garden, 'Light'	1/2 cup	50	11	0.0
garden harvest, 'Today's Recipe'	4 oz	50	8	1.0
'Gardenstyle Chunky'	1/2 cup	120	18	4.0
green and red pepper, 'Gardenstyle Chunky'	1/2 cup	120	19	4.0
'Homestyle'	4 oz	50	6	2.0
Italian garden combination, 'Chunky Gardenstyle'	4 oz	110	15	5.0
Italian tomato, 'Hearty'	1/2 cup	120	19	3.0
meat flavored, 'Old World Style'	1/2 cup	90	9	5.0
mushroom, 'Old World Style'	1/2 cup	80	10	3.5

Food Name	Serv. Size	Total Cal.	Carbs GMS	Fat GMS
mushroom, chunky, 'Light'	1/2 cup	50	11	0.0
mushroom, chunky, 'Today's Recipe'	4 oz	50	8	1.0
no sugar added, 'Light'	1/2 cup	60	9	1.5
Parmesan, 'Hearty'	1/2 cup	120	18	4.0
smooth, traditional 'Old World'	1/2 cup	80	12	2.6
spaghetti, 'Chunky Gardenstyle'	4 oz	70	10	3.0
spaghetti, 'Slow Cooked Homestyle'	4 oz	110	15	5.0
'Thick & Hearty'	4 oz	100	15	3.0
tomato, garlic, and onion, 'Gardenstyle Chunky'	1/2 cup	120	19	4.0
tomato, Italian, 100% natural,	1/2 cup	120	19	3.0
tomato and herbs, 'Today's Recipe'	4 oz	50	8	1.0
traditional, 'Old World Style'	1/2 cup	80	10	3.5
vegetable primavera, 'Gardenstyle Super'	1/2 cup	110	17	4.0
w/meat, 'Homestyle'	4 oz	110	15	5.0
w/mushrooms, 'Gardenstyle Super'	1/2 cup	120	19	4.0
w/mushrooms, 'Homestyle'	4 oz	110	15	2.0
w/mushrooms, 'Thick & Hearty'	4 oz	100	15	3.0
w/mushrooms and green peppers, 'Gardenstyle Chunky'	1/2 cup	120	18	4.0
w/mushrooms and onions, 'Gardenstyle Chunky'	1/2 cup	120	19	4.0
w/sautéed onion and garlic, 100% natural, 'Hearty'	1/2 cup	130	19	5.0
w/sautéed onion and mushroom, 'Hearty'	1/2 cup	110	17	4.0
w/tomato and herbs, 'Homestyle'	4 oz	110	15	5.0
w/tomato and herbs, 'Ragu Fine Italian'	4 oz	90	13	3.0
(S&W) 'Ready Cut'	1/4 cup	20	4	0.0
(Sutter Home) Zinfandel wine	1/2 cup	100	11	5.0
(Timpone's) fresh garlic and basil, 'Mom's Sauce'	4.5 oz	70	7	4.0
(Weight Watchers)				
meat flavor	1/3 cup	50	9	1.0
mushroom flavor, nonfat	1/3 cup	40	9	0.0
(Westbrae)				
primavera	4 oz	60	7	3.0
primavera, nonfat, no salt added	4 oz	40	7	0.0
PEANUT				
(Mr. Spice) Thai, nonfat, salt-free	1 tbsp	19	3	1.0
(San-J) Thai	1 tbsp	30	3	1.3
PEPPER DILL (Golden Dipt) 'Nature Bay'	2 grams	8	1	0.0
PEPPER				
(Hunt's) homestyle, hot	1 tsp	1	0	0.0
(Hunt's) orignal homestyle, original	1 tsp	1	0	0.0
PEPPER STEAK (Betty Crocker) 'Recipe Sauces'	3.8 oz	50	8	2.0
PEPPERCORN (McCormick/Schilling) green, blend	2 tsp	20	3	0.0
PESTO				
(Christopher Ranch) basil and garlic	1/4 cup	230	4	23.0
(Contadina)				
frozen, food service product	1 oz	66	2	5.4
refrigerated, 'Fresh'	2.33 oz	350	6	34.0
w/basil	1/4 cup	310	5	30.0
w/sun-dried tomatoes	1/4 cup	250	6	24.0
(DiGiorno) refrigerated	2.3 oz	340	5	32.0
PICANTE				
(Azteca) mild	1 tbsp	4	1	0.0
(Chi-Chi's)				
hot	1 oz	10	2	2.0
medium	1 oz	8	2	2.0
mild	1 oz	9	2	2.0
(Del Monte)				
hot	1/2 cup	20	4	0.0

Food Name	Serv. Size	Total Cal.	Carbs GMS	Fat GMS
hot, chunky	1/4 cup	15	3	0.0
(Estee)	2 tbsp	8	2	0.0
(Gebhardt)	1 tbsp	4	1	0.0
(Guiltless Gourmet)				
hot	2 tbsp	8	1	0.0
medium	2 tbsp	8	1	0.0
mild	2 tbsp	8	1	0.0
(Hunt's) mild, 'Homestyle'	1.09 oz	11	2	0.2
(La Victoria)				
medium	2 tbsp	5	1	0.0
mild	2 tbsp	10	2	0.0
(LaCasita) mild, chunky	2 oz	16	4	0.0
(Nestlé)				
'Que Bueno'	1 pkg	1311	257	8.9
'Que Bueno'	2 tbsp	10	2	0.1
(Old El Paso)				
'Thick 'n Chunky'	2 tbsp	6	1	0.0
all varieties, 'Chunky'	2 tbsp	7	2	0.0
all varieties	2 tbsp	8	2	1.0
hot	2 tbsp	10	2	0.0
hot, 'Thick n' Chunky'	2 tbsp	10	2	0.0
medium	2 tbsp	10	2	0.0
medium, 'Thick n' Chunky'	2 tbsp	10	2	0.0
mild	2 tbsp	10	2	0.0
mild, 'Thick n' Chunky'	2 tbsp	10	2	0.0
(Ortega) picante, can or jar	1 oz	10	2	0.0
(Pace)				
extra mild, 'Thick & Chunky'	2 tsp	3	1	0.1
hot, 'Thick & Chunky'	2 tsp	3	1	0.1
medium, 'Thick & Chunky'	2 tsp	3	1	0.1
mild, 'Thick & Chunky'	2 tsp	3	1	0.1
(Rosarita)				
	1.09 oz	7	1	0.1
hot, chunky	3 tbsp	18	4	1.0
jalapeño, hot, zesty	1.09 oz	8	2	0.2
jalapeño, medium, zesty	1.09 oz	9	2	0.2
jalapeño, mild, zesty	1.09 oz	8	2	0.1
jalapeño, zesty, 'de Mexico Style'	2 tbsp	12	3	0.0
mild	3.5 oz	45	9	1.0
mild, chunky	3 tbsp	25	5	1.0
(S&W) hot, 'Sun-Vista'	2 tbsp	10	2	0.0
(Santiago)	1 fl oz	10	2	0.1
(Sun Vista) hot	2 tbsp	10	2	0.0
(Sun Vista) mild	2 tbsp	5	2	0.0
(Wise)	2 tbsp	12	3	0.0
PIZZA				
(Angela Mia)				
food service product	1/4 cup	63	4	0.5
super heavy, food service product	1/4 cup	29	6	0.5
super heavy, 'Premium Choice'	2.26 oz	28	6	0.5
(Chef Boyardee)				
w/cheese	2.63 oz	70	7	4.0
w/cheese, 'Jars'	3.88 oz	90	10	6.0
(Contadina)				
	1/4 cup	25	4	0.5
deluxe	1/4 cup	34	5	0.7
original, 'Quick & Easy'	1/4 cup	30	5	1.0

Food Name	Serv. Size	Total Cal.	Carbs GMS	Fat GMS
pepperoni flavor	1/4 cup	30	4	1.0
'Pizza Squeeze'	1/4 cup	30	5	1.0
w/Italian cheese	1/4 cup	30	4	1.0
(Eden Foods) and pasta sauce, organic	4 oz	80	10	3.0
(Enrico's) all natural, no salt added, 'Homemade Style'	4 oz	60	9	1.0
(Hunt's)				
	2.36 oz	32	5	1.1
fully prepared	2.22 oz	21	4	0.5
(Nestlé) deluxe	1 pkg	1623	261	34.6
(Pastorelli) 'Italian Chef'	4 oz	90	12	3.0
(Pizza Quick) traditional	3 tbsp	35	3	2.0
PLUM				
(Dynasty) nonfat	2 tbsp	80	18	0.0
(La Choy)				
	1 tbsp	25	6	0.1
food service product	1 tbsp	25	6	0.0
PRIMAVERA				
(McCormick/Schilling) blend	1 tbsp	30	4	1.0
(Ragu) Italian, light, 'Chicken Tonight'	4 oz	50	9	1.0
RIB *(Dip n'Joy)* 'Saucy Rib'	1 oz	60	14	0.0
RIGOLETTO *(DiGiorno)* refrigerated	5 oz	110	9	8.0
ROBERT *(Escoffier)* 'Sauce Robert'	1 tbsp	20	5	0.0
SANDWICH				
(Hunt's)				
barbecue flavored, 'Manwich'	1/4 cup	60	14	0.0
bold flavor, 'Manwich'	2.22 oz	62	13	1.1
extra thick and chunky, 'Manwich'	2.5 oz	60	15	1.0
'Manwich'	2.26 oz	32	6	0.4
Mexican, 'Manwich'	2.26 oz	26	5	0.2
nonfat, 'Manwich'	2.5 oz	40	10	0.5
thick and chunky, 'Manwich'	2.29 oz	44	9	0.5
SAUSAGE AND BELL PEPPER *(Contadina)* spicy Italian	1/2 cup	100	9	5.0
SEAFOOD				
(Great Impressions)				
Creole	1 tbsp	21	5	0.1
dipping	1 tbsp	17	2	0.7
Polynesian, dipping	1 tbsp	38	10	1.0
(Progresso) mixed	1/2 cup	110	12	6.0
SEASONING				
(A Taste of Thai)	1 tbsp	15	1	0.0
(Cajun Sunshine) hot pepper	1 tsp	0	0	0.0
(Dragon Sauce) rice, vegetables, and stir fry	1 tsp	5	1	0.0
(Eden Foods)				
carob, 'EdenBlend'	8 oz	150	23	4.0
original, 'EdenBlend'	8 oz	120	16	3.0
original, 'Edensoy'	8 oz	130	13	4.0
original extra, 'EdenBlend'	8 oz	130	13	4.0
(Maggi) Asian	1 tbsp	0	0	0.0
(Tennessee Sunshine)	1 tsp	0	0	0.0
(Tiger Sauce) meat, seafood, and poultry	1 tsp	10	2	0.0
(Yucatan Sunshine) habanero pepper	1 tsp	0	0	0.0
SHRIMP *(Tone's)* 'Craboil'	1 tsp	10	1	0.6
SHOYU. See under Soy Sauce, below.				
SLOPPY JOE				
(Del Monte)				
hickory flavor	1/4 cup	70	18	0.0
Italian recipe	2.5 oz	60	14	0.0

Food Name	Serv. Size	Total Cal.	Carbs GMS	Fat GMS
original recipe	1/4 cup	70	16	0.0
(Hormel) 'Not-so-Sloppy-Sloppy Joe'	2.24 oz	70	16	1.0
(Libby's)	1/3 cup	45	10	0.0
SOY				
from hydrolyzed vegetable protein	1/4 cup	24	4	0.0
from hydrolyzed vegetable protein	1 tbsp	7	1	0.0
from hydrolyzed vegetable protein	1 tsp	2	0	0.0
shoyu, from soy and wheat	1 cup	150	20	0.1
shoyu, from soy and wheat	1 tbsp	9	1	0.0
shoyu, from soy and wheat	1 tsp	3	0	0.0
shoyu, from soy and wheat, low-sodium	1 cup	135	22	0.2
shoyu, from soy and wheat, low-sodium	1 tbsp	10	2	0.0
shoyu, from soy and wheat, low-sodium	1 tsp	3	0	0.0
tamari, from soy	1 tbsp	11	1	0.0
tamari, from soy	1 tsp	4	0	0.0
(Angostura)	1 tbsp	10	1	0.0
(Eden Foods)				
shoyu, from soy and wheat, organic	1/2 tsp	2	0	0.0
shoyu, naturally brewed	1/2 tsp	2	0	0.0
shoyu, reduced-sodium, organic	1/2 tsp	2	0	0.0
tamari, wheat-free, organic	1/2 tsp	2	0	0.0
(Golden Dipt) honey, 'Nature Bay'	1 oz	90	5	8.0
(Kikkoman)				
'Lite'	1 tbsp	10	1	0.0
naturally brewed	1 tbsp	10	0	0.0
(La Choy)				
	1 tbsp	11	1	0.0
food service product	1 tbsp	11	1	0.0
light	1 tbsp	15	2	0.0
light, food service product	1 tbsp	15	2	0.0
shoyu	1 tsp	1	0	0.0
shoyu, 'Lite'	1 tsp	1	0	0.0
(San-J) tamari, less salt	1 tbsp	16	1	0.0
(Westbrae)				
low-salt	1/2 tsp	2	1	0.0
mild	1/2 tsp	2	1	0.0
organic	1/2 tsp	2	1	0.0
wheat-free	1/2 tsp	3	1	0.0
STEAK				
(A.1.)				
bold	1 tbsp	18	4	0.0
regular	1 tbsp	18	4	0.0
(Adolph's) '100% Natural'	1/4 tsp	0	0	0.0
(Angostura)				
regular	1 tbsp	12	3	0.0
salsa flavor	1 tbsp	8	2	0.0
(Bullfighter) and burger	1 tbsp	15	4	0.0
(Heinz 57)				
hickory smoke, '57'	1 tbsp	16	4	0.0
traditional	1 tbsp	12	3	0.0
(Hunt's)	1 tbsp	10	2	0.1
(Kikkoman)	1 tbsp	20	5	0.0
(Lea & Perrins)	1 oz	40	10	1.0
STIR-FRY				
(Dynasty) Chinese	2 tbsp	60	5	3.0
(Flavor of the Rain Forest)				
ginger, curry	1 tbsp	15	2	1.0

Food Name	Serv. Size	Total Cal.	Carbs GMS	Fat GMS
honey hibiscus	1 tbsp	45	2	4.0
lime coconut, for seafood	1 tbsp	49	1	5.0
'Mango Grille'	1 tbsp	13	2	1.0
papaya pepper	1 tsp	3	1	0.0
savory	1 tsp	4	1	0.0
(Kikkoman)	1 tbsp	15	3	0.0
(La Choy)				
and marinade, food service product	1 tbsp	25	5	0.1
Mandarin soy	1/4 cup	35	8	0.1
Szechwan	1/4 cup	42	9	0.1
(Lawry's)	1/4 cup	120	20	3.8
(Mr. Spice) ginger, fat-free, salt-free	1 tbsp	11	3	0.0
(Nestlé) all-purpose, 'Chef-Mate'	1 tbsp	16	2	0.6
(S&W) Oriental	1 tbsp	20	5	0.0
STROGANOFF (Betty Crocker) 'Recipe Sauces'	4 oz	60	6	4.0
SUKIYAKI (Kikkoman)	1 tbsp	20	4	0.0
SWEET AND SOUR				
(A Taste of Thai) tangy, hot	2 tbsp	30	8	0.0
(Betty Crocker) 'Recipe Sauces'	4.1 oz	130	32	0.0
(Contadina)	2 tbsp	40	8	1.0
(Dynasty)	2 tbsp	70	14	1.0
(Great Impressions)				
Hawaiian	2 tbsp	102	26	0.0
hot	2 tbsp	102	26	0.0
regular	2 tbsp	102	26	0.0
(Hickory Farms)				
Hawaiian	2 tbsp	102	26	0.0
regular	2 tbsp	102	26	0.0
(Kikkoman)	2 tbsp	35	9	0.0
(La Choy)				
	1/4 cup	69	18	0.0
	1 tbsp	29	7	0.1
duck sauce	1 tbsp	31	7	0.1
food service product	2 tbsp	58	14	0.1
(Lawry's)	1/4 cup	549	12	7.5
(Nestlé) glaze, 'Chef-Mate'	2 tbsp	51	12	0.0
(Ragu) 'Chicken Tonight'	4 oz	80	19	0.0
(Sauceworks)	1 tbsp	25	5	0.0
(Simmer Chef) Oriental	1/2 cup	110	23	1.0
SZECHUAN				
(LaChoy) hot and spicy	1 oz	48	12	0.2
(Nestlé) 'Chef-Mate'	2 tbsp	42	6	1.8
(San-J)	1 tbsp	15	2	0.1
TACO				
(Chi-Chi's)				
hot	1 oz	18	4	2.0
thick, chunky	1 oz	12	3	2.0
(Del Monte)				
hot	1/4 cup	15	4	0.0
mild	1/2 cup	15	4	0.0
(El Molino) red, mild	2 tbsp	10	2	0.0
(Enrico's) mild, no salt added	2 tbsp	14	3	0.0
(Estee)	2 tbsp	14	3	0.0
(Hain) and dip	4 tbsp	25	5	1.0
(Heinz)				
medium	1 tbsp	6	1	0.0
mild	1 tbsp	6	1	0.0

Food Name	Serv. Size	Total Cal.	Carbs GMS	Fat GMS
(La Victoria)				
green	1 tbsp	0	1	0.0
green, medium	1 tbsp	5	1	0.1
green, mild	1 tbsp	5	1	0.1
mild	1 tbsp	7	1	0.1
red	1 tbsp	5	1	0.0
red, medium	1 tbsp	7	1	0.1
(Lawry's)				
chunky	1/4 cup	22	4	0.4
'Sauce'n Seasoner'	1/4 cup	40	8	0.6
(Manwich) seasoning	1/4 cup	30	6	0.0
(Old El Paso)				
canned	2 tbsp	15	3	0.0
hot	2 tbsp	10	2	1.0
medium	2 tbsp	10	2	1.0
mild or medium, extra chunky	1 tbsp	5	1	0.0
mild	2 tbsp	10	2	1.0
(Ortega)				
hot	1 oz	12	3	0.0
mild	1 oz	12	3	0.0
Western style	1 oz	8	2	0.0
(Pancho Villa) mild	2 tbsp	15	3	0.0
(Rosarita)				
	0.18 oz	2	0	0.0
food service product	1 tbsp	2	0	0.0
(Santiago)	1 fl oz	13	3	0.2
TAMARI. See under Soy Sauce, above.				
TANGY, nonfat, salt-free *(Mr. Spice)*	1 tsp	4	1	0.0
TARTAR				
(Best Foods)				
	2 tbsp	140	1	16.0
low-fat	2 tbsp	40	7	1.5
(Golden Dipt)				
	1 tbsp	70	2	7.0
'Lite'	1 tbsp	50	4	4.0
(Great Impressions)	1 tbsp	86	1	9.0
(Heinz)	1 tbsp	71	2	7.2
(Hellmann's)				
	1 tbsp	70	0	8.0
low-fat	2 tbsp	40	7	1.5
(Kraft) nonfat, 'Free'	1 tbsp	10	3	0.0
(Life) egg-free, all-natural	1 tbsp	38	1	4.0
(Sauceworks)				
	1 tbsp	50	2	5.0
lemon and herb flavor, natural	1 tbsp	70	0	8.0
(Weight Watchers)	1 tbsp	35	3	3.0
TEMPURA, dipping sauce *(Kikkoman)*	1 tsp	5	1	0.0
TERIYAKI				
(Angostura)	1 tbsp	10	2	0.0
(Betty Crocker) 'Recipe Sauces'	3.9 oz	60	13	1.0
(Golden Dipt) ginger	1 oz	120	12	7.0
(Kikkoman)				
baste and glaze	2 tbsp	50	11	0.0
baste and glaze, w/honey and pineapple	2 tbsp	80	18	0.0
(La Choy)				
	1/4 cup	47	11	0.1
	1 tbsp	17	3	0.1

Food Name	Serv. Size	Total Cal.	Carbs GMS	Fat GMS
basting	1.23 oz	37	8	0.0
hot	1 tbsp	17	3	0.4
light	1 tbsp	18	4	0.0
'Sauce & Marinade'	1 oz	30	5	0.0
thick and rich	1 oz	41	9	0.1
(Lawry's)				
barbecue	1/8 cup	82	14	1.1
w/pineapple juice	1/4 cup	72	11	0.4
(Nestlé) 'Chef-Mate'	1 tbsp	21	4	0.6
(S&W)				
and marinade	1 tbsp	25	5	0.0
and marinade, light	1 tbsp	25	5	0.0
TOMATO				
(S&W)				
herb and garlic, Italian	1 tbsp	15	2	1.0
original, 'Tomato Garden'	1/4 cup	20	4	0.0
(Simmer Chef) Mexicali, zesty	1/2 cup	90	16	3.0
TONKATSU (Kikkoman)	1 tbsp	20	5	0.0
VEGETABLE (Contadina) garden, 'Light'	0.5 oz	50	10	0.0
WHITE (Golden Dipt) French	1 oz	55	3	4.0
WORCESTERSHIRE				
(Angostura)	1 tsp	5	1	0.0
(French's)				
regular	1 tsp	0	1	0.0
smoky	1 tsp	0	1	0.0
(Heinz)	1 tbsp	6	1	0.0
(Lea & Perrins)				
	1 tsp	5	1	1.0
white wine	1 tsp	3	1	1.0
(Life) 'All Natural'	1/2 tbsp	5	1	1.0
(Wine & Pepper) w/sherry, hot pepper	1 tsp	0	1	0.0
SAUCE MIX				
ALFREDO				
(French's) 'Pasta Toss' mix only	2 tsp	25	2	2.0
(Knorr) CPC, mix only	2 tbsp	62	7	2.7
(Lawry's) 'Pasta Alfredo' mix only	1 pkg	226	19	13.3
(Schilling) 'Pasta Prima' mix only	1/4 envelope	40	3	2.5
BARBECUE				
(Blue Plate) concentrate	2 tbsp	110	19	4.0
(Woody's) concentrate, 'Cook-in' Sauce'.	2 tbsp	50	4	4.0
BEEF SAUCE				
(Lipton) sauté, golden, mix only	1/6 pkg	120	24	2.0
(Lipton) sauté, golden, prepared w/2 tsp butter	1/2 cup	180	24	8.0
CHEESE				
(Custom Foods)				
cheddar, 'Superb' mix only	1 serving	60	8	2.6
nacho, 'Superb' mix only	1 serving	60	8	2.6
(Durkee) mix only	1/4 cup	25	4	1.5
(French's) prepared w/whole milk	1/4 cup	80	7	4.0
(McCormick/Schilling)				
mix only	1/4 pkg	35	4	1.5
nacho, mix only	1/4 pkg	42	5	1.5
(Nestlé)				
nacho, 'Trio' mix only	2 tbsp	51	8	1.9
supreme, 'Trio' mix only	2 tbsp	54	7	2.4
'Trio' mix only	2 tbsp	54	7	2.3

Food Name	Serv. Size	Total Cal.	Carbs GMS	Fat GMS
CHICKEN				
(McCormick/Schilling)				
cacciatore 'Sauce Blends' mix only	1 pkg	132	28	4.8
Creole 'Sauce Blends' mix only	1 pkg	140	24	4.8
curry 'Sauce Blends' mix only	1 pkg	152	24	5.6
Dijon 'Sauce Blends' mix only	1 pkg	156	20	6.8
mesquite marinade, 'Sauce Blends' mix only	1 pkg	132	24	3.0
teriyaki, 'Sauce Blends' mix only	1 pkg	172	28	3.6
CURRY				
(S&B)				
golden, hot, mix only	1/5 pkt	120	11	7.0
golden, medium hot, mix only	1/5 pkt	120	10	7.0
ENCHILADA				
(Old El Paso) mix only	2 tsp	10	2	0.0
(Tio Sancho) 'Dinner Kit' mix only	3 oz	278	62	1.5
HOLLANDAISE				
(McCormick/Schilling) mix only	1/4 pkg	51	4	3.8
(Tone's) mix only	1 tsp	15	1	1.0
ITALIAN				
(Custom Foods) all purpose, 'Red Label' mix only	1 serving	19	4	0.2
LEMON BUTTER *(Weight Watchers)* mix only	1 tbsp	6	1	0.0
PASTA/spaghetti				
(Estee) preparedw/margarine and nonfat milk	4 oz	60	9	1.0
(Featherweight) preparedw/margarine and nonfat milk	4 oz	60	11	1.0
(French's)				
cheese and garlic, 'Pasta Toss' mix only	2 tsp	25	2	2.0
Italian, 'Pasta Toss' mix only	2 tsp	25	2	2.0
Romanoff 'Pasta Toss' mix only	2 tsp	30	1	2.0
w/mushrooms, prepared	5/8 cup	100	13	4.0
(Lawry's)				
'Rich & Thick' mix only	1 pkg	147	28	2.2
w/imported mushrooms, mix only	1 pkg	143	26	1.5
(McCormick/Schilling) mix only	1/4 pkg	32	6	0.3
(Prego) preparedw/margarine and nonfat milk	4 oz	130	20	5.0
(Ragu) preparedw/margarine and nonfat milk	4 oz	80	9	4.0
PEANUT *(A Taste of Thai)* mix only	2 tbsp	25	4	0.5
PESTO *(French's)* 'Pasta Toss' mix only	2 tsp	20	1	1.0
SANDWICH *(Manwich)* mix only	0.25 oz	22	5	0.1
SEAFOOD *(Old Bay)* 'Old Bay Seas'n' mix only	1/5 pkg	30	4	0.0
SOUR CREAM *(McCormick/Schilling)* mix only	1/4 pkg	44	4	2.8
SPAGHETTI. See SAUCE, PASTA.				
STROGANOFF				
(Lawry's) mix only	1 pkg	123	26	0.3
(McCormick/Schilling) mix only	2 tsp	15	3	0.0
(Natural Touch) prepared as directed	4 oz	90	10	3.0
SWEET AND SOUR				
(Kikkoman) mix only	1 1/2 tbsp	60	14	0.0
(Sun Bird) Oriental, mix only	1/2 tbsp	15	4	0.0
TACO *(Tio Sancho)* 'Dinner Kit' prepared	2 oz	62	13	0.2
TAHINI *(Casbah)* prepared	1/4 cup	160	10	13.0
TERIYAKI *(Kikkoman)* mix only	2 tsp	20	5	0.0
SAUERKRAUT				
Canned				
(A&P) w/liquid	1/2 cup	20	5	1.0
(Allens) shredded, w/liquid	1/2 cup	21	5	1.0
(Bush's Best)				
'Bavarian Kraut'	1/2 cup	60	15	0.0

Food Name	Serv. Size	Total Cal.	Carbs GMS	Fat GMS
chopped, 'Kraut'	1/2 cup	20	5	0.0
kosher, deli-style, 'Kraut'	1/2 cup	20	5	0.0
shredded, 'Kraut'	1/2 cup	20	5	0.0
(Del Monte)				
	2 tbsp	0	1	0.0
w/liquid	1/2 cup	25	6	0.0
(Eden Foods) organic	1/2 cup	25	4	1.0
(Finast) w/liquid	1/2 cup	30	6	0.0
(Libby's)				
Bavarian style, w/caraway seeds	2 tbsp	15	3	0.0
crispy	2 tbsp	5	1	0.0
(Pathmark) w/liquid	1/2 cup	20	4	0.0
(S&W)	2 tbsp	5	2	0.0
(Silver Floss) Bavarian style	1/2 cup	35	7	0.0
(Snow Floss) w/liquid	1/2 cup	28	4	0.0
(Stokely)				
Bavarian style, w/caraway seeds, mild	1/2 cup	35	7	0.0
Bavarian style, w/liquid	1/2 cup	30	7	0.0
shredded and chopped, w/liquid	1/2 cup	20	4	0.0
shredded, traditional	2 tbsp	5	1	0.0
extra mild	1/2 cup	80	18	0.0
(Vlasic) w/liquid, 'Old Fashioned'	1/2 cup	4	1	0.0
Frozen or refrigerated				
(Claussen)	1/4 cup	5	1	0.0
(S&W)	2 tbsp	5	1	0.0
SAUERKRAUT JUICE, canned or bottled *(Biotta)*	6 fl oz	21	4	0.1
SAUSAGE				
(Armour) links, 'Premium Smokee'	2 links	150	2	13.0
(Eckrich) minced, roll	1 oz slice	80	1	7.0
(Hickory Farms) 'Safari'	1 oz	98	1	9.0
(JM)				
patty, cooked	1 patty	70	1	6.0
patty, raw	1 oz	130	1	14.0
raw, 'Tasty Link'	2 links	220	1	21.0
(Jones Dairy Farm)				
patty	1 patty	155	0	14.4
patty, 'Golden Brown'	1 patty	155	0	14.7
patty, spicy, 'Golden Brown'	1 link	100	0	9.5
roll, 'Cello Roll'	1 slice	105	0	9.6
(Oscar Mayer) link, 'Smokie Links'	1 serving	130	1	11.7
BEEF				
(Eckrich)				
	1 oz	100	1	9.0
'Lean Supreme'	1 oz	80	1	7.0
'Smok-Y-Links'	2 links	160	2	14.0
(Hillshire Farm)				
'Flavorseal'	2 oz	180	2	16.0
hot links	1 serving	260	2	24.0
(Jones Dairy Farm) 'Golden Brown'	1 link	75	0	6.1
(Oscar Mayer) 'Smokies'	1 serving	128	1	11.5
(Pemmican) Tabasco	1.1 oz	120	2	10.0
BEERWURST				
beef, 4-inch diam, 1/8 inch slice	1 slice	76	0	6.9
beef, 2.5-inch diam, 1/4 inch slice	1 slice	20	0	1.8
pork, 4-inch diam, 1/8 inch slice	1 slice	55	0	4.3
pork, 2.5-inch diam, 1/4 inch slice	1 slice	14	0	1.1

Food Name	Serv. Size	Total Cal.	Carbs GMS	Fat GMS
BERLINER				
pork and beef	1 oz	65	1	4.9
pork and beef, 2.5-inch diam, 1/4 inch slice	1 slice	53	1	4.0
BLOOD SAUSAGE				
	1 oz	107	0	9.8
5 x 4 5/8 x 1/16 inch slice	1 slice	95	0	8.6
BOCKWURST				
pork, veal, milk, and eggs	1 oz	87	0	7.8
pork, veal, milk, and eggs, 7 links per lb.	1 link	200	0	17.9
BRATWURST				
pork, cooked	1 oz	85	1	7.3
pork, cooked, 4 per 12 oz pkg	1 link	256	2	22.0
(Eckrich)	1 link	310	1	30.0
(Hickory Farms)				
'Brotwurst'	1 oz	90	1	8.0
cheddar, 'Cheddy Brots'	1 oz	98	1	9.0
hot, 'Hot Brots'	1 oz	96	1	9.0
(Johnsonville) w/real Wisconsin beef	1 link	300	1	27.0
(Kahn's)	1 link	190	2	17.0
BRAUNSCHWEIGER				
	1 oz	102	1	9.1
2.5-Inch diam, 1/4-inch slice	1 slice	65	1	5.8
(Hormel)	1 oz	80	0	7.0
(JM)	1 oz	80	2	6.0
(Oscar Mayer)				
	1 oz	100	1	9.0
	1 slice	100	1	9.0
'German Brand'	1 oz	96	1	8.7
'Tube'	1 oz	97	1	8.7
BREAKFAST				
(Green Giant)				
links, frozen	3 links	110	5	5.0
patties, frozen	2 patties	100	5	4.0
(Healthy Choice)				
links	2 links	50	3	1.5
patties	2 patties	50	3	1.5
(Hudson) turkey, ground	1 oz	65	0	5.3
(Louis Rich)				
turkey, 85% fat-free	1 oz	55	1	3.0
turkey, ground, cooked	1 oz	56	0	3.5
(Mr. Turkey) turkey	2.5 oz	190	0	13.4
(The Turkey Store) links, mild	2 oz	140	1	11.0
BROWN AND SERVE				
(Eckrich) 'Lean Supreme'	2 links	120	1	10.0
(Hormel)				
link, uncooked	2 links	180	0	17.0
link, cooked	2 links	140	0	13.0
(Jones Dairy Farm) link, 'Light'	1 link	60	1	4.1
(Swift)				
link, 'Country Recipe'	1 link	130	1	12.0
link, 'Premium Original'	1 link	130	1	12.0
link, beef, 'Premium Brown 'N Serve'	1 link	120	1	12.0
link, maple flavored	1 link	120	1	12.0
link, microwave	1 link	120	1	12.0
link, smoked flavor	1 link	120	1	11.0
link, w/bacon	1 link	120	1	11.0
link, w/ham	1 link	130	1	13.0

Food Name	Serv. Size	Total Cal.	Carbs GMS	Fat GMS
patty, 'Country Recipe'	1 patty	130	1	12.0
patty, 'Premium Original'	1 patty	120	1	12.0
CAPOCOLLO *(Hormel)*	1 oz	80	0	6.0
CERVELAT				
(Hillshire Farm) Thuringer	2 oz	180	1	15.0
(Hormel)				
Thuringer, 'Old Smokehouse Chub'	1 oz	100	0	9.0
Thuringer, 'Old Smokehouse Sliced'	1 oz	100	0	9.0
Thuringer, 'Old Smokehouse'	1 oz	90	1	8.0
Thuringer, 'Viking Club Cervelat'	1 oz	90	0	8.0
(JM)				
Thuringer, beef	1 oz slice	80	1	7.0
Thuringer, 'Cervalot'	1 oz slice	70	1	6.0
(Oscar Mayer)				
Thuringer, beef	1 serving	142	1	12.4
Thuringer, beef, sliced	1 slice	71	0	6.2
Thuringer, beef and pork	1 oz	95	0	8.4
Thuringer, beef and pork, 4-inch diam, 1/8-inch slice	1 slice	77	0	6.8
CHEESE				
(Eckrich)				
'Smok-Y-Links'	2 links	160	2	14.0
hot, 'Smok-Y-Links'	2 links	150	1	14.0
maple flavored, 'Smok-Y-Links'	2 links	160	2	14.0
original, 'Smok-Y-Links'	2 links	160	2	14.0
w/ham, 'Smok-Y-Links'	2 links	160	2	15.0
(Hillshire Farm)				
bun size, 'Cheddarwurst'	2 oz	200	1	18.0
hot, 'Flavorseal'	2 oz	180	2	16.0
links, 'Cheddarwurst'	2 oz	190	1	17.0
smoked, 'Cheddarwurst'	1 serving	260	3	23.0
(Hormel) 'Smokie Cheezers'	2 links	168	1	15.0
(Louis Rich)				
turkey, and cheddar, smoked, 90% fat-free	1 oz	45	1	3.0
turkey, w/cheese, smoked	1 oz	47	1	2.8
(Oscar Mayer)				
pork and turkey, little, 'Smokies'	1 link	28	0	2.5
'Smokies'	1 serving	130	1	11.7
CHORIZO				
pork and beef	1 oz	129	1	10.8
pork and beef, 4-inch link	1 link	273	1	23.0
(Carmelita)				
beef	2.5 oz	250	5	23.0
pork	2.5 oz	250	3	23.0
GERMAN STYLE *(Hickory Farms)*	1 oz	100	1	8.0
HEAD CHEESE *(Oscar Mayer)*	1 slice	50	0	4.0
HONEY ROLL				
beef	1 oz	52	1	3.0
beef, 4-inch diam, 1/8-inch slice	1 slice	42	1	2.4
HOT				
(JM)				
patty, cooked	1 patty	70	1	6.0
patty, raw	1 oz	130	1	14.0
(OHSE) 'Hot Links'	1 oz	80	4	3.0
JALAPEÑO *(Bar-S)* smoked	2 oz	180	2	16.0
ITALIAN STYLE				
pork, cooked, 5 links per lb.	1 link	216	1	17.2
pork, cooked, 4 links per lb.	1 link	268	1	21.3

Food Name	Serv. Size	Total Cal.	Carbs GMS	Fat GMS
pork, raw, 7 links per lb	1 link	315	1	28.5
pork, raw, 4 links per lb	1 link	391	1	35.4
(Hillshire Farm) smoked, 'Flavorseal'	2 oz	200	1	18.0
(Johnsonville)				
hot	1 link	300	1	27.0
mild	1 link	300	1	27.0
(Shelton's) turkey	1 serving	160	0	16.0
(The Turkey Store) turkey, hot	3 oz	140	2	9.0
KIELBASA				
pork and beef	1 oz	88	1	7.7
(Eckrich)				
light, 'Lean Supreme Polska'	1 oz	72	1	6.0
w/o skin, 'Polska'	1 link	180	2	16.0
(Healthy Choice) low-fat	2 oz	70	6	1.5
(Hillshire Farm) bun size	1 serving	180	2	16.0
(Hormel)				
'Kolbase'	3 oz	220	1	19.0
w/o skin	1/2 link	180	1	14.0
(Louis Rich) turkey, smoked, 90% fat-free	1 oz	40	1	2.0
(Mr. Turkey) 'Polska Kielbasa'	1 oz	59	1	4.4
KNOCKWURST				
pork and beef	1 oz	87	0	7.9
pork and beef, 4-inch x 1 1/8 inch diam	1 link	209	1	18.9
(Hebrew National) beef, 1 link	3 oz	263	1	25.0
LIVER. See SAUSAGE, BRAUNSCHWEIGER.				
LUNCHEON				
pork and beef	1 oz	74	0	5.9
pork and beef, 4-inch diam, 1/8-inch slice	1 slice	60	0	4.8
MILD (Jones Dairy Farm) 'Golden Brown'	1 link	100	0	9.8
MORTADELLA				
beef and pork	1 oz	88	1	7.2
beef and pork, 15 per 8-oz pkg	1 slice	47	0	3.8
NEW ENGLAND STYLE				
pork and beef	1 oz	46	1	2.1
pork and beef, 4-inch diam, 1/8-inch slice	1 slice	37	1	1.7
(Eckrich) New England brand	1 oz slice	35	1	1.0
(Light & Lean) New England brand	2 slices	90	0	6.0
(Oscar Mayer)	1 slice	60	1	2.5
PEPPERONI				
pork and beef, 10 1/4 inch long x 1 3/8 inch diam	1 sausage	1247	7	110.4
pork and beef, 1 3/8 inch diam, 1/8-inch slice	1 slice	27	0	2.4
(Gallo Salame)				
deli style	11 slices	160	0	14.0
pizza style	9 slices	140	0	13.0
(Hickory Farms)	1 oz	140	1	13.0
(Hormel)				
	1 oz	140	0	13.0
bits	1 tbsp	35	0	3.0
'Chunk'	1 oz	140	0	12.0
'Leoni Brand'	1 oz	130	0	12.0
'Perma-Fresh'	2 slices	80	0	7.0
'Rosa'	1 oz	140	0	13.0
'Rosa Grande'	1 oz	140	0	13.0
turkey, 'Pillow Pak'	1 serving	74	1	3.5
(JM) sliced	8 slices	70	1	6.0
(Oscar Mayer)	15 slices	140	0	13.0

Food Name	Serv. Size	Total Cal.	Carbs GMS	Fat GMS
PICKLED				
(Penrose)				
beer	1 link	40	1	3.0
firecracker	1 link	40	1	3.0
firecracker, giant	1 link	170	1	14.0
hot	1 link	40	1	3.0
red hot	1 link	40	1	3.0
POLISH STYLE. See also KIELBASA.				
pork	1 oz	92	0	8.1
pork, 10-inch long x 1.25-inch diam	1 sausage	740	4	65.2
(Hormel)	2 links	170	0	14.0
(OHSE)				
hot	1 oz	70	3	5.0
	1 oz	80	1	7.0
(Penrose) pickled	1 link	40	1	3.0
(Pilgrim's Pride)	3 oz	131	2	7.7
PORK				
link, 4-inch long x 1 1/8 inch diam	1 link	265	1	21.6
link, fresh, cooked, 4-inch long x 7/8-inch diam before cooking	1 link	48	0	4.1
link, fresh, raw, 7/8-inch diam x 4-inch long	1 link	117	0	11.3
link, 2-inch long x 3/4-inch diam	1 link	62	0	5.1
patty, fresh, cooked, 3 7/8 inch diam x 1/4-inch thick				
before cooking	100	5	349	2.9
patty, fresh, raw 3 7/8 inch diam x 1/4-inch thick	1 patty	238	1	23.0
(Hormel)				
links, 'Midget Links'	2 links	143	0	13.0
links, 'Little Sizzlers'	2 links	103	0	9.0
(Jimmy Dean)				
hot	2 oz	250	0	24.0
'Light'	1.2 oz	80	1	7.0
links	2 links	180	1	17.0
patties	1 patty	140	1	13.0
regular, cooked	1 oz	120	1	11.0
sage	2 oz	250	0	24.0
(JM)				
and bacon, cooked, 'Tasty Link'	2 links	100	1	9.0
cooked, 'Tasty Link'	2 links	190	1	18.0
raw, 'Tasty Link'	2 links	260	1	26.0
(Jones Dairy Farm)				
	1 link	140	0	13.7
'Golden Brown Light'	1 link	55	1	4.2
'Light'	1 link	70	1	5.0
(Oscar Mayer)				
(Oscar Mayer) link	2 links	170	1	15.0
(Oscar Mayer) link, cooked	1 link	82	0	7.3
link, 'Little Friers' cooked	1 link	82	0	7.5
(Owens)				
country style	2 oz	290	0	27.0
country style, hot	2 oz	290	0	27.0
country style, sage	2 oz	250	1	23.0
(Pierre)				
link, all meat, product 3755	1 piece	85	0	5.3
patty, all meat, product 3750	1 piece	85	0	5.3
patty, all meat, product 3751	1 piece	174	1	10.8
patty, all meat, product 3850	1 piece	95	1	6.6
patty, all meat, product 3851	1 piece	193	1	13.4
(Tyson) country, whole hog	3.5 oz	320	1	29.0

Food Name	Serv. Size	Total Cal.	Carbs GMS	Fat GMS
PORK AND BEEF				
link, 4-inch long x 1 1/8 inch diam	1 link	228	1	20.6
link, fresh, cooked, 4-inch long x 7/8-inch diam before cooking	1 link	51	0	4.7
link, 2-inch long x 3/4-inch diam	1 link	54	0	4.9
patty, fresh, cooked, 3 7/8 inch diam x 1/4-inch thick before cooking	1 patty	107	1	9.8
PORK AND TURKEY (Oscar Mayer) little, 'Smokies'	1 link	27	0	2.4
SAGE (Jimmy Dean) cooked	1 oz	120	1	11.0
SALAMI. See also under LUNCHEON MEAT.				
beef and pork, cooked	1 oz	71	1	5.7
beef and pork, cooked, 4-inch diam, 1/8 inch slice	1 slice	58	1	4.6
beef, cooked	1 oz	74	1	5.9
beef, cooked, 4-inch diam, 1/8 inch slice	1 slice	60	1	4.8
pork, dry or hard, 3 1/8 inch diam, 1/16-inch slice	1 slice	41	0	3.4
pork and beef, dry or hard, 3 1/8 inch diam, 1/16-inch slice	1 slice	42	0	3.4
SCRAPPLE (Jones Dairy Farm)	1 slice	65	4	3.7
SMOKED				
(Eckrich)				
'Lean Supreme'	1 oz	70	1	6.0
'No skin'	1 link	180	2	16.0
(Healthy Choice) low-fat	2 oz	70	6	1.5
(Hillshire Farm)				
'Flavorseal'	2 oz	190	1	17.0
original, bun size	1 serving	180	2	16.0
(Hormel) 'Smokies'	2 links	160	2	14.0
(OHSE)	1 oz	80	1	7.0
(Oscar Mayer) link 'Big & Juicy'	2.7 oz	227	1	20.5
(Pilgrim's Pride)	3 oz	144	3	9.1
SUMMER				
(Eckrich)	1 oz slice	80	1	7.0
(Hormel)				
beef, 'Beefy'	1 oz	100	0	9.0
'Perma-Fresh'	2 slices	140	0	11.0
'Tangy, Chub'	1 oz	90	0	7.0
'Thuringer'	1 oz	90	0	9.0
(Lean & Lite)	1 oz	43	1	2.3
(Light & Lean)	2 slices	100	0	8.0
(Louis Rich)				
turkey	1 oz slice	55	0	3.9
turkey, 85% fat-free	1 oz slice	55	1	4.0
(OHSE)				
	1 oz	75	2	5.0
beef	1 oz	80	1	6.0
(Oscar Mayer) sliced	1 slice	69	0	6.1
SWEDISH STYLE (Hickory Farms)	1 oz	100	0	9.0
TURKEY				
(Butterball)	1 oz	50	1	4.0
(Jimmy Dean) 'Light'	1.2 oz	80	1	7.0
(Louis Rich)				
link, cooked	1 link	46	0	2.7
link, cooked, 85% fat-free	0.84 oz	45	1	3.0
original or hot	2.5 oz	120	1	8.0
smoked	1 serving	90	2	5.4
(Norbest) 'Tasti-Lean, Chub or Links'	1 oz	53	0	2.8
(Shelton's)				
links	1 serving	140	0	14.0
patty	1 serving	140	0	11.0

Food Name	Serv. Size	Total Cal.	Carbs GMS	Fat GMS
VEGETARIAN				
(Boca) breakfast patty, vegetarian	1 patty	70	4	3.0
(Garden Sausage) garden sausage, meatless, soy-free	1 oz	95	18	1.0
(Heartline)				
Italian style, cooked	2 oz	176	9	7.0
pepperoni style, lite	0.5 oz	22	1	0.0
(Loma Linda)				
breakfast links, vegetarian	2 links	93	3	5.6
'Linketts'	1 link	70	1	4.5
'Little Links'	2 links	90	1	6.0
(Morningstar Farms)				
'Breakfast Links'	2 links	60	2	2.0
'Breakfast Patties'	1 patty	80	3	3.0
'Sausage Style Recipe Crumbles'	2/3 cup	90	5	3.0
(Worthington)				
breakfast links, vegetarian	2 links	63	2	2.4
breakfast patty, vegetarian	1 pkg	8531	399	297.6
breakfast patty, vegetarian	1 patty	79	4	2.8
'Leanies'	1 link	100	2	7.0
'Low Fat Veja-Links'	1 link	40	1	1.5
'Prosage Links'	2 links	63	2	2.4
'Prosage Patties'	1 patty	96	3	3.2
'Prosage' roll, frozen	5/8-inch slice	142	2	10.4
'Saucettes'	2 slices	86	1	6.5
'Super Links'	1 link	110	2	8.0
'Veja-Links'	1 link	49	1	3.0
VIENNA				
beef and pork, canned, 7/8-inch diam x 2-inch long	1 sausage	45	0	4.0
(Armour)				
chicken, in beef stock, lite, canned, 'Premium'	2 oz	150	1	13.0
hot and spicy, canned	2.5 oz	190	3	17.0
in barbecue sauce, canned	2.5 oz	190	4	17.0
in beef stock, canned	2 oz	180	1	17.0
in beef stock, lite, canned	2 oz	150	1	13.0
smoked, canned	2 oz	180	1	17.0
(Hormel)				
canned	1 oz	69	2	7.0
chicken, canned	1 oz	56	1	5.0
no broth, canned	4 links	200	1	18.0
(Libby's)				
chicken, in beef broth, canned	2 oz	130	3	10.0
in barbecue sauce, canned	2.5 oz	180	2	15.0
in beef broth, canned, approx. 3 1/2 links	2 oz	160	1	15.0
SAUSAGE STICK				
(Hickory Farms) stick, 'Sportsman Stick'	1 oz	138	4	10.0
(Slim Jim) smoked, 'Giant Slim'	1.1 oz	180	2	16.0
(Slim Jim) smoked, 'Jumbo Jim'	1 oz	150	2	12.0
(Slim Jim) smoked, pepperoni 'Handi-Paks'	0.31 oz	50	1	4.0
(Slim Jim) smoked, spicy 'Handi-Paks'	0.31 oz	50	1	4.0
(Slim Jim) Tabasco, 'Handi-Paks'	0.31 oz	50	1	4.0
SAVORY				
ground	1 tbsp	12	3	0.3
ground	1 tsp	4	1	0.1
ground *(Durkee)*	1 tsp	5	0	0.0
ground *(Laurel Leaf)*	1 tsp	5	0	0.0
ground *(McCormick/Schilling)*	1 tsp	7	2	0.0
ground *(Spice Islands)*	1 tsp	5	1	0.1

Food Name	Serv. Size	Total Cal.	Carbs GMS	Fat GMS
summer, ground *(Tone's)*	1 tsp	4	1	0.1
SAVOY CABBAGE. See CABBAGE, SAVOY.				
SCALLION				
Fresh				
raw, chopped *(Dole)*	1 tbsp	2	0	0.1
raw, tops and bulb, chopped	1 cup	32	7	0.2
raw, tops and bulb, chopped	1 tbsp	2	0	0.0
raw, tops and bulb, whole, large, 5 1/4 inch long	1 scallion	8	2	0.0
raw, tops and bulb, whole, medium, 4 1/8-inch long	1 scallion	5	1	0.0
raw, tops and bulb, whole, small, 3-inch long	1 scallion	2	0	0.0
Freeze dried				
(McCormick/Schilling)	1 tsp	4	1	0.0
SCALLOP				
mixed species, breaded and fried	2 large	67	3	3.4
mixed species, raw	2 large	26	1	0.2
mixed species, raw	3 oz	75	2	0.6
SCALLOP SQUASH. See SQUASH, SCALLOP.				
SCALLOP SUBSTITUTE				
made from Surimi	3 oz	84	9	0.3
vegetarian, 'Skallops' *(Worthington)*	1/2 cup	86	3	1.4
SCORZONERA. See SALSIFY, BLACK.				
SCOTCH KALE. See KALE, SCOTCH.				
SCRAPPLE. See under SAUSAGE.				
SCROD ENTRÉE				
(Gorton's) frozen, baked 'Microwave Entrees'	1 pkg	320	17	18.0
SCUP/sea bream				
baked, broiled, grilled, or microwaved	3 oz	115	0	3.0
raw	1 cup	174	0	4.5
raw	3 oz	89	0	2.3
raw, boneless	1 oz	30	0	0.8
SEA BASS. See BASS, SEA.				
SEA BREAM. See SCUP.				
SEA DEVIL. See MONKFISH.				
SEA PERCH. See OCEAN PERCH, ATLANTIC.				
SEA TROUT. See under TROUT.				
SEA VEGETABLE				
AGAR, raw	2 tbsp	3	1	0.0
ALARIA, dry *(Maine Coast)*	1/3 cup	18	3	0.0
DULSE				
dry *(Maine Coast)*	1/3 cup	18	3	0.0
raw	3.5 oz	<1	0.0	3.2
HIZIKI, dry *(Eden Foods)*	1/2 cup	30	6	0.0
IRISH MOSS, raw	2 tbsp	5	1	0.0
KELP				
dry *(Maine Coast)*	1/3 cup	17	3	0.0
raw	2 tbsp	4	1	0.1
KOMBU, wild, 7-inch pieces *(Eden Foods)*	1/2 piece	10	2	0.0
LAVER				
raw	10 sheets	9	1	0.1
raw	2 tbsp	4	1	0.0
NORI				
dry *(Maine Coast)*	1/3 cup	22	3	0.0
dry *(Eden Foods)*	1 piece	10	1	0.0
dry, for sushi *(Eden Foods)*	1 sheet	10	1	0.0
WAKAME				
dry *(Eden Foods)*	1/2 cup	25	4	0.0
flakes, instant *(Eden Foods)*	1 tsp	3	0	0.0

Food Name	Serv. Size	Total Cal.	Carbs GMS	Fat GMS
raw	2 tbsp	5	1	0.1
SEA VEGETABLE CHIP *(Eden Foods)*	1 oz	130	22	5.0
SEAFOOD DINNER/ENTRÉE. See also individual listings.				
(Armour) w/natural herbs, frozen, 'Classics Lite'	10 oz	190	29	2.0
(Budget Gourmet)				
Newburg, frozen	10 oz	350	43	12.0
shrimp w/scallops, frozen, 'Mariner'	11.5 oz	320	43	9.0
(Cajun Cookin') gumbo, frozen	17 oz	330	51	7.0
(Mrs. Paul's)				
shrimp and clams, w/linguini, frozen, 'Light'	10 oz	240	36	5.0
(Pillsbury) casserole, frozen, 'Microwave Classic'	1 pkg	420	37	24.0
(Swanson) Creole, w/rice, frozen, 'Homestyle Recipe'	9 oz	240	40	6.0
SEAFOOD SEASONING. See under SEASONING MIX.				
SEASONING AND COATING MIX. See also MARINADE; MARINADE MIX.				
ALL-PURPOSE				
(Golden Dipt) breading	1 oz	90	20	0.0
(Shake 'N Bake) country mild recipe	1/4 pkt	80	10	4.0
CHICKEN				
(Don's Chuck Wagon) frying mix, super crispy	1/4 cup	95	21	0.0
(Golden Dipt)				
....	1 oz	90	20	0.0
frying mix	1 oz	90	20.0	0.0
(Luzianne) Cajun coating, bake, fry, or microwave	2 tbsp	100	20	0.5
(Oven Fry)				
extra crispy recipe	1 serving	60	10	1.0
home style flour recipe	1 serving	40	7	1.0
(Shake 'N Bake)				
barbecue	1 serving	45	9	1.0
hot and spicy	1/4 pkt	80	15	2.0
original	1 serving	40	7	1.0
'Original Barbecue Recipe'	1/4 pkt	90	18	2.0
(Tone's) Cajun, batter seasoning	1 tsp	12	3	0.1
FISH				
(Tone's) Cajun	1 tsp	12	3	0.1
(Don's Chuck Wagon) no MSG	1/4 cup	95	21	0.0
(Shake 'N Bake) original	1 serving	70	14	1.5
FLOUR, seasoned, all-purpose, dry *(Kentucky Kernel)*	1/4 cup	90	20	0.0
PORK				
(Oven Fry) extra crispy recipe	1 serving	60	11	1.5
(Shake 'N Bake)				
....	1 serving	45	9	1.0
hot and spicy	1/8 pkt	45	8	1.0
'Original Recipe'	1/8 pkt	40	8	1.0
SEAFOOD				
(Don's Chuck Wagon) seasoned, no MSG	1/4 cup	95	21	0.0
(Golden Dipt)				
fish fry, Cajun style, mix only	2/3 oz	60	14	0.0
fish fry, mix only	2/3 oz	60	14	0.0
mix only	2/3 oz	60	14	0.0
(Luzianne) bake, fry, or microwave, Cajun, mix only	2 tbsp	100	22	0.5
SEASONING MIX				
ALL-PURPOSE				
(Knorr)	1 gram	5	0	0.0
(Mrs. Dash) table blend	0.13 tsp	2	0	0.0
(Praise Allah) for steak, meats, stews, and gravies	1/4 tsp	0	0	0.0
(Spike All Purpose) all natural	1/4 tsp	1	0	0.0
(Trader Joe's) salt-free, '21 Seasoning Salute'	1/4 tsp	0	0	0.0

Food Name	Serv. Size	Total Cal.	Carbs GMS	Fat GMS
APPLE PIE SPICE *(Tone's)*	1 tsp	9	2	0.2
BARBECUE SPICE *(Tone's)*	1 tsp	9	1	0.4
BEEF				
(Adolph's) stew, 'Meal Makers'	1 tbsp	20	4	0.0
(Bag 'n Season)				
pot roast	1 tsp	10	1	0.0
Swiss steak	1 tsp	15	2	0.0
(French's) w/onions, ground	1/4 pkg	25	6	0.0
(Kikkoman) broccoli beef stir-fry	2 tsp	15	3	0.0
(Lawry's)				
pot roast, 'Seasoning Blends'	1 pkg	122	25	0.7
stew, 'Seasoning Blends'	1 pkg	131	26	0.7
(McCormick/Schilling) stew	2 tsp	15	3	0.0
(Schilling)				
pot roast, 'Bag'n Season'	1 pkg	55	9	0.6
steak, 'Montreal LaGrille'	1/4 tsp	0	0	0.0
steak, broiled, 'Spice Blends'	1/4 tsp	1	0	0.0
stew	1/2 pkg	33	6	0.3
stew, 'Bag'n Season'	1 pkg	87	11	1.0
stew, 'Bag'n Season'	1 tsp	15	1	0.0
Stroganoff	1/4 pkg	32	6	0.3
Swiss steak, 'Bag'n Season'	1 pkg	81	17	0.4
(Sun Bird) beef and broccoli, Oriental	3/4 tbsp	20	5	0.0
(Tone's) steak, blackened	1 tsp	9	2	0.3
BURRITO				
(Lawry's) 'Seasoning Blends'	1 pkg	132	23	1.7
(Old El Paso)	2 tsp	20	3	0.0
(Tio Sancho) 'Dinner Kit'	3.25 oz	265	49	2.1
CAJUN				
(Luzianne)	1/4 tsp	0	0	0.0
(Tone's)	1 tsp	9	2	0.2
CHICKEN				
(Featherweight)	1/4 pkg	18	8	0.0
(Kikkoman) roast	1 tbsp	25	4	0.0
(Lawry's) Southwest, 'Seasoning Blends'	1 pkg	71	16	0.3
(Schilling)				
'Bag'n Season'	1 pkg	134	19	5.0
barbecue, tangy	2 tsp	20	3	0.0
fried chicken	1/4 tsp	1	0	0.1
rotisserie style	3/4 tsp	0	1	0.0
CHILI				
(Carroll Shelby's) Texas brand, original	3 tbsp	80	14	1.5
(Gebhardt)				
'Chili Quik'	1 tbsp	14	3	0.3
'Chili Quik' food service product	1 tbsp	18	4	0.4
(Hain)				
hot	1/4 pkg	30	5	1.0
medium	1/4 pkg	30	5	1.0
mild	1/2 pkg	30	5	1.0
(Lawry's) 'Seasoning Blends'	1 pkg	143	27	1.8
(McCormick/Schilling) original	1 tbsp	25	4	0.5
(Old El Paso)	1 tbsp	25	4	0.5
(Schilling)	1/4 pkg	27	5	0.5
(Tio Sancho)	1.23 oz	109	6	2.2
(Tone's)	1 tsp	12	2	0.3
(Wick Fowler's)				
mild, 'False Alarm'	2 tbsp	50	9	1.5

Food Name	Serv. Size	Total Cal.	Carbs GMS	Fat GMS
'2 Alarm'	3 tbsp	60	10	1.5
CHILI POWDER				
	1 tbsp	24	4	1.3
	1 tsp	8	1	0.4
(Gebhardt)	1 tbsp	3	1	0.2
(Tone's)				
hot	1 tsp	8	1	0.4
mild	1 tsp	8	1	0.4
CHOP SUEY (Sun Bird) Oriental	1 tbsp	20	5	0.0
CHOW MEIN (Kikkoman)	1 tbsp	20	3	0.0
CREOLE, no MSG (Tony Chachere's)	1/4 tsp	0	0	0.0
CURRY				
(A Taste of Thai)				
panang curry base	1 tbsp	25	2	2.0
red curry base	1 tbsp	20	1	1.5
CURRY POWDER				
	1 tbsp	20	4	0.9
	1 tsp	7	1	0.3
(Tone's)	1 tsp	6	1	0.3
DILL (Schilling) 'Parsley Patch It's a Dilly'	1 tsp	11	2	0.4
ENCHILADA				
(Lawry's) 'Seasoning Blends'	1 pkg	152	30	1.2
(Old El Paso)	1/8 pkg	6	1	0.0
FAJITA				
(Crown Colony)	1/2 tsp	5	1	0.0
(Lawry's) 'Seasoning Blends'	1 pkg	63	14	0.4
FISH (Featherweight)	1/4 pkg	18	8	0.0
FIVE-SPICE (Tone's) Oriental	1 tsp	9	2	0.3
FRENCH FRY (Tone's)	1 tsp	5	1	0.1
GARLIC				
(Golden Dipt)	2 grams	8	1	0.0
(Lawry's) concentrate	1 tbsp	15	0	1.6
(Schilling)				
'Parsley Patch'	1 tsp	13	2	0.5
'Season All'	1/4 tsp	2	0	0.0
spread	1/2 tbsp	45	1	4.0
GARLIC AND HERB				
(Cook's Classics) spread	1 tbsp	100	0	11.0
(Mrs. Dash) seasoning	0.13 tsp	2	0	0.0
(Schilling) spread	1/2 tbsp	45	1	4.5
GARLIC BREAD				
(Gran' Mere's) spread, all-purpose	1 oz	90	2	9.0
(Lawry's) spread	1/2 tbsp	47	1	4.6
(Molly McButter) garlic butter flavored	1/2 tsp	3	1	0.0
(Schilling) 'Garlic Bread Sprinkle'	1/4 tsp	5	0	0.4
(Tone's) 'Garlic Bread Sprinkle'	1 tsp	17	1	1.6
GARLIC PEPPER (Lawry's)	1/4 tsp	0	0	0.0
GARLIC SALT				
(Good Day)	1/4 tsp	0	0	0.0
(Lawry's)	1/4 tsp	0	0	0.0
(Morton)	1 tsp	3	1	0.1
(Schilling)	1/4 tsp	0	0	0.0
(Tone's)	1 tsp	2	0	0.0
GREEK (Cavender's) all purpose	1/4 tsp	0	0	0.0
GUACAMOLE				
(Lawry's) 'Seasoning Blend'	1 pkg	60	13	0.4
(Old El Paso)	1/7 pkg	7	2	0.0

Food Name	Serv. Size	Total Cal.	Carbs GMS	Fat GMS
GUMBO *(Tone's)* file powder	1 tsp	8	2	0.2
HERB				
(Lawry's) mixed, 'Pinch of Herbs'	1 tsp	9	1	0.5
(Schilling) Italian, 'Bag'n Season'	1 pkg	94	21	0.2
ITALIAN				
(Tone's)	1 tsp	3	1	0.1
(Trader Joe's) salt-free	1/4 tsp	0	0	0.0
LEMON DILL *(Schilling)* 'Bag'n Season'	1 pkg	161	15	11.0
LEMON HERB				
(Mrs. Dash)	0.13 tsp	2	0	0.0
(Schilling) 'Spice Blends'	1/4 tsp	1	0	0.1
LEMON PEPPER				
(Lawry's)				
	1/4 tsp	<1	0	0.0
'Spice Blends'	1 tsp	6	1	0.1
(Schilling)				
'Parsley Patch'	1 tsp	13	1	0.6
salt-free	1/4 tsp	0	0	0.0
'Spice Blends'	1 tsp	7	1	0.0
(Tone's)				
	1 tsp	6	1	0.2
coarse ground, 'Mr. Pepper'	1 tsp	12	3	0.1
fine ground, 'Mr. Pepper'	1 tsp	12	3	0.1
(Trader Joe's) salt-free	1/4 tsp	0	0	0.0
KOTTERIN MIRIN *(Kikkoman)* sweet	1 tbsp	40	10	0.0
MEAT LOAF				
(Adolph's) 'Meal Makers'	1 tbsp	30	7	0.0
(Bag 'n Season)	2 tsp	15	2	0.0
(French's)	1/8 pkg	20	5	0.0
(Lawry's) 'Seasoning Blends'	1 pkg	355	65	1.2
(Schilling) 'Bag'n Season'	1 pkg	111	26	0.7
MEATBALL				
(French's)	1/4 pkg	35	7	0.0
(Schilling) Swedish	1/6 pkg	45	4	1.0
MENUDO *(Gebhardt)*	1 tsp	4	1	0.2
MESQUITE *(Tone's)*	1 tsp	13	3	0.1
MEXICAN *(Tone's)*	1 tsp	6	1	0.1
NACHO *(Lawry's)* 'Seasoning Blends'	1 pkg	141	15	6.8
ORIENTAL *(Schilling)* 'Bag'n Season'	1 pkg	152	31	8.0
PAD THAI *(Kikkoman)*	2 tsp	20	4	0.0
PARSLEY *(Schilling)* all purpose 'Parsley Patch'	1 tsp	6	1	0.0
PASTA				
(Tone's) spaghetti	1 tsp	11	3	0.1
(Trader Joe's) salt-free	1/4 tsp	0	0	0.0
PEPPER				
(Lawry's)	1/4 tsp	0	1	0.0
(Schilling) seasoned, 'All Pepper'	1/4 tsp	1	0	0.0
PEPPER DILL *(Golden Dipt)*	2 grams	8	1	0.0
PICKLING SPICE *(Tone's)*	1 tsp	10	1	0.6
POPCORN				
(McCormick/Schilling) 'Parsley Patch'	1 tsp	10	3	0.1
(Tone's)	1 tsp	0	0	0.0
PORK				
(Bag 'n Season)				
chop	2 tsp	15	4	0.0
spare rib	1 tbsp	30	6	0.0

Food Name	Serv. Size	Total Cal.	Carbs GMS	Fat GMS
(Schilling)				
chop, 'Bag'n Season'	1 pkg	103	24	0.4
spare rib, 'Bag'n Season'	1 pkg	185	42	1.5
POTATO				
(Perfect Potatoes) herb and garlic	1/6 pkt	20	5	0.0
(Potato Shakers)				
cheddar, zesty	8 grams	30	5	1.0
Parmesan and herb	8 grams	25	5	0.5
(Shake 'N Bake) herb and garlic	1/8 pkt	20	5	0.0
POTATO SALAD *(Tone's)*	1 tsp	5	0	0.2
PROTEIN *(Bragg)* liquid aminos	1/2 tsp	2	0	0.0
PUMPKIN PIE				
	1 tbsp	19	4	0.7
	1 tsp	6	1	0.2
RICE				
(Kikkoman) fried	1 1/3 tbsp	30	6	0.0
(Lawry's) Mexican, 'Seasoning Blends'	1 pkg	94	17	2.0
(McCormick/Schilling) fried, w/chicken	1 tbsp	35	6	0.0
(Sun Bird) fried	1/2 tbsp	12	3	0.0
SALAD				
(Lawry's) taco, 'Seasoning Blends'	1 pkg	124	25	0.9
(Schilling) 'Salad Supreme'	1 tsp	11	1	0.1
SALT				
(Estee) 'Seasoned Salt-It'	1/8 tsp	0	0	0.0
(Good Day)	1/4 tsp	0	0	0.0
(Lawry's)				
	1/4 tsp	0	0	0.0
'Hot n' Spicy'	1 tsp	3	2	0.1
no MSG	1/4 tsp	0	0	0.0
(Morton) seasoned	1 tsp	4	1	0.1
(Schilling)				
'California style'	1/4 tsp	0	0	0.0
no MSG, 'Home Style'	1/4 tsp	0	0	0.0
no MSG, 'Season All'	1/4 tsp	0	0	0.0
SAUSAGE *(Tone's)* pork	1 tsp	12	3	0.3
SEAFOOD				
(Golden Dipt)				
all purpose	1/4 tsp	2	0	0.0
blackened redfish	1/4 tsp	2	0	0.0
broiled fish	1/4 tsp	2	0	0.0
lemon pepper	1/4 tsp	8	1	0.0
shrimp and crab, Cajun style	1/4 tsp	2	0	0.0
(Old Bay) seafood, poultry, meat seasoning	1/2 tsp	0	0	0.0
(Schilling) Chesapeake Bay	1/2 tsp	2	0	0.1
(Tone's)				
	1 tsp	10	1	0.7
Chesapeake	1 tsp	8	1	0.3
SESAME				
(Eden Foods)				
garlic, shake, organic	1/2 tsp	10	0	1.5
shake, organic	1/2 tsp	10	0	0.5
seaweed, shake, organic	1/2 tsp	10	0	0.5
(Maranatha Natural) sesame salt	7 grams	200	7	16.0
(Schilling) all-purpose, 'Parsley Patch'	1 tsp	15	1	1.0
SLOPPY JOE *(Lawry's)* 'Seasoning Blends'	1 pkg	126	28	0.4
SOUR CREAM FLAVORED *(Molly McButter)*	1/2 tsp	4	1	0.1

Food Name	Serv. Size	Total Cal.	Carbs GMS	Fat GMS
STIR-FRY				
(Adolph's) teriyaki flavor, 'Meal Makers'	1 tbsp	30	7	0.0
(Gilroy)	1 tsp	6	1	0.0
(Kikkoman)				
	1 tbsp	30	6	0.0
shrimp, Szechwan	1 1/3 tbsp	30	5	0.5
tomato-beef	2 tsp	20	4	0.0
(McCormick/Schilling)	2 tsp	20	3	0.0
(Sun Bird) Oriental	1/2 tbsp	15	3	0.0
TACO				
(Hain)	1/10 pkg	10	2	0.0
(Lawry's) 'Seasoning Blends'	1 pkg	118	24	1.1
(McCormick/Schilling) mild	2 tsp	20	4	0.0
(Nabisco) mild, mix for one taco	1 serving	90	18	1.0
(Old El Paso)				
	2 tsp	20	5	0.0
40% less sodium	2 tsp	20	4	0.0
(Ortega) meat	1 oz	90	18	1.0
(Pancho Villa)	2 tsp	20	5	0.0
(Schilling)	1/4 pkg	31	6	0.5
(Tio Sancho)				
	1.25 oz	104	21	1.4
'Dinner Kit'	1.51 oz	132	26	1.7
TURKEY *(Schilling)* roast, 'Bag'n Season'	1 pkg	146	20	5.0
TERIYAKI *(Golden Dipt)* ginger	1 oz	120	12	7.0
SEAWEED. See SEA VEGETABLE.				
SEITAN				
Philly steak slices, vegetarian *(White Wave)*	3 slices	60	2	0.0
traditional, vegetarian *(White Wave)*	1 piece	140	4	0.0
turkey style, vegetarian, sandwich sliced *(White Wave)*	1 slice	80	7	0.0
SEITAN MIX				
quick, flavored *(Arrowhead Mills)* mix only	1/3 cup	150	14	1.0
SELTZER. See under SOFT DRINKS AND MIXERS.				
SEMOLINA				
enriched	1 cup	601	122	1.8
unenriched	1 cup	601	122	1.8
whole grain	1 cup	602	121.6	1.8
whole grain	1 oz	102	20.6	0.3
SERRANO PEPPER. See PEPPER, SERRANO.				
SESAME BUTTER/tahini. See also TAHINI MIX.				
	1 tbsp	95	4	8.1
made from raw and stone ground kernels	1 oz	162	7	13.6
made from raw and stone ground kernels	1 tbsp	86	4	7.2
made from roasted and toasted kernels	1 oz	169	6	15.2
made from roasted and toasted kernels	1 tbsp	89	3	8.1
made from unroasted kernels, hulls removed	1 oz	172	5	16.0
made from unroasted kernels, hulls removed	1 tbsp	85	3	7.9
(Arrowhead Mills) organic	1 oz	170	4	17.0
(Erewhon) 'Sesame Tahini'	2 tbsp	200	3	18.0
(Maranatha Natural)				
raw, 'Sesame Tahini'	2 tbsp	210	3	19.0
roasted, 'Sesame Tahini'	2 tbsp	210	3	19.0
(Roaster Fresh)				
gourmet	1 oz	168	6	15.0
roasted, w/o salt, creamy	1 oz	168	6	15.0
(Westbrae)				
Mid-Eastern, organic, no salt added	2 tbsp	220	3	20.0

Food Name	Serv. Size	Total Cal.	Carbs GMS	Fat GMS
organic, 'Natural'	2 tbsp	220	6	19.0
original, no salt added	2 tbsp	210	1	19.0
raw, organic	2 tbsp	210	1	19.0
toasted, organic, no salt added	2 tbsp	220	3	19.0
SESAME MEAL, partially defatted	1 oz	161	7	13.6
SESAME OIL				
	1 cup	1927	0	218.0
	1 tbsp	120	0	13.6
(Hain)	1 tbsp	120	0	14.0
100% pure (Dynasty)	1 tbsp	130	0	14.0
100% pure, extra virgin (Loriva')	1 tbsp	120	0	14.0
hot pepper (Eden Foods)	1 tbsp	120	0	14.0
pure pressed, organic (Spectrum)	1 tbsp	120	0	14.0
toasted (Eden Foods)	1 tbsp	130	0	14.0
toasted (International Collection)	1 tbsp	120	0	14.0
toasted, pure pressed, organic (Spectrum)	1 tbsp	120	0	14.0
unrefined (Eden Foods)	1 tbsp	120	0	14.0
SESAME SEED/sim sim				
Dried				
hulled	1 cup	882	14	82.2
hulled	1 tbsp	47	1	4.4
hulled	1 tsp	16	0	1.5
hulled (Arrowhead Mills)	1 oz	160	4	14.0
whole	1 cup	825	34	71.5
whole	1 tbsp	52	2	4.5
whole (Arrowhead Mills)	1 oz	160	6	14.0
Raw				
(McCormick/Schilling)	1 tsp	21	0	1.6
hulled, natural, unsalted (Flanigan Farms)	1/4 cup	160	7	14.0
whole (Durkee)	1 tsp	13	0	0.0
whole (Laurel Leaf)	1 tsp	13	0	0.0
whole (Spice Islands)	1 tsp	9	1	0.4
Roasted and toasted, whole	1 oz	160	7	13.6
Toasted				
hulled, salted	1 cup	726	33	61.4
hulled, salted	1 oz	161	7	13.6
hulled, unsalted	1 cup	726	33	61.4
hulled, unsalted	1 oz	161	7	13.6
SESAME STICKS				
wheat-based, unsalted	1 oz	153	13	10.4
wheat-based, unsalted	2 oz	307	26	20.8
SESBANIA FLOWER. See KATURAY.				
SHAD, AMERICAN				
baked, broiled, grilled, or microwaved	3 oz	214	0	15.0
raw	3 oz	167	0	11.7
SHALLOT				
Freeze-dried				
chopped	1/4 cup	13	3	0.0
chopped	1 tbsp	3	1	0.0
chopped (McCormick/Schilling)	1 tsp	2	0	0.0
Fresh				
raw	3.5 oz	72	16.8	0.1
raw, chopped	1 tbsp	7	2	0.0
raw, trimmed	1 oz	20	4.8	<.1
raw, untrimmed	1 lb	287	67.1	0.4
SHARK				
MAKO, frozen, steak, boneless, raw (Peter Pan Seafoods)	3.5 oz	87	0	1.2

Food Name	Serv. Size	Total Cal.	Carbs GMS	Fat GMS
MIXED SPECIES, fresh				
batter dipped, fried	3 oz	194	5	11.7
raw	3 oz	110	0.0	3.8
SHEA NUT OIL				
	1 cup	1927	0	218.0
	1 tbsp	120	0	13.6
SHEEPSHEAD/fathead				
baked, broiled, grilled, or microwaved	3 oz	107	0	1.4
raw	3 oz	92	0	2.0
SHELLIE BEAN. See BEAN, SHELLY.				
SHELLY BEAN. See BEAN, SHELLY.				
SHERBET. See also FRUIT BAR, FROZEN; ICE BAR/DESSERT; SHERBET BAR, FROZEN; SORBET.				
(Borden) orange	1/2 cup	110	25	1.0
(Darigold) orange	1/2 cup	120	26	1.0
(Dreyers)				
strawberry kiwi	1/2 cup	120	27	1.0
Swiss orange	1/2 cup	150	30	2.5
(Edys)				
strawberry kiwi	1/2 cup	120	27	1.0
Swiss orange	1/2 cup	150	30	2.5
(Sealtest) all flavors	1/2 cup	130	28	1.0
SHERBET BAR, FROZEN				
(Creamsicle) all flavors, w/cream, sugar-free	1 bar	25	5	1.0
(Fudgsicle)				
all flavors, fat-free	1 bar	70	14	0.0
all flavors, sugar-free	1 bar	35	6	1.0
chocolate	1 bar	70	12	1.0
chocolate, w/nuts, no sugar, 'Fudge Nut Dip'	1 bar	130	12	8.0
SHERRY				
(Gallo)				
	2 fl oz	64	2	0.0
cream, 'Livingston Cellars'	2 fl oz	78	6	0.0
very dry, 'Livingston Cellars'	2 fl oz	60	1	0.0
(Italian Swiss Colony)				
cream	2 fl oz	85	7	0.0
dry	2 fl oz	63	1	0.0
straight	2 fl oz	67	2	0.0
SHIITAKE. See MUSHROOM, SHIITAKE.				
SHIMEJI. See MUSHROOM, OYSTER.				
SHORTENING				
For baking				
hydrogenated soybean oil w/palm and cottonseed oils	1 cup	1812	0	205.0
hydrogenated soybean oil w/palm and cottonseed oils	1 tbsp	113	0	12.8
For bread				
hydrogenated soybean oil w/cottonseed oil	1 cup	1812	0	205.0
hydrogenated soybean oil w/cottonseed oil	1 tbsp	113	0	12.8
For cake and frosting				
hydrogenated soybean oil	1 cup	1812	0	205.0
hydrogenated soybean oil	1 tbsp	113	0	12.8
For cake mix				
hydrogenated soybean and cottonseed oils	1 cup	1812	0	205.0
hydrogenated soybean and cottonseed oils	1 tbsp	113	0	12.8
For confectionery				
fractionated palm oil	1 cup	1927	0	218.0
fractionated palm oil	1 tbsp	120	0	13.6
hydrogenated coconut and/or palm kernel oil	1 cup	1812	0	205.0
hydrogenated coconut and/or palm kernel oil	1 tbsp	113	0	12.8

Food Name	Serv. Size	Total Cal.	Carbs GMS	Fat GMS
For frying				
heavy-duty, beef tallow and cottonseed oil	1 cup	1845	0	205.0
heavy-duty, beef tallow and cottonseed oil	1 tbsp	115	0	12.8
heavy-duty, hydrogenated palm oil	1 cup	1812	0	205.0
heavy-duty, hydrogenated palm oil	1 tbsp	113	0	12.8
heavy-duty, hydrogenated soybean (under 1% linoleic)	1 cup	1812	0	205.0
heavy-duty, hydrogenated soybean (under 1% linoleic)	1 tbsp	113	0	12.8
heavy-duty, hydrogenated soybean (30% linoleic), w/stabilizers	1 cup	1812	0	205.0
heavy-duty, hydrogenated soybean (30% linoleic), w/stabilizers	1 tbsp	113	0	12.8
hydrogenated soybean and cottonseed oils	1 cup	1812	0	205.0
hydrogenated soybean and cottonseed oils	1 tbsp	113	0	12.8
Household				
hydrogenated soybean and cottonseed oils	1 cup	1812	0	205.0
hydrogenated soybean and cottonseed oils	1 tbsp	113	0	12.8
hydrogenated soybean oil w/palm oil	1 cup	1812	0	205.0
hydrogenated soybean oil w/palm oil	1 tbsp	113	0	12.8
lard and vegetable oil	1 cup	1845	0	205.0
lard and vegetable oil	1 tbsp	115	0	12.8
(Crisco)				
vegetable oil	1 tbsp	110	0	12.0
(Finast)				
vegetable oil	1 tbsp	110	0	13.0
vegetable oil, butter flavor	1 tbsp	110	0	12.0
(Wesson) vegetable oil	1 tbsp	109	0	12.1
Industrial				
hydrogenated soybean oil w/cottonseed oil	1 cup	1812	0	205.0
hydrogenated soybean oil w/cottonseed oil	1 tbsp	113	0	12.8
lard and vegetable oil	1 cup	1845	0	205.0
lard and vegetable oil	1 tbsp	115	0	12.8
(Wesson)				
'Crystal'	1 tbsp	122	0	13.5
low-melt	1 tbsp	122	0	13.5
'Super'	1 tbsp	122	0	13.5
'Wesgold'	1 tbsp	122	0	13.5
'Wespour'	1 tbsp	122	0	13.5
Multipurpose				
hydrogenated soybean and palm oils	1 cup	1812	0	205.0
hydrogenated soybean and palm oils	1 tbsp	113	0	12.8
(Quest)				
'Cirol'	1 oz	256	2	28.4
'Durola Select'	1 oz	256	0	28.4
'Duromel'	1 oz	256	0	28.4
SHOYU. See under SAUCE, SOY.				
SHRIMP. See also SHRIMP DISH/ENTRÉE.				
Canned				
medium, deveined, in water and salt (S&W)	1/4 cup	45	0	0.0
mixed species	1 cup	154	1	2.5
mixed species	10 medium	38	0	0.6
mixed species	3 oz	102	1	1.7
mixed species, cooked	1 oz	34	0	0.6
mixed species, drained (Louisiana Brand)	2 oz	58	0	1.0
mixed species, large, drained (ShopRite)	2 oz	50	0	1.0
peeled, broken (Crown Prince)	1/2 can	60	1	0.5
small, deveined, in water and salt (S&W)	1/4 cup	45	0	0.0
tiny, peeled (Crown Prince)	1/2 can	60	1	0.5
Fresh				
mixed species, boiled, poached, or steamed	3 oz	84	0	0.9

Food Name	Serv. Size	Total Cal.	Carbs GMS	Fat GMS
mixed species, large, boiled, poached, or steamed .... 4 shrimp		22	0	0.2
mixed species, raw .... 3 oz		90	1	1.5
mixed species, raw, large .... 4 shrimp		30	0	0.5
mixed species, raw, medium .... 1 shrimp		6	0	0.1
mixed species, raw, small .... 1 shrimp		5	0	0.1
Frozen				
butterfly, 'Specialty' (Gorton's) .... 4 oz		160	16	1.0
cooked, peeled, deveined, tail off, 250/300 count (Contessa) ...... 3 oz		40	0	0.0
w/tails (Harvest Of The Sea) .... 3 oz		70	0	0.0

SHRIMP COCKTAIL. See under SHRIMP DISH/ENTRÉE.

SHRIMP DISH/ENTRÉE

Food Name	Serv. Size	Total Cal.	Carbs GMS	Fat GMS
(Armour)				
baby bay, frozen, 'Classics Lite' .... 9.75 oz		220	31	6.0
Creole, frozen, 'Classics Lite' .... 11.25 oz		260	53	2.0
(Booth)				
Alfredo, w/fettucini, frozen .... 10 oz		260	28	8.0
cocktail, w/garlic butter sauce and vegetable rice .... 10 oz		400	40	25.0
New Orleans, w/wild rice, frozen .... 10 oz		230	35	5.0
Oriental, w/pineapple rice, frozen .... 10 oz		190	30	3.0
primavera, w/fettuccini, frozen .... 10 oz		200	28	3.0
w/garlic butter sauce and vegetable rice, frozen .... 10 oz		400	40	25.0
(Budget Gourmet)				
cocktail, w/fettuccine, frozen .... 9.5 oz		375	38	20.0
mariner, frozen, 'Light & Healthy' .... 1 dinner		230	40	6.0
(Cajun Cookin')				
Creole, frozen .... 12 oz		390	55	11.0
etouffée, frozen .... 17 oz		360	52	9.0
jambalaya, frozen .... 12 oz		450	43	20.0
(Gorton's)				
breaded, w/original seasoning .... 6 shrimp		229	18	13.0
crisps, frozen, 'Specialty' .... 4 oz		280	26	15.0
crunchy, frozen, microwave, 'Crunchy Shrimp' .... 1/2 pkg		160	12	9.0
crunchy, whole, frozen, 'Microwave Specialty' .... 5 oz		380	35	20.0
popcorn .... 1 cup		260	21	16.0
scampi, baked .... 6 shrimp		250	18	16.0
scampi, frozen, 'Microwave Entrees' .... 1 pkg		390	21	30.0
(Healthy Choice)				
Creole, frozen .... 11.25 oz		210	42	1.0
marinara .... 1 entree		250	44	4.0
w/vegetables .... 1 entree		270	39	6.0
(Hudson) stir-fry, complete meal kit, frozen .... 1 3/4 cup		210	35	2.0
(LaChoy)				
chow mein .... 1 cup		53	10	0.9
chow mein, canned .... 3/4 cup		35	4	1.0
cocktail, w/lobster sauce, 'Fresh & Lite' .... 10 oz		240	36.4	6.2
(Longacre)				
salad, 'Saladfest' .... 1 oz		45	2.0	3.0
salad, w/seafood, 'Saladfest' .... 1 oz		42	2.0	3.0
(Marie Callender's) over angel hair pasta, frozen .... 1 cup		300	37	12.0
(Mrs. Paul's)				
breaded, fried, frozen .... 3 oz		200	16	11.0
Cajun style, frozen, 'Light' .... 9 oz		230	37	5.0
cocktail, w/clams and linguini, 'Light' .... 10 oz		240	36	5.0
primavera, frozen 'Light' .... 9.5 oz		180	28	3.0
(Right Course) primavera, frozen .... 9 5/8 oz		240	32	7.0
(Sau-Sea) cocktail .... 4 oz		113	19	1.0

Food Name	Serv. Size	Total Cal.	Carbs GMS	Fat GMS
(SeaPak)				
battered, frozen, 'Shrimp 'n Batter'	4 oz	260	20	15.0
breaded, butterfly, frozen, 'Mikado'	4 oz	160	26	1.0
breaded, butterfly/round, frozen	4 oz	150	20	1.0
cocktail, 'Super Valu' heat and serve	4 oz	210	30	4.0
w/crab meat stuffing, battered, frozen	4 oz	260	27	13.0
(Shanghai) stir-fry, frozen	10.3 oz	170	19	2.0
(Smart Ones)				
marinara	1 entrée	200	37	2.0
marinara, w/linguini, frozen	8 oz	150	26	1.0
(Ultra Slim-Fast)				
Creole, frozen	12 oz	240	45	4.0
marinara, frozen	12 oz	290	53	3.0
SHRIMP PASTE, canned	1 tsp	13	0.1	0.7
SHRIMP SALAD. See under SHRIMP DISH/ENTRÉE.				
SHRIMP SUBSTITUTE, made from surimi	3 oz	86	8	1.3
SICAMA. See JICAMA				
SILVER HAKE. See WHITING.				
SILVER SALMON. See under SALMON.				
SIM SIM. See SESAME SEED.				
SISYMBRIUM SEED				
dried, whole	1 cup	235	43	3.4
dried, whole	1 oz	90	17	1.3
SKIL. See COD, ALASKAN.				
SKIPJACK. See under TUNA.				
SKUNK CABBAGE. See CABBAGE, SKUNK.				
SLIMEHEAD. See ORANGE ROUGHY.				
SLOPPY JOE MIX. See under SANDWICH FILLING MIX.				
SLOPPY JOE SEASONING. See under SEASONING MIX.				
SMELT, RAINBOW				
baked, broiled, grilled, or microwaved	3 oz	105	0	2.6
raw	3 oz	82	0	2.1
SNACK BAR. See also BREAKFAST BAR; CAKE, SNACK; FRUIT BAR; GRANOLA/CEREAL BAR; SPORTS AND DIET/NUTRITION BAR.				
(Barbara's Bakery)				
apple-filled, whole grain, organic	1.3 oz bar	120	29	0.0
blueberry-filled, whole grain, organic	1.3 oz bar	120	29	0.0
raspberry-filled, whole grain, organic, nonfat	1 bar	110	28	0.0
strawberry-filled, whole grain, organic, nonfat	1.3 oz bar	120	29	0.0
(Bear Valley)				
carob cocoa, food bar, 'Pemmican'	3.75 oz	440	68	12.0
coconut almond, food bar, 'Meal Pack'	3.75 oz	400	56	12.0
fruit and nut, food bar, 'Pemmican'	3.75 oz	420	59	13.0
sesame lemon, food bar, 'Meal Pack'	3.75 oz	410	57	13.0
(Clif)				
chocolate chip, '100% Natural Endurance'	2.4 oz	250	51	3.0
dark chocolate, '100% Natural Endurance'	2.4 oz	250	52	2.0
(Earth Grains)				
banana apple walnut, 'Bagel Power Bar'	1 bar	270	45	6.0
citrus almond, w/mixed fruit 'Bagel Power Bar'	1 bar	260	45	4.0
fruit and nut, 'Bagel Power Bar'	1 bar	240	48	3.0
(Edgebar) chocolate crunch	1 bar	234	46	2.0
(Fruit Boosters)				
apple, low-fat	1 bar	130	27	2.0
blueberry, low-fat	1 bar	130	27	2.0
(General Mills) date	1/32 pkg	60	9	2.0

Food Name	Serv. Size	Total Cal.	Carbs GMS	Fat GMS
(Glenny's)				
apple-cinnamon	1.25 oz	120	28	1.0
caramel	1.25 oz	120	29	1.0
chocolate	1.25 oz	120	28	1.0
raspberry	1.25 oz	120	29	1.0
(Golden Temple)				
original, 100% natural, 'Wha Guru Chew'	1.13 oz	166	14	9.0
sesame almond, 100% natural, 'Wha Guru Chew'	1.13 oz	162	11	11.0
(Great Cakes)				
all natural 'Summer Fruits'	3 oz	190	35	2.5
all natural 'Tropical Fruits'	3 oz	185	35	2.0
(Health Valley)				
apple, 'Bakes'	1 serving	100	16	3.0
'Date Bakes'	1 serving	100	16	3.0
fruit, 'Fruit & Fitness'	2 bars	200	39	3.0
fruit-nut, 'Oat Bran Jumbo Fruit Bars'	1 serving	150	29	4.0
oat bran, 'Fig & Nut Bakes'	1 serving	110	19	3.0
oat bran, 'Oat Bran Jumbo Fruit Bars'	1 serving	170	28	5.0
oat bran, raisin and cinnamon	1 serving	140	32	2.0
'Oat Bran Apricot Bakes'	1 serving	100	19	2.0
'Raisin Bakes'	1 serving	100	16	3.0
rice bran, almond, and date	1 serving	190	29	6.0
(Kellogg's)				
apple-cinnamon, wheat, whole-grain oats, fruit	1 bar	140	26	4.0
wheat, whole-grain oats, fruit	1 bar	140	26	4.0
(Kudos)				
peaches and cream, 'Pan Squares'	1 sq.	150	22	6.0
peanut butter and chocolate chip, 'Pan Squares'	1 sq.	170	20	9.0
strawberry and cream cheese, 'Pan Squares'	1 sq.	150	22	6.0
(Marin)				
fig, honey sweetened, organic	1 bar	120	21	3.0
fig, organic	1 bar	70	16	0.0
(Natural Nectar)				
almond, 'Treat Yourself Right'	1 bar	150	22	5.0
apple, 'Original Fruit Bar'	1 bar	100	15	3.0
apple-cinnamon, low-fat, 'Fi-Bar'	1 bar	90	22	1.0
apple-oatmeal spice 'Fi-Bar A.M.'	1 bar	150	27	3.0
banana nut, 'Fi-Bar A.M.'	1 bar	150	26	4.0
chocolate, 'Fi-Bar Lite'	2.5 oz	190	29	6.0
cocoa-almond crunch, 'Fi-Bar'	1 bar	130	21	4.0
cocoa-almond, whole grain, 'Fi-Bar Chewy & Nutty'	1 bar	140	23	4.5
cocoa peanut butter crunch, 'Chewy & Nutty'	1 bar	130	20	4.0
cocoa peanut, 'Fi-Bar Chewy & Nutty'	1 bar	130	20	1.0
coconut	1 bar	120	20	4.0
cranberry, w/wild berries, 'Original Fruit Bar'	1 bar	120	23	2.0
lemon, 'Original Fruit Bar'	1 bar	100	15	3.0
Mandarin orange 'Original Fruit Bar'	1 bar	100	15	3.0
peanut butter	1 bar	130	20	4.0
peanut butter, 'Treat Yourself Right'	1 bar	150	18	5.0
raisin nut bran, 'Fi-Bar A.M.'	1 bar	150	26	4.0
raspberry, 'Canadian'	1 bar	120	21	3.0
raspberry, 'Original Fruit Bar'	1 bar	120	23	2.0
strawberry, 'Canadian'	1 bar	120	21	3.0
strawberry, 'Original Fruit Bar'	1 bar	120	23	2.0
strawberry-oatmeal, w/almonds, 'Fi-Bar A.M.'	1 bar	150	24	4.0
vanilla almond, 'Fi-Bar Chewy & Nutty'	1 bar	130	21	4.0

Food Name	Serv. Size	Total Cal.	Carbs GMS	Fat GMS
vanilla almond crunch, 'Canadian Chewy & Nutty' .... 1 bar		130	21	4.0
vanilla peanut, 'Fi-Bar Chewy & Nutty' .... 1 bar		130	20	4.0
(Pemmican) carob cocoa, meatless .... 1 pkg		440	68	12.0
SNACK BAR MIX. See also CAKE, SNACK, MIX.				
(Betty Crocker)				
caramel oatmeal, 'Supreme Dessert' mix only .... 1/32 pkg		90	15	3.0
caramel oatmeal, 'Supreme Dessert' prepared w/margarine ...... 1 bar		110	15	5.0
chocolate and toffee, 'Supreme Dessert' mix only .... 1/32 pkg		90	17	2.0
chocolate and toffee, 'Supreme Dessert' prepared .... 1 bar		110	17	4.0
chocolate peanut butter 'Supreme Dessert' prepared .... 1 bar		110	14	5.0
chocolate peanut butter, 'Supreme Dessert' mix only .... 1/32 pkg		100	14	4.0
date, 'Classic' prepared .... 1 bar		60	9	2.0
M&M's cookie bars, 'Supreme Dessert' mix only .... 1/32 pkg		100	16	3.0
M&M's cookie bars, 'Supreme Dessert' prepared .... 1 bar		110	16	5.0
raspberry, 'Supreme Dessert' mix only .... 1/32 pkg		100	16	3.0
raspberry, 'Supreme Dessert' prepared .... 1/32 pkg		100	16	4.0
Sunkist lemon, 'Supreme Dessert' mix only .... 1/32 pkg		100	17	3.0
Sunkist lemon, 'Supreme Dessert' prepared w/4 eggs .... 1 bar		110	17	4.0
SNACK CHIP. See also BAGEL CHIPS, BANANA CHIPS; CARROT CHIPS; CORN CHIPS AND SNACKS; PASTA CHIPS; POTATO CHIPS AND SNACKS; RICE CHIPS; SEA VEGETABLE CHIPS; SNACK MIX; TARO CHIPS; TORTILLA CHIPS; VEGETABLE CHIPS; WASABI CHIPS.				
(Bake-Itos) pico de gallo .... 1 oz		110	23	0.9
(Bugles)				
nacho flavor .... 1 1/3 cup		160	18	9.0
original flavor .... 1 1/3 cup		160	18	9.0
ranch flavor .... 1 1/3 cup		160	18	9.0
(Frito-Lay's)				
'Funyuns' .... 1 oz		140	18	7.0
'Munchos' .... 1 oz		160	16	10.0
(Sun Chips)				
French onion .... 1 oz		140	19	6.0
harvest cheddar .... 1 oz		140	19	6.0
original .... 1 oz		140	19	6.0
SNACK MIX				
(Burns & Ricker) nonfat, 'Party Mix' .... 3/4 cup		120	23	0.0
(Eagle) 'Snack Mix' .... 1/2 cup		150	17	7.0
(Flavor Tree)				
no salt, 'Party Mix' .... 1 1/2 cups		163	13	10.8
original, 'Party Mix' .... 1/4 cup		163	12	11.0
(General Mills)				
barbecue flavor, 'Chex' .... 1 oz		130	18	5.0
cheese, 'Chex' .... 2/3 cup		120	18	4.9
cool sour cream and onion flavor,'Chex' .... 2/3 cup		130	19	5.0
golden cheddar, 'Chex' .... 2/3 cup		130	19	5.0
nacho cheese, 'Chex' .... 2/3 cup		130	19	5.0
(Harmony)				
Oriental, party mix .... 1/4 cup		150	11	10.0
'Swiss Mix' .... 1/4 cup		190	27	8.0
(Nabisco)				
original flavor, 'Doo Dads' .... 1/2 cup		129	18	5.2
traditional, baked, 'Ritz' .... 1 oz		130	18	6.0
(Pepperidge Farm)				
'Classic' .... 1 oz		140	14	8.0
lightly smoked .... 1 oz		150	13	9.0
spicy .... 1 oz		140	14	8.0
super cheddar, 'Goldfish Party Mix' .... 1 oz		140	15	7.0
w/cashews and almonds, 'Nutty Deluxe' 'Goldfish' .... 1/2 cup		180	20	9.0

Food Name	Serv. Size	Total Cal.	Carbs GMS	Fat GMS
w/honey roasted peanuts, original, 'Goldfish'	1/2 cup	170	21	8.0
(Super Snax)	1 oz	137	17	6.5
SNACK STICKS, sesame and cheese, 'Twigs' *(Nabisco)*	15 sticks	150	17	7.0
SNAP BEAN. See BEAN, GREEN.				
SNAP PEAS. See PEAS, SNAP.				
SNAPPER				
mixed species, baked, broiled, grilled, or microwaved	3 oz	109	0	1.5
mixed species, raw	3 oz	85	0	1.1
SOBA NOODLE. See under NOODLE, JAPANESE.				
SOCKEYE SALMON. See under SALMON.				
SODA. See under SOFT DRINKS AND MIXERS.				
SOFT DRINKS AND MIXERS. See also WATER, FLAVORED.				
(A&W)				
cream	1 fl oz	14	4	0.0
cream, diet	1 fl oz	1	0	0.1
root beer	1 fl oz	15	4	0.1
root beer, diet	1 fl oz	1	0	0.0
(Canada Dry)				
Collins mixer	8 fl oz	80	20	0.0
ginger ale	8 fl oz	90	21	0.0
ginger ale, 'Golden'	8 fl oz	100	24	0.0
grape, 'Concord'	8 fl oz	130	32	0.0
tonic water	8 fl oz	90	22	0.0
whiskey sour mixer	8 fl oz	90	22	0.0
(Coca-Cola)				
'Caffeine-Free Coke'	12 fl oz	145	41	0.0
'Caffeine-Free Diet Coke'	12 fl oz	2	0	0.0
'Classic Coke'	12 fl oz	145	41	0.0
'Coke'	6 fl oz	77	20	0.0
'Diet Cherry Coke'	6 fl oz	1	0	0.0
'Diet Coke'	12 fl oz	2	0	0.0
'Tab'	6 fl oz	1	0	0.0
(Dr. Diablo) cola	12 fl oz	140	38	0.0
(Dr Pepper)				
'Caffeine-Free Diet Dr Pepper'	12 fl oz	3	0	0.0
cola	12 fl oz	150	38	0.0
cola, caffeine-free	12 fl oz	150	38	0.0
'Diet 'Dr Pepper'	12 fl oz	3	0	0.0
(Fresca) citrus	6 fl oz	2	0	0.0
(Health Valley)				
ginger ale	12 fl oz	153	35	1.0
root beer, 'Old Fashioned'	12 fl oz	120	26	1.0
root beer, sarsaparilla	12 fl oz	153	35	1.0
wild berry	12 fl oz	142	33	1.0
(Hires)				
cream, caffeine-free	6 fl oz	90	24	1.0
cream, diet, caffeine-free	6 fl oz	2	1	1.0
root beer, caffeine-free	6 fl oz	90	23	1.0
root beer, caffeine-free, diet, w/NutraSweet	6 fl oz	2	1	1.0
(Jolt) cola	6 fl oz	85	21	0.0
(Mello Yello)				
citrus	6 fl oz	87	22	0.0
citrus, diet	6 fl oz	3	0	0.0
(Mug) root beer, diet	12 fl oz	4	1	0.0
(Natural 90 Diet) all flavors	6 fl oz	2	1	0.0
(Pathmark) cola, sugar-free, 'No Frills'	8 fl oz	0	0	0.0

Food Name	Serv. Size	Total Cal.	Carbs GMS	Fat GMS
(Pepsi-Cola)				
'Light'	12 fl oz	1	0	0.0
'Wild Cherry'	12 fl oz	163	43	0.0
'Diet Crystal'	6 fl oz	0	0	0.0
'Caffeine-Free Diet Pepsi'	12 fl oz	1	0	0.0
(Santa Cruz Natural) ginger ale, organic, 'Sparkling'	8 fl oz	155	36	1.0
(Schweppes)				
bitter lemon	6 fl oz	82	20	0.0
blackberry, 'Royal'	6 fl oz	35	8	0.0
citrus, tropical, 'Royal'	6 fl oz	35	8	0.0
club soda	6 fl oz	0	0	0.0
Collins mixer	6 fl oz	75	18	0.0
ginger ale	6 fl oz	65	16	0.0
ginger ale, sugar-free	6 fl oz	2	1	0.0
grape	6 fl oz	95	23	0.0
grapefruit	6 fl oz	80	20	0.0
kiwi-passionfruit, 'Royal'	6 fl oz	35	8	0.0
lemon-lime	6 fl oz	72	18	0.0
orange, sparkling	6 fl oz	88	22	0.0
peaches and cream, 'Royal'	6 fl oz	35	8	0.0
raspberry ginger ale, diet	6 fl oz	2	1	0.0
root beer	6 fl oz	76	19	0.0
seltzer, all flavors	6 fl oz	0	0	0.0
seltzer, low-sodium	6 fl oz	0	0	0.0
sour lemon	6 fl oz	79	19	0.0
strawberry-banana, 'Royal'	6 fl oz	35	8	0.0
tonic water	6 fl oz	64	16	0.0
tonic water, diet	6 fl oz	2	1	0.0
vanilla bean, 'Royal'	6 fl oz	35	8	0.0
Vichy water	6 fl oz	0	0	0.0
wild cherry, 'Royal'	6 fl oz	35	8	0.0
wild raspberry, 'Royal'	6 fl oz	35	8	0.0
(7-Up)				
cherry citrus	12 fl oz	148	39	0.0
cherry citrus, diet	12 fl oz	4	0	0.0
lemon-lime	12 fl oz	144	36	0.0
lemon-lime, diet	12 fl oz	4	0	0.0
(Shasta)				
black cherry	12 fl oz	162	44	0.0
cherry cola	12 fl oz	140	38	0.0
citrus mist	12 fl oz	170	46	0.0
club soda	12 fl oz	0	0	0.0
cola	12 fl oz	147	40	0.0
Collins mixer	12 fl oz	118	32	0.0
'Creme'	12 fl oz	154	42	0.0
fruit punch	12 fl oz	173	47	0.0
ginger ale	12 fl oz	120	33	0.0
grape	12 fl oz	177	48	0.0
lemon-lime	12 fl oz	146	39	0.0
'Luigi Berry'	8 fl oz	130	32	0.0
'Mario Punch'	8 fl oz	130	31	0.0
orange	12 fl oz	177	48	0.0
'Princess Toadstool Cherry'	8 fl oz	130	31	0.0
red berry	12 fl oz	158	43	0.0
root beer	12 fl oz	154	42	0.0
strawberry	12 fl oz	147	40	0.0
tonic water	12 fl oz	121	33	0.0

Food Name	Serv. Size	Total Cal.	Carbs GMS	Fat GMS
'Yoshi Apple'	8 fl oz	130	31	0.0
(Slice) orange, 'Diet'	12 fl oz	12	2	0.0
(Soda-Licious)				
cherry cola	1 pouch	100	22	1.0
fruit punch, red	1 pouch	100	22	1.0
grape	1 pouch	100	22	1.0
lemon-lime	1 pouch	100	22	1.0
orange	1 pouch	100	22	1.0
root beer	1 pouch	100	22	1.0
(Spree)				
cherry-lime	12 fl oz	158	43	0.0
cola	12 fl oz	147	40	0.0
ginger ale	12 fl oz	120	33	0.0
grapefruit	12 fl oz	154	42	0.0
lemon-lime	12 fl oz	154	42	0.0
lemon-tangerine	12 fl oz	165	45	0.0
lime, Mandarin	12 fl oz	154	42	0.0
root beer	12 fl oz	154	42	0.0
tropical blend	12 fl oz	146	41	0.0
(Squirt)				
citrus	1 fl oz	13	3	0.0
citrus, 'Diet'	1 fl oz	1	0	0.0
citrus berry, 'Ruby Red'	8 fl oz	120	30	0.0
(Vernors)				
ginger ale	3.5 fl oz	40	10	0.1
ginger ale, 'Diet'	3.5 fl oz	1	0	0.1
(Wink) grapefruit	8 fl oz	120	30	0.0
SOLE				
Fresh				
baked, broiled, grilled, or microwaved	3 oz	99	0.0	1.3
raw	3 oz	77	0.0	1.0
Frozen				
Atlantic *(Booth)*	4 oz	90	0	1.0
fillet *(SeaPak)*	4 oz	90	0	1.0
fillet, lightly breaded *(Van de Kamp's)*	1 serving	220	17	11.0
fillet, 'Natural' *(Van de Kamp's)*	4 oz	100	0	2.0
'Fishmarket Fresh' *(Gorton's)*	5 oz	110	1	1.0
SOLE DISH/ENTRÉE				
(Gorton's)				
fillet, stuffed, frozen, 'Select' approx 5 oz	1 fillet	160	18	3.0
in lemon butter, frozen, 'Microwave Entrees'	1 pkg	380	17	24.0
(Healthy Choice)				
au gratin, frozen	11 oz	270	40	5.0
w/lemon butter sauce, frozen	8.25 oz	230	33	4.0
SOMEN NOODLE. See under NOODLE, JAPANESE.				
SORBET. See also SHERBET.				
(Cascadian Farm)				
blackberry sorbet, all-fruit, organic, nonfat	1/2 cup	90	22	0.0
blackberry, nonfat	1 oz	25	21	0.1
blackberry, w/vanilla ice cream, organic	1/2 cup	110	21	2.0
orange, w/vanilla ice cream, organic	1/2 cup	110	21	2.0
raspberry, all-fruit, organic, nonfat	1/2 cup	90	21	0.0
raspberry, nonfat	1 oz	28	21	0.2
raspberry, w/vanilla ice cream, organic	1/2 cup	110	21	2.0
strawberry, all-fruit, organic, nonfat	1/2 cup	70	17	0.0
strawberry, nonfat	1 oz	26	22	0.1
(Diamond Crystal) lower calorie, all flavors	1 serving	30	7	0.0

Food Name	Serv. Size	Total Cal.	Carbs GMS	Fat GMS
(Dole)				
Mandarin orange, nonfat	4 oz	110	28	0.1
peach, nonfat	4 oz	120	28	0.6
pineapple, nonfat	4 oz	120	28	0.1
raspberry, nonfat	4 oz	110	28	0.1
strawberry, nonfat	4 oz	110	28	0.1
(Frusen Gladje) raspberry, nonfat	1/2 cup	140	36	0.0
(Haagen-Dazs)				
blueberry, w/vanilla ice cream	1/2 cup	190	25	8.0
key lime, w/vanilla ice cream	1/2 cup	200	29	7.0
lemon, 'Ice Cream Shop'	4 oz	140	34	0.0
orange, 'Ice Cream Shop'	4 oz	113	30	0.0
raspberry	1/2 cup	120	29	0.0
raspberry, nonfat, 'Ice Cream Shop'	4 oz	93	22	0.0
strawberry	1/2 cup	130	33	0.0
(Real Fruit)				
red raspberry, chunky, nonfat	1/2 cup	100	25	0.0
tropical blend, chunky, nonfat	1/2 cup	100	26	0.0
wildberry, chunky, nonfat	1/2 cup	100	25	0.0
(TCBY Treats) all flavors, soft serve, nonfat	1/2 cup	100	24	0.0
SORGHUM				
broomcorn, whole grain	3.5 oz	327	72.9	2.9
whole grain	1 cup	651	143.3	6.3
whole grain	1 oz	96	21.2	0.9
SORGHUM SYRUP. See under SYRUP.				
SORREL				
boiled, drained	4 oz	23	3.3	0.7
raw, trimmed	1 oz	6	0.9	0.2
raw, trimmed, chopped	1/2 cup	15	2.1	0.5
raw, untrimmed	1 lb	70	10.2	2.2
SOUP. See also SOUP MIX.				
ASPARAGUS, CREAM OF				
Canned, condensed				
prepared w/milk	1 cup	161	16	8.2
prepared w/water	1 cup	85	11	4.1
unprepared	10.75-oz can	210	26	9.9
unprepared	1 cup	173	21	8.2
Frozen				
(Kettle Ready)	3/4 cup	62	5	4.3
(Myers)	9.75 oz	152	10	8.0
(Soup Supreme)	1 cup	160	17	9.0
BARLEY W/MUSHROOM				
Canned, condensed *(Rokeach)* prepared	1 cup	85	17	0.2
BARLEY BEAN, frozen *(Tabatchnick)*	7.5 oz	130	22	2.0
BEAN AND HAM, heat and serve *(Healthy Choice)*	1 cup	160	29	1.5
BEAN				
Canned, condensed				
w/frankfurter, prepared	1 cup	188	22	7.0
w/frankfurter, unprepared	11.25-oz can	453	53	16.9
w/frankfurter, unprepared	1 cup	373	44	14.0
w/pork, prepared	1 cup	172	23	5.9
w/pork, unprepared	11.5-oz can	421	55	14.4
w/pork, unprepared	1 cup	347	46	11.9
(Campbell's)				
'Homestyle' prepared	1 cup	130	25	1.0
w/bacon, 'Healthy Request' unprepared	1/2 cup	150	26	2.0
(Stouffer's) navy bean, classic, food service product, prepared	1 cup	128	18	3.2

Food Name	Serv. Size	Total Cal.	Carbs GMS	Fat GMS
Canned, ready to use				
w/ham, chunky, commercial product	19.25-oz can	519	61	19.1
w/ham, chunky, commercial product	1 cup	231	27	8.5
(Grandma Brown's)	1 cup	190	31	3.4
(Health Valley) five bean vegetable, nonfat	7.5 oz	100	14	0.0
(Hormel) w/ham, 'Hearty Soups'	7.5 oz	190	29	4.0
Frozen				
(Kettle Ready)				
w/beef, vegetable	3/4 cup	85	11	3.0
w/ham	3/4 cup	113	20	3.6
(Soup Supreme)				
royal navy, food service product	1 cup	140	24	2.0
w/ham, food service product	1 cup	140	23	2.0
(Tabatchnick) Northern bean	7.5 oz	164	29	2.0
BEEF				
Canned, condensed				
(Campbell's)				
prepared	1 cup	80	10	2.0
w/bouillon, prepared	1 cup	16	1	0.0
w/broth, prepared	1 cup	16	1	0.0
Canned, ready to use				
chunky	19-oz can	303	44	11.5
chunky	1 cup	170	20	5.1
(Campbell's)				
'Chunky'	10 3/4 oz can	200	24	5.0
Stroganoff style, 'Chunky'	10 3/4 oz can	320	28	16.0
w/vegetables and pasta, 'Home Cookin'	10 3/4 oz can	140	18	2.0
(College Inn) w/broth, ready to serve	1 cup	18	1	0.0
(Health Valley) w/broth, no salt added	7.5 oz	17	2	1.0
(Healthy Choice) 'Hearty Beef'	7.5 oz	120	17	2.0
(Progresso)				
	10.5-oz can	180	17	6.0
hearty	9.5 oz	160	15	4.0
w/broth, seasoned	1/2 cup	10	1	1.0
w/minestrone	10.5-oz can	180	18	6.0
(Swanson) w/broth, ready to serve	7.25 oz	18	0	1.0
BEEF AND POTATO				
Canned, ready to use (Healthy Choice)	1 cup	110	17	1.0
BEEF BARLEY				
Canned, ready to use				
(Progresso)				
	10.5-oz can	150	16	5.0
low-fat, 'Healthy Classics'	1 cup	142	20	1.9
BEEF BROTH/BOUILLON				
Canned, condensed				
prepared	1 cup	23	0	1.3
unprepared	10.5-oz can	72	4	0.0
unprepared	1 cup	59	4	0.0
Canned, ready to use				
	14-oz can	28	0	0.9
	10.5-oz can	41	0	1.3
	1 cup	17	0	0.5
and tomato juice	5.5-oz can	62	14	0.2
and tomato juice	1 oz	11	3	0.0
(College Inn)	7 oz	16	1	0.0
(Health Valley)				
no salt added	6.9 oz	10	2	0.0

Food Name	Serv. Size	Total Cal.	Carbs GMS	Fat GMS
nonfat	1 cup	20	0	0.0
regular	6.9 oz	10	2	0.0
(Swanson) clear	1 cup	20	1	1.0
BEEF MUSHROOM				
Canned, condensed				
prepared	1 cup	73	6	3.0
unprepared	10.75-oz can	186	16	7.3
unprepared	1 cup	153	13	6.0
BEEF NOODLE				
Canned, condensed				
prepared	1 cup	83	9	3.1
unprepared	10.75-oz can	204	22	7.5
unprepared	1 cup	168	18	6.2
(Campbell's) 'Homestyle' prepared	1 cup	80	7	4.0
Canned, ready to use *(Progresso)*	9.5 oz	170	18	4.0
BEEF VEGETABLE				
Canned, condensed				
(Campbell's) 'Healthy Request' unprepared	1/2 cup	70	9	2.0
(Progresso) and rotini, prepared	1 cup	120	10	3.5
Canned, ready to use				
country, chunky	1 cup	153	16	4.4
w/barley, prepared	1 cup	77	10	1.8
(Healthy Choice) 'Vegetable Beef'	7.5 oz	130	21	1.0
(Hormel)				
'Hearty Soups'	7.5 oz	90	15	1.0
micro cup, 'Hearty Soups'	1 container	71	12	1.0
(Lipton) 'Hearty Ones'	11-oz container	229	40	3.0
(Progresso)	10.5-oz can	170	18	3.0
BERRY				
Canned, ready to use *(Great Impressions)* 'Three Berry'	3/4 cup	107	26	0.2
BLACK BEAN				
Canned, condensed				
prepared	1 cup	116	20	1.5
unprepared	11-oz can	284	48	4.1
unprepared	1 cup	234	40	3.4
(Stouffer's) prepared	1 cup	192	30	3.2
Canned, ready to use				
(Health Valley)				
	7.5 oz	160	24	3.0
and vegetable, nonfat	1 cup	110	24	0.0
no salt added	7.5 oz	160	24	3.0
Frozen				
(Kettle Ready) w/ham	3/4 cup	154	23	6.2
(Soup Supreme) Southern style, food service product	1 cup	150	23	3.0
BLUEBERRY, canned, ready to use *(Great Impressions)*	3/4 cup	95	23	0.3
BORSCHT				
Canned, ready to use				
(Gold's)				
	1 cup	100	21	0.0
low-calorie	1 cup	20	5	1.0
(Manischewitz)				
low-calorie	1 cup	20	4	0.0
w/beets	1 cup	80	20	0.0
(Rokeach)				
	1 cup	96	23	0.3
'Diet'	1 cup	29	6	0.2
'Unsalted'	1 cup	103	23	0.3

Food Name	Serv. Size	Total Cal.	Carbs GMS	Fat GMS
BROCCOLI				
Canned, ready to use *(Health Valley)* carotene, nonfat	1 cup	70	16	0.0
BROCCOLI, CREAM OF				
Canned, condensed				
(Campbell's)				
'Healthy Request' unprepared	1/2 cup	70	9	2.0
prepared w/whole milk	1 cup	140	14	7.0
unprepared	1/2 cup	80	12	3.0
(Stouffer's) prepared w/whole milk	1 cup	272	17	19.2
Canned, ready to use				
(Andersen's)	.5 oz	170	20	8.0
(Stouffer's) food service product	1 cup	288	13	21.6
(Progresso) 'Healthy Classics'	1 cup	88	13	2.8
Frozen				
(Kettle Ready)	6 oz	94	6	7.2
(Myers)	9.75 oz	174	11	11.0
(Soup Supreme)				
food service product	1 cup	180	16	11.0
w/cheese, food service product	1 cup	190	16	12.0
(Tabatchnick)	7.5 oz	90	10	4.0
CABBAGE SOUP, frozen *(Tabatchnick)*	7.5 oz	110	21	2.0
CAULIFLOWER, CREAM OF, frozen *(Kettle Ready)*	3/4 cup	93	6	7.0
CELERY, CREAM OF				
Canned, condensed				
unprepared	10.75-oz can	220	21	13.6
unprepared	1 cup	181	18	11.2
prepared w/milk	1 cup	164	15	9.7
prepared w/water	1 cup	90	9	5.6
(Campbell's)				
'Healthy Request' unprepared	1/2 cup	70	11	2.0
prepared w/water	1 cup	100	8	7.0
CHEDDAR CAULIFLOWER				
Frozen *(Soup Supreme)* food service product	1 cup	130	13	8.0
CHEDDAR VEGETABLE				
Frozen, *(Soup Supreme)* food service product	1 cup	140	14	8.0
CHEESE				
Canned, condensed				
prepared w/milk	1 cup	231	16	14.6
prepared w/water	1 cup	156	11	10.5
unprepared	11-oz can	378	26	25.4
unprepared	1 cup	311	21	20.9
(Campbell's)				
nacho, prepared w/water	1 cup	110	8	8.0
nacho, prepared w/whole milk	1 cup	180	13	12.0
Frozen				
(Kettle Ready)				
cheddar, cream of	3/4 cup	158	7	12.5
cheddar, cream of, w/broccoli	3/4 cup	137	5	11.3
(Myers) and broccoli	9.75 oz	325	19	23.0
(Soup Supreme) cheddar, club, food service product	1 cup	240	17	16.0
CHERRY, canned, ready to use *(Great Impressions)*	3/4 cup	123	30	0.2
CHICKEN				
Canned, condensed				
w/dumplings, prepared	10.5-oz can	234	15	13.4
w/dumplings, prepared	1 cup	96	6	5.5
w/dumplings, unprepared	10.5-oz can	235	15	13.4
w/dumplings, unprepared	1 cup	194	12	11.1

Food Name	Serv. Size	Total Cal.	Carbs GMS	Fat GMS
(Stouffer's) prepared	1 cup	104	12	4.8
Canned, ready to use				
chunky	19-oz can	383	37	14.2
chunky	10.75-oz can	217	21	8.1
chunky	1 cup	178	17	6.6
(Campbell's) 'Chunky Old Fashioned'	10-3/4 oz	180	21	5.0
(Healthy Choice) hearty	1 cup	130	18	2.5
(Progresso)				
'Homestyle'	9.5 oz	110	12	3.0
spicy, w/penne	1 cup	120	13	4.0
w/meatballs, 'Chickarina'	9.5 oz	130	13	5.0
Frozen *(Tabatchnick)*	7.5 oz	65	10	2.0
CHICKEN, CREAM OF				
Canned, condensed				
prepared w/milk	10.75-oz can	464	36	27.8
prepared w/milk	1 cup	191	15	11.5
prepared w/water	10.75-oz can	285	23	17.9
prepared w/water	1 cup	117	9	7.4
unprepared	10.75-oz can	284	23	17.9
unprepared	1 cup	233	19	14.7
(Campbell's)				
'Healthy Request' prepared w/water	1 cup	70	11	2.0
'Healthy Request' unprepared	1/2 cup	80	12	2.0
98% nonfat, unprepared	1/2 cup	80	9	3.0
Canned, ready to use *(Progresso)*	9.5 oz	190	12	11.0
Frozen				
(Kettle Ready)	3/4 cup	98	5	6.2
(Soup Supreme)	1 cup	160	14	8.0
CHICKEN AND BROCCOLI, CREAM OF				
Canned, condensed				
(Campbell's)				
'Healthy Request' unprepared	1/2 cup	80	10	2.5
prepared	1 cup	110	9	7.0
CHICKEN BARLEY				
Canned, condensed *(Campbell's)* prepared	1 cup	70	10	2.0
Canned, ready to use *(Progresso)*	9.25 oz	100	12	2.0
CHICKEN BROTH/BOUILLON				
Canned, condensed				
prepared	1 cup	38	1	1.4
unprepared	10.75-oz can	95	2	3.2
unprepared	1 cup	78	2	2.6
(Campbell's) prepared	1 cup	30	2	2.0
Canned, ready to use				
(Campbell's)				
'Healthy Request'	1 cup	16	1	0.0
low-salt	1 cup	40	2	2.0
nonfat, 'Healthy Request'	1 cup	16	1	0.0
(College Inn)				
	1 cup	35	0	3.0
lower salt	7 oz	20	0	2.0
(Hain)				
	8.75 oz	70	0	6.0
'No Salt Added'	8.75 oz	60	0	5.0
(Health Valley)				
	7.5 oz	35	1	2.0
no salt added	7.5 oz	35	1	2.0
nonfat	1 cup	30	0	0.0

Food Name	Serv. Size	Total Cal.	Carbs GMS	Fat GMS
(Pritikin) defatted	1 cup	18	1	1.0
(Progresso) nonfat	1/2 cup	8	0	0.0
(Shelton's)				
nonfat	1 cup	10	0	0.0
w/salt and pepper	1 cup	35	0	2.5
(Swanson) clear	1 cup	30	1	2.0
CHICKEN CORN CHOWDER				
Canned, ready to use *(Healthy Choice)*	1 cup	160	26	2.5
CHICKEN GUMBO				
Canned, condensed				
prepared	1 cup	56	8	1.4
unprepared	10.75-oz can	137	20	3.5
unprepared	1 cup	113	17	2.9
Frozen				
(Kettle Ready)	3/4 cup	94	12	3.5
(Soup Supreme)				
food service product	1 cup	90	11	2.5
spicy, Southern style, food service product	1 cup	110	14	3.0
Canned, ready to use				
(Campbell's) w/sausage, 'Home Cookin'	10.75-oz can	140	15	4.0
CHICKEN MINESTRONE				
Canned, ready to use				
(Campbell's) 'Home Cookin'	10.75 oz	180	17	6.0
(Progresso)	10.5 oz	140	14	4.0
CHICKEN MUSHROOM				
Canned, condensed				
prepared	1 cup	132	9	9.2
unprepared	10.75-oz can	332	23	22.3
unprepared	1 cup	274	19	18.3
Canned, ready to use				
chowder, chunky	1 cup	192	17	10.6
(Campbell's) creamy, 'Chunky'	10.5 oz	270	13	19.0
CHICKEN NOODLE				
Canned, condensed				
prepared	1 cup	75	9	2.5
unprepared	10.5-oz can	182	23	5.5
unprepared	1 cup	150	19	4.6
(Campbell's)				
creamy, prepared w/2% milk	1 cup	180	16	9.0
creamy, prepared w/water	1/2 cup	120	10	7.0
'Healthy Request' unprepared	1/2 cup	70	9	2.0
Teddy bear pasta in chicken broth, prepared	1 cup	60	11	1.0
unprepared	10.75-oz can	156	21	4.6
(Progresso) prepared	1 cup	80	8	2.0
Canned, ready to use				
chunky	19-oz can	393	38	13.5
chunky	1 cup	175	17	6.0
w/celery and carrots, homestyle	1 cup	95	9	3.4
w/meatballs, chunky	20-oz can	227	19	8.2
w/meatballs, chunky	1 cup	99	8	3.6
(Campbell's)				
'Chunky'	10.75 oz	200	20	7.0
hearty, 'Healthy Request'	1 cup	100	14	3.0
'Home Cookin'	10.75 oz	140	12	4.0
low-salt	1 cup	170	18	5.0
(Hain)				
	9.5 oz	120	11	4.0

Food Name	Serv. Size	Total Cal.	Carbs GMS	Fat GMS
low-salt, low-fat, 'Homestyle Naturals' .... 1 cup		80	8	2.0
(Healthy Choice)				
old-fashioned .... 1 cup		150	23	2.5
w/pasta .... 1 cup		120	17	2.5
(Hormel)				
'Hearty Soups' .... 7.5 oz		110	14	3.0
micro cup, 'Hearty Soups' .... 1 container		108	14	3.0
(Lipton) 'Hearty Ones Homestyle' .... 11 oz		227	37	4.0
(Lunch Bucket) microwave cup .... 7.25 oz		90	13	2.0
(Pritikin) w/ribbon pasta .... 1 cup		80	13	1.0
(Progresso)				
'Healthy Classics' .... 1 cup		76	9	1.6
w/rotini, hearty .... 1 cup		90	8	2.0
(Weight Watchers)				
.... 10.5 oz		80	9	2.0
microwave cup .... 7.5 oz		90	13	1.0
Frozen				
(Kettle Ready) .... 3/4 cup		94	12	3.0
(Myers) .... 9.75 oz		87	5	5.0
(Soup Supreme)				
food service product .... 1 cup		120	15	3.0
seasoned, food service product .... 1 cup		100	16	2.5
CHICKEN RICE				
Canned, condensed				
prepared .... 10.5-oz can		147	17	4.6
prepared .... 1 cup		60	7	1.9
unprepared .... 10.5-oz can		146	17	4.6
unprepared .... 1 cup		121	14	3.8
(Campbell's)				
'Healthy Request' unprepared .... 1/2 cup		60	10	2.5
'Healthy Request' prepared .... 1 cup		60	7	3.0
(Progresso) and vegetable, prepared .... 1 cup		110	12	3.0
Canned, ready to use				
chunky .... 19-oz can		286	29	7.2
chunky .... 1 cup		127	13	3.2
(Campbell's)				
hearty, 'Healthy Request' .... 1 cup		110	15	3.0
microwave .... 10.5 oz		120	20	2.5
(Healthy Choice) .... 7.5 oz		140	18	4.0
(Hormel) 'Hearty Soup' .... 7.5 oz		110	17	2.0
(Progresso)				
.... 10.5 oz		120	12	4.0
.... 9.5 oz		130	16	3.0
wild rice .... 9.5 oz		120	17	3.0
wild rice, w/vegetables .... 1 cup		93	12	2.2
w/vegetables, 'Healthy Classics' .... 1 cup		88	13	1.5
Frozen				
(Soup Supreme)				
w/white and wild rice, food service product .... 1 cup		210	17	12.0
CHICKEN VEGETABLE				
Canned, condensed				
prepared .... 10.5-oz can		182	21	6.9
prepared .... 1 cup		75	9	2.8
unprepared .... 10.5-oz can		182	21	6.9
unprepared .... 1 cup		150	17	5.7
(Campbell's) 'Healthy Request' unprepared .... 1/2 cup		80	12	2.0

Food Name	Serv. Size	Total Cal.	Carbs GMS	Fat GMS
Canned, ready to use				
chunky	19-oz can	372	42	10.8
chunky	1 cup	166	19	4.8
(Campbell's)				
'Chunky'	9.5 oz	170	19	6.0
hearty, 'Healthy Request'	1 cup	120	16	3.0
'Home Cookin'	10-3/4 oz	180	25	4.0
low-sodium, 'Chunky'	10-3/4 oz	240	21	11.0
(Hain)				
	9.5 oz	120	14	4.0
no salt added	9.5 oz	130	14	4.0
(Health Valley)				
chunky	7.5 oz	125	20	2.0
chunky, no salt added	7.5 oz	125	20	2.0
(Hormel) and rice, micro cup, 'Hearty Soups'	1 container	114	16	3.0
(Pritikin)	1 cup	70	12	1.0
(Progresso)	9.5 oz	140	17	4.0
CHILI BEEF				
Canned, condensed				
unprepared	11.25-oz can	412	52	16.0
unprepared	1 cup	339	43	13.2
prepared	1 cup	170	21	6.6
(Campbell's) prepared	1 cup	140	20	5.0
(Stouffer's) w/beans, food service product, prepared	1 cup	144	19	3.2
Canned, ready to use				
(Campbell's)				
'Chunky'	11 oz	290	37	7.0
'Microwave'	7.5 oz	190	32	4.0
(Healthy Choice)	1 cup	170	29	1.5
Frozen				
(Kettle Ready)				
jalapeño	3/4 cup	173	15	8.0
traditional	3/4 cup	161	14	6.5
(Soup Supreme)				
panhandle, food service product	1 cup	200	16	10.0
w/beans, classic, food service product	1 cup	250	23	10.0
w/beans, grande, food service product	1 cup	250	23	10.0
CLAM CHOWDER				
Canned, condensed				
Manhattan, prepared	10.75-oz can	190	30	5.4
Manhattan, prepared	1 cup	78	12	2.2
Manhattan, unprepared	10.75-oz can	186	30	5.4
Manhattan, unprepared	1 cup	153	24	4.4
New England, prepared w/milk	10.75-oz can	397	40	16.0
New England, prepared w/milk	1 cup	164	17	6.6
New England, prepared w/water	10.75-oz can	231	30	7.0
New England, prepared w/water	1 cup	95	12	2.9
New England, unprepared	10.75-oz can	214	27	6.1
New England, unprepared	1 cup	176	22	5.0
(Campbell's)				
Manhattan style, 'Seashore Soups' unprepared	1/2 cup	70	10	2.0
New England, prepared w/whole milk	1 cup	150	17	7.0
New England, 'Seashore Soups' unprepared	1/2 cup	80	12	3.0
(Doxsee) Manhattan, prepared	7.5 oz	70	11	2.0
(Gorton's)				
New England, prepared w/whole milk	1/4 can	140	17	5.0
New England, unprepared	3.75 oz	70	12	1.0

Food Name	Serv. Size	Total Cal.	Carbs GMS	Fat GMS
(Snow's)				
Manhattan, prepared	7.5 oz	70	11	2.0
Manhattan, unprepared	3.75 oz	70	9	2.0
New England, prepared w/whole milk	7.5 oz	140	13	6.0
New England, unprepared	3.75 oz	70	8	2.0
(Stouffer's)				
Boston, food service product, prepared w/milk	1 cup	208	20	10.4
Manhattan, food service product, prepared	1 cup	80	10	2.4
New England, food service product, prepared w/whole milk	1 cup	248	21	13.6
Canned, ready to use				
Manhattan, chunky	19-oz can	302	42	7.6
Manhattan, chunky	1 cup	134	19	3.4
(Campbell's)				
New England, 'Healthy Request'	1 cup	100	14	3.0
New England, 'Home Cookin''	10-3/4 oz	260	15	18.0
(Gorton's)	7.5 oz	140	17	5.0
(Hain) New England, ready to serve	9.25 oz	180	26	4.0
(Health Valley)				
Manhattan	7.5 oz	110	15	2.0
Manhattan, no salt added	7.5 oz	110	15	2.0
(Healthy Choice) New England	1 cup	120	22	1.0
(Hormel)				
New England, 'Hearty Soup'	7.5 oz	130	16	5.0
New England, micro cup, 'Hearty Soups'	1 container	118	15	5.0
(Progresso)				
Manhattan	1 cup	110	11	2.0
New England	1 cup	180	17	10.0
New England, 'Healthy Classics'	1 cup	117	20	2.0
(Stouffer's)				
Boston, food service product, 'Heat 'N Serve'	1 cup	192	20	8.0
New England, food service product, 'Heat 'N Serve'	1 cup	184	23	5.6
(Weight Watchers) New England	7.5 oz	90	16	0.0
Frozen				
(Kettle Ready)				
Boston	3/4 cup	131	13	7.3
Manhattan	3/4 cup	69	8	2.6
New England	3/4 cup	116	11	6.5
(Myers) New England	9.75 oz	152	21	5.0
(Soup Supreme)				
Boston, food service product	1 cup	200	17	10.0
New England, food service product	1 cup	180	22	6.0
(Stouffer's) New England	1 cup	180	16	9.0
(Tabatchnick) New England	3/4 cup	98	14	2.0
CONSOMMÉ				
Canned, condensed *(Campbell's)* beef, w/gelatin, prepared	1 cup	25	2	0.0
CORN AND BROCCOLI CHOWDER				
Frozen *(Kettle Ready)*	3/4 cup	102	13	5.0
CORN				
Canned, condensed				
(Campbell's)				
golden, cream, prepared w/2% milk	1 cup	160	23	5.0
golden, cream, prepared w/water	1 cup	110	18	3.0
golden, cream, unprepared	1/2 cup	110	18	3.0
Canned, ready to use				
(Health Valley)				
country, and vegetable	7.5 oz	70	13	0.0
country, and vegetable, nonfat	1 cup	70	17	0.0

Food Name	Serv. Size	Total Cal.	Carbs GMS	Fat GMS
CORN CHOWDER				
Canned, condensed				
(Snow's)				
New England, prepared w/milk	7.5 oz	150	18	6.0
New England, unprepared	3.75 oz	80	13	2.0
(Stouffer's) food service product, prepared w/whole milk	1 cup	264	28	13.6
Canned, ready to use				
(Progresso)	9.25 oz	200	22	10.0
(Stouffer's) 'Heat 'N Serve'	1 cup	280	21	20.0
Frozen *(Soup Supreme)* Captain's	1 cup	200	29	7.0
CRAB				
Canned, condensed				
(Stouffer's) Maryland, food service product, prepared	1 cup	80	10	2.4
Canned, ready to use				
	13-oz can	114	16	2.3
	1 cup	76	10	1.5
CREOLE				
Canned, ready to use *(Campbell's)* 'Chunky'	10 3/4 oz	240	31	8.0
Frozen *(Soup Supreme)* Southern style	1 cup	110	20	3.0
ESCAROLE				
Canned, ready to use				
	10.5 oz can	61	4	4.0
	1 cup	27	2	1.8
(Progresso) in chicken broth	9.25 oz	30	2	1.0
FISH CHOWDER				
Canned, condensed				
(Snow's)				
New England, prepared w/whole milk	7.5 oz	130	11	6.0
New England, unprepared	3.75 oz	60	6	2.0
GARLIC AND PASTA				
Canned, ready to use *(Progresso)* 'Healthy Classics'	1 cup	100	18	1.3
GAZPACHO				
Canned, ready to use				
	13-oz can	70	7	0.4
	1 cup	46	4	0.2
GREEN PEA				
Canned, condensed				
prepared w/milk	11.25-oz can	579	78	17.1
prepared w/milk	1 cup	239	32	7.0
prepared w/water	1 cup	165	27	2.9
unprepared	11.25-oz can	399	64	7.1
unprepared	1 cup	329	53	5.9
HAM AND BEAN				
Canned, ready to use				
(Campbell's) w/butter beans, 'Chunky'	10 3/4 oz	280	34	10.0
(Progresso)	9.5 oz	140	28	2.0
ITALIAN STYLE WEDDING				
Canned, condensed				
(Stouffer's) food service product, prepared	1 cup	216	25	8.0
LEMON, canned, ready to use *(Great Impressions)*	3/4 cup	90	22	1.0
LENTIL				
Canned, ready to use				
w/ham	20-oz can	318	46	6.3
w/ham	1 cup	139	20	2.8
(Hain)				
	9.5 oz	160	25	3.0
no salt added	9.5 oz	160	24	3.0
(Health Valley)				
	7.5 oz	170	28	2.0

Food Name	Serv. Size	Total Cal.	Carbs GMS	Fat GMS
and carrot, nonfat	1 cup	90	25	0.0
no salt added	7.5 oz	170	28	2.0
(Healthy Choice)	1 cup	140	28	1.0
(Progresso)				
	1 cup	140	22	2.0
'Healthy Classics'	1 cup	126	20	1.5
w/sausage	9.5 oz	170	21	8.0
Frozen *(Tabatchnick)*	7.5 oz	170	27	2.0
MACARONI AND BEAN				
Canned, ready to use *(Progresso)*	10 1/2 oz	150	27	4.0
MENUDO, canned, ready to use *(Old El Paso)*	1/2 can	476	14	52.0
MINESTRONE				
Canned, condensed				
prepared	10.5-oz can	199	27	6.1
prepared	1 cup	82	11	2.5
unprepared	10.5-oz can	203	27	6.1
unprepared	1 cup	167	23	5.0
(Campbell's) 'Healthy Request' unprepared	1/2 cup	90	17	1.0
(Stouffer's) food service product, prepared	1 cup	104	16	2.4
Canned, ready to use				
chunky	19-oz can	286	47	6.3
chunky	1 cup	127	21	2.8
(Campbell's) hearty, 'Healthy Request'	1 cup	120	24	2.0
(Hain)				
	9.5 oz	170	27	2.0
no salt added	9.5 oz	160	28	4.0
(Health Valley)				
	7.5 oz	130	19	3.0
no salt added	7.5 oz	130	19	3.0
nonfat	1 cup	80	21	0.0
(Healthy Choice)	1 cup	110	24	1.0
(Hormel)				
'Hearty Soups'	7.5 oz	100	17	1.0
micro cup, 'Hearty Soups'	1 container	104	15	2.0
(Lipton) 'Hearty Ones'	11 oz	189	36	3.2
(Progresso)				
	1 cup	130	22	2.5
chunky, hearty	9.25 oz	110	16	2.0
chunky, zesty	9.5 oz	150	19	8.0
'Healthy Classics'	1 cup	123	20	2.5
(Stouffer's) food service product, 'Heat 'N Serve'	1 cup	80	10	2.4
Frozen				
(Kettle Ready) hearty	3/4 cup	104	15	4.4
(Soup Supreme) food service product	1 cup	70	11	2.5
(Tabatchnick)	7.5 oz	137	24	2.0
MUSHROOM				
Canned, condensed				
w/beef stock, prepared	10.75-oz can	208	23	9.8
w/beef stock, prepared	1 cup	85	9	4.0
w/beef stock, unprepared	10.75-oz can	207	23	9.8
w/beef stock, unprepared	1 cup	171	19	8.1
(Campbell's)				
beefy, prepared	1 cup	60	5	3.0
w/ground beef, prepared	1 cup	90	10	4.0
MUSHROOM, CREAM OF				
Canned, condensed				
prepared w/milk	10.75-oz can	494	36	33.0

Food Name	Serv. Size	Total Cal.	Carbs GMS	Fat GMS
prepared w/milk	1 cup	203	15	13.6
prepared w/water	10.75-oz can	314	23	21.8
prepared w/water	1 cup	129	9	9.0
unprepared	10.75-oz can	314	23	23.1
unprepared	1 cup	259	19	19.0
(Campbell's)				
'Healthy Request' unprepared	1/2 cup	70	10	2.5
98% nonfat, unprepared	1/2 cup	70	9	3.0
Canned, ready to use				
(Campbell's) low-sodium	10 1/2 oz	210	18	14.0
(Hain) creamy	9.25 oz	110	16	4.0
(Progresso)	9.25 oz	160	14	10.0
(Weight Watchers)	10 1/2 oz	90	14	2.0
Frozen				
(Kettle Ready)	3/4 cup	85	6	6.4
(Soup Supreme) food service product	1 cup	200	13	15.0
(Tabatchnick)	3/4 cup	75	11	2.0
MUSHROOM BARLEY				
Canned, condensed				
prepared	10.75-oz can	178	28	5.5
prepared	1 cup	73	12	2.3
unprepared	10.75-oz can	186	29	5.5
unprepared	1 cup	153	24	4.5
Canned, ready to use				
(Hain)	9.5 oz	100	17	2.0
(Health Valley)				
	7.5 oz	100	16	2.0
no salt added	7.5 oz	100	16	2.0
Frozen				
(Tabatchnick)				
	7.5 oz	92	16	2.0
'No Salt'	7.5 oz	97	18	1.0
ONION				
Canned, condensed				
prepared	10.5-oz can	141	20	4.2
prepared	1 cup	58	8	1.7
unprepared	10.5-oz can	137	20	4.2
unprepared	1 cup	113	16	3.5
(Stouffer's) French, food service product, prepared	1 cup	72	9	2.4
Frozen				
(Kettle Ready) French	3/4 cup	42	5	2.2
(Soup Supreme) French, food service product	1 cup	80	11	4.0
ONION, CREAM OF				
Canned, condensed				
prepared w/milk	10.75-oz can	452	45	22.8
prepared w/milk	1 cup	186	18	9.4
prepared w/water	10.75-oz can	261	31	12.8
prepared w/water	1 cup	107	13	5.3
unprepared	10.75-oz can	268	32	12.8
unprepared	1 cup	221	26	10.5
(Campbell's)				
prepared w/4 oz soup, 2 oz whole milk, 2 oz water	1 cup	140	15	7.0
PEA				
Frozen				
(Kettle Ready) tortellini, in tomato	3/4 cup	122	15	5.4
(Tabatchnick)				
	7.5 oz	175	31	1.0

Food Name	Serv. Size	Total Cal.	Carbs GMS	Fat GMS
'No Salt'	7.5 oz	175	31	1.0
PEPPER POT				
Canned, condensed				
prepared	10.5-oz can	252	23	11.3
prepared	1 cup	104	9	4.6
unprepared	10.5-oz can	250	23	11.3
unprepared	1 cup	207	19	9.3
POT ROAST				
Frozen *(Soup Supreme)* Yankee, food service product	1 cup	90	13	1.5
POTATO, CREAM OF				
Canned, condensed				
prepared w/milk	10.75-oz can	361	42	15.7
prepared w/milk	1 cup	149	17	6.4
prepared w/water	10.75-oz can	178	28	5.8
prepared w/water	1 cup	73	11	2.4
unprepared	10.75-oz can	180	28	5.7
unprepared	1 cup	148	23	4.7
(Campbell's) prepared w/tofu, 1 tbsp oil	1 cup	120	15	4.0
(Stouffer's) food service product, prepared w/whole milk	1 cup	264	28	12.8
Frozen *(Soup Supreme)* food service product	1 cup	190	22	9.0
Canned, ready to use				
(Andersen's)	7.5 oz	200	25	10.0
(Stouffer's) food service product, 'Heat 'N Serve'	1 cup	240	28	9.6
POTATO-LEEK				
Canned, ready to use				
(Health Valley)				
	7.5 oz	130	23	2.0
no salt added	7.5 oz	130	23	2.0
RED BEAN AND RICE, *(Norpac)* lowfat, 'Soup Supreme'	1 cup	130	26	1.5
SCHAV, canned, ready to serve *(Gold's)*	1 cup	25	4	0.0
SCOTCH BROTH				
Canned, condensed				
prepared	10.5-oz can	193	23	6.4
prepared	1 cup	80	9	2.6
unprepared	10.5-oz can	197	23	6.4
unprepared	1 cup	162	19	5.3
(Campbell's) prepared	1 cup	80	9	3.0
SEAFOOD BISQUE, frozen *(Myers)*	9.75 oz	163	13	8.0
SEAFOOD CHOWDER				
Canned, condensed				
(Snow's)				
New England, prepared w/whole milk	7.5 oz	140	14	6.0
New England, unprepared	3.75 oz	60	6	2.0
SEAFOOD GUMBO				
Frozen *(Soup Supreme)* food service product	1 cup	90	14	1.5
SHRIMP AND OKRA GUMBO				
Frozen				
(Soup Supreme) Southern style, food service product	1 cup	110	16	3.0
SHRIMP, CREAM OF				
Canned, condensed				
prepared w/milk	10.75-oz can	397	34	22.6
prepared w/milk	1 cup	164	14	9.3
unprepared	10.75-oz can	220	20	12.6
unprepared	1 cup	181	16	10.4
(Campbell's)				
'Seashore Soups' prepared w/2% milk	1/2 cup	140	13	10.0
'Seashore Soups' prepared w/whole milk	1 cup	160	13	10.0

Food Name	Serv. Size	Total Cal.	Carbs GMS	Fat GMS
'Seashore Soups' unprepared	1/2 cup	90	8	6.0
SIRLOIN BURGER				
Canned, ready to use *(Campbell's)* 'Chunky'	10 3/4 oz	220	23	9.0
SPINACH, CREAM OF				
Frozen				
(Myers)	9.75 oz	174	10	11.0
(Stouffer's)	3/4 cup	210	12	15.0
(Tabatchnick)	3/4 cup	85	12	2.0
SPLIT PEA				
Canned, condensed				
w/ham, prepared w/milk	11.5-oz can	461	68	10.7
w/ham, prepared w/water	1 cup	190	28	4.4
w/ham, unprepared	11.5-oz can	460	68	10.7
w/ham, unprepared	1 cup	379	56	8.8
(Campbell's) w/ham and bacon, prepared w/water	1 cup	160	24	4.0
(Rokeach) w/egg barley, prepared w/water	1 cup	132	24	0.5
(Stouffer's) w/ham, food service product, prepared w/water	1 cup	176	29	1.6
Canned, ready to use				
w/ham, chunky	19-oz can	415	60	8.9
w/ham, chunky	1 cup	185	27	4.0
(Andersen's) nonfat	7.5 oz	130	24	0.0
(Campbell's) low-salt	1 cup	240	38	4.0
(Grandma Brown's)	1 cup	208	31	4.1
(Hain)				
	9.5 oz	170	28	1.0
no salt added	9.5 oz	170	29	1.0
(Health Valley)				
and carrot, nonfat	1 cup	110	17	0.0
green	7.5 oz	190	34	0.3
no salt added	7.5 oz	190	34	0.3
(Healthy Choice) and ham	1 cup	160	25	1.5
(Progresso)				
green	10 1/2 oz	201	31	3.0
'Healthy Classics'	1 cup	180	30	2.3
w/ham	1 cup	160	20	4.0
Frozen				
(Kettle Ready) w/ham	3/4 cup	155	25	4.4
(Soup Supreme) w/ham, food service product	1 cup	120	18	1.5
STOCKPOT				
Canned, condensed				
prepared	11-oz can	240	28	9.5
prepared	1 cup	99	11	3.9
unprepared	11-oz can	243	28	9.5
unprepared	1 cup	200	23	7.8
TOMATO				
Canned, condensed				
prepared w/milk	10.75-oz can	391	54	14.6
prepared w/milk	1 cup	161	22	6.0
prepared w/water	10.75-oz can	208	40	4.7
prepared w/water	1 cup	85	17	1.9
unprepared	10.75-oz can	207	40	4.7
unprepared	1 cup	171	33	3.8
(Campbell's)				
'Healthy Request' unprepared	1/2 cup	90	18	1.5
'Healthy Request' prepared w/1/2 cup 2% milk	1 cup	140	22	3.0
'Healthy Request' prepared w/water	1 cup	90	17	2.0
'Healthy Request' prepared w/whole milk	1 cup	150	22	4.0

Food Name	Serv. Size	Total Cal.	Carbs GMS	Fat GMS
(Stouffer's)				
hearty, food service product, prepared w/water . . . . 1 cup	96	13	3.2
Canned, ready to use				
(Campbell's) w/tomato pieces, low-salt . . . . 1 cup	170	28	6.0
(Health Valley)				
. . . . 7.5 oz	100	17	3.0
no salt added . . . . 7.5 oz	100	17	3.0
(Healthy Choice) garden . . . . 1 cup	100	19	1.5
(Progresso)				
. . . . 9.5 oz	120	20	3.0
garden, 'Healthy Classics' . . . . 1 cup	99	19	1.0
(Stouffer's)				
garden, food service product, 'Heat 'N Serve' . . . . 1 cup	112	10	7.2
Frozen				
(Soup Supreme)				
basil, vegetarian, low-fat, food service product . . . . 1 cup	100	15	3.0
Florentine, food service product . . . . 1 cup	90	16	1.5
TOMATO, CREAM OF				
Canned, condensed				
(Campbell's)				
'Healthy Request' prepared w/nonfat milk . . . . 1/2 cup	130	22	2.0
'Homestyle' prepared w/water . . . . 1 cup	110	20	3.0
'Homestyle' prepared w/whole milk . . . . 1 cup	180	25	7.0
prepared w/whole milk . . . . 1 cup	150	22	4.0
zesty, prepared w/water . . . . 1 cup	100	20	2.0
TOMATO BEEF				
Canned, condensed				
w/noodles, prepared . . . . 10.75-oz can	338	51	10.4
w/noodles, prepared . . . . 1 cup	139	21	4.3
w/noodles, unprepared . . . . 10.75-oz can	342	51	10.4
w/noodles, unprepared . . . . 1 cup	281	42	8.6
Canned, ready to use *(Progresso)* w/rotini . . . . 9.5 oz	170	18	6.0
TOMATO BISQUE				
Canned, condensed				
prepared w/milk . . . . 11-oz can	481	71	16.0
prepared w/milk . . . . 1 cup	198	29	6.6
unprepared . . . . 11-oz can	300	58	6.1
unprepared . . . . 1 cup	247	47	5.0
TOMATO RICE				
Canned, condensed				
prepared . . . . 11-oz can	288	53	6.6
prepared . . . . 1 cup	119	22	2.7
unprepared . . . . 1 cup	239	44	5.4
unprepared . . . . 11-oz can	290	53	6.6
Frozen *(Tabatchnick)* . . . . 3/4 cup	73	14	1.0
TOMATO TORTELLINI, canned, ready to use *(Progresso)* . . . . 1 cup	120	13	5.0
TOMATO VEGETABLE				
Canned, ready to use *(Health Valley)* nonfat . . . . 1 cup	80	17	0.0
TORTELLINI				
Canned, ready to use				
(Progresso)				
. . . . 9.5 oz	90	11	3.0
creamy . . . . 9.25 oz	240	17	16.0
TURKEY				
Canned, condensed				
prepared . . . . 10.75-oz can	166	21	4.9
prepared . . . . 1 cup	68	9	2.0

Food Name	Serv. Size	Total Cal.	Carbs GMS	Fat GMS
unprepared	10.75-oz can	168	21	4.8
unprepared	1 cup	138	17	4.0
Canned, ready to use				
chunky	18.75-oz can	303	32	9.9
chunky	1 cup	135	14	4.4
TURKEY RICE				
Canned, ready to use				
(Hain)				
	9.5 oz	100	10	3.0
no salt added	9.5 oz	120	13	4.0
(Healthy Choice) white and wild rice	1 cup	90	14	2.0
TURKEY VEGETABLE				
Canned, condensed				
prepared	10.5-oz can	176	21	7.4
prepared	1 cup	72	9	3.0
unprepared	10.5-oz can	179	21	7.4
unprepared	1 cup	148	17	6.1
Canned, ready to use				
(Campbell's) 'Chunky'	9 1/3 cup	150	16	6.0
(Weight Watchers)	10 1/2 oz	70	10	2.0
VEGETABLE				
Canned, condensed				
(Campbell's)				
'Healthy Request' unprepared	1/2 cup	90	16	1.0
'Homestyle' prepared	1 cup	60	9	2.0
vegetarian	1/2 cup	60	14	0.0
w/pasta, 'Healthy Request' unprepared	1/2 cup	90	18	1.0
w/pasta, hearty, prepared	1 cup	70	15	1.0
(Stouffer's) vegetarian, food service product, prepared	1 cup	96	14	2.4
Canned, ready to use				
chunky	19-oz can	275	43	8.3
chunky	1 cup	122	19	3.7
(Campbell's)				
hearty, 'Healthy Request'	1 cup	100	20	1.0
Mediterranean, 'Chunky' ready to serve	9.5 oz	170	24	6.0
(Hain)				
Italian, w/pasta	9.5 oz	160	25	5.0
Italian, w/pasta, low-sodium	9.5 oz	140	22	6.0
vegetarian	9.5 oz	140	22	4.0
vegetarian, no salt added	9.5 oz	150	23	5.0
(Health Valley)				
	7.5 oz	110	20	1.0
5-bean, chunky, no salt added	7.5 oz	110	21	2.0
5-bean, nonfat	1 cup	140	32	0.0
no salt added	7.5 oz	110	20	1.0
power carotene	1 cup	70	17	0.0
(Healthy Choice)				
country	1 cup	100	22	0.5
garden	1 cup	120	24	1.0
(Hormel)				
country, 'Hearty Soups'	7.5 oz	90	14	2.0
country, micro cup, 'Hearty Soups'	1 container	89	13	2.0
(Lunch Bucket) country, microwave cup	7.25 oz	70	15	1.0
(Norpac) vegerarian, low-fat, 'Soup Supreme'	1 cup	70	13	1.5
(Progresso)				
	9.5 oz	80	15	2.0
'Healthy Classics'	1 cup	81	13	1.3

Food Name	Serv. Size	Total Cal.	Carbs GMS	Fat GMS
(Stouffer's)				
vegetarian, food service product, 'Heat 'N Serve'	1 cup	96	16	2.4
(Westbrae)				
Sante Fe, nonfat	1 cup	115	23	0.0
Southwest, spicy, nonfat	1 cup	70	15	0.0
(Weight Watchers)				
vegetarian, chunky	10 1/2 oz	100	18	2.0
w/beef stock	10 1/2 oz	90	13	2.0
Frozen				
(Kettle Ready) garden	3/4 cup	85	12	3.0
(Soup Supreme)				
harvest, food service product	1 cup	90	17	1.5
Italian, zesty, food service product	1 cup	70	14	1.0
(Tabatchnick)				
	7.5 oz	97	18	1.0
no salt	7.5 oz	92	16	2.0
VEGETABLE BARLEY				
Canned, ready to use *(Health Valley)* nonfat	1 cup	90	19	0.0
VEGETABLE BEEF				
Canned, condensed				
prepared	10.5-oz can	199	32	4.6
prepared	1 cup	82	13	1.9
unprepared	10.5-oz can	197	32	4.6
unprepared	1 cup	162	26	3.8
(Campbell's)				
'Healthy Request' prepared	1 cup	70	10	2.0
'Healthy Request' unprepared	1/2 cup	80	11	2.0
(Stouffer's) w/barley, food service product, prepared	1 cup	144	12	8.8
Canned, ready to use				
(Campbell's)				
hearty, 'Healthy Request'	1 cup	140	20	2.5
low-salt, 'Chunky'	1 cup	160	11	4.5
old-fashioned, 'Chunky'	10-3/4 oz	190	20	6.0
(Stouffer's) w/barley, 'Heat 'N Serve'	1 cup	144	11	8.8
(Weight Watchers) microwave cup	7.5 oz	90	13	1.0
Frozen				
(Myers)	9.75 oz	120	8	6.0
(Soup Supreme)				
food service product	1 cup	80	14	1.5
w/barley, food service product	1 cup	90	14	2.0
VEGETABLE BROTH				
Canned, ready to use				
(Hain)				
	9.5 oz	45	10	0.0
low-sodium	9.5 oz	40	8	1.0
(Swanson) canned	1 cup	20	3	1.0
WILD RICE				
Canned, ready to use				
(Hain) 99% fat free, 'Healthy Naturals'	1 cup	80	15	2.0
ZUCCHINI, frozen *(Tabatchnick)*	3/4 cup	80	12	2.0
SOUP MIX				
ASPARAGUS, CREAM OF, prepared	1 cup	58	9	1.7
BEAN				
w/bacon, prepared	1 cup	106	16	2.1
(Bean Cuisine)				
'Island Black Bean' bag, prepared	1 cup	160	29	1.0
'Island Black Bean' box, prepared	1 cup	126	24	1.0

Food Name	Serv. Size	Total Cal.	Carbs GMS	Fat GMS
'Mesa Maise & Bean' prepared	1 cup	180	32	1.5
'Rocky Mountain Red Bean' prepared	1 cup	190	35	1.5
13-bean bouillabaisse, bag, prepared	I cup	110	19	0.5
13-bean bouillabaisse, box, prepared	1 cup	99	18	1.0
'White Bean Provencal' bag, prepared	1 cup	180	32	1.0
'White Bean Provencal' box, prepared	1 cup	103	19	1.0
(Fantastic Foods) 5-bean, 'Hearty Soups' mix only	2.3 oz	230	43	1.0
(Hodgson Mill) choice, no barley, mix only	1/4 cup	150	27	0.0
(Hormel) w/ham, chowder 'Micro-Cup Hearty Soups' prepared	1 container	191	31	3.0
BEEF				
broth, cubed, mix only	1 cube	9	1	0.3
broth, dried, prepared	1 cup	19	2	0.7
(American Institutional) stock, concentrated, mix only	2 tsp	20	2	0.0
(Soup Starter) hearty, 'Homestyle' mix only	27 grams	90	20	1.0
(Tone's) base, mix only	1 tsp	11	1	0.6
(Ultra Slim-Fast) w/noodles, prepared	6 oz	45	7	1.0
BEEF NOODLE				
prepared	1 cup	40	6	0.8
(Campbell's)				
w/vegetables, prepared	6 oz	220	44	2.0
microwave cup, prepared	1.35 oz	130	23	2.0
'Ramen Noodle' prepared	6 oz	160	32	1.0
(Estee) prepared	6 oz	20	3	1.0
(Lipton)				
'Cup-A-Soup' prepared	6 oz	44	8	0.7
hearty, prepared	6 oz	107	20	1.4
BEEF VEGETABLE (Soup Starter) 'Homestyle' mix only	26 grams	90	18	1.0
BOUILLON				
Beef flavor				
(Diamond Crystal) dried, instant, low-salt, mix only	1 serving	10	2	0.0
(Featherweight) dried, instant, mix only	1 tsp	18	2	1.0
(Herb-Ox)				
cubed, mix only	1 cube	5	1	0.0
cubed, low-salt, mix only	1 cube	10	2	0.0
granulated, mix only	1 tsp	5	1	0.0
(Lite-Line) dried, instant, low-sodium, mix only	1 tsp	12	2	1.0
(Steero)				
cubed, mix only	1 cube	6	1	1.0
dried, instant, mix only	1 tsp	6	1	1.0
(Weight Watchers) dried, instant, 'Broth Mix' mix only	1 pkt	8	1	0.0
(Wyler's)				
cubed, mix only	1 cube	6	1	1.0
dried, mix only	1 tsp	5	1	0.0
dried, instant, mix only	1 tsp	6	1	1.0
dried, low-salt, mix only	1 tsp	10	2	0.0
Brown				
(G. Washington's) dried, 'Seasoning & Broth' mix only	0.14 oz	6	1	0.0
Chicken flavor				
(Diamond Crystal) dried, instant, low-salt, mix only	1 serving	10	2	0.0
(Featherweight) dried, instant, mix only	1 tsp	18	2	1.0
(Herb-Ox)				
cubed, mix only	1 cube	5	1	0.0
cubed, low-salt	1 cube	10	2	0.0
granulated, mix only	1 tsp	5	1	0.0
(Lite-Line) dried, instant, low-sodium, mix only	1 tsp	12	2	1.0

Food Name	Serv. Size	Total Cal.	Carbs GMS	Fat GMS
(Steero)				
cubed, mix only	1 cube	8	1	1.0
dried, instant, mix only	1 tsp	8	1	1.0
(Weight Watchers) dried, instant 'Broth Mix' mix only	1 pkt	8	1	0.0
(Wyler's)				
cubed, mix only	1 cube	8	1	1.0
dried, instant, mix only	1 tsp	8	1	1.0
dried, low-salt, mix only	1 tsp	10	2	0.0
Golden				
(G. Washington's)				
dried, kosher, 'Seasoning & Broth' mix only	0.13 oz	6	1	0.0
dried, 'Seasoning & Broth' mix only	0.13 oz	6	1	0.0
Onion flavor				
(G. Washington's) dried, 'Seasoning & Broth' mix only	0.11 cup	12	2	0.0
(Wyler's) dried, instant, mix only	1 tsp	10	1	1.0
Vegetable				
(G. Washington's) dried, 'Seasoning & Broth' mix only	0.11 cup	12	2	0.0
(Herb-Ox) cubed, mix only	1 cube	5	1	0.0
(Wyler's) dried, instant, mix only	1 tsp	6	1	1.0
BROCCOLI				
(Fantastic Foods) and cheddar, creamy, mix only	1.4 oz	160	26	3.0
(Lipton)				
and cheese, 'Cup-A-Soup' mix only	1 serving	67	9	2.9
creamy, 'Cup-A-Soup Food Service' prepared	6 oz	62	9	2.3
creamy, 'Cup-A-Soup' prepared	6 oz	62	9	2.4
golden, 'Cup-A-Soup Lite' prepared	6 oz	42	16	1.2
(Ultra Slim-Fast) creamy, prepared	6 oz	75	14	1.0
CAULIFLOWER, prepared	1 cup	69	11	1.7
CELERY, prepared	1 cup	64	10	1.6
CHEESE				
(Fantastic Noodles) cheddar, creamy, w/noodles, prepared	6 oz	178	21	8.0
(Hain)				
'Savory Soup & Sauce Mix' prepared	6 oz	250	20	16.0
and broccoli, prepared	6 oz	310	19	22.0
CHICKEN				
broth, cubed, mix only	1 cube	11	1	0.6
broth, dried, mix only	1 tsp	5	0	0.3
broth, dried, prepared	6 fl oz	16	1	0.8
(American Institutional) stock, concentrated, mix only	2 tsp	15	1	0.0
(Campbell's) w/white meat, creamy, prepared	6 oz	90	12	4.0
(Lipton)				
broth, 'Cup-A-Soup' prepared	1 serving	18	3	0.1
Florentine, 'Lite' prepared	6 oz	42	8	0.5
lemon, 'Cup-A-Soup Lite' prepared	6 oz	48	9	0.4
w/pasta, fat-free, 'Cup-A-Soup' prepared	1 serving	44	8	0.3
w/pasta, beans, 'Kettle Creations' prepared	1 serving	106	19	1.3
w/corn, 'Country' prepared	6 oz	133	18	5.5
hearty, supreme, 'Cup-A-Soup' prepared	1 serving	90	14	3.8
CHICKEN, CREAM OF				
(Lipton)				
'Cup-A-Soup' mix only	1 envelope	68	12	2.2
'Food Service' prepared	6 oz	84	9	4.4
w/vegetables, prepared	6 oz	93	14	3.1
hearty, 'Country Style' prepared	6 oz	69	11	1.1
CHICKEN LEEK *(Ultra Slim Fast)* creamy, prepared	6 oz	50	7	1.0
CHICKEN NOODLE				
prepared	1 cup	58	9	1.4

Food Name	Serv. Size	Total Cal.	Carbs GMS	Fat GMS
(Campbell's)				
'Lowfat Block' prepared	1 cup	160	32	1.0
microwave cup, mix only	1.35 oz	140	22	3.0
'Ramen Noodle' prepared	1 cup	190	26	8.0
w/vegetables, prepared	1 cup	270	38	10.0
w/vegetables, low-fat, prepared	1 cup	220	44	2.0
w/white meat, prepared	6 oz	90	12	2.0
(Estee) 'Instant' prepared	6 oz	25	4	1.0
(Lipton)				
and rice, prepared	6 oz	47	8	0.8
'Cup-A-Soup' prepared	6 oz	48	7	1.1
hearty, 'Cup-A-Soup' mix only	1 envelope	61	10	1.2
prepared w/water	1 cup	81	12	1.8
real chicken broth, 'Soup Secrets' prepared	1 serving	62	9	1.9
'Soup Secrets' prepared	1 serving	77	11	2.0
supreme, prepared	6 oz	107	12	5.9
w/diced white meat, prepared	1 cup	81	12	1.8
w/meat, 'Cup-A-Soup' prepared	1 serving	381	62	8.0
w/vegetables, 'Cup' prepared	6 oz	47	8	0.6
w/vegetable, hearty, prepared	1 cup	75	12	1.6
(Mrs. Grass) 'Chickeny Rich' mix only	1/4 pkg	70	10	2.0
(Soup Starter) 'Homestyle' mix only	21 grams	70	15	1.0
(Ultra Slim-Fast) prepared	6 oz	45	6	1.0
CHICKEN RICE, prepared w/water	1 cup	58	9	1.4
CHICKEN VEGETABLE, prepared w/water	1 cup	49	8	0.8
CHILI *(Fantastic Foods)* 'Cha Cha Chili' 'Hearty Soups' mix only	2.4 oz	220	37	1.0
CHILI PEPPER *(A Taste of Thai)* hot and sour, prepared	1 cup	40	5	2.0
CLAM CHOWDER				
(Golden Dipt)				
Manhattan, mix only	1/4 pkg	80	13	2.0
Manhattan, prepared	1 cup	95	13	3.7
New England, mix only	1/4 pkg	70	12	2.0
CONSOMMÉ w/gelatin, prepared	1 cup	17	2	0.0
CORN CHOWDER				
(Bean Cuisine) 'Sante Fe' prepared	1 cup	112	21	1.0
(Fantastic Foods) and potato, creamy, mix only	1.6 oz	170	34	2.0
COUSCOUS-LENTIL				
(Fantastic Foods) 'Hearty Soups' mix only	2.3 oz	230	44	1.0
CRAB *(Kikkoman)* Chinese style, mix only	1 tbsp	25	5	0.0
EGG FLOWER				
(Kikkoman)				
corn, Chinese style, mix only	1 tbsp	50	11	0.0
hot and sour, Chinese style, mix only	2 tsp	30	6	0.0
vegetable, Chinese style, mix only	1 1/2 tbsp	45	7	2.0
GINGER *(A Taste of Thai)* tangy coconut, prepared	1 cup	250	3	1.5
GREEN PEA				
prepared w/water	1 cup	133	23	1.6
(Hain) 'Savory Soup Mix' prepared	6 oz	310	16	10.0
(Lipton)				
'Cup-A-Soup' prepared	6 oz	113	14	4.2
'Cup-A-Soup Food Service' prepared	6 oz	115	15	4.5
Virginia, 'Country Style' prepared	6 oz	148	17	6.4
Virginia, prepared	6 oz	113	15	4.1
HERB				
(Lipton)				
Fiesta, 'Recipe Secrets' prepared	1 serving	29	6	0.3
savory, w/garlic 'Recipe Secrets' prepared	1 serving	31	6	0.4

Food Name	Serv. Size	Total Cal.	Carbs GMS	Fat GMS
LEEK				
prepared	1 cup	71	11	2.1
(Ultra Slim Fast) creamy, prepared	6 oz	80	15	1.0
LENTIL				
(Bean Cuisine) 'Lots of Lentil' prepared	1 cup	230	20	0.0
(Fantastic Foods) country, 'Hearty Soups' mix only	2.3 oz	230	41	1.0
(Hain) 'Savory Soup Mix' prepared w/water	6 oz	130	20	2.0
(Legumes Plus)				
Cajun, w/brown rice, mix only	1/5 cup	190	34	1.0
meatless, mix only	1/4 cup	190	31	1.0
minestrone style, mix only	1/3 cup	150	28	0.5
pasta-pasta, mix only	1/3 cup	180	33	1.0
red curry, mix only	1/5 cup	200	34	1.0
robust bacon flavor, mix only	1/4 cup	170	26	2.0
subtly seasoned, mix only	1/3 cup	190	31	1.0
w/barley, hearty, mix only	1/4 cup	140	26	1.0
w/country vegetable, mix only	1/3 cup	180	34	0.0
w/herbs and rice, mix only	1/6 cup	150	29	1.0
w/wagon wheel pasta, mix only	1/3 cup	190	34	0.5
w/wild rice and herbs, mix only	1/4 cup	160	31	1.0
zesty tomato, mix only	1/4 cup	180	29	1.0
(Lipton) homestyle, 'Kettle Creations' prepared	1 serving	127	22	1.2
LOBSTER BISQUE *(Golden Dipt)* mix only	1/4 pkg	30	5	1.0
MINESTRONE				
(Cous-cous) tomato, prepared	10 oz	200	41	0.0
(Fantastic Foods) hearty, mix only	1.5 oz	150	29	1.0
(Hain) 'Savory Soup Mix' prepared	6 oz	110	20	1.0
(Manischewitz) prepared	6 oz	50	9	1.0
MISO				
(Kikkoman)				
red, prepared	1 serving	35	4	1.0
shiro, white, prepared	1 serving	35	4	1.0
tofu, prepared	1 serving	35	4	1.0
tofu-spinach	1 serving	35	4	1.0
MUSHROOM				
(Estee) 'Instant' prepared	6 oz	40	3	2.0
(Fantastic Foods) garlic, creamy, mix only	1.5 oz	160	28	3.0
(Hain)				
no salt added, 'Savory Soup & Recipe Mix' prepared	6 oz	250	15	20.0
'Savory Soup & Recipe Mix' prepared	6 oz	210	11	15.0
(Lipton)				
beef flavor, prepared	1 cup	38	7	0.5
beefy, 'Recipe Secrets' prepared	1 serving	33	7	0.4
MUSHROOM, CREAM OF				
(Lipton) 'Cup-A-Soup' prepared	6 oz	71	9	3.2
NOODLE				
(Campbell's)				
double noodle, in chicken broth, mix only	1.71 oz	200	36	2.0
hearty, 'Quality Soup & Recipe' prepared	1 cup	90	15	1.0
Oriental, 'Ramen Noodle Lowfat Block' prepared	1 cup	150	31	1.0
Oriental, 'Ramen Noodle' prepared	1 cup	190	26	8.0
'Quality Soup & Recipe' prepared	1 cup	110	19	2.0
w/chicken broth, microwave cup, mix only	1.35 oz	130	23	2.0
w/vegetables, Oriental, 'Cup-A-Ramen Lowfat' prepared	1 cup	220	44	2.0
w/vegetables, Oriental, 'Cup-A-Ramen' prepared	1 cup	270	38	10.0
(Fantastic Foods)				
curry ramen, mix only	1.5 oz	140	28	1.0

Food Name	Serv. Size	Total Cal.	Carbs GMS	Fat GMS
vegetable miso ramen, mix only	1.3 oz	130	25	1.0
(Kikkoman) memmi, noodle soup base, mix only	2 tbsp	40	7	0.0
(Lipton)				
giggle noodle, 'Soup Secrets' prepared	1 serving	74	11	2.1
ring noodle, 'Cup-A-Soup' prepared	1 serving	53	9	1.1
ring noodle, 'Soup Secrets' prepared	1 serving	66	10	2.0
w/extra noodle, 'Soup Secrets' prepared	1 serving	86	15	1.6
(Oodles of Noodles) Oriental, prepared	1 cup	390	49	18.0
(Top Ramen) Oriental, mix only	1 serving	190	28	7.2
Beef flavor				
(Cup O'Noodles) prepared	1 cup	290	33	14.0
(Oodles of Noodles) prepared	1 cup	390	49	18.0
(Top Ramen) prepared	1 cup	390	49	18.0
Chicken flavor				
(Campbell's)				
'Cup 2 Minute Soup' prepared	6 oz	90	15	2.0
double noodle, prepared	1 cup	200	36	2.0
(Cup O'Noodles)				
country, 'Hearty' prepared	1 cup	300	35	14.0
prepared	1 cup	300	32	16.0
(Oodles of Noodles) prepared	1 cup	400	48	18.0
(Top Ramen) individual package, mix only	1 container	296	37	14.1
Pork flavor				
(Campbell's)				
'Ramen Noodle' prepared	1 cup	200	26	8.0
'Ramen Noodle Lowfat Block' prepared	1 cup	150	31	1.0
w/vegetables, microwave, mix only	1.7 oz	180	32	2.0
(Cup O'Noodles)				
vegetable beef, 'Hearty' prepared	1 cup	290	36	15.0
w/old fashioned vegetables, 'Hearty' prepared	6 oz	290	34	15.0
w/seafood, savory, 'Hearty' prepared	1 cup	300	34	15.0
w/shrimp, prepared	1 cup	300	32	14.0
(Oodles of Noodles) prepared	1 cup	390	51	20.0
(Top Ramen) prepared	1 cup	390	51	20.0
ONION				
prepared	1 cup	27	5	0.6
(Estee) prepared	6 oz	25	4	1.0
(Hain)				
'Savory Soup, Dip & Recipe Mix' no salt, prepared	6 oz	50	9	1.0
'Savory Soup, Dip & Recipe Mix' prepared	6 oz	50	6	2.0
(Lipton)				
'Recipe Secrets' prepared	1 serving	18	4	0.1
beefy, 'Recipe Secrets' prepared	1 serving	25	5	0.6
(Mrs. Grass) 'Soup & Dip Mix' mix only	1/4 pkg	35	6	1.0
(Ultra Slim-Fast) creamy, prepared	6 oz	45	7	1.0
ONION MUSHROOM (Lipton) 'Recipe Secrets' prepared	1 serving	32	6	0.8
ORIENTAL (Lipton) 'Cup-A-Soup Lite' prepared	6 oz	45	6	1.7
OSUIMONO (Kikkoman) Japanese clear broth, prepared	1 serving	0	1	0.0
OXTAIL, prepared	1 cup	71	9	2.6
PASTA (Lipton) spirals, 'Soup Secrets' prepared	1 serving	64	11	0.9
PASTA AND BEAN				
(Bean Cuisine)				
'Ultima Pasta E Fagioli' bag, prepared	1 cup	190	34	1.0
'Ultima Pasta E Fagioli' box, prepared	1 cup	117	22	1.0
(Lipton) homestyle, 'Kettle Creations' prepared	1 serving	125	23	1.4
POTATO LEEK (Hain) 'Savory Soup Mix' prepared	6 oz	260	20	18.0
SCALLOP (Kikkoman) Chinese style, mix only	1 tbsp	35	7	0.0

Food Name	Serv. Size	Total Cal.	Carbs GMS	Fat GMS
SEAFOOD CHOWDER *(Golden Dipt)* mix only .... 1/4 pkg		70	12	2.0
SHRIMP				
(Campbell's)				
w/vegetables 'Cup-A-Ramen' prepared .... 1 cup		280	40	10.0
w/vegetables, low-fat, prepared .... 1 cup		230	45	2.0
(Kikkoman) Chinese style, mix only .... 1 tbsp		30	5	0.5
SHRIMP BISQUE *(Golden Dipt)* mix only .... 1/4 pkg		30	5	1.0
SPLIT PEA				
(Bean Cuisine)				
'Thick As Fog Split Pea' bag, prepared .... 1 cup		140	24	0.5
'Thick As Fog Split Pea' box, prepared .... 1 cup		116	21	1.0
(Legumes Plus)				
green, traditional, mix only .... 1/4 cup		180	32	1.0
yellow, mix only .... 1/4 cup		170	30	2.5
(Manischewitz) green, prepared w/water .... 6 oz		45	9	1.0
TOMATO				
prepared .... 1 cup		103	19	2.4
(Estee) 'Instant' prepared .... 6 oz		40	5	1.0
(Hain) 'Savory Soup & Recipe Mix' prepared .... 6 oz		220	19	14.0
(Lipton) 'Cup-A-Soup' mix only .... 1 envelope		95	20	0.9
(Ultra Slim-Fast) creamy, prepared .... 6 oz		60	10	1.0
TOMATO RICE PARMESANO				
(Fantastic Foods) creamy, mix only .... 1 serving		200	41	2.0
TOMATO VEGETABLE				
prepared .... 1 cup		56	10	0.9
(Fantastic Foods)				
ramen noodle, mix only .... 1.5 oz		150	31	1.0
w/noodles, prepared .... 7 oz		158	20	8.0
VEGETABLE				
(American Institutional) stock, concentrated, mix only .... 2 tsp		15	3	0.0
(Campbell's) nonfat, 'Quality Soup & Recipe' prepared .... 1 cup		40	8	0.0
(Cous-cous) parmesan, prepared .... 10 oz		200	35	3.0
(Hain)				
no salt added, 'Savory Soup Mix' prepared .... 6 oz		80	13	1.0
'Savory Soup Mix' prepared .... 6 oz		80	13	1.0
(Lipton)				
'Cup-A-Soup' mix only .... 1 serving		52	10	1.0
'Recipe Secrets' mix only .... 1 serving		28	6	0.2
spring, 'Cup-A-Soup' mix only .... 1 envelope		47	8	1.0
(Manischewitz) prepared .... 6 oz		50	9	1.0
(Ultra Slim-Fast) hearty, prepared .... 6 oz		45	5	1.0
VEGETABLE, CREAM OF, prepared .... 1 cup		107	12	5.7
VEGETABLE BARLEY				
(Fantastic Foods) hearty, mix only .... 1.5 oz		150	29	0.5
VEGETABLE BEEF, prepared .... 1 cup		57	9	1.2
WAKAME *(Kikkoman)* prepared .... 1 serving		15	3	0.0
SOUR CREAM				
cultured .... 1 cup		493	10	48.2
cultured .... 1 tbsp		26	1	2.5
half and half, less fat, cultured .... 1 cup		326	10	29.0
half and half, less fat, cultured .... 1 tbsp		20	1	1.8
(Alta Dena) pasteurized, 100% natural .... 1 oz		60	1	6.0
(Bison) .... 2 tbsp		50	1	5.0
(Breakstone's)				
half and half, 'Light Choice' .... 1 tbsp		25	1	2.0
less fat .... 2 tbsp		47	2	3.7
nonfat .... 2 tbsp		29	5	0.4

Food Name	Serv. Size	Total Cal.	Carbs GMS	Fat GMS
regular	1 tbsp	30	1	3.0
(Crowley)				
French onion	2 tbsp	50	1	5.0
light	2 tbsp	30	2	2.0
regular	2 tbsp	50	1	5.0
(Darigold)	1 tbsp	23	1	2.8
(Friendship)				
low-fat, 'Lite Delite'	2 tbsp	35	2	2.0
regular	2 tbsp	55	1	5.0
(Knudsen)				
light	2 tbsp	40	2	3.0
nonfat	2 tbsp	35	6	0.0
regular, 'Hampshire'	2 tbsp	60	1	6.0
(Land O'Lakes)				
'Light'	2 tbsp	40	4	2.0
nonfat	2 tbsp	30	5	0.0
w/chives, 'Light'	2 tbsp	40	4	2.0
(Naturally Yours) no fat, 'Real Dairy'	2 tbsp	15	1	0.0
(Sealtest)				
half and half, 'Light'	1 tbsp	25	1	2.0
regular	1 tbsp	30	1	3.0
(Tone's) w/chives, topping	1 tsp	16	1	1.2
(Weight Watchers) light	2 tbsp	35	2	2.0
SOUR CREAM SUBSTITUTE				
cultured	1 cup	479	15	44.9
cultured	1 oz	59	2	5.5
(Crowley) nondairy	1 oz	40	1	4.0
(IMO)	1 tbsp	30	0	3.0
(Light n' Lively) nonfat, cultured	1 tbsp	10	1	0.0
(Pet)	1 tbsp	25	1	2.0
(Tofutti) no cholesterol, 'Sour Supreme'	1 tbsp	25	1	2.5
SOURSOP. See GUANABANA.				
SOY BEVERAGE				
(Ah-Soy)				
carob	6 fl oz	160	30	3.0
chocolate	6 fl oz	160	29	3.0
vanilla	6 fl oz	160	23	5.0
(Eden Foods)				
'Edensoy'	8 fl oz	150	23	3.0
'Edensoy' carob, natural	8.45 fl oz	160	30	5.0
'Edensoy' original, natural, organic, dairy-free	8.45 fl oz	140	14	4.0
'Edensoy' vanilla, natural	8.45 fl oz	150	25	3.0
'Edensoy Extra'	8 fl oz	150	24	3.0
'Edensoy Extra' vanilla, dairy-free	8.45 fl oz	150	25	3.0
(Health Valley) nonfat, 'Soy Moo'	8 fl oz	110	22	0.0
(Pacific Foods)				
'Pacific Lite' plain	8 fl oz	100	14	2.5
'Pacific Lite' vanilla	8 fl oz	110	18	2.0
'Pacific Select' plain	8 fl oz	100	14	3.0
'Pacific Select' vanilla	8 fl oz	120	17	3.0
(Sovex) 'Better Than Milk' original, premixed	8 fl oz	90	15	2.0
(Vitasoy)				
carob supreme	8 fl oz	210	32	6.0
cocoa, light	8 fl oz	130	25	2.0
cocoa, rich	8 fl oz	210	32	6.0
original, creamy	8 fl oz	160	14	7.0
original, light	8 fl oz	90	15	2.0

Food Name	Serv. Size	Total Cal.	Carbs GMS	Fat GMS
vanilla delite	8 fl oz	190	27	6.0
vanilla, light	8 fl oz	110	20	2.0
(Westbrae Natural Foods)				
'WestSoy' almond malted, lite	6 fl oz	160	26	4.0
'WestSoy' almond malted, natural	6 fl oz	250	31	11.0
'WestSoy' banana, creamy, lite	6 fl oz	160	26	3.0
'WestSoy' carob malted, natural	6 fl oz	270	37	11.0
'WestSoy' carob, malted, lite	6 fl oz	160	27	3.0
'WestSoy' cocoa, lite	8 fl oz	140	27	2.0
'WestSoy' cocoa-mint malted, nondairy, frozen	6 fl oz	270	37	11.0
'WestSoy' cocoa-mint, lite	6 fl oz	160	26	3.0
'WestSoy' java malted, natural	6 fl oz	270	37	11.0
'WestSoy' original, natural	8 fl oz	150	18	5.0
'WestSoy' plain, lite	8 fl oz	100	16	2.0
'WestSoy' unsweetened, natural	8 fl oz	100	5	5.0
'WestSoy' vanilla malted, natural	6 fl oz	250	31	11.0
'WestSoy' vanilla royale, lite	6 fl oz	160	26	3.0
'WestSoy' vanilla, lite	8 fl oz	110	20	2.0
'WestSoy' vanilla, natural	8 fl oz	120	22	2.5
'WestSoy Plus' carob	8 fl oz	160	21	5.0
'WestSoy Plus' plain	8 fl oz	150	18	5.0
'WestSoy Plus' vanilla	8 fl oz	150	20	5.0
SOY BEVERAGE MIX				
(Better Than Milk)				
(Darifree) fat free	3 tbsp	90	21	0.0
(Snoe Tofu) lactose & cholesterol free	3 tbsp	90	10	5.0
(Solait)				
chocolate	2 tbsp	114	18	3.0
original	3 tbsp	90	13	2.0
vanilla bean	3 tbsp	98	16	2.0
(Sovex)				
'Better Than Milk'	2 tbsp	98	19	2.0
'Better Than Milk' carob, nondairy	1 fl oz	130	20	5.0
'Better Than Milk' light	2 tbsp	70	14	0.5
'Better Than Milk' natural, light, nondairy	2 tbsp	80	15	1.0
'Better Than Milk' original	2 tbsp	100	16	2.5
(Soy Moo)	8 fl oz	125	11	5.0
SOY CHEESE. See under CHEESE SUBSTITUTE.				
SOY MEAL				
defatted, raw	1 cup	414	49	2.9
defatted, raw, crude protein basis Nx6.25	1 cup	411	44	2.9
SOY PROTEIN CONCENTRATE				
produced by acid wash	1 oz	94	9	0.1
produced by alcohol extraction	1 oz	94	9	0.1
SOY PROTEIN ISOLATE				
	1 oz	96	2	1.0
K type	1 oz	92	3	0.1
K type, crude protein basis Nx6.25	1 oz	91	1	0.1
(Protein Technologies)				
'ProPlus'	1 oz	108	0	1.1
'Supro'	1 oz	110	0	1.1
SOY SAUCE. See under SAUCE.				
SOYBEAN				
Dried				
mature, boiled	1 cup	298	17	15.4
mature, boiled	1 tbsp	19	1	1.0
mature, dry-roasted	1 cup	774	56	37.2

Food Name	Serv. Size	Total Cal.	Carbs GMS	Fat GMS
mature, raw	1 cup	774	56	37.1
mature, roasted	1 cup	810	58	43.7
mature, sprouted, raw	1/2 cup	43	3	2.3
mature, sprouted, raw	10 sprouts	12	1	0.7
mature, sprouted, steamed	1 cup	76	6	4.2
raw *(Arrowhead Mills)*	2 oz	230	19	10.0
roasted halves *(Solnuts)*	1 oz	146	8	6.8
Green				
boiled, drained	1 cup	254	20	11.5
raw	1 cup	376	28	17.4
SOYBEAN, FERMENTED/natto	1 cup	371	25	19.3
SOYBEAN CURD. See TOFU.				
SOYBEAN FLAKES *(Arrowhead Mills)*	2 oz	250	18	11.0
SOYBEAN OIL				
salad or cooking	1 cup	1927	0	218.0
salad or cooking	1 tbsp	120	0	13.6
salad or cooking, hydrogenated	1 cup	1927	0	218.0
salad or cooking, hydrogenated	1 tbsp	120	0	13.6
(Crisco)	1 tbsp	120	0	14.0
(Hain) salad or cooking	1 tbsp	120	0	14.0
(IGA) salad or cooking	1 tbsp	120	0	14.0
SOYBEAN-COTTONSEED OIL				
salad or cooking, hydrogenated	1 cup	1927	0	218.0
salad or cooking, hydrogenated	1 tbsp	120	0	13.6
SOYBEAN-LECITHIN OIL				
	1 cup	1663	0	218.0
	1 tbsp	104	0	13.6
SOYMILK				
	1 cup	81	4	4.7
	1 fl oz	10	1	0.6
SOYMILK MIX, powder *(Soyamel)*	8 oz	130	10	7.0
SOYNUT				
dry-roasted *(Karen's Kitchen)*	1 oz	90	7	4.0
dry-roasted, honey-coated *(Nature's Select)*	1 oz	130	13	4.0
SPAGHETTI. See under PASTA				
SPAGHETTI DISH/ENTRÉE. See under PASTA DISH/ENTRÉE.				
SPAGHETTI SQUASH. See SQUASH, SPAGHETTI.				
SPANISH MACKEREL. See under MACKEREL.				
SPANISH PEANUT. See under PEANUT.				
SPEARMINT				
dried	1 tbsp	5	1	0.1
dried	1 tsp	1	0	0.0
dried *(McCormick/Schilling)*	1 tsp	2	0	0.0
fresh	2 tbsp	5	1	0.1
SPINACH. See also SPINACH DISH/ENTRÉE.				
Canned				
(Allens)	1/2 cup	28	3	1.0
(Finast)	1/2 cup	25	4	0.0
(Stokely)	1/2 cup	30	3	0.0
chopped *(Allens)*	1/2 cup	28	3	1.0
chopped *(Bush's Best)*	1/2 cup	25	4	0.0
chopped, w/liquid *(Del Monte)*	1/2 cup	25	4	0.0
cut *(Freshlike)*	1/2 cup	20	4	0.0
cut *(Veg-All)*	1/2 cup	20	4	0.0
cut, w/butter sauce *(Green Giant)*	1/2 cup	40	5	1.5
cut, water packed, no salt added *(Freshlike)*	1/2 cup	20	4	0.0
cut, water packed, no sugar or salt added *(Freshlike)*	1/2 cup	20	4	0.0

Food Name	Serv. Size	Total Cal.	Carbs GMS	Fat GMS
drained . . . . 1 cup	1 cup	49	7	1.1
no salt, w/liquid . . . . 1 cup	1 cup	44	7	0.9
no salt added *(Finast)* . . . . 1/2 cup	1/2 cup	25	4	0.0
no salt added *(Pathmark)* . . . . 1/2 cup	1/2 cup	30	4	1.0
'Premium Northwest' *(S&W)* . . . . 1/2 cup	1/2 cup	25	3	0.0
regular pack, w/liquid . . . . 1 cup	1 cup	44	7	0.9
sliced *(Allens)* . . . . 1/2 cup	1/2 cup	28	3	1.0
whole leaf *(Allens)* . . . . 1/2 cup	1/2 cup	28	3	1.0
whole leaf *(Featherweight)* . . . . 1/2 cup	1/2 cup	35	4	1.0
whole leaf *(Pathmark)* . . . . 1/2 cup	1/2 cup	30	4	1.0
whole leaf, 'No Frills' *(Pathmark)* . . . . 1 cup	1 cup	45	8	1.0
whole leaf, w/liquid *(Del Monte)* . . . . 1/2 cup	1/2 cup	25	4	0.0
whole leaf, w/liquid, no salt added *(Del Monte)* . . . . 1/2 cup	1/2 cup	25	4	0.0
Fresh				
raw . . . . 1 cup	1 cup	7	1	0.1
raw . . . . 1 med leaf	1 med leaf	2	0	0.0
raw *(Dole)* . . . . 3 oz	3 oz	9	0	0.3
Frozen				
chopped *(A&P)* . . . . 3.3 oz	3.3 oz	20	4	1.0
chopped *(Birds Eye)* . . . . 3.3 oz	3.3 oz	20	3	0.0
chopped *(C&W)* . . . . 1/3 cup	1/3 cup	20	2	0.0
chopped *(Finast)* . . . . 3.3 oz	3.3 oz	20	3	0.0
chopped *(Flav-R-Pac)* . . . . 1/3 cup	1/3 cup	20	2	0.0
chopped *(Frosty Acres)* . . . . 3.3 oz	3.3 oz	20	3	0.0
chopped *(Seabrook)* . . . . 3.3 oz	3.3 oz	20	3	0.0
chopped *(Southern)* . . . . 3.5 oz	3.5 oz	25	4	0.3
chopped or leaf, boiled, drained . . . . 10-oz pkg	10-oz pkg	62	12	0.5
chopped or leaf, boiled, drained . . . . 1/2 cup	1/2 cup	27	5	0.2
chopped or leaf, no salt added, drained . . . . 10-oz pkg	10-oz pkg	62	12	0.5
chopped or leaf, no salt added, drained . . . . 1/2 cup	1/2 cup	27	5	0.2
chopped or leaf, unprepared . . . . 10-oz pkg	10-oz pkg	68	11	0.9
chopped or leaf, unprepared . . . . 1 cup	1 cup	37	6	0.5
cut *(Freshlike)* . . . . 3.3 oz	3.3 oz	20	4	0.0
cut *(Green Giant)* . . . . 3/4 cup	3/4 cup	25	3	0.0
cut *(Seabrook)* . . . . 3.3 oz	3.3 oz	20	4	0.0
cut *(Veg-All)* . . . . 3.3 oz	3.3 oz	20	4	0.0
'Harvest Fresh' *(Green Giant)* . . . . 1/2 cup	1/2 cup	25	3	0.0
'Plain Polybag' *(Green Giant)* . . . . 1/2 cup	1/2 cup	25	6	0.0
whole leaf *(A&P)* . . . . 3.3 oz	3.3 oz	25	4	1.0
whole leaf *(Birds Eye)* . . . . 3.3 oz	3.3 oz	20	4	0.0
whole leaf *(Finast)* . . . . 3.3 oz	3.3 oz	20	4	0.0
whole leaf *(Flav-R-Pac)* . . . . 1/3 cup	1/3 cup	20	2	0.0
whole leaf *(Frosty Acres)* . . . . 3.3 oz	3.3 oz	20	4	0.0
whole leaf *(Southern)* . . . . 3.5 oz	3.5 oz	25	4	0.3
whole leaf, 'Portion Pack' *(Birds Eye)* . . . . 3.2 oz	3.2 oz	20	3	0.0
SPINACH, MALABAR				
cooked . . . . 1 med bunch	1 med bunch	4	0	0.1
cooked . . . . 1 cup	1 cup	10	1	0.3
SPINACH, NEW ZEALAND				
boiled, drained, chopped . . . . 1 cup	1 cup	22	4	0.3
raw, chopped . . . . 1 cup	1 cup	8	1	0.1
SPINACH, VINE/basella				
raw . . . . 1 lb	1 lb	86	15.4	1.4
raw . . . . 3.5 oz	3.5 oz	19	3.4	0.3
SPINACH DISH/ENTRÉE				
(Birds Eye) creamed, 'Combination Vegetables' . . . . 3 oz	3 oz	60	5	4.0
(Budget Gourmet) au gratin, frozen . . . . 1 pkg	1 pkg	222	11	16.6

Food Name	Serv. Size	Total Cal.	Carbs GMS	Fat GMS
(Green Giant) creamed	1/2 cup	80	10	3.0
(Stouffer's)				
cream of, side dish	1/2 cup	160	8	12.0
creamed	1 pkg	336	18	26.3
creamed, food service product	1 oz	46	2	3.8
soufflé, side dish	1/2 cup	150	9	10.0
SPINY LOBSTER. See under LOBSTER.				
SPIRULINA. See under ALGAE.				
SPLIT PEAS. See PEAS, SPLIT.				
SPONGE GOURD. See GOURD, DISHCLOTH.				
SPORTS AND DIET/NUTRITION BARS				
(Advantage Bar)				
almond brownie, 'Atkins Diet Food Bar'	1 bar	230	3	10.0
chocolate coconut, 'Atkins Diet Food Bar'	1 bar	250	2	13.0
chocolate peanut butter, 'Atkins Diet Food Bar'	1 bar	218	3	13.0
praline crunch, 'Atkins Diet Food Bar'	1 bar	221	3	13.0
(Bally BFIT)				
chocolate-covered chocolate energy bar	1 bar	240	37	5.0
chocolate-covered peanut energy bar	1 bar	240	37	5.0
wafer snack, 'Trim Fat'	2 wafers	25	5	0.0
(Bear Valley)				
coconut almond food bar, 'Meal Pack'	1 pkg	400	56	12.0
sesame lemon food bar, 'Meal Pack'	1 pkg	410	57	13.0
(Biochem Ultimate)				
chocolate brownie nut food bar, low-carbohydrate	1 bar	240	2	7.0
chocolate chip protein bar	1 bar	290	19	5.0
honey almond food bar, low-carbohydrate	1 bar	240	2	7.0
(BIOX)				
chocolate and peanut butter protein bar	1 bar	300	37	7.0
chocolate chip protein bar	1 bar	330	48	3.0
chocolate protein bar	1 bar	290	40	5.0
triple chocolate chip protein bar	1 bar	330	48	4.0
(Biozone) 'Food Bar'	1 bar	180	20	4.0
(Boulder Bar)				
apple cinnamon energy bar	1 bar	190	37	2.0
berry energy bar	1 bar	190	37	2.0
chocolate energy bar	1 bar	200	40	3.0
peanut butter energy bar	1 bar	210	37	4.0
(Clif)				
apple cherry, '100% Natural Endurance'	2.4 oz	250	52	2.0
apricot, '100% Natural Endurance'	2.4 oz	250	50	2.0
(Clif Bar)				
apple cherry energy bar	1 bar	250	52	2.0
apricot energy bar	1 bar	250	50	2.0
carrot cake energy bar	1 bar	240	42	4.0
chocolate almond fudge energy bar	1 bar	250	39	5.0
chocolate chip energy bar	1 bar	250	51	3.0
chocolate chip peanut energy bar	1 bar	250	40	6.0
chocolate espresso energy bar	1 bar	250	51	3.0
chocolate pecan nutrition bar, for women, 'Luna'	1 bar	180	24	5.0
cookies 'n cream energy bar	1 bar	250	42	5.0
lemon zest nutrition bar, for women, 'Luna'	1 bar	180	26	4.0
peanut butter energy bar, crunchy	1 bar	250	45	4.0
real berry energy bar	1 bar	250	52	2.0
(Complete Bar)				
chocolate, '40/30/30 Bar'	1 bar	190	21	6.0
graham, '40/30/30 bar'	1 bar	190	21	6.0

Food Name	Serv. Size	Total Cal.	Carbs GMS	Fat GMS
peanut butter, '40/30/30 Bar'	1 bar	190	21	6.0
(Complete Protein Diet) 'Complete Protein Diet Bar'	1 bar	190	2	5.0
(Energx)				
chocolate protein cookie, all natural	2 cookies	200	28	3.0
oatmeal raisin protein cookie, all natural	2 cookies	200	31	2.0
peanut butter protein cookie, all natural	2 cookies	200	31	3.0
(Fi-Bar) strawberry, oatmeal, almond 'A.M. snack bar'	1 bar	150	24	4.0
(Figurines)				
chocolate caramel, '100'	1 bar	100	10	6.0
chocolate caramel, w/8 oz nonfat milk	2 bars	280	33	12.0
chocolate peanut butter, w/8 oz nonfat milk	2 bars	290	31	12.0
chocolate, w/8 oz nonfat milk	2 bars	280	34	11.0
S'mores, w/8 oz nonfat milk	2 bars	290	34	11.0
vanilla, w/8 oz nonfat milk	2 bars	290	33	12.0
(Gatorade Bar) peanut butter energy bar	1 bar	260	47	5.0
(Genisoy)				
apple spice protein bar, yogurt-coated, soy	1 bar	220	32	4.0
café mocha protein bar, soy	1 bar	220	34	3.5
café mocha protein bar, soy	1 bar	220	34	4.0
chocolate-coated protein bar, soy	1 bar	220	33	3.5
chocolate mint protein bar, soy	1 bar	220	33	4.0
chocolate protein bar, uncoated, soy	1 bar	210	36	0.0
peanut butter fudge protein bar, soy	1 bar	230	31	5.0
(Jenny Craig)				
chocolate peanut nutrition meal	1 bar	220	33	5.0
lemon meringue nutrition meal	1 bar	210	31	5.0
oatmeal raisin nutrition meal	1 bar	210	35	3.0
(Jog Mate) muscle recovery protein supplement	1 tube	100	8	3.0
(Kashi) chocolate and peanut butter high-protein bar, 'Golean'	1 bar	280	50	6.0
(Lean Body)				
coconut cream meal replacement	1 bar	300	19	7.0
mint chocolate chip meal replacement	1 bar	300	19	7.0
(Maxxbar) chocolate chip energy bar	1 bar	170	25	4.0
(MET-RX)				
apple caramel energy bar, 'Sourceone'	1 bar	190	30	3.0
apple cinnamon oatmeal cereal bar, 'Caffe'	1 pkt	290	43	3.0
chocolate cheesecake energy bar, 'Sourceone'	1 bar	190	30	3.0
chocolate chip cookie dough energy bar	1 bar	340	50	4.0
chocolate chip graham cracker energy bar	1 bar	320	48	3.0
chocolate peanut energy bar, 'Sourceone'	1 bar	190	30	3.0
chocolate raspberry energy bar, 'Sourceone'	1 bar	180	31	3.0
devil's food energy bar, 'Sourceone'	1 bar	190	30	3.0
extreme chocolate nutrition bar	1 bar	240	18	8.0
extreme vanilla nutrition bar	1 bar	320	48	3.0
fudge brownie nutrition bar	1 bar	320	52	3.0
high-protein bar, 'Protein Plus'	1 bar	290	15	8.0
oatmeal raisin energy bar, iced, 'Sourceone'	1 bar	180	33	3.0
peanut butter cookie dough energy bar	1 bar	340	50	4.0
traditional flavor oatmeal cereal bar, 'Caffe'	1 pkt	280	35	4.0
(MLO Hardbody)				
chocolate truffle energy bar, 'Vita-Ox Formula'	1 bar	280	41	7.0
honey almond energy bar, 'Vita-Ox Formula'	1 bar	280	46	7.0
peanut butter energy bar, 'Vita-Ox Formula'	1 bar	290	46	7.0
pineapple coconut energy bar, 'Vita-Ox Formula'	1 bar	280	46	7.0
(Myoplex)				
chocolate fudge food bar	1 bar	340	44	7.0
chocolate nutrition bar, deluxe, 'Plus'	1 bar	340	42	7.0

Food Name	Serv. Size	Total Cal.	Carbs GMS	Fat GMS
chocolate peanut butter nutrition bar, deluxe, 'Plus'	1 bar	340	45	7.0
chocolate peanut butter precision nutrition bar, deluxe, 'Plus'	1 bar	340	44	7.0
chocolate precision nutrition bar, deluxe	1 bar	340	43	7.0
(Nature's Plus) high-protein wafers, all flavors 'Spirutein'	6 wafers	99	9	1.0
(Nextra) apple protein crunch energy bar	1 pkg	140	14	2.0
(Nutrablast) 'Nutrablast Her for Women'	1 bar	190	27	6.0
(Odwalla Bar)				
'C Monster Food Bar'	1 bar	230	52	2.0
carrot raisin food bar, organic	1 bar	230	51	2.0
chocolate raspberry food bar	1 bar	240	45	5.0
cranberry citrus food bar	1 bar	240	52	2.0
peanut crunch food bar	1 bar	260	44	7.0
'Super Protein Food Bar'	1 bar	260	44	7.0
(Peak Bar)				
chocolate chip energy bar	1 bar	314	58	6.0
chocolate malt energy bar	1 bar	290	62	4.0
fruit mania energy bar	1 bar	284	58	5.0
peanut chocolate chunk energy bar	1 bar	295	56	7.0
(PowerBar)				
apple crisp, 'Harvest'	1 bar	240	45	4.0
apple-cinnamon	1 bar	230	45	3.0
banana	1 bar	230	45	2.0
blueberry, 'Harvest'	1 bar	240	45	4.0
cherry crunch, 'Harvest'	1 bar	240	45	4.0
chocolate energy gel	1 pack	120	28	2.0
chocolate	1 bar	230	45	2.0
chocolate, 'Essentials'	1 bar	180	28	4.0
chocolate, 'Harvest'	1 bar	240	45	4.0
chocolate, 'Protein Plus'	1 bar	290	38	5.0
lemon lime energy gel	1 pack	110	28	0.0
malt nut	1 bar	230	45	3.0
mocha	1 bar	230	45	3.0
oatmeal raisin	1 bar	230	45	3.0
peanut butter	1 bar	230	45	3.0
peanut butter w/chocolate chips, 'Harvest'	1 bar	240	45	5.0
strawberry, 'Harvest'	1 bar	240	45	4.0
tropical fruit energy gel	1 pack	110	28	0.0
vanilla energy gel	1 pack	110	28	0.0
vanilla yogurt, 'Protein Plus'	1 bar	290	38	5.0
wild berry	1 bar	230	45	3.0
(PR Bar)				
Bavarian mint nutrition bar, '40-30-30'	1 bar	190	21	7.0
carrot cake food bar	1 bar	200	23	6.0
chocolate peanut nutrition bar	1 bar	190	19	6.0
granola food bar	1 bar	180	21	6.0
iced brownie food bar	1 bar	200	22	6.0
strawberry yogurt food bar	1 bar	200	23	6.0
(Pure Protein Bar)				
chocolate chip protein bar	1 bar	190	11	4.0
white chocolate protein bar	1 bar	180	11	3.0
(Sci Fit)				
chocolate protein bar	1 bar	334	22	5.0
cinnamon protein bar	1 bar	334	22	6.0
oatmeal protein bar	1 bar	330	24	6.0
(Shaklee)				
'Carbo Crunch'	1 bar	180	27	4.0
'Fiber Blend Tablets'	5 tablets	6	1	0.5

Food Name	Serv. Size	Total Cal.	Carbs GMS	Fat GMS
(Slim-Fast)				
chocolate chip crunch	1 bar	120	16	4.0
Dutch chocolate	1 bar	140	20	5.0
peanut butter	1 bar	150	19	5.0
(Sportpharma Promax)				
double fudge brownie protein bar	1 bar	270	34	5.0
Dutch chocolate protein bar	2 scoops	270	2	2.0
lemon chiffon protein bar	1 bar	270	41	4.0
(Sweet Success) oatmeal raisin, chewy	1 bar	120	23	4.0
(Tiger's Milk)				
peanut butter and honey snack, carob coated	1 bar	160	23	5.0
(Trek Barr)				
apple raisin cinnamon energy bar	1 bar	130	29	1.0
chocolate extreme energy bar	1 bar	130	29	2.0
java express energy bar	1 bar	130	29	2.0
mountain berry energy bar	1 bar	130	29	2.0
peach apricot energy bar	1 bar	130	29	1.0
peanut butter chocolate chip energy bar	1 bar	130	26	2.0
(Twinlab)				
apple sports bar, 'Protein Fuel'	1 bar	340	12	5.0
chocolate food bar, 'Soy Sensations'	1 bar	180	22	6.0
chocolate sports bar, 'Protein Fuel'	1 bar	320	12	5.0
lemon food bar, 'Soy Sensations'	1 bar	180	23	5.0
peanut butter sports bar, 'Protein Fuel'	1 bar	340	12	5.0
peanut food bar, 'Soy Sensations'	1 bar	170	23	5.0
peanut nutrition bar, creamy, 'Ironman'	1 bar	230	23	8.0
(Ultra Slim-Fast)				
apple breakfast	1 bar	160	38	0.0
blueberry breakfast	1 bar	170	39	0.0
brownie	1 bar	120	20	4.0
caramel crunch, chewy	1 bar	120	22	3.5
choco almond crunch	1 bar	120	20	4.0
chocolate chip crunch snack	1 bar	120	19	4.0
fig breakfast	1 bar	160	37	0.0
peanut butter crunch	1 bar	120	19	4.0
peanut caramel crunch	1 bar	120	22	4.0
strawberry breakfast	1 bar	170	39	0.0
vanilla crunch	1 bar	120	20	4.0
(Viactiv) apple crunch, 'Energy Bar for Women'	1 bar	180	29	5.0
(Weider)				
'Sportsfood Enerquench Bar'	1 bar	200	44	1.0
chewable, 'Victory Explosive Workout'	6 wafers	30	6	0.0
protein bar, 'Sportsfood'	1 bar	160	21	4.0
(Weight Watchers)				
chocolate brownie, chewy, 'Sweet Success'	1 bar	120	23	4.0
chocolate chip, chewy 'Sweet Success'	1 bar	120	23	4.0
chocolate peanut butter, chewy 'Sweet Success'	1 bar	120	23	4.0
(Zone Perfect)				
apple cinnamon crunch nutrition bar, '40-30-30'	1 bar	210	23	7.0
strawberry yogurt nutrition bar, '40-30-30'	1 bar	210	24	7.0

SPORTS AND DIET/NUTRITION DRINKS. See SPORTS AND DIET/NUTRITION DRINK MIX.

(All Sport)				
fruit punch	8 fl oz	70	20	0.0
grape, caffeine-free, 'Thirst Quencher'	8 fl oz	70	20	0.0
lemon-lime, 'Thirst quencher, caffeine-free	8 fl oz	70	19	0.0
orange, caffeine-free, 'Thirst Quencher'	8 fl oz	70	19	0.0
(Clinical Resource) yogurt, flavored	8 fl oz	250	44	4.2

Food Name	Serv. Size	Total Cal.	Carbs GMS	Fat GMS
(Dannon) yogurt drink, all flavors, 'Dan'up'	8 fl oz	190	32	4.0
(Endurox) 'Endurox R4'	12 fl oz	280	53	2.0
(Ensure)				
black walnut flavor liquid nutrition	8 fl oz	250	34	8.8
chocolate liquid nutrition	8 fl oz	250	34	8.8
chocolate liquid nutrition, 'Plus'	8 fl oz	355	47	12.6
chocolate liquid nutrition, w/fiber	8 fl oz	260	38	8.8
eggnog flavor liquid nutrition	8 fl oz	250	34	8.8
strawberry flavor liquid nutrition	8 fl oz	250	34	8.8
strawberry flavor liquid nutrition, 'Plus'	8 fl oz	355	47	12.6
vanilla liquid nutrition	8 fl oz	250	34	8.8
vanilla liquid nutrition, 'Plus'	8 fl oz	355	47	12.6
vanilla liquid nutrition, w/fiber	8 fl oz	260	38	8.8
(Gatorade)				
fruit punch, low-sodium, no caffeine	8 fl oz	50	14	0.0
grape, low-sodium, no caffeine	8 fl oz	50	14	0.0
lemon and tea	8 fl oz	50	14	0.0
lemon-lime, 'Thirst Quencher'	8 fl oz	50	14	0.0
lemon-lime, 'Thirst Quencher Light'	8 fl oz	25	7	0.0
orange, 'Thirst Quencher'	8 fl oz	50	14	0.0
original, 'Thirst Quencher'	8 fl oz	50	14	0.0
pineapple-citrus, 'Thirst Quencher Light'	8 fl oz	25	7	0.0
tropical fruit, 'Thirst Quencher'	8 fl oz	50	14	0.0
(Genesis Nutrition)				
'Super Carbo Charge'	1 serving	348	87	0.0
'Super Metabolic Optimizer'	1 serving	260	48	1.0
'Super Weight Gain 1800'	1 serving	1800	284	24.0
'Super Workout Pak'	1 serving	0	0	0.0
(Go Healthy)				
chocolate nutrition drink	8 fl oz	235	40	3.0
mocha nutrition drink	8 fl oz	235	40	3.0
orange cream nutrition drink	8 fl oz	220	36	3.0
strawberry-banana nutrition drink	8 fl oz	220	36	3.0
vanilla nutrition drink	8 fl oz	220	36	3.0
(Knudsen)				
fruit juice sweetened, all flavors	8 fl oz	70	18	0.0
'Lemon Recharge'	1 cup	70	18	0.0
'Orange Recharge'	1 cup	70	18	0.0
'Tropical Recharge'	1 cup	70	18	0.0
'Vita Juice Fortified Blend'	8 fl oz	120	29	0.0
(Nutra/Balance)				
'Nutra/Shake Free'	4 fl oz	200	25	8.0
'Nutra/Shake with Fiber'	4 fl oz	200	40	1.3
'Nutra/Shake'	4 fl oz	229	35	6.9
(Nutrament)				
chocolate shake, meal replacement	12 fl oz	360	52	10.0
vanilla shake, meal replacement	12 fl oz	360	52	10.0
(Opti-Carb 140)				
grape	16 fl oz	140	35	0.0
orange	16 fl oz	140	35	0.0
(Power Burst)				
lemonade, advanced performance beverage	8 fl oz	50	14	0.0
(Powerade)				
fruit punch	16 fl oz	144	38	0.0
grape	16 fl oz	146	38	0.0
lemon-lime	16 fl oz	144	38	0.0
'Mountain Blast'	16 fl oz	146	38	0.0

Food Name	Serv. Size	Total Cal.	Carbs GMS	Fat GMS
orange	16 fl oz	144	38	0.0
(Pro-formance)				
fruit punch	8 fl oz	99	26	0.0
grape	8 fl oz	99	26	0.0
lemon-lime	8 fl oz	99	26	0.0
orange	8 fl oz	99	26	0.0
(Resource)				
chocolate health shake	4 fl oz	190	32	4.0
vanilla health shake	4 fl oz	190	32	4.0
(Sego)				
chocolate, 'Lite'	10 fl oz	150	20	3.0
chocolate, 'Very Chocolate'	10 fl oz	225	43	1.0
chocolate malt, 'Very Chocolate'	10 fl oz	225	43	1.0
Dutch chocolate, 'Lite'	10 fl oz	150	20	3.0
French vanilla, 'Lite'	10 fl oz	150	17	4.0
strawberry, 'Lite'	10 fl oz	150	17	4.0
strawberry, 'Very Strawberry'	10 fl oz	225	34	5.0
vanilla, plain, 'Lite'	10 fl oz	150	17	4.0
vanilla, 'Very Vanilla'	10 fl oz	225	34	5.0
(Shasta)				
lemon-lime, caffeine-free, 'Body Works'	8 fl oz	60	15	0.0
orange, caffeine-free, 'Body Works'	8 fl oz	60	15	0.0
(Slim-Fast)				
chocolate shake	8 fl oz	190	33	1.3
chocolate shake, 'Nutra Start'	1 shake	210	40	2.5
strawberry shake	8 fl oz	190	33	0.7
vanilla shake, 'Nutra Start'	1 shake	210	38	2.5
(Sustacal)				
chocolate, liquid food, nutritionally complete	8 fl oz	240	33	5.5
vanilla, liquid food, nutritionally complete	8 fl oz	240	33	5.5
(Weight Watchers)				
chocolate mocha, w/phenylalanine, 'Sweet Success'	10 fl oz	200	32	3.0
chocolate, w/phenylalanine, 'Sweet Success'	10 fl oz	200	38	3.0
dark chocolate fudge, 'Sweet Success'	10 fl oz	200	32	3.0
milk chocolate, creamy, 'Sweet Success'	10 fl oz	200	32	3.0
vanilla, w/phenylalanine, 'Sweet Success'	10 fl oz	200	32	3.0
(Ultra Slim-Fast)				
'Chocolate Fantasy'	8 fl oz	270	51	1.9
chocolate fudge shake	1 shake	220	42	3.0
chocolate royale shake	1 shake	220	38	3.0
coffee shake	1 shake	220	38	3.0
French vanilla	12 fl oz	220	38	1.0
milk chocolate shake	1 shake	220	42	3.0
strawberry shake	1 shake	220	42	3.0
vanilla shake	1 shake	220	38	3.0
(Yogloo)				
yogurt, fruit basket, nonfat	10 fl oz	170	40	0.0
yogurt, original, nonfat	10 fl oz	170	40	0.0
yogurt, peach, nonfat	10 fl oz	170	40	0.0
yogurt, strawberry, nonfat	10 fl oz	170	40	0.0
SPORTS AND DIET/NUTRITION DRINK MIX				
(Alba)				
milkshake mix, double fudge, sugar-free, mix only	0.75 oz	60	10	0.0
milkshake mix, strawberry, sugar-free, mix only	0.75 oz	60	11	0.0
milkshake mix, vanilla flavor, no sugar, mix only	0.75 oz	70	11	0.0
(Alba '77)				
'Fit'N' chocolate marshmallow, prepared	6 fl oz	346	52	3.6

Food Name	Serv. Size	Total Cal.	Carbs GMS	Fat GMS
'Fit'N' chocolate, prepared	6 fl oz	346	56	2.5
'Fit'N' frosty double fudge, prepared	6 fl oz	346	52	3.3
'Fit'N' strawberry, prepared	6 fl oz	333	55	1.7
'Fit'N' vanilla, prepared	6 fl oz	333	55	1.4
(Amerifit) 'Heavy Weight Bulk Up' prepared	12 fl oz	71	14	0.3
(Balance Drink) meal replacement, '40-30-30' mix only	2 scoops	180	19	6.0
(Bally)				
muscle growth supplement, whey, mix only	1 scoop	100	3	2.0
protein supplement, soy	2 scoops	80	1	1.0
'Mass Builder' vanilla	4 scoops	750	163	1.0
(BFIT-RX)				
meal replacement, chocolate, light, mix only	1 pkt	190	26	1.0
meal replacement, vanilla, mix only	1 pkt	290	27	2.0
meal replacement for women, mix only	1 pkt	220	33	1.0
(Bio-Design X) vanilla, whey, mix only	20 grams	77	1	1.0
(BIOX) protein drink, chocolate, mix only	1 pkg	130	12	1.0
(Champion Nutrition)				
'Heavyweight Gainer 900' prepared	1 serving	650	105	12.0
(Complete Protein Diet)				
complete protein diet, chocolate, mix only	1 pkt	200	3	5.0
(EAS Precision)				
whey protein, 'Muscle Builder' mix only	3 tbsp	100	3	1.0
(Gatorade)				
'Thirst Quencher' fruit punch, prepared	8 fl oz	60	15	0.0
'Thirst Quencher' lemonade, prepared	8 fl oz	60	15	0.0
'Thirst Quencher' lemon-lime, mix only	3/4 scoop	58	15	0.0
(Genesis Nutrition)				
milk and egg protein drink, mix only	1 tbsp	39	2	0.0
'Super Trim Fast' mix only	1 serving	90	15	0.5
'Super Trim Fast' prepared	1 serving	198	27	2.0
(Genisoy)				
protein shake, chocolate, ultra soy protein, mix only	1 scoop	120	16	0.0
(Knox)				
gelatin drink, orange flavor, mix only	1 envelope	39	4	0.1
gelatin drink, orange flavor, w/aspartame, mix only	1 envelope	41	3	0.1
(Labrada)				
'Kwik Size XXXL' mix only	5 scoops	740	150	2.0
'Proplex+' mix only	1 scoop	90	3	1.0
(Lean Body)				
chocolate peanut butter, mix only	1 pkt	300	28	2.0
vanilla, mix only	1 pkt	300	28	2.0
(MET-RX)				
apple pie a la mode, mix only	1 pkt	250	22	2.0
extreme chocolate, mix only	1 pkt	240	18	1.0
milk chocolate, w/protein, mix only	3 scoops	220	7	2.0
original flavor, mix only	1 pkt	250	22	2.0
peach, mix only	1 pkt	250	22	2.0
strawberry cream, w/protein, mix only	3 scoops	210	3	1.0
vanilla butter cream, w/protein, mix only	3 scoops	210	3	1.0
white chocolate mocha, mix only	1 pkt	250	22	2.0
(MLO)				
'MUS-L Blast 2000' chocolate, mix only	4 scoops	580	118	3.0
'MUS-L Blast 2000' strawberry and banana, mix only	4 scoops	570	118	3.0
'MUS-L Blast 2000' vanilla, mix only	4 scoops	570	118	3.0
(Myoplex)				
'Mass Drink' chocolate cream, mix only	1 pkt	500	75	7.0
'Mass Drink' strawberry cream, light, mix only	1 pkt	280	24	2.0

Food Name	Serv. Size	Total Cal.	Carbs GMS	Fat GMS
'Mass Drink' strawberry cream, mix only	1 pkt	500	76	7.0
'Mass Drink' vanilla cream, light, mix only	1 pkt	280	24	2.0
'Mass Drink' vanilla cream, mix only	1 pkt	500	75	7.0
nutrition drink, chocolate cream, light, mix only	1 pkt	190	20	2.0
nutrition drink, chocolate cream, mix only	1 pkt	280	24	2.0
nutrition drink, chocolate, deluxe, mix only	1 pkt	280	24	2.0
(Nature's Plus)				
'Carrot-tein' mix only	1 scoop	97	11	0.0
'Fruitein' mix only	1 scoop	96	14	0.0
high-protein drink, banana, mix only	1 scoop	94	10	0.0
high-protein drink, cappuccino, mix only	1 scoop	100	11	0.0
high-protein drink, chocolate, vanilla, mix only	1 scoop	87	8	0.0
'Oxy-Nectar' mix only	1 scoop	107	17	0.0
(Olympian Labs)				
carbohydrate loading recovery drink, mix only	3 scoops	336	80	1.0
100% egg white w/complex carbs, vanilla, mix only	2 scoops	120	15	1.0
(Opti-Lean)				
chocolate, mix only	1 pkt	170	20	1.0
vanilla, mix only	1 pkt	170	20	1.0
(Scandishake)				
chocolate shake, instant, mix only	3 oz	440	58	21.0
chocolate shake, instant, lactose-free, mix only	3 oz	190	55	21.0
weight-gain shake, instant, lactose-free, mix only	3 oz	440	55	21.0
weight-gain shake, instant, sweetened w/aspartame, mix only	3 oz	440	55	21.0
weight-gain shake, instant, vanilla or strawberry, mix only	3 oz	440	58	21.0
(Shaklee)				
'After Exercise Energizer'	1/3 cup	180	33	0.5
'Daily Blend' mix only	1 1/2 tbsp	40	13	0.0
'Fiber Blend' 25% soluble/75% insoluble, mix only	1 tbsp	20	5	1.0
'Fiber Plan' fruit-flavored, mix only	2 tbsp	90	22	0.0
'Fiber Plan' unflavored, mix only	2 tsp	20	5	0.0
'Meal Shake' Bavarian cocoa, mix only	1/4 cup	120	23	0.5
'Meal Shake' Bavarian cocoa, prepared w/low-fat milk	8 fl oz prep	230	32	5.0
'Meal Shake' French vanilla, mix only	1/4 cup	120	23	0.5
'Meal Shake' French vanilla, prepared w/low-fat milk	8 fl oz	230	32	5.0
'Physique' mix only	1/2 cup	210	38	0.5
'Physique' prepared w/2 oz mix, 8 oz nonfat milk	1 serving	300	50	1.0
'Physique' prepared w/3 oz mix, 8 oz water	1 serving	320	57	1.0
protein drink, cocoa flavor, mix only	1/2 cup	110	8	1.0
protein drink, instant, mix only	1/4 cup	100	8	0.5
'Slim Plan' high fiber, low-fat, low-sodium, mix only	1/2 cup	210	33	3.0
(Slim-Fast)				
chocolate malt shake, prepared w/skim milk	8 fl oz	190	33	1.0
vanilla shake, prepared w/skim milk	1 cup	190	33	0.7
(Sportpharma)				
'Actisyn' strawberry flavor, mix only	1 pkt	150	8	1.0
'Just Whey' vanilla cream, mix only	1 oz	110	2	1.0
'Musclemax' chocolate, mix only	3 scoops	450	85	1.0
'Nutriforce' chocolate royale, mix only	1 pkt	250	21	2.0
'Nutriforce' French vanilla, mix only	1 pkt	260	21	2.0
(Strength Systems) 'USA Diet Octane' prepared	8 fl oz	127	9	1.0
(Weight Watchers)				
'Sweet Success' chocolate almond, mix only	1 scoop	90	12	2.0
'Sweet Success' chocolate almond, prepared	8 fl oz	180	24	2.0
'Sweet Success' chocolate, mix only	1 scoop	90	19	1.5
'Sweet Success' dark chocolate fudge, mix only	1 scoop	90	11	2.0
'Sweet Success' dark chocolate fudge, prepared	8 fl oz	180	23	2.0

Food Name	Serv. Size	Total Cal.	Carbs GMS	Fat GMS
(Tiger's Milk)				
'Breakfast Booster' mix only	2 tbsp	70	14	1.0
'Energy Booster' mix only	3 round tbsp	120	28	1.0
'Energy Booster' prepared w/8 oz nonfat milk	8 fl oz	200	40	1.0
'Protein Booster' Dutch chocolate, mix only	3 round tbsp	90	12	1.0
'Protein Booster' Dutch chocolate, prepared w/skim milk	8 fl oz	200	28	1.0
'Protein Booster' vanilla-orange creme, mix only	3 round tbsp	90	12	1.0
'Protein Booxter' vanilla-orange creme, prepared w/nonfat milk	8 fl oz	200	28	1.0
(Turbo Nutrition)				
protein powder, chocolate, prepared w/low-fat milk	8 fl oz	330	34	6.0
protein powder, strawberry flavored, mix only	2 oz	210	22	1.0
protein powder, strawberry flavored, prepared w/whole milk	8 fl oz	360	33	9.0
weight gain protein powder, chocolate, mix only	2 oz	210	22	1.0
(Twinlab)				
'Fuel Plex' whey protein, chocolate, mix only	1 pkt	300	25	2.0
'Fuel Plex' whey protein, strawberry, mix only	1 pkt	300	25	2.0
'Fuel Plex' whey protein, vanilla, mix only	1 pkt	300	25	2.0
(Ultra Slim-Fast)				
'Cafe Mocha' mix only	1 scoop	100	24	1.0
'Cafe Mocha' prepared w/nonfat milk	8 fl oz	200	38	1.0
'Chocolate Fantasy' 'Plus' mix only	1.41 oz	120	33	1.0
chocolate fudge shake, prepared w/skim milk	8 fl oz	200	36	2.6
chocolate malt shake, prepared w/skim milk	8 fl oz	200	36	1.3
'Chocolate Royale' shake, prepared w/skim milk	8 fl oz	200	36	1.3
French vanilla, mix only	1 scoop	100	24	1.0
French vanilla, prepared w/8 oz nonfat milk	1 serving	190	36	1.0
milk chocolate shake, prepared w/skim milk	8 fl oz	210	36	1.3
'Mixes w/Fruit Juice' mix only	1 scoop	90	17	0.0
'Mixes w/Fruit Juice' prepared w/orange juice	8 fl oz	200	43	1.0
'Plus' chocolate, mix only	1 scoop	120	33	1.0
'Plus' chocolate, prepared w/nonfat milk	12 fl oz	250	50	2.0
'Plus' piña colada flavor, mix only	1.16 oz	90	24	1.0
'Plus' piña colada flavor, prepared w/nonfat milk	8 fl oz	190	38	1.0
'Plus' strawberry jubilee, mix only	1 scoop	110	32	1.0
'Plus' strawberry jubilee, prepared w/nonfat milk	12 fl oz	240	50	2.0
strawberry shake, prepared w/skim milk	8 fl oz	200	36	1.3
vanilla shake, prepared w/skim milk	8 fl oz	200	33	0.7
(Weider)				
beef protein drink, mix only	1 cup	420	39	0.0
beef protein drink, prepared w/nonfat milk	8 fl oz	165	19	0.0
'Big' chocolate malt, sugar-free, mix only	4 scoops	320	58	2.0
'Big' chocolate malt, sugar-free, prepared w/milk	16 fl oz	620	81	18.0
'Carbo Energizer' orange flavor, mix only	4 scoops	230	58	0.0
'Crash Weight Gain No. 7' vanilla, mix only	4 round tbsp	300	61	3.0
'Crash Weight Gain No. 7' vanilla, prepared w/milk	16 fl oz	610	83	21.0
'Dynamic Body Shaper' Dutch chocolate, mix only	2 scoops	110	12	1.0
'Dynamic Body Shaper' Dutch chocolate, mix only	2 scoops	190	24	1.0
'Dynamic Body Shaper' mix only	1 cup	420	66	1.5
'Dynamic Body Shaper' prepared w/nonfat milk	8 fl oz	173	26	0.7
'Dynamic Muscle Builder' chocolate, mix only	2 scoops	200	21	1.0
'Dynamic Muscle Builder' chocolate, natural, mix only	2 scoops	120	9	1.0
'Dynamic Muscle Builder' chocolate, prepared	11 fl oz	220	36	1.0
'Dynamic Muscle Builder' mix only	1/3 cup	190	27	0.0
'Dynamic Muscle Builder' mix only	3 heaping tbsp	100	6	0.0
'Dynamic Muscle Builder' prepared w/whole milk	8 fl oz	250	17	9.0
'Dynamic Muscle Builder' prepared w/skim milk	8 fl oz	206	29	0.3
'Dynamic Muscle Builder' vanilla, natural, mix only	2 scoops	120	9	1.0

Food Name	Serv. Size	Total Cal.	Carbs GMS	Fat GMS
'Dynamic Protein' vanilla, mix only	2 scoops	100	10	0.0
'Dynamic Protein' vanilla, prepared w/skim milk	8 fl oz	190	22	1.0
'Dynamic Weight Gainer 1250' milkshake, prepared w/water	16 fl oz	330	61	1.0
'Dynamic Weight Gainer 1250' milkshake, prepared w/whole milk	16 fl oz	630	84	17.0
'Dynamic Weight Gainer 1250' milkshake, prepared w/whole milk	32 fl oz	1250	168	34.0
'Dynamic Weight Gainer' chocolate, prepared	11 fl oz	280	48	2.0
'Dynamic Weight Gainer' Dutch chocolate, mix only	4 scoops	320	61	1.0
'Dynamic Weight Gainer' mix only	1 cup	660	124	1.0
'Dynamic Weight Gainer' peanut butter, mix only	4 scoops	330	61	2.0
'Dynamic Weight Gainer' prepared w/whole milk	1 cup	252	34	6.6
'Dynamic Weight Gainer' vanilla, mix only	4 tbsp	310	54	2.0
'Dynamic Weight Gainer' vanilla, prepared w/milk	16 fl oz	630	76	20.0
'Dynamic' vanilla, natural, prepared w/skim milk	16 fl oz	200	21	1.0
egg protein drink, mix only	1 cup	360	27	0.0
egg protein drink, prepared w/nonfat milk	8 fl oz	150	16	0.0
'Fat Burner System' mix only	1/3 cup	110	11	1.0
'Fat Burner System' prepared w/skim milk	8 fl oz	146	17	1.1
'Giant Mega Mass 4000' mix only	1 cup	547	106	1.3
'Giant Mega Mass 4000' prepared w/low-fat milk	8 fl oz	336	59	3.0
'Mass 1000' mix only	1 cup	513	104	0.7
'Mass 1000' prepared w/low-fat milk	8 fl oz	290	51	2.9
'90% Plus Protein' chocolate malt, mix only	3 heaping tbsp	180	12	1.0
'90% Plus Protein' chocolate malt, sugar-free, mix only	3 heaping tbsp	100	0	0.0
'90-Plus Protein' vanilla, sugar-free, mix only	2 scoops	100	1	0.0
'90-Plus Protein' vanilla, sugar-free, prepared w/skim milk	8 fl oz	190	13	1.0
'Nitro-Fire' protein blend, mix only	2 tbsp	110	17	1.0
'Nitro-Fire' protein blend, prepared w/skim milk	8 fl oz	190	29	1.0
'Performance Builder' mix only	1 cup	601	93	3.0
'Performance Builder' prepared w/skim milk	8 fl oz	218	32	1.1
'Performance Shaper' mix only	1 cup	450	66	1.5
'Performance Shaper' prepared w/skim milk	1 cup	180	26	0.7
'Performance Weight Gainer' mix only	1 cup	585	117	1.5
'Performance Weight Gainer' prepared w/low-fat milk	8 fl oz	306	54	0.9
'Protein Blast' chocolate, prepared	11.5 fl oz	270	44	1.0
'Signature Line Dynamic Muscle Builder' mix only	2 scoops	120	9	1.0
'Sports Food Enerquench' lemon-lime, prepared	8 fl oz	60	15	0.0
'Sports Food Enerquench' orange flavor, prepared	8 fl oz	60	15	0.0
'Sports Foods Gainer' chocolate supreme, prepared w/water	1 serving	300	53	3.0
'Sports Foods Gainer' chocolate, prepared w/skim milk	1 serving	460	77	3.0
'Sports Foods Gainer' vanilla frost, prepared w/water	1 serving	300	53	3.0
'Sports Foods Gainer' vanilla, prepared w/skim milk	1 serving	460	77	3.0
'Sports Foods Gainer' wild strawberry, prepared w/skim milk	1 serving	460	77	3.0
'Sports Foods Gainer' wild strawberry, prepared w/water	1 serving	300	53	3.0
'Sports Gainer' French vanilla, prepared w/skim milk	12 fl oz	460	77	3.0
'Sports Gainer' French vanilla, prepared w/water	12 fl oz	300	53	3.0
'Sports Gainer' strawberry, prepared w/skim milk	16 fl oz	460	77	3.0
'Sports Gainer' strawberry, prepared w/water	12 fl oz	300	53	3.0
'Sports Line Power Shake' Dutch chocolate, prepared	11 fl oz	220	37	1.0
'Super Mega Mass 2000' banana, mix only	1 cup	547	106	1.5
'Super Mega Mass 2000' banana, prepared w/low-fat milk	8 fl oz	334	59	3.1
'Super Mega Mass 2000' chocolate, mix only	1 cup	547	106	1.5
'Super Mega Mass 2000' chocolate, prepared w/low-fat milk	8 fl oz	334	59	3.1
'Super Mega Mass 2000' strawberry, mix only	1 cup	547	106	1.5
'Super Mega Mass 2000' strawberry, prepared w/low-fat milk	8 fl oz	334	59	3.1
'Super Mega Mass 2000' vanilla, mix only	1 cup	547	106	1.5

Food Name	Serv. Size	Total Cal.	Carbs GMS	Fat GMS
'Super Mega Mass 2000' vanilla, prepared w/low-fat milk	8 fl oz	334	59	3.1
vegetable protein drink, mix only	1 cup	390	42	0.0
vegetable protein drink, prepared w/nonfat milk	8 fl oz	158	20	0.0
'Victory CarboFire' prepared w/water	8 fl oz	250	62	0.0
'Victory Explosive Workout' citrus, mix only	4 tbsp	190	48	0.0
'Victory Mass 1000' vanilla, prepared w/low-fat milk	16 fl oz	1020	180	11.0
'Victory Mass 1000' vanilla, prepared w/water	16 fl oz	770	156	1.0
'Victory Mega Mass 2000' prepared w/low-fat milk	24 fl oz	2000	351	19.0
'Victory Mega Mass 2000' prepared w/water	16 fl oz	1090	211	3.0
'Victory Mega Mass 2000' prepared w/water	24 fl oz	1640	317	5.0
'Victory Mega Mass 2000' prepared w/water	8 fl oz	550	106	2.0
(Weight Watchers)				
'Sweet Success' chocolate raspberry, mix only	1 scoop	90	11	2.0
'Sweet Success' vanilla flavor, mix only	1 scoop	90	20	0.5
SPOT				
baked, broiled, grilled, or microwaved	3 oz	134	0	5.3
raw	3 oz	105	0	4.2
SPRING ONION. See SCALLION.				
SQUAB				
average of all parts, meat and skin, raw	3 oz	252	0	20.4
average of all parts, meat only, raw	3 oz	122	0	6.4
light meat, meat only, raw	3 oz	115	0	3.9
SQUASH. See also ZUCCHINI.				
ACORN				
baked, cubed	1 cup	115	30	0.3
boiled, mashed	1 cup	83	22	0.2
raw, approx 4-inch diam	1 squash	172	45	0.4
raw, cubed	1 cup	56	15	0.1
raw, cubed (Frieda of California)	1 oz	16	4	0.1
BANANA, baked (Frieda of California)	1 oz	18	4	0.1
BUTTERNUT				
Fresh				
baked, cubed	1 cup	82	22	0.2
raw, cubed	1 cup	63	16	0.1
Frozen				
boiled, mashed	1 cup	94	24	0.2
unprepared	12-oz pkg	194	49	0.3
unprepared	4-lb pkg	1034	261	1.8
unprepared (Flav-R-Pac)	1/3 cup	30	8	0.0
CROOKNECK				
Canned, yellow (Allens)	1/2 cup	16	3	1.0
Frozen				
cooked (Kohl's)	4 oz	45	11	1.0
yellow (Seabrook)	3.3 oz	18	4	0.0
yellow (Southern)	3.5 oz	21	4	0.1
HUBBARD				
Fresh				
baked, cubed	1 cup	103	22	1.3
boiled, mashed	1 cup	71	15	0.9
raw, cubed	1 cup	46	10	0.6
MARROW/vegetable marrow				
raw, trimmed	1 oz	4	1.0	<.1
SCALLOP				
boiled, mashed	1 cup	38	8	0.4
boiled, sliced	1 cup	29	6	0.3
raw, sliced	1 cup	23	5	0.3

Food Name	Serv. Size	Total Cal.	Carbs GMS	Fat GMS
SPAGHETTI				
boiled or baked, drained	1 cup	42	10	0.4
raw, cubed	1 cup	31	7	0.6
SUMMER. See also ZUCCHINI.				
Canned				
crookneck or straightneck, no salt added, mashed, drained	1 cup	31	7	0.2
crookneck or straightneck, no salt added, diced, drained	1 cup	27	6	0.1
crookneck or straightneck, no salt added, drained	1 cup	28	6	0.2
Fresh				
all varieties, boiled, drained, sliced	1 cup	36	8	0.6
all varieties, raw, sliced	1 cup	23	5	0.2
all varieties, raw, whole	1 large	65	14	0.7
all varieties, raw, whole	1 medium	39	9	0.4
all varieties, raw, whole	1 small	24	5	0.2
crookneck or straightneck, boiled, drained, sliced	1 cup	36	8	0.6
crookneck or straightneck, drained, solid, sliced	1/2 cup	18	4	0.3
crookneck or straightneck, raw, sliced	1 cup	25	5	0.3
Frozen				
crookneck or straightneck, drained, sliced	1 cup	48	11	0.4
crookneck or straightneck, sliced, unprepared	1 cup	26	6	0.2
WINTER				
Fresh				
all varieties, baked, cubed	1 cup	80	18	1.3
all varieties, raw, cubed	1 cup	43	10	0.3
Frozen				
cooked *(Birds Eye)*	4 oz	45	11	0.0
cooked *(Seabrook)*	4 oz	45	11	0.0
YELLOW, frozen, sliced *(Flav-R-Pac)* sliced	2/3 cup	15	2	0.0
SQUASH DISH/ENTRÉE				
(Stouffer's) casserole, frozen, food service product	1 oz	35	2	2.1
SQUASH SEED				
dried, kernels	1 cup	747	25	63.3
dried, kernels, hulled, approx 142 seeds	1 oz	153	5	13.0
roasted, kernels	1 cup	1185	30	95.6
roasted, kernels	1 oz	148	4	11.9
roasted, whole	1 cup	285	34	12.4
roasted, whole, approx 85 seeds	1 oz	126	15	5.5
SQUID/calamari				
mixed species, fried	3 oz	149	7	6.4
mixed species, raw	3 oz	78	3	1.2
mixed species, raw, boneless	1 oz	26	1	0.4
SQUIRREL				
raw	1 oz	34	0	0.9
roasted	3 oz	147	0	4.0
STAR FRUIT/carambola				
raw, cubed	1 cup	45	11	0.5
raw, sliced	1 cup	36	8	0.4
raw, whole, large, approx 4.5-inch long	1 fruit	42	10	0.4
raw, whole, medium, approx 3 5/8 inch long	1 fruit	30	7	0.3
raw, whole, small, approx 3-inch long	1 fruit	23	5	0.2
STEAK SAUCE. See under SAUCE.				
STEW. See also under individual types of dinner/entrée listings.				
(Stouffer's) Cajun seasoned, frozen, food service product	1 oz	24	2	1.4
STIR-FRY ENTRÉE KIT				
(Tyson)				
	9 oz	230	15	9.0
'Yoshida Oriental Sauce'	1.6 oz	100	22	1.0

Food Name	Serv. Size	Total Cal.	Carbs GMS	Fat GMS
STIR-FRY SEASONING. See under SEASONING MIX.				
STRAW MUSHROOM. See MUSHROOM, STRAW.				
STRAWBERRY				
Canned, in heavy syrup, w/liquid	1 cup	234	60	0.7
Fresh				
raw, halved	1 cup	46	11	0.6
raw, puréed	1 cup	70	16	0.9
raw, sliced	1 cup	50	12	0.6
raw, trimmed	1 pint	107	25	1.3
raw, whole	1 cup	43	10	0.5
raw, whole, extra large, approx 1 5/8 inch diam.	1 berry	8	2	0.1
raw, whole, large, approx 1 3/8 inch diam.	1 berry	5	1	0.1
raw, whole, medium, approx 1 1/4 inch diam	1 berry	4	1	0.0
raw, whole, small, approx 1 inch diam	1 berry	2	0	0.0
Frozen				
sliced *(Flav-R-Pac)*	1/2 cup	150	33	1.5
sliced, sweetened	10-oz pkg	273	74	0.4
sliced, sweetened, thawed	1 cup	245	66	0.3
whole *(Flav-R-Pac)*	1 cup	50	13	1.0
whole, sweetened	10-oz pkg	222	60	0.4
whole, sweetened, thawed	1 cup	199	54	0.4
whole, unsweetened	1 med berry	4	1	0.0
whole, unsweetened	20-oz pkg	198	52	0.6
whole, unsweetened, thawed	1 cup	77	20	0.2
whole, unsweetened, unthawed	1 cup	52	14	0.2
STRAWBERRY COLADA. See under COCKTAIL MIX.				
STRAWBERRY DRINK. See under FRUIT DRINK; FRUIT JUICE BLEND; FRUIT JUICE DRINK.				
STRAWBERRY GUAVA. See GUAVA, STRAWBERRY.				
STRAWBERRY TOPPING				
	1 cup	864	225	0.3
	2 tbsp	107	28	0.0
(Flav-R-Pac)	2 tbsp	40	10	0.0
(Kraft) nonfat	1 tbsp	50	14	0.0
(Smucker's)				
nonfat	2 tbsp	120	30	0.0
nonfat, 'Light'	2 tbsp	55	14	0.0
STRAWBERRY TOPPING, pourable *(Knudsen)*	1 oz	75	18	1.0
STRING BEAN. See BEAN, GREEN.				
STRIPED BASS. See BASS, STRIPED.				
STRIPED MULLET. See MULLET, STRIPED.				
STROGANOFF ENTRÉE. See under BEEF DINNER/ENTRÉE; BEEF SUBSTITUTE DINNER/ENTRÉE MIX.				
STUFFING				
(Stouffer's) frozen, food service product, 'Old Fashion Stuff'n'	1 oz	70	7	4.0
STUFFING MIX				
(Brownberry) sage and onion, mix only	1 serving	255	47	3.4
(Pepperidge Farm)				
apple and raisin, mix only	1/2 cup	140	27	1.5
country garden and herb, mix only	1/2 cup	150	22	5.0
harvest vegetable and herb, mix only	1/2 cup	140	23	3.0
(Stove Top)				
chicken-flavored, 'Flexible Serving' prepared	1/2 cup	120	19	3.0
chicken flavored, 'Flexible Serving' prepared w/margarine	1/2 cup	170	20	9.0
cornbread, 'Flexible Serving' prepared	1/2 cup	110	19	2.5
cornbread, 'Flexible Serving' prepared w/margarine	1/2 cup	170	21	8.0
for beef, prepared w/margarine	1/2 cup	180	22	9.0
for turkey, prepared w/margarine	1/2 cup	170	20	9.0

Food Name	Serv. Size	Total Cal.	Carbs GMS	Fat GMS
STURGEON				
mixed species, baked, broiled, grilled, or microwaved	3 oz	115	0	4.4
mixed species, baked, broiled, grilled, or microwaved, flaked	1 cup	184	0	7.0
mixed species, raw	3 oz	89	0	3.4
mixed species, smoked	3 oz	147	0	3.7
mixed species, smoked	1 oz	49	0	1.2
SUCCOTASH. See under VEGETABLE DISH/ENTRÉE.				
SUCKER, WHITE				
baked, broiled, grilled, or microwaved	3 oz	101	0	2.5
raw	3 oz	78	0	2.0
SUET				
beef, raw	4 oz	965	0	106.2
beef, raw	1 oz	242	0	26.6
SUGAR				
BEET				
granulated *(Crystal)*	1 tsp	16	4	0.0
granulated juice, organic *(Sucanat)*	1 tsp	12	3	0.0
CANE				
Brown				
dark brown 'Old Fashioned' *(Domino)*	1 tsp	16	4	0.0
golden brown, Hawaiian *(C&H)*	1 tsp	16	4	0.0
granulated	1 tsp	12	3	0.0
light brown, golden, packed *(Domino)*	1 tsp	16	4	0.0
light brown, granulated, 'Brownulated' *(Domino)*	1 tsp	12	3	0.0
packed	1 cup	827	214	0.0
packed	1 tsp	17	4	0.0
unpacked	1 cup	545	141	0.0
unpacked	1 tsp	11	3	0.0
White				
confectioner's, sifted, 10-X powdered *(Domino)*	1/2 cup	240	60	0.0
confectioner's/powdered	1 tsp	10	2	0.0
confectioner's/powdered, unsifted	1 cup	467	119	0.1
confectioner's/powdered, unsifted	1 tbsp	31	8	0.0
cubes	1 cube	19	5	0.0
cubes, 'Dots' *(Domino)*	1 cube	8	2	0.0
granulated	1 cup	774	200	0.0
granulated	1 tsp	16	4	0.0
granulated *(Crystal)*	1 tsp	16	4	0.0
granulated *(Domino)*	1 tsp	16	4	0.0
granulated, 'Packets' *(Domino)*	1 pkt	16	4	0.0
granulated juice, organic *(Succanat)*	1 tsp	12	3	0.0
superfine, instant-dissolving *(Domino)*	1 tsp	16	4	0.0
MAPLE				
	1 oz	100	26	0.1
	1 tsp	11	3	0.0
approx 1.75 x 1.25 x 1/2 inch pieces	1 piece	99	25	0.1
TURBINADO *(Hain)*	1 tbsp	50	12	0.0
SUGAR APPLE/sweetsop				
raw, pulp	1 cup	235	59	0.7
raw, whole, approx 2 7/8 inch diam	1 fruit	146	37	0.4
SUGAR CANE BATON				
(Frieda of California)	1 oz	21	50	0.1
(Sprinkle Sweet)	1 tsp	2	1	0.0
SUGAR SNAP PEAS. See PEAS, SNAP.				
SUGAR SUBSTITUTE				
(Featherweight)				
liquid	3 drops	0	0	0.0

Food Name	Serv. Size	Total Cal.	Carbs GMS	Fat GMS
saccharin grain tablet	1/4 tablet	0	0	0.0
(Nutra Taste) w/o saccharin	1 pkt	4	1	0.0
(NutraSweet)				
w/aspartame, 'Equal'	1 pkt	4	1	0.0
w/aspartame, 'Equal'	1 tsp	12	3	0.0
(S&W) liquid, 'Nutradiet'	1/8 tsp	0	0	0.0
(Splenda)	1 tsp	2	1	0.0
(Sprinkle Sweet)	1 tsp	2	1	0.0
(Sucanat) juice, organic	1 tsp	12	3	0.0
(Sugar Twin)				
w/saccharin	1 pkt	4	1	0.0
w/saccharin, 'Plus'	1 pkt	3	1	0.0
(Superose)				
liquid	1 tsp	0	0	0.0
	1 tsp	4	1	0.0
(Sweet 'n Low) saccharin-based	1 pkt	4	1	0.0
(Sweet 10)				
	1/8 tsp	0	0	0.0
liquid	1 tsp	0	0	0.0
(Sweet One)	1 pkt	4	1	0.0
(Sweet Plus) w/saccharin, equivalent to 2 tsp sugar	1 pkt	4	1	0.0
(TKI Foods) w/aspartame, 'Superose Plus'	1 serving	0	1	0.0
(Weight Watchers) 'Sweet'ner'	1 pkt	4	1	0.0

SUMMER SQUASH. See under SQUASH. See also ZUCCHINI.

SUNCHOKE. See JERUSALEM ARTICHOKE.

SUNDAE. See under ICE CREAM BAR/DESSERT; ICE CREAM SUBSTITUTE BAR/DESSERT.

SUNFISH/calico bass/crappie/pumpkinfish

baked, broiled, grilled, or microwaved	3 oz	97	0	0.8
raw	3 oz	76	0	0.6

SUN-DRIED TOMATO. See under TOMATO.

SUNFLOWER BUTTER

	1 oz	164	8	13.5
	1 tbsp	93	4	7.6
unsalted	1 oz	164	8	13.5
unsalted	1 tbsp	93	4	7.6
(Maranatha Natural) roasted	2 tbsp	170	8	14.0
(Roaster Fresh)				
gourmet	1 oz	160	5	13.6
roasted, w/o salt, creamy	1 oz	160	5	14.0

SUNFLOWER SEED

Dried

(Frito-Lay's)	1 oz	160	6	14.0
kernels *(Arrowhead Mills)*	1 oz	160	6	13.0
kernels	1 cup	821	27	71.4
kernels, in shell	1 cup	262	9	22.8
kernels, shelled *(National Sunflower)*	1/4 cup	205	6	18.0
natural, unsalted *(Flanigan Farms)*	1/4 cup	160	5	14.0
salted, in shell *(Fisher)*	1 oz	170	6	14.0
salted, in shell, 15–16 shelled seeds *(Fisher)*	1 oz	160	6	14.0
unsalted *(Fisher)*	1 oz	170	6	14.0

Dry-roasted

(Fisher)	1 oz	170	6	15.0
(Planters)	1 oz	160	6	14.0
in shell *(Fisher)*	1 oz	170	6	15.0
kernels *(Flavor House)*	1 oz	180	4	15.0
kernels *(Pathmark)*	1 oz	180	7	14.0
kernels, hulled, unsalted	1 cup	745	31	63.7

Food Name	Serv. Size	Total Cal.	Carbs GMS	Fat GMS
kernels, salted	1 cup	745	31	63.7
kernels, salted	1 oz	165	7	14.1
kernels, shelled (Pathmark)	1 oz	180	7	14.0
kernels, unsalted	1 oz	165	7	14.1
w/tamari (Eden Foods)	1 oz	170	9	11.0
Oil-roasted				
(Fisher)	1 oz	170	4	16.0
(Planters)	1 oz	170	5	15.0
kernels, salted	1 cup	830	20	77.6
kernels, salted	1 oz	174	4	16.3
kernels, shelled, salted	1 cup	830	20	77.6
kernels, unsalted	1 cup	830	20	77.6
kernels, unsalted	1 oz	174	4	16.3
Roasted				
barbecue, salted, w/shell (David's)	3/4 cup	190	5	15.0
barbecue, salted, shelled (David's)	3/4 cup	190	5	15.0
salted, shelled (David's)	3/4 cup	190	5	15.0
salted, w/shell (David's)	3/4 cup	190	5	15.0
salted (Harmony)	1/4 cup	170	11	13.0
Toasted				
kernels, salted	1 cup	829	28	76.1
kernels, salted	1 oz	175	6	16.1
kernels, unsalted	1 cup	829	28	76.1
kernels, unsalted	1 oz	175	6	16.1
SUNFLOWER SEED OIL				
(Hain)	1 tbsp	120	0	14.0
(IGA)	1 tbsp	120	0	14.0
(Kroger)	1 tbsp	122	0	13.6
(Pathmark)	1 tbsp	130	0	14.0
at least 60% linoleic	1 cup	1927	0	218.0
at least 60% linoleic	1 tbsp	120	0	13.6
less than 60% linoleic	1 cup	1927	0	218.0
less than 60% linoleic	1 tbsp	120	0	13.6
linoleic, hydrogenated	1 cup	1927	0	218.0
linoleic, hydrogenated	1 tbsp	120	0	13.6
pure pressed, organic (Spectrum)	1 tbsp	120	0	14.0

SURIMI. See under CRAB SUBSTITUTE; SCALLOP SUBSTITUTE.
SURINAM CHERRY. See PITANGA.
SWAMP CABBAGE. See CABBAGE, SKUNK.
SWEET CHESTNUT. See CHESTNUT, EUROPEAN.
SWEET PEPPER. See PEPPER, BELL.
SWEET POTATO

Food Name	Serv. Size	Total Cal.	Carbs GMS	Fat GMS
Fresh				
baked in skin	1 cup	206	49	0.2
baked in skin	1 large	185	44	0.2
baked in skin	1 medium	117	28	0.1
baked in skin	1 small	62	15	0.1
boiled, w/o skin	1 medium	159	37	0.5
boiled, w/o skin, mashed	1 cup	344	80	1.0
raw, approx 5-inch long	1 potato	137	32	0.4
raw, cubed	1 cup	140	32	0.4
Canned				
cut, in water (Allens)	1/2 cup	70	16	1.0
mashed	1 cup	258	59	0.5
mashed (Joan of Arc)	1/2 cup	90	24	0.0
mashed (Princella)	1/2 cup	90	24	0.0
mashed (Royal Prince)	1/2 cup	90	24	0.0

Food Name	Serv. Size	Total Cal.	Carbs GMS	Fat GMS
mashed, vacuum pack	1 cup	232	54	0.5
pieces, vacuum pack	1 cup	182	42	0.4
syrup pack, drained	1 cup	212	50	0.6
syrup pack, w/liquid	1 cup	203	48	0.5
whole, vacuum pack *(Taylor's Brand)*	1 cup	210	55	0.0
Frozen				
cubes	1 cup	169	39	0.3
whipped, food service product *(Stouffer's)*	1 oz	40	7	1.4
SWEET POTATO LEAF				
Fresh				
raw, whole, 12.25-inch leaf	1 leaf	6	1	0.0
raw, chopped	1 cup	12	2	0.1
steamed, chopped	1 cup	22	5	0.2

SWEETBREAD. See BEEF, PANCREAS; BEEF THYMUS; LAMB, PANCREAS; VEAL, PANCREAS; VEAL, THYMUS.

SWEETENER. See BARLEY MALT; CORN SYRUP; HONEY; SUGAR, BEET; SUGAR, CANE BATON; SUGAR, MAPLE; SUGAR SUBSTITUTE; SYRUP.

SWEETSOP. See SUGAR APPLE.

Food Name	Serv. Size	Total Cal.	Carbs GMS	Fat GMS
SWISS CHARD/chard				
Fresh				
boiled, drained, chopped	1 cup	35	7	0.1
raw, chopped	1 cup	7	1	0.1
raw, whole	1 med leaf	9	2	0.1
SWORDFISH				
Fresh				
baked, broiled, grilled, or microwaved	3 oz	132	0	4.4
raw	3 oz	103	0	3.4
Frozen				
steaks, boneless, raw *(Peter Pan Seafoods)*	3.5 oz	118	0	4.0
steaks, w/o seasoning mix *(SeaPak)*	6-oz pkg	210	0	7.0
SYRUP				
BLACKBERRY *(Knott's Berry Farm)*	1 oz	120	30	0.0
BLUEBERRY				
(Estee) 'Breakfast'	1 tbsp	12	3	0.0
(Featherweight)	1 tbsp	16	4	0.0
(Knott's Berry Farm)				
	1 oz	120	30	0.0
'Light'	1 oz	50	12	0.0
(Knudsen)	1 oz	75	19	1.0
(S&W) lower calorie	1/4 cup	60	15	0.0
BOYSENBERRY				
(Knott's Berry Farm)				
	1 oz	120	30	0.0
'Light'	1 oz	50	12	0.0
BUTTER FLAVOR *(S&W)* lower calorie	1/4 cup	60	15	0.0
CHOCOLATE				
(Estee) 'Choco-Syp'	1 tbsp	20	5	0.0
(Hershey's) light, genuine chocolate	2 tbsp	50	12	0.1
(Nestlé) 'Quik'	2 tbsp	100	23	0.5
(Smucker's)	2 tbsp	130	27	2.0
FRUIT *(Smucker's)* all flavors	2 tbsp	100	26	0.0
MALT				
	1 cup	1221	273.8	0.0
	1 tbsp	76	17.1	0.0
(Eden Foods) barley, organic, w/sprouted barley	1 tbsp	60	14	0.0
MAPLE				
	1 cup	825	212	0.6
	1 tbsp	52	13	0.0

Food Name	Serv. Size	Total Cal.	Carbs GMS	Fat GMS
(Estee) 'Breakfast'	1 tbsp	12	3	0.0
(Knudsen) 'Fruit 'N Maple'	1 oz	105	26	1.0
(Maple House)				
100% pure	1 oz	100	61	0.0
no sugar	2 tbsp	110	27	0.0
(Maple Valley) no sugar, 'Lite'	2 tbsp	60	16	0.0
(Pillsbury)				
butter	1/4 cup	210	52	0.0
butter, lite	1/4 cup	100	24	0.0
lite	1/4 cup	100	24	0.0
regular	1/4 cup	210	52	0.0
(S&W) no sugar, saccharin sweetened	1 tsp	4	1	0.0
MAPLE FLAVOR *(S&W)* lower calorie	1/4 cup	60	15	0.0
PANCAKE				
cane and maple, 15% maple	1 cup	879	237	0.3
cane and maple, 15% maple	1 tbsp	56	15	0.0
cane and maple, 2% maple	1 cup	835	219	0.3
cane and maple, 2% maple	1 tbsp	53	14	0.0
(Aunt Jemima)				
'Butter Rich'	1/4 cup	210	52	0.0
'Butterlite'	1/4 cup	100	26	0.0
'Lite'	1 oz	54	13	0.1
lite, lower calorie, 3% real maple syrup	1/4 cup	100	27	0.0
'Original' rich maple taste	1 oz	100	26	0.0
pancake/waffle	1/4 cup	210	53	0.0
(Br'er Rabbit)				
dark	1 oz	120	31	0.0
light	1 oz	120	31	0.0
(Cary's) sugar-free, lower calorie, artificial maple	1/4 cup	35	9	0.0
(Estee)	1 tbsp	4	1	0.0
(Featherweight)	1 tbsp	16	4	0.0
(Hungry Jack)				
	2 tbsp	100	26	0.0
light, microwaveable	1/4 cup	100	24	0.0
lite	2 tbsp	50	14	0.0
microwaveable	1/4 cup	210	52	0.0
(Karo)	4 tbsp	234	59	0.0
(Knott's Berry Farm)				
	1 oz	110	28	0.0
'Country'	1 oz	110	27	0.0
'Light' microwaveable	1 oz	45	11	0.0
lower calorie, microwave, 'Heat & Pour'	1 oz	45	11	0.0
microwave, 'Heat & Pour'	1 oz	110	28	0.0
w/30% real maple, microwaveable	1 oz	110	28	0.0
(Log Cabin)				
butter flavor, 'Country Kitchen'	1 oz	100	27	0.0
'Country Kitchen'	1 oz	100	26	0.0
lite, lower calorie	1 oz	50	13	0.0
'Pancake & Waffle'	1 oz	100	26	0.0
syrup product 'Country Kitchen Lite'	1 oz	50	13	0.0
(Mrs. Butterworth's)				
lower calorie	1/4 cup	100	25	0.0
thick and rich, 'Lite'	2 tbsp	60	15	0.0
(S&W)				
butter flavor, reduced calorie	1/4 cup	60	15	0.0
maple flavor, reduced calorie	1/4 cup	60	15	0.0
(Vermont Maid)	1 tbsp	50	13	0.0

Food Name	Serv. Size	Total Cal.	Carbs GMS	Fat GMS
(Weight Watchers) lower calorie	1 tbsp	25	7	0.0
RASPBERRY *(Knudsen)*	1 oz	75	18	1.0
RICE *(Lundberg Family)* organic 'Sweet Dreams'	1 tbsp	42	10	1.0
SORGHUM				
	1 cup	957	247	0.0
	1 tbsp	61	16	0.0
STRAWBERRY				
(Knott's Berry Farm)	1 oz	120	30	0.0
(Knudsen & Sons)	1 oz	75	18	1.0
(Nestlé) 'Quik'	2 tbsp	110	27	0.0
(S&W)				
lower calorie	1/4 cup	60	15	0.0
w/Saccharin	1 tsp	4	1	0.0

T

Food Name	Serv. Size	Total Cal.	Carbs GMS	Fat GMS
TABBOULEH MIX. See under RICE DISH/ENTRÉE MIX.				
TACO				
(Owens)				
ham, refrigerated, 'Border Breakfasts'	2.17 oz	90	13	6.0
sausage, refrigerated, 'Border Breakfasts'	2.17 oz	190	11	12.0
TACO DINNER/ENTRÉE KIT				
(Pancho Villa)				
w/2 shells, seasoning, and sauce, mix only	1 serving	150	20	8.0
prepared	2 tacos	270	20	13.0
(Tio Sancho)				
taco sauce, 'Dinner Kit'	2 oz	62	13	0.2
taco seasoning, 'Dinner Kit'	1.25 oz	104	21	1.4
taco shell, 'Dinner Kit'	1 shell	64	8	3.1
TACO FILLING				
(Hunt's) 'Manwich'	1/4 cup	31	7	0.1
(Chili Bowl) beef	1/4 cup	150	4	11.0
(McCarty) chicken	1.29 oz	80	1	5.1
TACO MIX				
(Del Monte) starter	8 oz	140	28	1.0
(Natural Touch				
	3 tbsp	60	5	0.9
vegetarian	2 tbsp	90	6	2.0
(Old El Paso) prepared	1 taco	67	8	3.0
(Ortega) meat, prepared	1 oz	60	1	4.0
(Tio Sancho) 'Dinner Kit'	1 shell	64	8	3.1
TACO SALAD SEASONING. See under SEASONING MIX.				
TACO SEASONING MIX. See under SEASONING MIX.				
TACO SHELL				
baked	1 oz	133	18	6.4
baked, large, 6.5-inch dia.	1 shell	98	13	4.7
baked, medium, 5-inch diam	1 shell	62	8	3.0
baked, mini, 3-inch diam	1 shell	23	3	1.1
baked, no salt added	1 oz	133	18	6.4
baked, no salt added, medium, 5-inch diam	1 shell	61	8	2.9
baked, no salt added, mini, 3-inch diam	1 shell	23	3	1.1
(Aztoca)				
corn	1 shell	60	7	3.0
flour, for salad	1 shell	200	18	12.0

Food Name	Serv. Size	Total Cal.	Carbs GMS	Fat GMS
(Bearitos) blue corn	1 serving	130	17	7.0
(Chi-Chi's)	0.96 oz	140	17	7.0
(Gebhardt)	1 shell	52	6	2.8
(Lawry's)				
	1 shell	50	8	2.1
'Super'	1 shell	86	13	3.6
(Old El Paso)				
mini	3 shells	70	7	4.0
'Super'	2 shells	190	21	12.0
'Super Size'	1 shell	100	11	6.0
(Ortega)	1 shell	50	8	2.0
(Pancho Villa)	3 shells	190	19	11.0
(Rosarita)	1 serving	52	6	2.8
(Tio Sancho)				
	1 shell	64	8	3.1
'Super'	1 shell	94	11	4.7
TAFFY. See under CANDY.				
TAHINI. See SESAME BUTTER.				
TAHINI MIX				
(Arrowhead Mills) organic	1 oz	170	4	17.0
(Westbrae)				
Mid-Eastern, organic	2 tbsp	220	3	20.0
raw, organic	2 tbsp	210	1	19.0
toasted, organic	2 tbsp	220	3	19.0
TAMALE DINNER/ENTRÉE				
(Amy's Kitchen) pie, organic, frozen, 'Mexican'	8-oz pie	220	41	3.0
(Dennison's) in chili gravy, canned, 'Tamalito'	7.5 oz	310	37	16.0
(Derby)				
beef, canned	6.561 oz	253	21	17.4
beef, canned	2 tamales	160	15	7.0
(Gebhardt)				
	2 tamales	290	19	22.0
canned	5.75 oz	269	19	20.7
jumbo, canned	6.949 oz	332	24	25.2
jumbo, canned	1 serving	166	12	12.6
(Hormel)				
beef, canned	2 pieces	140	8	10.0
beef, canned, 'Hot'N Spicy'	2 pieces	140	9	10.0
beef, frozen	1 piece	140	13	7.0
canned	7.5 oz	280	19	20.0
hot-spicy, canned	7.5 oz	280	19	20.0
(Libby's) beef, w/sauce, canned	7.5 oz	408	26	30.2
(Old El Paso) canned	2 pieces	190	16	12.0
(Patio) frozen	13 oz	470	58	21.0
(Van Camp's) w/sauce, canned	1 cup	293	29	16.2
(Wolf Brand) canned	7.75 oz	328	25	24.5
TAMARI. See under SAUCE.				
TAMARIND/Indian date				
Fresh				
raw, pulp	1 cup	287	75	0.7
raw, whole, approx 1 x 3 inches	1 fruit	5	1	0.0
'Tamarindos' (Frieda of California)	3.5 oz	239	63	0.6
TANGERINE. See also MANDARIN ORANGE				
Fresh				
raw, sections	1 cup	86	22	0.4
raw, whole, large, approx 2.5-inch diam	1 fruit	43	11	0.2
raw, whole, medium, approx 2 3/8 inch diam	1 fruit	37	9	0.2

Food Name	Serv. Size	Total Cal.	Carbs GMS	Fat GMS
raw, whole, small, approx 2.25 inch diam	1 fruit	31	8	0.1
TANGERINE JUICE				
canned, sweetened	1 cup	125	30	0.5
canned, sweetened	1 fl oz	16	4	0.1
chilled, 'Pure & Light Mandarin Tangerine' (Dole)	6 fl oz	97	25	0.1
fresh, raw	1 cup	106	25	0.5
fresh, raw	1 fl oz	13	3	0.1
frozen concentrate, diluted	1 cup	111	27	0.3
frozen concentrate, diluted	1 fl oz	14	3	0.0
frozen concentrate, undiluted	6 fl oz	345	83	0.8
frozen or chilled (Minute Maid)	6 fl oz	90	23	0.0
TANNIA. See YAUTIA.				
TAPIOCA. See also under PUDDING.				
pearl, dry	1 cup	544	135	0.0
pearl, dry	1 oz	97	25.1	tr
TAQUITO beef, crispy, shredded				
(Prima Rosa by Ruiz)	5 taquitos	330	35	15.0
TARO				
cooked, sliced	1 cup	187	46	0.1
raw, sliced	1 cup	116	28	0.2
Tahitian, cooked, sliced	1 cup	60	9	0.9
Tahitian, raw, sliced	1 cup	55	9	1.2
TARO CHIPS				
	1 oz	141	19	7.1
	10 chips	115	16	5.7
salted (Ray's)	1 oz	139	20	6.0
unsalted (Ray's)	1 oz	139	20	6.0
TARO LEAF				
raw, chopped	1 cup	12	2	0.2
raw, whole, 11x6.5-inch leaf	1 leaf	4	1	0.1
steamed, chopped	1 cup	35	6	0.6
TARO SHOOT				
cooked, sliced	1 cup	20	4	0.1
raw, whole	1 med shoot	9	2	0.1
raw, sliced	1/2 cup	5	1	0.0
TARRAGON				
dried (McCormick/Schilling)	1 tsp	2	0	0.0
ground	1 tbsp	14	2	0.3
ground	1 tsp	5	1	0.1
ground (Spice Islands)	1 tsp	5	1	0.1
ground, fresh (Durkee)	1 tsp	10	0	0.0
ground, fresh (Laurel Leaf)	1 tsp	10	0	0.0
TEA				
BLACK				
Brewed				
decaffeinated, prepared w/tap water	6 fl oz	2	1	0.0
decaffeinated, prepared w/tap water	8 fl oz	2	1	0.0
regular, prepared w/distilled water	6 fl oz	2	1	0.0
regular, prepared w/tap water	6 fl oz	2	1	0.0
regular, prepared w/tap water	8 fl oz	2	1	0.0
(Bigelow)				
Darjeeling	5.25 fl oz	1	0	0.0
'Earl Grey'	5.25 fl oz	1	0	0.0
'English Teatime'	5.25 fl oz	1	0	0.0
(Celestial Seasonings)				
'Classic English Breakfast'	8 fl oz	3	0	0.0
decaffeinated	8 fl oz	4	1	0.0

Food Name	Serv. Size	Total Cal.	Carbs GMS	Fat GMS
'Extraordinary Earl Grey'	8 fl oz	3	1	0.0
(Exotica)				
'Assam Breakfast'	8 fl oz	0	0	0.0
'Ceylon Earl Grey'	8 fl oz	0	0	0.0
'Champagne Oolong'	8 fl oz	0	0	0.0
'China White'	8 fl oz	0	0	0.0
'Darjeeling'	8 fl oz	0	0	0.0
'Dragonwell'	8 fl oz	0	0	0.0
'Osmanthus'	8 fl oz	0	0	0.0
'Reserve Blend'	8 fl oz	0	0	0.0
'Silver Jasmine'	8 fl oz	0	0	0.0
(Lipton)				
black, regular	6 fl oz	0	0	0.0
black, w/lemon flavor	6 fl oz	3	1	0.0
(Stash's)				
'American'	8 fl oz	0	0	0.0
'China Black'	8 fl oz	0	0	0.0
'Earl Grey' decaffeinated	8 fl oz	0	0	0.0
'English Breakfast' decaffeinated	8 fl oz	0	0	0.0
'English Breakfast'	8 fl oz	0	0	0.0
'Oolong'	8 fl oz	0	0	0.0
'Orange Pekoe'	8 fl oz	0	0	0.0
Instant				
powder, unsweetened	1 tsp	2	0	0.0
powder, unsweetened, prepared	8 fl oz	2	0	0.0
(Lipton) decaffeinated, prepared	6 fl oz	0	0	0.0
GREEN, brewed *(Bigelow)* 'Chinese Fortune'	5.25 fl oz	1	0	0.0
HERBAL/FLAVORED				
Bagged				
(Good Earth)				
'Good Night' caffeine-free	1 bag	1	1	0.0
apple and spice, caffeine-free	1 bag	1	1	0.0
chamomile, caffeine-free	1 bag	1	0	0.0
fruit and spice, caffeine-free	1 bag	1	1	0.0
ginseng, caffeine-free	1 bag	1	0	0.0
lemon twist, caffeine-free	1 bag	2	1	0.0
orange spice, caffeine-free	1 bag	1	1	0.0
original flavor, caffeine-free	1 bag	4	0	0.0
original spice, caffeine-free	1 bag	4	1	0.0
(Super Dieters Tea)				
apricot, caffeine-free	1 bag	3	1	1.0
cinnamon spice, caffeine-free	1 bag	3	1	1.0
lemon mint, caffeine-free	1 bag	0	0	0.0
original flavor, caffeine-free	1 bag	3	1	1.0
peppermint, caffeine-free	1 bag	3	1	1.0
Brewed				
chamomile, brewed	6 fl oz	2	0	0.0
chamomile, brewed	8 fl oz	2	0	0.0
herbal, all types, except chamomile, brewed	6 fl oz	2	0	0.0
herbal, all types, except chamomile, brewed	8 fl oz	2	0	0.0
(Bigelow)				
almond orange	5 fl oz	1	0	0.0
'Apple Orchard'	5.25 fl oz	5	1	0.0
apple spice	5 fl oz	1	0	0.0
chamomile	5 fl oz	1	0	0.0
chamomile mint	5 fl oz	1	0	0.0
cinnamon orange	5 fl oz	1	0	0.0

Food Name	Serv. Size	Total Cal.	Carbs GMS	Fat GMS
'Cinnamon Stick'	5.25 fl oz	1	0	0.0
'Constant Comment'	5.25 fl oz	1	0	0.0
cranberry apple	5 fl oz	1	0	0.0
'Fruit & Almond'	5.25 fl oz	1	0	0.0
grains, roasted, w/carob	5 fl oz	3	1	0.0
hibiscus, w/rose hips	5 fl oz	1	0	0.0
'I Love Lemon'	5.25 fl oz	1	0	0.0
'Lemon & C'	5 fl oz	1	0	0.0
'Lemon Lift'	5.25 fl oz	1	0	0.0
'Mint Blend'	5 fl oz	1	0	0.0
'Mint Medley'	5.25 fl oz	1	0	0.0
'Orange & C'	5 fl oz	1	0	0.0
'Orange & Spice'	5.25 fl oz	1	0	0.0
peppermint	5 fl oz	1	0	0.1
'Plantation Mint'	5.25 fl oz	1	0	0.0
'Raspberry Royale'	5.25 fl oz	1	0	0.0
red raspberry	5 fl oz	1	0	0.0
spearmint	5 fl oz	1	0	0.0
'Specially Strawberry'	5 fl oz	1	0	0.0
'Sweet Dreams'	5.25 fl oz	1	0	0.0
'Take-A-Break'	5.25 fl oz	1	1	0.0
(Celestial Seasonings)				
'Almond Sunset'	8 fl oz	3	1	0.0
'Amaretto Nights'	8 fl oz	3	1	0.0
apple spice, 'Fruit & Tea'	8 fl oz	3	0	0.0
'Bavarian Chocolate Orange'	8 fl oz	7	2	0.0
chamomile	8 fl oz	2	1	0.0
'Cinnamon Apple Spice'	8 fl oz	3	0	0.0
'Cinnamon Rose'	8 fl oz	2	1	0.0
'Cinnamon Vienna'	8 fl oz	2	0	0.0
'Country Peach Spice'	8 fl oz	3	1	0.0
'Cranberry Cove'	8 fl oz	3	1	0.0
'Darjeeling Gardens'	8 fl oz	3	1	0.0
'Emperor's Choice'	8 fl oz	4	1	0.1
'Ginseng Plus'	8 fl oz	3	1	0.0
'Grandma's Tummy Mint'	8 fl oz	2	0	0.0
'Irish Cream Mist'	8 fl oz	3	1	0.0
lemon, 'Fruit & Tea'	8 fl oz	3	1	0.0
'Lemon Mist'	8 fl oz	2	1	0.0
'Lemon Zinger'	8 fl oz	4	1	0.0
'Mandarin Orange Spice'	8 fl oz	5	1	0.0
'Mellow Mint'	8 fl oz	2	0	0.0
'Mint Magic'	8 fl oz	1	0	0.0
'Mo's 24'	8 fl oz	2	0	0.0
'Morning Thunder'	8 fl oz	3	0	0.0
orange spice, 'Fruit & Tea'	8 fl oz	3	0	0.0
'Orange Zinger'	8 fl oz	5	1	0.0
peppermint	8 fl oz	2	1	0.0
raspberry, 'Fruit & Tea'	8 fl oz	2	1	0.0
'Raspberry Patch'	8 fl oz	4	1	0.0
'Red Zinger'	8 fl oz	4	1	0.0
'Roastaroma'	8 fl oz	11	2	0.1
'Sleepytime'	8 fl oz	5	1	0.0
spearmint	8 fl oz	5	0	0.1
'Strawberry Fields'	8 fl oz	4	1	0.0
'Sunburst C'	8 fl oz	3	1	0.0
'Swiss Mint'	8 fl oz	3	0	0.0

Food Name	Serv. Size	Total Cal.	Carbs GMS	Fat GMS
'Wild Forest Blackberry'	8 fl oz	2	2	0.0
(Glenny's) ginseng, 100% natural	42 grams	180	58	7.0
(Lipton)				
'Almond Pleasure'	8 fl oz	4	1	0.0
chamomile	8 fl oz	4	1	0.0
cinnamon apple	8 fl oz	2	1	0.0
'Citrus Sunset'	8 fl oz	4	1	0.0
'Gentle/Tangy Orange'	8 fl oz	4	1	0.0
'Lemon Soother'	8 fl oz	4	1	0.0
'Toasty Spice'	8 fl oz	6	1	0.0
(Stash's)				
'Apple Cinnamon'	8 fl oz	0	0	0.0
'Black Currant Ice'	8 fl oz	0	0	0.0
'Caravan'	8 fl oz	0	0	0.0
'Chamomile'	8 fl oz	0	0	0.0
'Citrus Spice'	8 fl oz	0	0	0.0
'Crepe Faire'	8 fl oz	0	0	0.0
'Estate'	8 fl oz	0	0	0.0
'Herbal Peach'	8 fl oz	0	0	0.0
'Irish Breakfast'	8 fl oz	0	0	0.0
'Jasmine Spice'	8 fl oz	0	0	0.0
'Lemon Blossom'	8 fl oz	0	0	0.0
'Lemon Spice'	8 fl oz	0	0	0.0
'Licorice Spice'	8 fl oz	0	0	0.0
'Moroccan Mint'	8 fl oz	0	0	0.0
'Orange Spice' decaffeinated	8 fl oz	0	0	0.0
'Orange Spice'	8 fl oz	0	0	0.0
'Oregon Mint'	8 fl oz	0	0	0.0
'Oriental Rose'	8 fl oz	0	0	0.0
'Peach'	8 fl oz	0	0	0.0
'Peppermint'	8 fl oz	0	0	0.0
'Premium Green'	8 fl oz	0	0	0.0
'Ruby Mist'	8 fl oz	0	0	0.0
'Sandman'	8 fl oz	0	0	0.0
'Tangerine'	8 fl oz	0	0	0.0
'Tropical Fruit'	8 fl oz	0	0	0.0
'Tropical Mist'	8 fl oz	0	0	0.0
'Wild Black Currant'	8 fl oz	0	0	0.0
'Wild Raspberry'	8 fl oz	0	0	0.0
'Wintermint'	8 fl oz	0	0	0.0
(Tetley)				
'Apple Freeze'	8 fl oz	79	20	0.0
'Classic'	8 fl oz	69	17	0.0
'Classic Lemon'	8 fl oz	108	27	0.0
'Diet Lemon Frost'	8 fl oz	10	2	0.0
'Diet Raspberry Blizzard'	8 fl oz	10	2	0.0
'Lemon Frost'	8 fl oz	89	22	0.0
'Orange Glazier'	8 fl oz	79	20	0.0
'Peach Chiller'	8 fl oz	79	20	0.0
'Raspberry Blizzard'	8 fl oz	95	24	0.0
Instant				
(Nature's Plus)				
Chinese herbal, citrus-flavored	1 tsp	24	6	0.0
Chinese herbal, decaffeinated, citrus-flavored, 'Chi'	1 tsp	24	6	0.0
TEA, ICED				
BLACK				
(Clinical Resource) 'Lemon Iced Tea'	8 fl oz	180	36	0.0

Food Name	Serv. Size	Total Cal.	Carbs GMS	Fat GMS
(Lipton)				
regular, w/natural lemon flavor	8.45 fl oz	96	24	0.3
w/lemon, sugar-free	8 fl oz	1	0	0.0
(Nestea)				
diet	8 fl oz	4	1	0.0
regular	8 fl oz	90	22	0.0
sweetened	16 fl oz	97	27	0.0
w/lemon, sugar-free	8 fl oz	2	1	0.0
w/lemon, sugar-sweetened	8 fl oz	70	17	0.0
natural	16 fl oz	180	44	0.0
natural	6 fl oz	66	17	0.0
(Shasta)	12 fl oz	124	34	0.0
(10-K)	8 fl oz	60	15	0.0
(Tetley)				
regular	8 fl oz	74	19	0.0
sweetened	8 fl oz	74	19	0.0
w/lemon	8 fl oz	74	19	0.0
(Thick & Easy)				
honey consistency	1/2 cup	70	17	0.0
nectar consistency	1/2 cup	60	16	0.0
(Veryfine) w/lemon	8 fl oz	80	16	0.0
HERBAL/FLAVORED				
(Fruitopia)				
'Born Raspberry'	16 fl oz	162	44	0.0
'Lemon Berry Intuition'	16 fl oz	166	44	0.0
'Peaceable Peach'	16 fl oz	162	44	0.0
(Knudsen)				
hibiscus, 'Iced Tea Cooler'	1 cup	90	23	0.0
blacklemon, 'Iced Tea Cooler'	1 cup	90	23	0.0
blackmango, 'Iced Tea Cooler'	1 cup	90	23	0.0
blackorange, 'Iced Tea Cooler'	1 cup	90	23	0.0
blackraspberry, 'Iced Tea Cooler'	1 cup	90	23	0.0
(Nestea)				
apple spice	16 fl oz	180	44	0.0
apple spice	6 fl oz	66	17	0.0
peach	16 fl oz	180	44	0.0
peach	6 fl oz	66	17	0.0
raspberry	16 fl oz	180	44	0.0
raspberry	6 fl oz	66	17	0.0
tropical	16 fl oz	180	44	0.0
tropical	6 fl oz	66	17	0.0
(Wyler's) 'Fruit Tea Punch'	12 fl oz	118	30	0.0
TEA, ICED, MIX				
BLACK				
(Crystal Light)				
decaffeinated, sugar-free, prepared	8 fl oz	4	0	0.0
sugar-free, prepared	8 fl oz	4	0	0.0
(Lipton)				
decaffeinated, sugar-free, prepared	8 fl oz	1	0	0.0
lemon flavor, decaffeinated, prepared	6 fl oz	55	14	0.0
lemon flavor, prepared	6 fl oz	55	14	0.0
lemon flavor, w/NutraSweet, prepared	8 fl oz	5	1	0.0
sugar-free, prepared	8 fl oz	1	0	0.0
sweet, no lemon, mix only	1 2/3 tbsp	70	17	0.0
sweet, sugar-free, no lemon, mix only	1 tbsp	0	1	0.0
(Nestea)				
decaffeinated, '100%' prepared	8 fl oz	0	0	0.0

Food Name	Serv. Size	Total Cal.	Carbs GMS	Fat GMS
lemon flavor, decaffeinated, sugar-free, mix only	2 tsp	6	1	0.0
lemon flavor, sugar-free, prepared	8 fl oz	4	1	0.0
'100%' mix only	1 tsp	2	0	0.0
'100%' prepared	8 fl oz	2	0	0.0
sugar-free, prepared	8 fl oz	6	1	0.0
w/sugar and lemon, prepared	8 fl oz	70	19	0.0
(Pathmark)				
lemon flavor, mix only	1 tsp	6	1	0.0
lemon flavor, artificially sweetened, mix only	1 tsp	4	1	0.0
lemon flavor, decaffeinated, low-calorie, prepared	8 fl oz	4	1	0.0
lemon flavor, decaffeinated, sugar-sweetened, mix only	2 tbsp	80	20	0.0
lemon flavor, low-calorie, prepared	8 fl oz	4	1	0.0
'No Frills' mix only	0.75 oz	70	21	0.0
HERBAL/FLAVORED				
(Lipton)				
tropical flavor, sugar-free, mix only	1 tbsp	5	1	0.0
tropical flavor, w/sugar, mix only	1 2/3 tbsp	90	22	0.0
(Nestea) all flavors, 'Ice Teasers' prepared	8 fl oz	6	1	0.0
(Soothing Moments)				
cinnamon apple, caffeine-free, mix only	1/2 tsp	5	1	0.0
gentle orange, caffeine-free, mix only	1/2 tsp	5	1	0.0
lemon soother, caffeine-free, mix only	1/2 tsp	5	1	0.0
TEASEED OIL				
	1 cup	1927	0	218.0
	1 tbsp	120	0	13.6
TEFF FLOUR. See under FLOUR.				
TEFF SEED *(Arrowhead Mills)*	2 oz	200	41	1.0
TEMPEH				
	1 cup	320	16	17.9
(White Wave)				
5-grain, vegetarian	1 piece	140	15	4.0
original, soy, vegetarian	1 piece	150	10	6.0
sea veggie, vegetarian	1 piece	120	11	3.0
soy rice, vegetarian	1 piece	140	13	5.0
wild rice, vegetarian	1 piece	140	12	4.0
TENDERGREEN. See MUSTARD SPINACH.				
TEQUILA				
80 proof	1 fl oz	65	0	0.0
86 proof	1 fl oz	70	0	0.0
90 proof	1 fl oz	74	0	0.0
94 proof	1 fl oz	77	0	0.0
100 proof	1 fl oz	83	0	0.0
TERIYAKI STIR-FRY ENTRÉE *(Lunch Express)*	1 entrée	260	39	5.0
TERRAPIN, diamondback, raw	100 gm	111	0.0	3.5
THYME, DRIED				
dried *(McCormick/Schilling)*	1 tsp	17	1	0.0
fresh	1 tsp	1	0	0.0
fresh	1/2 tsp	0	0	0.0
ground *(Spice Islands)*	1 tsp	5	1	0.1
ground	1 tbsp	12	3	0.3
ground	1 tsp	4	1	0.1
ground, fresh *(Durkee)*	1 tsp	5	0	0.0
ground, fresh *(Laurel Leaf)*	1 tsp	5	0	0.0
TILEFISH				
baked, broiled, grilled, or microwaved	3 oz	125	0	4.0
raw	3 oz	82	0	2.0
TOASTER BISCUIT. See BISCUIT, TOASTER.				

Food Name	Serv. Size	Total Cal.	Carbs GMS	Fat GMS
TOASTER PASTRY. See PASTRY, TOASTER.				
TOFU				
fried	1 oz	77	3	5.7
fuyu, salted and fermented	1 block	13	1	0.9
fuyu, salted and fermented, prepared w/calcium sulfate	1 block	13	1	0.9
okara	1 cup	94	15	2.1
(Nasoya)				
five-spice	1 piece	70	0	4.0
French country	1 piece	70	0	4.0
(White Wave) less fat	1 piece	90	4	4.0
EXTRA FIRM				
w/nigari	1/5 block	87	2	5.7
(Azumaya) Chinese style	3.5 oz	0	2	4.0
(Mori-Nu)				
silken	1 slice	46	2	1.6
silken	3 oz	55	2	2.0
silken, light	1 slice	32	1	0.6
silken, light	3 oz	35	1	1.0
(Nasoya)	1 piece	93	1	5.0
FIRM				
nigan	1/2 cup	97	4	5.6
prepared w/calcium sulfate	1/2 cup	183	5	11.0
(Azumaya) Japanese style	3.5 oz	70	4	2.5
(Kikkoman)	3 oz	50	2	2.5
(Mori-Nu)				
silken	1/2 pkg	90	4	4.0
silken	1 slice	52	2	2.3
silken	3 oz	50	2	2.5
silken, light	3 oz	35	1	1.0
silken, light	1 slice	31	1	0.7
(Nasoya)	1 piece	76	2	3.8
FREEZE-DRIED/koyadofu	1 oz	136	4.1	8.6
REGULAR, prepared w/calcium sulfate	1/2 cup	94	2	5.9
SOFT				
(Azumaya) Kinugoshi	3.5 oz	50	5	4.0
(Kikkoman)	3 oz	45	2	2.5
(Mori-Nu)				
silken	1/2 pkg	80	4	4.0
silken	1 slice	46	2	2.3
silken	3 oz	45	2	2.5
(Nasoya)				
	1 piece	64	2	3.0
silken	1 piece	48	2	2.2
nigan	1 cubic inch	11	0	0.6
TOFU SPREAD				
(Natural Touch)				
green chili, canned, 'Tofu Topper'	2 tbsp	50	2	4.0
herb and spice, canned, 'Tofu Topper'	2 tbsp	50	2	4.0
Mexican, canned, 'Tofu Topper'	2 tbsp	60	2	5.0
TOM COLLINS. See under COCKTAIL; COCKTAIL MIX.				
TOMATILLO/ground husk tomato				
raw, chopped or diced	1/2 cup	21	4	0.7
raw, whole	1 medium	11	2	0.3
TOMATO. See also TOMATO DISH.				
Canned				
(A&P)	1/2 cup	25	6	1.0
(Featherweight)	1/2 cup	20	4	0.0

Food Name	Serv. Size	Total Cal.	Carbs GMS	Fat GMS
'Choice Cut' *(Hunt's)*	1/2 cup	22	5	0.2
chopped, food service product *(Angela Mia)*	1/2 cup	24	4	0.4
crushed *(Angela Mia)*	1/2 cup	27	6	0.2
crushed *(Contadina)*	1/4 cup	20	4	0.0
crushed *(Hunt's)*	1/2 cup	29	7	0.3
crushed *(Pathmark)*	1/2 cup	40	9	0.0
crushed *(Progresso)*	1/4 cup	20	4	0.0
crushed *(S&W)*	1/4 cup	20	4	0.0
crushed, 'No Frills' *(Pathmark)*	1 cup	90	20	0.0
crushed, chunky, food service product *(Angela Mia)*	1/2 cup	26	5	0.3
crushed, concentrated, food service product *(Angela Mia)*	1/4 cup	30	6	0.4
crushed, food service product *(Angela Mia)*	1/2 cup	32	7	0.4
crushed, Italian flavored *(Hunt's)*	1/2 cup	40	9	1.0
crushed, organic, no salt added *(Eden Foods)*	1/2 cup	35	6	0.0
cut, peeled, 'Ready-Cut' *(S&W)*	1/2 cup	25	6	0.0
diced, in juice *(Hunt's)*	1/2 cup	20	4	0.1
diced, in juice, no salt added *(Hunt's)*	1/2 cup	20	4	0.1
diced, in purée, food service product *(Hunt's)*	1/2 cup	23	5	0.1
diced, in rich purée *(S&W)*	1/2 cup	35	8	0.0
diced, Italian style *(Muir Glen)*	1/2 cup	25	4	0.0
diced, organic *(Eden Foods)*	1/2 cup	30	6	0.0
diced, peeled *(Libby's)*	1/2 cup	25	4	0.0
diced, w/green chilies *(Eden Foods)*	1/2 cup	30	5	0.0
diced, w/green chilies *(Ro-Tel)*	1/2 cup	20	4	0.0
diced, w/Italian herbs, 'Choice Cut' *(Hunt's)*	1/2 cup	24	5	0.0
diced, w/roasted garlic, 'Choice Cut' *(Hunt's)*	1/2 cup	24	5	0.0
dried, chopped, marinated *(Parmalat)*	3 pieces	35	3	2.5
in aspic, supreme *(S&W)*	1/2 cup	60	16	0.0
in juice, no salt added *(S&W)*	1/2 cup	25	4	0.0
Italian style *(Contadina)*	1/2 cup	35	8	1.0
Mexican style *(S&W)*	1/2 cup	40	8	0.0
'No Frills' *(Pathmark)*	1 cup	50	11	0.0
organic, diced *(Muir Glen)*	1/2 cup	25	4	0.0
'Pasta Ready' *(Contadina)*	1/2 cup	40	5	2.0
pear-shaped *(Hunt's)*	1/2 cup	20	4	0.1
pear-shaped, Italian flavored *(Hunt's)*	1/2 cup	20	5	1.0
peeled *(Contadina)*	1/2 cup	25	4	0.0
peeled, 'Choice Cut' *(Hunt's)*	1/2 cup	20	5	1.0
peeled, whole, in juice *(DiNapoli)*	1/2 cup	25	6	0.0
plum, w/basil sauce *(Contadina)*	1/2 cup	70	8	3.0
primavera 'Pasta Ready' *(Contadina)*	1/2 cup	50	8	1.5
'Recipe Ready' *(Contadina)*	1/2 cup	25	5	0.0
sliced *(A&P)*	1/2 cup	35	8	1.0
sliced *(Finast)*	1/2 cup	35	9	0.0
sliced *(Pathmark)*	1/2 cup	35	9	0.0
sliced *(S&W)*	1/2 cup	35	9	0.0
sliced, Italian *(S&W)*	1/2 cup	35	9	0.0
w/basil, peeled *(Progresso)*	1/2 cup	25	4	0.0
w/crushed red pepper 'Pasta Ready' *(Contadina)*	1/2 cup	60	8	3.0
w/green chilies *(Old El Paso)*	1/4 cup	14	3	0.0
w/jalapeños *(Contadina)*	1/2 cup	35	8	1.0
w/jalapeños *(Ortega)*	1 oz	8	1	0.0
w/mushrooms 'Pasta Ready' *(Contadina)*	1/2 cup	50	9	1.5
w/olives 'Pasta Ready' *(Contadina)*	1/2 cup	60	8	3.0
w/three cheeses 'Pasta Ready' *(Contadina)*	1/2 cup	70	8	4.0
wedges, w/liquid *(Del Monte)*	1/2 cup	30	8	0.0
whole *(Hunt's)*	2 tomatoes	22	4	0.1

Food Name	Serv. Size	Total Cal.	Carbs GMS	Fat GMS
whole *(Stokely)*	1/2 cup	25	5	0.0
whole, 'Nutradiet' *(S&W)*	1/2 cup	25	5	0.0
whole, Italian flavored *(Hunt's)*	1/2 cup	25	6	1.0
whole, no salt added *(Hunt's)*	2 tomatoes	22	5	0.5
whole, peeled *(Finast)*	1/2 cup	25	6	0.0
whole, peeled *(Hunt's)*	4.83 oz	21	4	0.1
whole, peeled *(Libby's)*	1/2 cup	25	4	0.0
whole, peeled *(Progresso)*	1/2 cup	25	4	0.0
whole, peeled *(S&W)*	1/2 cup	20	4	0.0
whole, peeled, food service product *(Hunt's)*	1 serving	11	2	0.1
whole, peeled, no salt added *(Hunt's)*	4.83 oz	21	4	0.1
whole, peeled, no salt added *(Pathmark)*	1/2 cup	25	6	0.0
whole, peeled, organic *(Muir Glen)*	1/2 cup	30	5	0.0
whole, peeled, w/liquid *(Del Monte)*	1/2 cup	25	5	0.0
whole, peeled, w/tomato juice *(Pathmark)*	1/2 cup	25	6	0.0
Dried *(Melissa's)*	5 pieces	55	10	0.5
Fresh, raw, ripe				
cherry, red, ripe, June–October	1 cup	31	7	0.5
cherry, red, ripe, June–October, medium	1 tomato	4	1	0.1
cherry, red, ripe, November–May	1 cup	31	7	0.5
cherry, red, ripe, November–May, medium	1 tomato	4	1	0.1
cherry, red, ripe, year-round average	1 cup	31	7	0.5
cherry, red, ripe, year-round average, medium	1 tomato	4	1	0.1
green, raw, chopped	1 cup	43	9	0.4
green, raw, whole, large	1 tomato	44	9	0.4
green, raw, whole, medium	1 tomato	30	6	0.2
green, raw, whole, small	1 tomato	22	5	0.2
orange, raw, chopped	1 cup	25	5	0.3
orange, raw, whole, medium	1 tomato	18	4	0.2
plum, red, ripe, raw, June–October, medium	1 tomato	13	3	0.2
plum, red, ripe, raw, November–May, medium	1 tomato	13	3	0.2
plum, red, ripe, raw, year-round average, whole, medium	1 tomato	13	3	0.2
plum/Italian, raw, June–October, medium	1 tomato	13	3	0.2
red, ripe, boiled	1 cup	65	14	1.0
red, ripe, boiled, medium	2 tomatoes	66	14	1.0
red, ripe, raw, June–October, chopped	1 cup	38	8	0.6
red, ripe, raw, June–October, medium	1 tomato	26	6	0.4
red, ripe, raw, June–October, 1/2-inch slices, medium	1 slice	6	1	0.1
red, ripe, raw, June–October, 1/4-inch slices, medium	1 slice	4	1	0.1
red, ripe, raw, June–October, quartered, medium	1/4 tomato	7	1	0.1
red, ripe, raw, June–October, whole, 3 inch diam	1 tomato	38	8	0.6
red, ripe, raw, June–October, whole, 2 3/5 inch diam	1 tomato	26	6	0.4
red, ripe, raw, June–October, whole, 2 2/5 inch diam	1 tomato	19	4	0.3
red, ripe, raw, November–May, chopped or sliced	1 cup	38	8	0.6
red, ripe, raw, November–May, medium	1 tomato	26	6	0.4
red, ripe, raw, November–May, quartered, medium	1/4 tomato	7	1	0.1
red, ripe, raw, November–May, 1/2 inch slices, medium	1 slice	6	1	0.1
red, ripe, raw, November–May, 1/4 inch slices, medium	1 slice	4	1	0.1
red, ripe, raw, November–May, whole, 3 inch diam	1 large	38	8	0.6
red, ripe, raw, November–May, whole, 2 3/5 inch diam	1 tomato	26	6	0.4
red, ripe, raw, year-round average, chopped or sliced	1 cup	38	8	0.6
red, ripe, raw, year-round average, quartered, medium	1/4 tomato	7	1	0.1
red, ripe, raw, year-round average, 1/2 inch slices, medium	1 slice	6	1	0.1
red, ripe, raw, year-round average, 1/4 inch slices, medium	1 slice	4	1	0.1
red, ripe, raw, year-round average, whole, 3-inch diam	1 large	38	8	0.6
red, ripe, raw, year-round average, whole, 2 3/5 inch diam	1 tomato	26	6	0.4
red, ripe, raw, year-round average, whole, 2 2/5 inch diam	1 tomato	19	4	0.3

Food Name	Serv. Size	Total Cal.	Carbs GMS	Fat GMS
red, ripe, stewed	1 cup	80	13	2.7
yellow, raw, chopped	1 cup	21	4	0.4
yellow, raw, whole, medium	1 tomato	32	6	0.6
Pickled *(Claussen)* kosher, in jars, approx. 1.7 oz	1 piece	9	2	0.0
Sun-dried				
	1 cup	139	30	1.6
	1 piece	5	1	0.1
in oil and herbs *(Bella Sun Luci)*	2/3 oz	60	6	3.0
packed in oil, drained	1 cup	234	26	15.5
packed in oil, drained	1 piece	6	1	0.4
sun-ripened, 2-3 pieces *(Mezzetta)*	1/5 oz	15	3	0.0
yellow, in olive oil, 3 pieces *(Trader Joe's)*	1/5 oz	15	3	0.0
TOMATO DISH				
(Contadina)				
stewed, canned	1/2 cup	40	9	0.0
stewed, Italian style, canned	1/2 cup	40	8	0.0
stewed, Mexican style, canned	1/2 cup	40	9	0.0
(Del Monte)				
stewed, canned	1/2 cup	35	8	0.0
stewed, no salt added, canned	1/2 cup	35	8	0.0
stewed, original recipe, no salt added, canned	1/2 cup	35	9	0.0
(Green Giant)				
stewed, classic recipe, canned	1/2 cup	35	7	0.0
stewed, Italian recipe, canned	1/2 cup	30	7	0.0
stewed, Mexican recipe, canned	1/2 cup	35	7	0.0
(Hunt's)				
stewed, canned	1/2 cup	33	7	0.3
stewed, canned, food service product	1/2 cup	29	7	0.1
stewed, Italian flavored, canned	1/2 cup	35	8	1.0
stewed, no salt added, canned	1/2 cup	29	7	0.1
(Muir Glen) whole, stewed, organic, canned	1/2 cup	25	4	0.0
(S&W)				
stewed, 50% reduced salt, canned	1/2 cup	35	9	0.0
stewed, no salt	1/2 cup	35	7	0.0
(Stokely) stewed, canned	1/2 cup	35	8	0.0
TOMATO JUICE. See also FRUIT JUICE BLEND.				
canned	1 cup	41	10	0.1
canned	6 fl oz	31	8	0.1
canned, no salt added	1 cup	41	10	0.1
canned, no salt added	6 fl oz	31	8	0.1
canned, no salt added	1 fl oz	5	1	0.0
(A&P)	6 fl oz	30	7	0.0
(Biotta)	6 fl oz	28	6	0.1
(Campbell's)	8 fl oz	50	9	0.0
(Del Monte)				
	8 fl oz	40	7	0.0
from concentrate	8 fl oz	50	10	0.0
(Featherweight)	6 fl oz	35	8	0.0
(Hunt's)				
	8 fl oz	34	8	0.3
food service product	8 fl oz	35	7	0.1
no salt added	8 fl oz	34	8	0.3
(Knudsen) organic	8 fl oz	50	10	0.0
(Libby's)				
bottled or canned	6 fl oz	35	7	0.0
canned	5.5 fl oz	35	6	0.0

Food Name	Serv. Size	Total Cal.	Carbs GMS	Fat GMS
(Pathmark)				
.... 6 fl oz		30	6	0.0
frozen, diluted .... 6 fl oz		35	8	0.0
(S&W)				
.... 5.5 fl oz		30	5	0.0
'California' .... 6 fl oz		35	8	0.0
'Nutradiet' .... 6 fl oz		35	8	0.0
(Stokely) .... 4 fl oz		20	4	0.0
(Welch's) .... 6 fl oz		35	7	0.0
TOMATO PASTE				
.... 6-oz can		139	33	0.9
.... 1/2 cup		107	25	0.7
no salt added .... 1 cup		215	51	1.4
no salt added .... 6-oz can		139	33	0.9
no salt added .... 1 tbsp		13	3	0.1
(Contadina)				
.... 2 tbsp		30	6	0.0
Italian style .... 2 tbsp		40	7	1.0
(Hunt's) no salt added .... 2 tbsp		30	6	0.5
(Progresso) .... 2 tbsp		30	6	0.0
(S&W) .... 2 tbsp		30	6	0.0
TOMATO PURÉE				
.... 1 cup		100	24	0.4
no salt added .... 1 cup		100	24	0.4
(Angela Mia) .... 2.19 oz		16	3	0.3
(Contadina)				
.... 1/4 cup		20	4	0.0
w/crushed tomatoes .... 1/2 cup		30	6	1.0
(Hunt's)				
.... 1/4 cup		24	5	0.3
food service product .... 1/4 cup		26	5	0.4
(Progresso) thick style .... 1/4 cup		25	5	0.0
TOMATO SAUCE				
(A&P) canned .... 1/2 cup		45	9	1.0
(Buitoni) marinara .... 1/2 cup		70	11	3.0
(Contadina)				
.... 1/4 cup		20	4	0.0
chunky, light .... 1/2 cup		45	8	0.5
four-cheese .... 4 oz		300	7	27.0
garden vegetable .... 5 oz		80	9	3.0
Italian sausage .... 5 oz		110	8	6.0
Italian style .... 1/4 cup		15	4	0.0
marinara, refrigerated, 'Fresh' .... 7.5 oz		100	12	4.0
pesto .... 2.33 oz		350	5	34.0
plum .... 5 oz		80	8	4.0
plum, w/basil, refrigerated, 'Fresh' .... 7.5 oz		100	14	4.0
refrigerated, 'Light' .... 0.5 oz		50	9	0.0
thick and zesty .... 1/4 cup		20	3	0.0
(Del Monte)				
canned .... 1 cup		70	16	1.0
no salt added .... 1 cup		70	16	1.0
no salt added .... 1/4 cup		20	4	0.0
w/onions .... 1 cup		100	23	1.0
(Eden Foods) lightly seasoned, organic .... 1/4 cup		25	5	0.0
(Finast)				
.... 1/2 cup		45	9	0.0
no salt added .... 8 oz		90	18	0.0

Food Name	Serv. Size	Total Cal.	Carbs GMS	Fat GMS
(Health Valley)				
.... 1 cup		70	13	0.5
no salt added .... 1 cup		70	13	0.5
(Hunt's)				
.... 1/4 cup		16	3	0.2
canned 'Special' .... 4 oz		35	8	0.0
canned .... 4 oz		30	7	0.0
'Casera' .... 2.19 oz		22	5	0.1
chunky tomato .... 2.19 oz		13	3	0.1
food service product .... 1/4 cup		15	3	0.2
hot, 'Maya'.. 1.06 oz		6	1	0.2
Italian style .... 1/4 cup		33	5	1.2
Italian style .... 4 oz		60	11	2.0
'Meatloaf Fixin's' .... 2 oz		20	5	1.0
no salt added .... 1/4 cup		16	3	0.2
w/garlic .... 4 oz		70	10	2.0
w/herbs.. 1/4 cup		32	5	1.0
w/mushrooms .... 4 oz		25	6	1.0
w/onions .... 4 oz		40	9	1.0
w/tomato bits .... 4 oz		30	7	1.0
(Old El Paso)				
w/green chilies .... 1/4 cup		14	3	1.0
w/jalapeños.. 1/4 cup		11	2	1.0
(Pathmark)				
.... 1/2 cup		40	9	0.0
marinara, 'No Frills' .... 1/2 cup		80	12	3.0
no salt added .... 1/2 cup		45	9	0.0
(Progresso) .... 1/4 cup		20	4	0.0
(Rokeach)				
Italian style.. 3 oz		60	8	2.0
low-sodium .... 3 oz		50	8	2.0
marinara .... 3 oz		60	9	2.0
(S&W) .... 1/4 cup		20	4	0.0
(Stokely) .... 1/2 cup		30	7	0.0

TOMATOSEED OIL

Food Name	Serv. Size	Total Cal.	Carbs GMS	Fat GMS
.... 1 cup		1927	0	218.0
.... 1 tbsp		120	0	13.6

TONIC WATER. See under SOFT DRINKS AND MIXERS.
TOPPING. See individual listings.
TORSK. See CUSK.
TORTELLINI DISH/ENTRÉE

Food Name	Serv. Size	Total Cal.	Carbs GMS	Fat GMS
(Bernardi)				
cheese .... 1 cup		260	40	6.0
cheese, w/spinach pasta .... 1 cup		280	40	8.0
cheese, tortelloni .... 1 cup		260	40	6.0
meat filled, precooked .... 1 cup		250	38	6.0
meat filled, w/raw pasta .... 1 cup		280	41	8.0
(Contadina)				
cheese .... 3/4 cup		261	39	6.0
cheese and basil .... 1 cup		360	49	11.0
chicken and prosciutto, tortelloni .... 1 cup		360	46	13.0
chicken and vegetable .... 3/4 cup		259	39	7.0
garlic and cheese, light .... 1 cup		280	50	5.0
sausage and bell pepper, tortelloni, spicy .... 1 cup		330	47	10.0
(Mona's) cheese, frozen.................................... 1 cup		370	50	11.0
(Stouffer's) cheese, w/Alfredo sauce, frozen .... 8 7/8 oz		580	35	37.0
(Tofutti) meatless, frozen .... 2 oz		220	38	2.0

Food Name	Serv. Size	Total Cal.	Carbs GMS	Fat GMS
(Weight Watchers) cheese, frozen	9 oz	310	50	6.0
TORTELLONI ENTRÉE. See under TORTELLINI DISH/ENTRÉE.				
TORTILLA				
corn, no salt added, ready to bake or fry	1 oz	63	13	0.7
corn, no salt added, ready-to-bake or fry, 6-inch diam	1 tortilla	58	12	0.7
corn, ready-to-bake or fry	1 oz	63	13	0.7
corn, ready-to-bake or fry, 6-inch diam	1 tortilla	58	12	0.7
flour, ready to bake or fry, 12-inch diam	1 tortilla	380	65	8.3
flour, ready to bake or fry, 10-inch diam	1 tortilla	234	40	5.1
flour, ready to bake or fry, 7–8-inch diam	1 tortilla	159	27	3.5
flour, ready to bake or fry, 6-inch diam	1 tortilla	104	18	2.3
flour, ready to bake or fry	1 oz	92	16	2.0
(Azteca)				
corn	1 tortilla	45	9	0.0
flour, 7-inch diam	1 tortilla	80	14	2.0
flour, 9-inch diam	1 tortilla	130	23	3.0
(Fry's) flour, fajita style, extra soft	1 tortilla	100	17	2.0
(Garcia's)				
flour, burrito style	1 tortilla	220	37	5.0
flour, fajita style	1 tortilla	100	17	2.5
wheat, 8-inch diam	1 tortilla	160	24	5.0
(LA LA'S) flour	1 tortilla	160	28	3.0
(La Tortilla)				
flour, burrito sized, 99% fat free	1 tortilla	120	25	0.5
flour, fat free	1 tortilla	60	13	0.0
whole wheat, 99% fat free	1 tortilla	60	12	0.0
(Mission)				
flour, burrito size 'Premium'	1 tortilla	230	40	6.0
flour, light	1 tortilla	70	16	1.0
flour, soft, taco size, 8-inch diam	1 tortilla	146	25	3.1
(Old El Paso)				
corn	1 tortilla	60	10	1.0
flour	1 tortilla	150	27	3.0
(Tyson)				
flour, burrito style	1 tortilla	173	29	4.0
flour, burrito style, large, heat pressed	1 tortilla	182	33	4.0
flour, burrito style, small, hand stretched	1 tortilla	106	19	2.0
flour, fajita style	1 tortilla	84	18	2.0
flour, soft, taco size	1 tortilla	121	20	3.0
TORTILLA CHIPS. See also CORN CHIPS AND SNACKS.				
(Bachman)				
	1 oz	140	19	6.0
nacho cheese	1 oz	140	18	6.0
no salt	1 oz	140	19	6.0
(Barbara's Bakery)				
yellow corn, no salt added, organic	1 oz	140	18	7.0
yellow corn, regular, organic	1 oz	140	18	7.0
(Bearitos)				
blue corn, organic	1 oz	146	17	7.0
blue corn, organic, unsalted'	1 oz	137	17	6.5
no salt added	1 oz	140	16	7.0
yellow corn, no salt added, organic	1 oz	148	17	7.2
yellow corn, organic	1 oz	143	18	6.4
(Bravos)				
nacho cheese flavored, round	1 oz	150	18	8.0
nacho cheese flavored, strips	1 oz	140	18	7.0
nacho cheese and jalapeño	1 oz	150	19	7.0

Food Name	Serv. Size	Total Cal.	Carbs GMS	Fat GMS
(Buenitos)				
no salt added	1 oz	150	18	8.0
'Tortilla Chips'	1 oz	150	18	8.0
(Doritos)				
approx 18 chips	1 oz	140	19	6.0
cool ranch	1 oz	140	18	7.0
cool ranch, approx 16 chips	1 oz	140	18	7.0
cool ranch, light	1 oz	120	21	4.0
'Jumpin' Jack' approx 16 chips	1 oz	140	18	7.0
nacho, spicy	1 oz	140	18	7.0
nacho cheese, approx 15 chips	1 oz	140	18	7.0
nacho cheese 'Light'	1 oz	120	21	4.0
'Nacho Cheesier'	1 oz	140	17	7.0
salsa and cheese, 'Thins'	1 oz	150	17	8.0
'Salsa Rio' approx 16 chips	1 oz	140	18	7.0
salsa verde	1 oz	150	20	7.0
taco, approx 16 chips	1 oz	140	18	7.0
'Taco Bell'	1 oz	150	21	7.0
toasted corn, approx 16 chips	1 oz	140	19	7.0
toasted	1 oz	140	18	7.0
white corn, lightly salted, 'Thins'	1 oz	140	19	7.0
(Eagle) ranch	1 oz	140	17	8.0
(Featherweight)				
low-salt, round	1 oz	150	18	8.0
nacho cheese, low-salt	1 oz	150	18	8.0
(Garden of Eden)				
black bean, organic	10 chips	150	18	7.0
blue corn and sunflower seed, organic	10 chips	160	16	8.0
blue corn, hot and spicy, organic	10 chips	140	3	7.0
blue corn, organic, no salt added	10 chips	150	18	7.0
blue corn, salted, organic	10 chips	150	18	7.0
chipotle, hot and smoky, organic	10 chips	120	23	2.0
unsalted, no oil added, organic	10 chips	110	23	1.0
w/jalapeño, organic	10 chips	140	18	7.0
yogurt and green onion, organic	10 chips	120	23	2.0
(Guiltless Gourmet)				
baked, original	1 oz	110	22	1.0
blue corn	1 oz	110	22	1.0
chili lime	1 oz	110	22	1.0
nacho, baked	1 oz	110	22	1.0
original, no salt added	1 oz	110	22	1.0
ranch	1 oz	110	22	1.0
white corn	1 oz	110	22	1.0
yellow corn, baked, no salt added, approx 24 chips	1 oz	110	22	1.0
yellow corn, baked, w/salt, approx 24 chips	1 oz	110	22	1.0
(Hain)				
sesame	1 oz	140	19	7.0
sesame, cheese	1 oz	160	20	8.0
sesame, no salt added	1 oz	140	19	7.0
taco	1 oz	160	15	11.0
(Keebler)				
cinnamon crispana, flour, 'Chacho's'	1 oz	140	19	7.0
original, restaurant style 'Chacho's'	1 oz	140	18	7.0
(Kettle Tias)				
blue corn, lightly salted	1 oz	140	18	6.0
blue corn, no salt added	1 oz	140	18	6.0
yellow corn, lightly salted	1 oz	140	19	7.0

Food Name	Serv. Size	Total Cal.	Carbs GMS	Fat GMS
yellow corn, no salt added	1 oz	140	19	7.0
(La Famous)				
no salt added	1 oz	140	18	7.0
regular	1 oz	140	18	7.0
(Laura Scudder's)				
nacho cheese, jalapeño, 'Strips'	1 oz	150	19	7.0
nacho cheese, 'Triangles'	1 oz	140	18	7.0
picante, 'Restaurant Style Strips'	1 oz	150	19	7.0
restaurant style, lightly salted	1 oz	140	18	7.0
(Louise's) 95% nonfat	1 oz	120	23	1.5
(Mexi-Snax)				
hot	12 chips	140	21	5.0
no salt added	12 chips	140	21	6.0
vegetable medley	12 chips	140	21	5.0
(Mi Ranchito)				
jalapeño cheddar	10 chips	140	20	7.0
spicy red chili, 'Rojo's'	10 chips	140	20	7.0
(Michael Season's)				
white corn, lightly salted	1 oz	135	17	6.0
yellow corn, lightly salted, organic	1 oz	135	19	5.0
yellow corn, organic	1 oz	135	19	5.0
(Old El Paso)				
crispy, approx 16 chips	1 oz	150	17	8.0
'NaChips' approx 9 chips	1 oz	150	18	7.0
white corn, low-sodium, round, 'NaChips'	1 oz	160	17	9.0
(Planters)				
nacho cheese	1 oz	150	18	8.0
traditional	1 oz	150	18	8.0
(Santitas)				
food service product, 'Restaurant Strips'	1 oz	140	19	6.0
100% white corn	1 oz	140	19	6.0
restaurant style	1 oz	140	19	6.0
(Slimchips) nonfat, approx 10 chips	0.4 oz	44	10	0.5
(Tio Sancho) 'Microwave Snacks'	4 oz	567	74	26.1
(Tostitos)				
approx 11 chips	1 oz	140	18	8.0
baked	1 oz	110	24	1.0
bite-size	1 oz	140	17	8.0
lime and chile	1 oz	150	17	7.0
nacho cheese, sharp, approx 11 chips	1 oz	150	17	8.0
restaurant style	1 oz	140	19	6.0
rounds	1 oz	150	18	8.0
unsalted	1 oz	110	24	1.0
white corn, baked, 'Cool Ranch'	1 oz	130	21	3.0
(Vera Cruz)				
tortilla rounds, baked	1 oz	120	22	1.5
tortilla rounds, baked, unsalted	1 oz	120	22	1.5
(Wise) nacho cheese flavored, crispy, round	1 oz	150	18	8.0
TOSTACO SHELL (Old El Paso)	1 shell	100	11	5.0
TOSTADA CHIPS				
(Michael Season's) yellow corn, lightly salted, bite-sized	1 oz	135	19	5.0
TOSTADA SHELL				
(Bearitos) yellow corn	1 shell	140	17	7.0
(Lawry's)	1 shell	73	10	3.5
(Ortega)	1 shell	50	8	2.0
(Pancho Villa)	1 shell	55	6	3.0

Food Name	Serv. Size	Total Cal.	Carbs GMS	Fat GMS
(Rosarita)				
. . . .	1 shell	63	9	2.4
1-oz shell	2 shells	138	17	7.6
(Tio Sancho)	1 shell	67	8	3.2
TOWELGOURD. See GOURD, DISHCLOTH.				
TRAIL MIX SNACK				
(Harmony)				
'Deluxe Super'	1/4 cup	150	23	7.0
nut and berry mix	1/4 cup	160	21	8.0
(Maranatha Natural)				
'Deluxe'	1/4 cup	150	13	9.0
'Mountain Delight'	1/4 cup	140	15	8.0
'Nature Trail'	1/4 cup	150	15	9.0
'Snack Attack'	1/4 cup	140	16	8.0
(Pacific Shores) all fruit	1/4 cup	110	21	2.0
(Pilgram Joe's) cranberry	1/4 cup	150	12	9.0
(Trader Joe's)				
'Muir Trail Mix'	1/4 cup	180	11	13.0
w/carob chips, 'Mt. Baldy Mix'	1/4 cup	190	15	14.0
TREE FERN				
cooked, chopped	1/2 cup	28	8	0.1
cooked, whole, 6.5-inch long	1 frond	12	3	0.0
TREE MUSHROOM. See MUSHROOM, OYSTER.				
TRITICALE	1 cup	645	138	4.0
TROUT				
MIXED SPECIES				
baked, broiled, grilled, or microwaved	3 oz	162	0	7.2
raw	3 oz	126	0	5.6
RAINBOW				
farmed, baked, broiled, grilled, or microwaved	3 oz	144	0	6.1
farmed, raw	3 oz	117	0	4.6
wild, baked, broiled, grilled, or microwaved	3 oz	128	0	4.9
wild, raw	3 oz	101	0	2.9
SEA				
mixed species, baked, broiled, grilled, or microwaved	3 oz	113	0	3.9
mixed species, raw	3 oz	88	0	3.1
TUNA				
Canned				
in oil, drained	3 oz	158	0	6.9
in water, drained	3 oz	99	0	0.7
in water, no salt added, drained	3 oz	99	0	0.7
solid, in olive oil *(Progresso)*	1/4 cup	160	0	12.0
very low sodium *(Chicken of the Sea)*	2 oz	60	0	0.5
Frozen, steak, w/o seasoning mix *(SeaPak)*	6-oz pkg	180	0	2.0
ALBACORE				
Canned				
solid white, in soybean oil, drained *(Bumble Bee)*	2 oz	100	0	8.0
solid white, in soybean oil, drained *(Finast)*	2 oz	145	1	10.0
solid white, in soybean oil, drained *(S&W)*	2 oz	160	0	12.0
solid white, in soybean oil, drained *(Star-Kist)*	2 oz	140	1	10.0
solid white, in spring water, fancy *(Chicken of the Sea)*	2 oz	60	1	1.0
solid white, in water, drained *(A&P)*	2 oz	70	1	1.0
solid white, in water, drained *(Bumble Bee)*	2 oz	60	0	2.0
solid white, in water, drained *(Finast)*	2 oz	70	1	1.0
solid white, in water, drained *(Pathmark)*	2 oz	70	0	2.0
solid white, in water, drained *(Star-Kist)*	2 oz	70	1	1.0
solid white, in water, drained *(Weight Watchers)*	2 oz	70	1	1.0

Food Name	Serv. Size	Total Cal.	Carbs GMS	Fat GMS
Frozen				
steak, white, boneless/skinless, raw *(Peter Pan Seafoods)*	3.5 oz	102	0	4.9
BLUEFIN				
Fresh				
baked, broiled, grilled, or microwaved	3 oz	156	0	5.3
raw	3 oz	122	0	4.2
CHUNK LIGHT				
Canned				
in Canola oil *(Chicken of the Sea)*	2 oz	110	0	6.0
in oil *(S&W)*	3 oz	167	0	9.1
in soybean oil, drained *(Bumble Bee)*	2 oz	110	0	12.0
in soybean oil, drained *(Finast)*	2 oz	150	1	13.0
in soybean oil, drained *(Star-Kist)*	2 oz	150	1	13.0
in soybean oil, drained, 'Fancy' *(S&W)*	2 oz	140	0	10.0
in vegetable oil, w/liquid *(Chicken of the Sea)*	2 oz	160	1	12.0
in water *(Captains Choice)*	3 oz	90	0	2.0
in water *(Chicken of the Sea)*	2 oz	60	0	0.5
in water *(S&W)*	3 oz	106	0	0.8
in water, diet, drained *(Star-Kist)*	2 oz	65	1	1.0
in water, drained *(Bumble Bee)*	2 oz	50	0	1.0
in water, drained *(Featherweight)*	2 oz	60	0	1.0
in water, drained *(Finast)*	2 oz	60	1	1.0
in water, drained *(Pathmark)*	2 oz	70	0	2.0
in water, drained *(Star-Kist)*	2 oz	60	1	1.0
in water, drained, 'Fancy' *(S&W)*	2 oz	60	0	1.0
in water, low-sodium *(Chicken of the Sea)*	2 oz	60	0	0.5
in water, no salt added, drained *(Weight Watchers)*	2 oz	60	1	1.0
in water, 60% less salt, drained *(Star-Kist)*	2 oz	65	1	1.0
CHUNK WHITE				
Canned				
in soybean oil, drained *(Bumble Bee)*	2 oz	110	0	12.0
in water *(Chicken of the Sea)*	2 oz	60	0	1.0
in water, diet, drained *(Star-Kist)*	2 oz	70	1	1.0
in water, drained *(A&P)*	2 oz	100	1	5.0
in water, drained *(Bumble Bee)*	2 oz	60	0	2.0
in water, 60% less salt, drained *(Star-Kist)*	2 oz	70	1	1.0
LIGHT				
Canned				
in oil, drained	3 oz	168	0	7.0
in oil, no salt added, drained	3 oz	168	0	7.0
in soybean oil, drained *(A&P)*	2 oz	150	1	13.0
in water, drained *(A&P)*	2 oz	60	1	1.0
in water, drained *(Empress)*	2 oz	60	0	1.0
SKIPJACK/aku/katsuo/oceanic bonito				
Fresh				
baked, broiled, grilled, or microwaved	3 oz	112	0	1.1
raw	3 oz	88	0	0.9
SOLID LIGHT				
Canned				
in Canola oil *(Chicken of the Sea)*	2 oz	90	0	3.0
in oil *(S&W)*	3 oz	121	0	2.3
in soybean oil, drained *(Star-Kist)*	2 oz	150	1	13.0
in soybean oil, drained, solid *(Progresso)*	1/3 cup	150	1	13.0
in water *(Chicken of the Sea)*	2 oz	70	0	1.0
in water, drained *(Star-Kist)*	2 oz	60	1	1.0
in water, drained, 'Prime Catch' *(Star-Kist)*	2 oz	60	1	1.0

Food Name	Serv. Size	Total Cal.	Carbs GMS	Fat GMS
SOLID WHITE				
Canned				
in soybean oil, drained *(Star-Kist)*	2 oz	140	1	10.0
in water *(Captains Choice)*	2 oz	70	0	1.0
WHITE				
Canned				
in oil, no salt added, drained	3 oz	158	0	6.9
in soybean oil, drained *(A&P)*	2 oz	150	1	10.0
in water, drained	3 oz	109	0	2.5
in water, no salt added, drained	3 oz	109	0	2.5
YELLOWFIN/ahi				
Fresh				
baked, broiled, grilled, or microwaved	3 oz	118	0	1.0
raw	3 oz	92	0	0.8
raw boneless	1 oz	31	0	0.3
Frozen				
steak, boneless, skinless, raw *(Peter Pan Seafoods)*	3.5 oz	131	0	4.1
TUNA DISH/ENTRÉE				
(Banquet) pie, frozen	7 oz	540	44	33.0
(Marie Callender's) chunky tuna and noodles	12 oz	960	43	35.0
(Stouffer's)				
tuna-noodle casserole	1 entrée	320	37	10.0
tuna-noodle casserole, frozen, food service product	1 oz	35	3	1.9
(Weight Watchers) tuna-noodle casserole	1 entrée	270	39	7.0
TUNA DISH/ENTRÉE MIX				
(Tuna Helper)				
au gratin meal, mix only	1/2 cup	190	34	3.5
au gratin meal, prepared	1 cup	300	37	11.0
buttery rice, prepared	1/5 pkg	160	32	2.0
cheesy pasta meal, mix only	3/4 cup	170	29	3.0
cheesy pasta meal, prepared	1 cup	280	32	11.0
creamy broccoli, prepared	1/5 pkg	200	35	4.0
creamy mushroom, prepared	1/5 pkg	140	28	1.0
creamy pasta meal, mix only	3/4 cup	190	29	6.0
creamy pasta meal, prepared	1 cup	300	31	13.0
fettuccine Alfredo meal, mix only	3/4 cup	170	30	3.5
fettuccine Alfredo meal, prepared	1 cup	310	32	14.0
pasta salad, prepared	1/5 pkg	140	28	1.0
pot pie, prepared	1/2 cup	340	35	20.0
pot pie, prepared	1/6 pkg	290	31	17.0
Romanoff meal, mix only	2/3 cup	210	38	3.0
Romanoff meal, prepared	1 cup	280	38	8.0
tetrazzini meal, mix only	2/3 cup	180	32	3.0
tetrazzini meal, prepared	1 cup	310	33	12.0
TUNA SALAD SPREAD *(Libby's)* 'Spreadables'	1/3 cup	130	6	8.0
TUNA SUBSTITUTE				
(Natural Touch) vegetarian, 'Tuno'	1/3 cup drained	60	2	2.0
(Worthington)				
vegetarian, 'Tuno' 12-oz can	1/3 cup drained	80	4	4.0
vegetarian, 'Tuno' 12-oz roll	1/2 cup drained	80	2	6.0
TUNKA. See GOURD, WHITE.				
TURBOT, EUROPEAN				
baked, broiled, grilled, or microwaved	3 oz	104	0	3.2
raw	3 oz	81	0	2.5
TURKEY				
BACK				
Fresh				
all classes, meat and skin, raw	1 lb	896	0.0	59.2

Food Name	Serv. Size	Total Cal.	Carbs GMS	Fat GMS
all classes, meat and skin, raw	1 oz	56	0.0	3.7
all classes, meat and skin, roasted	4 oz	276	0.0	16.3
fryer/roaster, meat and skin, raw	4 oz	173	0	8.3
fryer/roaster, meat and skin, roasted	4 oz	233	0	11.7
fryer/roaster, meat only, raw	4 oz	137	0	4.0
fryer/roaster, meat only, roasted	4 oz	194	0	6.5
young hen, meat and skin, raw	4 oz	252	0	18.4
young hen, meat and skin, roasted	4 oz	290	0	17.9
young tom, meat and skin, raw	4 oz	205	0	12.7
young tom, meat and skin, roasted	4 oz	272	0	15.6
BREAST				
Fresh				
all classes, meat and skin, raw	1 lb	720	0.0	32.0
all classes, meat and skin, raw	1 oz	45	0.0	8.4
all classes, meat and skin, roasted	4 oz	214	0.0	8.4
fryer/roaster, meat and skin, raw	4 oz	152	0	3.0
fryer/roaster, meat and skin, roasted	4 oz	175	0	3.7
fryer/roaster, meat and skin, pre-basted, roasted	4 oz	114	0	4.0
young hen, meat and skin, raw	4 oz	191	0	9.5
young hen, meat and skin, roasted	4 oz	222	0	9.0
young tom, meat and skin, raw	4 oz	173	0	7.2
young tom, meat and skin, roasted	4 oz	216	0	8.4
Frozen or refrigerated				
barbecue, quartered (Mr. Turkey)	3.5 oz	95	1	0.8
cooked (Land O'Lakes)	3 oz	100	0	1.0
cooked (Louis Rich)	1 oz	47	0	1.5
cooked, 'Cook-N-Bag' (Longacre)	1 oz	38	1	1.0
cooked, 'Fresh Turkey Cuts' (Louis Rich)	1 oz	45	1	2.0
8% self-basting solution (Jennie-O)	4 oz	160	0	8.0
hen, cooked, w/o wings (Louis Rich)	1 oz	50	0	2.0
hickory smoked, cooked (Louis Rich)	1 oz	33	1	1.0
honey roasted, cooked (Louis Rich)	1 oz	33	1	0.8
oven-roasted, cooked (Louis Rich)	1 oz	31	0	0.9
raw, 'Cook-N-Bag' (Longacre)	1 oz	27	1	1.0
raw, 'Ready-to-Cook' (Longacre)	1 oz	39	0	1.0
raw, 'Tasti-Lean Tenders' (Norbest)	4 oz	135	0	2.0
roast, cooked (Louis Rich)	1 oz	42	0	0.8
roast, cooked, 'Fresh Turkey Cuts' (Louis Rich)	1 oz	40	1	1.0
slices, cooked (Louis Rich)	1 oz	39	0	0.5
smoked, cooked (Louis Rich)	1 oz	33	0	1.0
smoked, cooked, no bone (Norbest)	1 oz	42	0	1.6
steaks, cooked (Louis Rich)	1 oz	39	0	0.5
steaks, cooked, 'Fresh Turkey Cuts' (Louis Rich)	1 oz	40	1	1.0
steaks, cubed, raw (Norbest)	4 oz	135	0	2.0
strips and tips, raw, 'Tasti-Lean' (Norbest)	4 oz	135	0	2.0
tenderloins, cooked (Louis Rich)	1 oz	39	0	0.5
tenderloins, cooked, 'Fresh Turkey Cuts' (Louis Rich)	1 oz	40	1	1.0
COMPOSITE CUTS				
Canned				
chunk (Hormel)	6 3/4 oz	230	0	10.0
chunk (Swanson)	1 cup	360	16	8.0
in broth, drained	5-oz can	231	0	9.7
puréed (Bryan Foods)	1/3 cup	160	0	11.0
CUTLET				
Frozen or refrigerated, raw, 'Tasti-Lean' (Norbest)	4 oz	135	0	2.0
DARK MEAT				
Fresh				
all classes, meat and skin, raw	1 lb	720	0.0	40.0

Food Name	Serv. Size	Total Cal.	Carbs GMS	Fat GMS
all classes, meat and skin, raw	1 oz	45	0.0	2.5
all classes, meat and skin, roasted	1 4 oz	251	0.0	13.1
all classes, meat only, raw	1 lb	560	0.0	19.2
all classes, meat only, raw	1 oz	35	0.0	1.2
all classes, meat only, roasted	4 oz	212	0.0	8.2
all classes, meat only, roasted, chopped or diced	1 cup	262	0.0	10.1
fryer/roaster, meat and skin, raw	4 oz	147	0	5.5
fryer/roaster, meat and skin, roasted	4 oz	208	0	8.1
fryer/roaster, meat only, raw	4 oz	114	0	3.1
fryer/roaster, meat only, roasted	4 oz	184	0	5.0
fryer/roaster, meat only, roasted, chopped or diced	1 cup	227	0	6.0
young hen, meat and skin, raw	4 oz	196	0	11.7
young hen, meat and skin, roasted	4 oz	265	0	14.6
young hen, meat only, raw	4 oz	149	0	5.5
young hen, meat only, roasted	4 oz	220	0	6.3
young hen, meat only, roasted, chopped or diced	1 cup	269	0	10.9
young tom, meat and skin, raw	4 oz	174	0	9.0
young tom, meat and skin, roasted	4 oz	235	0	12.4
young tom, meat only, raw	4 oz	141	0	4.7
young tom, meat only, roasted	4 oz	212	0	8.0
GIBLETS				
Fresh				
all classes, raw	4 oz	150	2.4	4.8
all classes, raw	1/2 oz	21	0	0.7
all classes, w/fat, simmered	0.35 oz	17	0	0.5
all classes, w/fat, simmered, chopped or diced	1 cup	242	3	7.4
GIZZARD				
Fresh				
all classes, raw	1 med gizzard	132	1	4.2
all classes, raw	1/4 oz	8	0	0.3
all classes, simmered	0.14 oz	7	0	0.2
all classes, simmered, chopped or diced	1 cup	236	1	5.6
GROUND				
Fresh				
all classes, breaded, battered, fried	3.33-oz patty	266	15	16.9
all classes, breaded, battered, fried	2.25-oz patty	181	10	11.5
all classes, cooked	4-oz patty	193	0	10.8
all classes, raw	4-oz patty	170	0	9.4
Frozen or refrigerated				
(Louis Rich)	4 oz	190	0	12.0
(Mr. Turkey)	1 oz	54	0	4.0
burger patty (Shelton's)	1 serving	170	0	10.0
cooked (Hudson)	1 oz	55	0	3.7
cooked (Longacre)	1 oz	60	0	4.0
extra lean, 97% fat-free (Turkey Store)	4 oz	120	0	1.5
lean, 7% fat, w/natural flavorings (Turkey Store)	4 oz	160	0	8.0
raw (Norbest)	1 oz	45	0	2.6
w/natural flavoring (Louis Rich)	1 oz	50	0	2.2
HEART				
Fresh				
all classes, raw	1 med heart	41	0	2.0
all classes, simmered, chopped or diced	1 cup	257	3	8.8
HINDQUARTER				
Frozen or refrigerated, roast (Land O'Lakes)	3 oz	140	0	8.0
LEG				
Fresh				
all classes, meat and skin, raw	1 lb	656	0.0	30.4

Food Name	Serv. Size	Total Cal.	Carbs GMS	Fat GMS
all classes, meat and skin, raw	1 oz	41	0.0	1.9
all classes, meat and skin, roasted	4 oz	236	0.0	11.1
fryer/roaster, meat and skin, raw	4 oz	135	0	4.0
fryer/roaster, meat and skin, roasted	4 oz	194	0	6.2
fryer/roaster, meat only, raw	4 oz	123	0	2.7
fryer/roaster, meat only, roasted	4 oz	182	0	4.3
young hen, meat and skin, raw	4 oz	173	0	8.6
young hen, meat and skin, roasted	4 oz	235	0	11.0
Frozen or refrigerated				
(Land O'Lakes).	3 oz	120	0	5.0
cooked (Louis Rich)	1 oz	56	0	2.6
cooked, 'Fresh Turkey Cuts' (Louis Rich)	1 oz	55	1	3.0
LIGHT MEAT				
Canned				
chunk white, in water, 97% fat-free (Valley Fresh)	2 oz	80	0	1.5
white meat (Swanson)	2.5 oz	80	1	1.0
Fresh				
all classes, meat and skin, raw	1 lb	720	0.0	33.6
all classes, meat and skin, raw	1 oz	45	0.0	2.1
all classes, meat and skin, roasted	4 oz	223	0.0	9.4
all classes, meat only, raw	1 lb	528	0.0	6.4
all classes, meat only, raw	1 oz	33	0.0	0.4
all classes, meat only, roasted	4 oz	178	0.0	3.7
all classes, meat only, roasted, chopped or diced	1 cup	220	0.0	4.5
fryer/roaster, meat and skin, raw	4 oz	152	0	4.4
fryer/roaster, meat and skin, roasted	4 oz	188	0	5.2
fryer/roaster, meat only, raw	4 oz	123	0	0.6
fryer/roaster, meat only, roasted	4 oz	160	0	1.3
fryer/roaster, meat only, roasted, chopped or diced	1 cup	196	0	1.7
young hen, meat and skin, raw	4 oz	189	0	9.3
young hen, meat and skin, roasted	4 oz	237	0	10.8
young hen, meat only, raw	4 oz	133	0	1.9
young hen, meat only, roasted	4 oz	184	0	4.3
young hen, meat only, roasted, chopped or diced	1 cup	225	0	5.2
young tom, meat and skin, raw	4 oz	179	0	8.0
young tom, meat and skin, roasted	4 oz	218	0	8.8
young tom, meat only, raw	4 oz	131	0	1.8
young tom, meat only, roasted	4 oz	176	0	3.3
LIVER				
Fresh				
all classes, raw	3.5 oz	140	4	4.0
all classes, raw	0.25 oz	10	0	0.3
all classes, simmered	0.18 oz	8	0	0.3
all classes, simmered, chopped or diced	1 cup	237	5	8.3
NECK				
Fresh				
all classes, raw	1 lb	608	0.0	24.0
all classes, raw	1 oz	38	0.0	1.5
all classes, simmered	4 oz	204	0.0	8.2
PATTY				
Frozen or refrigerated, kosher (Empire Kosher)	1 patty	200	14	10.0
SKIN				
Fresh				
all classes, raw	1 lb	1760	0.0	168.0
all classes, raw	1 oz	110	0.0	10.5
all classes, roasted	1 oz	125	0.0	11.2
fryer/roaster, raw	4 oz	325	0	26.8

Food Name	Serv. Size	Total Cal.	Carbs GMS	Fat GMS
fryer/roaster, roasted	4 oz	343	0	26.6
young hen, raw	4 oz	476	0	46.4
young hen, roasted	4 oz	551	0	50.8
young tom, raw	4 oz	421	0	39.4
young tom, roasted	4 oz	482	0	42.5
THIGH				
Frozen or refrigerated				
(Land O'Lakes)	3 oz	150	0	10.0
cooked (Louis Rich)	1 oz	64	0	3.7
cooked, 'Fresh Turkey Cuts' (Louis Rich)	1 oz	65	1	4.0
WHOLE				
Frozen or refrigerated				
barbecue, kosher (Empire Kosher)	5 oz	250	0	12.0
cooked, excluding giblets, 'Fresh Whole Turkey' (Louis Rich)	1 oz	50	1	2.0
cooked, no bone (Norbest)	1 oz	42	0	1.5
cooked, w/o giblets (Louis Rich)	1 oz	52	0	2.3
young (Land O'Lakes) frozen/refrig., young	3 oz	130	1	7.0
young, butter-basted (Land O'Lakes)	3 oz	140	1	8.0
young, self-basting, broth (Land O'Lakes)	3 oz	120	1	5.0
young, 3% self-basting solution, 'Natural Choice' (Jennie-O)	4 oz	170	0	8.0
WING				
Fresh				
all classes, meat and skin, raw	1 lb	896	0.0	56.0
all classes, meat and skin, raw	1 oz	56	0.0	3.5
all classes, meat and skin, roasted	4 oz	260	0.0	14.1
fryer/roaster, meat and skin, raw	3 oz	136	0	6.7
fryer/roaster, meat and skin, roasted	3 oz	178	0	8.6
fryer/roaster, meat only, raw	3 oz	92	0	1.0
fryer/roaster, meat only, roasted	3 oz	141	0	3.0
young hen, meat and skin, raw	3 oz	181	0	11.9
young hen, meat and skin, roasted	3 oz	205	0	11.6
young tom, meat and skin, raw	3 oz	160	0	9.7
young tom, meat and skin, roasted	3 oz	188	0	9.8
Frozen or refrigerated				
(Land O'Lakes)	3 oz	120	0	5.0
cooked (Louis Rich)	1 oz	54	0	2.7
cooked, 'Drumettes' (Louis Rich)	1 oz	51	0	2.2
cooked, 'Fresh Turkey Cuts' (Louis Rich)	1 oz	55	1	3.0
portions, cooked (Louis Rich)	1 oz	54	0	2.9
TURKEY DINNER/ENTRÉE				
(Armour) w/dressing and gravy, frozen, 'Classics'	11.5 oz	320	34	12.0
(Banquet)				
pie, frozen	7 oz	510	39	31.0
pie, frozen, 'Supreme Microwave'	7 oz	430	30	27.0
sliced, w/gravy, frozen, 'Cookin' Bags'	5 oz	100	5	6.0
sliced, w/gravy, frozen, 'Family Entrées'	8 oz	150	8	8.0
turkey entrée, frozen	1 entrée	280	34	10.0
turkey entrée, frozen	10.5 oz	390	35	20.0
turkey entrée, frozen, 'Extra Helping'	19 oz	750	68	42.0
w/dressing, potatoes, corn, in sauce	1 entrée	280	34	9.9
w/gravy and dressing, frozen, 'Healthy Balance'	11.25 oz	270	41	5.0
w/mashed potatoes and corn, in seasoned sauce	1 serving	280	34	9.9
(Budget Gourmet)				
breast, Dijon, frozen	11.2 oz	340	37	12.0
breast, sliced, frozen	11.1 oz	290	36	9.0
turkey à la king, w/rice, frozen	10 oz	390	36	18.0
turkey entrée, glazed, frozen, 'Light'	1 entrée	250	38	4.0

Food Name	Serv. Size	Total Cal.	Carbs GMS	Fat GMS
w/escalloped noodles 'Special Selections'	1 entrée	440	44	20.0
(Butterball)				
breast, hickory-smoked, no skin, 99% fat-free	3 oz	80	1	1.0
breast, roasted, no skin, 99% fat-free	3 oz	80	2	1.0
breast, roasted, w/honey, no skin, 99% fat-free	3 oz	90	3	1.0
(Dinty Moore)				
w/dressing and gravy, 'Micro Meal'	1 bowl	280	32	7.0
w/dressing and gravy, packaged, 'American Classics'	10 oz	290	33	5.0
(Empire Kosher) pie, kosher	1 pie	470	46	23.0
(Freezer Queen)				
croquettes, breaded, w/gravy, frozen	7 oz	250	19	13.0
sliced, frozen	10 oz	280	36	8.0
sliced, w/gravy and dressing, frozen, 'Single Serve'	9 oz	230	32	5.0
sliced, w/gravy, frozen, 'Cook-In-Pouch'	5 oz	70	6	2.0
sliced, w/gravy, frozen, 'Family Suppers'	7 oz	110	8	5.0
w/gravy and dressing, frozen, 'Deluxe Family'	7 oz	160	18	5.0
(Healthy Choice)				
breast medallions and vegetables, frozen, 'Classics'	12.5 oz	350	45	6.0
breast, 'Traditional'	1 entrée	290	40	4.5
breast, sliced, w/gravy and dressing, frozen	10 oz	270	30	4.0
breast, traditional, frozen	1 meal	280	40	3.0
'Country Inn Roast'	1 entrée	250	28	6.0
country roast, w/mushrooms, gravy, rice	1 entrée	223	28	3.9
roasted, w/mushrooms and gravy, frozen	8.5 oz	200	26	3.0
tetrazzini, frozen	12.6 oz	340	49	6.0
turkey and vegetables, 'Hearty Handfuls'	1 entrée	320	51	5.0
w/mushrooms, 'Country Roast'	1 entrée	230	26	5.0
w/vegetables, lowfat, frozen, 'Homestyle'	9.5 oz	230	28	3.0
(Hormel) w/vegetable, microwave, 'Health Selections'	7.25 oz	220	35	2.0
(Hudson) sliced, extra lean	1 slice	30	0	0.5
(Hungry Man)				
pot pie	1 pie	650	65	34.0
turkey entrée, mostly white meat, frozen	1 entrée	510	64	15.0
(Jennie-O)				
white and dark meat, roasted, w/gravy	4 oz	150	3	7.0
white meat, roasted, w/gravy	4 oz	150	3	7.0
(Le Menu)				
breast, sliced, w/mushroom gravy, frozen	10.5 oz	300	38	7.0
glazed, frozen, 'LightStyle'	8.25 oz	260	34	6.0
sliced, frozen, 'LightStyle'	10 oz	210	21	5.0
turkey divan, frozen, 'LightStyle'	10 oz	260	23	7.0
white meat, w/gravy and stuffing, frozen	8 oz	200	19	5.0
(Lean Cuisine)				
breast, sliced, in mushroom sauce w/rice, frozen	8 oz	230	24	7.0
breast, sliced, w/dressing, frozen	7 7/8 oz	200	23	5.0
Dijon, frozen	9.5 oz	210	20	6.0
homestyle	1 entrée	230	26	6.0
homestyle, w/vegetables and pasta, frozen	9 3/8 oz	230	25	5.0
pot pie	1 entrée	300	34	9.0
tenderloins, glazed	1 entrée	240	37	5.0
(Libby's) w/gravy and dressing, microwave, 'Diner'	7 oz	170	15	7.0
(Louis Rich)				
breast, roasted, 99 fat-free	2 oz	50	1	0.5
breast, roasted, dinner slices, 99% fat-free	1 slice	70	1	1.0
nuggets/sticks, breaded	1 serving	235	13	14.9
nuggets/sticks, breaded	1 piece	77	4	4.9
patty, white meat, breaded	1 serving	220	13	13.0

Food Name	Serv. Size	Total Cal.	Carbs GMS	Fat GMS
(Marie Callender's)				
grilled breast and rice pilaf	11.7 oz	320	34	10.0
pot pie	1 pie	610	57	36.0
turkey w/gravy and dressing, frozen	14 oz	500	52	19.0
w/gravy and dressing, w/broccoli	1 entrée	504	52	19.0
(Morton) turkey entrée, frozen	10 oz	230	28	6.0
(Mountain House) tetrazzini, freeze-dried, prepared	1 cup	200	20	8.0
(Mrs. Paterson's)				
pie, w/broccoli, hand held, frozen, 'Aussie Pie'	5.5 oz	460	42	26.0
(Norbest)				
breast, w/gravy, raw	4 oz	115	1	2.4
w/gravy, raw	4 oz	115	1	2.7
(Pierre)				
nuggets, product 1936	1 piece	70	2	5.2
nuggets, product 1937	1 piece	49	1	3.7
patty, breaded, flame-broiled, product 1939	1 piece	287	8	21.3
patty, flame-broiled, frozen, product 9719	1 piece	86	0	3.9
patty, flame-broiled, frozen, product 9721	1 piece	105	0	4.8
patty, strip-shaped, frozen, product 1938	1 piece	94	3	7.0
(Pillsbury) casserole, frozen, 'Microwave Classic'	1 pkg	430	31	25.0
(Right Course)				
sliced, in mild curry sauce, w/rice pilaf, frozen	8.75 oz	320	40	8.0
(Shelton's)				
pot pie, white flour crust	1 serving	220	18	10.0
pot pie, whole wheat crust	1 serving	220	18	10.0
(Stouffer's)				
breast, roasted, w/gravy and stuffing, frozen	7 7/8 oz	270	27	9.0
pot pie	1 entrée	530	36	33.0
roasted, w/stuffing, 'Homestyle'	1 entrée	280	25	11.0
tetrazzini	1 entrée	360	33	17.0
tetrazzini, frozen, food service product	1 oz	36	3	2.0
(Sunday House)				
young turkey, w/broth and caramel color	3 oz	110	0	5.0
(Swanson)				
breast, w/pasta, frozen	11.25 oz	310	36	9.0
pot pie	1 pie	400	42	21.0
turkey and dressing, mostly white meat, w/gravy	1 entrée	240	30	9.0
turkey entrée, frozen	11.5 oz	350	42	11.0
turkey entrée, frozen, 'Hungry Man'	17 oz	550	61	18.0
turkey entrée, mostly white meat, frozen	1 entrée	320	42	8.0
(Turkey By George)				
hickory barbecue, packaged	5 oz	190	8	5.0
Italian Parmesan, packaged	5 oz	170	3	5.0
lemon pepper, packaged	5 oz	160	4	4.0
mustard tarragon, packaged	5 oz	180	3	6.0
(Tyson)				
pie, frozen	9 oz	370	39	18.0
turkey entrée, frozen, 'Gourmet Selection'	11.5 oz	380	51	11.0
w/dressing, frozen, 'Elmer Fudd'	6.55 oz	260	40	7.0
w/gravy, frozen, 'Gourmet Selections'	9.5 oz	320	34	12.0
(Ultra Slim-Fast)				
glazed, w/dressing, frozen	10.5 oz	340	49	5.0
medallions, in herb sauce, frozen	12 oz	280	33	6.0
(Weight Watchers)				
breast, stuffed	1 entrée	230	28	5.0
medallions, roasted, w/mushroom sauce, frozen, 'Smart Ones'	8.5 oz	200	35	1.0
medallions, 'Smart Ones'	1 entrée	190	34	2.0
w/mushroom, rice, vegetable, 'Smart Ones'	1 entrée	214	35	1.7

Food Name	Serv. Size	Total Cal.	Carbs GMS	Fat GMS
(Wonderbites)				
fajita, flame-broiled, product 2196, 'Dippers' .... 1 piece		34	1	1.3
TURKEY FAT				
.... 1 cup		1846	0	204.6
.... 1 tbsp		115	0	12.8
.... 1 tsp		39	0	4.3
TURKEY JERKY *(Shelton's)* .... 1/2 oz		50	1	0.5
TURKEY SEASONING. See under SEASONING MIX.				
TURKEY SNACK STICKS				
(Turkey Store)				
breast meat, cheese, 'Gobble Stix' .... 1 stick		30	1	0.8
breast meat, smoked, 'Gobble Stix' .... 1 stick		25	0	0.2
TURKEY SPREAD				
(Libby's) turkey salad, 'Spreadables' .... 1/3 cup		150	7	10.0
(Underwood) chunky 'Light' .... 2 1/8 oz		75	2	2.0
TURKEY SUBSTITUTE				
(Worthington)				
canned, drained .... 2 slices		120	3	8.0
slices .... 3 slices		193	3	14.0
smoked, roll, frozen .... 4 slices		180	5	12.0
vegetarian, 'Meatless Smoked Turkey' .... 3 slices		140	3	10.0
vegetarian, 'Turkee Slices' .... 3 slices		170	3	12.0
TURMERIC				
dried *(McCormick/Schilling)* .... 1 tsp		8	2	0.0
ground .... 1 tbsp		24	4	0.7
ground .... 1 tsp		8	1	0.2
ground *(Durkee)* .... 1 tsp		9	0	0.0
ground *(Laurel Leaf)* .... 1 tsp		9	0	0.0
ground *(Spice Islands)* .... 1 tsp		7	1	0.2
TURNIP. See also RUTABAGA.				
Canned				
(Stokely) .... 1/2 cup		20	3	0.0
diced *(Allens)* .... 1/2 cup		16	2	1.0
Fresh				
boiled, drained, cubed .... 1 cup		33	8	0.1
boiled, drained, mashed .... 1 cup		48	11	0.2
raw, cubed .... 1 cup		35	8	0.1
Frozen				
cubes, boiled, drained .... 1 cup		33	8	0.1
diced *(Southern)* .... 3.5 oz		17	3	0.2
mashed, boiled, drained .... 1 cup		48	11	0.2
mashed, unprepared .... 10-oz pkg		45	8	0.5
w/greens, boiled, drained .... 1 cup		28	5	0.3
w/greens, unprepared .... 10-oz pkg		60	10	0.5
TURNIP, CABBAGE. See KOHLRABI.				
TURNIP-ROOTED PARSLEY. See PARSLEY ROOT.				
TURNIP GREENS				
Canned				
chopped *(Allens)* .... 1/2 cup		21	3	1.0
chopped *(Bush's Best)* .... 1/2 cup		20	3	0.0
chopped, w/diced turnips *(Allens)* .... 1/2 cup		19	1	1.0
seasoned w/pork *(Luck's)* .... 1 cup		35	5	1.5
w/diced turnips *(Bush's Best)* .... 1/2 cup		25	4	0.0
w/diced turnips *(Stokely)* .... 1/2 cup		20	0	0.0
w/liquid .... 1/2 cup		16	3	0.4
Fresh				
boiled, drained, chopped .... 4 oz		23	4.9	0.3
boiled, drained, chopped .... 1/2 cup		14	3.1	0.2

Food Name	Serv. Size	Total Cal.	Carbs GMS	Fat GMS
raw, chopped .... 1 cup		15	3	0.2
Frozen				
boiled, drained .... 10-oz pkg		66	11	0.9
chopped *(Flav-R-Pac)* .... 1/3 cup		30	2	0.0
chopped *(Frosty Acres)* .... 3.3 oz		20	4	0.0
chopped *(Seabrook)* .... 3.3 oz		20	4	0.0
chopped *(Southern)* .... 3.5 oz		25	4	0.3
chopped, boiled, drained .... 1 cup		29	6	0.3
chopped, unprepared .... 10-oz pkg		62	10	0.9
chopped, w/diced turnips *(Flav-R-Pac)* .... 1/3 cup		30	2	0.0
chopped or diced, unprepared .... 1/2 cup		18	3	0.3
w/diced turnips *(Seabrook)* .... 3.3 oz		20	3	0.0
TURNOVER. See under PASTRY.				
TURTLE, GREEN				
canned .... 3.5 oz		106	0.0	0.7
raw .... 3.5 oz		89	0.0	0.5
TUSCAN PEPPER. See PEPPER, TUSCAN.				
TUSK. See CUSK.				

U

Food Name	Serv. Size	Total Cal.	Carbs GMS	Fat GMS
UCUHUBA BUTTER OIL				
.... 1 cup		1927	0	218.0
.... 1 tbsp		120	0	13.6
UDON. See under NOODLE, JAPANESE.				
UMEBOSHI/Japanese plum				
peeled and seeded .... 1 oz		13	3.4	0.1
raw, approx 0.6 oz .... 1 medium		5	1.2	<0.1
untrimmed .... 1 lb		132	34.1	0.6

V

Food Name	Serv. Size	Total Cal.	Carbs GMS	Fat GMS
VANILLA EXTRACT				
.... 1 cup		599	26	0.1
.... 1 tbsp		37	2	0.0
.... 1 tsp		12	1	0.0
pure *(Virginia Dare)* .... 1 tsp		10	0	0.0
VANILLA EXTRACT SUBSTITUTE				
imitation .... 1 tbsp		7	2	0.0
imitation .... 1 tsp		2	1	0.0
imitation, w/alcohol .... 1 tbsp		31	0	0.0
imitation, w/alcohol .... 1 tsp		10	0	0.0
VANILLA, BAKING chips, vanilla milk *(Hershey's)* .... 1/4 cup		240	25	14.0
VEAL				
(NOTE: TRIMMED = Lean; separable fat removed after cooking. UNTRIMMED = Separable fat not removed.)				
BRAIN				
braised .... 3 oz		116	0	8.2
pan-fried .... 3 oz		181	0	14.2
raw .... 4 oz		134	0	9.3
BREAST				
Trimmed, whole, boneless, braised .... 3 oz		185	0	8.3

Food Name	Serv. Size	Total Cal.	Carbs GMS	Fat GMS
Untrimmed				
plate half, boneless, braised	3 oz	240	0	16.1
point half, boneless, braised	3 oz	211	0	12.0
whole, boneless, braised	3 oz	226	0	14.3
GROUND				
broiled	3 oz	146	0	6.4
raw	4 oz	163	0	7.7
HEART				
braised	3 oz	158	0	5.7
raw	4 oz	125	0	4.5
KIDNEY				
braised	3 oz	139	0	4.8
raw	4 oz	112	1	3.5
LEG				
Trimmed				
top round, braised	3 oz	173	0	4.3
top round, breaded, pan-fried	3 oz	175	8	5.3
top round, pan-fried	3 oz	156	0	3.9
top round, raw	1 oz	30	0	0.5
top round, roasted	3 oz	128	0	2.9
Untrimmed				
top round, braised	3 oz	179	0	5.4
top round, breaded, pan-fried	3 oz	194	8	7.8
top round, pan-fried	3 oz	179	0	7.1
top round, raw	1 oz	33	0	0.9
top round, roasted	3 oz	136	0	4.0
LEG AND SHOULDER				
Trimmed				
cubed for stew, braised	3 oz	160	0	3.7
cubed for stew, raw	1 oz	31	0	0.7
LIVER				
braised	3 oz	140	2	5.9
pan-fried	3 oz	208	3	9.7
raw	4 oz	152	5	5.0
LOIN				
Trimmed				
braised	3 oz	192	0	7.8
raw	1 oz	33	0	0.9
roasted	3 oz	149	0	5.9
Untrimmed				
braised	3 oz	241	0	14.6
raw	1 oz	46	0	2.6
roasted	3 oz	184	0	10.5
LUNGS				
braised	3 oz	88	0	2.2
raw	4 oz	102	0	2.6
PANCREAS				
braised	3 oz	218	0	12.4
raw	4 oz	206	0	14.9
RIB				
Trimmed				
braised	3 oz	185	0	6.6
raw	1 oz	34	0	1.1
roasted	3 oz	150	0	6.3
Untrimmed				
braised	3 oz	213	0	10.7
raw	1 oz	46	0	2.6

Food Name	Serv. Size	Total Cal.	Carbs GMS	Fat GMS
roasted	3 oz	194	0	11.9
SHANK				
Trimmed				
fore and hind, braised	3 oz	150	0	3.7
fore and hind, raw	1 oz	31	0	0.8
Untrimmed				
fore and hind, braised	3 oz	162	0	5.3
fore and hind, raw	1 oz	32	0	1.0
SHOULDER				
Trimmed				
arm, braised	3 oz	171	0	4.5
arm, raw	1 oz	30	0	0.6
arm, roasted	3 oz	139	0	4.9
blade, braised	3 oz	168	0	5.5
blade, raw	1 oz	32	0	0.9
blade, roasted	3 oz	145	0	5.8
whole, arm and blade, braised	3 oz	169	0	5.2
whole, arm and blade, raw	1 oz	32	0	0.9
whole, arm and blade, roasted	3 oz	145	0	5.6
Untrimmed				
arm, braised	3 oz	201	0	8.7
arm, raw	1 oz	37	0	1.5
arm, roasted	3 oz	156	0	7.0
blade, braised	3 oz	191	0	8.6
blade, raw	1 oz	37	0	1.5
blade, roasted	3 oz	158	0	7.4
whole, arm and blade, braised	3 oz	194	0	8.6
whole, arm and blade, raw	1 oz	37	0	1.5
whole, arm and blade, roasted	3 oz	156	0	7.2
SIRLOIN				
Trimmed				
braised	3 oz	173	0	5.5
raw	1 oz	31	0	0.7
roasted	3 oz	143	0	5.3
Untrimmed				
braised	3 oz	214	0	11.2
raw	1 oz	43	0	2.2
roasted	3 oz	172	0	8.9
SPLEEN				
braised	3 oz	110	0	2.5
raw	4 oz	111	0	2.5
THYMUS				
braised	3 oz	148	0	3.6
raw	4 oz	112	0	2.8
TONGUE				
braised	3 oz	172	0	8.6
raw	4 oz	149	2	6.2
VEAL DINNER/ENTRÉE				
(Armour) Parmigiana, frozen, 'Classics'	11.25 oz	400	34	22.0
(Banquet)				
Parmigiana	1 entrée	360	35	19.0
Parmigiana, breaded patty, frozen, 'Cookin' Bags'	4 oz	230	20	11.0
Parmigiana, w/tomato sauce, potato. peas in sauce	1 entrée	362	35	19.0
(Contadina) Parmigiana, frozen	1 oz	42	3	2.3
(Freezer Queen)				
Parmigiana, breaded, frozen, 'Cook-In-Pouch'	5 oz	220	17	12.0
Parmigiana, breaded, frozen, 'Deluxe Family Suppers'	7 oz	300	22	15.0

Food Name	Serv. Size	Total Cal.	Carbs GMS	Fat GMS
Parmigiana, platter, frozen	10 oz	400	32	20.0
(Hormel)				
steak, breaded, frozen	4 oz	240	13	13.0
steak, frozen	4 oz	130	2	4.0
(Le Menu)				
Marsala, frozen, 'LightStyle'	10 oz	230	28	3.0
Parmigiana, frozen	11.5 oz	390	36	17.0
(Morton) Parmigiana, frozen	10 oz	260	35	8.0
(Pierre) veal and beef patty, Italian, frozen, product 1905	1 piece	279	12	19.6
(Stouffer's) Parmigiana, w/spaghetti, 'Homestyle'	1 entrée	420	43	19.0
(Swanson)				
Parmigiana	1 entrée	390	40	18.0
Parmigiana, 'Hungry Man'	1 entrée	640	74	23.0
Parmigiana, frozen, 'Homestyle Recipe'	10 oz	330	33	13.0
(Weight Watchers)				
Parmigiana, breaded patty, frozen, 'Ultimate 200'	8.2 oz	150	5	4.0
VEGETABLE CHIPS				
(Eden Foods)	1-oz bag	130	22	4.0
sea vegetable *(Eden Foods)*	1-oz bag	130	22	5.0
VEGETABLE DISH/ENTRÉE See also individual listings.				
(Amy's Kitchen)				
pot pie	1 serving	360	44	18.0
shepherd's pie	1 serving	160	27	4.0
(Budget Gourmet)				
w/chicken, Chinese style, frozen	10 oz	280	47	7.0
w/chicken, Italian style, frozen	10.25 oz	310	50	8.0
(Dinty Moore) stew, canned	8 oz	155	20	6.0
(Flav-R-Pac)				
stir-fry w/asparagus, frozen	1 cup	25	4	0.0
stir-fry w/noodles, frozen	1 cup	50	9	0.0
stir-fry w/rice, frozen	1 cup	80	18	0.0
succotash, frozen	2/3 cup	100	22	1.0
vegetarian dinner blend	3/4 cup	25	4	0.0
(Frosty Acres) succotash, frozen	3.3 oz	100	19	0.0
(Gardenburger)				
vegetable patty, vegetarian, roasted, 'Gourmet'	2.5 oz	120	17	2.8
(Green Giant)				
broccoli, cauliflower, carrots, in cheese sauce	2/3 cup	80	11	2.5
four vegetables in butter sauce w/pasta *(Green Giant)*	3/4 cup	70	11	2.0
w/sauce, 'Garden Gourmet Fettuccine Primavera'	9.5 oz serving	307	34	13.3
(Hanover) rice and vegetables w/soy sauce, 'Stir Fry 2'	1 cup	130	27	0.4
(La Choy)				
chow mein, contains no meat	3/4 cup	35	6	0.4
chow mein, meatless, canned	1 cup	55	10	0.7
chow mein, vegetable, frozen, food service product	1 cup	108	20	2.3
(Morningstar Farms)				
vegetarian, 'Garden Grille'	1 patty	120	18	2.5
vegetarian, 'Garden Veggie Patties'	1 patty	100	3	2.5
(Morton)				
w/beef, frozen	7 oz	430	27	31.0
w/chicken, frozen	7 oz	420	27	28.0
w/turkey, frozen	7 oz	420	27	28.0
(Mountain House) stew, w/beef, freeze-dried, prepared	1 cup	230	27	7.0
(Natural Touch)				
vegetarian, 'Dinner Entrée'	1 pattie	220	2	15.0
vegetarian, 'Garden Veggie Pattie'	1 pattie	100	8	2.5
vegetarian, 'Okara Patties'	1 pattie	110	4	5.0

Food Name	Serv. Size	Total Cal.	Carbs GMS	Fat GMS
(S&W) succotash, canned, 'Country Style'	1/2 cup	80	16	1.0
(Seabrook) succotash, frozen	3.3 oz	100	19	0.0
(Shanghai) stir-fry, frozen	5.1 oz	75	11	1.0
(Stokely) succotash, canned	1/2 cup	90	20	0.0
(Stouffer's)				
chow mein, frozen, food service product	1 oz	14	2	0.7
lasagna, frozen, food service product	1 oz	45	4	2.6
(Tofu Classics) chow mein, Mandarin, prepared w/tofu	1/2 cup	110	14	6.0
(Ultra Slim-Fast) and beef tips, country style	12 oz	230	26	5.0
(Worthington)				
vegetarian, 'Multigrain Cutlets' 50-oz can	1 slice	80	4	1.5
vegetarian, 'Multigrain Cutlets' 20-oz can	2 slices	100	5	2.0
vegetarian, 'Vegetarian Cutlets'	1 slice	70	3	1.0
VEGETABLE FLAKES (French's) dehydrated	1 tbsp	12	3	0.0
VEGETABLE JUICE DRINK				
(Biotta)				
'Breuss Juice'	6 fl oz	67	13	0.1
'Cocktail'	6 fl oz	50	10	0.1
(Knudsen)				
'Very Veggie' blend, low-salt	8 fl oz	50	10	1.0
'Very Veggie' fruit juice sweetened	8 fl oz	50	10	1.0
'Very Veggie' low-sodium	8 fl oz	40	8	0.0
'Very Veggie' organic	8 fl oz	40	8	0.0
'Very Veggie' original	8 fl oz	40	8	0.0
'Very Veggie' spicy	8 fl oz	40	8	0.0
(Sacramento)	8 fl oz	30	9	0.0
(Smucker's)				
hearty	8 fl oz	58	13	0.1
hot and spicy	8 fl oz	58	13	0.1
(V8)				
low-salt	8 fl oz	60	11	0.0
100% juice	8 fl oz	50	10	0.0
100% juice, lightly tangy	8 fl oz	60	11	0.0
picante	11.5 fl oz	70	14	0.0
spicy hot	8 fl oz	50	10	0.0
(Veryfine) '100%'	6 fl oz	32	6	0.0
VEGETABLE OIL. See also individual listings.				
salad or cooking	1 cup	1927	0	218.0
salad or cooking	1 tbsp	120	0	13.6
(Blue Plate)	1 tbsp	130	0	14.0
(Crisco) Canola and corn oil blend	1 tbsp	120	0	14.0
(Finast)	1 tbsp	120	0	14.0
(Hain)				
'All Blend'	1 tbsp	120	0	14.0
w/garlic, 'Garlic & Oil'	1 tbsp	120	0	14.0
(Kroger)	1 tbsp	122	0	13.6
(Mazola) Canola and corn oil blend, 'Right Blend'	1 tbsp	120	0	14.0
(Pathmark)				
	1 tbsp	120	0	14.0
'No Frills'	1 tbsp	130	0	14.0
(Puritan)	1 tbsp	120	0	14.0
(Wesson)				
	1 tbsp	122	0	13.6
butter flavor	1 tbsp	122	0	13.6
Canola and vegetable oil blend, 'Best Blend'	1 tbsp	120	0	14.0

VEGETABLE OIL SPREAD. See MARGARINE; MARGARINE SPREAD; MARGARINE SUBSTITUTE.
VEGETABLE OYSTER. See SALSIFY.

Food Name	Serv. Size	Total Cal.	Carbs GMS	Fat GMS
VEGETABLE SPONGE. See GOURD, DISHCLOTH.				
VEGETABLES, MIXED				
Canned				
(A&P)				
'Eastern'	1/2 cup	45	8	1.0
no salt added	1/2 cup	40	9	1.0
'Western'	1/2 cup	40	9	1.0
(Bush's Best) greens, mixed	1/2 cup	20	3	0.0
(Chun King) chow mein	1/2 cup	10	2	0.0
(Featherweight)	1/2 cup	40	8	0.0
(Finast)				
	1/2 cup	40	8	0.0
no salt added	1/2 cup	40	8	0.0
(Freshlike)				
water packed, no salt added	1/2 cup	35	8	0.0
water packed, no sugar or salt added	1/2 cup	35	8	0.0
(Green Giant)				
	1/2 cup	60	12	0.0
'Garden Medley'	1/2 cup	35	9	0.0
'Pantry Express'	1/2 cup	35	8	1.0
(La Choy)				
Chinese	1/2 cup	12	2	0.1
Chinese, food service product	2/3 cup	15	3	0.1
chop suey	1/2 cup	9	2	0.1
chop suey vegetables	1/2 cup	14	3	0.1
chop suey vegetables, food service product	1/2 cup	11	2	0.4
fancy	2/3 cup	9	1	0.1
(P&Q)				
'Chunky Eastern'	1/2 cup	40	8	1.0
'Chunky Western'	1/2 cup	40	9	1.0
(Pathmark)				
	1/2 cup	35	8	0.0
no salt added	1/2 cup	35	7	0.0
(S&W) 'Old Fashioned Harvest'	1/2 cup	35	6	0.0
(Stokely)				
	1/2 cup	40	8	0.0
no salt or sugar added	1/2 cup	40	8	0.0
(Veg-All)				
large cut, 'Homestyle'	1/2 cup	35	9	0.0
lite	1/2 cup	35	8	0.0
original	1/2 cup	35	8	0.0
Frozen				
(A&P)				
	3.3 oz	65	13	1.0
California blend	3.3 oz	25	5	1.0
Italian style blend	3.3 oz	40	8	1.0
Oriental style blend	3.3 oz	25	5	1.0
winter blend	3.3 oz	24	6	1.0
(Birds Eye)				
	3.3 oz	60	13	0.0
broccoli, cauliflower, carrots, 'Farm Fresh'	4 oz	35	7	0.0
broccoli, cauliflower, red peppers, 'Farm Fresh'	4 oz	30	5	0.0
broccoli, corn, red peppers, 'Farm Fresh'	4 oz	60	14	1.0
broccoli, green beans, pearl onions, red peppers	4 oz	35	7	0.0
broccoli, red peppers, bamboo shoots, mushrooms	4 oz	30	5	0.0
Brussels sprouts, cauliflower, carrots	4 oz	40	8	0.0

Food Name	Serv. Size	Total Cal.	Carbs GMS	Fat GMS
cauliflower, baby carrots, snow pea pods	4 oz	40	8	0.0
cauliflower, whole baby carrots, snow pea pods	4 oz	40	8	0.0
cauliflower, zucchini, carrots, red peppers	4 oz	30	6	0.0
Chinese style, 'Stir-Fry'	3.3 oz	35	8	0.0
Italian style, 'International Recipes'	3.3 oz	100	11	5.0
Japanese style, 'International Recipes'	3.3 oz	90	10	5.0
Japanese style, 'Stir-Fry'	3.3 oz	30	7	0.0
New England style, 'International Recipes'	3.3 oz	130	14	7.0
Oriental style, 'International Recipes'	3.3 oz	70	8	4.0
pepper stir-fry, 'Farm Fresh Mixtures'	1 cup	25	5	0.0
San Francisco style, 'International Recipes'	3.3 oz	100	11	5.0
sugar snap peas, baby carrots, water chestnuts	3.2 oz	50	11	0.0
(C&W)				
corn, broccoli, red peppers, 'Vegetable Stand'	2/3 cup	60	14	0.5
peas, corn, green beans, baby carrots	3/4 cup	60	11	0.0
petite peas and baby carrots, 'Early Harvest'	3.3 oz	60	12	0.0
red, green, and yellow bell pepper strips	1/2 cup	20	4	0.0
(Flav-R-Pac)				
Capri	3/4 cup	25	4	0.0
fajita blend	3/4 cup	20	5	0.0
fiesta	2/3 cup	60	10	0.0
five vegetables	2/3 cup	60	12	0.5
four vegetables	2/3 cup	50	9	0.0
Italian, frozen	2/3 cup	30	5	0.0
Italian, w/buttery sauce	1/2 cup	50	8	2.0
Mexicali	2/3 cup	80	18	0.5
omelette blend	3/4 cup	25	5	0.0
Oriental	3/4 cup	25	4	0.0
Scandinavian	3/4 cup	40	7	0.0
stew vegetables	2/3 cup	40	9	0.0
stew/soup vegetables	2/3 cup	40	9	0.0
stir-fry blend, frozen	3/4 cup	25	5	0.0
stir-fry blend, frozen, deluxe	3/4 cup	30	5	0.0
w/buttery sauce, frozen	1/2 cup	90	16	2.5
winter	1 cup	25	4	0.0
(Freshlike)				
	3.3 oz	70	13	0.0
'California Blend'	3.3 oz	30	6	0.0
'Chuckwagon Blend'	3.3 oz	70	16	1.0
'Country Blend'	3.3 oz	50	12	0.0
for soup	3.3 oz	50	11	0.0
for stew, 4-ways	3.3 oz	50	11	0.0
for stew, 5-ways	3.3 oz	50	12	0.0
'Italian Blend' food service product	3.3 oz	25	5	0.0
'Italian Blend'	3.3 oz	30	7	0.0
'Midwestern Blend'	3.3 oz	40	8	0.0
'Oriental Blend'	3.3 oz	25	5	0.0
'Scandinavian Blend'	3.3 oz	45	9	0.0
'Winter Blend'	3.3 oz	25	5	0.0
(Frosty Acres)				
	3.3 oz	65	13	0.0
Dutch style	3.2 oz	30	5	0.0
Italian style	3.2 oz	40	8	0.0
Oriental style	3.2 oz	25	5	0.0
(Green Giant)				
	1/2 cup	40	9	0.0

Food Name	Serv. Size	Total Cal.	Carbs GMS	Fat GMS
broccoli, cauliflower, carrots 'One Serving'	1 pkg	30	7	0.0
California style, 'American Mixtures'	1/2 cup	25	6	0.0
five vegetables in butter sauce	3/4 cup	60	8	2.0
heartland style, 'American Mixtures'	1 cup	30	6	0.0
LeSueur style, 'Valley Combinations'	1/2 cup	70	12	2.0
Manhattan style, 'American Mixtures'	1 cup	25	4	0.0
New England style, 'American Mixtures'	2/3 cup	70	13	1.5
'Plain Polybag'	1/2 cup	40	9	0.0
'Portion Pack'	3 oz	50	12	0.0
San Francisco style, 'American Mixtures'	3/4 cup	30	6	0.0
Santa Fe style, 'American Mixtures'	3/4 cup	60	13	0.0
Seattle style, 'American Mixtures'	3/4 cup	25	5	0.0
Western style, 'American Mixtures'	3/4 cup	50	9	1.5
(Health Valley)	1/2 cup	68	14	0.0
(La Choy) stir-fry vegetables, food service product	1/2 cup	34	6	0.1
(Pictsweet)				
'California'	3/4 cup	20	4	0.0
'Cantonese'	3.2 oz	35	7	0.0
'Chinese Stir-Fry'	3/4 cup	30	5	0.0
'Del Sol'	3.2 oz	30	6	0.0
'Grande'	3/4 cup	45	10	0.5
'Japanese'	3.2 oz	15	5	1.0
low-sodium, vitamins A and C	3.2 oz	60	12	0.0
'Oriental Stir-Fry'	3/4 cup	30	5	0.0
peas, carrots	2/3 cup	50	9	0.0
(Seabrook)	3.3 oz	65	13	0.0
(Southern)	3.5 oz	69	14	0.0
(Stokely)				
broccoli, cauliflower, baby carrots 'Singles'	3 oz	25	5	1.0
'Singles'	3 oz	60	12	1.0
(Trader Joe's) red, yellow, and green pepper strips, 'Melange a Trois'	1/3 cup	20	4	0.0
(Veg-All)				
	3.3 oz	70	13	0.0
'California Blend'	3.3 oz	30	6	0.0
'Chuckwagon Blend'	3.3 oz	70	16	1.0
'Country Blend'	3.3 oz	50	12	0.0
for soup	3.3 oz	50	11	0.0
for stew, 4-ways	3.3 oz	50	11	0.0
for stew, 5-ways	3.3 oz	50	12	0.0
'Italian Blend' food service product	3.3 oz	25	5	0.0
'Italian Blend'	3.3 oz	30	7	0.0
large cut	1/2 cup	45	9	0.0
'Midwestern Blend'	3.3 oz	40	8	0.0
'Oriental Blend'	3.3 oz	25	5	0.0
'Scandinavian Blend'	3.3 oz	45	9	0.0
'Winter Blend'	3.3 oz	25	5	0.0

VEGETARIAN FOODS. See individual listings.
VEGGIE BURGER. See under BEEF SUBSTITUTE DINNER/ENTRÉE.
VENISON. See CARIBOU; DEER; ELK; MOOSE.
VERMOUTH

(Gallo)				
dry	2 fl oz	56	1	0.0
sweet	2 fl oz	90	9	0.0
(Gambarelli & Davitto)				
dry	2 fl oz	64	2	0.0

Food Name	Serv. Size	Total Cal.	Carbs GMS	Fat GMS
sweet	2 fl oz	77	8	0.0
(Lejon)				
dry	2 fl oz	64	2	0.0
sweet	2 fl oz	77	8	0.0

VICHY WATER. See under SOFT DRINKS AND MIXERS.
VIENNA SAUSAGE. See under SAUSAGE.
VINE SPINACH. See SPINACH, VINE.
VINEGAR
APPLE CIDER

Food Name	Serv. Size	Total Cal.	Carbs GMS	Fat GMS
	1 cup	34	14	0.0
	1 tbsp	2	1	0.0
(Hain)	1 tbsp	2	4	0.0
(Heinz)	0.51 oz	2	0	0.0
(Indian Summer)	1 cup	40	14	1.0
(Lucky Leaf) pure	1 oz	4	2	0.0
(Musselman's) pure	1 oz	4	2	0.0
(S&W)	1 tbsp	0	0	0.0
(White House) distilled, colored or white, distilled	1 oz	4	2	0.0
MALT				
(Heinz) gourmet, 'Decanter'	0.51 oz	4	0	0.0
(S&W) malt ale, 'International'	1 tbsp	0	0	0.0
FLAVORED				
(Great Impressions)				
basil wine	1 tbsp	7	1	0.0
garlic wine	1 tbsp	7	1	0.0
hot paprika wine	1 tbsp	6	1	0.0
raspberry wine	1 tbsp	7	1	0.0
red wine	1 tbsp	6	1	0.0
(Heinz)				
garlic wine, gourmet, 'Decanter'	0.51 oz	4	0	0.0
tarragon, gourmet, 'Decanter'	0.51 oz	2	0	0.0
(S&W)				
garlic wine, 'International'	1 tbsp	0	0	0.0
Italian herb, 'International'	1 tbsp	0	0	0.0
tarragon, 'International'	1 tbsp	0	0	0.0
SALAD *(Heinz)* gourmet, 'Decanter'	0.51 oz	2	0	0.0
WHITE				
(Heinz) white, distilled	1 tbsp	2	0	0.0
(Indian Summer) white, distilled	1 cup	30	12	1.0
(Lucky Leaf) white, distilled	1 oz	4	2	0.0
(Musselman's) white, distilled	1 oz	4	2	0.0
(S&W) white, distilled	1 tbsp	0	0	0.0
WINE				
(Heinz) gourmet wine 'Decanter'	0.51 oz	4	0	0.0
(Lucky Leaf) red	1 oz	0	0	0.0
(Musselman's) red	1 oz	0	0	0.0
(Regina)				
all varieties	1 oz	4	0	0.0
red	1 oz	4	0	0.0
(S&W) red, 'International'	1 tbsp	0	0	0.0
VODKA				
80 proof	1 fl oz	64	0	0.0
86 proof	1 fl oz	70	0	0.0
90 proof	1 fl oz	73	0	0.0
94 proof	1 fl oz	76	0	0.0
100 proof	1 fl oz	82	0	0.0

W

Food Name	Serv. Size	Total Cal.	Carbs GMS	Fat GMS
WAFFLE				
(Aunt Jemima)				
apple cinnamon, frozen	1 waffle	176	29	5.6
buttermilk, frozen	1 waffle	179	29	5.8
low-fat, frozen	2 waffles	160	32	1.5
oat bran, frozen	2.5 oz	154	29	2.8
original, frozen, 2.5 oz	1 waffle	173	28	5.6
Quaker Oats, original, frozen	1 serving	197	30	6.0
whole-grain wheat, frozen	5-oz waffle	154	29	2.8
(Downyflake)				
apple and cinnamon, frozen 'Crisp & Healthy'	1 waffle	80	16	1.0
butter, frozen, 'Hot-N-Buttery'	2 waffles	180	27	6.0
buttermilk, frozen	2 waffles	190	32	5.0
buttermilk, frozen, 'Jumbo'	2 waffles	170	30	4.0
frozen, 'Jumbo'	2 waffles	170	30	4.0
frozen, blueberry, frozen	2 waffles	180	32	4.0
multigrain, frozen	2 waffles	250	28	4.0
oat bran, frozen	2 waffles	260	30	13.0
plain, frozen, 'Crisp & Healthy'	1 waffle	80	16	1.0
regular, frozen	2 waffles	120	20	3.0
rice bran, frozen	2 waffles	210	25	11.0
(Eggo)				
apple, 'Fruit Top'	3.1 oz	190	32	6.0
apple cinnamon	1 waffle	130	18	5.0
banana bread, 'Kellogg's Nutri-Grain'	1 serving	212	32	7.4
blueberry, frozen	1 waffle	130	18	5.0
blueberry, frozen, 'Fruit Top'	3.1 oz	190	32	6.0
blueberry, low-fat, 'Kellogg's Nutri-Grain'	1 serving	146	30	2.0
blueberry, low-fat, round, 'Kellogg's Nutri-Grain'	1 waffle	73	15	1.0
buttermilk, frozen	1 waffle	120	16	5.0
cinnamon toast, mini, sets of four	3 sets	280	45	9.0
golden oat	1 serving	139	26	2.3
golden oat, round	1 waffle	69	13	1.1
homestyle	1 waffle	120	16	5.0
homestyle, low-fat	1 serving	165	31	2.5
homestyle, mini, frozen, sets of four	3 sets	240	34	8.0
homestyle, round	1 waffle	83	15	1.2
'Kellogg's Nutri-Grain'	1 waffle	130	18	5.0
low-fat, 'Kellogg's Nutri-Grain'	1 serving	142	28	2.2
low-fat, round, 'Kellogg's Nutri-Grain'	1 waffle	71	14	1.1
multi-bran, 'Kellogg's Nutri-Grain'	2 waffles	180	32	6.0
nonfat, 'Kellogg's Special K'	2 waffles	140	29	0.0
nut and honey, frozen	2 waffles	240	32	10.0
oat bran, 'Common Sense'	1 waffle	110	16	4.0
oat bran, w/fruit and nut, 'Common Sense'	1 waffle	120	17	5.0
peach, 'Fruit Top'	3.1 oz	190	30	6.0
raisin and bran, 'Kellogg's Nutri-Grain'	1 waffle	130	18	5.0
strawberry	1 waffle	130	18	5.0
strawberry, 'Fruit Top'	1 waffle	190	31	6.0
wheat, whole grain, 'Kellogg's Nutri-Grain'	2 waffles	190	30	6.0
(Krusteaz)				
blueberry, frozen	1 waffle	110	19	3.0
buttermilk, frozen	1 waffle	100	16	2.0
buttermilk, frozen	1 waffle	100	16	2.0

Food Name	Serv. Size	Total Cal.	Carbs GMS	Fat GMS
golden, frozen	1 waffle	100	16	2.0
(Med Diet) Belgian, low-protein	1 serving	237	46	7.0
(Roman Meal) frozen	2 waffles	280	33	14.0
(Van's)				
apple cinnamon, frozen	1 waffle	75	8	2.0
Belgian, 7-grain, frozen	1 waffle	88	10	2.0
Belgian, oat bran, frozen	1 waffle	89	11	2.0
Belgian, original, frozen	1 waffle	86	14	2.0
honey almond, frozen	1 waffle	75	8	2.0
multigrain, frozen	1 waffle	75	8	2.0
WAFFLE DISH/MEAL				
(Swanson)				
Belgian, w/sausage, frozen, 'Great Starts'	2.85 oz	280	21	19.0
Belgian, w/sausage and strawberries, frozen	3.5 oz	210	31	8.0
w/bacon, frozen, 'Great Starts'	2.2 oz	230	19	14.0
WAFFLE MIX. See also PANCAKE/WAFFLE MIX.				
(Krusteaz) Belgian, prepared, 4-inch diam.	1 waffle	170	22	7.0
WAKAME. See under SEA VEGETABLE.				
WALLEYE. See under PIKE; POLLACK				
WALNUT				
ALL TYPES				
chopped, natural, unsalted *(Flanigan Farms)*	1 oz	180	4	19.0
halves and pieces *(Azar)*	2 oz	360	10	35.0
halves and pieces, natural, unsalted *(Flanigan Farms)*	1/4 cup	180	5	18.0
BLACK				
Dried				
	1 oz	172	3	16.0
	1 tbsp	47	1	4.4
(Planters)	1 oz	180	3	17.0
chopped	1 cup	759	15	70.7
shelled *(Fisher)*	1 oz	170	3	16.0
Raw *(Planters)*	1 oz	180	3	17.0
ENGLISH				
Dried				
in shell, whole, 7 med nuts	1 cup	183	4	18.3
shelled *(Diamond)*	1 oz	192	4	19.0
shelled, chopped *(Fisher)*	1 oz	180	5	18.0
shelled, chopped	1 cup	785	16	78.3
shelled, ground	1 cup	523	11	52.2
shelled, ground *(Fisher)*	1 oz	180	5	18.0
shelled, halved *(Planters)*	1 oz	190	3	20.0
shelled, halved, 50 halves	1 cup	654	14	65.2
shelled, pieces *(Planters)*	1 oz	190	3	20.0
shelled, pieces or chips	1 cup	785	16	78.3
shelled, whole *(Planters)*	1 oz	190	3	20.0
Raw *(Fisher)*	1 oz	180	5	18.0
PERSIAN				
Dried				
shelled *(Diamond)*	1 oz	192	4	19.0
shelled, halves *(Planters)*	1 oz	190	3	20.0
shelled, pieces *(Planters)*	1 oz	190	3	20.0
shelled, whole *(Planters)*	1 oz	190	3	20.0
WALNUT OIL				
	1 cup	1927	0	218.0
	1 tbsp	120	0	13.6
(Hain)	1 tbsp	120	0	14.0
(International Collection)	1 tbsp	120	0	14.0

Food Name	Serv. Size	Total Cal.	Carbs GMS	Fat GMS
California, 100% pure *(Loriva')*	1 tbsp	125	0	14.0
pure pressed, organic *(Spectrum)*	1 tbsp	120	0	14.0
WASABI CHIPS				
(Eden Foods)				
	1-oz bag	130	22	4.0
hot and spicy	1-oz bag	130	22	4.0
WASABI ROOT/Japanese horseradish				
raw, sliced	1 cup	142	31	0.8
raw, whole	1 med root	184	40	1.1
WATER				
FLAVORED. See also under SOFT DRINKS AND MIXERS.				
(Cascadia)				
cherry blackberry, sparkling, w/juice	6 fl oz	2	0	0.0
grapefruit, sparkling, w/juice	6 fl oz	2	0	0.0
guava berry, sparkling, w/juice	6 fl oz	2	0	0.0
lemonade, sparkling, w/juice	6 fl oz	2	0	0.0
(Clearly Canadian)				
sparkling, 'Coastal Cranberry'	6 fl oz	70	16	0.0
sparkling, 'Country Raspberry' sparkling	6 fl oz	70	16	0.0
sparkling, 'Mountain Blackberry'	6 fl oz	70	16	0.0
sparkling, 'Orchard Peach'	6 fl oz	70	16	0.0
sparkling, 'Western Loganberry'	6 fl oz	70	16	0.0
sparkling, 'Wild Cherry'	6 fl oz	70	16	0.0
(H2OH!)				
lemon-lime, sparkling	6 fl oz	0	0	0.0
natural berry, sparkling	6 fl oz	0	0	0.0
(Quest)				
black cherry, sparkling, 'Refresher'	8 fl oz	2	0	0.0
peach citrus, sparkling, 'Refresher'	8 fl oz	2	0	0.0
raspberry, sparkling, 'Refresher'	8 fl oz	2	0	0.0
red raspberry, sparkling, 'Refresher'	8 fl oz	2	0	0.0
strawberry-kiwi, sparkling, 'Refresher'	8 fl oz	2	0	0.0
tangerine lime, sparkling, 'Refresher'	8 fl oz	2	0	0.0
UNFLAVORED				
(Perrier)	8 fl oz	0	0	0.0
(Poland Spring)	8 fl oz	0	0	0.0
distilled *(Arrowhead)*	1 liter	0	0	0.0
drinking *(Arrowhead)*	1 liter	0	0	0.0
fluoridated *(Arrowhead)*	1 liter	0	0	0.0
mineral *(Perrier)*	1 liter	0	0	0.0
municipal	8 fl oz	0	0	0.0
sparkling, natural *(Clearly Canadian)*	6 fl oz	0	0	0.0
spring *(Arrowhead)*	1 liter	0	0	0.0
spring, 'Arizona Tule' *(Arrowhead)*	1 liter	0	0	0.0
Vichy *(Schweppes)*	6 fl oz	0	0	0.0
WATER BUFFALO				
raw	1 oz	28	0	0.4
roasted	3 oz	111	0	1.5
roasted, diced	1 cup	183	0.0	2.5
WATER CHESTNUT				
Canned				
Chinese *(LaChoy)*	1.28 oz	18	5	0.1
Chinese, sliced, w/liquid	1/2 cup	35	9	0.0
Chinese, whole, w/liquid	4 medium	14	3	0.0
chopped *(LaChoy)*	0.63 oz	9	2	0.1
sliced *(China Boy)*	1/2 cup	45	11	0.0
sliced *(Chun King)*	1 oz	12	2	1.0

Food Name	Serv. Size	Total Cal.	Carbs GMS	Fat GMS
sliced *(La Choy)*	2 tbsp	11	3	0.1
sliced, food service product *(La Choy)*	2 tbsp	11	3	0.1
whole *(La Choy)*	2 medium	10	2	0.1
whole, food service product *(La Choy)*	2 medium	10	2	0.1
Fresh				
Chinese, matai, raw, sliced	1/2 cup	60	15	0.1
Chinese, matai, raw, whole	4 medium	35	9	0.0
WATER CONVOLVULUS. See CABBAGE, SKUNK.				
WATERCRESS				
Fresh				
raw, chopped	1 cup	4	0	0.0
raw, whole sprigs	10 medium	3	0	0.0
raw, whole sprigs	1 medium	0	0	0.0
WATERMELON				
raw, balls	1 cup	49	11	0.7
raw, balls	10 balls	39	9	0.5
raw, diced	1 cup	49	11	0.7
raw, sliced, 1/16 of 10-inch diam melon	1 slice	92	21	1.2
WATERMELON SEED				
dried, kernels	1 cup	602	17	51.2
dried, kernels	1 oz	158	4	13.4
WAX BEAN. See BEAN, WAX.				
WAX GOURD. See GOURD, WAX.				
WELSH RAREBIT. See under CHEESE DISH/ENTRÉE.				
WEST INDIAN CHERRY. See ACEROLA.				
WESTERN ENTRÉE				
(Banquet) frozen	11 oz	630	40	41.0
(Morton) frozen	10 oz	290	29	14.0
(Swanson) frozen	11.5 oz	430	43	19.0
WHEAT				
BULGAR, gluten-free, 'Old World' *(Ener-G Foods)*	1/4 cup	181	39	0.6
DURUM	1 cup	651	137	4.7
HARD RED				
spring	1 cup	632	131	3.7
spring or winter, whole grain *(Arrowhead Mills)*	2 oz	190	41	1.0
winter	1 cup	628	137	3.0
HARD WHITE	1 cup	657	146	3.3
SOFT RED				
whole grain, for pastry *(Arrowhead Mills)*	2 oz	190	41	1.0
winter	1 cup	556	125	2.6
SOFT WHITE	1 cup	571	127	3.3
SPROUTED	1 cup	214	46	1.4
WHEAT BRAN				
crude	1 cup	125	37	2.5
crude *(Arrowhead Mills)*	2 oz	50	30	2.0
unprocessed *(Quaker)*	2 tbsp	8	4	0.2
unprocessed, miller's bran, dry *(Hodgson Mill)*	1/4 cup	30	10	0.0
unprocessed, natural *(Miller's)*	6 tbsp	70	17	1.0
WHEAT CAKE *(Quaker)* lightly salted	1 cake	35	7	0.0
WHEAT FLOUR. See under FLOUR.				
WHEAT GERM				
crude	1 cup	414	60	11.2
toasted, plain, ready to eat	1 cup	432	56	12.1
toasted, plain, ready to eat	1 oz	108	14	3.0
(Arrowhead Mills) raw	2 oz	210	26	6.0
(Hodgson Mill) untoasted, 25% protein, dry	2 tbsp	55	7	1.0

Food Name	Serv. Size	Total Cal.	Carbs GMS	Fat GMS
(Kretschmer)				
....	2 tbsp	50	6	1.0
honey crunch	1 2/3 tbsp	52	8	1.1
honey crunch, sodium-free, cholesterol-free	1 oz	110	15	3.0
sodium-free, cholesterol-free	2 tbsp	50	6	1.0
WHEAT GERM NUTS *(Anacon Foods)*	1/2 oz	100	2	9.3
WHEAT GERM OIL				
....	1 cup	1927	0	218.0
....	1 tbsp	120	0	13.6
WHEAT GLUTEN				
(Arrowhead Mills) Vita 1	1 oz	100	9	1.0
(Hodgson Mill) Vital w/Vit-C	1 tbsp	30	2	0.0
WHEAT SNACKS				
wheat nuts, flavored, no salt added, all flavors except macadamia ...	1 oz	183	6	17.7
wheat nuts, formulated, unflavored, salted	1 oz	176	7	16.4
(Ralston)				
'Delicious'	16 crackers	140	23	4.0
full fat, 'Delicious'	16 crackers	140	20	6.0
full fat, 'Grand Union'	16 crackers	140	20	6.0
full fat, 'Stop & Shop'	16 crackers	140	20	6.0
full fat, unsalted, 'Stop & Shop'	16 crackers	140	20	6.0
'Grand Union'	16 crackers	140	23	4.0
less fat	16 crackers	140	23	4.0
unsalted tops, 'Stop & Shop'	16 crackers	140	23	4.0
WHEATGRASS				
powder *(Pines)*	1 tsp	13	2	0.0
tablets *(Pines)*	7 tablets	13	2	0.0
WHELK				
boiled, poached, or steamed	3 oz	234	13	0.7
raw	3 oz	116	7	0.3
WHEY				
acid, dried	1 cup	193	42	0.3
acid, dried	1 tbsp	10	2	0.0
acid, fluid	1 quart	235	50	0.9
acid, fluid	1 cup	59	13	0.2
sweet, dried	1 cup	512	108	1.6
sweet, dried	1 tbsp	26	6	0.1
sweet, fluid	1 quart	263	51	3.5
sweet, fluid	1 cup	66	13	0.9
WHIPPED TOPPING. See CREAM TOPPING.				
WHISKEY				
80 proof	1 fl oz	64	0	0.0
86 proof	1 fl oz	70	0	0.0
90 proof	1 fl oz	73	0	0.0
94 proof	1 fl oz	76	0	0.0
100 proof	1 fl oz	82	0	0.0
WHISKEY SOUR. See under COCKTAIL; COCKTAIL MIX.				
WHITE ACRE PEAS, canned, fresh *(Allens)*	1/2 cup	90	14	1.0
WHITE BEAN. See BEAN, WHITE.				
WHITE CURRANT. See under CURRANT.				
WHITE GOURD. See CHINESE WATERMELON.				
WHITE MUSHROOM. See MUSHROOM, WHITE.				
WHITE PEPPER. See under PEPPER, GROUND.				
WHITE RICE. See under RICE.				
WHITE SUCKER. See SUCKER, WHITE.				
WHITEFISH				
mixed species, baked, broiled, grilled, or microwaved	3 oz	146	0	6.4

Food Name	Serv. Size	Total Cal.	Carbs GMS	Fat GMS
mixed species, raw	3 oz	114	0	5.0
mixed species, smoked	3 oz	92	0	0.8
mixed species, smoked, flaked	1 cup	147	0	1.3
WHITE-FLOWERED GOURD. See GOURD, BOTTLE.				
WHITING/silver hake				
Fresh				
mixed species, baked, broiled, grilled, or microwaved	3 oz	99	0	1.4
mixed species, raw	3 oz	77	0	1.1
Frozen, 'Individually Wrapped' *(Booth)*	4 oz	80	0	1.0
WILD RICE. See RICE, WILD.				
WINE. See also SHERRY; VERMOUTH; WINE, COOKING; WINE COOLER.				
(Mission Bell)				
'Arriba'	2 fl oz	95	7	0.0
'Diamond Red'	2 fl oz	95	7	0.0
'Silver Satin'	2 fl oz	83	5	0.0
'Silver Satin Bitter Lemon'	2 fl oz	83	6	0.0
'Swiss Up'	2 fl oz	84	6	0.0
BARBERA, white *(Colony)*	4 fl oz	91	4	0.0
BURGUNDY				
(Bravo) red	4 fl oz	91	2	0.0
(Carlo Rossi) red.	4 fl oz	92	2	0.0
(Colony)				
red 'Classic'	4 fl oz	90	1	0.0
white, 'Classic'	4 fl oz	80	1	0.0
(Gallo)				
red	4 fl oz	88	1	0.0
red, 'Hearty'	4 fl oz	92	2	0.0
(Gambarelli & Davitto) red 'Parma'	4 fl oz	91	2	0.0
(Petri) red.	4 fl oz	91	2	0.0
CABERNET SAUVIGNON				
(Colony)	4 fl oz	88	1	0.0
(Gallo)	4 fl oz	88	0	0.0
CARBONATED				
(Jacques Bonet)				
almond	4 fl oz	104	8	0.0
apricot	4 fl oz	111	10	0.0
cherry	4 fl oz	106	8	0.0
(Carlo Rossi) 'Paisano'	4 fl oz	92	2	0.0
(Jacques Bonet)				
peach	4 fl oz	111	10	0.0
raspberry	4 fl oz	106	8	0.0
CHABLIS				
(Bravo)	4 fl oz	86	2	0.0
(Carlo Rossi)				
pink	4 fl oz	92	4	0.0
white	4 fl oz	84	2	0.0
(Colony)				
	4 fl oz	98	5	0.0
'Classic'	4 fl oz	84	2	0.0
emerald	4 fl oz	102	5	0.0
gold	4 fl oz	97	4	0.0
ruby	4 fl oz	104	6	0.0
(Gallo)				
	4 fl oz	80	4	0.0
'Blanc'	4 fl oz	80	1	0.0
(Petri)				
	4 fl oz	98	5	0.0

Food Name	Serv. Size	Total Cal.	Carbs GMS	Fat GMS
'Chablis Blanc'	4 fl oz	86	2	0.0
(Gambarelli & Davitto) 'Parma'	4 fl oz	86	2	0.0
CHAMPAGNE				
(Jacques Bonet)				
brut	4 fl oz	92	2	0.0
extra dry	4 fl oz	97	3	0.0
pink	4 fl oz	98	4	0.0
(Lejon)				
brut	4 fl oz	92	3	0.0
extra dry	4 fl oz	97	2	0.0
pink	4 fl oz	98	4	0.0
CHENIN BLANC				
(Colony)	4 fl oz	86	2	0.0
(Gallo)	4 fl oz	88	2	0.0
CHIANTI				
(Carlo Rossi) 'Light'	4 fl oz	92	2	0.0
(Petri)	4 fl oz	91	2	0.0
COLD DUCK				
(Jacques Bonet)	4 fl oz	108	6	0.0
(Lejon)	4 fl oz	108	6	0.0
FRENCH COLOMBARD				
(Colony)	4 fl oz	84	2	0.0
(Gallo)	4 fl oz	88	2	0.0
GEWÜRZTRAMINER (Gallo)	4 fl oz	88	2	0.0
MARSALA (Gambarelli & Davitto).	4 fl oz	77	4	0.0
MOSELLE (Colony) 'Rhineskeller'	4 fl oz	97	4	0.0
MUSCATEL (Italian Swiss Colony)	2 fl oz	122	6	0.0
PASTOSO (Petri)	4 fl oz	92	2	0.0
PORT				
(Gallo)				
	2 fl oz	64	2	0.0
tawny, 'Livingston Cellars'	2 fl oz	86	6	0.0
white	2 fl oz	86	6	0.0
(Italian Swiss Colony)				
	2 fl oz	85	6	0.0
white	2 fl oz	86	6	0.0
RED TABLE	3.5 fl oz	74	2	0.0
RHINE				
(Bravo)	4 fl oz	97	4	0.0
(Carlo Rossi)	4 fl oz	84	4	0.0
(Colony) 'Classic'	4 fl oz	89	4	0.0
(Gallo)	4 fl oz	80	4	0.0
(Gambarelli & Davitto) 'Parma'	4 fl oz	92	1	0.0
(Petri)	4 fl oz	97	4	0.0
RIESLING (Gallo) 'Johannisberg'	4 fl oz	84	2	0.0
ROSÉ				
(Bravo)	4 fl oz	92	3	0.0
(Carlo Rossi) 'Vin Rose'	4 fl oz	88	3	0.0
(Colony) 'Classic'	4 fl oz	89	3	0.0
(Gallo)				
'Grenache'	4 fl oz	88	2	0.0
'Red Rose'	4 fl oz	112	6	0.0
'Vin Rose'	4 fl oz	88	3	0.0
(Gambarelli & Davitto) 'Parma'	4 fl oz	92	3	0.0
(Petri)	4 fl oz	92	3	0.0
SAUVIGNON BLANC (Gallo)	4 fl oz	80	1	0.0
TOKAY (Italian Swiss Colony)	2 fl oz	82	5	0.0

Food Name	Serv. Size	Total Cal.	Carbs GMS	Fat GMS
WHITE TABLE	3.5 fl oz	70	1	0.0
WINE, COOKING				
(Holland House)				
Marsala	1 fl oz	9	2	0.0
red	1 fl oz	6	2	0.0
sherry	1 fl oz	5	1	0.0
vermouth	1 fl oz	2	1	0.0
white	1 fl oz	2	1	0.0
(Regina)				
Burgundy	1/4 cup	2	1	1.0
Sauternes	1/4 cup	2	1	1.0
sherry	1/4 cup	20	5	1.0
WINE COOLER				
(Bartles & Jaymes)				
berry cooler, 'Light'	12 fl oz	150	32	0.0
black cherry cooler, 'Light'	12 fl oz	139	30	0.0
citrus cooler, 'Light'	6 fl oz	67	12	1.0
tropical cooler, 'Light'	12 fl oz	151	32	0.0
WINGED BEAN. See BEAN, WINGED.				
WINTER RADISH. See under RADISH, BLACK.				
WINTER SQUASH. See SQUASH, WINTER.				
WOLF FISH/ocean catfish				
Fresh				
Atlantic, baked, broiled, or grilled	3 oz	105	0	2.6
Atlantic, raw	3 oz	82	0	2.0
Frozen *(Booth)*	4 oz	115	0	20.0
WONTON WRAPPER				
including egg roll wrappers	1 oz	82	16	0.4
including egg roll wrappers, 7-inch square	1 wrapper	93	19	0.5
including egg roll wrappers, 3.5-inch square	1 wrapper	23	5	0.1
(Nasoya)	1 wrapper	23	5	0.0

Y

Food Name	Serv. Size	Total Cal.	Carbs GMS	Fat GMS
YAM				
Fresh				
boiled, drained, cubed	1 cup	158	38	0.2
boiled, drained, cubed	1/2 cup	79	19	0.1
raw, cubed	1 cup	177	42	0.3
Canned				
(Bush's Best)	1/2 cup	120	28	0.0
cut, in light syrup *(Princella)*	2/3 cup	160	40	0.5
orange pineapple *(Royal Prince)*	1/2 cup	210	43	0.5
CHINESE. See JICAMA.				
MOUNTAIN/HAWAIIAN				
Fresh				
raw, whole	1 medium	281	69	0.4
raw, cubed	1/2 cup	46	11	0.1
steamed, cubed	1 cup	119	29	0.1
YAM DISH				
(Flav-R-Pac) yam patties	2 pieces	150	33	1.0
(Stouffer's) yam and apples, frozen, food service product	1 oz	37	8	0.7
YAMBEAN TUBER. See JICAMA.				
YARDLONG BEAN. See BEAN, YARDLONG.				

Food Name	Serv. Size	Total Cal.	Carbs GMS	Fat GMS
YAUTIA/tannia				
Fresh				
raw, sliced .... 1 cup		132	32	0.5
raw, whole .... 1 med root		299	72	1.2
YEAST				
BAKER'S				
active, dry .... 1 tbsp		35	5	0.6
active, dry .... 1 tsp		12	2	0.2
active dry *(Red Star)*............................. 0.25 oz		15	2	0.0
active dry, 'RapidRise' *(Fleischmann's)*............ 0.25 oz		20	3	0.0
compressed .... 0.6-oz cake		18	3	0.3
BREWER'S				
debittered .... 1 oz		79	10.8	0.3
debittered .... 1 tbsp		23	3.1	0.1
torula .... 1 oz		78	10.4	0.3
YELLOW BEAN. See BEAN, YELLOW.				
YELLOW MOMBIN. See JOBO.				
YELLOW PEPPER. See PEPPER, BANANA; PEPPER, BELL.				
YELLOW SQUASH. See under SQUASH.				
YELLOW EYE BEANS. See under BAKED BEANS, CANNED.				
YELLOWFIN TUNA. See under TUNA.				
YELLOWTAIL				
mixed species, baked, broiled, grilled, or microwaved .... 3 oz		159	0	5.7
mixed species, raw .... 3 oz		124	0	4.5
YOGURT				
(Crowley) all flavors, 'Swiss Style' .... 1 cup		240	48	2.0
(Light n' Lively) all flavors except strawberry, nonfat, 'Free' .... 4.4 oz		50	8	0.0
(Ripple) all flavors, fat-free, '70' .... 6 oz		70	13	0.0
(Yoplait)				
all fruit flavors, custard style .... 6 oz		190	32	3.5
all fruit flavors, light .... 6 oz		90	16	0.0
all fruit flavors, nonfat .... 6 oz		90	16	0.0
all fruit flavors, original, 99% fat-free .... 6 oz		180	34	1.5
APPLE CINNAMON *(Dannon)* low-fat .... 1 container		240	46	3.0
APPLE CRISP *(New Country)* low-fat .... 6 oz		150	30	2.0
BANANA				
(Yoplait) custard style .... 6 oz		180	30	3.0
(Dannon) lowfat, 'Sprinkl'ins' .... 4.1 oz		140	24	2.0
BANANA BERRY				
(Light n' Lively) berry, low-fat, 1% milk fat, cultured .... 4.4 oz		130	24	1.0
BERRY *(Yoplait)* w/wheat, raisins, walnuts, 'Breakfast' .... 6 oz		200	39	2.0
BLACK CHERRY				
(Alta Dena)				
blended .... 8 oz		190	38	1.0
fruit on the bottom .... 1 cup		240	40	4.0
(Breyers) low-fat... 8 oz		260	49	3.0
(Knudsen) nonfat, 'Cal 70' .... 6 oz		70	12	0.0
(Light n' Lively)				
.... 8 oz		230	44	2.0
nonfat, '100' .... 8 oz		100	17	0.0
(Mountain High) natural, 'Honey Light' .... 8 oz		190	35	1.0
BLUEBERRY				
(Alta Dena) fruit on the bottom, 'Maya' .... 1 cup		280	39	9.0
(Breyers) low-fat.. 8 oz		250	48	2.0
(Dannon)				
low-fat .... 1 container		240	46	3.0
nonfat, blended .... 3/4 cup		160	33	0.0

Food Name	Serv. Size	Total Cal.	Carbs GMS	Fat GMS
nonfat, light	8 oz	100	19	0.0
(Knudsen) nonfat, 'Cal 70'	6 oz	70	11	0.0
(Light n' Lively)				
	8 oz	240	46	2.0
nonfat, 'Free'	4.4 oz	50	8	0.0
nonfat, '100'	8 oz	90	15	0.0
(Mountain High) natural, 'Honey Light'	8 oz	190	35	1.0
(New Country) 'Supreme'	6 oz	150	31	2.0
(White Wave) nondairy	1 serving	150	31	1.0
(Yoplait)				
fruit on the bottom	6 oz	170	35	0.0
light	6 oz	90	16	0.0
99% fat-free, original	6 oz	180	32	2.0
BLUEBERRIES AND CREAM				
(Weight Watchers) 'Ultimate 90'	1 cup	90	14	0.0
BLUEBERRY AND VANILLA *(Yoplait)* parfait style	6 oz	200	34	3.0
BLUEBERRY CHEESECAKE *(Yogi)* w/gelatin, 'Sundae'	5.6 oz	50	14	1.0
BOYSENBERRY				
(Dannon) low-fat	1 container	240	45	3.0
(Yoplait) 99% fat-free, original	6 oz	180	32	2.0
CAPPUCCINO				
(Dannon) light	8 oz	100	16	0.0
(Weight Watchers) 'Ultimate 90'	1 cup	90	14	0.0
CHERRIES JUBILEE *(Weight Watchers)* 'Ultimate 90'	1 cup	90	14	0.0
CHERRY				
(Dannon)				
low-fat	1 container	240	45	3.0
low-fat, 'Sprinkl'ins'	4.1 oz	140	24	2.0
(Light n' Lively)	4.4 oz	140	27	1.0
(New Country) 'Supreme'	6 oz	150	32	2.0
(Yoplait)				
custard style	6 oz	180	30	4.0
light	6 oz	90	16	0.0
99% fat-free, original	6 oz	180	32	2.0
triple cherry, 'Trix'	6 oz	190	31	3.0
w/almonds, 'Breakfast'	6 oz	200	38	3.0
CHERRY VANILLA				
(Dannon)				
'Light'	8 oz	100	18	0.0
low-fat, 'Sprinkl'ins'	4.1 oz	140	24	2.0
nonfat, light	8 oz	100	18	0.0
(Lite-Line) 1% fat, 'Swiss Style'	1 cup	240	45	2.0
(Yogi) w/gelatin, 'Sundae'	5.6 oz	50	14	1.0
(Yoplait)				
light, custard style	6 oz	90	17	0.0
parfait style	6 oz	200	34	3.0
COFFEE				
(Bison) low-fat	1 cup	210	33	4.0
(Dannon)	8 oz	200	34	3.0
(Friendship) low-fat	1 cup	210	35	3.0
CRANBERRY RASPBERRY				
(Weight Watchers) 'Ultimate 90'	1 cup	90	14	0.0
FRUIT CRUNCH *(New Country)* low-fat	6 oz	150	30	2.0
GRAPE				
(Dannon) lowfat, 'Sprinkl'ins'	4.1 oz	140	24	2.0
(Light n' Lively)	4.4 oz	130	24	1.0
LEMON				
(Alta Dena) fruit on the bottom	1 cup	240	40	4.0

Food Name	Serv. Size	Total Cal.	Carbs GMS	Fat GMS
(Bison) low-fat	1 cup	210	33	4.0
(Dannon)				
	8 oz	200	34	3.0
low-fat	1 container	210	36	3.0
(Knudsen) nonfat, 'Cal 70'	6 oz	70	12	0.0
(Light n' Lively) nonfat, '100'	8 oz	100	16	0.0
(Mountain High) natural	8 oz	220	31	6.0
(New Country) 'Supreme'	6 oz	150	31	2.0
(Yoplait) 99% fat-free, original	6 oz	180	32	2.0
LEMON CHIFFON				
(Dannon)				
blended	6 oz	150	30	0.0
'Light'	8 oz	100	15	0.0
(Weight Watchers) 'Ultimate 90'	1 cup	90	14	0.0
(Yogi) w/gelatin, 'Sundae'	5.6 oz	50	14	1.0
MIXED BERRIES				
(Alta Dena) blended	8 oz	190	39	1.0
(Breyers) low-fat	8 oz	250	48	2.0
(New Country) low-fat	6 oz	150	31	2.0
(Yoplait) custard style	6 oz	180	30	4.0
ORANGE				
(Dannon) low-fat	1 container	240	45	3.0
(New Country) 'Supreme'	6 oz	150	31	2.0
ORANGE-PINEAPPLE *(Yogi)* w/gelatin, 'Sundae'	5.6 oz	50	14	1.0
PEACH				
(Alta Dena) fruit on the bottom	1 cup	240	40	4.0
(Breyers) low-fat	8 oz	250	48	2.0
(Carnation) fruit on the bottom, 'Smooth'n Creamy'	8 oz	250	47	3.0
(Dannon)				
low-fat	1 container	240	45	3.0
nonfat, light	8 oz	100	17	0.0
(Knudsen) nonfat, 'Cal 70'	6 oz	70	11	0.0
(Light n' Lively)				
	8 oz	240	46	2.0
nonfat, '100'	8 oz	100	16	0.0
(Lite-Line) 1% fat, 'Swiss Style'	1 cup	230	42	2.0
(Mountain High) natural	8 oz	220	31	6.0
(Weight Watchers) 'Ultimate 90'	1 cup	90	14	0.0
(Yogi) peachy, w/gelatin, 'Sundae'	5.6 oz	50	14	1.0
(Yoplait)				
99% fat-free, original	6 oz	180	32	2.0
nonfat, light, custard style	6 oz	90	17	0.0
nonfat, fruit on the bottom	6 oz	170	35	0.0
nonfat, w/granola, 'Crunch 'N Yogurt'	7 oz	220	43	2.0
PEACH AND VANILLA *(Yoplait)* parfait style	6 oz	200	34	3.0
PEACHES AND CREAM *(New Country)* low-fat	6 oz	150	31	2.0
PIÑA COLADA *(Yoplait)* 99% fat-free, original	6 oz	180	32	2.0
PINEAPPLE				
(Breyers) low-fat	8 oz	250	50	2.0
(Knudsen) nonfat, 'Cal 70'	6 oz	70	12	0.0
(Light n' Lively)	8 oz	230	47	2.0
(Yoplait) 99% fat-free, original	6 oz	180	32	2.0
PLAIN				
(Alta Dena)	1 cup	100	13	1.0
(Bison)				
low-fat	1 cup	150	17	4.0
nonfat	1 cup	120	16	0.0
(Breyers) low-fat	8 oz	140	16	3.0

Food Name	Serv. Size	Total Cal.	Carbs GMS	Fat GMS
(Crowley)				
....	1 cup	160	14	8.0
low-fat	1 cup	140	17	2.0
nonfat	1 cup	120	17	1.0
(Dannon)				
low-fat	8 oz	140	16	4.0
nonfat	8 oz	110	16	0.0
(Friendship) low-fat, 1.5% fat	1 cup	150	17	3.0
(Knudsen)				
....	8 oz	200	16	9.0
low-fat	8 oz	160	17	5.0
(Lite-Line) 1.5% fat, 'Swiss Style'	1 cup	140	18	2.0
(Meadow Gold) low-fat, 2% milk fat	1 cup	160	16	5.0
(Mountain High) plain	1 cup	200	16	9.0
(Weight Watchers) 'Ultimate 90'	1 cup	90	14	0.0
(White Wave) nondairy	1 serving	180	18	7.0
(Yoplait)				
98% fat-free, original	6 oz	120	15	2.0
nonfat	8 oz	120	18	0.0
RAINBOW PUNCH *(Yoplait)* 'Trix'	6 oz	190	31	3.0
RASPBERRIES AND CREAM				
(Weight Watchers) 'Ultimate 90'	1 cup	90	14	0.0
RASPBERRY				
(Alta Dena)				
blended	8 oz	180	37	1.0
fruit on the bottom	1 cup	240	40	4.0
(Breyers) low-fat	8 oz	250	48	2.0
(Dannon)				
low-fat	1 container	240	45	3.0
nonfat, blended	6 oz	150	30	0.0
nonfat, 'Light'	8 oz	100	18	0.0
(Knudsen) nonfat, 'Cal 70'	6 oz	70	11	0.0
(Light n' Lively)				
nonfat, '100'	8 oz	90	15	0.0
red	8 oz	230	43	2.0
red, nonfat, 'Free'	4.4 oz	50	8	0.0
(Meadow Gold)				
low-fat, natural, 'Sundae Style'	1 cup	250	42	4.0
red, low-fat, 1.5% milk fat	1 cup	250	42	4.0
(Mountain High) natural, 'Honey Light'	8 oz	190	35	1.0
(New Country) red, 'Supreme'	6 oz	150	31	2.0
(Yoplait)				
light	6 oz	90	16	0.0
99% fat-free, original	6 oz	180	32	2.0
nonfat, fruit on the bottom	6 oz	170	35	0.0
STRAWBERRY				
(Alta Dena)				
blended	8 oz	180	37	1.0
fruit on the bottom	1 cup	240	40	4.0
fruit on the bottom, 'Maya'	1 cup	280	39	9.0
(Breyers)				
....	8 oz	218	41	1.8
low-fat	8 oz	250	48	2.0
nonfat, w/aspartame and fructose sweeteners	8-oz container	125	22	0.5
'Smooth & Creamy'	8 oz	232	45	2.0
(Carnation) 'Smooth 'n Creamy'	8 oz	230	44	3.0
(Crowley) nonfat	1 cup	190	35	1.0

Food Name	Serv. Size	Total Cal.	Carbs GMS	Fat GMS
(Dannon)				
low-fat	1 container	240	46	3.0
low-fat, 'Sprinkl'ins'	4.1 oz	140	24	2.0
nonfat, blended	6 oz	150	30	0.0
nonfat, light	8 oz	100	17	0.0
(Knudsen)				
low-fat	8 oz	250	45	4.0
nonfat, 'Cal 70'	6 oz	70	11	0.0
(Light n' Lively)				
	8 oz	240	45	2.0
	4.4 oz	135	27	1.0
nonfat	4.4 oz	70	12	0.0
nonfat, '100'	8 oz	90	15	0.0
(Lite-Line) low-fat, 1% fat	1 cup	240	46	2.0
(Mountain High) natural, 'Honey Light'	8 oz	190	35	1.0
(New Country) 'Supreme'	6 oz	150	30	2.0
(Sara Lee) 'Free & Light'	1/10 pkg	120	26	1.0
(Weight Watchers) 'Ultimate 90'	1 cup	90	14	0.0
(White Wave) nondairy	1 serving	150	30	1.0
(Yoplait) custard style	6 oz	180	30	3.0
99% fat-free, original	6 oz	180	32	2.0
nonfat, fruit on the bottom	6 oz	170	35	0.0
nontat, light	6 oz	90	16	0.0
nonfat, light, custard style	6 oz	90	17	0.0
STRAWBERRY AND VANILLA *(Yoplait)* parfait style	6 oz	200	34	3.0
STRAWBERRY CHEESECAKE				
(Yogi) w/gelatin, 'Sundae'	5.6 oz	50	14	1.0
STRAWBERRY FRUIT BASKET				
(Knudsen) nonfat, 'Cal 70'	6 oz	70	11	0.0
STRAWBERRY FRUIT CUP				
(Dannon) light	8 oz	100	17	0.0
(Light n' Lively)				
	8 oz	240	47	2.0
nonfat, 'Free'	4.4 oz	50	8	0.0
'100'	8 oz	90	15	0.0
(New Country) low-fat	6 oz	150	30	2.0
STRAWBERRY-ALMOND *(Yoplait)* 'Breakfast Yogurt'	6 oz	200	38	3.0
STRAWBERRY-BANANA				
(Alta Dena) fruit on the bottom	1 cup	180	35	1.0
(Breyers) low-fat	8 oz	250	50	2.0
(Carnation) 'Smooth 'n Creamy'	8 oz	240	42	4.0
(Dannon)				
light	8 oz	100	17	0.0
low-fat	1 container	240	43	3.0
low-fat, 'Sprinkl'ins'	4.1 oz	140	24	2.0
(Knudsen) nonfat, 'Cal 70'	6 oz	70	12	0.0
(Light n' Lively)				
	8 oz	260	52	2.0
nonfat, 'Free'	4.4 oz	50	8	0.0
(Mountain High) natural, 'Honey Light'	8 oz	190	35	1.0
(New Country)	6 oz	150	31	2.0
(Weight Watchers) 'Ultimate 90'	1 cup	90	14	0.0
(Yoplait)				
bash, 'Trix'	6 oz	190	31	3.0
fruit on the bottom	6 oz	170	35	0.0
light	6 oz	90	16	0.0
99% fat-free, original	6 oz	180	32	2.0

Food Name	Serv. Size	Total Cal.	Carbs GMS	Fat GMS
w/wheat and walnuts, 'Breakfast'	6 oz	200	40	2.0
STRAWBERRY-RHUBARB *(Yoplait)*	6 oz	190	32	3.0
TROPICAL FRUIT				
(Dannon) nonfat, light	8 oz	100	18	0.0
(Weight Watchers) nonfat, 'Ultimate 90'	1 cup	90	13	0.0
(Yoplait) w/wheat, raisin, nuts, 'Breakfast'	6 oz	200	41	3.0
VANILLA				
(Bison) low-fat	1 cup	210	33	4.0
(Breyers) low-fat	8 oz	230	41	3.0
(Crowley) low-fat	1 cup	200	33	2.0
(Dannon)				
French, fat-free, blended	3/4 cup	150	31	0.0
low-fat	1 container	210	36	3.0
nonfat, light	8 oz	100	16	0.0
w/wheat, 'Hearty Nuts & Raisins'	8 oz	270	48	5.0
(Friendship) low-fat	1 cup	210	35	3.0
(Knudsen)				
low-fat	8 oz	240	43	4.0
nonfat, 'Cal 70'	6 oz	70	11	0.0
(New Country) French, low-fat	6 oz	150	31	2.0
(Weight Watchers) 'Ultimate 90'	1 cup	90	14	0.0
(White Wave) nondairy	1 serving	140	23	2.5
(Yoplait)				
	6 oz	180	29	3.0
custard style	6 oz	180	30	4.0
fat-free	6 oz	150	28	0.0
nonfat, light, custard style	6 oz	90	17	0.0
nonfat, w/granola, 'Crunch 'N Yogurt'	7 oz	220	43	2.0
WILD BERRY				
(Light n' Lively) low-fat, 1% milk fat, cultured	4.4 oz	140	28	1.0
YOGURT, FROZEN				
(Alta Dena) apricot mango	4 oz	90	20	0.0
(Ben & Jerry's)				
black raspberry swirl	1/2 cup	150	32	0.0
cappuccino	1/2 cup	140	30	0.0
chocolate	1/2 cup	130	29	0.0
vanilla fudge swirl	1/2 cup	140	31	0.0
(Bison) chocolate	3.5 oz	94	18	2.0
(Breyers)				
black cherry	1/2 cup	120	24	1.0
chocolate	1/2 cup	120	24	1.0
peach	1/2 cup	110	22	1.0
red raspberry	1/2 cup	120	23	1.0
strawberry	1/2 cup	110	22	1.0
strawberry-banana	1/2 cup	110	22	1.0
vanilla	1/2 cup	120	23	1.0
(Cascadian Farm)				
chocolate, organic	1/2 cup	105	20	2.0
strawberry, organic	1/2 cup	102	19	1.0
vanilla, organic	1/2 cup	109	20	2.0
(Crowley)				
banana, soft-serve, 'Peaks of Perfection'	1/2 cup	100	19	2.0
cherry	3 oz	80	16	1.0
chocolate	3 oz	80	15	2.0
chocolate, soft-serve, 'Peaks of Perfection'	1/2 cup	100	19	2.0
lemon, soft-serve, 'Peaks of Perfection'	1/2 cup	100	19	2.0
peach	3 oz	80	16	1.0

Food Name	Serv. Size	Total Cal.	Carbs GMS	Fat GMS
plain, 'Peaks of Perfection'	1/2 cup	90	20	1.0
raspberry	3 oz	80	16	1.0
raspberry, soft-serve, 'Peaks of Perfection'	1/2 cup	100	19	2.0
strawberry	3 oz	80	16	1.0
strawberry, soft-serve, 'Peaks of Perfection'	1/2 cup	100	19	2.0
vanilla	3 oz	80	15	2.0
vanilla, soft-serve, 'Peaks of Perfection'	3.5 oz	100	19	2.0
(Dannon)				
blueberry, soft-serve	1/2 cup	100	18	2.0
butter pecan, soft-serve	1/2 cup	100	18	2.0
cappuccino, light	4 oz	80	19	0.0
cappuccino, soft-serve	1/2 cup	100	18	2.0
caramel pecan, 'Pure Indulgence'	4 oz	180	22	8.0
cheesecake, soft-serve	1/2 cup	100	18	2.0
chocolate, light	4 oz	80	19	1.0
chocolate, 'Pure Indulgence'	3 oz	130	24	3.0
chocolate, soft-serve	1/2 cup	120	23	2.0
chocolate nut, chunky, 'Pure Indulgence'	4 oz	190	24	9.0
cookies and cream, 'Pure Indulgence'	4 oz	180	18	7.0
Heath Bar crunch, 'Pure Indulgence'	4 oz	170	25	7.0
lemon meringue, soft-serve	1/2 cup	100	18	2.0
mixed berry, low-fat	1 container	240	45	3.0
peach, light	4 oz	80	19	0.0
peach, soft-serve	1/2 cup	100	18	2.0
piña colada, soft-serve	1/2 cup	100	18	2.0
raspberry soft-serve	1/2 cup	100	18	2.0
red raspberry	4 oz	90	21	0.0
red raspberry, soft-serve, nonfat	1/2 cup	90	21	0.0
strawberry, light	4 oz	80	19	0.0
strawberry-banana	1/2 cup	100	18	2.0
vanilla, 'Pure Indulgence'	3 oz	130	25	3.0
vanilla, light	4 oz	80	20	0.0
(Dreyers)				
blueberry, 'Inspirations'	3 oz	80	15	1.0
cherry, 'Inspirations'	3 oz	80	15	1.0
cherry vanilla, fat-free	1/2 cup	90	19	0.0
cherry vanilla, nonfat, 'Inspirations'	4 oz	90	19	0.0
chocolate, 'Inspirations'	3 oz	80	15	1.0
(Dreyers) chocolate fudge, fat-free	1/2 cup	100	22	0.0
'Perfectly Peach' 'Inspirations'	3 oz	80	15	1.0
raspberry, 'Inspirations'	3 oz	80	15	1.0
strawberry, 'Inspirations'	3 oz	80	15	1.0
strawberry-banana, 'Inspirations'	3 oz	80	15	1.0
vanilla, fat-free	1/2 cup	80	18	0.0
vanilla and chocolate, fat-free	1/2 cup	80	18	0.0
vanilla chocolate swirl, 'Inspirations'	4 oz	90	19	0.0
vanilla raspberry swirl, 'Inspirations'	3 oz	80	15	1.0
(Edys)				
cherry vanilla	1/2 cup	90	19	0.0
chocolate fudge	1/2 cup	100	22	0.0
vanilla	1/2 cup	80	18	0.0
vanilla and chocolate	1/2 cup	80	18	0.0
(Elan) chocolate almond	1/2 cup	160	23	7.0
(Haagen-Dazs)				
banana, soft-serve, nonfat	1 oz	25	5	0.0
chocolate, soft-serve	1 oz	30	4	1.0
chocolate, soft-serve, nonfat	1 oz	30	6	0.0

Food Name	Serv. Size	Total Cal.	Carbs GMS	Fat GMS
peach	3 oz	120	20	3.0
'Praline Pandemonium' 'Extras'	4 oz	240	33	9.0
raspberry, soft-serve	1 oz	30	5	1.0
strawberry	3 oz	120	21	3.0
strawberry, soft-serve	1 oz	25	5	0.0
strawberry, soft-serve, nonfat	1 oz	25	5	0.0
'Strawberry Cheesecake Craze' 'Extras'	4 oz	210	31	7.0
vanilla almond crunch	3 oz	150	22	5.0
(Sealtest)				
black cherry, nonfat, 'Free'	1/2 cup	110	24	0.0
chocolate, nonfat, 'Free'	1/2 cup	110	24	0.0
peach, nonfat, 'Free'	1/2 cup	100	23	0.0
red raspberry, nonfat, 'Free'	1/2 cup	100	23	0.0
strawberry, nonfat, 'Free'	1/2 cup	100	22	0.0
(Stars)				
butter pecan	1/2 cup	210	18	14.0
cappuccino fudge, fruit-sweetened	1/2 cup	110	22	0.0
carob-peppermint, nonfat, fruit-sweetened	1/2 cup	110	22	0.0
chocolate	1/2 cup	170	20	8.0
dark chocolate, nonfat, fruit sweetened	1/2 cup	110	23	0.0
espresso almond fudge	1/2 cup	200	23	10.0
fruit, nonfat, fruit-sweetened, 'Black Leopard'	1/2 cup	100	20	0.0
mango raspberry, nonfat, fruit sweetened	1/2 cup	100	23	0.0
mint chip	1/2 cup	210	18	14.0
peanut butter cup	1/2 cup	200	23	10.0
'Vanilla Bean'	1/2 cup	170	20	8.0
'Very Berry Blueberry' nonfat,	1/2 cup	110	23	0.0
(Stonyfield Farm)				
apricot mango, nonfat, natural	4 oz	110	22	0.0
(Stonyfield Farm)				
chocolate mint chip	4 oz	140	24	3.0
chocolate peanut butter swirl	4 oz	210	20	10.0
chocolate walnut amaretto	4 oz	150	21	5.0
coffee, French roast, decaffeinated	4 oz	100	20	0.0
coffee hazelnut fudge	4 oz	150	23	4.0
'Double Raspberry'	4 oz	120	25	0.0
'Double Strawberry'	4 oz	100	21	0.0
Dutch chocolate, nonfat	4 oz	110	21	0.0
mocha fudge, nonfat	4 oz	120	24	0.0
'Very Vanilla'	4 oz	100	20	0.0
(TCBY Treats)				
all flavors, regular	1/2 cup	140	23	3.0
all flavors, hand-dipped, 96% nonfat	1/2 cup	110	22	2.5
all flavors, hand-dipped, nonfat	1/2 cup	100	22	0.0
all flavors, nonfat, no sugar added	1/2 cup	80	20	0.0
all flavors, soft-serve, nonfat	1/2 cup	110	23	0.0
(Yoplait)				
caramel turtle fudge	1/2 cup	120	24	2.0
chocolate fudge brownie	1/2 cup	110	24	1.5
mixed berry	6 oz	180	32	2.0
vanilla	1/2 cup	100	20	1.5
YOGURT BAR, FROZEN				
(Cascadian Farm)				
blackberry, organic	1 bar	80	14	1.0
chocolate, organic	1 bar	80	15	1.5
vanilla, organic	1 bar	80	15	1.0

Food Name	Serv. Size	Total Cal.	Carbs GMS	Fat GMS
(Dole)				
cherry, 'Fruit & Yogurt'	1 bar	80	17	1.0
raspberry, 'Fruit & Yogurt'	1 bar	70	17	1.0
strawberry, 'Fruit & Yogurt'	1 bar	70	17	1.0
(Haagen-Dazs)				
peach	1 bar	100	18	1.0
'Strawberry Daiquiri'	1 bar	100	20	1.0
'Tropical Orange Passion'	1 bar	100	21	1.0
(Yoplait)				
'Vanilla Orange Creme', lowfat	1 bar	30	8	0.5
vanilla/chocolate/strawberry, w/dark chocolate coating	1 bar	110	11	6.0
YOGURT DRINK. See under SPORTS AND DIET/NUTRITION DRINKS.				
YOKAN	1 oz	74	17.2	(tr)
YUCA. See CASSAVA.				

Z

Food Name	Serv. Size	Total Cal.	Carbs GMS	Fat GMS
ZANTE CURRANT. See under CURRANT.				
ZITI. See under PASTA.				
ZITI DISH/ENTRÉE. See under PASTA DISH/ENTRÉE.				
ZUCCHINI				
Canned, Italian style *(Progresso)*	1/2 cup	50	8	2.0
Fresh				
baby, raw, whole	1 large	3	0	0.1
baby, raw, whole	1 medium	2	0	0.0
w/skin, boiled, drained, mashed	1/2 cup	19	5	0.1
w/skin, boiled, drained, sliced	1 cup	29	7	0.1
w/skin, raw, chopped	1 cup	17	4	0.2
w/skin, raw, sliced	1 cup	16	3	0.2
w/skin, raw, whole	1 large	45	9	0.5
w/skin, raw, whole	1 medium	27	6	0.3
w/skin, raw, whole	1 small	17	3	0.2
Frozen				
(Seabrook)	3.3 oz	16	3	0.0
(Southern)	3.5 oz	18	4	0.1
breaded, kosher *(Empire Kosher)*	1 piece	100	18	0.0
breaded, 'Quick Krisp' *(Stilwell)*	3.3 oz	200	24	10.0
sliced *(Flav-R-Pac)*	2/3 cup	15	2	0.0
w/skin, boiled, drained	1 cup	38	8	0.3
w/skin, unprepared	3-lb pkg	231	49	1.8
w/skin, unprepared	10-oz pkg	48	10	0.4

Fast-Food/Chain
Restaurant Values

Food Name	Serv. Size	Total Cal.	Carbs GMS	Fat GMS
ARBY'S				
BACON	2 strips	90	0	7.0
BISCUIT				
w/margarine	2.8 oz	270	26	16.0
CATSUP/KETCHUP	1 pkt	10	3	0.0
CHEESE				
Swiss	1 slice	45	0	3.0
CROISSANT				
	2.2 oz	260	28	16.0
DRESSING				
bleu cheese	2.5 oz	390	3	39.0
buttermilk ranch	2.5 oz	210	2	49.0
buttermilk ranch, reduced calorie	2 oz	50	12	0.0
honey French	2.5 oz	350	24	27.0
Italian, lower calorie	2.19 oz	20	4	1.0
Thousand Island	2.5 oz	350	11	33.0
EGG				
scrambled	1.8 oz	70	0	5.0
FINGER MEAL				
chicken	10.7 oz	880	81	47.0
FINGER SNACK				
chicken	7.4 oz	610	62	32.0
jalapeño bites	3.9 oz	330	29	21.0
mozzarella sticks	4.8 oz	470	34	29.0
onion petals	4 oz	410	43	24.0
FRENCH FRIES				
cheddar curly	6 oz	450	52	25.0
curly, large	7 oz	600	75	30.0
curly, medium	4.5 oz	380	49	19.0
curly, small	3.8 oz	320	40	16.0
homestyle, large	7.5 oz	630	86	29.0
homestyle, medium	5 oz	420	57	19.0
homestyle, small	4 oz	340	46	15.0
FRENCH TOASTIX, w/o powdered sugar or syrup	3 hotcakes	370	48	17.0
HAM.	1.5 oz	50	1	3.0
HOT CHOCOLATE	8.6 oz	110	23	1.0
MAPLE SYRUP	1.5 oz	220	54	0.0
MUSTARD				
German	1 pkt	5	0	0.0
honey	1 oz	130	5	12.0
ORANGE JUICE.	10 oz	140	34	0.0
SAUCE				
Arby's	1 pkt	15	3	0.0
barbecue dipping	1 oz	40	10	0.0
beef stock aus jus	2 oz	10	0	0.0
bronco berry	1.5 oz	90	23	0.0
horsey	1 pkt	60	3	5.0
marinara sauce	1.5 oz	35	4	1.5
tangy Southwest	1.52 oz	250	3	25.0
SANDWICH				
Arby-Q	6.6 oz	380	42	15.0
Beef 'N Cheddar	7 oz	510	45	28.0
chicken, bacon 'n Swiss	7.8 oz	610	52	30.0
chicken breast fillet	7.6 oz	560	49	28.0
chicken cordon bleu	8.9 oz	650	50	34.0
fish fillet sandwich	7.9 oz	540	51	27.0
French dip sub	7.1 oz	490	43	22.0

Food Name	Serv. Size	Total Cal.	Carbs GMS	Fat GMS
grilled chicken, lowfat	6.3 oz	280	33	5.0
grilled chicken deluxe	8.7 oz	420	42	16.0
hot ham 'n Swiss sub	9.7 oz	570	47	31.0
Italian sub.	10.3 oz	800	49	54.0
Philly beef 'n Swiss sub	11.1 oz	780	52	48.0
roast beef, big Montana.	11 oz	720	44	40.0
roast beef, giant.	8.1 oz	550	43	28.0
roast beef, junior.	4.6 oz	340	36	16.0
roast beef, regular.	5.6 oz	400	36	20.0
roast beef, super.	8.7 oz	530	50	27.0
roast beef melt w/cheddar.	5.4 oz	380	38	19.0
roast beef sub.	10.7 oz	770	48	49.0
roast chicken club.	8.4 oz	540	39	29.0
roast chicken deluxe, low-fat.	7 oz	260	32	5.0
roast turkey deluxe, lowfat.	6.9 oz	230	33	5.0
turkey sub	10.7 oz	670	49	39.0
POTATO, BAKED				
broccoli 'n cheddar	13.6 oz	550	71	25.0
chicken broccoli	15.8 oz	830	68	47.0
cool ranch	12.3 oz	500	67	23.0
deluxe	12.3 oz	610	68	31.0
jalapeño	14.6 oz	660	72	36.0
Philly chicken	15.8 oz	880	75	53.0
w/butter and sour cream	11.3 oz	500	65	24.0
POTATO CAKES	2 cakes	220	21	14.0
SALAD				
garden, w/one crouton packet, 2 saltine crackers	10.2 oz	110	16	3.0
grilled chicken, low-fat	14.2 oz	190	16	4.0
roast chicken, lowfat	14.2 oz	200	16	5.0
w/one crouton packet, 2 saltine crackers	5.4 oz	90	12	3.0
SAUSAGE PATTY	1.4 oz	200	1	19.0
SHAKE				
CHOCOLATE	10.3 oz	390	69	9.0
jamocha	10.3 oz	380	66	9.0
strawberry	10.3 oz	380	67	9.0
vanilla	10.3 oz	380	67	9.0
TURNOVER				
iced apple	3.4 oz	360	54	14.0
iced cherry	3.5 oz	350	53	14.0
ARTHUR TREACHER'S				
CHICKEN PATTIES				
	2 patties	369	17	21.6
SANDWICH				
chicken	1 sandwich	413	44	19.2
fish	1 sandwich	440	39	24.0
COD FILLET, 'Bake'n Broil' tail shape	5 oz	245	10	14.2
COLESLAW				
	3 oz	123	11	8.2
DESSERT, Lemon Luv	1 serving	276	35	13.9
FISH FILLET	5.2 oz	355	25	19.8
FRENCH FRIES, chips	4 oz	276	35	13.2
HUSHPUPPY, 'Krunch Pup'	1 piece	203	12	14.8
SHRIMP	7 pieces	381	27	24.4
AU BON PAIN				
BAGEL				
cinnamon.	1 bagel	395	86	2.0

Food Name	Serv. Size	Total Cal.	Carbs GMS	Fat GMS
onion	1 bagel	390	81	2.0
plain	1 bagel	380	79	2.0
sesame.	1 bagel	425	81	5.0
BREAD				
baguette	1 loaf	810	166	2.0
cheese	1 loaf	1670	269	29.0
four-grain	1 loaf	1420	262	11.0
multigrain	2 slices	391	77	3.0
onion herb	1 loaf	1430	263	13.0
pita pocket.	2 slices	80	18	1.0
ponsienne	1 loaf	1490	166	4.0
rye	2 slices	374	73	4.0
CHICKEN POT PIE	1 serving	440	46	21.0
COOKIE				
chocolate chip	1 cookie	280	37	15.0
chocolate chunk, w/pecan, 'Gourmet'	1 cookie	290	37	17.0
cookie, oatmeal, oatmeal raisin, 'Gourmet'	1 cookie	250	41	9.0
peanut butter, 'Gourmet'	1 cookie	290	33	15.0
shortbread, 'Gourmet'	1 cookie	425	46	26.0
white chocolate chunk, w/pecan, 'Gourmet'	1 cookie	300	37	17.0
CROISSANT				
almond	1 croissant	420	41	25.0
apple	1 croissant	250	38	10.0
blueberry cheese	1 croissant	380	44	20.0
chocolate	1 croissant	400	46	24.0
cinnamon raisin	1 croissant	390	60	13.0
coconut pecan	1 croissant	440	51	23.0
hazelnut chocolate	1 croissant	480	56	28.0
croissant, plain	1 croissant	220	29	10.0
raspberry cheese	1 croissant	400	49	20.0
strawberry cheese	1 croissant	400	49	20.0
sweet cheese	1 croissant	420	45	23.0
MUFFIN				
blueberry, gourmet	1 muffin	390	66	4.0
bran, gourmet	1 muffin	390	73	11.0
carrot, gourmet	1 muffin	450	58	22.0
corn, gourmet	1 muffin	460	71	17.0
cranberry walnut, gourmet	1 muffin	350	53	13.0
oat bran apple gourmet	1 muffin	400	71	2.0
pumpkin gourmet	1 muffin	410	63	16.0
whole grain, gourmet	1 muffin	440	68	16.0
PASTRY				
cheese Danish	1 Danish	390	43	22.0
cherry Danish.	1 Danish	335	42	16.0
cherry dumpling Danish	1 Danish	360	59	13.0
raspberry Danish	1 Danish	335	43	16.0
ROLL				
'Alpine'	1 roll	220	43	3.0
braided.	1 roll	387	64	11.0
country seed	1 roll	220	37	4.0
croissant.	1 roll	300	38	14.0
French.	1 roll	320	65	1.0
hearth	1 roll	370	69	3.0
'Petit Pain'	1 roll	220	44	1.0
pumpernickel	1 roll	210	42	2.0
raisin	1 roll	250	46	4.0
rye	1 roll	230	44	2.0
soft	1 roll	310	50	8.0

Food Name	Serv. Size	Total Cal.	Carbs GMS	Fat GMS
vegetable	1 roll	230	40	5.0
SALAD				
garden, small	1 salad	20	5	1.0
garden w/grilled chicken	1 salad	110	9	2.0
garden w/shrimp	1 salad	102	8	2.0
garden w/tuna.	1 salad	350	11	25.0
Italian, low-calorie	1 salad	68	3	6.0
SANDWICH				
chicken, cracked pepper, on French roll	1 sandwich	440	66	3.0
chicken, cracked pepper, on hearth roll	1 sandwich	490	70	5.0
chicken, cracked pepper, on soft roll	1 sandwich	430	51	10.0
chicken, grilled, on French roll	1 sandwich	450	66	5.0
chicken, grilled, on hearth roll	1 sandwich	500	70	7.0
chicken, grilled, on soft roll	1 sandwich	440	51	12.0
chicken, tarragon, on French roll	1 sandwich	590	68	16.0
chicken, tarragon, on hearth roll	1 sandwich	640	72	18.0
chicken, tarragon, on soft roll	1 sandwich	580	53	23.0
ham, on French roll	1 sandwich	470	68	8.0
ham, on hearth roll	1 sandwich	520	72	10.0
ham, on soft roll	1 sandwich	460	53	15.0
ham and cheese croissant, hot, filled	1 sandwich	370	38	20.0
roast beef, on French roll	1 sandwich	500	66	9.0
roast beef, on hearth roll	1 sandwich	550	70	11.0
roast beef, on soft roll	1 sandwich	490	51	16.0
spinach and cheese croissant, hot, filled	1 sandwich	290	29	16.0
turkey and cheddar croissant, hot, filled	1 sandwich	410	38	22.0
turkey and havarti croissant, hot, filled	1 sandwich	410	38	21.0
turkey sandwich, smoked, on French roll	1 sandwich	420	65	2.0
turkey sandwich, smoked, on hearth roll	1 sandwich	470	69	4.0
turkey sandwich, smoked, on soft roll	1 sandwich	410	50	9.0
SANDWICH FILLING				
boursin cheese	1 serving	290	2	29.0
brie cheese	1 serving	300	3	24.0
provolone cheese	1 serving	155	1	12.6
SOUP				
beef barley	1 bowl	112	15	3.0
beef barley	1 cup	75	10	2.0
broccoli, cream of	1 bowl	302	18	26.0
broccoli, cream of	1 cup	201	12	17.0
chicken, w/noodle	1 bowl	119	14	1.7
chicken, w/noodle.	1 cup	79	9	1.0
chili, vegetarian	1 bowl	208	37	4.0
chili, vegetarian.	1 cup	139	24	3.0
clam chowder	1 bowl	433	36	27.0
clam chowder.	1 cup	289	24	18.0
minestrone.	1 cup	105	20	2.0
split pea.	1 bowl	264	45	2.0
split pea.	1 cup	176	30	1.0
tomato Florentine	1 bowl	92	15	1.7
tomato Florentine	1 cup	61	10	1.0
vegetarian, garden	1 bowl	44	9	1.0
vegetarian, garden.	1 cup	29	6	1.0

BASKIN-ROBBINS
ICE

	Serv. Size	Total Cal.	Carbs GMS	Fat GMS
grape	1/2 cup	100	27	0.0
margarita.	1/2 cup	110	28	0.0

Food Name	Serv. Size	Total Cal.	Carbs GMS	Fat GMS
ICE CREAM				
'Berries 'n Banana,' sugarless	1/2 cup	80	15	1.0
'Call Me Nuts,' sugarless	1/2 cup	110	21	2.0
'Cappuccino Blast,' w/whipped cream	1 serving	160	22	7.0
'Caramel Banana Surprise,' nonfat	1/2 cup	110	24	0.0
caramel praline, soft serve, nonfat	1/2 cup	120	25	0.0
'Cherry Cordial,' sugarless	1/2 cup	100	18	2.0
chocolate chip, 'Chillyburger'	1 serving	220	27	11.0
chocolate chip, sugarless	1/2 cup	100	17	2.5
chocolate chip, sugarless, 'Low, Lite 'n Luscious'	1 serving	100	20	2.0
chocolate marshmallow, nonfat	1/2 cup	110	26	0.0
chocolate vanilla twist, nonfat	1/2 cup	100	21	0.0
'Chocolate Wonder,' nonfat.	1/2 cup	90	20	0.0
'Chunky Banana,' sugarless	1/2 cup	90	16	1.5
coconut fudge, sugarless	1/2 cup	110	20	1.5
'Double Raspberry,' light	1/2 cup	90	16	2.0
espresso, light	1/2 cup	110	18	4.0
'Jamoca Swirl,' nonfat	1/2 cup	110	23	0.0
'Jamoca Swiss Almond,' sugarless	1/2 cup	100	16	2.5
'Just Chocolate Vanilla' dairy, nonfat	1/2 cup	100	21	0.0
'Just Peachy' dairy, nonfat	1/2 cup	100	22	0.0
'Kookaberry Kiwi,' nonfat.	1/2 cup	90	20	0.0
'Mocha Cappuccino Blast,' nonfat	1 serving	120	26	0.0
peach, nonfat.	1/2 cup	100	22	0.0
peanut butter cream, nonfat.	1/2 cup	100	21	0.0
pineapple cheesecake, nonfat.	1/2 cup	110	24	0.0
pineapple coconut, sugarless.	1/2 cup	90	16	1.5
'Pistachio Creme Chip,' light.	1/2 cup	120	17	4.0
'Pralines 'n Cream'	1 scoop	280	35	14.0
praline, light.	1/2 cup	120	18	4.0
'Raspberry Revelation' sugarless	1/2 cup	100	20	1.0
'Rocky Path,' light.	1/2 cup	130	19	4.0
strawberry, sugarless, 'Low, Lite 'n Luscious'	1 serving	80	17	1.0
'Strawberry Royal,' light	1/2 cup	110	19	3.0
vanilla, soft serve, nonfat.	1/2 cup	120	25	0.0
'Thin Mint,' sugarless.	1/2 cup	100	16	2.5
'Vanilla Bean,' nonfat.	1/2 cup	100	20	0.0
'Vanilla Swiss Almond,' sugarless	1/2 cup	110	20	2.0
ICE CREAM BAR				
'Sundae Bars' chocolate, caramel ribbon, light	1 bar	150	24	5.0
'Cappuccino Blast'	1 bar	120	18	5.0
ICE CREAM CONE				
waffle, cone and cup, plain	1 cone	140	28	2.0
sugar, cone and cup, plain	1 cone	60	11	1.0
SHERBET				
orange	1/2 cup	120	26	1.5
rainbow	1/2 cup	120	26	1.5
SORBET				
fruit whip, nonfat	1 serving	80	24	0.0
raspberry cranberry	1/2 cup	110	29	0.0
red raspberry	1/2 cup	120	30	0.0
strawberry, soft-serve, nonfat	1 serving	100	20	0.0
TOPPING				
butterscotch	1 oz	100	24	1.0
hot fudge	1 oz	100	17	3.0
hot fudge, nonfat, sugar-free	1 oz	90	20	0.0
praline caramel	1 oz	90	19	0.0

Food Name	Serv. Size	Total Cal.	Carbs GMS	Fat GMS
strawberry	1 oz	60	14	0.0
YOGURT, FROZEN				
black cherry, nonfat	1/2 cup	110	24	0.0
blueberry, lowfat	1/2 cup	120	24	1.5
cheesecake, lowfat	1/2 cup	120	21	1.5
chocolate, lowfat	1/2 cup	120	23	1.5
chocolate, lowfat, large	9 oz	315	54	9.0
chocolate, lowfat, medium	7 oz	246	42	7.0
chocolate mint, nonfat	1/2 cup	100	23	0.0
coconut, nonfat, large	9 oz	180	45	0.0
coconut, nonfat, medium	7 oz	140	35	0.0
coconut, nonfat, small	5 oz	100	25	0.0
Dutch chocolate, nonfat	1/2 cup	100	23	0.0
'For Heaven's Cake,' low-fat	1/2 cup	120	24	2.0
'Have Your Cake,' low-fat	1/2 cup	110	22	1.0
Kahlua frozen, nonfat	1/2 cup	100	21	0.0
key lime nonfat	1/2 cup	100	22	0.0
'Mango in Paradise,' nonfat	1/2 cup	130	28	0.0
maple walnut, nonfat	1/2 cup	100	22	0.0
peach, nonfat	1/2 cup	100	22	0.0
'Peppermint Twist,' nonfat	1/2 cup	100	22	0.0
pina colada, nonfat	1/2 cup	110	22	0.0
raspberry, nonfat	1/2 cup	100	22	0.0
raspberry, nonfat, large	9 oz	225	45	0.0
raspberry, nonfat, medium	7 oz	164	35	0.0
raspberry, nonfat, small	5 oz	125	25	0.0
strawberry, low-fat, large	9 oz	270	54	9.0
strawberry, low-fat, medium	7 oz	211	42	7.0
strawberry, low-fat, small	5 oz	150	30	5.0
strawberry, nonfat	1/2 cup	100	23	0.0
strawberry, nonfat, large	9 oz	225	45	0.0
strawberry, nonfat, medium	7 oz	176	35	0.0
vanilla, low-fat	1/2 cup	120	22	2.0
vanilla, low-fat, large	9 oz	270	54	9.0
vanilla, low-fat, medium	7 oz	211	42	7.0
vanilla, nonfat	1/2 cup	110	23	0.0

BIG BOY RESTAURANT
DESSERT

Food Name	Serv. Size	Total Cal.	Carbs GMS	Fat GMS
'No-no' frozen	1 serving	75	17	0.0
yogurt, frozen, nonfat	1 serving	72	16	0.0
ENTRÉE				
chicken and vegetable stir-fry	1 serving	562	68	14.0
chicken breast, w/salad, no dressing, oat bran bread	1 serving	349	20	13.0
chicken breast, w/mozzarella, salad, no dressing, bread	1 serving	370	24	12.0
chicken, Cajun, w/salad, no dressing, oat bran bread	1 serving	349	20	13.0
cod, baked, w/salad, no dressing, oat bran bread	1 serving	364	20	12.0
cod, Dijon, baked, w/salad, no dressing, bread	1 serving	427	21	18.0
cod, broiled, w/salad, no dressing, oat bran bread	1 serving	364	20	12.0
cod, Dijon, broiled, w/salad, no dressing, bread	1 serving	427	21	18.0
cod, Cajun, w/salad, no dressing, oat bran bread	1 serving	364	20	12.0
spaghetti marinara, w/salad, no dressing, oat bran bread	1 serving	450	87	6.0
vegetable stir-fry	1 serving	408	74	10.0
SALAD				
chicken breast, Dijon	1 salad	391	31	11.0
dinner, no dressing	1 salad	19	4	0.0
SALAD DRESSING, buttermilk	1 serving	36	4	2.0

Food Name	Serv. Size	Total Cal.	Carbs GMS	Fat GMS
SANDWICH				
chicken w/mozzarella, on pita, 'Heart Smart'	1 sandwich	404	26	13.0
turkey, on pita, 'Heart Smart'	1 sandwich	224	24	5.0
SIDE DISH				
corn	1 serving	90	21	1.0
mixed vegetables	1 serving	27	5	0.0
potato, baked	1 serving	163	37	0.0
rice	1 serving	114	25	0.0
roll	1 roll	139	30	0.0
SOUP				
cabbage	1 bowl	43	9	1.0
cabbage	1 cup	37	8	0.0
BOJANGLES				
BISCUIT	1 serving	239	30	11.0
CHICKEN				
breast, no skin, 'Southern'	3.5 oz	239	10	11.5
breast, no skin, 'Southern'	4 oz	271	11	13.0
leg, no skin, 'Southern'	1.8 oz	128	5	12.0
leg, no skin, 'Southern'	3.5 oz	251	10	23.5
thigh, no skin, 'Southern'	3.5 oz	291	11	18.7
thigh, no skin, 'Southern'	3.2 oz	264	10	17.0
SANDWICH, chicken fillet, grilled, no mayo	1 sandwich	329	37	7.0
SIDE DISH				
coleslaw	1 serving	105	19	4.0
dirty rice	1 serving	167	21	7.0
pinto bean, Cajun	1 serving	124	25	0.0
BONANZA RESTAURANTS				
HALIBUT FILLET				
	6 oz	139	3	2.0
	3.5 oz	82	2	1.2
RIBEYE STEAK				
	5.5 oz	196	1	8.0
	3.5 oz	126	1	5.1
BOSTON MARKET				
CHICKEN				
drumstick, Tabasco barbecue	1 drumstick	130	4	6.0
1/4 chicken, dark meat, w/o skin	1/4 chicken	190	1	10.0
1/4 chicken, dark meat, w/skin	1/4 chicken	320	2	21.0
1/4 chicken, teriyaki, dark meat, w/skin	1/4 chicken	380	17	21.0
1/4 chicken, w/skin	1/4 chicken	590	4	33.0
1/4 chicken, w/wing, white meat, w/skin	1/4 chicken	280	2	12.0
1/4 chicken, w/o wing, white meat, w/o skin	1/4 chicken	170	2	4.0
Southwest, savory	1 portion	400	26	15.0
triple topped	1 portion	470	20	22.0
wing, Tabasco barbecue	1 wing	110	4	7.0
CHICKEN POT PIE	1 pie	780	61	46.0
CORNBREAD	1 loaf	200	33	6.0
DESSERT				
brownie	1 piece	450	47	27.0
chocolate chip cookie	1 cookie	340	48	17.0
cinnamon apple pie	1/5 pie	390	46	23.0
GRAVY, chicken	1 oz	15	2	1.0
HAM, Boston hearth, lean	5 oz	210	9	9.0
MEAT LOAF				
w/brown gravy	7 oz	390	19	22.0

Food Name	Serv. Size	Total Cal.	Carbs GMS	Fat GMS
w/chunky tomato sauce	8 oz	370	22	18.0
SALAD				
Caesar, entrée	10 oz	510	17	42.0
Caesar, side	4 oz	200	7	17.0
Caesar, w/o dressing	8 oz	230	14	12.0
chicken, chunky	3/4 cup	370	3	27.0
chicken Caesar	13 oz	650	17	45.0
tossed, individual, w/Caesar dressing	1 salad	380	18	31.0
tossed, individual, w/fat-free ranch dressing	1 salad	160	29	2.5
tossed, individual, w/old Venice dressing	1 salad	340	20	27.0
SANDWICH				
barbecue chicken	1 sandwich	540	84	9.0
barbecue chicken pastry	1 sandwich	640	56	39.0
broccoli chicken cheddar pastry	1 sandwich	690	45	47.0
chicken, w/cheese and sauce sandwich.	1 sandwich	750	72	33.0
chicken, w/o cheese and sauce	1 sandwich	430	62	4.5
chicken salad.	1 sandwich	680	63	30.0
ham, w/cheese and sauce	1 sandwich	750	72	34.0
ham and cheddar pastry.	1 sandwich	640	47	41.0
ham sub, w/o cheese and sauce	1 sandwich	440	66	8.0
Italian chicken pastry.	1 sandwich	630	43	41.0
meatloaf, w/cheese	1 sandwich	860	95	33.0
meatloaf, w/o cheese	1 sandwich	690	86	21.0
turkey, open faced	1 sandwich	500	61	12.0
turkey, w/cheese and sauce.	1 sandwich	710	68	28.0
turkey club	1 sandwich	650	64	26.0
turkey sub, w/o cheese and sauce	1 sandwich	400	61	3.5
SIDE DISH				
applesauce, cinnamon	3/4 cup	250	56	4.5
applesauce, cinnamon, low-fat, chunky	3/4 cup	250	62	0.0
barbecue baked beans.	3/4 cup	270	48	5.0
black rice and beans.	1 cup	300	45	10.0
broccoli cauliflower au gratin	3/4 cup	200	14	11.0
broccoli rice casserole.	3/4 cup	240	26	12.0
broccoli w/red peppers.	3/4 cup	60	5	3.5
butternut squash, low-fat.	3/4 cup	160	25	6.0
carrots, honey glazed.	3/4 cup	280	35	15.0
chili, chicken	1 cup	220	21	7.0
coleslaw.	3/4 cup	300	30	19.0
corn, whole kernel	3/4 cup	180	30	4.0
coyote bean salad	3/4 cup	190	24	9.0
cranberry relish, low-fat.	3/4 cup	370	84	5.0
fruit salad	3/4 cup	70	15	0.5
green beans	3/4 cup	80	5	6.0
green bean casserole	3/4 cup	130	10	9.0
macaroni and cheese	3/4 cup	280	32	11.0
potato, baked, sweet low-fat	1 potato	460	94	7.0
potato, mashed, homestyle	2/3 cup	190	24	9.0
potato, mashed, homestyle, w/gravy	3/4 cup	210	26	10.0
potato, new, low-fat	3/4 cup	130	25	2.5
potato planks, oven-roasted, low-fat.	5 planks	180	32	5.0
potato salad, old-fashioned	3/4 cup	340	30	24.0
red beans and rice, low-fat	1 cup	260	45	5.0
rice pilaf.	2/3 cup	180	32	5.0
spinach, creamed.	3/4 cup	260	11	20.0
squash casserole.	3/4 cup	330	20	24.0
stuffing, savory.	3/4 cup	310	44	12.0
sweet potato casserole.	3/4 cup	280	39	18.0

Food Name	Serv. Size	Total Cal.	Carbs GMS	Fat GMS
vegetables, steamed, low-fat	2/3 cup	35	7	0.5
zucchini marinana, low-fat.	3/4 cup	60	7	3.0
SOUP				
chicken noodle	1 cup	130	12	4.5
chicken tortilla	1 cup	220	19	11.0
potato.	1 cup	270	24	16.0
tomato bisque	1 cup	280	16	23.0
TURKEY, breast, rotisserie, skinless, low-fat	5 oz	170	1	1.0

BRAUM'S

Food Name	Serv. Size	Total Cal.	Carbs GMS	Fat GMS
	1 serving	180	16	3.0
diet, sugarless, w/NutraSweet	1 serving	90	13	3.0
nonfat	1 serving	90	20	0.0
'Premium Light'	1 serving	102	15	3.0

BRAZIER. See DAIRY QUEEN/BRAZIER.

BRESLER'S

Food Name	Serv. Size	Total Cal.	Carbs GMS	Fat GMS
ICE CREAM, 'Royal Lites,' all flavors	1 serving	132	9	5.0
SHERBET, all flavors.	1 serving	160	34	2.0
YOGURT, FROZEN				
gourmet, all flavors	1 serving	116	22	2.0
nonfat, all flavors.	1 serving	108	24	0.0

BURGER CHEF
BREAKFAST

Food Name	Serv. Size	Total Cal.	Carbs GMS	Fat GMS
sausage biscuit.	1 serving	418	33	25.0
scrambled eggs and bacon platter.	1 serving	567	50	31.0
scrambled eggs and sausage platter.	1 serving	668	50	40.0
'Sunrise' w/bacon	1 serving	392	30	21.0
'Sunrise' w/sausage	1 sandwich	526	30	33.0
CHEESEBURGER				
regular.	1 serving	278	28	12.0
double patty	1 serving	402	28	22.0
DESSERT, apple turnover.	1 serving	237	38	9.0
HAMBURGER				
'Big Chef'.	1 serving	556	37	36.0
mushroom, single patty	1 serving	520	34	29.0
regular	1 serving	235	27	9.0
'Super Chef'	1 serving	604	35	39.0
'Top Chef'	1 serving	541	29	33.0
HAMBURGER MEAL, 'Funmeal'	1 serving	514	85	19.0
SANDWICH				
chicken club.	1 sandwich	521	33	25.0
'Fisherman's Fillet'	1 sandwich	534	41	32.0
SIDE DISH				
french fries, large.	1 serving	285	36	14.0
french fries, regular.	1 serving	204	26	10.0
'Hash Rounds'	1 serving	235	26	14.0
salad, lettuce	1 salad	11	3	0.0

BURGER KING
BEVERAGE

Food Name	Serv. Size	Total Cal.	Carbs GMS	Fat GMS
chocolate shake, medium.	1 serving	440	75	10.0
chocolate shake, medium, syrup added	1 serving	570	105	10.0
chocolate shake, small	1 serving	330	58	7.0
chocolate shake, small, syrup added	1 serving	390	72	7.0
'Coca-Cola Classic,' medium	22 fl oz	280	70	0.0

Food Name	Serv. Size	Total Cal.	Carbs GMS	Fat GMS
coffee	12 fl oz	5	1	0.0
'Diet Coke,' medium.	22 fl oz	1	0	0.0
orange juice,'Tropicana'	10 fl oz	140	33	0.0
milk, 2%.	8 fl oz	130	12	5.0
'Sprite,' medium.	22 fl oz	260	66	0.0
strawberry shake, medium, syrup added	1 medium	550	104	9.0
strawberry shake, small, syrup added	1 serving	390	72	7.0
vanilla shake, medium.	1 medium	430	73	9.0
vanilla shake, small.	1 small	330	56	7.0
BREAKFAST				
bacon.	3 pieces	40	0	3.0
biscuit.	1 serving	300	35	15.0
biscuit w/egg.	1 sandwich	380	37	21.0
biscuit w/sausage.	1 sandwich	490	36	33.0
biscuit w/sausage, egg and cheese.	1 sandwich	620	37	43.0
'Cini-Minis' w/vanilla icing	1 serving	110	20	3.0
'Cini-Minis' w/o vanilla icing	4 rolls	440	51	23.0
'Croissan'wich' w/sausage and cheese.	1 sandwich	450	21	35.0
'Croissan'wich' w/sausage, egg, and cheese.	1 sandwich	530	23	41.0
French toast sticks.	5 sticks	440	51	23.0
ham.	1 serving	35	0	1.0
hash brown rounds, large.	1 serving	410	42	26.0
hash brown rounds, small.	1 serving	240	25	15.0
BUN				
hamburger.	1 serving	130	24	2.0
'Whopper'.	1 serving	220	39	4.0
CHEESE, American, processed	2 slices	90	0	8.0
CHEESEBURGER				
bacon double	1 serving	620	28	38.0
bacon	1 serving	400	27	22.0
double patty	1 serving	580	27	36.0
regular	1 serving	360	27	19.0
'Double Whopper'	1 serving	1010	47	67.0
'Double Whopper' w/o mayo	1 serving	850	47	50.0
'Whopper'	1 serving	760	47	48.0
'Whopper' w/o mayo	1 serving	600	47	31.0
'Whopper Jr.'	1 serving	450	28	28.0
'Whopper Jr.' w/o mayo	1 serving	370	28	19.0
CHICKEN BREAST PATTY, 'BK Broiler'.	1 serving	140	4	4.0
CHICKEN TENDERS				
	5 pieces	230	11	14.0
	4 pieces	180	9	11.0
CONDIMENTS				
barbecue sauce, 'Bull's Eye'	1/2 oz	20	5	0.0
butter, whipped, 'Land O' Lakes Classic Blend'	1 serving	65	0	7.0
catsup.	1/2 oz	15	4	0.0
dip, 'A.M. Express'.	1 serving	80	21	0.0
dipping sauce	1 serving	170	2	17.0
dipping sauce, barbecue	1 serving	35	9	0.0
dipping sauce, honey flavored	1 serving	90	23	0.0
dipping sauce, honey mustard	1 serving	90	10	6.0
dipping sauce, sweet and sour.	1 serving	45	11	0.0
jam, grape, 'A.M. Express'.	1 serving	30	7	0.0
jam, strawberry, 'A.M. Express'.	1 serving	30	8	0.0
'King Sauce'.	1/2 oz	70	2	7.0
mustard.	1/9 oz	0	0	0.0
tartar sauce.	1.5 oz	260	0	29.0
DESSERT, Dutch apple pie.	1 serving	300	39	15.0

Food Name	Serv. Size	Total Cal.	Carbs GMS	Fat GMS
HAMBURGER				
'Big King'	1 burger	640	28	42.0
'Double Whopper' w/o mayo	1 serving	760	47	42.0
'Double Whopper'	1 serving	920	47	59.0
regular	1 serving	320	27	15.0
'Whopper Jr.' w/o mayo	1 serving	320	28	15.0
'Whopper Jr.'	1 serving	400	28	24.0
'Whopper' w/o mayo	1 serving	510	47	23.0
'Whopper'	1 serving	660	47	40.0
HAMBURGER PATTY				
regular	1 serving	170	0	13.0
'Whopper'.	1 serving	250	0	19.0
LETTUCE.	3/4 oz	0	0	0.0
ONION.	1/2 oz	5	1	0.0
PICKLE.	4 slices	0	0	0.0
SANDWICH				
'Chick 'N Crisp'	1 sandwich	460	37	27.0
'Chick 'N Crisp' w/o mayo.	1 sandwich	360	37	16.0
chicken	1 sandwich	710	54	43.0
chicken, w/o mayo	1 sandwich	500	54	20.0
chicken, 'BK Broiler'	1 sandwich	530	45	26.0
chicken, 'BK Broiler' w/o mayo	1 sandwich	370	45	9.0
fish, 'BK Big'	1 sandwich	720	59	43.0
SIDE DISH				
French fries, king size, salted	1 serving	590	74	30.0
French fries, medium, salted	1 serving	400	50	21.0
French fries, medium, unsalted	1 serving	400	50	21.0
French fries, small, salted	1 serving	250	32	13.0
French fries, small, unsalted	1 serving	250	32	13.0
onion rings, king size, salted	1 serving	600	74	30.0
onion rings, medium.	1 serving	380	46	19.0
TOMATO.	2 slices	5	1	0.0
CAPTAIN D'S				
CONDIMENTS				
salad dressing, Italian, nonfat, low-calorie	2 tbsp	9	2	0.0
sweet and sour sauce	2 tbsp	52	13	0.0
ENTRÉE				
chicken, w/rice, green beans, breadstick, salad	1 serving	414	55	8.0
fish, baked, w/rice, green beans, breadstick, coleslaw	1 serving	659	62	30.0
orange roughy, w/rice, green beans, breadstick, salad	1 serving	537	56	19.0
shrimp, w/rice, green beans, breadstick, salad	1 serving	457	34	10.0
SIDE DISH				
breadstick, plain	1 stick	91	17	1.0
green beans, seasoned	1 serving	46	5	2.0
rice	serving	124	28	0.0
salad, dinner, no dressing	1 salad	27	3	1.0
white bean	1 serving	126	22	1.0
CARL'S JR.				
BACON.	2 strips	50	0	4.0
BEVERAGE				
chocolate shake.	13.5 fl oz	390	74	7.0
'Coca-Cola Classic' regular.	16 fl oz	200	54	0.0
coffee.	12 fl oz	5	1	0.0
'Diet Coke,' regular.	16 fl oz	0	0	0.0
'Diet 7-Up,' regular.	16 fl oz	0	0	0.0
'Dr. Pepper,' regular.	16 fl oz	200	52	0.0
hot chocolate.	12 fl oz	110	22	2.0

Food Name	Serv. Size	Total Cal.	Carbs GMS	Fat GMS
iced tea, regular	16 fl oz	5	0	0.0
lemonade, 'Minute Maid' original style, regular	16 fl oz	190	52	0.0
milk, 1%.	10 fl oz	150	18	3.0
'Nestea,' raspberry, regular.	16 fl oz	160	42	0.0
orange juice.	10 fl oz	140	33	0.0
orange soda, 'Minute Maid' regular	16 fl oz	210	58	0.0
root beer, 'Barq's,' regular	16 fl oz	220	60	0.0
'Sprite,' regular	16 fl oz	190	54	0.0
strawberry shake.	13.5 fl oz	400	77	7.0
vanilla shake.	13.5 fl oz	330	54	8.0
BREADSTICK.	1 stick	35	7	0.5
BREAKFAST				
burrito	1 burrito	480	26	30.0
cheese Danish	1 serving	400	49	22.0
English muffin, w/margarine.	1 muffin	210	27	9.0
French toast dips, w/o syrup	1 serving	370	42	20.0
hash brown nuggets.	1 serving	330	32	21.0
quesadilla	1 quesadilla	310	27	16.0
scrambled egg.	1 egg	160	1	11.0
'Sunrise Sandwich' no bacon or sausage	1 sandwich	360	28	21.0
CHEESE				
American.	1 slice	60	0	5.0
Swiss.	1 slice	50	0	3.5
CHEESEBURGER				
double Western bacon.	1 burger	900	64	49.0
Western bacon.	1 burger	650	63	30.0
CHICKEN STARS.	1 serving	280	15	19.0
CONDIMENTS. See also Salad Dressing.				
barbecue sauce.	1 pkt	50	11	0.0
croutons, salad bar item	1 crouton	35	5	1.0
honey sauce.	1 pkt	90	22	0.0
jam, strawberry.	1 pkt	35	9	0.0
jelly, grape.	1 pkt	35	9	0.0
mustard sauce.	1 serving	50	11	0.0
salsa	1 serving	10	2	0.0
sweet and sour sauce	1 serving	50	12	0.0
syrup, table	1 serving	90	21	0.0
DESSERT				
chocolate cake.	1 cake	300	49	10.0
chocolate chip cookie.	1 cookie	370	49	19.0
strawberry swirl cheesecake	1 serving	290	30	17.0
HAMBURGER				
'Famous Star'.	1 burger	580	49	32.0
'Jr.'.	1 burger	330	34	13.0
'Super Star'.	1 burger	790	50	46.0
SALAD				
'Salad-To-Go,' charbroiled chicken.	1 salad	200	12	7.0
'Salad-To-Go,' gardeb	1 salad	50	4	2.5
SALAD DRESSING				
blue cheese.	1 pkt	320	1	35.0
French, nonfat.	1 pkt	60	16	0.0
house.	1 pkt	220	3	22.0
Italian, nonfat.	1 pkt	15	4	0.0
Thousand Island.	1 pkt	230	5	23.0
SANDWICH				
bacon Swiss crispy chicken	1 sandwich	690	60	36.0
barbecue chicken	1 sandwich	280	37	3.0
chicken club	1 sandwich	460	33	22.0
fish, 'Carl's Catch'.	1 sandwich	510	50	27.0

Food Name	Serv. Size	Total Cal.	Carbs GMS	Fat GMS
ranch crispy chicken.	1 sandwich	590	59	29.0
Santa Fe chicken.	1 sandwich	510	32	31.0
SAUSAGE PATTY.	1 patty	200	2	19.0
SIDE DISH				
baked potato, w/bacon and cheese.	1 serving	630	76	29.0
baked potato, w/broccoli and cheese.	1 serving	530	74	21.0
baked potato, plain.	1 serving	290	68	0.0
baked potato, w/sour cream and chives.	1 serving	430	70	14.0
French fries.	1 serving	290	37	14.0
French fries, criss cut.	1 serving	410	43	24.0
onion rings.	1 serving	430	53	21.0
zucchini.	1 serving	340	37	19.0
CARVEL				
ICE CREAM				
'Caravella'.	1 serving	164	16	8.0
'Thinny-Thin'	1 serving	92	16	0.0
ICE CREAM CONE				
plain.	1 cone	25	5	0.0
sugar	1 cone	45	10	1.0
YOGURT, FROZEN				
'Lo-Yo'	1 serving	124	20	4.0
sugarless, low-fat	I serving	104	20	4.0
CHICK-FIL-A				
BEVERAGE				
'Coca-Cola Classic' small	1 serving	110	28	0.0
'Diet Coke' small	1 serving	0	0	0.0
iced tea, sweetened, small	1 serving	150	38	0.0
iced tea, unsweetened, small	1 serving	0	0	0.0
lemonade, small	1 serving	90	23	0.0
lemonade, diet, small	1 serving	5	2	0.0
CHICKEN PIECES				
'Chick-N-Strips' 4 per serving	1 strip	230	10	8.0
nuggets, fried, 8 per serving	1 serving	290	12	14.0
DESSERT				
brownie, fudge nut	1 brownie	350	41	16.0
cheesecake	1 slice	300	23	21.0
'Ice Dream Cone' small	1 serving	140	16	4.0
lemon pie	1 slice	280	19	22.0
SALAD				
chargrilled chicken garden	1 salad	190	12	5.0
'Chick-N-Strips'	1 salad	370	21	17.0
chicken Caesar	1 salad	230	5	10.0
side	1 salad	70	13	0.0
SANDWICH				
chicken	1 sandwich	290	29	9.0
chicken, chargrilled	1 sandwich	280	36	3.0
chicken club	1 sandwich	390	38	12.0
chicken salad	1 sandwich	320	42	5.0
SIDE DISH				
carrot and raisin salad	1 cup	150	28	2.0
coleslaw	1 cup	130	11	6.0
French fries, potato waffle, small	1 serving	290	49	10.0
SOUP, breast of chicken, hearty	1 cup	110	10	1.0
CHURCH'S FRIED CHICKEN				
CHICKEN				
breast, fried	4.3 oz serving	278	9	17.0

Food Name	Serv. Size	Total Cal.	Carbs GMS	Fat GMS
breast, fried	3.5 oz	228	7	13.9
breast, w/o bone	3.5 oz	252	5	15.6
breast, w/o bone	2.8 oz	200	4	12.4
breast fillet	1 serving	608	46	34.0
breast fillet, w/cheese	1 serving	661	47	38.0
leg	3.5 oz	179	6	10.9
leg	2.9-oz serving	147	5	9.0
leg, w/o bone	3.5 oz	247	4	16.1
leg, w/o bone	2 oz	140	2	9.1
thigh	4.2-oz serving	306	9	22.0
thigh	3.5 oz	257	8	18.5
thigh, w/o bone	3.5 oz	290	7	20.4
thigh, w/o bone	2.8 oz	230	5	16.2
wing, fried	4.8-oz serving	303	9	20.0
wing, fried	3.5 oz	223	7	14.7
wing, w/o bone	3.5 oz	284	9	18.3
wing, w/o bone	3.1 oz	250	8	16.1
DESSERT				
apple pie	3.1 oz	280	41	12.3
frozen dessert	1 serving	180	27	6.0
FISH				
fillet	1 serving	430	45	18.0
fillet, w/cheese	1 serving	483	46	22.0
HOT DOG				
super	1 serving	520	44	27.0
w/cheese	1 serving	330	21	21.0
w/cheese, super	1 serving	580	45	34.0
w/chili	1 serving	320	23	20.0
w/chili, super	1 serving	570	47	32.0
SIDE DISH				
biscuit	2.1 oz	250	26	16.4
Cajun rice	3.5 oz	148	18	8.0
Cajun rice	3.1 oz	130	16	7.0
coleslaw	3 oz	92	8	5.5
corn on the cob	5.7 oz	190	32	5.4
corn on the cob, w/butter oil	1 med ear	237	33	9.0
French fries	2.7 oz	210	29	10.5
French fries, large	1 serving	320	40	16.0
hushpuppy	2 pieces	156	23	6.0
mashed potatoes, w/gravy	3.7 oz	90	14	3.3
mashed potatoes, w/gravy	3.5 oz	86	13	3.1
okra	2.8 oz	210	19	16.1
onion rings	1 serving	280	31	16.0
COLOMBO				
YOGURT, FROZEN				
French vanilla	8 oz	215	30	7.0
'Gourmet'				
Bavarian chocolate chunk	3 oz	120	18	4.0
caramel pecan chunk	3 oz	120	19	3.0
dream	3 oz	90	16	2.0
'Heath Bar Crunch'	3 oz	130	19	5.0
mocha Swiss almond	3 oz	120	17	5.0
peanut butter cup	3 oz	140	16	7.0
'Strawberry Passion'	3 oz	100	18	2.0
wild raspberry cheesecake	3 oz	100	18	2.0
low-fat	4 oz	99	18	2.0
nonfat.	4 oz	95	21	0.0
'Sundae Style'				

Food Name	Serv. Size	Total Cal.	Carbs GMS	Fat GMS
banana split, 'Sundae Style'	3 oz	100	20	1.0
caramel fudge sundae, low-fat, 'Sundae Style'	3 oz	100	21	1.0
chocolate peanut butter twist, 'Sundae Style'	3 oz	110	18	3.0

COUSIN'S SUBS

Food Name	Serv. Size	Total Cal.	Carbs GMS	Fat GMS
BACON	3 strips	50	1	4.0
BREAD				
Italian	1 oz	85	12	2.0
wheat, 2 3/4 oz per half sub	1 oz	85	11	2.0
CONDIMENT, tzatziki sauce	1 serving	50	1	4.0
DESSERT				
chocolate chip cookie	1 cookie	210	25	11.0
cranberry walnut cookie	1 cookie	187	24	8.4
PEPPERONI	6 slices	70	0	6.0
SALAD				
chef, low-fat	1 salad	194	6	7.9
garden, low-fat	1 salad	136	6	5.9
Italian	1 salad	288	6	17.9
seafood, low-fat	1 salad	176	12	5.9
side, low-fat	1 salad	71	0	4.2
tuna	1 salad	306	6	19.9
SANDWICH				
Cold				
bacon, lettuce, and tomato sub	1/2 sub	593	34	39.8
bacon, lettuce, and tomatoy sub, w/o mayo	1/2 sub	337	34	13.5
cheese sub	1/2 sub	664	30	46.3
cheese sub, mini	1/2 sub	354	16	24.7
cheese sub, mini, w/o mayo	1/2 sub	228	16	10.7
cheese sub, w/o mayo	1/2 sub	427	30	20.1
club sub	1/2 sub	730	30	45.4
club sub, w/o mayo	1/2 sub	494	30	19.2
'Cousins Special' sub, mini	1/2 sub	290	25	14.0
ham and cheese sub	1/2 sub	622	30	40.1
ham and cheese sub, mini	1/2 sub	332	16	21.4
ham and cheese sub, mini, w/o mayo	1/2 sub	206	16	7.4
ham and cheese sub, w/o mayo	1/2 sub	386	30	13.8
ham sub	1/2 sub	547	30	34.3
ham sub, low-fat, mini, w/o mayo	1/2 sub	167	16	4.3
ham sub, low-fat, w/o mayo	1/2 sub	311	30	8.0
ham sub, mini	1/2 sub	292	16	18.3
Italian cappacolla and cheese sub	1/2 sub	567	30	33.9
Italian cappacolla and Genoa sub	1/2 sub	567	30	35.5
Italian Cousins Special sub	1/2 sub	731	30	48.6
Italian Genoa and cheese sub	1/2 sub	668	30	44.5
Italian sub, regular	1/2 sub	622	30	40.0
meatball and cheese sub, mini	1/2 sub	365	16	23.1
roast beef sub	1/2 sub	598	30	34.8
roast beef sub, w/o mayo	1/2 sub	361	30	8.5
seafood w/crab sub	1/2 sub	555	38	33.6
seafood w/crab sub, mini	1/2 sub	296	20	17.9
tuna sub	1/2 sub	756	32	54.3
tuna sub, made w/o added mayo on bread	1/2 sub	500	32	28.0
tuna sub, mini	1/2 sub	495	22	37.0
tuna sub, mini, made w/o added mayo on bread	1/2 sub	290	22	16.0
turkey sub	1/2 sub	561	30	34.8
turkey sub, low-fat, mini, w/o mayo	1/2 sub	172	16	4.4
turkey sub, low-fat, w/o mayo	1/2 sub	325	30	8.5
turkey sub, mini	1/2 sub	299	16	18.5
veggie sub	1/2 sub	360	33	14.3

Food Name	Serv. Size	Total Cal.	Carbs GMS	Fat GMS
Hot				
cheese steak sub	1/2 sub	470	46	17.0
chicken breast sub	1/2 sub	556	30	31.8
chicken breast sub, w/o mayo	1/2 sub	320	30	5.5
double cheese steak sub	1/2 sub	550	35	26.0
gyro sub	1/2 sub	550	57	23.0
Italian sausage sub	1/2 sub	816	30	57.5
meatball and cheese sub	1/2 sub	685	30	43.3
pepperoni melt sub	1/2 sub	702	30	46.1
pepperoni melt sub, w/o mayo	1/2 sub	466	30	19.8
Philly cheese steak sub	1/2 sub	510	43	23.0
steak sub	1/2 sub	425	51	12.0
veggie sub	1/2 sub	380	48	11.0
SIDE DISH				
French fries, large	1 serving	525	72	24.5
French fries, medium	1 serving	400	55	18.7
French fries, small	1 serving	275	38	12.8
SOUP				
cheese, large	1 serving	330	23	22.0
cheese, regular	1 serving	210	15	14.0
cheese broccoli, large	1 serving	261	22	16.5
cheese broccoli, regular	1 serving	166	14	10.5
chicken noodle, low-fat, large	1 serving	165	21	4.1
chicken noodle, low-fat, regular	1 serving	105	13	2.6
chicken w/wild rice, large	1 serving	289	23	16.5
chicken w/wild rice, regular	1 serving	184	15	10.5
chili, large	1 serving	344	32	13.8
chili, low-fat, regular	1 serving	219	20	8.8
clam chowder, low-fat, large	1 serving	248	30	8.3
clam chowder, low-fat, regular	1 serving	158	19	5.3
potato, cream of, large	1 serving	261	30	12.4
potato, cream of, low-fat, regular	1 serving	166	19	7.9
red rice and beans, low-fat, large	1 serving	179	36	2.1
red rice and beans, low-fat, regular	1 serving	114	23	1.3
tomato basil, low-fat, large	1 serving	138	21	4.1
tomato basil, low-fat, regular	1 serving	88	13	2.6
vegetable beef, low-fat, large	1 serving	110	19	2.1
vegetable beef, low-fat, regular	1 serving	70	12	1.3

DAIRY QUEEN/BRAZIER

Food Name	Serv. Size	Total Cal.	Carbs GMS	Fat GMS
BEVERAGE				
chocolate milkshake, large	1 serving	990	168	26.0
chocolate milkshake, regular	14 fl oz	540	94	14.0
malted, 'Queen' large	21 fl oz	889	157	21.0
milkshake, 'Queen' large	21 fl oz	831	140	22.0
vanilla malt	14.7 fl oz	610	106	14.0
vanilla malt milkshake	14.7 fl oz	610	106	14.0
vanilla milkshake, large	16.3 fl oz	600	101	16.0
vanilla milkshake, regular	14 fl oz	520	88	14.0
DESSERT				
Banana split	1 serving	510	96	12.0
'Blizzard'				
Heath	14.3 oz	820	114	36.0
Heath	10.3 oz	560	79	23.0
Heath	3.5 oz	202	28	8.9
strawberry	13.5 oz	740	92	16.0
strawberry	9.4 oz	500	64	12.0
strawberry	3.5 oz	193	24	4.2

Food Name	Serv. Size	Total Cal.	Carbs GMS	Fat GMS
'Brownie Delight'				
hot fudge	10.8-oz serving	710	102	29.0
hot fudge	3.5 oz	232	33	9.5
'Breeze'				
Heath	13.4 oz	680	113	21.0
Heath	9.6 oz	450	78	12.0
Heath	3.5 oz	179	30	5.5
strawberry	12.5 oz	590	90	1.0
strawberry	8.7 oz	400	63	1.0
strawberry	3.5 oz	166	25	0.3
'Buster Bar'				
	3.5 oz	299	27	19.3
	5.3 oz	450	40	29.0
'Chipper Sandwich'	1 serving	318	56	7.0
'Dilly Bar'				
	3.5 oz	247	25	15.3
	3 oz	210	21	13.0
'Double Delight'	1 serving	490	69	20.0
'DQ Frozen Cake'				
undecorated	3.5 oz	231	30	10.9
undecorated	5.8 oz	380	50	18.0
'DQ Sandwich'	1 serving	140	24	4.0
'Fudge Nut Bar'	1 serving	406	40	25.0
Ice cream cone				
chocolate	3.5 oz	162	25	4.9
chocolate	5 oz	230	36	7.0
chocolate	7.5 oz	350	54	11.0
chocolate, chocolate dipped	1 serving	525	61	24.0
chocolate, chocolate dipped	5.5 oz	330	40	16.0
chocolate, 'Queen's Choice'	1 serving	326	40	16.0
vanilla	3 oz	140	22	4.0
vanilla	3.5 oz	162	25	4.9
vanilla	5 oz	230	36	7.0
vanilla	7.5 oz	340	53	10.0
vanilla, 'Queen's Choice'	1 serving	322	40	16.0
'Mr. Misty Float'	1 serving	390	74	7.0
'Mr. Misty Freeze'	1 serving	500	91	12.0
'Mr. Misty'				
large	1 serving	340	84	0.0
regular	11.6 oz serving	250	63	0.0
'Nutty Double Fudge'				
	3.5 oz	211	31	8.0
	9.7 oz	580	85	22.0
'Peanut Buster Parfait'				
	10.8 oz	710	94	32.0
	3.5 oz	232	31	10.4
'QC Big Scoop'				
chocolate	4.5 oz	310	40	14.0
chocolate	3.5 oz	243	31	11.0
vanilla	4.5 oz	300	39	14.0
vanilla	3.5 oz	235	31	11.0
Strawberry shortcake	1 serving	540	100	11.0
Sundae				
chocolate	6.2 oz	300	54	7.0
chocolate	3.5 oz	171	31	4.0
chocolate, large	1 serving	440	78	10.0
strawberry, waffle cone	3.5 oz	202	32	6.9

Food Name	Serv. Size	Total Cal.	Carbs GMS	Fat GMS
strawberry, waffle cone	6.1 oz	350	56	12.0
Yogurt, frozen				
	7 oz	230	49	1.0
cone, large	7.5 oz	260	56	1.0
cone, regular	5 oz	180	38	1.0
cup, regular	5 oz	170	35	1.0
strawberry sundae	12.5 oz	200	43	1.0
CHEESEBURGER				
double patty	3.5 oz	251	14	15.0
double patty	8 oz	570	31	34.0
regular	3.5 oz	234	19	11.5
regular	5.5 oz	365	30	18.0
triple patty	1 serving	820	34	50.0
CHICKEN NUGGETS, all white meat	1 serving	276	13	18.0
HAMBURGER				
double patty	3.5 oz	232	15	12.6
double patty	7 oz	460	29	25.0
'Homestar Ultimate'	3.5 oz	255	11	17.1
'Homestar Ultimate'	9.7 oz	700	30	47.0
regular	3.5 oz	219	20	9.2
regular	5 oz	310	29	13.0
triple patty	1 serving	710	33	45.0
HOT DOG				
'DQ Hounder' w/cheese	1 serving	533	22	40.0
'DQ Hounder' w/chili	1 serving	575	25	41.0
'DQ Hounder'	1 serving	480	21	36.0
'Super Dog' w/cheese	1 serving	580	45	34.0
'Super Dog' w/chili	1 serving	570	47	32.0
'Super Dog'	3.5 oz	297	21	19.1
'Super Dog'	7 oz	590	41	38.0
SALAD				
garden, w/o dressing	10 oz	200	7	13.0
side, w/o dressing	4.8 oz	25	4	0.0
SALAD DRESSING				
French, diet	2 oz	90	11	5.0
Thousand Island	2 oz	225	10	21.0
SANDWICH				
barbecue beef	3.5 oz	176	27	3.1
barbecue beef	4.5 oz	225	34	4.0
chicken fillet, breaded	3.5 oz	226	19	10.5
chicken fillet, breaded	6.7 oz	430	37	20.0
chicken fillet, breaded, w/cheese	3.5 oz	235	19	12.3
chicken fillet, breaded, w/cheese	7.2 oz	480	38	25.0
chicken fillet, grilled	6.5 oz	300	33	8.0
chicken fillet, grilled	3.5 oz	163	18	4.3
fish fillet	3.5 oz	218	23	9.4
fish fillet	6 oz	370	39	16.0
fish fillet, w/cheese	3.5 oz	228	22	11.4
fish fillet, w/cheese	6.5 oz	420	40	21.0
SIDE DISH				
French fries	3.5 oz	300	40	14.0
French fries, large	4.5 oz	390	52	18.0
onion rings	3 oz	240	29	12.0

DEL TACO
BURRITO

Food Name	Serv. Size	Total Cal.	Carbs GMS	Fat GMS
beef, deluxe	1 serving	440	43	20.0
'Big Del'	1 serving	453	49	20.0

Food Name	Serv. Size	Total Cal.	Carbs GMS	Fat GMS
breakfast	1 burrito	256	30	11.0
chicken	1 serving	264	32	10.0
chicken, spicy	1 serving	480	65	16.0
chicken fajita, 'Deluxe'	1 serving	435	41	22.0
combination	1 serving	413	46	17.0
combo	1 serving	490	53	21.0
combo, deluxe	1 serving	530	56	25.0
'Del Beef'	1 serving	590	45	33.0
'Del Beef' deluxe	1 serving	550	42	30.0
green	1 serving	229	32	8.0
green, large	1 serving	330	46	11.0
red	1 serving	235	32	8.0
red, large	1 serving	342	46	11.0
'The Works'	1 serving	480	69	18.0
CHEESEBURGER	1 serving	284	26	13.0
CONDIMENTS				
guacamole	2 tbsp	60	2	6.0
hot sauce	1 tbsp	2	1	0.0
salsa	4 tbsp	14	3	0.0
HAMBURGER	1 serving	231	26	8.0
QUESADILLA				
cheese	1 serving	260	24	12.0
chicken	1 serving	580	41	31.0
SALAD				
chicken, deluxe	1 serving	710	75	32.0
taco, deluxe	1 salad	760	76	37.0
SIDE DISH				
French fries	1 serving	242	32	11.0
refried beans, w/cheese	1 serving	122	17	7.0
TACO				
	1 serving	160	11	10.0
beef	1 serving	210	11	13.0
beef, double, deluxe	1 serving	240	13	16.0
beef, double, soft, deluxe	1 serving	250	18	14.0
beef, soft	1 serving	210	16	11.0
chicken fajita, deluxe	1 serving	211	18	10.0
chicken fajita, soft, deluxe	1 serving	210	16	12.0
regular	1 serving	211	19	10.0
soft	1 serving	146	17	6.0
TOSTADA	1 serving	210	24	9.0

DENNY'S
APPETIZER

Food Name	Serv. Size	Total Cal.	Carbs GMS	Fat GMS
"Kids Heads N' Tails Cracker'	0.5 oz	70	9	3.0
mozzarella sticks, 8 sticks	8 oz	710	49	41.0
sampler	17 oz	1405	124	80.0
BEVERAGE				
'Blender Blaster' Butterfinger	13 oz	768	97	38.0
'Blender Blaster' kids jr.	7 oz	370	46	18.0
apple juice	10 fl oz	125	33	0.0
coffee, French vanilla flavored	8 fl oz	76	16	1.0
coffee, hazelnut flavored	8 fl oz	66	14	1.0
coffee, Irish cream flavored	8 fl oz	73	16	1.0
cola float	12 oz	280	47	10.0
grapefruit juice	10 fl oz	115	29	0.0
hot chocolate	8 fl oz	90	18	2.0
iced tea, raspberry flavored	16 fl oz	78	21	0.0
lemonade, w/ice	16 fl oz	150	35	0.0

Food Name	Serv. Size	Total Cal.	Carbs GMS	Fat GMS
milk, chocolate, whole milk	10 fl oz	235	30	9.0
milk, 2%	5 fl oz	90	7	5.0
milkshake, malted, vanilla, or chocolate	12 oz	583	82	26.0
milkshake, vanilla or chocolate	12 oz	560	76	26.0
orange juice	10 fl oz	125	31	0.0
orange-strawberry-banana juice drink, 10% juice	10 fl oz	137	38	0.0
root beer float	12 oz	280	47	10.0
tomato juice	10 fl oz	55	11	0.0
BREAKFAST MEAL. See also individual listings.				
'All American Slam' w/o bread, choice of potato or grits	13 oz	712	9	62.0
'Cinnamon Swirl Slam'	13 oz	1105	68	78.0
'Country Slam'	18 oz	1000	61	66.0
'Farmer's Slam'	19 oz	1200	82	80.0
'French Slam'	14 oz	1029	58	71.0
'Kids Frenchtastic Slam' w/o bread, potato, or meat	6 oz	452	22	33.0
'Kids Junior Grand Slam' w/o bread, potato, or meat	5 oz	397	33	25.0
'Moons Over My Hammy' w/o bread, choice of potato or grits	12 oz	807	46	48.0
'Original Grand Slam'	10 oz	795	65	50.0
'Play It Again Slam'	15 oz	1192	98	75.0
'Sausage Lover's Slam'	17 oz	960	33	68.0
'Scram Slam'	18 oz	740	14	62.0
'Senior Belgian Waffle Slam' w/o syrup, margarine	6 oz	399	12	33.0
'Senior Triple Play' w/o bread, potato, or meat	8 oz	537	64	25.0
sirloin steak and eggs, w/o bread, choice of potato or grits	9 oz	622	1	49.0
'Slim Slam' w/o topping	12 oz	495	98	12.0
'Southern Slam'	13 oz	1065	47	84.0
T-bone steak and eggs, w/o bread, choice of potato or grits	14 oz	991	1	77.0
BREAD AND ROLLS. See also French Toast.				
bagel, w/o added condiments	3 oz	235	46	1.0
biscuit, w/butter	3 oz	272	39	11.0
English muffin, 1 muffin, w/o added condiments	4 oz	125	24	1.0
toast, dry, 1 slice	1 oz	90	17	1.0
toast, herb	2 oz	170	15	11.0
BUFFALO CHICKEN BURGER				
burger only, w/o added condiments	13 oz	803	67	45.0
BUFFALO WINGS, 12 wings	15 oz	940	3	68.0
CEREAL, ready to eat, 'Kellogg's' average dry	1 oz	100	23	0.0
CHEESE	8 oz	293	13	23.0
CHEESEBURGER				
classic, burger only, w/o added condiments	13 oz	836	43	53.0
'Kids The Big Cheese' w/o fries or substitute	3 oz	334	28	20.0
w/bacon, burger only, w/o added condiments	14 oz	875	58	52.0
CHICKEN DINNER				
breast, grilled, w/o salad dressing, bread	4 oz	130	0	4.0
Charleston, w/o choice of side dishes	6 oz	327	16	18.0
'Senior Grilled Chicken Breast Dinner' w/o bread, soup, salad, fruit, vegetable	6 oz	200	15	5.0
CHICKEN NUGGETS				
'Kids Dennysaur' w/o fries or substitute	2 oz	190	9	13.0
CHICKEN STRIPS DINNER				
5 strips, w/o choice of side dishes	10 oz	720	56	33.0
Buffalo, 5 strips, w/o choice of side dishes	10 oz	734	43	42.0
CHILI, with cheese topping	11 oz	401	21	19.0
CONDIMENTS				
bacon, 4 strips	1 oz	162	1	18.0
bacon, peppered, 4 strips	1 oz	175	2	13.0
barbecue sauce	1.5 oz	47	11	1.0

Food Name	Serv. Size	Total Cal.	Carbs GMS	Fat GMS
cream cheese	1 oz	100	1	10.0
guacamole	1.5 oz	74	4	6.0
honey	0.5 oz	40	12	0.0
margarine, whipped	0.5 oz	87	0	10.0
marinara sauce	1.5 oz	48	7	2.0
mushroom, grilled	2 oz	14	2	0.0
raisins	0.75 oz	65	17	0.0
salsa	1.5 oz	14	1	0.0
sour cream	1.5 oz	91	2	9.0
sugar, brown	1 oz	110	30	0.0
syrup, blueberry flavored	1.5 oz	102	26	0.0
syrup, maple favored, 3 tbsp	1.5 oz	143	36	0.0
syrup, maple favored, sugar free	1.5 oz	23	9	0.0
syrup, strawberry flavored	1.5 oz	91	23	0.0
tartar sauce	1.5 oz	230	5	24.0
tomato, sliced, 3 slices	2 oz	13	3	0.0
DESSERT				
apple pie, 1/6 pie	7 oz	470	64	24.0
banana royale	10 oz	548	80	25.0
banana split	19 oz	894	121	43.0
'Butterfinger Hot Fudge Sundae'	9 oz	700	106	38.0
cheescako, w/o topping	4 oz	470	48	27.0
cherry pie, 1/6 pie	7 oz	630	101	25.0
chocolate layer cake	3 oz	275	42	12.0
chocolate peanut butter pie, 1/6 pie	6 oz	653	64	39.0
chocolate silk pie, 1/6 pie	6 oz	650	60	43.0
Dutch apple pie, 1/6 pie	7 oz	440	65	19.0
hot fudge cake	7 oz	620	73	35.0
key lime pie, 1/6 pie	6 oz	600	79	27.0
'Kids Jr. Butterfinger Hot Fudge Sundae'	4 oz	341	46	17.0
Oreo cookies and creme pie, 1/6 pie	6 oz	590	73	30.0
rainbow sherbet	4 oz	120	25	1.5
sundae, double scoop, w/o topping	6 oz	375	29	27.0
sundae, single scoop, w/o topping, 'Delicious Dip'	3 oz	188	14	14.0
yogurt, frozen, chocolate chocolate chip, low-fat	4 oz	110	19	2.0
EGGS BENEDICT, w/o choice of potato or grits	15 oz	695	34	46.0
FISH DINNER				
	9 oz	732	48	47.0
'Senior Fish Dinner' w/o bread, soup, salad, fruit, vegetable	5 oz	465	25	34.0
FRENCH TOAST				
plain, w/o choice of meat, fruit topping or syrup, margarine	2 pieces	507	54	24.0
cinnamon swirl, w/o choice of meat, fruit topping or syrup, margarine	12 oz	1030	124	49.0
GARDEN BURGER, burger only, w/o added condiments	11 oz	665	75	33.0
GRAVY				
biscuit and sausage	7 oz	398	45	21.0
brown	1 oz	13	2	0.0
chicken	1 oz	14	2	0.5
country	1 oz	17	2	1.0
sausage	4 oz	126	6	10.0
HAM, grilled, grilled slice	3 oz	94	2	3.0
HAMBURGER				
'Big Texas Barbecue' burger only, w/o added condiments	14 oz	929	53	58.0
'Classic' burger only, w/o added condiments	11 oz	673	42	40.0
'Double Decker' burger only, w/o added condiments	15 oz	1247	82	80.0
'Garlic Mushroom Swiss' burger only, w/o added condiments	15 oz	872	58	51.0
'Kid's Burgerlicious' w/cheese, w/o fries or substitute	4 oz	341	24	20.0

Food Name	Serv. Size	Total Cal.	Carbs GMS	Fat GMS
'Kid's Burgerlicious' w/o fries or substitute	4 oz	296	24	17.0
HOT DOG MEAL, 'Kids Pig in a Blanket'	5 oz	479	63	21.0
HOTCAKES				
buttermilk, w/o choice of meat, fruit topping or syrup, margarine	3 hotcakes	491	95	7.0
'Kids Smiley-Face Hotcakes' w/meat, w/o syrup, margarine	6 oz	463	63	22.0
'Kids Smiley-Face Hotcakes' w/omeat, w/o syrup, margarine	4 oz	344	62	9.0
OATMEAL				
'Quaker'	4 oz	100	18	2.0
and fixings, w/o juice, bread	20 oz	535	115	6.0
OMELET				
farmer's, w/o bread, choice of potato or grits	14 oz	650	17	51.0
ham and cheddar, w/o bread, choice of potato or grits	10 oz	581	4	45.0
'Senior Omelette' w/o bread, potato, or meat	9 oz	429	8	20.0
'Ultimate' w/o bread, choice of potato or grits	13 oz	564	9	47.0
'Veggie-Cheese' w/o bread, choice of potato or grits	12 oz	480	9	39.0
PIZZA MEAL, 'Kids Pizza Party'	6 oz	400	47	15.0
POT ROAST DINNER				
w/gravy	7 oz	292	5	11.0
'Senior Pot Roast Dinner' w/o bread, soup, salad, fruit, vegetable	4 oz	160	3	6.0
POTATO PANCAKE, w/o meat, w/o choice of fruit topping or syrup, margarine	13 oz	530	59	27.0
SALAD				
Buffalo chicken, w/o dressing, bread	16 oz	516	26	35.0
Caesar, side, w/dressing, w/o bread	6 oz	362	20	26.0
California grilled chicken, w/o dressing, bread	13 oz	277	10	12.0
fried chicken, w/o dressing, bread	15 oz	438	26	26.0
garden, side, w/o dressing, bread	7 oz	113	16	4.0
'Garden Chicken Delight' w/o dressing, bread	16 oz	277	30	5.0
grilled chicken Caesar, w/dressing, w/o bread	13 oz	600	19	41.0
SALAD DRESSING				
blue cheese	1 oz	163	1	18.0
Caesar	1 oz	133	1	14.0
French	1 oz	106	3	10.0
honey mustard, nonfat	1 oz	38	9	0.0
Italian, lower calorie, reduced calorie	1 oz	15	3	0.5
ranch	1 oz	101	1	11.0
Thousand Island	1 oz	118	5	11.0
SALMON DINNER				
Alaskan salmon, grilled, w/o salad dressing, bread	6 oz	210	1	4.0
SANDWICH				
bacon, lettuce and tomato, sandwich only, w/o added condiments	6 oz	634	37	46.0
Charleston chicken, sandwich only, w/o added condiments	11 oz	632	53	32.0
club, sandwich only, w/o added condiments	11 oz	718	62	38.0
grilled cheese, sandwich only	7 oz	510	40	30.0
grilled chicken, fit-fare, sandwich only	14 oz	434	56	9.0
grilled chicken, sandwich only, w/o added condiments	11 oz	520	64	14.0
ham and swiss, on rye, sandwich only, w/o added condiments	9 oz	533	40	31.0
ham and swiss, sandwich only, w/o added condiments	9 oz	497	34	30.0
Reuben, sandwich only, w/o added condiments	9 oz	580	37	35.0
'Super Bird' sandwich only, w/o added condiments	9 oz	620	48	32.0
turkey breast, on multigrain bread, sandwich only, w/o added condiments	9 oz	476	39	26.0
turkey sub, sandwich only	9 oz	476	39	26.0
SHRIMP DINNER				
'Kids Shrimpsational Basket' w/o fries or substitute	5 oz	291	27	16.0

Food Name	Serv. Size	Total Cal.	Carbs GMS	Fat GMS
fried	8 oz	558	49	32.0
SIDE DISH				
applesauce, 'Musselmans'	3 oz	60	15	0.0
banana, slices	4 oz	100	27	0.0
banana, whole	4 oz	110	29	0.0
baked potato, plain, w/skin	7 oz	220	51	0.0
broccoli, w/butter	4 oz	65	7	3.0
carrots, w/honey glaze	4 oz	80	12	3.0
corn, w/butter	4 oz	120	19	4.0
cottage cheese	3 oz	72	2	3.0
country fried potato	6 oz	515	23	35.0
French fries, chili cheese	12 oz	816	77	44.0
French fries, unsalted	4 oz	323	44	14.0
fries, seasoned	4 oz	261	35	12.0
fries, smothered cheese	9 oz	767	69	48.0
fruit mix	3 oz	36	9	0.0
grapefruit, 1/2 grapefruit	5 oz	60	16	0.0
grapes	3 oz	55	15	1.0
green beans, w/bacon	4 oz	60	6	4.0
green peas, w/butter	4 oz	100	14	3.0
grits	4 oz	80	18	0.0
hash browns	4 oz	218	20	14.0
hash browns, covered	6 oz	318	21	23.0
hash browns, covered and smothered	8 oz	359	26	26.0
hash browns, doubled, covered, smothered	13 oz	460	48	26.0
mashed potato, plain	6 oz	105	21	1.0
melon, cantaloupe, 1/4 melon	3 oz	32	8	0.0
melon, honeydew, 1/4 melon	3 oz	31	8	0.0
onion rings	4 oz	381	38	23.0
sausage link, 1 link	3 oz	354	0	32.0
sausage patty, 2 patties	3 oz	300	1	28.0
strawberry-banana medley	4 oz	108	27	1.0
stuffing, bread, plain	3 oz	100	19	1.0
vegetable rice pilaf	3 oz	85	16	1.0
SKILLET MEAL				
'Big Texas Chicken Fajita' w/o bread	17 oz	1217	25	70.0
'Meat Lover's' w/o bread	15 oz	1147	24	93.0
'Sausage Supreme' w/o bread	16 oz	1054	30	83.0
SOUP				
broccoli, cream of	8 oz	193	15	12.0
chicken noodle	8 oz	60	8	2.0
clam chowder	8 oz	214	22	11.0
potato, cream of	8 oz	222	23	12.0
split pea	8 oz	146	18	6.0
vegetable beef	8 oz	79	11	1.0
STEAK MEAL				
chicken-fried steak and eggs, w/o choice of bread, potato or grits	8 oz	430	9	36.0
'Senior Chicken-Fried Steak Dinner' w/o bread, soup, salad, fruit, or vegetable	8 oz	341	29	18.0
sirloin	6 oz	271	0	21.0
T-bone	12 oz	642	1	50.0
chicken-fried steak	7 oz	495	24	32.0
steak and shrimp dinner	9 oz	645	31	42.0
STIR-FRY				
grilled chicken, w/o bread	18 oz	524	72	11.0
vegetable, w/o bread	20 oz	470	90	6.0

Food Name	Serv. Size	Total Cal.	Carbs GMS	Fat GMS
TOPPING				
blueberry	3 oz	106	26	0.0
blueberry	2 oz	71	17	0.0
cherry	3 oz	86	21	0.0
cherry	2 oz	57	14	0.0
chocolate	2 oz	317	27	25.0
fudge	2 oz	201	30	10.0
nut, 1 tsp	0.3 oz	42	1	4.0
strawberry	3 oz	115	26	1.0
strawberry	2 oz	77	17	1.0
whipped cream, 2 tbsp	0.3 oz	23	2	2.0
TURKEY DINNER				
roast turkey and stuffing, w/gravy, w/o salad dressing, bread	14 oz	388	38	3.0
'Senior Turkey and Stuffing Dinner' w/o bread, soup, salad, fruit, vegetable	8 oz	220	25	2.0
WAFFLE				
'Kids Wacky Waffles' w/o syrup or margarine	5 oz	215	23	12.0
w/o choice of meat, fruit topping or syrup, and margarine	1 waffle	304	23	21.0
D'LITES OF AMERICA				
CHEESE, light	1 slice	53	2	3.0
CHEESEBURGER				
w/bacon, on multigrain bun	1 serving	370	20	18.0
w/bacon, on sesame seed bun	1 serving	370	20	18.0
CONDIMENTS				
salad dressing, lower calorie	1 tbsp	40	1	4.0
salad dressing, mayonnaise type				
mayonnaise, light	1 tbsp	40	1	4.0
tartar sauce, light	1 tbsp	60	2	6.0
DESSERT				
frozen, 'Chocolate D'Lite'	1 serving	203	36	4.0
HAMBURGER				
'Double D'Lite' on multigrain bun	1 serving	450	19	22.0
'Double D'Lite' on sesame seed bun	1 serving	450	19	22.0
'Junior D'Lite' on multigrain bun	1 serving	200	19	7.0
'Junior D'Lite' on sesame seed bun	1 serving	200	19	7.0
'Quarter Pound D'Lite' on multigrain bun	1 serving	280	19	12.0
'Quarter Pound D'Lite' on sesame seed bun	1 serving	280	19	12.0
SANDWICH				
chicken fillet, on multigrain bun	1 sandwich	280	24	11.0
chicken fillet, on sesame seed bun	1 sandwich	280	24	11.0
fish fillet, on multigrain bun	1 sandwich	390	29	21.0
fish fillet, on sesame seed bun	1 sandwich	390	29	21.0
ham and cheese, on multigrain bun	1 sandwich	280	26	8.0
ham and cheese, on sesame seed bun	1 sandwich	280	26	8.0
vegetarian, 'Vegetarian D'Lite'	1 sandwich	270	20	14.0
SIDE DISH				
baked potato	10-oz serving	230	50	1.0
baked potato	3.5 oz	81	18	0.3
baked potato, 'Mexican'	1 serving	510	61	18.0
baked potato, w/bacon and cheddar	1 serving	490	52	20.0
baked potato, w/broccoli and cheddar	1 serving	410	51	16.0
French fries, large	1 serving	320	42	15.0
French fries, regular	1 serving	260	34	12.0
potato skin, 'Mexi-Skins'	1 piece	99	6	7.0
salad bar platter	1 salad	130	9	6.0
SOUP				
broccoli, cream of	1 serving	180	21	7.0
'D'Lite'	1 serving	130	10	4.0

Food Name	Serv. Size	Total Cal.	Carbs GMS	Fat GMS
DOMINO'S				
BREADSTICK	1 piece	116	18	4.0
BUFFALO WINGS				
barbecue	1 piece	50	2	2.0
hot	1 piece	45	1	2.0
CHEESY BREAD	1 piece	142	18	6.0
PIZZA				
Deep-dish				
cheese, individual, 6-inch	1 serving	598	68	28.0
cheese, large, 14-inch diam	2 slices	677	80	30.0
cheese, medium, 12-inch diam	2 slices	482	56	22.0
ham, individual, 6-inch diam	1 serving	615	69	28.0
ham, large, 14-inch diam	2 slices	708	81	31.0
ham, medium, 12-inch diam	2 slices	505	57	23.0
pepperoni, individual, 6-inch diam	1 serving	647	69	32.0
pepperoni, large, 14-inch diam	2 slices	775	81	38.0
pepperoni, medium, 12-inch diam	2 slices	556	56	28.0
sausage, individual, 6-inch diam	1 serving	642	70	31.0
sausage, large, 14-inch diam	2 slices	787	83	38.0
sausage, medium, 12-inch diam	2 slices	559	58	28.0
vegetable, w/mushrooms, green peppers, onions, olives, individual, 6-inch diam	1 serving	616	70	29.0
vegetable, w/mushrooms, green peppers, onions, olives, large, 14-inch diam	2 slices	697	83	31.0
vegetable, w/mushrooms, green peppers, onions, olives, medium, 12-inch diam	2 slices	498	58	23.0
Hand-tossed				
cheese, medium, 12-inch diam	2 slices	375	55	11.0
cheese, large, 14-inch diam	2 slices	516	75	15.0
ham, medium, 12-inch diam	2 slices	398	55	12.0
ham, large, 14-inch diam	2 slices	547	76	17.0
pepperoni, medium, 12-inch diam	2 slices	448	55	17.0
pepperoni, large, 14-inch diam	2 slices	614	75	24.0
sausage, medium, 12-inch diam	2 slices	452	57	17.0
sausage, large, 14-inch diam	2 slices	626	78	24.0
vegetable, w/mushrooms, green peppers, onions, olives, medium, 12-inch diam	2 slices	391	57	12.0
vegetable, w/mushrooms, green peppers, onions, olives, large, 14-inch diam	2 slices	536	77	17.0
Thin crust				
cheese, medium, 12-inch diam	1/4 of pizza	273	31	12.0
cheese, large, 14-inch diam	1/4 of pizza	382	43	17.0
ham, medium, 12-inch diam	1/4 of pizza	296	31	13.0
ham, large, 14-inch diam	1/4 of pizza	414	44	18.0
pepperoni, medium, 12-inch diam	1/4 of pizza	347	31	18.0
pepperoni, large, 14-inch diam	1/4 of pizza	481	44	25.0
sausage, medium, 12-inch diam	1/4 of pizza	350	33	18.0
sausage, large, 14-inch diam	1/4 of pizza	492	47	25.0
vegetable, w/mushrooms, green peppers, onions, olives, medium, 12-inch diam	1/4 of pizza	289	33	13.0
vegetable, w/mushrooms, green peppers, onions, olives, large, 14-inch diam	1/4 of pizza	402	46	18.0
DRUTHER'S				
BISCUITS AND GRAVY	8.1-oz servings	331	42	14.7
BREAKFAST MEAL				
bacon and fried egg platter	1 serving	721	62	41.9
bacon and scrambled egg platter	1 serving	742	64	43.0

Food Name	Serv. Size	Total Cal.	Carbs GMS	Fat GMS
biscuit, bacon, and egg	3.1-oz serving	258	15	16.3
biscuit, ham, and egg	3.5-oz serving	217	15	11.2
ham and fried egg platter	1 serving	681	62	35.3
ham and scrambled egg platter	1 serving	762	64	44.6
sausage and biscuit platter, two of each	3.4-oz serving	358	26	22.3
sausage and egg biscuit	3.3-oz serving	246	15	15.1
sausage and fried egg platter	1 serving	741	63	43.4
sausage and scrambled egg platter	1 serving	742	64	43.0
CHEESEBURGER				
'Deluxe Quarter'	8.7 oz	660	46	37.6
double patty	6.4 oz	500	35	26.1
regular	4.7 oz	380	35	17.8
CHICKEN				
12 pieces	3.9 lbs	5496	637	171.2
8 pieces	2.6 lbs	3664	425	114.1
breast, w/wing, dinner or snack	2 pieces	595	28	30.7
leg, w/thigh, dinner or snack	2 pieces	549	29	29.8
thigh and leg, dinner or snack	3 pieces	1281	90	66.9
thigh and wing, dinner or snack	3 pieces	1309	87	70.3
CHICKEN ENTREE				
breast and wing, w/potatoes and coleslaw	2 pieces	970	76	49.9
leg and thigh, w/potatoes and coleslaw	2 pieces	925	77	49.0
FISH ENTREE				
	13.3-oz entrée	770	79	31.3
fried, w/fries	11.2 oz	729	71	29.8
FISH SANDWICH	4.8 oz	349	33	14.4
HAMBURGER	4.4 oz	327	35	13.4

DUNKIN' DONUTS

Food Name	Serv. Size	Total Cal.	Carbs GMS	Fat GMS
BAGEL				
blueberry	1 bagel	340	75	1.0
cinnamon raisin	1 bagel	340	74	1.0
egg	1 bagel	350	72	1.5
everything	1 bagel	360	74	2.0
garlic	1 bagel	360	76	1.0
onion	1 bagel	330	70	1.0
plain	1 bagel	340	73	1.0
poppyseed	1 bagel	360	74	2.5
pumpernickel	1 bagel	350	75	1.5
salt	1 bagel	340	73	1.0
sesame	1 bagel	380	74	4.5
wheat	1 bagel	330	73	1.5
BEVERAGE				
'Coolatta' coffee w/cream	16 fl oz	410	51	22.0
'Coolatta' coffee w/milk	16 fl oz	260	52	4.0
'Coolatta' coffee w/skim milk	16 fl oz	230	52	0.0
'Coolatta' coffee w/2% milk	16 fl oz	240	52	2.0
'Coolatta' orange mango fruit	16 fl oz	290	71	0.0
'Coolatta' pink lemonade	16 fl oz	350	88	0.0
'Coolatta' raspberry lemonade	16 fl oz	280	68	0.0
'Coolatta' strawberry fruit	16 fl oz	280	70	0.0
'Coolatta' vanilla	16 fl oz	450	94	7.0
'Dunkaccino'	18.75 fl oz	480	67	22.0
'Dunkaccino'	10 fl oz	250	34	11.0
'Dunkaccino'	14 fl oz	360	51	17.0
'Dunkaccino'	20 fl oz	510	71	23.0
hot cocoa	18.75 fl oz	440	75	15.0
hot cocoa	10 fl oz	230	38	8.0
hot cocoa	14 fl oz	330	57	11.0

Food Name	Serv. Size	Total Cal.	Carbs GMS	Fat GMS
hot cocoa	20 fl oz	470	79	16.0
BREAKFAST SANDWICH				
'Omwich' bagel, w/bacon and cheddar	1 sandwich	600	79	21.0
'Omwich' bagel, Spanish, cheese	1 sandwich	570	79	18.0
'Omwich' bagel, three cheese	1 sandwich	610	78	22.0
'Omwich' croissant, w/bacon and cheddar	1 sandwich	560	33	38.0
'Omwich' croissant, Spanish, cheese	1 sandwich	530	33	36.0
'Omwich' croissant, three cheese	1 sandwich	560	33	39.0
'Omwich' English muffin, w/bacon and cheddar	1 sandwich	400	33	21.0
'Omwich' English muffin, Spanish, cheese	1 sandwich	370	34	18.0
'Omwich' English muffin, three cheese	1 sandwich	400	33	22.0
'Omwich' ham, egg, cheese	1 sandwich	320	31	12.0
CINNAMON BUN	1 bun	510	85	15.0
COOKIE				
chocolate chocolate chunk	1 cookie	210	26	11.0
chocolate chunk	1 cookie	220	28	11.0
chocolate chunk w/nuts	1 cookie	230	27	12.0
chocolate-white chocolate chunk	1 cookie	230	28	12.0
oatmeal raisin pecan	1 cookie	220	29	10.0
peanut butter chocolate chunk w/nuts	1 cookie	240	24	14.0
peanut butter w/nuts	1 cookie	240	24	14.0
CREAM CHEESE				
chive	1 packet	190	3	19.0
garden vegetable	1 packet	180	3	17.0
lite	1 packet	130	3	11.0
plain	1 packet	200	3	19.0
salmon	1 packet	180	2	17.0
CROISSANT				
almond	1 croissant	350	34	22.0
chocolate	1 croissant	400	37	25.0
plain	1 croissant	290	26	18.0
DOUGHNUT				
apple crumb	1 donut	230	34	10.0
apple fritter	1 donut	300	41	14.0
apple n' spice	1 donut	200	29	8.0
Bavarian kreme	1 donut	210	30	9.0
bismark, chocolate-iced	1 donut	340	50	15.0
black raspberry	1 donut	210	32	8.0
blueberry cake	1 donut	290	35	16.0
blueberry crumb	1 donut	240	36	10.0
Boston kreme	1 donut	240	36	9.0
bow tie	1 donut	300	34	17.0
butternut cake ring	1 donut	300	36	16.0
cake, glazed	1 donut	270	33	15.0
chcolate cake glazed	1 donut	290	33	16.0
chocolate coconut cake	1 donut	300	31	19.0
chocolate cruller, glazed	1 donut	280	35	15.0
chocolate kreme filled	1 donut	270	35	13.0
chocolate-frosted	1 donut	200	29	9.0
chocolate-frosted cake	1 donut	300	38	16.0
cinnamon cake	1 donut	270	31	15.0
coconut cake	1 donut	290	33	17.0
coffee roll	1 donut	270	33	14.0
coffee roll, chocolate-frosted	1 donut	290	36	15.0
coffee roll, maple frosted	1 donut	290	36	14.0
cruller, glazed	1 donut	290	37	15.0
double chocolate cake	1 donut	310	37	17.0
dunkin'	1 donut	240	25	15.0
éclair	1 donut	270	39	11.0

Food Name	Serv. Size	Total Cal.	Carbs GMS	Fat GMS
fritter, glazed	1 donut	260	31	14.0
glazed	1 donut	180	25	8.0
jelly stick	1 donut	290	44	12.0
jelly-filled	1 donut	210	32	8.0
lemon	1 donut	200	28	9.0
maple frosted	1 donut	210	30	9.0
marble frosted	1 donut	200	29	9.0
old-fashioned cake	1 donut	250	26	15.0
plain cruller	1 donut	240	25	15.0
powdered cake	1 donut	270	32	15.0
powdered cruller	1 donut	270	30	15.0
strawberry	1 donut	210	32	8.0
strawberry-frosted	1 donut	210	30	9.0
sugar cruller	1 donut	250	27	15.0
sugar raised	1 donut	170	22	8.0
sugared cake	1 donut	250	27	15.0
toasted coconut cake	1 donut	300	35	17.0
vanilla kreme filled	1 donut	270	36	13.0
vanilla-frosted	1 donut	210	30	9.0
whole wheat glazed cake	1 donut	310	32	19.0
DOUGHNUT HOLE				
'Munchkin' cake butternut	3 munchkins	200	25	11.0
'Munchkin' cake chocolate glazed	3 munchkins	200	26	10.0
'Munchkin' cake cinnamon	4 munchkins	250	30	14.0
'Munchkin' cake coconut	3 munchkins	200	23	12.0
'Munchkin' cake glazed	3 munchkins	200	27	10.0
'Munchkin' cake plain	4 munchkins	220	22	14.0
'Munchkin' cake powdered	4 munchkins	250	29	14.0
'Munchkin' cake sugared	4 munchkins	240	28	14.0
'Munchkin' cake toasted coconut	3 munchkins	200	24	11.0
'Munchkin' yeast glazed	5 munchkins	200	27	9.0
'Munchkin' yeast jelly filled	5 munchkins	210	30	9.0
'Munchkin' yeast lemon filled	4 munchkins	170	23	8.0
'Munchkin' yeast sugar raised	7 munchkins	220	26	12.0
MUFFIN				
apple and spice, low-fat	1 muffin	240	54	1.5
apple cinnamon pecan	1 muffin	510	74	21.0
apple n' spice	1 muffin	350	57	12.0
banana nut	1 muffin	360	52	15.0
banana, low-fat	1 muffin	250	57	1.5
blueberry, 4-oz muffin	1 muffin	320	49	12.0
blueberry, 6-oz muffin	1 muffin	490	76	17.0
blueberry, lower fat reduced fat	1 muffin	450	77	12.0
blueberry, low-fat	1 muffin	250	55	1.5
bran	1 muffin	390	60	12.0
bran, low-fat	1 muffin	240	57	1.0
cherry	1 muffin	340	53	12.0
cherry, low-fat	1 muffin	250	56	1.5
chocolate chip, 4-oz muffin	1 muffin	400	58	17.0
chocolate chip, 6-oz muffin	1 muffin	590	88	24.0
chocolate hazelnut chunk	1 muffin	610	87	26.0
chocolate, low-fat	1 muffin	250	53	2.5
corn, 4-oz muffin	1 muffin	390	57	15.0
corn, 6-oz muffin	1 muffin	500	78	16.0
corn, low-fat	1 muffin	240	52	2.5
corn, reduced fat	1 muffin	460	79	11.0
cranberry orange	1 muffin	470	76	15.0
cranberry orange nut	1 muffin	350	52	15.0

Food Name	Serv. Size	Total Cal.	Carbs GMS	Fat GMS
cranberry orange, low-fat	1 muffin	240	55	1.5
honey bran raisin	1 muffin	490	84	16.0
lemon poppyseed	1 muffin	360	56	13.0
oat bran	1 muffin	370	55	13.0

EL POLLO LOCO
BEANS
pinto	6 oz	185	29	4.0
black, smoky	5 oz	255	29	13.0
black, smoky, bowl	16 oz	604	75	23.0

BEVERAGE
smoothie, kiwi strawberry	9.5 oz	357	66	7.0
smoothie, 'Minute Maid' orange	20 oz	526	99	4.0
smoothie, 'Minute Maid' orange	16 oz	457	84	4.0
smoothie, strawberry banana	11 oz	367	68	7.0

BURRITO
black bean, smoky	8 oz	515	71	20.0
'BRC'	7 oz	440	64	14.0
chicken, classic	11 oz	580	66	22.0
chicken, Southwest	12 oz	627	69	27.0
chicken Caesar, Mexican	11 oz	734	65	35.0
'Chicken Grande'	14 oz	648	72	26.0
'Chicken Lovers'	9 oz	476	47	19.0
'Ultimate Chicken'	12.8 oz	633	66	23.0

CHICKEN
breast, flame-broiled, w/o bone	3 oz	160	0	6.0
leg, flame-broiled, w/o bone	1.75 oz	90	0	5.0
thigh, flame-broiled, w/o bone	2 oz	180	0	12.0
wing, flame-broiled, w/o bone	1.5 oz	110	0	6.0
CHICKEN NUGGETS, 'Dinosaur Chicken Bites' 4 oz	4 pieces	185	11	10.4
CHURROS	1.75 oz	179	18	11.0

CONDIMENTS. See also Salad Dressing.
gravy	1 oz	14	2	0.0
guacamole	1.75 oz	52	5	3.0
jalapeño hot sauce, 0.5 oz	1 pkt	5	1	0.0
salsa, avocado	1 oz	12	1	1.0
salsa, house	1 oz	6	1	0.0
salsa, pico de gallo	1 oz	11	2	0.5
salsa, spicy chipotle	1 oz	7	1	0.0
sour cream, light	1 oz	45	2	3.0

DESSERT
banana split	15 oz	717	107	28.0
cheesecake	3.5 oz	310	30	18.0
'Foster's Freeze' w/o topping	4.6 oz	180	30	5.0

SALAD
'Pollo Bowl'	17 oz	469	66	11.0
bowl, flame-broiled chicken	12 oz	357	39	13.0
bowl, Mexican Caesar chicken	11 oz	491	32	30.0
bowl, Southwest chicken	13 oz	529	40	31.0
garden, large	14 oz	225	17	13.0
garden, regular	4 oz	105	7	7.0
tostada, w/o shell and sour cream	14 oz	304	28	11.0

SALAD DRESSING
blue cheese	2 oz	300	2	32.0
cilantry, creamy	1.75 oz	266	1	29.0
Italian, light	2 oz	25	3	1.0
ranch	2 oz	350	2	39.0
Southwest	1.75 oz	301	2	32.0
Thousand Island	2 oz	270	9	27.0

Food Name	Serv. Size	Total Cal.	Carbs GMS	Fat GMS
SIDE DISH. See also Beans.				
coleslaw	5 oz	206	12	16.0
corn cobbette	3 oz	80	18	1.0
French fries	5.5 oz	444	61	19.0
macaroni and cheese	1 serving	330	32	16.0
mashed potato	5 oz	97	21	1.0
potato salad	6 oz	256	30	14.0
Spanish rice	4 oz	130	24	3.0
vegetables, fresh	4 oz	57	8	2.0
TACO				
'Al Carbon'	3 oz	164	14	6.0
chicken, soft	4.5 oz	237	15	12.0
taquito, chicken	5 oz	370	43	17.0
TORTILLA				
corn, 6-inch diam	1 oz	70	14	1.0
corn, 4.5-inch diam	0.5 oz	32	6	0.5
flour, 11-inch diam	3 oz	260	42	7.0
flour, 6-inch diam	1 oz	90	13	3.0
spicy tomato	3 oz	254	42	6.0
TORTILLA CHIPS, no salt	5 oz	760	86	42.0
TOSTADA SHELL	5.6 oz	440	42	27.0

EVERYTHING YOGURT
YOGURT, FROZEN

Food Name	Serv. Size	Total Cal.	Carbs GMS	Fat GMS
low-fat	1 serving	95	18	1.0
nonfat	1 serving	80	17	0.0

GODFATHER'S PIZZA
PIZZA
Cheese

Food Name	Serv. Size	Total Cal.	Carbs GMS	Fat GMS
golden crust, large	1/10 pizza	261	31	11.0
golden crust, medium	1/8 pizza	229	28	9.0
golden crust, small	1/6 pizza	213	27	8.0
original crust, large	1/10 pizza	271	37	8.0
original crust, medium	1/8 pizza	242	35	7.0
original crust, mini	1/4 pizza	138	20	4.0
original crust, small	1/6 pizza	239	32	7.0
thin crust, large	1/10 pizza	228	28	7.0
thin crust, medium	1/8 pizza	210	26	7.0
thin crust, small	1/6 pizza	180	21	6.0
Combo				
golden crust, large	1/10 pizza	322	33	15.0
golden crust, medium	1/8 pizza	283	30	13.0
golden crust, small	1/6 pizza	273	29	12.0
original crust, large	1/10 pizza	332	39	12.0
original crust, medium	1/8 pizza	318	37	12.0
original crust, mini	1/4 pizza	164	21	5.0
original crust, small	1/6 pizza	299	34	11.0
thin crust, large	1/10 pizza	336	31	16.0
thin crust, medium	1/8 pizza	310	29	14.0
thin crust, small	1/6 pizza	270	23	13.0
STUFFED PIZZA				
cheese, large	1/10 pizza	381	44	16.0
cheese, medium	1/8 pizza	350	42	13.0
cheese, small	1/6 pizza	310	38	11.0
combo, large	1/10 pizza	521	47	26.0
combo, medium	1/8 pizza	480	45	23.0
combo, small	1/6 pizza	430	41	20.0

Food Name	Serv. Size	Total Cal.	Carbs GMS	Fat GMS
GOLDEN CORRAL				
BREAD, 'Texas Toast'	1 serving	170	26	6.0
CHICKEN				
fillet, 'Golden Fried'	1 serving	370	14	19.0
fillet, 'Golden Grilled'	1 serving	170	0	5.0
POTATO, baked	1 serving	220	46	2.0
RIBEYE STEAK, regular	1 serving	450	0	35.0
SHRIMP, 'Golden Fried'	1 serving	250	24	12.0
SIRLOIN STEAK				
	5-oz serving	230	0	14.0
chopped	4-oz serving	320	0	23.0
tips, w/onions and pepper	8.2-oz serving	290	8	13.0
HARDEE'S				
BEVERAGE				
chocolate shake	12.3 fl oz	370	67	5.0
orange juice	10 fl oz	140	34	0.0
vanilla shake	12.3 fl oz	350	65	5.0
BISCUIT				
and gravy	1 serving	530	56	30.0
apple cinnamon n' raisin	1 serving	250	42	8.0
jelly	1 serving	440	57	21.0
chicken	1 sandwich	590	62	27.0
country ham	1 sandwich	440	44	22.0
egg and cheese	1 sandwich	520	45	30.0
ham	1 sandwich	410	45	20.0
'Made From Scratch'	1 serving	390	44	21.0
omelet	1 sandwich	550	45	32.0
plain or buttermilk	1 biscuit	353	47	16.0
sausage and egg	1 sandwich	620	45	41.0
sausage biscuit	1 sandwich	550	44	36.0
steak	1 sandwich	580	56	32.0
CHICKEN				
breast, w/o bone	1 serving	370	29	15.0
leg, w/o bone	1 serving	170	15	7.0
thigh, w/o bone	1 serving	330	30	15.0
wing, w/o bone	1 serving	200	23	8.0
DESSERT				
apple turnover	1 serving	270	38	12.0
cone, twist	1 serving	180	34	2.0
peach cobbler	1 serving	310	60	7.0
GRAVY	1 serving	20	3	0.0
HAMBURGER				
'All-Star'	1 burger	660	41	43.0
'Famous Star'	1 burger	570	41	35.0
'Frisco Burger'	1 burger	720	37	49.0
'Monster Burger'	1 burger	1060	37	79.0
regular	1 burger	270	29	11.0
'Super Star'	1 burger	790	41	53.0
HOT DOG, w/condiments	1 serving	450	25	32.0
SANDWICH				
bacon Swiss crispy chicken	1 sandwich	670	45	44.0
chicken fillet	1 sandwich	480	44	23.0
chicken, grilled	1 sandwich	350	28	16.0
'Fisherman's Fillet'	1 sandwich	530	45	28.0
'Frisco Ham'	1 sandwich	450	42	22.0
ham and cheese, hot	1 sandwich	300	34	12.0
roast beef, big	1 sandwich	410	26	24.0
roast beef, monster	1 sandwich	610	26	39.0

Food Name	Serv. Size	Total Cal.	Carbs GMS	Fat GMS
roast beef, regular	1 sandwich	310	26	16.0
SIDE DISH				
coleslaw	1 serving	240	13	20.0
crispy curl potatoess, large	1 serving	520	62	28.0
crispy curl potatoes, medium	1 serving	340	41	18.0
crispy curl potatoes, monster	1 serving	590	70	31.0
French fries, large	1 serving	440	59	21.0
French fries, monster	1 serving	510	67	24.0
French fries, regular	1 serving	340	45	16.0
hash rounds, regular	1 serving	230	24	14.0
mashed potato, small	1 serving	70	14	0.0

HARVEY'S FOODS
BREAKFAST

Food Name	Serv. Size	Total Cal.	Carbs GMS	Fat GMS
pancake	1 serving	89	17	1.0
sausage	1 serving	167	3	14.0
toast, plain	1 serving	250	48	3.0
CHEESEBURGER	1 serving	415	41	18.0
CHICKEN FINGERS	1 serving	240	18	12.0
DESSERT, apple turnover	1 serving	179	28	7.0
HAMBURGER				
double	1 burger	530	44	26.0
regular	1 burger	355	40	14.0
super	1 burger	477	38	19.0
HOT DOG	1 serving	332	32	15.0
MUFFIN				
blueberry	1 muffin	254	45	6.0
bran	1 muffin	301	42	13.0
SANDWICH				
chicken	1 sandwich	419	46	16.0
'Western'	1 sandwich	347	58	10.0
SIDE DISH				
French fries	1 serving	478	56	24.0
hash browns	1 serving	146	15	9.0
onion rings	1 serving	288	36	14.0

HUNGRY HUNTER

Food Name	Serv. Size	Total Cal.	Carbs GMS	Fat GMS
CHICKEN, breast, teriyaki, boneless, charbroiled	1 serving	413	9	8.0
CRAB				
Alaskan king, w/1 tbsp butter	1 serving	432	0	13.0
Alaskan king, w/o butter	1 serving	332	0	2.0
STEAK				
filet mignon	8 oz	539	0	27.0
filet mignon, choice	3.5 oz	238	0	11.9
LOBSTER				
cooked, w/o butter	1 serving	139	2	1.0
cooked, w/1 tbsp. butter	1 serving	241	2	12.0
SIDE DISH				
baked potato	1 serving	185	43	0.0
rice pilaf	1 serving	142	26	2.0
SNAPPER, RED, fresh, cooked in 1/2 oz. butter	1 serving	329	0	15.0

IN-N-OUT
BEVERAGE

Food Name	Serv. Size	Total Cal.	Carbs GMS	Fat GMS
chocolate shake	15 fl oz	690	83	36.0
'Coca-Cola Classic'	16 fl oz	198	54	0.0
coffee	10 fl oz	5	1	0.0
'Diet Coke'	16 fl oz	0	0	0.0
'Dr. Pepper'	16 fl oz	200	52	0.0

Food Name	Serv. Size	Total Cal.	Carbs GMS	Fat GMS
iced tea	16 fl oz	0	0	0.0
lemonade	16 fl oz	180	40	0.0
milk	10 fl oz	180	18	6.0
root beer	16 fl oz	222	60	0.0
'Seven-Up'	16 fl oz	220	52	0.0
strawberry shake	15 fl oz	690	91	33.0
vanilla shake	15 fl oz	680	78	37.0
CHEESEBURGER				
'Protein Style' w/lettuce leaves, w/o bun	1 serving	330	11	25.0
regular	1 serving	480	39	27.0
w/o spread, w/mustard and ketchup	1 serving	400	41	18.0
HAMBURGER				
'Double Double'	1 serving	670	40	41.0
'Double Double' protein style, w/lettuce leaves, w/o bun	1 serving	520	11	39.0
'Double Double' w/o spread, w/mustard and ketchup	1 serving	590	42	32.0
regular	1 serving	390	39	19.0
regular, protein style, w/lettuce leaves, w/o bun	1 serving	240	10	17.0
regular, w/o spread, w/mustard and ketchup	1 serving	310	41	10.0
SIDE DISH, French fries	1 serving	400	54	18.0

JACK IN THE BOX

Food Name	Serv. Size	Total Cal.	Carbs GMS	Fat GMS
BEVERAGE				
cappuccino ice cream shake, regular	16 fl oz	630	80	29.0
chocolate ice cream shake, regular	16 fl oz	630	85	27.0
'Coca Cola Classic' regular	20 fl oz	170	46	0.0
coffee, regular	12 fl oz	5	1	0.0
'Diet Coke' regular	20 fl oz	0	0	0.0
'Dr. Pepper' regular	20 fl oz	190	49	0.0
iced tea, regular	20 fl oz	0	0	0.0
lemonade, 'Minute Maid' regular	20 fl oz	190	65	0.0
milk, 2%	8 fl oz	130	14	5.0
orange juice	10 fl oz	150	34	0.0
Oreo cookie ice cream shake, regular	16 fl oz	740	91	36.0
root beer, 'Barq's' regular	20 fl oz	180	50	0.0
'Sprite' regular	20 fl oz	160	41	0.0
BREAKFAST				
'Breakfast Jack'	1 sandwich	280	28	12.0
French toast sticks, w/bacon	1 serving	470	53	23.0
pancake, w/bacon	1 serving	370	59	9.0
sausage croissant	1 sandwich	700	38	51.0
'Supreme Croissant'	1 sandwich	530	37	32.0
'Ultimate Breakfast Sandwich'	1 sandwich	600	39	34.0
CHEESE				
American	1 slice	45	1	4.0
Swiss style	1 slice	40	1	4.0
CHEESEBURGER				
'Bacon Ultimate'	1 burger	1020	37	71.0
double patty	1 burger	460	32	27.0
'Jumbo Jack'	1 burger	680	39	45.0
regular	1 burger	320	30	16.0
'Ultimate'	1 burger	950	37	66.0
CHICKEN, breast pieces	5 pieces	360	24	17.0
CHICKEN MEAL				
chicken teriyaki bowl	1 serving	670	128	4.0
4 chicken pieces, w/French fries	1 serving	730	79	34.0
CONDIMENTS. See also Salad Dressing.				
barbecue dipping sauce	1 serving	45	11	0.0
buttermilk dipping house sauce	1 serving	130	3	13.0
catsup	1 serving	10	2	0.0

Food Name	Serv. Size	Total Cal.	Carbs GMS	Fat GMS
croutons, salad bar item	1 serving	50	8	2.0
jelly, grape	1 serving	40	10	0.0
margarine-like spread, 'Country Crock'	1 serving	25	0	2.5
salsa	1 serving	10	2	0.0
sour cream	1 serving	60	1	6.0
soy sauce	1 serving	5	1	0.0
sweet and sour sauce	1 serving	45	11	0.0
syrup	1 serving	130	30	0.0
tartar sauce	1 serving	210	2	22.0
DESSERT				
apple turnover, hot	1 serving	340	41	18.0
carrot cake	1 serving	370	54	16.0
double fudge cake	1 serving	300	50	10.0
cheesecake	1 serving	320	32	18.0
strawberry ice cream, regular	16 fl oz	640	85	28.0
vanilla ice cream, regular	16 fl oz	610	73	31.0
FISH AND CHIPS	1 serving	780	86	39.0
HAMBURGER				
'Jumbo Jack'	1 burger	590	39	37.0
regular	1 burger	280	30	12.0
'Sourdough Jack'	1 burger	690	37	45.0
SALAD				
chicken garden	1 salad	200	8	9.0
side	1 salad	50	3	3.0
SALAD DRESSING				
blue cheese	1 serving	210	11	15.0
house, buttermilk	1 serving	290	6	30.0
Italian, low-calorie	1 serving	25	2	1.5
Thousand Island	1 serving	250	10	24.0
SANDWICH				
chicken	1 sandwich	420	39	23.0
chicken, 'Jack's Spicy'	1 sandwich	570	52	29.0
'Chicken Fajita Pita'	1 sandwich	280	25	9.0
chicken fillet, grilled	1 sandwich	480	39	24.0
'Chicken Supreme'	1 sandwich	830	67	48.0
'Philly Cheesesteak'	1 sandwich	580	56	16.0
'Sourdough Breakfast'	1 sandwich	450	36	24.0
SIDE DISH				
eggroll	3 egg rolls	440	40	24.0
French fries, curly, chili cheese	1 serving	650	60	41.0
French fries, curly, seasoned	1 serving	410	45	23.0
French fries, jumbo	1 serving	430	58	20.0
French fries, regular	1 serving	350	46	16.0
French fries, super scoop	1 serving	610	82	28.0
hash browns	1 serving	170	14	12.0
jalapeños, stuffed	7 jalapeños	530	46	31.0
onion rings	1 serving	410	45	23.0
potato, bacon cheddar wedges	1 serving	800	49	58.0
TACO				
monster	1 serving	270	19	17.0
regular	1 serving	170	12	10.0
KENTUCKY FRIED CHICKEN				
BISCUIT	1 biscuit	180	20	10.0
CHICKEN				
breast, extra crispy, w/o bone, 5.9 oz	1 breast	470	17	28.0
breast, hot and spicy, w/o bone, 6.5 oz	1 breast	505	23	29.0

Food Name	Serv. Size	Total Cal.	Carbs GMS	Fat GMS
breast, original recipe, w/o bone, 5.4 oz	1 breast	400	16	24.0
drumstick, extra crispy, w/o bone, 2.4 oz	1 drumstick	195	7	12.0
drumstick, hot and spicy, w/o bone, 2.3 oz	1 drumstick	175	9	10.0
drumstick, original recipe, w/o bone, 2.2 oz	1 drumstick	140	4	9.0
popcorn, large	6.0 oz	620	36	40.0
popcorn, small	3.5 oz	362	21	23.0
thigh, extra crispy, w/o bone, 4.2 oz	1 thigh	380	14	27.0
thigh, hot and spicy, w/o bone, 3.8 oz	1 thigh	355	13	26.0
thigh, original recipe, w/o bone, 3.2 oz	1 thigh	250	6	18.0
wing, honey barbecue	6 pieces	607	33	38.0
wing, hot	6 pieces	471	18	33.0
wing, whole, extra crispy, w/o bone, 1.9 oz	1 wing	220	10	15.0
wing, whole, hot and spicy, w/o bone, 1.9 oz	1 wing	210	9	15.0
wing, whole, original recipe, w/o bone, 1.6 oz	1 wing	140	5	10.0
CHICKEN POT PIE, chunky	13 oz	770	69	42.0
CHICKEN SANDWICH				
honey barbecue, w/sauce, 5.3 oz	1 sandwich	310	37	6.0
original recipe, w/o sauce, 6.6 oz	1 sandwich	360	3	13.0
original recipe, w/sauce, 7.3 oz	1 sandwich	450	33	22.0
'Tender Roast' w/o sauce, 6.2 oz	1 sandwich	270	26	5.0
'Tender Roast' w/sauce, 7.4 oz	1 sandwich	350	23	15.0
'Triple Crunch Zinger' w/o sauce, 6.2 oz	1 sandwich	390	39	15.0
'Triple Crunch Zinger' w/sauce, 7.4 oz	1 sandwich	550	36	32.0
'Triple Crunch' w/o sauce, 6.2 oz	1 sandwich	390	39	15.0
'Triple Crunch' w/o sauce, 6.6 oz	1 sandwich	490	29	29.0
CHICKEN STRIPS				
crispy	3 strips	300	18	16.0
crispy, spicy	3 strips	335	23	15.0
DESSERT				
apple pie, 4.0 oz	1 slice	310	44	14.0
double chocolate chip, 2.7 oz	1 serving	320	41	16.0
'Little Bucket Parfait' chocolate creme, 4.0 oz	1 serving	290	37	15.0
'Little Bucket Parfait' fudge brownie, 3.5 oz	1 serving	280	44	10.0
'Little Bucket Parfait' lemon creme, 4.5 oz	1 serving	410	62	14.0
'Little Bucket Parfait' strawberry shortcake, 3.5 oz	1 serving	200	33	7.0
pecan pie, 4.0 oz	1 slice	490	66	23.0
strawberry creme pie, 2.7 oz	1 slice	280	32	15.0
SIDE DISH				
barbecue baked beans	5.5 oz	190	33	3.0
coleslaw	5 oz	232	26	13.5
corn on the cob	5.7 oz	150	35	1.5
macaroni and cheese	5.4 oz	180	21	8.0
mashed potato, w/gravy	4.8 oz	120	17	6.0
potato salad	5.6 oz	230	23	14.0
potato wedges	4.8 oz	280	28	13.0

KRYSTAL

BREAKFAST

Food Name	Serv. Size	Total Cal.	Carbs GMS	Fat GMS
bacon biscuit	3.6 oz	355	36	20.0
egg biscuit	4.8 oz	372	36	21.0
gravy biscuit	8.2 oz	445	43	26.0
plain biscuit	3.2 oz	289	35	14.0
sausage biscuit	4.3 oz	429	37	27.0
'Sunriser'	3.6 oz	264	17	17.0
CHEESEBURGER				
regular	1 serving	189	16	10.0
w/bacon	6.4 oz	583	34	35.0

Food Name	Serv. Size	Total Cal.	Carbs GMS	Fat GMS
'Burger Plus'	7 oz	545	37	31.0
double patty	1 serving	214	22	8.0
CHILI				
large	12-oz serving	322	33	11.0
regular	8-oz serving	214	22	8.0
CORN DOG, 'Corn Pup'	2.3 oz	214	17	14.0
DESSERT				
apple pie	4.5 oz	320	45	14.0
lemon meringue pie	4 oz	340	60	9.0
pecan pie	4 oz	450	61	24.0
DOUGHNUT				
plain	1.3 oz	100	17	9.0
w/chocolate icing	1.8 oz	162	27	11.0
w/vanilla icing	1.8 oz	148	29	9.0
HAMBURGER				
'Big K'	7.3 oz	608	35	36.0
'Burger Plus'	6.4 oz	488	36	27.0
double patty	4 oz serving	276	24	14.0
small	2.2 oz serving	158	15	7.0
HOT DOG				
'Chili Cheese Pup'	2.6 oz	203	15	13.0
'Chili Pup'	2.5 oz	184	14	12.0
plain	1.9 oz	164	14	10.0
MILKSHAKE, chocolate	12.8 fl oz	271	41	10.0
SANDWICH				
chicken, 6.4 oz	1 sandwich	392	44	16.0
country ham, 4.5 oz	1 sandwich	379	36	19.0
SIDE DISH				
French fries, crisscut, 'Krys Kross'	2.6 oz	242	33	11.0
French fries, crisscut, 'Krys Kross' w/cheese	3.6 oz	292	35	15.0
French fries, regular, large	5 oz serving	615	111	17.0
French fries, regular, medium	3.9 oz serving	474	86	13.0
French fries, regular, small	2.8 oz serving	338	61	9.0
LITTLE CAESARS				
BREAD, 'Crazy Bread'	1 serving	98	18	1.0
CONDIMENTS, 'Crazy Sauce'	1 serving	63	11	1.0
PIZZA				
'Baby Pan! Pan!'	1 serving	525	53	22.0
cheese, single slice, 2.2 oz	1 slice	170	20	6.0
pepperoni combination, single slice	1 serving	190	20	7.0
'Pizza! Pizza!!' large	1 serving	169	18	6.0
'Pizza! Pizza!!' medium	1 serving	154	16	5.0
'Pizza! Pizza!!' small	1 serving	138	14	5.0
'Pizza! Pizza!!' square, large	1 serving	188	22	6.0
'Pizza! Pizza!!' square, medium	1 serving	185	22	6.0
PIZZA MEAL				
cheese pizza, hand-tossed, w/individual tossed salad	1 serving	600	73	21.0
vegetable pizza, w/individual tossed salad	1 serving	640	76	22.0
SALAD				
antipasto, w/low-calorie dressing	12 oz serving	170	12	9.0
Greek, w/low-calorie dressing	11 oz serving	140	8	8.0
tossed, small	1 serving	37	7	1.0
tossed, w/low-calorie dressing	11 oz serving	80	11	2.0
SANDWICH				
ham and cheese	1 sandwich	520	55	21.0
submarine, Italian	1 sandwich	590	55	28.0

Food Name	Serv. Size	Total Cal.	Carbs GMS	Fat GMS
tuna melt	1 sandwich	700	58	37.0
turkey	1 sandwich	450	49	17.0
vegetarian	1 sandwich	620	58	30.0

LONG JOHN SILVER'S
CHICKEN
batter-dipped, 2 oz	1 piece	120	11	6.0
'FlavorBaked'	2.6 oz	110	1	3.0
CLAMS, batter-dipped	3 oz	300	31	17.0

CONDIMENTS. See also Salad Dressing.

catsup	0.32 oz	10	2	0.0
honey mustard sauce	0.42 oz	20	5	0.0
malt vinegar	0.28 oz	0	0	0.0
margarine	0.18 oz	35	0	4.0
shrimp sauce	0.42 oz	15	3	0.0
sour cream	1 oz	60	1	6.0
sweet and sour sauce	0.42 oz	20	5	0.0
tartar sauce	0.42 oz	35	5	1.5

FISH
batter-dipped, 2.98 oz	1 piece	170	12	11.0
'Flavorbaked' 2.3 oz	1 piece	90	1	2.5

SALAD
garden	1 salad	45	9	0.0
grilled chicken	1 salad	140	10	2.5
ocean chef	1 salad	130	15	2.0
side	4.3 oz	25	4	0.0

SALAD DRESSING
Thousand Island	1 oz	110	5	10.0
French, fat-free	1.5 oz	50	14	0.0
Italian	1 oz	130	2	14.0
ranch	1 oz	170	1	18.0
ranch, nonfat	1.5 oz	50	13	0.0

SANDWICH
fish, batter-dipped, no sauce	5.4 oz	320	40	13.0
fish, 'Ultimate'	6.4 oz	430	44	21.0
chicken, 'Flavorbaked'	5.8 oz	290	27	10.0
fish, 'Flavorbaked'	6 oz	320	28	14.0
SHRIMP, batter-dipped, 0.4 oz	1 piece	35	2	2.5

SIDE DISH
baked potato	8 oz	210	49	0.0
cheese sticks	1.6 oz	160	12	9.0
coleslaw	3.4 oz	140	20	6.0
corn cobbette, w/butter	3.3 oz	140	19	8.0
corn cobbette w/o butter	3.05 oz	80	19	0.5
French fries	3 oz	250	28	15.0
green beans	3.5 oz	30	5	0.5
hushpuppy, 0.8 oz	1 piece	60	9	2.5
rice pilaf	3 oz	140	26	3.0

MAZZIO'S
CHICKEN PARMESAN, noodles chicken Parmesan	17.5 oz	590	68	19.0
FETTUCCINE ALFREDO, small	1 serving	440	34	28.0
GARLIC BREAD, w/cheese	2 slices	700	74	35.0
LASAGNA, meat, small	1 serving	460	26	25.0
NACHOS, meat	4.5 oz	500	21	37.0
PIZZA				
cheese, deep pan	1 serving	350	42	8.0

Food Name	Serv. Size	Total Cal.	Carbs GMS	Fat GMS
cheese, original, medium	2 slices	260	33	8.0
cheese, thick crust	1 serving	220	22	9.0
combination, deep pan, medium	1 slice	410	42	18.0
combination, original, medium	1 slice	320	34	13.0
'Light' medium	1 slice	240	30	8.0
pepperoni, deep pan, medium	1 slice	380	38	17.0
pepperoni, original, medium	1 slice	280	30	11.0
sausage, deep pan, medium	1 slice	430	41	21.0
sausage, original, medium	1 slice	350	34	16.0
SANDWICH				
barbecue beef and cheddar	1 sandwich	580	53	24.0
chicken and cheddar	1 sandwich	570	56	24.0
ham and cheese sandwich	1 sandwich	790	71	39.0
SPAGHETTI ENTRÉE, small	1 serving	290	39	10.0

MCDONALD'S
BEVERAGE

Food Name	Serv. Size	Total Cal.	Carbs GMS	Fat GMS
apple bran muffin, low-fat	1 serving	300	61	3.0
chocolate shake, small	1 small	360	60	9.0
'Coca Cola Classic' medium	21 fl oz	310	58	0.0
'Diet Coke' medium	21 fl oz	0	0	0.0
English muffin	1 serving	140	25	2.0
orange drink, 'Hi-C' medium	21 fl oz	240	64	0.0
milk, 1%	8 fl oz	100	13	2.5
orange juice	6 fl oz	80	20	0.0
'Sprite' medium	21 fl oz	210	56	0.0
strawberry shake, small	1 serving	360	60	9.0
vanilla shake, small	1 serving	360	59	9.0
BREAKFAST				
apple Danish	1 serving	340	47	15.0
biscuit, plain or buttermilk	1 serving	262	35	11.9
bacon, egg, and cheese biscuit	1 sandwich	540	36	34.0
cheese Danish	1 serving	400	45	21.0
cinnamon roll	1 serving	390	50	18.0
hash browns	1 serving	130	14	8.0
hotcakes, plain	1 serving	340	58	8.0
hotcakes, w/margarine and syrup	1 serving	600	104	17.0
sausage biscuit	1 sandwich	470	35	31.0
sausage and egg biscuit	1 sandwich	550	35	37.0
breakfast burrito	1 serving	320	21	20.0
'Egg McMuffin'	1 sandwich	290	27	12.0
ham, egg, and cheese bagel	1 sandwich	550	58	23.0
sausage	1 serving	170	0	16.0
'Sausage McMuffin'	1 sandwich	360	26	23.0
'Sausage w/Egg McMuffin'	1 sandwich	440	27	28.0
scrambled eggs	2 eggs	160	1	11.0
Spanish omelette bagel	1 sandwich	690	59	38.0
steak egg and cheese bagel	1 sandwich	660	57	31.0
CHEESEBURGER				
'Big Xtra!'	1 burger	810	52	55.0
'Quarter Pounder with Cheese'	1 burger	530	38	30.0
regular	1 burger	320	35	13.0
CHICKEN NUGGETS				
'Chicken McNuggets'	4 pieces	190	13	11.0
'Chicken McNuggets'	6 piece	290	20	17.0
'Chicken McNuggets'	9 piece	430	29	25.0

CONDIMENTS. See also Salad Dressing.

Food Name	Serv. Size	Total Cal.	Carbs GMS	Fat GMS
barbecue sauce	1 pkg	45	10	0.0
croutons, salad bar item	1 pkg	50	9	1.0
honey	1 pkg	45	12	0.0
honey mustard sauce	1 pkg	50	3	4.5
hot mustard sauce	1 pkg	60	7	3.5
mayonnaise, light	1 pkg	40	0	4.0
sweet and sour sauce	1 pkg	50	11	0.0
DESSERT				
apple pie, baked	1 serving	260	34	13.0
chocolate chip cookie	1 serving	170	22	10.0
ice cream cone, vanilla, reduced fat	1 serving	150	23	4.5
'McDonaldland'	1 pkg	180	32	5.0
'McFlurry' Butterfinger	1 serving	620	90	22.0
'McFlurry' M&M	1 serving	630	90	23.0
'McFlurry' Nestlé Crunch	1 serving	630	89	24.0
'McFlurry' Oreo	1 serving	570	82	20.0
nut topping, for sundae	1 serving	40	2	3.5
sundae, hot caramel	1 serving	360	61	10.0
sundae, hot fudge	1 serving	340	52	12.0
sundae, strawberry	1 serving	290	50	7.0
HAMBURGER				
'Big Mac'	1 burger	570	45	32.0
'Big Xtra!'	1 burger	710	51	46.0
'Quarter Pounder'	1 burger	430	37	21.0
regular	1 burger	270	35	8.0
SALAD				
shaker, chef	1 salad	150	5	8.0
shaker, garden	1 salad	100	4	6.0
shaker, grilled chicken Caesar	1 salad	100	3	2.5
SALAD DRESSING				
Caesar	1 pkg	150	5	13.0
herb vinaigrette, nonfat	1 pkg	30	7	0.0
honey mustard	1 pkg	150	13	11.0
ranch	1 pkg	170	2	18.0
red ranch, reduced calorie	1 pkg	130	18	6.0
Thousand Island	1 pkg	130	11	9.0
SANDWICH				
chicken, crispy	1 sandwich	550	54	27.0
'Chicken McGrill'	1 sandwich	450	46	18.0
'Chicken McGrill' w/o mayo	1 sandwich	340	45	7.0
'Fillet-O-Fish'	1 sandwich	470	45	26.0
SIDE DISH				
French fries, large	1 serving	540	68	26.0
French fries, medium	1 serving	450	57	22.0
French fries, small	1 serving	210	26	10.0
French fries, super size	1 serving	610	77	29.0

MRS. WINNER
BISCUIT

	Serv. Size	Total Cal.	Carbs GMS	Fat GMS
	1 serving	245	45	5.0
CHICKEN				
breast, fried, no skin	4 oz	280	14	15.0
fillet, baked	1 serving	120	0	2.0
leg, fried, no skin	1.7 oz	110	5	6.0
HAM, country	1 serving	60	0	1.0
ROLL, honey yeast	1 roll	200	35	4.0

Food Name	Serv. Size	Total Cal.	Carbs GMS	Fat GMS
SALAD				
chicken	1 salad	583	39	8.0
seafood	1 salad	553	41	9.0
tossed	1 salad	6	1	0.0
SANDWICH				
chicken, breaded	1 sandwich	203	12	10.0
chicken fillet	1 sandwich	379	45	7.0
chicken salad	1 sandwich	313	33	6.0
steak	1 sandwich	429	43	11.0
SAUSAGE, patty	1 serving	200	0	10.0
SIDE DISH				
coleslaw	1 serving	188	9	16.0
French fries	1 serving	225	27	9.0
mashed potato, w/gravy	1 serving	148	22	3.0
potato wedges, oven roasted	1 serving	139	31	1.0
STEAK ENTRÉE, country fried	1 serving	220	0	14.0
PERKINS				
BROCCOLI, raw	4 oz	31	6	0.4
CHICKEN ENTRÉE				
lemon pepper, w/rice pilaf, broccoli, salad	1 serving	620	60	12.5
FRUIT CUP, w/cantaloupe, honeydew, blueberries	4.5 oz serving	48	12	0.3
HASH BROWNS	3 oz	101	17	2.6
MUFFIN				
apple	1 muffin	543	76	24.0
banana nut	1 muffin	586	75	29.0
blueberry	1 muffin	506	71	23.0
bran	1 muffin	478	83	17.0
carrot	1 muffin	560	88	23.0
chocolate chocolate chip	1 muffin	546	73	26.0
corn	1 muffin	683	121	17.0
cranberry nut	1 muffin	558	71	28.0
oat bran	1 muffin	513	87	16.0
plain	1 muffin	586	81	26.0
plain, low-fat	1 muffin	495	111	1.2
OMELET				
'Country Club'	1 serving	932	6	79.1
'Country Club' w/3 oz hash browns	1 serving	1033	23	81.7
'Deli Ham and Lotsa Cheese'	1 serving	962	8	79.1
'Deli Ham and Lotsa Cheese' w/3 oz hash browns	1 serving	1063	25	81.7
'Denver' w/fruit cup	1 serving	235	22	6.5
'Everything'	1 serving	697	9	53.4
'Everything' w/3 oz hash browns	1 serving	798	25	56.0
'Granny's Country'	1 serving	941	7	81.5
'Granny's Country' w/9 oz hash browns	1 serving	1245	57	89.2
ham and cheese	1 serving	644	3	51.3
ham and cheese, w/3 oz hash browns	1 serving	745	19	53.9
mushroom and cheese	1 serving	687	5	59.9
mushroom and cheese, w/3 oz hash browns	1 serving	788	22	62.5
seafood, w/fruit cup	1 serving	271	28	5.7
ORANGE ROUGHY ENTRÉE				
w/rice pilaf, broccoli, salad	1 serving	467	60	7.0
PANCAKE				
buttermilk	3 pancakes	442	70	12.0
'Harvest Grain' w/1.5 oz low-cal syrup	5 pancakes	473	93	3.4
'Short Stack Harvest Grain'	3 pancakes	268	56	2.0
PIE				
apple	1 slice	521	72	26.0

Food Name	Serv. Size	Total Cal.	Carbs GMS	Fat GMS
apple, w/Equal sugar substitute	1 slice	420	55	24.0
cherry	1 slice	571	84	26.0
cherry, w/Equal sugar substitute	1 slice	425	55	24.0
coconut cream	1 slice	437	56	33.0
French silk	1 slice	551	59	37.0
lemon meringue	1 slice	395	63	16.0
peanut butter brownie	1 slice	455	44	35.0
pecan	1 slice	669	106	26.0
SALAD				
chef, mini	1 salad	214	7	11.0
dinner, 'Lite and Healthy'	1 salad	103	15	2.1
SYRUP, low-calorie	1.5 oz	26	7	0.0
TOAST, w/.5 oz margarine, grape jelly	0.75-oz slice	219	28	12.2
VEGETABLE STIR-FRY, w/mixed vegetables	6 oz	49	10	0.4
VEGETABLE SANDWICH				
stir-fry, on pita	1 sandwich	308	41	9.2
stir-fry, on pita, w/coleslaw	1 sandwich	441	54	17.8
stir-fry, on pita, w/coleslaw and pasta salad	1 sandwich	626	63	32.5
stir-fry, on pita, w/pasta salad	1 sandwich	493	50	23.9

PETER PIPER PIZZA
PIZZA
  Beef

Food Name	Serv. Size	Total Cal.	Carbs GMS	Fat GMS
extra large	1 slice	280	36	8.0
large	1 slice	296	39	8.0
express lunch	1 slice	165	21	5.0
medium	1 slice	222	29	6.0
small	1 slice	194	25	5.0
Cheese				
extra large	1 pizza	3078	437	73.0
extra large	1 slice	257	36	6.1
large	1 pizza	2159	311	49.4
large	1 slice	270	39	6.2
express lunch pizza	1 pizza	608	83	16.0
express lunch pizza	1 slice	152	21	4.0
medium	1 pizza	1622	235	37.0
medium	1 slice	203	29	5.0
small	1 pizza	1059	152	25.0
small	1 slice	177	25	4.0
w/black olive, large	1 slice	259	22	8.0
w/black olive, medium	1 slice	193	17	6.0
w/black olive, small	1 slice	171	15	6.0
w/green pepper, large	1 slice	245	22	7.0
w/green pepper, medium	1 slice	183	17	5.0
w/green pepper, small	1 slice	163	15	4.0
w/ham, large	1 slice	258	22	7.0
w/ham, medium	1 slice	194	16	6.0
w/ham, small	1 slice	172	15	5.0
w/jalapeño, large	1 slice	244	22	7.0
w/jalapeño, medium	1 slice	183	17	5.0
w/jalapeño, small	1 slice	163	15	4.0
w/mushroom, large	1 slice	245	22	7.0
w/mushroom, medium	1 slice	183	17	5.0
w/mushroom, small	1 slice	162	15	4.0
w/onion, large	1 slice	243	22	7.0
w/onion, medium	1 slice	183	17	5.0
w/onion, small	1 slice	162	15	4.0
w/pineapple, large	1 slice	246	23	7.0

Food Name	Serv. Size	Total Cal.	Carbs GMS	Fat GMS
w/pineapple, medium	1 slice	185	17	5.0
w/pineapple, small	1 slice	164	15	4.0
Salami				
express lunch	1 slice	164	21	5.0
extra large	1 slice	273	37	7.5
large	1 slice	288	39	8.0
medium	1 slice	216	29	6.0
small	1 slice	189	25	5.0

PIZZA HUT

Food Name	Serv. Size	Total Cal.	Carbs GMS	Fat GMS
BREADSTICK	1 serving	130	20	4.0
BREADSTICK DIPPING SAUCE	1 serving	30	5	0.5
CHICKEN				
Buffalo wings, hot	4 pieces	210	4	12.0
Buffalo wings, mild	5 pieces	200	1	12.0
GARLIC BREAD	1 slice	150	16	8.0
PASTA				
cavatini	1 serving	480	66	14.0
'Cavatini Supreme'	1 serving	560	73	19.0
spaghetti, w/marinara sauce	1 serving	490	91	6.0
spaghetti, w/meat sauce	1 serving	600	98	13.0
spaghetti, w/meatballs	1 serving	850	120	24.0
PIZZA				
Apple, dessert	1 slice	250	48	4.5
Beef				
hand-tossed, medium	1 slice	347	44	12.0
pan, medium	1 slice	399	45	18.0
Sicilian, medium	1 slice	282	31	12.0
stuffed crust, medium	1 slice	466	46	22.0
thin and crispy, medium	1 slice	305	28	15.0
Cheese				
'Big New Yorker'	1 slice	393	42	16.6
hand-tossed, medium	1 slice	309	43	9.0
pan, medium	1 slice	361	44	15.0
pan, personal	1 pizza	813	110	27.0
Sicilian, medium	1 slice	295	32	13.0
stuffed crust, medium	1 slice	445	46	19.0
thin and crispy, medium	1 slice	243	27	10.0
Cherry, dessert	1 slice	250	47	4.5
'Chicken Supreme'				
hand-tossed, medium	1 slice	291	44	6.0
pan, medium	1 slice	343	45	12.0
Sicilian, medium	1 slice	269	32	10.0
stuffed crust, medium	1 slice	432	47	17.0
'The New Edge' medium	1 slice	90	9	3.5
thin and crispy, medium	1 slice	232	29	7.0
Ham				
hand-tossed, medium	1 slice	279	43	6.0
pan, medium	1 slice	331	44	12.0
Sicilian, medium	1 slice	257	30	10.0
stuffed crust, medium	1 slice	404	45	22.0
thin and crispy, medium	1 slice	212	27	7.0
Italian sausage				
hand-tossed, medium	1 slice	363	44	14.0
pan, medium	1 slice	415	45	20.0
Sicilian, medium	1 slice	333	31	18.0
stuffed crust, medium	1 slice	478	46	23.0
thin and crispy, medium	1 slice	325	28	18.0

Food Name	Serv. Size	Total Cal.	Carbs GMS	Fat GMS
'Meat Lover's'				
thin and crispy, medium	1 slice	339	28	19.0
hand-tossed, medium	1 slice	376	44	15.0
pan, medium	1 slice	428	45	21.0
Sicilian, medium	1 slice	344	31	18.0
stuffed crust, medium	1 slice	543	46	29.0
'The New Edge' medium	1 slice	160	8	11.0
Pepperoni				
'Big New Yorker'	1 slice	380	42	16.0
hand-tossed, medium	1 slice	301	43	8.0
pan, medium	1 slice	353	44	14.0
pan, personal	1 pizza	810	111	28.0
Sicilian, medium	1 slice	227	31	113.0
stuffed crust, medium	1 slice	438	45	19.0
thin and crispy, medium	1 slice	235	27	10.0
'Pepperoni Lover's'				
hand-tossed, medium	1 slice	372	43	14.0
pan, medium	1 slice	370	44	16.0
Sicilian, medium	1 slice	321	31	16.0
stuffed crust, medium	1 slice	525	46	26.0
thin and crispy, medium	1 slice	289	28	14.0
Pork				
hand-tossed, medium	1 slice	342	44	12.0
pan, medium	1 slice	394	45	18.0
Sicilian, medium	1 slice	314	31	16.0
stuffed crust, medium	1 slice	461	46	21.0
thin and crispy, medium	1 slice	298	28	15.0
'Super Supreme'				
hand-tossed, medium	1 slice	359	45	12.0
pan, medium	1 slice	401	46	18.0
Sicilian, medium	1 slice	323	32	16.0
stuffed crust, medium	1 slice	505	46	25.0
thin and crispy, medium	1 slice	304	29	15.0
'Supreme'				
'Big New Yorker'	1 slice	459	44	22.3
hand-tossed, medium	1 slice	333	44	11.0
pan, medium	1 slice	385	45	17.0
pan, personal	1 pizza	808	111	27.0
Sicilian, medium	1 slice	307	32	15.0
stuffed crust, medium	1 slice	487	47	23.0
thin and crispy, medium	1 slice	284	29	13.0
Taco				
beef, hand-tossed, medium	1 slice	270	35	8.0
beef, pan, medium	1 slice	300	36	12.0
beef, thin and crispy, medium	1 slice	260	29	10.0
chicken, hand-tossed, medium	1 slice	290	35	11.0
chicken, pan, medium	1 slice	320	36	15.0
chicken, thin and crispy, medium	1 slice	260	26	12.0
hand-tossed, medium	1 slice	280	34	11.0
meatless, hand-tossed, medium	1 slice	250	35	8.0
meatless, pan, medium	1 slice	290	36	12.0
meatless, thin and crispy, medium	1 slice	230	27	8.0
pan, medium	1 slice	310	36	13.0
pan, personal	1 pizza	780	90	35.0
thin and crispy, medium	1 slice	260	27	11.0
'The Works' 'The New Edge' medium	1 slice	110	9	6.0
'Veggie Lover's'				
hand-tossed, medium	1 slice	281	45	6.0

Food Name	Serv. Size	Total Cal.	Carbs GMS	Fat GMS
pan, medium	1 slice	333	46	12.0
Sicilian, medium	1 slice	252	32	10.0
stuffed crust, medium	1 slice	421	48	17.0
'The New Edge' medium	1 slice	70	9	3.0
thin and crispy, medium	1 slice	222	30	8.0
SANDWICH				
ham and cheese	1 sandwich	550	57	21.0
'Supreme'	1 sandwich	640	62	28.0
PONDEROSA				
CHICKEN ENTRÉE				
breast	5.5 oz	98	1	2.1
wing	2 pieces	213	11	9.0
CONDIMENTS. See also Salad Bar Items; Salad Dressing.				
cheese sauce	2 oz	52	6	2.0
cheese topping, herb and garlic	1 tbsp	100	0	10.0
gravy, brown	2 oz	25	4	1.0
gravy, turkey	2 oz	25	5	0.2
margarine, liquid	1 tbsp	100	0	11.0
margarine, whipped	1 tbsp	34	0	1.2
tartar sauce	1 oz	85	11	10.9
DESSERT				
dougnut, winter mix	3.5 oz	25	4	0.0
gelatin dessert, plain, nonfat	4 oz	71	17	0.0
ice milk, chocolate	3.5 oz	152	30	3.0
ice milk, vanilla	3.5 oz	150	30	3.0
mousse, chocolate	4 oz	312	28	18.0
mousse, chocolate	1 oz	78	7	4.4
mousse, strawberry	4 oz	297	25	18.0
mousse, strawberry	1 oz	74	6	4.6
pudding, banana	4 oz	207	27	10.0
vanilla wafer cookie, peanut butter	2 wafers	35	6	1.0
DESSERT TOPPING				
caramel	1 oz	100	26	0.7
chocolate	1 oz	89	24	0.3
peanut, granulated	.2 oz	30	1	2.3
strawberry	1 oz	71	24	0.2
strawberry glaze	1 oz	37	10	0.0
whipped	1 oz	80	5	7.0
FISH. See also individual listings.				
nuggets	1 piece	31	2	1.7
baked, 'Bake 'R Broil' baked	5.2 oz	230	10	13.0
fried	3.2 oz	190	17	9.0
HALIBUT, broiled	6 oz	170	0	2.4
HOT DOG	1.6 oz	144	1	13.0
MEATBALLS	2 pieces	115	2	4.0
ORANGE ROUGHY, broiled	5 oz	139	21	5.0
ROLL				
dinner	1 piece	184	33	3.0
sourdough	1 piece	110	22	1.0
SALAD BAR ITEMS				
banana chips	.2 oz	25	3	1.3
banana	1 medium	87	23	0.2
breadstick, Italian	1 stick	100	19	1.0
breadstick, sesame	2 sticks	35	6	0.0
broccoli, raw	1 oz	9	2	0.9
cabbage, green	1 oz	9	2	0.0
cheese, imitation, shredded	1 oz	90	1	7.0

Food Name	Serv. Size	Total Cal.	Carbs GMS	Fat GMS
chicken macaroni salad	3.5 oz	335	49	12.0
chicken salad	3.5 oz	212	8	15.0
chow mein noodles	.2 oz	25	3	1.2
coconut, shredded	.2 oz	25	2	1.9
croutons	1 oz	115	18	4.0
fruit cocktail	4 oz	97	25	0.2
granola	.2 oz	24	3	1.0
grapes	10 grapes	34	9	0.2
ham, diced	2 oz	120	1	10.0
lemon	1 wedge	3	1	0.1
macaroni salad	3.5 oz	335	49	11.7
onion, green	1 piece	7	2	0.1
onion, yellow	1 oz	11	3	0.0
orange	1 piece	45	11	0.1
pasta salad	3.5 oz	268	34	12.0
pickle chips, sweet	.14 oz	4	1	0.0
pickle spear, dill	.14 oz	1	0	0.0
potato salad	3.5 oz	126	16	6.0
turkey ham salad	3.5 oz	186	10	13.0
turkey, julienne	1 oz	29	1	1.0
yogurt, frozen, fruit flavor	4 oz	115	23	1.0
yogurt, frozen, vanilla	4 oz	110	18	2.0
SALAD DRESSING				
blue cheese	1 oz	130	1	14.0
coleslaw	1 oz	150	6	14.0
creamy Italian	1 oz	103	3	10.0
cucumber, lower calorie	1 oz	69	3	6.0
Italian, lower calorie	1 oz	31	1	3.0
oil	1 tbsp	120	0	14.0
Parmesan pepper	1 oz	150	2	15.0
ranch	1 oz	147	1	15.0
sweet-n-tangy	1 oz	122	8	10.0
Thousand Island	1 oz	113	8	10.0
SALMON, broiled	6 oz	192	3	3.0
SCROD, baked	7 oz	120	0	1.0
SHRIMP				
fried	7 pieces	230	31	1.0
mini	6 pieces	47	6	1.0
SIDE DISH				
baked beans	4 oz	170	21	6.0
baked potato	7.2 oz	145	33	0.0
corn	3.5 oz	90	21	0.4
French fries	3 oz	120	17	4.0
green beans	3.5 oz	20	3	0.0
macaroni and cheese	1 oz	17	4	0.5
macaroni salad	3.5 oz	335	49	11.7
mashed potato	4 oz	62	13	0.0
okra, breaded	4 oz	124	23	1.0
onion rings, breaded	4 oz	213	30	9.0
pasta/noodles	2 oz	78	16	0.3
potato wedges	3.5 oz	130	16	6.0
rice pilaf	4 oz	160	26	4.0
spinach	1 oz	7	1	0.1
stuffing	4 oz	230	27	11.0
SPAGHETTI, w/sauce	6 oz	188	33	5.0
STEAK				
chopped	4 oz	225	1	16.0
kabobs, meat only	3 oz	153	2	5.0

Food Name	Serv. Size	Total Cal.	Carbs GMS	Fat GMS
Kansas City strip	5 oz	138	1	5.7
New York strip, choice	8 oz	314	1	10.5
Porterhouse, choice	16 oz	640	3	30.9
Porterhouse, non-graded	13 oz	440	1	30.0
ribeye, choice	6 oz	282	1	14.0
ribeye, non-graded	5 oz	219	1	13.0
sirloin, choice	7 oz	241	1	11.0
sirloin tips, choice	5 oz	197	1	8.0
T-bone, choice	10 oz	444	2	18.0
T-bone, non-graded	8 oz	178	2	8.5
teriyaki	5 oz	174	5	3.0
STEAK SANDWICH	4 oz	208	2	11.0
SWORDFISH, broiled	5.9 oz	271	0	10.0
TROUT	5 oz	228	1	4.0

POPEYES

Food Name	Serv. Size	Total Cal.	Carbs GMS	Fat GMS
BISCUIT, plain or buttermilk	1 biscuit	233	31	10.6
CHICKEN				
breast, mild, w/o bone	3.7 oz	270	9	15.9
breast, spicy, w/o bone	3.7 oz	270	9	15.9
leg, mild, w/o bone	1.7 oz	120	4	7.3
leg, spicy, w/o bone	1.7 oz	120	4	7.3
nuggets, fried	4.2 oz	410	18	31.9
thigh, mild, w/o bone	3.1 oz	300	9	22.7
thigh, spicy, w/o bone	3.1 oz	300	9	22.7
wing, mild, w/o bone	1.6 oz	160	7	10.7
wing, spicy, w/o bone	1.6 oz	160	7	10.7
DESSERT				
apple pie	3.1 oz	290	37	15.8
SHRIMP	2.8 oz	250	13	16.4
SIDE DISH				
Cajun rice	3.9 oz	150	17	5.4
coleslaw	4 oz	149	14	11.2
corn on the cob	5.2 oz	90	21	2.9
French fries	3 oz	240	31	12.2
mashed potato, w/gravy	3.8 oz	100	11	6.0
onion rings	3.1 oz	310	31	19.3
red beans and rice	5.9 oz	270	30	16.9

QUINCY'S

Food Name	Serv. Size	Total Cal.	Carbs GMS	Fat GMS
CATFISH, fillet, 2 pieces	6.9-oz serving	309	19	12.0
CHEESEBURGER, 1/4 lb precooked	1 serving	451	32	23.0
CHICKEN				
breast, grilled	5-oz serving	145	0	0.4
strips, 4 pieces	4.5 oz	318	4	15.0
CHILI, w/beans	9.2-oz serving	346	32	16.0
CORNBREAD	1.9-oz serving	178	28	6.0
HAMBURGER, 1/4 lb precooked	1 serving	403	32	19.0
MUSHROOM SAUCE	3-oz serving	27	5	1.0
SHRIMP, 7 pieces	3.9-oz serving	248	11	12.0
SIDE DISH				
baked potato, w/o butter	8.8-oz serving	181	41	1.0
coleslaw	2.1-oz serving	60	4	5.0
green beans	4.3-oz serving	40	7	1.0
peppers and onions	4-oz serving	80	8	5.0
steak fries	5.5-oz serving	426	56	21.0
SOUP				
broccoli, cream of	9.2-oz serving	193	13	14.0

Food Name	Serv. Size	Total Cal.	Carbs GMS	Fat GMS
clam chowder	9.2-oz serving	198	15	14.0
vegetable beef soup	8.6-oz serving	78	10	2.0
STEAK				
chopped, luncheon	4-oz serving	350	0	25.0
country style, w/mushroom sauce	6-oz serving	288	17	19.0
fillet	5.6-oz serving	331	0	12.0
ribeye	7.3-oz serving	665	0	60.0
sirloin club	4.8-oz serving	283	0	10.0
sirloin tips	4-oz serving	236	0	9.0
sirloin	5.9-oz serving	649	0	54.0
sirloin, large	7.7-oz serving	852	0	70.0
sirloin, petite	4-oz serving	446	0	37.0
T-bone	7.8-oz serving	1045	0	95.0

RALLY'S
CHEESEBURGER

Food Name	Serv. Size	Total Cal.	Carbs GMS	Fat GMS
'Rallyburger w/Cheese'	1 burger	486	33	29.4
'Bacon Cheeseburger'	1 burger	622	35	40.3
'Double Cheeseburger'	1 burger	733	34	49.1
CHEESEBURGER MEAL				
'Large Combo' w/soft drink	1 meal	1018	129	45.0
'Small Combo' w/soft drink	1 meal	764	85	37.2
CHICKEN SANDWICH	1 sandwich	531	40	30.8
CHILI	8 oz	340	21	19.0
FRENCH FRIES				
large	1 serving	317	39	15.6
regular	1 serving	158	20	7.8
HAMBURGER 'Rallyburger'	1 burger	436	33	24.9
HAMBURGER MEAL				
'Large Combo' w/soft drink	1 meal	968	129	40.5
'Small Combo' w/soft drink	1 meal	714	84	32.7
SAUSAGE				
'Smokin' Sausage'	1 serving	724	31	55.0
'Smokin' Sausage' w/chili	1 serving	830	35	62.0
TACO, soft	1 taco	223	17	9.9

RAX

Food Name	Serv. Size	Total Cal.	Carbs GMS	Fat GMS
BEEF, roast beef	2.8 oz	140	1	9.0
BREADSTICK, sesame, salad bar item	1 oz	150	13	10.0
CHEESE, American, processed, slices	0.5 oz	60	1	5.0
CONDIMENTS. See also SALAD DRESSING.				
Alfredo sauce, pasta bar item	3.5 oz	80	12	3.0
banana pepper, Mexican bar item	1 tbsp	2	1	1.0
barbecue meat topping	3.25 oz	140	13	4.0
celery, salad bar item	1 tbsp	1	1	1.0
cheese sauce, regular, Mexican bar item	3.5 oz	420	58	17.0
chili topping	3 oz	80	8	2.0
chow mein noodles, salad bar item	1 oz	140	17	6.0
coconut, salad bar item	1 oz	160	15	11.0
croutons, salad bar item	0.5 oz	40	8	1.0
green onion, Mexican bar item	1/4 cup	10	2	1.0
margarine, liquid	1 tbsp	100	1	11.0
mushroom sauce	1 oz	16	1	1.0
nacho cheese sauce, Mexican bar item	3.5 oz	470	57	22.0
onion, diced	0.5 oz	10	1	1.0
pickle	1 spear	8	2	1.0
sour topping	3.5 oz	130	5	11.0
spaghetti sauce, pasta bar item	3.5 oz	80	19	1.0

Food Name	Serv. Size	Total Cal.	Carbs GMS	Fat GMS
spaghetti sauce, w/meat, pasta bar item	3.5 oz	150	12	8.0
spicy meat sauce, Mexican bar item	3.5 oz	80	6	4.0
sunflower seeds and raisins, salad bar item	1 oz	130	6	10.0
taco sauce, Mexican bar item	3.5 oz	30	6	1.0
taco shell, Mexican bar item	1 shell	40	6	2.0
turkey bits, salad bar item	2 oz	70	1	3.0
DESSERT				
butterscotch pudding, salad bar item	3.5 oz	141	20	6.0
chocolate chip cookie	1 cookie	130	17	6.0
chocolate pudding, salad bar item	3.5 oz	141	20	6.0
lime gelatin, salad bar item	1/2 cup	90	20	1.0
strawberry gelatin, salad bar item	1/2 cup	90	20	1.0
vanilla pudding, salad bar item	3.5 oz	141	20	6.0
DESSERT TOPPING, whipped	1 dollop	50	4	4.0
PASTA				
rainbow rotini, pasta bar item	3.5 oz	180	30	4.0
shells, pasta bar item	3.5 oz	170	27	4.0
spaghetti, pasta bar item	3.5 oz	140	23	4.0
vegetable, pasta bar item	3.5 oz	100	12	4.0
SALAD				
chef, w/o dressing	12.5-oz serving	230	4	14.0
garden, gourmet, 'Lighterside'	1 serving	134	13	6.0
garden, w/o dressing	10.5-oz serving	160	4	11.0
SALAD DRESSING				
blue cheese	1 tbsp	50	1	5.0
blue cheese, 'Lite'	1 tbsp	35	2	3.0
French	1 tbsp	60	6	4.0
Italian	1 tbsp	50	3	4.0
Italian, 'Lite'	1 tbsp	30	1	3.0
oil	1 tbsp	130	1	14.0
poppyseed	1 tbsp	60	5	4.0
ranch	1 tbsp	45	1	5.0
Thousand Island	1 tbsp	70	6	6.0
Thousand Island, 'Lite'	1 tbsp	40	3	3.0
vinegar	1 tbsp	2	1	1.0
SANDWICH				
barbecue	5.7-oz serving	420	53	14.0
beef, bacon, and chicken, 'BBC'	8-oz serving	720	40	49.0
fish	7-oz serving	460	58	17.0
ham and Swiss	7.9-oz serving	430	42	23.0
Philly beef and cheese	8.25-oz serving	480	44	22.0
roast beef, large	8-oz serving	570	41	35.0
roast beef, regular	5.25-oz serving	320	33	11.0
roast beef, 'Uncle Al' small	3.1-oz serving	260	21	14.0
turkey bacon club	9-oz serving	670	41	43.0
SIDE DISH				
baked potato, barbecue, w/2 oz cheese	1 serving	730	104	24.0
baked potato, cheese and bacon	3-oz serving	780	110	28.0
baked potato, cheese and broccoli	3-oz serving	760	112	26.0
baked potato, chili, w/2 oz cheese	1 serving	700	101	23.0
baked potato, plain	8.8-oz serving	270	60	1.0
baked potato, w/margarine	9.3-oz serving	370	60	11.0
baked potato, w/sour cream topping	1 serving	400	65	11.0
broccoli, salad bar item	1/2 cup	16	2	1.0
coleslaw, salad bar item	3.5 oz	70	8	4.0
French fries, large, salted	4.5-oz serving	390	50	20.0
French fries, large, unsalted	4.5-oz serving	390	50	20.0
French fries, regular, salted	3-oz serving	260	33	13.0

Food Name	Serv. Size	Total Cal.	Carbs GMS	Fat GMS
French fries, regular, unsalted	3-oz serving	260	33	13.0
grapefruit sections, salad bar item	1 cup	80	18	1.0
grapes, salad bar item	1 cup	100	25	1.0
kale, salad bar item	1 oz	16	2	1.0
kidney beans, salad bar item	1 cup	220	40	1.0
macaroni salad, salad bar item	3.5 oz	160	21	7.0
pasta salad, salad bar item	3.5 oz	80	16	1.0
potato salad, salad bar item	1 cup	260	41	7.0
refried beans, Mexican bar item	3 oz	120	16	4.0
Spanish rice, Mexican bar item	3.5 oz	90	20	1.0
three-bean salad	1/2 cup	100	23	1.0
SOUP				
broccoli, cream of	3.5 oz	50	6	2.0
chicken soup w/noodles, pasta bar item	3.5 oz	40	8	1.0

RED LOBSTER

Food Name	Serv. Size	Total Cal.	Carbs GMS	Fat GMS
CALAMARI				
breaded, fried, dinner portion	10 oz	720	60	42.0
breaded, fried, lunch portion	5 oz	360	30	21.0
CATFISH				
dinner portion	10 oz	340	0	20.0
lunch portion	5 oz	170	0	10.0
CHICKEN, breast	4 oz serving	120	0	3.0
CLAMS				
cherrystone, dinner portion	10 oz	260	22	4.0
cherrystone, lunch portion	5 oz	130	11	2.0
COD				
Atlantic, fillet, dinner portion	10 oz	200	0	2.0
Atlantic, fillet, lunch portion	5 oz	100	0	1.0
CRAB				
king, legs, 1 lb.	1 serving	170	6	2.0
snow, legs, 1 lb.	1 serving	150	1	2.0
FLOUNDER				
dinner portion	10 oz	200	2	2.0
lunch portion	5 oz	100	1	1.0
GROUPER				
dinner portion	10 oz	220	0	2.0
lunch portion	5 oz	110	0	1.0
HADDOCK				
dinner portion	10 oz	220	4	2.0
lunch portion	5 oz	110	2	1.0
HALIBUT				
dinner portion	10 oz	220	2	2.0
lunch portion	5 oz	110	1	1.0
HAMBURGER, 1/3 lb before cooked	1 serving	320	0	23.0
LANGOSTINO				
dinner portion	10 oz	240	4	2.0
lunch portion	5 oz	120	2	1.0
LOBSTER				
Maine, cooked, 1 1/4 lb	1 serving	240	5	8.0
rock, tail, cooked	1 serving	230	2	3.0
MACKEREL				
dinner portion	10 oz	380	40	24.0
raw weight	5 oz	190	20	12.0
MONKFISH				
dinner portion	10 oz	220	48	2.0
lunch portion	5 oz	110	24	1.0
MUSSELS	3-oz serving	70	3	2.0

Food Name	Serv. Size	Total Cal.	Carbs GMS	Fat GMS
OCEAN PERCH				
Atlantic, dinner portion	10 oz	260	2	8.0
Atlantic, lunch portion	5 oz	130	1	4.0
OYSTERS, on half shell	6 oysters	110	11	4.0
POLLACK				
dinner portion	10 oz	240	2	2.0
lunch portion	5 oz	120	1	1.0
RED ROCKFISH				
dinner portion	10 oz	180	0	2.0
lunch portion	5 oz	90	0	1.0
RED SNAPPER				
dinner portion	10 oz	220	0	2.0
lunch portion	5 oz	110	0	1.0
SALMON				
Norwegian, dinner portion	10 oz	460	6	24.0
Norwegian, lunch portion	5 oz	230	3	12.0
sockeye, dinner portion	10 oz	320	6	8.0
sockeye, lunch portion	5 oz	160	3	4.0
SCALLOPS				
calico, dinner portion	10 oz	360	16	4.0
calico, lunch portion	5 oz	180	8	2.0
deep sea, dinner portion	10 oz	260	4	4.0
deep sea, lunch portion	5 oz	130	2	2.0
SHARK				
blacktip, dinner portion	10 oz	300	0	2.0
blacktip, lunch portion	5 oz	150	0	1.0
mako, dinner portion	10 oz	280	0	2.0
mako, lunch portion	5 oz	140	0	1.0
SHRIMP, 8–12 pieces	1 serving	120	0	2.0
SOLE				
w/lemon, dinner portion	10 oz	240	2	2.0
w/lemon, lunch portion	5 oz	120	1	1.0
STEAK, strip	7 oz	690	0	64.0
SWORDFISH				
dinner portion	10 oz	200	0	8.0
lunch portion	5 oz	100	0	4.0
TILEFISH				
dinner portion	10 oz	200	0	4.0
lunch portion	5 oz	100	0	2.0
TROUT				
rainbow, dinner portion	10 oz	340	0	18.0
rainbow, lunch portion	5 oz	170	0	9.0
TUNA				
yellowfin, dinner portion	10 oz	360	0	12.0
yellowfin, lunch portion	5 oz	180	0	6.0
ROUND TABLE				
PIZZA				
'Alfredo Contempo'				
pan crust	1 slice	220	27	7.4
thin crust	1 slice	170	17	6.5
'Bacon Super Deli'				
pan crust	1 slice	260	26	13.5
thin crust	1 slice	200	16	12.6
Cheese				
pan	1 slice	210	26	7.2
thin crust	1 slice	170	17	5.6

Food Name	Serv. Size	Total Cal.	Carbs GMS	Fat GMS
Chicken and garlic				
pan, gourmet	1 slice	230	27	8.1
thin crust, gourmet	1 slice	170	17	7.2
'Classic Pesto'				
pan	1 slice	230	27	8.8
thin crust	1 slice	170	18	7.9
'Garden Delight'				
pan crust	1 slice	200	27	6.2
thin crust	1 slice	150	18	5.6
'Garden Pesto'				
pan crust	1 slice	230	28	8.6
thin crust	1 slice	170	18	7.7
'Gourmet Veggie'				
pan crust	1 slice	220	28	7.4
thin crust	1 slice	160	18	6.5
Italian Garlic Supreme'				
pan crust	1 slice	250	27	10.5
thin crust	1 slice	200	17	10.4
'King Arthur's Supreme'				
pan crust	1 slice	240	27	9.8
thin crust	1 slice	200	18	10.1
Pepperoni				
pan crust	1 slice	220	26	8.1
thin crust	1 slice	170	17	8.0
'Salute Chicken Cashew'				
pan crust	1 slice	200	31	4.5
thin crust	1 slice	150	21	4.1
'Salute Chicken and Garlic'				
pan crust	1 slice	200	28	5.8
thin crust	1 slice	150	18	5.4
'Salute Veggie'				
pan crust	1 slice	190	28	5.1
thin crust	1 slice	140	19	4.7
'Santa Fe Chicken'				
pan crust	1 slice	240	27	9.2
thin crust	1 slice	180	17	7.8

ROY ROGERS

Food Name	Serv. Size	Total Cal.	Carbs GMS	Fat GMS
BISCUIT	1 serving	231	26	12.0
BREAKFAST				
crescent, regular	1 serving	408	28	27.0
crescent, w/bacon	1 serving	446	28	30.0
crescent, w/ham	1 serving	456	29	29.0
crescent, w/sausage	1 serving	564	28	42.0
apple swirl Danish	1 serving	328	62	7.0
cheese swirl Danish	1 serving	383	54	15.0
cinnamon rod pastry,	1 serving	376	55	15.0
egg platter, w/bacon and biscuit	1 serving	607	44	39.0
egg platter, w/biscuit, regular	1 serving	557	44	34.0
egg platter, w/ham and biscuit,	1 serving	605	44	36.0
egg platter, w/sausage and biscuit	1 serving	713	44	49.0
pancake platter, regular, w/syrup and butter, regular	1 serving	386	63	13.0
pancake platter, w/bacon, w/syrup and butter	1 serving	436	63	17.0
pancake platter, w/ham, w/syrup and butter	1 serving	434	64	15.0
pancake platter, w/sausage, w/syrup and butter	1 serving	542	63	28.0
CHEESEBURGER				
'Express'	1 serving	613	42	37.0
'Express' w/bacon	1 serving	641	36	41.0

Food Name	Serv. Size	Total Cal.	Carbs GMS	Fat GMS
regular	1 serving	525	37	29.0
regular, w/bacon	1 sandwich	520	32	33.0
small	1 serving	275	24	13.0
CHICKEN				
breast, fried	1 serving	412	17	24.0
breast and wing, fried	1 serving	604	25	37.0
breast and wing, w/o skin, 'Roy's Roaster'	1 serving	190	2	6.0
dark meat, 1/4 'Roy's Roaster'	1 serving	490	2	34.0
dark meat, w/o skin, 1/4 'Roy's Roaster'	1 serving	190	1	10.0
leg, fried	1 serving	140	6	8.0
leg and thigh, fried	1 serving	436	17	28.0
nuggets, fried, 9 pieces	9 pieces	435	30	27.0
nuggets, fried, 6 pieces	6 pieces	290	20	18.0
thigh, fried	1 serving	296	12	20.0
white meat, 1/4 'Roy's Roaster'	1 serving	500	3	29.0
white meat, w/o skin, '1/4 'Roy's Roaster'	1 serving	190	2	6.0
wing, fried	1 serving	192	9	13.0
CONDIMENTS. See also Salad Dressing.				
Chinese noodles, salad bar item	1/4 cup	55	7	3.0
croutons, salad bar item	2 tbsp	14	3	0.0
granola, salad bar item	1/4 cup	65	9	3.0
grapes, salad bar item	5 grapes	20	5	0.0
onion, chopped, salad bar item	2 tbsp	7	2	0.0
DESSERT				
caramel sundae	1 serving	293	52	9.0
chocolate sundae	1 serving	358	61	10.0
gelatin parfait, salad bar item	1/4 cup	50	10	2.0
hot fudge sundae	1 serving	337	53	13.0
strawberry shortcake	1 serving	440	39	19.0
strawberry sundae	1 serving	216	33	7.0
vanilla sundae	1 serving	306	45	11.0
HAMBURGER				
'Express'	1 serving	561	42	32.0
regular	1 serving	472	37	25.0
'Roy Rogers Bar'	1 serving	573	38	31.0
small	1 serving	222	23	9.0
ROLL, crescent	1 serving	287	27	18.0
SALAD, grilled chicken	1 salad	120	2	4.0
SALAD DRESSING				
bacon and tomato	2 tbsp	136	6	12.0
blue cheese	2 tbsp	150	2	16.0
Italian, low-calorie	2 tbsp	70	2	6.0
ranch	2 tbsp	155	4	14.0
Thousand Island	2 tbsp	160	4	16.0
SANDWICH				
chicken, 'Gold Rush'	1 sandwich	558	51	30.0
fish	1 sandwich	514	58	24.0
roast beef	1 sandwich	329	29	10.0
roast beef, large	1 sandwich	373	31	12.0
roast beef, w/cheese	1 sandwich	403	37	15.0
roast beef, w/cheese, large	1 sandwich	427	31	17.0
SIDE DISH				
baked potato, plain, 'Hot Topped'	1 serving	211	48	0.0
broccoli, salad bar item	1/4 cup	6	1	0.0
coleslaw	1 serving	110	11	7.0
French fries, large	5.5-oz serving	440	54	22.0
French fries, regular	4-oz serving	320	39	16.0

Food Name	Serv. Size	Total Cal.	Carbs GMS	Fat GMS
French fries, small	3-oz serving	238	29	12.0
fruit cocktail, salad bar item	1/4 cup	46	12	0.0
Greek noodles, salad bar item	1/4 cup	159	19	9.0
lettuce, Romaine, salad bar item	1 cup	9	1	0.0
macaroni salad, salad bar item	1/4 cup	93	10	5.0
potato salad, salad bar item	1/4 cup	54	5	3.0

SCHLOTZSKY'S DELI
BEVERAGE

Food Name	Serv. Size	Total Cal.	Carbs GMS	Fat GMS
'Coca-Cola' regular	20 fl oz	248	68	0.0
'Diet Coke' regular	20 fl oz	0	0	0.0
iced tea, regular	20 fl oz	na	na	na
lemonade, 'All Natural' regular	20 fl oz	183	43	0.0
'Mr. Pibb' regular	20 fl oz	243	65	0.0
orange, 'Minute Maid' regular	20 fl oz	265	73	0.0
root beer, 'Barq's' regular	20 fl oz	278	75	0.0
'Sprite' regular	20 fl oz	243	65	na
CHILI, 'Timberline'	8 oz cup	210	24	7.0

CONDIMENTS. See also Salad Dressing.

Food Name	Serv. Size	Total Cal.	Carbs GMS	Fat GMS
croutons, garic cheese, salad bar item	1 crouton	46	5	2.0
chow mein noodles	1 serving	74	9	4.0

DESSERT

Food Name	Serv. Size	Total Cal.	Carbs GMS	Fat GMS
fudge brownie cake	1 serving	410	46	25.0
cookies and creme cheesecake	1 serving	330	36	18.0
New York style cheesecake	1 serving	310	31	18.0
strawberry swirl cheesecake	1 serving	300	30	17.0
chocolate chip cookie	1 cookie	160	23	7.0
chocolate chunk cookie	1 cookie	160	23	7.0
chocolate pecan chunk cookie	1 cookie	170	23	8.0
fudge chocolate chunk cookie	1 cookie	170	22	8.0
oatmeal raisin cookie	1 cookie	150	1	1.0
peanut butter cookie	1 cookie	170	21	8.0
peanut butter chocolate cookie	1 cookie	170	21	8.0
sugar cookie	1 cookie	160	23	6.0
white chocolate macadamia cookie	1 cookie	170	22	8.0

PIZZA

Food Name	Serv. Size	Total Cal.	Carbs GMS	Fat GMS
bacon, tomato, and mushroom, sourdough crust, 8-inch	1 pizza	635	78	24.0
barbecue chicken, sourdough crust, 8-inch	1 pizza	653	78	20.0
chicken and pesto, sourdough crust, 8-inch	1 pizza	649	78	19.0
double cheese and pepperoni, sourdough crust, 8-inch	1 pizza	744	77	34.0
double cheese, sourdough crust, 8-inch	1 pizza	603	77	21.0
fresh tomato and pesto, sourdough crust, 8-inch	1 pizza	539	76	16.0
Mediterranean, sourdough crust, 8-inch	1 pizza	564	84	19.0
New Orleans, sourdough crust, 8-inch	1 pizza	666	79	20.0
original combination, sourdough crust, 8-inch	1 pizza	648	79	25.0
smoked turkey and jalapeño, sourdough crust, 8-inch	1 pizza	647	81	19.0
Southwestern, sourdough crust, 8-inch	1 pizza	635	76	19.0
Thai chicken, sourdough crust, 8-inch	1 pizza	681	88	19.0
vegetarian special, sourdough crust, 8-inch	1 pizza	551	76	17.0

SALAD

Food Name	Serv. Size	Total Cal.	Carbs GMS	Fat GMS
Caesar, w/o dressing, croutons, chow mein noodles	1 salad	152	11	8.0
chef's, ham and turkey, dressing, croutons, chow mein noodles	1 salad	248	15	11.0
chef's, smoked turkey, w/o dressing, croutons, chow mein noodles	1 salad	243	15	10.0
chicken Caesar, w/o dressing, croutons, chow mein noodles	1 salad	254	13	10.0
chicken, Chinese, w/o dressing, croutons, chow mein noodles	1 salad	150	11	3.0
garden, small, w/o dressing, croutons, chow mein noodles	1 salad	25	3	1.0

Food Name	Serv. Size	Total Cal.	Carbs GMS	Fat GMS
garden, w/o dressing, croutons, chow mein noodles .... 1 salad		61	8	1.0
Greek, w/o dressing, croutons, chow mein noodles .... 1 salad		220	25	12.0
SALAD DRESSING				
Caesar, 'Olde World' .... 1 pkt		260	1	27.0
Greek balsamic vinaigrette .... 1 pkt		170	2	17.0
Italian, light .... 1 pkt		90	3	8.0
ranch, spicy .... 1 pkt		230	2	25.0
ranch, spicy, light .... 1 pkt		140	9	11.0
ranch, traditional .... 1 pkt		270	1	29.0
sesame ginger vinaigrette .... 1 pkt		170	8	15.0
Thousand Island .... 1 pkt		220	6	21.0
SANDWICH				
Bacon, lettuce and tomato				
large, on sourdough bun .... 1 sandwich		1141	140	46.0
regular, on sourdough bun .... 1 sandwich		578	70	24.0
small, on sourdough bun .... 1 sandwich		379	47	15.0
Cheese				
large, on sourdough bun .... 1 sandwich		1857	159	98.0
regular, on sourdough bun .... 1 sandwich		854	79	44.0
small, on sourdough bun .... 1 sandwich		596	53	31.0
Chicken				
breast, large, on sourdough bun .... 1 sandwich		1008	158	15.0
breast, regular, on sourdough bun .... 1 sandwich		535	81	10.0
breast, small, on sourdough bun .... 1 sandwich		363	55	7.0
Chicken club				
large, on sourdough bun .... 1 sandwich		1351	149	45.0
medium on sourdough bun .... 1 sandwich		686	75	23.0
small, on sourdough bun .... 1 sandwich		458	50	15.0
Corned beef				
large, on sourdough bun .... 1 sandwich		1134	139	25.0
regular, on dark rye bun .... 1 sandwich		587	70	15.0
small, on dark rye bun .... 1 sandwich		388	47	10.0
'Deluxe Original'				
large, on sourdough bun .... 1 sandwich		2638	173	152.0
regular, on sourdough bun .... 1 sandwich		1296	87	75.0
small, on sourdough bun .... 1 sandwich		1044	60	65.0
Dijon chicken				
large, on sourdough bun .... 1 sandwich		972	150	10.0
regular, on wheat bun .... 1 sandwich		497	74	6.0
small, on wheat bun .... 1 sandwich		330	50	4.0
Ham and cheese				
original, large, on sourdough bun .... 1 sandwich		1625	163	67.0
original, regular, on sourdough bun .... 1 sandwich		789	82	32.0
original, small, on sourdough bun .... 1 sandwich		537	55	22.0
'Original'				
large, on sourdough bun .... 1 sandwich		1917	161	102.0
regular, on sourdough bun .... 1 sandwich		941	81	50.0
small, on sourdough bun .... 1 sandwich		713	55	41.0
Pastrami and Swiss				
large, on sourdough bun .... 1 sandwich		1681	148	69.0
regular, on dark rye bun .... 1 sandwich		861	74	37.0
small, on dark rye bun .... 1 sandwich		570	49	24.0
Pesto chicken				
large, on sourdough bun .... 1 sandwich		999	145	15.0
regular, on sourdough bun .... 1 sandwich		512	73	9.0
small, on sourdough bun .... 1 sandwich		346	49	6.0

Food Name	Serv. Size	Total Cal.	Carbs GMS	Fat GMS
Philly				
large, on sourdough bun	1 sandwich	1709	157	66.0
regular, on sourdough bun	1 sandwich	824	78	32.0
small, on sourdough bun	1 sandwich	559	52	22.0
Reuben				
corned beef, large, on sourdough bun	1 sandwich	1594	147	62.0
corned beef, regular, on dark rye bun	1 sandwich	833	74	35.0
corned beef, small, on dark rye bun	1 sandwich	528	50	21.0
pastrami, large, on sourdough bun	1 sandwich	1777	152	77.0
pastrami, regular, on dark rye bun	1 sandwich	924	77	43.0
pastrami, small, on dark rye bun	1 sandwich	619	51	29.0
turkey, large, on sourdough bun	1 sandwich	1656	159	69.0
turkey, regular, on dark rye bun	1 sandwich	863	80	39.0
turkey, small, on dark rye bun	1 sandwich	579	54	26.0
Roast beef				
large, on sourdough bun	1 sandwich	1185	145	28.0
regular, on sourdough bun	1 sandwich	617	73	17.0
small, on sourdough bun	1 sandwich	413	49	11.0
Roast beef and cheese				
large, on sourdough bun	1 sandwich	1749	163	70.0
regular, on sourdough bun	1 sandwich	848	82	34.0
small, on sourdough bun	1 sandwich	580	55	24.0
Santa Fe chicken				
large, on sourdough bun	1 sandwich	1182	155	29.0
regular, on jalapeño cheese bun	1 sandwich	642	77	19.0
small, on jalapeño cheese bun	1 sandwich	431	52	13.0
'Texas Schlotzsky's'				
large, on sourdough bun	1 sandwich	1544	155	65.0
regular, on jalapeño cheese bun	1 sandwich	816	76	37.0
small, on jalapeño cheese bun	1 sandwich	561	51	26.0
Tuna				
albacore, large, on sourdough bun	1 sandwich	1000	147	26.0
albacore, regular, on wheat bun	1 sandwich	533	74	16.0
albacore, small, on wheat bun	1 sandwich	361	50	11.0
Tuna melt				
albacore, large, on sourdough bun	1 sandwich	1631	158	77.0
albacore, regular, on wheat bun	1 sandwich	818	79	40.0
albacore, small, on wheat bun	1 sandwich	562	53	28.0
Turkey				
breast, smoked, large, on sourdough bun	1 sandwich	988	150	13.0
breast, smoked, regular, on sourdough bun	1 sandwich	498	75	7.0
breast, smoked, small, on sourdough bun	1 sandwich	335	50	5.0
original, large, on sourdough bun	1 sandwich	2083	166	104.0
original, regular, on sourdough bun	1 sandwich	1017	83	51.0
original, small, on sourdough bun	1 sandwich	763	56	41.0
Turkey bacon club				
large, on sourdough bun	1 sandwich	1790	161	80.0
regular, on wheat bun	1 sandwich	874	79	40.0
small, on wheat bun	1 sandwich	596	53	27.0
Turkey guacamole				
large, on sourdough bun	1 sandwich	1317	166	42.0
regular, on sourdough bun	1 sandwich	683	84	24.0
small, on sourdough bun	1 sandwich	448	56	15.0
Vegetable club				
large, on sourdough bun	1 sandwich	1112	151	41.0
regular, on sourdough bun	1 sandwich	584	76	24.0
small, on sourdough bun	1 sandwich	393	50	16.0

Food Name	Serv. Size	Total Cal.	Carbs GMS	Fat GMS
Vegetarian				
large, on sourdough bun	1 sandwich	966	150	26.0
regular, on wheat bun	1 sandwich	519	75	17.0
small, on wheat bun	1 sandwich	351	51	11.0
Western, large, on sourdough bun	1 sandwich	1261	150	61.0
Western, regular, on sourdough bun	1 sandwich	651	75	33.0
Western, small, on sourdough bun	1 sandwich	449	51	23.0
SIDE DISH				
coleslaw, country style	5 oz	225	16	16.0
coleslaw, shredded	5 oz	225	16	16.0
macaroni salad	5 oz	338	23	23.0
potato salad, 'Choice'	5 oz	253	18	18.0
potato salad, diced, w/egg	5 oz	216	18	13.0
potato salad, mustard/egg	5 oz	225	17	15.0
seven bean medley	8 oz cup	145	24	2.0
SOUP				
Boston clam chowder	8 oz cup	233	24	15.0
broccoli cheese	8 oz cup	252	23	17.0
broccoli, cream of	8 oz cup	206	25	13.0
cauliflower cheese	8 oz cup	252	24	19.0
chicken gumbo	8 oz cup	110	13	5.0
chicken noodle, old-fashioned	8 oz cup	122	18	2.0
chicken tortilla	8 oz cup	167	24	3.0
chicken, w/wild rice	8 oz cup	378	24	28.0
corn chowder	8 oz cup	284	38	17.0
creamy turkey vegetable	8 oz cup	218	21	14.0
French onion	8 oz cup	78	9	3.0
minestrone	8 oz cup	89	17	1.0
potato, cream of, w/bacon	8 oz cup	226	31	13.0
ravioli tomato	8 oz cup	111	21	2.0
red beans and rice	8 oz cup	167	32	1.0
tomato Florentine	8 oz cup	100	19	1.0
vegetable beef barley	8 oz cup	100	12	3.0
vegetable cheese	8 oz cup	289	24	19.0
vegetable, lumberjack	8 oz cup	133	19	6.0
vegetable, vegetarian	8 oz cup	138	20	6.0
Wisconsin cheese	8 oz cup	319	26	25.0
SHAKEY'S PIZZA				
CHICKEN ENTRÉE				
fried, w/potatoes	3 pieces	947	51	56.0
fried, w/potatoes	5 pieces	1700	130	90.0
PIZZA				
Cheese				
homestyle pan crust, 12-inch pie	1/10 pie	303	31	13.7
thick crust, 'Shakey's Special' 12-inch pie	1/10 pie	208	22	8.3
thick crust, regular, 12-inch pie	1/10 pie	170	22	4.8
thin crust, 'Shakey's Special' 12-inch pie	1/10 pie	171	14	8.7
thin crust, regular, 12-inch pie	1/10 pie	133	13	5.2
Ham and cheese, 'Hot Ham and Cheese'	1 serving	550	56	21.0
Pepperoni				
homestyle pan crust 12-inch pie	1/10 pie	343	31	15.4
thick crust, 12-inch pie	1/10 pie	185	22	6.4
thin crust, 12-inch pie	1/10 pie	148	13	6.9
Sausage and mushroom				
homestyle pan crust, 12-inch pie	1/10 pie	343	31	16.9
thick crust, 12-inch pie	1/10 pie	179	22	5.6
thin crust, 12-inch pie	1/10 pie	141	13	6.0

Food Name	Serv. Size	Total Cal.	Carbs GMS	Fat GMS
Sausage and pepperoni				
homestyle pan crust, 12-inch pie	1/10 pie	374	31	19.9
thick crust, 12-inch pie	1/10 pie	177	22	8.0
thin crust, 12-inch pie	1/10 pie	166	13	8.4
'Sausage Supreme'				
homestyle pan crust, vegetable, 12-inch pie	1/10 pie	320	32	14.7
'Special' homestyle pan crust, 12-inch pie	1/10 pie	384	32	20.7
'Thai Chicken' thick crust, 12-inch pie	1/10 pie	162	22	4.1
POTATO, wedges	15 pieces	950	120	36.0
SANDWICH				
'Hot Ham and Cheese'	1 sandwich	550	56	21.0
'Super Hot Hero'	1 sandwich	810	67	44.0
SPAGHETTI ENTRÉE, w/meat sauce and garlic bread	1 serving	940	134	33.0
SHONEY'S				
BISCUIT	1 serving	170	22	8.1
BREAD, Grecian	1 serving	80	13	2.2
BREAKFAST				
bacon	3 strips	109	0	9.4
croissant, plain	1 serving	260	22	16.0
egg, fried	1 egg	159	1	14.7
ham	2 slices	59	1	2.1
honey bun	1 bun	265	32	14.0
pancake, 6-inch	1 cake	91	20	0.2
sausage	1 patty	103	0	9.6
syrup, low calorie	2.2 oz	98	24	0.0
toast, w/butter	2 slices	163	25	5.2
CHEESEBURGER, 'Mushroom/Swiss Burger'	1 burger	616	29	41.7
CHICKEN ENTRÉE				
charbroiled, 'LightSide'	1 serving	239	1	7.0
tenders, 'America's Favorites'	1 serving	388	17	20.4
COMBINATION ENTRÉE				
'Fish N' Shrimp'	1 serving	487	37	25.5
'Italian Feast'	1 serving	500	44	19.6
ribeye steak and chicken, charbroiled	1 serving	605	0	50.5
sirloin and chicken, charbroiled	1 serving	357	0	24.5
steak and chicken, charbroiled	8-oz serving	435	0	34.4
'Steak N' Shrimp' charbroiled shrimp	1 serving	361	1	22.6
'Steak N' Shrimp' fried shrimp	1 serving	507	15	32.7
CONDIMENTS. See also Salad dressing.				
gravy, country	3 oz	114	6	9.8
onion, sauteed	2.5-oz serving	37	4	2.1
sweet and sour sauce, souffle cup	1 cup	58	15	0.0
tartar sauce, souffle cup	1 cup	84	4	7.7
DESSERT				
apple pie, à la mode	1 serving	492	67	23.0
brownie, walnut, à la mode	1 serving	576	61	33.7
carrot cake	1 serving	500	56	26.0
hot fudge cake	1 serving	522	82	19.7
hot fudge sundae	1 serving	451	60	22.0
strawberry pie	1 serving	332	45	16.7
strawberry sundae	1 serving	380	48	19.0
FISH				
baked, 'LightSide'	1 serving	170	2	1.0
fried, 'Light'	1 serving	297	22	14.4
FISH ENTRÉE, fried, wfries	1 serving	639	50	34.8
HAMBURGER				
'All-American'	1 burger	501	27	32.6

Food Name	Serv. Size	Total Cal.	Carbs GMS	Fat GMS
'Old Fashioned'	1 burger	470	26	28.2
'Shoney Burger'	1 burger	498	22	35.7
w/bacon	1 burger	591	29	40.0
HAMBURGER PATTY, beef, light	1 serving	289	0	22.9
LASAGNA ENTRÉE				
'America's Favorites'	1 serving	297	45	9.8
light, 'LightSide'	1 serving	297	45	10.0
LIVER ENTRÉE, w/onions, 'America's Favorites'	1 serving	411	15	22.9
SALAD DRESSING				
Thousand Island	2 tbsp	130	2	13.0
Biscayne, low-calorie	2 tbsp	62	1	1.0
blue cheese	2 tbsp	113	0	13.0
French	2 tbsp	124	2	12.0
French rue	2 tbsp	122	2	10.0
honey mustard	2 tbsp	165	2	17.0
Italian, creamy	2 tbsp	135	1	15.0
Italian, golden	2 tbsp	141	1	15.0
Italian, nonfat	2 tbsp	10	2	0.0
Ranch	2 tbsp	95	0	10.0
SANDWICH				
cheese and bacon, grilled	1 sandwich	440	28	28.2
cheese, grilled	1 sandwich	454	29	29.0
chicken fillet	1 sandwich	464	39	21.2
chicken, charbroiled	1 sandwich	451	28	17.0
fish	1 sandwich	323	41	12.7
ham club, on whole wheat	1 sandwich	642	45	35.5
ham, baked	1 sandwich	290	28	10.3
patty melt	1 sandwich	640	30	41.7
Philly steak	1 sandwich	673	37	44.0
Reuben	1 sandwich	596	32	34.7
'Slim Jim'	1 sandwich	484	40	23.9
steak, country fried	1 sandwich	588	67	25.8
turkey club, on whole wheat	1 sandwich	635	44	32.7
SEAFOOD PLATTER ENTRÉE	1 serving	566	46	28.0
SHRIMP				
bite-sized	1 serving	387	25	24.7
charbroiled	1 serving	138	3	3.0
SHRIMP ENTRÉE				
boiled	1 serving	93	0	1.0
sampler	1 serving	412	26	22.7
'Shrimper's Feast' regular	1 serving	383	30	22.2
'Shrimper's Feast' large	1 serving	575	45	33.3
SIDE DISH				
ambrosia salad	1/4 cup	75	12	3.3
apple grape surprise salad	1/4 cup	19	5	0.0
baked potato	10-oz serving	264	61	0.3
beet-onion salad	1/4 cup	25	3	1.3
broccoli-cauliflower-ranch salad	1/4 cup	65	2	6.4
carrot-apple salad	1/4 cup	99	4	9.1
coleslaw	1/4 cup	69	5	5.1
cucumber salad, lite	1/4 cup	12	3	0.1
'Don's Pasta Salad'	1/4 cup	82	9	4.6
French fries	3-oz serving	189	29	7.5
French fries	4-oz serving	252	39	9.9
'Fruit Delight Salad'	1/4 cup	54	10	1.6
grits	3 oz	57	6	3.2
grits, instant	100 grams	67	7	3.8

Food Name	Serv. Size	Total Cal.	Carbs GMS	Fat GMS
hash browns	3 oz	90	14	3.1
home fries	3 oz	115	19	3.7
Italian vegetable salad	1/4 cup	11	3	0.1
kidney bean salad	1/4 cup	55	7	2.1
macaroni salad	1/4 cup	207	17	13.9
mixed squash salad	1/4 cup	49	2	4.1
mushroom, sauteed	3-oz serving	75	4	6.5
onion rings	1 ring	52	5	3.1
Oriental salad	1/4 cup	79	13	2.7
pea salad	1/4 cup	73	4	5.5
rice	3.5-oz serving	137	23	3.7
rotelli pasta	1/4 cup	78	9	4.0
seigan salad	1/4 cup	72	8	3.6
snow salad	1/4 cup	72	9	4.1
spaghetti salad	1/4 cup	81	9	4.6
spring salad	1/4 cup	38	2	2.9
summer salad	1/4 cup	114	2	11.6
three-bean salad	1/4 cup	96	12	5.1
Waldorf salad	1/4 cup	81	9	5.2
SOUP				
bean	6 oz	63	10	1.1
beef, w/cabbage	6 oz	86	9	3.0
broccoli, cream of	6 oz	75	11	4.6
cauliflower	6 oz	124	12	9.2
Cheddar chowder	6 oz	91	14	2.3
cheese Florentine, w/ham	6 oz	110	12	7.8
chicken, cream of	6 oz	136	14	8.9
chicken gumbo	6 oz	60	7	2.0
chicken noodle	6 oz	62	9	1.4
chicken vegetable, cream of	6 oz	79	13	1.3
chicken w/rice	6 oz	72	13	0.5
clam chowder	6 oz	94	10	5.4
corn chowder	6 oz	148	22	4.7
onion	6 oz	29	2	2.0
potato	6 oz	102	17	3.4
tomato, w/vegetable	6 oz	46	10	0.3
tomato Florentine	6 oz	63	11	1.1
vegetable beef	6 oz	82	14	1.5
SPAGHETTI ENTRÉE				
'America's Favorites'	1 serving	496	63	16.3
SPAGHETTI ENTRÉE, LIGHT				
light, 'LightSide'	1 serving	248	32	8.0
STEAK, sirloin, charbroiled	6 oz	357	0	24.5
STEAK ENTRÉE, country fried steak 'America's Favorites'	1 serving	449	34	27.2
SIZZLER				
BEEF				
roast beef, sliced	2/3 oz	17	0	0.3
steak, New York strip	12 oz	600	5	35.0
steak, sirloin	6.25 oz	447	0	34.0
BEEF PATTY	8 oz	530	0	38.0
BREAD, focaccia	2 pieces	108	9	7.0
BREADSTICK, garlic, soft	1 oz	75	15	0.5
CHICKEN				
breast, lemon herb	5 oz	151	27	4.0
wing	1 oz	73	4	4.0
wing, Cajun	3 oz	201	2	14.4
wing, Southern	1 oz	73	4	6.0

Food Name	Serv. Size	Total Cal.	Carbs GMS	Fat GMS
wing, whole, Southern	1 oz	74	4	4.8
CHICKEN ENTRÉE, w/noodles	6 oz	164	20	4.0
CHICKEN PATTY, 'Malibu'	1 patty	368	12	25.0
CHILI, 'Grande' w/beans	6 oz	100	18	1.0
CONDIMENTS				
buttery dipping sauce	1.5 oz	330	0	37.0
guacamole	1 oz	42	2	4.0
guacamole, extra chunky	3.5 oz serving	285	7	18.4
hibachi sauce	1.5 oz	57	11	0.0
Malibu sauce	1.5 oz	283	0	31.0
margarine, whipped	1.5 tbsp	105	0	12.0
marinade	1 oz	13	3	0.0
nacho cheese sauce	2 oz	120	3	10.0
pepper, bell, salad bar item	2 oz	8	2	0.0
salsa	1 oz	7	2	0.0
tartar sauce	1.5 oz	170	6	17.0
turkey ham, salad bar item	1 oz	62	0	5.0
CORNED BEEF, sliced	1 oz	45	0	1.5
CRAB, snow, legs and claws,	3.5 oz	91	0	1.1
CRAB, IMITATION, shredded	3.5 oz serving	104	14	1.0
CROISSANT, mini	1 croissant	120	12	8.0
DESSERT				
'Parfait Salad'	3.5 oz serving	84	17	1.7
yogurt, frozen, chocolate, soft-serve	4 oz	136	24	4.0
yogurt, frozen, vanilla, soft-serve	4 oz	136	24	4.0
DESSERT TOPPING				
chocolate syrup	1 oz	90	21	0.0
strawberry, nonfat	1 oz	70	18	0.0
whipped	1 tbsp	12	1	1.0
FISH NUGGETS	1 oz	40	5	0.0
HALIBUT, steak	6 oz	180	0	2.0
HAMBURGER, w/lettuce and tomato	1 serving	626	36	33.0
LASAGNA				
w/meat	8 oz	327	23	13.0
vegetable	8 oz	245	29	8.0
MACARONI AND CHEESE	6 oz	214	22	9.0
MEATBALL	4 meatballs	157	5	11.0
PASTA				
fettuccine	2 oz	80	15	1.0
fettuccine, whole egg, dry	2 oz	210	40	1.0
ravioli, cheese	4 oz	260	47	4.0
spaghetti	2 oz	80	16	0.0
POLLACK, breaded	4 oz	140	18	1.0
SALAD DRESSING				
bacon, hot	1 tbsp	40	58	20.0
blue cheese	1 oz	111	1	12.0
honey mustard	1 oz	160	4	16.0
Italian, lite	1 oz	14	2	0.0
Italian, Parmesan	1 oz	100	2	10.0
Japanese rice vinegar, nonfat	1 oz	10	2	0.0
Malibu	1 tbsp	100	0	11.0
ranch	1 oz	120	2	12.0
ranch, lower calorie	1 oz	90	4	8.0
sour	1.5 oz	89	0	9.0
sour	2 tbsp	60	0	6.0
Thousand Island	1 oz	143	3	15.0
SALMON	8 oz	247	0	12.0

Food Name	Serv. Size	Total Cal.	Carbs GMS	Fat GMS
SCALLOP, breaded, approx 30-40	4 oz	160	24	1.0
SHRIMP				
broiled	5 oz	150	0	6.0
butterfly, breaded, approx 16–20	3.5 oz	220	16	13.0
butterfly, breaded, approx 10–12	3.5 oz	145	14	0.1
butterfly, Cajun, breaded, approx 16–20	3.5 oz	145	24	0.1
butterfly, lemon pepper, breaded, approx 21–25	2 oz	190	38	1.0
Cajun, breaded, approx 80–90	3.5 oz	140	22	0.9
mini, breaded, approx 50–60	3.5 oz	140	22	0.9
mini, Cajun, breaded, approx 40–50	3.5 oz	141	22	0.9
scampi	5 oz	143	0	3.0
tempura-battered, approx 21–25	3 oz	155	13	8.0
SIDE DISH				
avocado, salad bar item	1/2 avocado	153	6	15.0
baked potato, flesh only	4 oz	105	24	0.0
broccoli, salad bar item	1/2 cup	12	2	0.0
carrot-raisin salad	2 oz	130	10	10.0
cauliflower, battered, not fried	3.5 oz serving	184	21.1	10.3
cheese toast	1 piece	273	16	21.0
Chinese chicken salad	2 oz	54	6	2.0
corn nuggets	3 oz	117	22	8.4
cottage cheese, low-fat	1/2 oup	100	4	2.0
four-bean salad	3.5 oz serving	104	19	2.5
French fries	4 oz	358	45	12.0
grapes, salad bar item	1/2 cup	29	8	0.0
jicama, salad bar item	2 oz	13	3	0.0
jicama salad, spicy	2 oz	16	4	0.0
kidney beans, salad bar item	1/4 cup	52	10	0.0
kiwifruit, salad bar item	2 oz	35	8	0.0
lettuce, Romaine, salad bar item	1 cup	9	1	0.0
macaroni and cheddar salad	3.5 oz serving	185	16	12.5
Mediterranean Minted fruit salad	2 oz	29	7	0.0
'Mexican Fiesta Salad'	2 oz	54	10	1.0
okra, breaded, not fried	3.5 oz serving	105	24	0.5
onion rings, steak cut, breaded, not fried	.5 oz serving	395	39	24.4
'Oriental Pasta Salad'	3.5 oz serving	114	23	1.6
potato and egg salad	3.5 oz serving	140	16	7.8
potato salad, 'Old Fashioned'	2 oz	84	10	5.0
potato salad, red, herb	2 oz	121	9	9.0
potato salad, red, herb	3.5 oz serving	213	15	16.2
potato skin	2 oz	160	22	8.0
refried beans	3 oz	120	16	4.0
rice pilaf	6 oz	256	47	5.0
'Seafood Louis' pasta salad	2 oz	64	9	2.0
seafood salad	2 oz	56	4	3.0
shell pasta salad	3.5 oz serving	112	19	2.7
spinach, salad bar item	1/2 cup	6	1	0.0
teriyaki beef salad	2 oz	49	5	2.0
tuna pasta salad	2 oz	133	6	10.0
tuna salad	3.5 oz serving	353	7	32.9
SOUP				
broccoli cheese soup	4 oz	139	10	9.0
chicken w/noodle	4 oz	31	4	1.0
clam chowder	4 oz	118	11	6.0
minestrone, nonfat	4 oz	36	7	0.0
vegetable, vegetarian	6 oz	50	6	1.0
vegetable sirloin soup	4 oz	60	6	2.0

Food Name	Serv. Size	Total Cal.	Carbs GMS	Fat GMS
SWORDFISH	8 oz	315	0	14.0
TACO SHELL	1 shell	50	7	2.0
TUNA, yellowfin	3.5 oz serving	125	0	4.0

SKIPPER'S

CHICKEN ENTRÉE

'Lite Catch' 3 pieces, w/small green salad	1 serving	305	17	15.0
tenderloin strips, 5 pieces, w/fries	1 serving	793	69	38.0
CHICKEN STRIPS, 'Create A Catch'	1 serving	82	4	4.0
CLAM ENTRÉE, 'Basket' strips w/fries	1 serving	1003	90	70.0

COD ENTRÉE

3 pieces, thick cut, w/fries	1 serving	665	68	32.0
4 pieces, thick cut w/fries	1 serving	759	74	36.0
5 pieces, thick cut, w/fries	1 serving	853	80	41.0

COMBINATION ENTRÉE

'Combos' clam strips, 1 piece fish, fries	1 serving	868	81	54.0
'Combos' jumbo shrimp, 1 piece fish, fries	1 serving	720	75	36.0
'Combos' original shrimp, 1 piece fish, fries	1 serving	728	77	37.0
'Combos' oysters, 1 piece fish, fries	1 serving	885	95	44.0
'Lite Catch' 1 piece fish, 2 pieces chicken, small green salad	1 serving	399	24	21.0
3-piece, chicken strip, fish, fries	1 serving	805	72	40.0
3-piece, chicken strip, shrimp, fries	1 serving	800	77	39.0

DESSERT

gelatin, nonfat, 'Jell-O' 'Create A Catch'	1 serving	55	12	0.0
root beer float	1 serving	302	33	10.0

FISH

fillet, 'Create A Catch'	1 serving	175	11	10.0

FISH ENTRÉE

1 fish fillet, w/fries	1 serving	558	51	28.0
2 fish fillets, w/fries	1 serving	733	71	38.0
3 fish fillets, w/fries	1 serving	908	82	48.0
'Lite Catch' 2 pieces, w/small green salad	1 serving	409	27	23.0

FISH SANDWICH

'Create A Catch'	1 sandwich	524	43	33.0
'Create A Catch' double	1 sandwich	698	54	73.0
OYSTER ENTRÉE, w/fries 'Basket'	1 serving	1038	118	51.0

SALAD

green, small, 'Lite Catch'	1 salad	59	6	3.0
shrimp and seafood	1 salad	167	15	3.0
side	1 salad	24	4	0.0

SALAD DRESSING

salad dressing, blue cheese, premium	1 pouch	222	4	23.0
salad dressing, Italian, gourmet	1 pouch	140	2	15.0
salad dressing, Italian, low-calorie	1 pouch	17	2	1.0
salad dressing, ranch house	1 pouch	188	2	20.0
salad dressing, Thousand Island	1 pouch	160	8	14.0
tartar sauce	1 tbsp	65	0	7.0
SALMON, baked	4.4 oz	270	1	11.0
SEAFOOD ENTRÉE, w/fries 'Skipper's Platter Basket'	1 serving	1038	97	63.0

SHRIMP ENTRÉE

w/fries, 'Basket'	1 serving	723	82	36.0
w/fries, jumbo, 'Basket'	1 serving	707	79	35.0
w/seafood salad, 'Lite Catch'	1 serving	167	15	3.0

SIDE DISH

baked potato	1 serving	145	32	0.0
coleslaw	.5 oz serving	289	10	27.0
French fries, 'Create A Catch'	1 serving	383	50	18.0

Food Name	Serv. Size	Total Cal.	Carbs GMS	Fat GMS
SOUP				
clam chowder, 'Create A Catch' cup	1 serving	100	14	3.5
clam chowder, 'Create A Catch' pint	1 serving	200	19	7.0
salmon chowder, 'Alder Smoked Salmon'	6 oz	166	14	7.0
SONIC				
CHEESEBURGER				
#1	1 serving	70	0	5.8
#2	1 serving	70	0	5.8
w/bacon	1 serving	548	23	38.6
jalapeño, double meat and cheese	1 serving	638	22	40.6
mini	1 serving	281	20	14.4
CHILI PIE	1 serving	327	20	22.6
CORN DOG	1 sandwich	280	30	15.0
HAMBURGER				
#1	1 serving	409	23	26.6
#2	1 serving	323	23	15.7
hickory	1 serving	314	23	15.7
mini	1 serving	246	20	11.5
'Super Sonic' double meat and cheese, w/mayo	1 serving	730	24	51.5
'Super Sonic' double meat and cheese, w/mustard	1 serving	644	24	40.7
HOT DOG				
'Cheese Coney' extra long	1 serving	635	45	39.0
'Cheese Coney' w/onions, extra long	1 serving	640	47	39.2
'Cheese Coney' regular	1 serving	358	23	23.3
regular	1 serving	258	21	15.3
'Cheese Coney' regular, w/onions	1 serving	361	24	23.3
SANDWICH				
bacon, lettuce, tomato	1 sandwich	327	27	19.3
cheese, grilled	1 sandwich	288	25	17.0
chicken	1 sandwich	319	41	9.0
chicken, breaded	1 sandwich	455	36	24.7
chicken, grilled, no dressing	1 sandwich	215	23	4.3
fish	1 sandwich	277	38	7.0
steak	1 sandwich	631	46	41.6
SIDE DISH				
French fries, large	1 serving	315	50	11.2
French fries, regular	1 serving	233	37	8.0
French fries, w/cheese, large	1 serving	420	51	20.2
onion rings, large	1 serving	577	54	37.8
onion rings, regular	1 serving	404	38	26.5
potato pieces, 'Tater Tots'	1 serving	150	19	7.0
potato pieces, 'Tater Tots' w/cheese	1 serving	220	19	13.0
SPAGHETTI WAREHOUSE				
MARINADE, dinner serving	1 serving	403	75	5.0
MINESTRONE SOUP	1 serving	56	8	1.0
TOMATO SAUCE, dinner serving	1 serving	410	76	5.0
STEAK 'N SHAKE				
CHEESEBURGER				
'Steakburger'	1 serving	353	33	13.0
'Steakburger' super	1 serving	451	33	18.0
'Steakburger' triple patty	1 serving	626	34	30.0
CHILI				
'Chili Mac' w/4 saltines	1 serving	310	34	12.0
'Chili 3 Ways' w/4 saltines	1 serving	411	45	16.0
w/oyster crackers	1 serving	337	37	14.0

Food Name	Serv. Size	Total Cal.	Carbs GMS	Fat GMS
DESSERT				
apple Danish	1 piece	391	35	24.0
apple pie à la mode	1 serving	549	76	25.0
brownie	1 brownie	258	39	12.0
cheesecake	1 serving	368	61	11.0
cheesecake, w/strawberries	1 serving	386	65	11.0
cherry pie à la mode'	1 serving	476	63	22.0
'Coca-Cola Float'	1 serving	514	76	17.0
fudge brownie sundae	1 serving	645	81	35.0
hot fudge nut sundae	1 serving	530	51	34.0
'Lemon Float'	1 serving	555	82	19.0
'Lemon Freeze'	1 serving	548	69	25.0
'Orange Float'	1 serving	502	74	17.0
'Orange Freeze'	1 serving	516	63	24.0
'Root Beer Float'	1 serving	529	78	17.0
strawberry sundae	1 serving	330	29	22.0
HAMBURGER				
'Steakburger'	1 serving	277	33	7.0
'Steakburger' super	1 serving	375	33	12.0
'Steakburger' triple patty	1 serving	474	33	17.0
SALAD				
chef	1 salad	313	6	18.0
lettuce and tomato, w/1 oz Thousand Island dressing	1 salad	168	7	15.0
SANDWICH				
cheese, toasted	1 sandwich	250	24	13.0
egg	1 sandwich	275	33	10.0
ham, baked	1 sandwich	451	37	22.0
ham and egg	1 sandwich	434	33	17.0
SIDE DISH				
baked beans	1 serving	173	27	4.0
French fries	1 serving	211	28	10.0
STEAK PLATTER, low calorie	1 serving	293	3	14.0
SUBWAY				
BEVERAGE				
'Berry 'Lishus Fruizle Smoothie'	12 oz	154	40	0.3
'Berry Blitz Fruizle Smoothie'	12 oz	129	37	0.0
'Berry Breeze Fruizle Smoothie'	12 oz	120	32	0.1
'Island Berry Fruizle Smoothie'	12 oz	120	32	0.1
'Island Fever Fruizle Smoothie'	12 oz	137	36	0.2
'Peach Paradise Fruizle Smoothie'	12 oz	119	32	0.1
'Peach Pizazz Fruizle Smoothie'	12 oz	126	33	0.0
'Pineapple Delite Fruizle Smoothie'	12 oz	142	38	0.3
'Pineapple Passion Fruizle Smoothie'	12 oz	140	38	0.2
'Sunrise Energizer Fruizle Smoothie'	12 oz	160	42	0.3
'Tropical Trio Fruizle Smoothie'	12 oz	138	36	0.2
'Wild Berries Fruizle Smoothie'	12 oz	130	36	0.1
BREAD				
Italian, 12-inch	1 large	380	76	2.0
Italian, 6-inch	1 small	190	38	1.0
wheat, 12-inch	1 serving	420	78	5.0
wheat, 6-inch	1 serving	210	39	3.0
wrap, 10.5-inch	1 wrap	200	45	2.0
CONDIMENTS				
bacon, 'Optional Fixin's'	2 slices	42	0	3.0
cheese	2 triangles	41	0	3.0
lettuce, deli style, 'Standard Fixin's'	1 serving	2	0	0.0
lettuce, 'Standard Fixin's'	1 serving	4	1	0.0

Food Name	Serv. Size	Total Cal.	Carbs GMS	Fat GMS
mayonnaise, regular, 'Optional Fixin's'	1 tsp	37	0	4.0
mayonnaise, light, 'Optional Fixin's'	1 tsp	18	0	2.0
vinegar, 'Optional Fixin's'	1 tsp	1	0	0.0
mustard, 'Optional Fixin's'	2 tsp	7	1	0.0
oil, 'Optional Fixin's'	1 tsp	45	0	5.0
olives, deli style, 'Standard Fixin's'	2 rings	2	0	0.0
olives, 'Standard Fixin's'	2 rings	2	0	0.0
onion, deli style, 'Standard Fixin's'	1 serving	2	1	0.0
onion 'Standard Fixin's'	1 serving	5	1	0.0
peppers, deli style 'Standard Fixin's'	2 strips	1	0	0.0
peppers, 'Standard Fixin's'	2 strips	1	0	0.0
pickle, deli style 'Standard Fixin's'	2 chips	1	0	0.0
pickle, 'Standard Fixin's'	3 chips	2	0	0.0
tomato, deli style, 'Standard Fixin's'	2 slices	8	2	0.0
tomato, 'Standard Fixin's'	2 slices	6	1	0.0
COOKIE				
Brazil nut	1 cookie	215	29	10.0
chocolate chip, 'M&M's"	1 cookie	212	29	10.0
chocolate chip	1 cookie	214	29	10.0
chocolate chunk	1 cookie	215	29	10.0
macadamia nut	1 cookie	222	28	11.0
oatmeal raisin	1 cookie	199	29	8.0
oatmeal raisin, low-fat	1 cookie	168	33	3.0
peanut butter	1 cookie	223	27	12.0
sugar	1 cookie	225	28	12.0
ROLL, deli style	1 serving	170	31	2.0
SALAD				
chicken breast, roasted, w/o dressing, cheese, condiments	1 salad	162	13	4.0
'Classic Italian BMT, w/o dressing, cheese, condiments	1 salad	269	11	19.0
'Cold Cut Trio' w/o dressing, cheese, condiments	1 salad	193	12	12.0
ham, w/o dressing, cheese, condiments	1 salad	112	11	3.0
meatball, w/o dressing, cheese, condiments	1 salad	232	17	13.0
roast beef, w/o dressing, cheese, condiments	1 salad	115	11	3.0
seafood and crab, w/light mayo, w/o dressing	1 salad	157	17	7.0
steak and cheese, w/o dressing	1 salad	182	13	8.0
'Subway Club' w/o dressing, cheese, condiments	1 salad	123	12	3.0
'Subway Melt' w/o dressing	1 salad	190	12	9.0
tuna, made w/light mayo, w/o dressing, cheese, condiments	1 salad	198	11	12.0
turkey and ham, w/o dressing, cheese, condiments	1 salad	107	11	2.0
turkey breast, w/o dressing, cheese, condiments	1 salad	101	12	2.0
'Veggie Delite, w/o dressing, cheese, condiments	1 salad	51	10	1.0
SANDWICH				
Bacon and egg				
deli style sub	1 sandwich	323	33	14.0
6-inch sub	1 sandwich	363	41	15.0
wrap	1 sandwich	353	47	14.0
Bologna, deli style sub, w/o cheese, condiments	1 sandwich	283	37	10.0
Cheese and egg				
deli style sub	1 sandwich	323	33	14.0
6-inch sub	1 sandwich	363	41	15.0
wrap	1 sandwich	353	47	14.0
Chicken breast				
roasted, 6-inch hot sub, w/o cheese, condiments	1 sandwich	342	46	6.0
roasted, super, 6-inch hot sub, w/o cheese, condiments	1 sandwich	453	49	9.0
Chicken Parmesan wrap	1 sandwich	333	56	5.0
'Classic Italian BMT'				
6-inch sub, w/o cheese, condiments	1 sandwich	450	45	21.0
super, 6-inch sub, w/o cheese, condiments	1 sandwich	668	47	39.0

Food Name	Serv. Size	Total Cal.	Carbs GMS	Fat GMS
'Cold Cut Trio'				
6-inch sub, w/o cheese, condiments	1 sandwich	374	45	14.0
super, 6-inch sub, w/o cheese, condiments	1 sandwich	517	47	24.0
Ham and egg				
deli style sub	1 sandwich	312	33	12.0
6-inch sub	1 sandwich	352	41	13.0
wrap	1 sandwich	342	47	12.0
Ham				
deli style sub, w/o cheese, condiments	1 sandwich	224	37	3.0
6-inch sub, w/o cheese, condiments	1 sandwich	293	45	5.0
super, 6-inch sub, w/o cheese, condiments	1 sandwich	354	47	7.0
Meatball				
6-inch hot sub, w/o cheese, condiments	1 sandwich	413	50	15.0
super, 6-inch hot sub, w/o cheese, condiments	1 sandwich	594	58	27.0
Roast beef				
deli style sub, w/o cheese, condiments	1 sandwich	236	37	4.0
6-inch sub, w/o cheese, condiments	1 sandwich	296	45	5.0
super, 6-inch sub, w/o cheese, condiments	1 sandwich	360	47	7.0
Seafood and crab				
super, w/light mayo, 6-inch sub	1 sandwich	444	58	15.0
w/light mayo, 6-inch sub	1 sandwich	338	51	9.0
Steak and cheese				
6-inch hot sub	1 sandwich	363	47	10.0
super, 6-inch sub	1 sandwich	495	50	17.0
wrap	1 sandwich	353	53	9.0
'Subway Club'				
6-inch sub, w/o cheese, condiments	1 sandwich	304	46	5.0
super, 6-inch sub, w/o cheese, condiments	1 sandwich	377	48	7.0
'Subway Melt'				
6-inch hot sub	1 sandwich	370	46	11.0
super, 6-inch hot sub	1 sandwich	509	48	19.0
Tuna				
w/light mayo, deli style sub, w/o cheese, condiments	1 sandwich	267	37	8.0
w/light mayo, 6-inch sub, w/o cheese, condiments	1 sandwich	378	45	14.0
w/light mayo, super, 6-inch sub, w/o cheese, condiments	1 sandwich	525	46	26.0
Turkey and ham				
6-inch sub, w/o cheese, condiments	1 sandwich	288	45	4.0
super, 6-inch sub, w/o cheese, condiments	1 sandwich	343	47	6.0
Turkey bacon wrap, deluxe	1 sandwich	355	52	10.0
Turkey breast				
deli style sub, w/o cheese, condiments	1 sandwich	227	37	4.0
6-inch sub, w/o cheese, condiments	1 sandwich	282	45	4.0
super, 6-inch sub, w/o cheese, condiments	1 sandwich	333	47	4.0
'Veggie Delite' 6-inch sub, w/o cheese, condiments	1 sandwich	232	43	3.0
Western egg				
deli style sub	1 sandwich	311	36	12.0
6-inch sub	1 sandwich	351	44	12.0
wrap	1 sandwich	341	50	12.0

SWENSEN'S
ICE CREAM

Food Name	Serv. Size	Total Cal.	Carbs GMS	Fat GMS
'Almond Praline Delight' low-fat	1/2 cup	130	25	2.0
caramel apple crisp, low-fat	1/2 cup	130	26	1.0
caramel turtle fudge, light	1 serving	120	18	4.0
caramel turtle fudge, low-fat	1/2 cup	140	26	2.5
chocolate chocolate chip cheesecake, low-fat	1/2 cup	130	26	2.5
chocolate fudge brownie, low-fat	1/2 cup	120	24	2.5
cookies and cream, light	1 serving	130	20	4.0

Food Name	Serv. Size	Total Cal.	Carbs GMS	Fat GMS
ice cream, cookies and cream, low-fat	1/2 cup	130	25	2.5
vanilla, light	1 serving	110	15	4.0
YOGURT, FROZEN				
Black Forest cake	1 serving	95	21	1.0
Black Forest cake, low-fat	1/2 cup	110	22	1.5
blueberry and cream, gourmet, sugar-free	1 serving	110	17	4.0
butter pecan, low-fat	1/2 cup	120	20	3.0
cherry, nonfat	1/2 cup	90	20	0.0
chocolate raspberry truffle, gourmet, sugar-free	1 serving	130	18	5.0
coconut pineapple	1 serving	120	26	1.0
hazelnut amaretto, low-fat	1/2 cup	120	20	3.0
mocha chip, low-fat	1/2 cup	110	22	1.5
strawberry banana and cream, nonfat	1/2 cup	90	20	0.0
triple chocolate, low-fat	1/2 cup	120	24	1.5
triple chocolate, nonfat	1 serving	100	21	0.0
vanilla Swiss almond, gourmet, sugar-free	1 serving	140	15	7.0
vanilla, nonfat	1/2 cup	90	20	0.0

SWISS CHALET

Food Name	Serv. Size	Total Cal.	Carbs GMS	Fat GMS
CHICKEN	1/2 chicken	634	1	38.0
DESSERT				
apple pie	1 serving	394	45	23.0
Black Forest cake	1 piece	278	36	14.0
chocolate éclair	1 serving	205	27	10.0
coconut pie	1 serving	292	40	14.0
fudge nut cake	1 piece	346	48	16.0
vanilla ice cream	1 serving	195	16	14.0
GRAVY, sandwich	1 serving	35	5	1.0
ROLL	1 roll	116	24	1.0
SALAD, chicken	1 salad	500	23	42.0
SANDWICH				
chicken	1 sandwich	360	42	5.0
chicken, hot	1 sandwich	310	30	6.0
SIDE DISH				
baked potato	1 serving	227	52	0.0
coleslaw, 'Chalet'	1 serving	56	10	1.0
French fries	1 serving	478	57	24.0
SOUP, chicken, 'Chalet'	1 serving	97	11	2.0

TCBY

Food Name	Serv. Size	Total Cal.	Carbs GMS	Fat GMS
YOGURT, FROZEN				
nonfat, giant	31.6 oz	869	182	0.0
nonfat, kiddie	3.2 oz	88	18	0.0
nonfat, large	10.5 oz	289	60	0.0
nonfat, medium	8.2 oz	226	47	0.0
nonfat, small	5.9 oz	162	34	0.0
nonfat, super	15.2 oz	418	87	0.0
regular, giant	31.6 oz	1027	182	24.0
regular, kiddie	3.2 oz	104	18	2.0
regular, large	10.5 oz	342	60	8.0
regular, medium	8.2 oz	267	47	6.0
regular, small	5.9 oz	192	34	4.0
regular, super	15.2 oz	494	87	11.0
strawberry	8 oz	220	43	2.0
sugarless, nonfat, giant	31.6 oz	632	142	0.0
sugarless, nonfat, kiddie	3.2 oz	64	14	0.0
sugarless, nonfat, large	10.5 oz	210	47	0.0
sugarless, nonfat, medium	8.2 oz	164	37	0.0

Food Name	Serv. Size	Total Cal.	Carbs GMS	Fat GMS
sugarless, nonfat, small	5.9 oz	118	27	0.0
sugarless, nonfat, super	15.2 oz	304	68	0.0

TACO BELL
BURRITO
Food Name	Serv. Size	Total Cal.	Carbs GMS	Fat GMS
bacon and egg, double, 6.25 oz	1 serving	480	39	27.0
bean, 7 oz	1 serving	370	54	12.0
'Big Beef Supreme' 10.5 oz	1 serving	510	52	23.0
'Big Beef' 7 oz	1 serving	400	43	17.0
'Big Chicken Supreme' 9 oz	1 serving	460	50	17.0
chicken, grilled, 7 oz	1 serving	390	49	13.0
chili cheese, 5 oz	1 serving	330	40	13.0
'Country Breakfast' 4 oz	1 serving	270	26	14.0
'Fiesta Breakfast' 3.5 oz	1 serving	280	25	16.0
'Grande Breakfast' 6.25 oz	1 serving	420	43	22.0
7-layer, 10 oz	1 serving	520	65	22.0
'Supreme' 9 oz	1 serving	430	50	18.0

CHALUPA
Food Name	Serv. Size	Total Cal.	Carbs GMS	Fat GMS
'Baja Beef' 5.5 oz	1 serving	420	30	27.0
'Baja Chicken' 5.5 oz	1 serving	400	28	24.0
'Baja Steak' 5.5 oz	1 serving	400	27	24.0
beef, supreme, 5.5 oz	1 serving	380	29	23.0
chicken, supreme, 5.5 oz	1 serving	360	28	20.0
'Santa Fe Beef' 5.5 oz	1 serving	440	31	29.0
'Santa Fe Chicken' 5.5 oz	1 serving	420	30	26.0
'Santa Fe Steak' 5.5 oz	1 serving	430	29	27.0
steak, supreme, 5.5 oz	1 serving	360	27	20.0

Food Name	Serv. Size	Total Cal.	Carbs GMS	Fat GMS
CINNAMON TWIST, 1 oz	1 serving	180	25	8.0
DESSERT, chaco taco ice cream, 4 oz	1 serving	310	37	17.0

GORDITA
Food Name	Serv. Size	Total Cal.	Carbs GMS	Fat GMS
'Baja Beef' 5.5 oz	1 serving	360	29	21.0
'Baja Chicken' 5.5 oz	1 serving	340	28	18.0
'Baja Steak' 5.5 oz	1 serving	340	27	18.0
beef, supreme, 5.5 oz	1 serving	300	27	14.0
chicken, supreme, 5.5 oz	1 serving	300	28	13.0
'Santa Fe Beef' 5.5 oz	1 serving	380	31	23.0
'Santa Fe Chicken' 5.5 oz	1 serving	370	30	20.0
'Santa Fe Steak' 5.5 oz	1 serving	370	29	20.0
steak, supreme, 5.5 oz	1 serving	300	27	14.0

Food Name	Serv. Size	Total Cal.	Carbs GMS	Fat GMS
MEXIMELT, big beef, 4.75 oz	1 serving	290	22	15.0

NACHOS
Food Name	Serv. Size	Total Cal.	Carbs GMS	Fat GMS
'Bellegrande' 11 oz	1 serving	760	83	39.0
'Big Beef Supreme' 7 oz	1 serving	440	44	24.0
chicken, 'Bellegrande' 11 oz	1 serving	740	82	36.0
regular, 3.5 oz	1 serving	320	34	18.0
steak, 'Bellegrande' 11 oz	1 serving	740	81	37.0

PIZZA
Food Name	Serv. Size	Total Cal.	Carbs GMS	Fat GMS
Mexican, 7.75 oz	1 serving	540	42	35.0
Mexican beef, 7.75 oz	1 serving	530	39	33.0
Mexican chicken, 7.75 oz	1 serving	520	41	32.0

QUESADILLA
Food Name	Serv. Size	Total Cal.	Carbs GMS	Fat GMS
cheese, 4.25 oz	1 serving	350	31	18.0
cheese, breakfast, 5.5 oz	1 serving	380	33	21.0
chicken, 6 oz	1 serving	400	33	19.0
w/bacon, breakfast, 6 oz	1 serving	450	33	27.0
w/sausage, breakfast, 6 oz	1 serving	430	33	25.0

SALAD
Food Name	Serv. Size	Total Cal.	Carbs GMS	Fat GMS
taco, w/salsa, 19 oz	1 salad	850	69	52.0

Food Name	Serv. Size	Total Cal.	Carbs GMS	Fat GMS
taco, w/salsa, w/o shell, 16.5 oz	1 salad	430	36	22.0
SIDE DISH				
hash brown nuggets, 3.5 oz	1 serving	280	29	18.0
Mexican rice, 4.75 oz	1 serving	190	23	9.0
pintos and cheese, 4.5 oz	1 serving	180	18	8.0
TACO				
'Double Decker' 5.75 oz	1 serving	330	37	15.0
'Double Decker Supreme' 7 oz	1 serving	380	39	18.0
'Supreme' 4 oz	1 serving	210	14	14.0
grilled chicken, soft, 4.5 oz	1 serving	200	20	7.0
grilled steak, soft, 4.5 oz	1 serving	200	19	7.0
grilled steak, soft, 'Supreme' 5.75 oz	1 serving	240	21	11.0
regular, 2.75 oz	1 serving	170	12	10.0
soft, 'Supreme' 5 oz	1 serving	260	22	13.0
soft, 3.5 oz	1 serving	210	20	10.0
TOSTADA, 6.25 oz	1 serving	250	27	12.0

TACO JOHN'S

Food Name	Serv. Size	Total Cal.	Carbs GMS	Fat GMS
BURRITO				
bean	5 oz	249	36	6.0
beef	5 oz	355	25	18.0
chicken, super, w/o sour cream, cheese	1 serving	366	40	14.0
chicken, w/o sour cream, cheese	1 serving	227	19	10.0
combination	5 oz	302	30	12.0
super	8.3 oz	434	66	11.0
super, w/o sour cream, cheese	1 serving	389	51	16.0
Texas chili	12.3 oz	518	48	24.0
w/green chili	12.3 oz	405	38	24.0
w/green chili, w/o sour cream, cheese	1 serving	367	40	18.0
CHILI, Texas	9.5 oz	430	35	22.0
CHIMICHANGA	12 oz	487	54	19.0
ENCHILADA	7 oz	379	33	18.0
NACHOS				
regular	4 oz	407	42	19.0
super	11.25 oz	657	57	34.0
PASTRY				
'Apple Grande' Danish	3 oz	257	44	8.0
churro	1.2 oz	122	12	7.0
SALAD				
chicken taco, super, w/o dressing, sour cream	1 salad	377	56	15.0
taco, w/o shell, dressing, sour cream, cheese	1 salad	228	30	13.0
taco, super	12.3 oz	450	48	18.0
SANDWICH, chicken fillet, 'Sierra'	8.5 oz	500	46	21.0
SIDE DISH				
'Potato Ole' large	6 oz	414	96	6.0
refried beans	9.5 oz	331	79	6.0
Mexican rice	1 serving	340	59	8.0
TACO				
'Taco Bravo' w/o sour cream	1 serving	319	42	14.0
'Taco Bravo' super	8 oz	485	51	20.0
chicken, soft shell	1 serving	180	20	8.0
regular	4.3 oz	228	15	13.0
soft	5 oz	276	23	13.0
TACOBURGER	6 oz	332	31	14.0
TOSTADA	4.3 oz	228	15	13.0

TACO TIME

Food Name	Serv. Size	Total Cal.	Carbs GMS	Fat GMS
BEEF, shredded	2.5 oz	70	1	0.0

Food Name	Serv. Size	Total Cal.	Carbs GMS	Fat GMS
BURRITO				
bean, crisp	5.25 oz	427	53	18.0
bean, soft, double	9.5 oz	506	77	12.0
bean, soft, single, 'Value'	6.75 oz	380	58	10.0
chicken, crisp	4.75 oz	422	32	25.0
combination, soft, double	9.5 oz	617	66	23.0
meat, 'Casita'	12 oz	647	54	31.0
meat, crisp	5.25 oz	552	39	30.0
meat, soft, double	9.5 oz	726	55	33.0
meat, soft, single, 'Value'	6.75 oz	491	48	21.0
veggie	11 oz	491	70	16.0
CHEESE, Cheddar	0.75 oz	86	0	7.0
CHEESEBURGER, taco, meat	7.5 oz	633	48	36.0
CHICKEN	2.5 oz	109	2	6.0
CHIPS	2 oz	266	35	12.0
CRUSTOS	3.5 oz	373	47	15.0
CONDIMENTS				
enchilada sauce	1 oz	12	3	0.0
guacamole	1 oz	29	2	2.0
hot sauce	1 oz	10	2	0.0
salad dressing, sour cream	1.5 oz	137	2	14.0
salad dressing, Thousand Island	1 oz	160	4	16.0
salsa, ranchero	2 oz	21	3	1.0
sour cream	1 oz	55	1	5.0
EMPANADA, cherry	4 oz	250	37	9.0
LETTUCE	0.5 oz	2	0	0.0
NACHOS				
deluxe	15.25 oz	1048	91	57.0
regular	10.5 oz	680	61	38.0
QUESADILLA, cheese	3.25 oz	205	17	11.0
SALAD				
chicken taco, w/o dressing	9 oz	370	27	21.0
taco, regular, w/o dressing	7.5 oz	479	30	28.0
'Tostada Delight' w/meat	9.75 oz	628	48	33.0
SIDE DISH				
French fries, 'Mexi'	8 oz	532	54	34.0
French fries, 'Mexi' regular	4 oz	266	27	17.0
Refritos	7 oz	326	44	10.0
Mexican rice	4 oz	159	30	2.0
TACO				
chicken, soft	7 oz	387	41	16.0
crisp	4 oz	295	16	17.0
flour, soft, rolled	7 oz	512	46	23.0
meat	2.5 oz	208	7	11.0
meat, natural, 'Super'	11.25 oz	627	60	27.0
shredded beef, soft, 'Super'	8 oz	368	38	11.0
soft, 'Value'	5.25 oz	316	23	15.0
TACO SHELL, 6-inch	1.25 oz	110	14	6.0
TOMATO	0.5 oz	3	1	0.0
TORTILLA				
flour, 10-inch	2.75 oz	213	31	4.0
flour, 8-inch	1.25 oz	107	16	3.0
flour, 7-inch	1.75 oz	88	16	1.0
flour, fried, 10-inch	2.75 oz	318	37	16.0
flour, fried, 8-inch	1.3 oz	205	24	11.0
wheat, 11-inch	3.5 oz	175	33	3.0

Food Name	Serv. Size	Total Cal.	Carbs GMS	Fat GMS
WENDY'S				
BACON	1 slice	20	0	1.5
BEVERAGE				
coffee	6 fl oz	0	1	0.0
coffee, decaffeinated	6 fl oz	0	1	0.0
cola, diet, small	8 fl oz	0	0	0.0
cola, small	8 fl oz	90	24	0.0
'Frosty' large	20 oz	540	91	14.0
'Frosty' medium	16 oz	440	73	11.0
'Frosty' small	12 oz	330	56	8.0
hot chocolate	6 fl oz	80	15	3.0
lemonade, small	8 fl oz	90	24	0.0
lemon-lime soft drink	8 fl oz	90	24	0.0
milk, 2%	8 fl oz	110	11	4.0
tea, hot or iced	6 fl oz	0	0	0.0
BREAD, pita, 'Classic Greek'	1 pita	440	50	20.0
BREADSTICK, soft	1 stick	130	23	3.0
BUN				
Kaiser	1 bun	190	36	3.0
sandwich	1 bun	160	29	2.5
CHEESE				
American	1 slice	70	1	5.0
American, junior	1 slice	45	0	3.5
Cheddar, shredded	2 tbsp	70	1	6.0
imitation, shredded, salad bar item	2 tbsp	50	1	4.0
CHEESEBURGER				
junior	1 burger	320	34	13.0
bacon, junior	1 burger	380	34	19.0
deluxe, junior	1 burger	360	36	17.0
kid's meal	1 burger	320	33	13.0
CHICKEN				
fillet, breaded	1 piece	230	10	12.0
fillet, grilled	1 fillet	110	0	3.0
fillet, spicy	1 piece	210	10	9.0
nuggets, fried	5 pieces	210	7	14.0
nuggets, fried	4 pieces	170	5	11.0
CHILI				
large	12 oz	310	32	10.0
small	8 oz	210	21	7.0
CONDIMENTS. See also Salad Dressing.				
bacon bits, salad bar item	2 tbsp	45	0	2.5
barbecue sauce	1 packet	45	10	0.0
buffalo wing sauce, spicy	1 packet	25	4	1.0
catsup	1 tsp	10	2	0.0
croutons, salad bar item	2 tbsp	14	4	1.0
honey mustard sauce	1 packet	130	6	12.0
honey mustard, lower calorie	1 tsp	25	2	1.5
lettuce	1 leaf	0	0	0.0
lettuce, iceberg/Romaine, salad bar item	1 cup	10	2	0.0
margarine, whipped	1 packet	60	0	7.0
mayonnaise	1 tsp	30	1	3.0
mustard	1 tsp	0	0	0.0
onion, red, sliced, salad bar item	3 rings	0	1	0.0
onion, sliced	4 rings	5	1	0.0
Parmesan blend, grated, salad bar item	2 tbsp	70	5	4.0
pepperoni, sliced, salad bar item	6 slices	30	0	3.0
pickle	4 slices	0	0	0.0

Food Name	Serv. Size	Total Cal.	Carbs GMS	Fat GMS
salad oil	1 tbsp	120	0	14.0
sour cream	1 packet	60	1	6.0
sunflower seeds and raisins, salad bar item	2 tbsp	80	5	5.0
sweet and sour sauce	1 packet	50	12	0.0
tomato, sliced	1 slice	5	1	0.0
tomato, wedges, salad bar item	1 piece	5	1	0.0
turkey ham, diced, salad bar item	2 tbsp	50	0	4.0
COOKIE, chocolate chip	1 cookie	270	36	13.0
CRACKERS, saltine	2 crackers	25	4	0.5
HAMBURGER				
'Big Bacon Classic'	1 burger	580	46	30.0
junior	1 burger	270	34	10.0
kid's meal	1 burger	270	33	10.0
single, plain	1 burger	360	31	16.0
w/everything	1 burger	420	37	20.0
HAMBURGER PATTY				
regular	2 oz	100	0	7.0
quarter-pound	0.25 lb	200	0	14.0
SALAD				
Caesar, side	1 salad	100	8	4.0
chicken Caesar	1 salad	260	17	9.0
chicken, grilled	1 salad	200	9	8.0
garden, deluxe	1 salad	110	9	6.0
side	1 salad	60	5	3.0
taco	1 salad	380	28	19.0
SALAD DRESSING				
blue cheese	2 tbsp	180	0	19.0
Caesar vinaigrette, pita dressing	1 tbsp	70	1	7.0
French	2 tbsp	120	6	10.0
French, nonfat	2 tbsp	35	8	0.0
garden ranch, pita dressing	1 tbsp	50	1	4.5
Italian Caesar	2 tbsp	150	1	16.0
Italian, reduced fat	2 tbsp	40	2	3.0
ranch, 'Hidden Valley'	2 tbsp	100	1	10.0
ranch, reduced fat, 'Hidden Valley'	2 tbsp	60	2	5.0
Thousand Island	2 tbsp	90	2	8.0
wine vinegar	1 tbsp	0	0	0.0
SANDWICH				
chicken, breaded	1 sandwich	440	44	18.0
chicken, grilled	1 sandwich	310	35	8.0
chicken, spicy	1 sandwich	410	43	15.0
chicken Caesar pita	1 pita	490	48	18.0
chicken club	1 sandwich	470	44	20.0
'Garden Ranch Chicken Pita'	1 pita	480	51	18.0
'Garden Veggie Pita'	1 pita	400	52	17.0
SIDE DISH				
applesauce, salad bar item	2 tbsp	30	7	0.0
baked potato, plain	10 oz	310	71	0.0
baked potato, w/bacon and cheese	1 serving	530	78	18.0
baked potato, w/broccoli and cheese	1 serving	470	80	14.0
baked potato, w/cheese	1 serving	570	78	23.0
baked potato, w/chili and cheese	1 serving	630	83	24.0
baked potato, w/sour cream and chives	1 serving	380	74	6.0
cantaloupe, sliced, salad bar item	1 piece	15	4	0.0
chicken salad, salad bar item	2 tbsp	70	2	5.0
cottage cheese, salad bar item	2 tbsp	30	1	1.5
cucumbers, salad bar item	2 slices	0	0	0.0
egg, hard cooked, salad bar item	2 tbsp	40	0	3.0

Food Name	Serv. Size	Total Cal.	Carbs GMS	Fat GMS
French fries, 'Biggie'	5.6 oz	470	61	23.0
French fries, 'Great Biggie'	6.7 oz	570	73	27.0
French fries, small	3.2 oz	270	35	13.0
green peas, salad bar item	2 tbsp	15	3	0.0
green peppers, salad bar item	2 pieces	0	1	0.0
orange, sliced, salad bar item	2 slices	15	4	0.0
pasta salad, salad bar item	2 tbsp	35	4	1.5
peaches, sliced, salad bar item	1 piece	15	4	0.0
potato salad, salad bar item	2 tbsp	80	5	7.0
watermelon, wedges, salad bar item	1 piece	20	4	0.0
TACO CHIPS	15 chips	210	24	11.0
WHATABURGER				
BACON	1 slice	38	0	3.3
BEVERAGE				
'Cherry Coke' medium	1 serving	227	60	0.0
chocolate shake, junior	1 serving	364	61	9.3
'Coca Cola Classic' medium	1 serving	211	56	0.0
coffee, small	1 serving	5	1	0.0
'Diet Coke' medium	1 serving	2	1	0.0
'Dr. Pepper' medium	1 serving	207	52	0.0
iced tea, 'Lipton' medium	1 serving	5	2	0.0
orange juice, 'Tropicana'	10 fl oz	140	33	0.0
milk, 2%	1 serving	113	11	4.3
'Sprite' medium	1 serving	211	48	0.0
strawberry shake, junior	1 serving	352	60	8.9
root beer, medium	1 serving	237	63	0.0
vanilla shake, junior	1 serving	325	51	9.5
BISCUIT, plain	1 serving	280	37	13.4
BREAKFAST				
bacon biscuit	1 sandwich	359	37	20.2
bacon, egg, and cheese biscuit	1 sandwich	511	38	32.9
'Breakfast on a Bun' w/bacon biscuit	1 sandwich	365	29	19.4
Breakfast on a Bun' w/sausage biscuit	1 sandwich	455	30	28.1
cinnamon roll	1 serving	320	39	16.0
egg and cheese biscuit	1 sandwich	434	38	26.3
egg omelet sandwich	1 sandwich	288	29	12.8
pancake	3 pancakes	259	40	5.8
pancake, 3 pancakes w/2 slices bacon	1 serving	335	40	12.4
pancake, 3 pancakes w/1 sausage patty	1 serving	426	40	21.1
platter, w/bacon, scrambled eggs, biscuit, hash browns	1 serving	695	54	44.0
platter, w/sausage, scrambled eggs, biscuit, hash browns	1 serving	785	54	52.7
sausage and gravy biscuit	1 sandwich	479	48	27.4
sausage biscuit	1 sandwich	446	37	28.7
sausage, egg, and cheese biscuit	1 sandwich	601	38	41.6
toast, Texas	1 slice	147	22	4.5
CHEESE, large slice	1 slice	89	0	7.4
CHICKEN STRIPS	2 strips	300	15	20.0
COOKIE				
chocolate chunk	1 serving	247	28	16.0
white chocolate macadamia nut	1 serving	269	31	16.0
FAJITA				
beef	1 serving	326	34	11.9
chicken, grilled	1 serving	272	35	6.7
GRAVY, peppered	3 oz	75	8	4.5
HAMBURGER				
'Justaburger'	1 burger	298	30	13.0
'Whataburger'	1 burger	598	61	26.0

Food Name	Serv. Size	Total Cal.	Carbs GMS	Fat GMS
'Whataburger' double meat	1 burger	823	62	42.4
'Whataburger' on small bun, w/o oil	1 burger	407	34	18.8
'Whataburger Jr.'	1 burger	322	35	13.3
MUFFIN, blueberry	1 serving	239	36	7.9
SALAD				
garden	1 salad	56	11	0.6
chicken, grilled	1 salad	150	14	1.2
SANDWICH				
chicken, grilled	1 sandwich	442	48	14.2
chicken, grilled, on small white bun, w/mustard, w/o oil, dressing	1 sandwich	300	35	3.2
chicken, grilled, w/o dressing	1 sandwich	385	46	8.5
chicken, grilled, w/o dressing, oil	1 sandwich	358	46	5.5
fish, 'Whatacatch'	1 sandwich	467	43	25.0
SIDE DISH				
French fries, junior	1 serving	221	25	12.1
French fries, large	1 serving	442	49	24.2
French fries, regular	1 serving	332	37	18.1
onion rings, large	1 serving	498	51	28.7
onion rings, regular	1 serving	329	34	19.1
TAQUITO				
bacon and egg	1 serving	335	32	16.1
potato and egg	1 serving	446	48	21.8
sausage and egg	1 serving	443	32	25.9
TURNOVER, apple, fried	1 serving	215	27	10.8

WHITE CASTLE

Food Name	Serv. Size	Total Cal.	Carbs GMS	Fat GMS
BEVERAGE				
chocolate shake	14 fl oz	220	32	7.0
'Coca Cola Classic'	14 fl oz	120	32	0.0
coffee, black, small	1 serving	6	1	0.0
'Diet Coke'	14 fl oz	1	0	0.0
tea, iced	14 fl oz	45	12	0.0
vanilla shake	14 fl oz	230	35	7.0
BREAKFAST, egg, sausage, cheese on bun	1 sandwich	340	17	25.0
CHEESEBURGER				
double patty	1 sandwich	285	16	18.0
regular	1 sandwich	160	11	9.0
w/bacon	1 sandwich	200	12	13.0
CHICKEN RINGS	6 rings	310	14	21.0
CHILI	12 oz	375	45	15.0
HAMBURGER				
double	1 burger	235	16	14.0
regular	1 burger	135	11	7.0
SANDWICH				
chicken	1 sandwich	190	21	8.0
fish	1 sandwich	160	18	6.0
SIDE DISH				
cheese sticks	3 sticks	290	19	17.0
French fries, small	1 serving	115	15	6.0
onion rings	8 rings	540	69	26.0

Nutrition and Fitness Software
for Your Windows PC

Looking to save time and effort managing your nutrition and exercise? If you have a Windows computer (Win 95 and up), you're in luck.

NutriBase nutrition and fitness software provides you with a research-quality nutrient database that gives you instant access to more than 100 nutrients. In fact, the data used in the NutriBase series of books is a subset of the data contained in the NutriBase software.

The software will allow you to view, rank, query, and perform food name searches on the nutrient data. You can track your dietary intake; create and analyze recipes; record and track your exercise; count calories, carbs, protein, or any other nutrient; add new food items; create meals; generate meal plans; graph results; generate reports; and monitor your progress on a daily basis.

**For complete product information, free downloads,
and links to our competitors, visit us at:**

NutriBase EZ Edition (easy-to-use edition)   imchubby.com

NutriBase Personal Plus Edition (robust personal edition)   dietsoftware.com

NutriBase Clinical Edition (professional nutrition software)   nutribase.com

Cybersoft, Inc. (800)959-4849